WITHDRAWN

Audiology
Treatment

Audiology Treatment

Edited by

Michael Valente, Ph.D.
Professor of Clinical Otolaryngology
Division of Audiology
Department of Otolaryngology–Head and Neck Surgery
Washington University School of Medicine
St. Louis, Missouri

Holly Hosford-Dunn, Ph.D.
President
Tucson Audiology Institute, Inc.
Managing Member
Arizona Audiology Network, LLC
Tucson, Arizona

Ross J. Roeser, Ph.D.
Professor and Director
Callier Center for Communication Disorders
School of Human Development
University of Texas at Dallas
Dallas, Texas

2000
Thieme
New York • Stuttgart

Thieme New York
333 Seventh Avenue
New York, NY 10001

Audiology: Treatment
Michael Valente, Ph.D.
Holly Hosford-Dunn, Ph.D.
Ross J. Roeser, Ph.D.

Senior Medical Editor: Andrea Seils
Editorial Director: Avé McCracken
Editorial Assistant: Thomas Soper
Director, Production and Manufacturing: Anne Vinnicombe
Senior Production Editor: Eric L. Gladstone
Marketing Director: Phyllis Gold
Sales Manager: Ross Lumpkin
Chief Financial Officer: Seth S. Fishman
President: Brian D. Scanlan
Cover Designer: Kevin Kall
Compositor: V&M Graphics, Inc.
Printer: Maple-Vail

Library of Congress Cataloging-in-Publication Data

Audiology : treatment / edited by Michael Valente, Holly Hosford-Dunn, Ross J. Roeser.
    p. ; cm.
  Includes bibliographical references and index.
  ISBN 0-86577-859-0 (TNY)—ISBN 3131164212 (GTV)
    1. Audiology. 2. Hearing disorders—Treatment. I. Valente, Michael. II. Hosford-Dunn,
Holly. III. Roeser, Ross J.
  [DNLM: 1. Hearing Disorders—therapy. 2. Hearing Aids. WV 270 A9125 2000]
RF290 .A926 2000
617.8—dc21
                                                                  99-051912

Contents

Principles of Treatmemt

Applications in Treatment

Future Directions

Preface

This book is on the topic of treatment in audiology, and is one in a series of three texts prepared to represent the breadth of knowledge covering the multi-faceted profession of audiology in a manner that has not been attempted before. The companion books to this volume are *Diagnosis* and *Practice Management*. In total, the three books provide a total of 73 chapters covering material on the range of subjects and current knowledge audiologists must have to practice effectively. Because many of the chapters in the three books relate to each other, our readers are encouraged to have all three of them in their libraries, so that the broad scope of the profession of audiology is made available to them.

A unique feature of all three books is the insertion of highlighted boxes (pearls, pitfalls, special considerations, and controversial points) in strategic locations. These boxes emphasize key points authors are making and expand important concepts that are presented.

This volume is intended to provide a comprehensive overview of the numerous treatment options available to help patients relieve the clinical symptoms (and others) described above. The intended audience is either an audiology graduate student or a practicing clinician.

To accomplish this task, this volume is divided into three sections. The first section underscores the **Principles of Treatment**. This section is designed to provide the graduate student and practitioner with a solid background before going into the specifics of available treatment options. First, Dave Preves and Jim Curran provide an excellent overview of the instrumentation and procedures involved in measuring the *electroacoustic* performance of hearing aids. The chapter by Michael Valente, Maureen Valente, Lisa Potts and Edward Lybarger illustrates the numerous ways that the amplified sound can be modified by the manner in which the hearing aids are connected to the coupler or real-ear. A chapter by Larry Revit follows on the instrumentation and procedures used to accurately measure the *real-ear* performance of hearing aids when worn on the individual ear(s) of the patient. Dawna Lewis provides the reader with an overview of the numerous issues to consider when fitting hearing aids to children, while Carol Sammeth and Harry Levitt provide similar information that must be considered when fitting the adult population.

Over the past few years there have been a large number of manufacturers introducing hearing aids whose performance changes in reaction to the intensity and spectrum of the input signals (i.e., nonlinear signal processing). The introduction of this technology created the need for new approaches for selecting, fitting and verifying the performance of hearing aids. Prior to this, signal processing provided by hearing aids was predominantly linear. That is, the gain provided by the hearing aids remained constant as the level of the input signal changed. Thus, the early prescriptive formulas were appropriate when fitting hearing aids with linear signal processing. However, with the proliferation of hearing aids with nonlinear signal processing, new prescriptive procedures needed to be developed so that a different prescriptive target was available for different input levels. Francis Kuk presents an overview on recently introduced approaches to selecting and fitting nonlinear hearing aids.

The appropriate fitting of hearing aids is only one step in the rehabilitation/habilitation process. Once the hearing aids are fit, the patient requires counseling on realistic expectations and other important aspects of what amplification can and cannot provide. This information is provided in the chapter by Jane Madell. In addition, audiologists need to be aware of the numerous state and federal regulations dealing with dispensing hearing aids and assistive listening devices (ALDs). Holly Kaplan and John Hesse do a masterful job in providing this vital information.

The second section deals with the **Applications in Treatment**. The first three chapters provide information on current medical and surgical treatments available for patients with conductive (Elizabeth Dinces and Richard Wiet), cochlear or neural hearing loss (J. Gail Neeley and Mark Wallace). Assuming that amplification is an appropriate treatment option for the hearing loss, Catherine Palmer, George Lindley and Elaine Mormer provide information on the procedures to follow for selecting, fitting and verifying the performance of conventional hearing aids. The chapter by Robert Sweetow provides similar information for those who are considering selecting, fitting and verifying the performance of programmable (analog signal processing) and recently introduced digital hearing aids. Selecting, fitting and verifying the performance of hearing aids is an important step in providing amplification. However, the patient needs to be counseled on the use and care of the hearing aids. This information is provided in the chapter by David Citron. A relatively recent trend in amplification is the surgical implantation of hearing aids for patients whose hearing loss is severe enough that they receive little or no benefit from conventional or digital hearing aids. Doug Miller and John Fredrickson provide an excellent chapter on the recent trend of implanting hearing aids into the middle ear or brain stem. A chapter by Pat Chute and Mary Ellen Nevins follows on cochlear implants in children, while Susan Waltzman and William Shapiro provide similar information for cochlear implantation in the adult population. As is well known by experienced dispensers, hearing aids alone cannot solve all the listening problems experienced by the user. This is especially true when the user is attempting to hear optimally in a noisy environment or when using a telephone. The chapter by Jean-Pierre Gagné and

Mary Beth Jennings provides information on the role contributed by aural rehabilitation in improving the listening skills of patients with reduced hearing. This is followed by the chapter by Peter Bengtsson and Preben Brunved which contributes a wealth of information on the numerous assistive listening devices that can be coupled to the patient's hearing aids or used alone. Another population to consider is those patients who have hearing sensitivity within normal limits, but are easily distracted by the environment surrounding them. Carl Crandell and Joe Smaldino provide the reader with an excellent chapter on methods to improve the acoustical environment within the classroom. Another patient population is those reporting dizziness and vertigo. Aside from the medical and surgical treatment options outlined in the chapter by J. Gail Neely and Mark Wallace, Alan Desmond reports on the relatively new treatment option of eliminating the sensations of dizziness through vestibular rehabilitation. For those patients whose hearing loss has been a result of excessive exposure to loud sounds (or for those who currently have normal hearing but are exposing themselves to loud sounds), Elliott Berger and John Casali offer insightful information on protective devices that are used to prevent hearing loss or further decrease in hearing. Still another population to consider are those who experience tinnitus or report hypersensitivity to typical environmental sounds. Robert Sandlin and Robert Olsson present an excellent chapter on the evaluation and treatment options for these patients.

The final section of this volume, hopefully, will serve to help the reader understand what may be arriving in the future in terms of treatment options. Christopher Schweitzer presents a wonderful chapter on what may lie ahead in amplification treatment options. His chapter leaves the promising impression that in the near future it will be possible for listeners with hearing loss to actually hear better in noisy environments than persons with normal hearing. Denis Byrne and Harvey Dillon present a thought-provoking chapter on what may lie ahead for the practitioner as he selects, fits and verifies the performance of hearing aids. Finally, Brenda Ryals presents a fascinating chapter on procedures that may result in the regeneration of hair cells in the cochlea that will restore hearing to normal. If this approach proves successful, then much of the information presented in this volume concerning treatment options will become obsolete!

The three of us were brought together by Ms. Andrea Seils, Senior Medical Editor at Thieme Medical Publishers, Inc. During the birthing stage of the project Andrea encouraged us to think progressively—out of the box. She reminded us repeatedly to shed our traditional thinking and concentrate on the new developments that have taken place in audiology in recent years and that will occur in the next 5 to 10 years. With Andrea's encouragement and guidance, each of us set out what some would have considered to be the impossible—to develop a series of three cutting-edge books that would cover the entire profession of audiology *in a period of less than 2 years*. Not only did we accomplish our goal, but as evidenced by the comprehensive nature of the material covered in the three books, we exceeded our expectations! We thank Andrea for her support throughout this 2-year project.

The authors who were willing to contribute to this book series have provided outstanding material that will assist audiologists in-training and practicing audiologists in their quest for the most up-to-date information on the areas that are covered. We thank them for their diligence in following our guidelines for preparing their manuscripts and their promptness in following our demanding schedule.

The consideration of our families for their endurance and patience with us throughout the duration of the project must be recognized. Our spouses and children understood our mission when we were away at editorial meetings; they were patient when we stayed up late at night and awoke in the wee hours of the morning to eke out a few more paragraphs; they tolerated the countless hours we were away from them. Without their support and encouragement we would never have finished our books in the timeframe we did.

Finally, each of us thanks our readers for their support of this book series. We would welcome comments and suggestions on this book, as well as the other two books in the series. Our email addresses are below.

Michael Valente—*valentem@msnotes.wustl.edu*
Holly Hosford-Dunn—*tucsonaud@aol.com*
Ross J. Roeser—*roeser@callier.utdallas.edu*

Acknowledgments

The editors of this book series, Ross J. Roeser, Ph.D., Michael Valente, Ph.D., and Holly Hosford-Dunn, Ph.D., would like to extend their deepest gratitude to the following companies and manufacturers who, through the generosity of their financial support, helped defray the costs incurred by our hard-working authors in the development of their contributions.

Beltone Electronics
Oticon
Siemens
Sonus USA, Inc.
Starkey Labs
Widex Hearing Aid Company

Contributors

Peter O. Bengtsson, M.S.E.E.
Centrum Sound Systems
Sunnyvale, CA

Elliott H. Berger, M.S.
Senior Scientist, Auditory Research
E.A.R. Hearing Protection Products
Indianapolis, IN

Preben B. Brunved, M.S.E.E.
Technical Management Department
Oticon, Inc.
Somerset, NJ

Dennis Byrne, Ph.D.
Research Director
National Acoustic Laboratories
Chatswood, NSW
Australia

John G. Casali, Ph.D.
John Grado Professor
Department of Industrial and Systems Engineering
Virginia Polytechnic Institute and State University
Blacksburg, VA

Patricia M. Chute, Ed.D.
Cochlear Implant Center
Lenox Hill Hospital
New York, NY

David Citron, III, Ph.D.
Director
South Shore Hearing Center, Inc.
South Weymouth, MA

Carl C. Crandell, Ph.D.
Associate Professor
Department of Communication Sciences and Disorders
University of Florida
Gainesville, FL

James R. Curran, M.S.
Director
Professional Support Services
Starkey Laboratories, Inc.
Eden Prairie, MN

Alan L. Desmond, M.S.
Director
Blue Ridge Hearing and Balance Clinic
Princeton, WV

Harvey Dillon, Ph.D.
Principal Research Scientist
National Acoustic Laboratories
Chatswood, NSW
Australia

Elizabeth A. Dinces, M.D.
Assistant Professor
Department of Otolaryngology
Albert Einstein College of Medicine
Montefiore Medical Center
Bronx, NY

John M. Fredrickson, M.D., Ph.D.
Professor
Department of Otolaryngology–Head and Neck Surgery
Washington University School of Medicine
St. Louis, MO

Jean-Pierre Gagné, Ph.D.
Professor and Director
École d'orthophonie et d'audiologie
Université de Montréal
Montreal, Quebec
Canada

John W. Hesse, II, J.D.
American Speech–Language–Hearing Association
Rockville, MD

Holly Hosford-Dunn, Ph.D.
President
Tucson Audiology Institute, Inc.
Managing Member
Arizona Audiology Network, LLC
Tucson, AZ

Mary Beth Jennings, M.Sc. (Applied)
Audiologist
Department of Audiology and Speech-Language Pathology
The Canadian Hearing Society
Toronto, Ontario
Canada

Holly S. Kaplan, Ph.D., CCC-A
Clinical Supervisor
Department of Communication Sciences and Disorders
University of Georgia
College of Education
Athens, GA

Francis K. Kuk, Ph.D.
Director of Audiology
Widex Hearing Aid Company
Long Island City, NY

Dawna E. Lewis, M.A.
Senior Audiologist
Boys Town National Research Hospital
Omaha, NE

Harry Levitt, B.Sc., Ph.D.
Professor
Center for Research in Speech and Hearing Sciences
City University of New York Graduate School
New York, NY

George A. Lindley, IV, M.S.
Assistant Professor
Department of Communication Science and Disorders
Towson University
Towson, MD

Edward H. Lybarger, B.A.
Allegheny Hearing Association, Inc.
Pittsburgh, PA

Jane R. Madell, Ph.D.
Director
Hearing and Learning Center
Department of Otolaryngology–Head and Neck Surgery
Beth Israel Medical Center
New York, NY

Douglas A. Miller, B.S.E.E.
Research Associate
Department of Otolaryngology
Washington University School of Medicine
St. Louis, MO
Currently: Engineering Research and Development
Otologics, LLC
Boulder, CO

Elaine A. Mormer, M.A.
Clinical Coordinator, Audiology
Department of Communication Science and Disorders
University of Pittsburgh
Audiology Coordinator
Center for Assistive Technology
University of Pittsburgh Medical Center
Pittsburgh, PA

J. Gail Neely, M.D.
Professor and Director of Otology, Neurotology, and Skull Base Surgery
Director of Research
Department of Otolaryngology–Head and Neck Surgery
Washington University School of Medicine
St. Louis, MO

Mary Ellen Nevins, Ed.D.
Program in Education of Hearing Impaired Children
Kean University
Union, NJ

Robert T. Olsson, M.A.
Senior Audiologist
Sonus Center for Tinnitus
San Diego, CA

Catherine V. Palmer, Ph.D.
Director
Audiology and Hearing Aid Services
Eye and Ear Institute
University of Pittsburgh Medical Center
Pittsburgh, PA

Lisa G. Potts, M.S.
Washington University School of Medicine
St. Louis, MO

David A. Preves, Ph.D., M.S.E.E., B.S.E.E.
Vice President
Research and Development
Songbird Medical
Cranbury, NJ

Lawrence J. Revit, M.A.
President
Revitronix
Brownsville, VT

Ross J. Roeser, Ph.D.
Professor and Director
Callier Center for Communication Disorders
School of Human Development
University of Texas at Dallas
Dallas, TX

Brenda M. Ryals, Ph.D.
Professor of Audiology
Department of Communication Sciences and Disorders
James Madison University
Harrisonburg, VA

Carol A. Sammeth, Ph.D., CCC-A
Associate Professor
Department of Audiology
Roudebush V.A. Medical Center
Indiana University School of Medicine
Indianapolis, IN
Currently: Research and Development
Otologics, LLC
Boulder, CO

Robert E. Sandlin, Ph.D.
Adjunct Professor of Audiology
Department of Communication Disorders
San Diego State University
San Diego, CA

H. Christopher Schweitzer, Ph.D.
Executive Director
HEAR 4-U International
Lafayette, CO

William H. Shapiro, M.A.
Clinical Assistant Professor
Department of Otolaryngology
New York University School of Medicine
New York, NY

Joseph J. Smaldino, Ph.D.
Department of Communicative Disorders
University of Northern Iowa
Cedar Falls, IA

Robert W. Sweetow, Ph.D.
Director, Division of Audiology
Professor–Department of Otolaryngology
University of California, San Francisco
San Francisco, CA

Maureen Valente, Ph.D.
Assistant Clinical Professor
Department of Communication Disorders
St. Louis University
St. Louis, MO

Michael Valente, Ph.D.
Professor of Clinical Otolaryngology
Division of Audiology
Department of Otolaryngology–Head and Neck Surgery
Washington University School of Medicine
St. Louis, MO

Mark S. Wallace, M.D.
Assistant Professor
Department of Otolaryngology–Head and Neck Surgery
Washington University School of Medicine
St. Louis, MO

Susan B. Waltzman, Ph.D.
Professor
Department of Otolaryngology
New York University School of Medicine
New York, NY

Richard J. Wiet, M.D.
Department of Otolaryngology–Head and Neck Surgery
Section of Otology/Neurotology
Northwestern University
Chicago, IL

Chapter 1

Hearing Aid Instrumentation and Procedures for Electroacoustic Testing

David A. Preves and James R. Curran

One way to characterize the history of electronic hearing aids is an unrelenting demand for contraction in physical size, accompanied by persistent pressure for improvement in electroacoustic performance. These two forces, often synergistic in effect but sometimes diametrically opposed in terms of their ability to be realized at the same moment, have been responsible for contributing both stunning advances and for holding back progress. The beneficial outcome of the search for ever smaller instrumentation by the industry and its suppliers is the development of today's components and circuits of minuscule size without sacrificing performance. An obvious example is the transducers used in hearing aids; the microphone used in the first successful headworn hearing aids in 1955 was about 60 times larger in volume than the smallest microphones available for use today (Knowles, 1966). Remarkably, the bandwidth, power-handling capacity, and robustness of current microphones far surpasses those of the mid 1950s.

Today's patients are the beneficiaries of the constant search for smaller circuitry and components. We are at a point where the smallest hearing aids (completely in-the-canal or CIC) contain incredibly advanced digital and multimemory programmable circuits that provide excellent, low-distortion, wide-band amplification. But the process of refining and decreasing instrument size has not been smooth; the downside of the ever present insistence to develop smaller hearing aids is seen, for example, in the incorporation of amplifier circuitry having low component count rather than larger, more elaborate, and better performing designs. Similarly, when custom in-the-ear (ITE) instruments became popular in the late 1970s, their small size disallowed the use of external trimmer controls, while at the same time larger, more conspicuous behind-the-ear (BTE) aids with excellent performance (and greater interior space availability) featured as many as six trimmers for performance changes.

EARLY INSTRUMENTATION

The genesis of the modern (wearable) electronic hearing aid took root in the 1930s (Carver, 1978). In those days, design engineers were faced with an unfavorable set of circumstances. Hearing aids consisted of two or more rather large and cumbersome parts, the battery pack and the amplifier, plus the external receiver, and sometimes, an external (crystal) microphone. Large vacuum tubes were used, which had enormous appetites for current and voltage. Even the "midget" vacuum tubes that spurred the development of one piece body worn aids in the mid 1940s (Berger, 1984) were as big as, or bigger than, a thimble; no components such as the transistor existed. Transducers were restricted in bandwidth compared with today, and gain and output were limited. Most importantly, the batteries that were available were relatively short lived and large, as large as or larger than a walk-around portable tape player. In fact, two were needed to operate a hearing aid: one to supply power for amplification, the other to supply the filament(s) on the vacuum tube(s).

The manufacturers' sales and marketing departments exerted constant pressure on the engineers to reduce the size of the instruments. Although one might believe the size of a hearing aid should not stop people from seeking help, then

Audiology: Treatment. Edited by Valente, Hosford-Dunn, and Roeser. Thieme Medical Publishers, Inc., New York © 2000

and today (Kochkin, 1993, 1994a,b), the size of the aid and its cosmetic appearance definitely constitutes one impediment to acceptance. Earlier generations disliked to advertise their disability by wearing a conspicuous hearing aid, even more than today (Watson & Tolan, 1949). Consequently, the engineers of the 1930s and 1940s were forced to make difficult decisions in order to reconcile their basic design objectives. They had to (1) guarantee adequate battery life, within (2) as small a package as possible, with (3) relatively acceptable gain and output. Given the limitations of available technology and the unsatisfactory performance of the components and parts at their disposal, these were nearly impossible demands (Watson & Tolan, 1949).

The need to constantly miniaturize hearing aids compelled adverse design compromises. If the impetus for reduction in size had not been such an operative force over the years, hearing aids with substantially better performance might have been available much earlier, but they would have been markedly larger in size. Each time advances in component or circuit miniaturization occurred, the pressure to reduce size increased. Hearing aid engineers scarcely finished with one design, before new, smaller and better performing technology would arrive. Smaller vacuum tubes, the first transistors, printed circuit boards, integrated circuits, hybrid circuits, smaller transducers, smaller controls and switches, smaller and smaller battery sizes: each new development forced redesign and style changes.

Leland Watson, the founder of Maico, commenting on the industry's progesss, in 1959 said:

> We introduced and pioneered miniaturization and sub-miniaturization of electronic chassis and components. We made the first civilian use of printed and potted circuits. In 1937, we initiated the development of sub-miniature vacuum tubes. In 1948, we made the first civilian use of the mercury-type cell as a source of power. In 1953, two years ahead of the radio and electronics industry generally, and even before their use in the military, we pioneered the application of the transistor and thereby, introduced the most revolutionary change in the electronic field in 40 years. (Skafte, 1990)

The march of miniaturization has continued without letup, from body aids, through eyeglass and BTE aids, to custom aids, and culminated in today's CIC instruments. Throughout the spiral of miniaturization, as mentioned, there was another constant: consumers and professionals alike were disappointed in the instruments' performance.

It can be suggested that much of the discontent, but definitely not all, can be attributed to the class A, peak clipping amplifier. It continued to be used in hearing aids long after it was expedient. Faced with batteries having quite limited life and having to use large components that used up current at an incredible rate, engineers of the 1930s and 1940s developed the simple, unrefined precursors of today's class A circuits (Berger, 1984). Ingenious circuits were developed that operated with one, two, and three or more vacuum tubes and, later, with transistors. Circuit complexity was kept to a minimum to keep size and current drain to a minimum; high emphasis was placed on designing circuits with low component count. The manufacturers also knew early on they had to provide instruments with battery life that did not put exorbitant strains on the pocketbook; this was an extremely important consideration then, and remains so today.

One of the distinguishing characteristics of the class A circuit is its rate of current drain: It is a constant and fairly predictable independent of where the volume control is set. As a result, by using class A circuits, the engineer could design an aid where battery life expectancy could be easily calculated and guaranteed, that had sufficient gain and output, and whose unwieldy components and parts could be fitted within the space available. Unfortunately, the very low current drain that the circuits had to operate under severely compromised the circuit's ability to amplify cleanly at moderately high input levels. An inexpedient characteristic of "current-starved" class A amplifiers is that as frequency increases, so too does impedance. Not enough voltage or current is available from the battery to follow the rapid oscillations of high-frequency signals, leading to excessive harmonic and intermodulation distortion.

The result of using low current–drain class A amplifiers is the unsatisfactory degree of distortion encountered when the aid is forced into saturation. As long as the patient is in an environment with relatively low signal levels, the quality of amplification provided by the class A circuit is acceptable. But at higher input levels, class A circuits peak clip, producing objectionable levels of harmonic and intermodulation distortion, to the point where many refuse to wear their instruments in high noise levels.

PEARL

Because of the necessity to control instrument size and battery life, the engineers continued over the years to use class A peak clipping (linear) circuits because they were understood, predictable in performance, small in size, and low in component count (Watson & Tolan, 1949). This continued even and especially when the changeover from body to headworn BTE and custom instruments occurred. Class A peak clipping circuitry, in its many variations and despite its known limitations, remained the workhorse hearing aid circuit throughout the industry in both Europe and North America for nearly 60 years, not because it was the best available but because battery deficiencies and size exigencies necessitated its use.

Notwithstanding, substantial improvement in hearing aid electroacoustic performance has taken place over the years, but usually in incremental steps that are often not obvious to the casual observer. The shape and appearance of the body, BTE, and custom aids of the 1970s in many respects look quite similar to present-day models. It is only when one looks "under the skin" that it becomes apparent what changes have occurred. For example, early magnetic microphones with their lack of sensitivity, bandwidth deficiencies, and susceptibility to feedback and shock eventually gave way to ceramic microphones and then later to today's rugged and superior performing electret microphones. Each was a distinct improvement on the last, but their exteriors looked virtually identical, except perhaps for size.

Each year the ability of the industry to package better performance into smaller spaces has increased. Advances flow from many sources, primarily from the various suppliers who provide components such as volume and trimmer controls, prefabricated circuits, electronic parts, cords, rubber parts, and transducers to the manufacturers. Many very early manufacturers were vertically integrated initially, (i.e., they manufactured their own components and the parts used in building their instruments). In time, more and more manufacturers became dependent on specialized suppliers to the industry to furnish these parts. Competition between manufacturers and between suppliers eventually became the natural engine for significant improvement in function and form. Now, as new styles are introduced to the marketplace, any hesitance about quality usually disappears quickly as the field has realized that modern advances in circuitry and assembly techniques have made electroacoustic performance decidedly less of an issue than it has been previously. Despite earlier skepticism and concern (e.g., see Berger, 1984, p. 130), any systematic relationship between size and performance no longer exists today.

STYLES OF INSTRUMENTATION

Body-Worn Hearing Aids

The earliest electronic hearing aids were based on the radios, telephones, and public address systems of the time and varied in size from portable units about the size of small suitcases to rather large desklike contrivances that could weigh up to 125 lb. Most were powered by wall current or storage batteries. It was not until the mid 1930s that battery-operated wearable electronic aids began to enter the marketplace. These multipack instruments were worn by men in the pockets of their shirts or coats and by women under their dresses, using special garment carriers. The batteries were contained in separate packs and were as large or larger than the amplifier/transmitter and were strapped to the leg or otherwise concealed under clothing. The first wearable vacuum tube hearing aids of the 1930s used vacuum tubes measuring almost 3 inches high, but by the 1940s the height of the tubes had diminished to approximately an inch (Berger, 1984). The tubes burned out and glass for the tubes was easily broken. With high-level inputs, the vacuum tubes generated microphonics, a faint but audible sound representing the signals they were processing. As late as the mid 1940s, persons with vacuum tube hearing aids continued to wear separate battery packs. After World War II the availability of smaller batteries, advanced, miniature vacuum tubes, and later, transistorized circuits, led to the one-piece (monopack) body aid that dominated the marketplace for the next 10 to 12 years. Although more than one battery was required with these more modern vacuum tube aids, their size was markedly diminished by comparison to those previously available. Later, body aids with transistor amplifiers required batteries of considerably lower voltage than those used with vacuum tube amplifiers;

eventually many body aids required only one battery for appropriate performance.

Another way to characterize the history of hearing aids, other than advances in miniaturization, is to note the effect that the position of the microphone and, to a lesser degree, the receiver has had on patient performance as each new style has been introduced. It turns out that the position of the microphone in the aids and where the aids are worn on the patient strongly influences, in either a positive or negative way, the amplification provided. In body aids the microphones are located at the top of the instruments to minimize the effect of clothing noise. When worn, the patient's body serves as an acoustic baffle and produces a significant increase in the low frequencies with an accompanying roll-off in the high frequencies (Byrne, 1983; Erber, 1973; Watson & Tolan, 1949). (see Fig. 1–1). A body aid that shows a relatively flat frequency response when measured in a test box becomes a low-frequency emphasis amplifier when worn, with a substantive decrement in the frequencies greater than 1000 Hz because of the body baffle effect. This is not an altogether negative outcome for patients with profound hearing loss who usually need a strong boost in the low frequencies or for certain patients with mixed or conductive loss. However, for mild to moderately severe sensorineural losses, where the higher frequencies are important and where upward spread of masking caused by overamplification in the low frequencies is a potential problem (Gagne, 1988; Klein et al, 1990; Trees & Turner, 1986), the effect can be detrimental.

Figure 1–2 shows a comparison of the average field-to-microphone transfer functions at 0 degrees for four styles of hearing aids (BTE, ITE, ITC, and CIC). Note the systematic

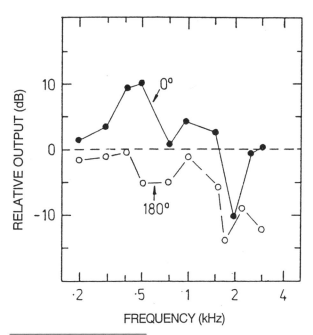

Figure 1–1 The average increase in the low-frequency gain and roll-off in the high-frequency gain for signals coming from the front (0 degrees) because of the body baffle effect. The body also acts as a barrier to the transmission of signals from behind (180 degrees) the wearer. (From Byrne [1983], with permission.)

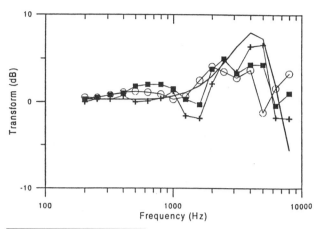

Figure 1–2 Field-to-microphone functions at 0 degrees azimuth for BTE aid (o), ITE (■), ITC (+), and CIC *(solid line)* hearing aids. Note the successive increases in gain above 2000 Hz that are obtained as the microphone position for each style of hearing aid moves closer to the concha-meatal junction. (From Cornelisse & Seewald [1997], with permission.)

increase in sound pressure in the high frequencies as the position of the microphone is changed across alternative styles, as well as the changes in the low frequencies. The striking differences in response are solely due to the differences in the location of the microphone, irrespective of the frequency/gain characteristic within the hearing aids, illustrating vividly the outstanding role microphone placement has played in improving wearable amplification (Cornelisse & Seewald, 1997).

The frequency response and other performance features of the early body aids could be changed by set screws and by interchanging external receivers, but the response changes available, especially for the high frequencies, could be quite limited. An example of the adjustments provided by one fairly high-quality body aid of the 1940s is shown in Figure 1–3 (Watson & Tolan, 1949). It is interesting to note that the useful frequency response range was primarily from 300 Hz to 3000 Hz, reflecting the restricted response provided by the external receivers of the time.

Current modern body aids provide the highest amount of gain and OSPL90 (output sound pressure level with a 90 dB sound pressure level [SPL] input signal)* available in hearing aids; they are capable of providing 2-cc coupler gain as high as 90 dB (peak), with OSPL90 values up to 155 dB SPL (peak). Concealed trimmer controls and switches provide a very wide selection of performance. A flexible wire cord is used to attach the main chassis to either a button-type air conduction receiver or to a bone conduction receiver. The separation of the chassis from the receiver allows very high

---

*The term *SSPL90* (saturation sound pressure level with 90 dB input) has traditionally been used to suggest that with a 90 dB SPL input signal that the hearing aid is in saturation. However, because many instruments incorporate compression circuitry and do not saturate as a result, the term *OSPL90* is recommended for use in the most recent revision of ANSI Standard S3.22, 1996.

CONTROVERSIAL POINT

In 1947 the influential "Harvard Report" (Davis et al, 1947) was published that suggested that either a flat (uniform response) or 6 dB/octave rise in the frequency response shape was optimal for all hearing losses and that additional response shapes were unnecessary. The data were collected using an experimental rack-mounted master hearing aid. Word tests were delivered to listeners by live talkers through PDR-10 supra-aural earphones rather than button receivers, with the result that the low frequencies were attenuated by comparison to actual use conditions (Cox & Studebaker, 1977). Furthermore, the microphone was free standing on a table and had no baffle behind it. The combined effect of the highly probable low-frequency roll-off caused by slit leak (Ciechanowski & Cooper, 1976; Cox & Studebaker, 1977) that occurred as the subjects listened under earphones and the essential elimination of body baffle because of the free-standing microphone resulted, in effect, that the subjects were most likely listening to stimuli having essentially higher frequency emphasis responses instead of the flat or 6 dB/octave rise responses intended. The Harvard Report discredited the idea of selective amplification (i.e., providing maximum amplification in the areas most needed) as "fallacious" and termed individual fitting sessions/protocols "futile and illusory." The report was such an authoritative and prestigious document that its effect was to retard progress and research in the area of hearing aid fitting for many years. However, with a few exceptions, manufacturers of the time (and up to the present) continued to design and sell instruments having the capability of multiple response adjustments because they disagreed with the report's conclusions (Watson & Tolan, 1949). Their experience suggested that the usual result in more than half the fittings, especially where a high-frequency loss was present, was that neither of the report's recommended responses would be beneficial.

amounts of effective gain to be achieved before feedback occurs. Body aids were considered the first choice for children at one time, but this no longer applies because current ear level instruments afford excellent signal processing and are rugged enough to withstand substantial abuse. The popularity of body aids has decreased steadily to less than 1% of the total sold in North America (Kirkwood, 1998), but they do afford special beneficial advantages for many individuals

<table>
<tr><td>

PEARL

It is important to remember that the body baffle effect will always affect the frequency response when a body aid is worn and will cause it to operate essentially as a low-pass filter, unless precautions are taken to adjust the frequency response to overcome the low-frequency boost and high-frequency de-emphasis. Audiologists should be sure to take this fact into account when fitting this type of aid. It is important to obtain a real-ear aided response (REAR) to establish the shape of the frequency response to which the patient is being exposed.

</td></tr>
</table>

with extremely severe or profound hearing loss or for those who need the availability of large controls.

During the early 1930s, bone conduction receivers for body hearing aids were introduced and grew in popularity over the next decade and a half. The bone conduction path to the cochlea was well known for years before being exploited for hearing aid amplification. Routine surgical intervention for the correction of middle ear problems had not yet been established, with the result that persons with conductive loss and adequate cochlear reserve benefited substantially from bone conduction amplification with body aids.

The early bone vibrators were quite bulky and cumbersome and were held in place on a lorgnette or by hand. Subsequent designs reduced the size of the vibrator substantially, and head bands were introduced to hold the smaller bone conduction oscillators in place. In terms of bandwidth, the bone conduction receiver acts as a low-pass filter, providing little or no amplification in the high frequencies. In addition, because it is designed to set the bones of the skull into oscillation, it requires considerable power to operate.

For some time, bone conduction hearing aids were the first choice for persons with conductive loss, whereas air conduction instruments were recommended and fitted to those with sensorineural losses. Today bone conduction amplification is rarely considered the first choice for either conductive or sensorineural losses. It is usually recommended for children or others having deformed or absent outer or middle ears or for those with intractable middle ear disease. Modern bone conduction hearing aids are not only available with body aids but are also constructed within a headband configuration or within the temples of eyeglass hearing aids. Usually, only patients with bone conduction thresholds within normal limits benefit, but occasionally, extremely powerful body aids can be used for those with poorer bone conduction thresholds.

Ear-Level Hearing Aids
Eyeglass

The advent of the junction transistor in 1952 (Berger, 1984) was the impetus for the introduction of three new styles of hearing aids in the 1950s, the eyeglass, BTE, and the custom ITE (Fig. 1–4). Of the three, the style that made the most impact initially was the air conduction eyeglass aid. The entire aid, including the receiver, was built into the eyeglass temples, with sound delivered to the ear through clear plastic tubing and a custom-fabricated earmold. Its introduction resulted in an avalanche of ads proclaiming that eyeglass hearing aids had "no wires and no buttons," even though the presence of the polyvinyl tubing and earmold probably called as much attention to the aids as the external button receiver and cord of body aids. The earliest versions were very large, bulky, and heavy, and the components were split between each of the two eyeglass temples, connected together by wires or electrical contacts concealed within the eyeglass frames. By the late 1950s downsizing of components had progressed so rapidly that all were housed solely in one temple.

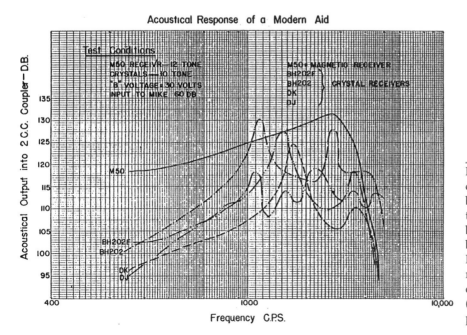

Figure 1–3 Frequency response curves for a "high-quality" monopack body hearing aid of the 1940s showing the variations in response that could be obtained by changing receivers or by adjusting tone screws and switches. Note the difference of the frequency response shape of the magnetic compared with the crystal receivers. (From Watson & Tolan [1949], with permission.)

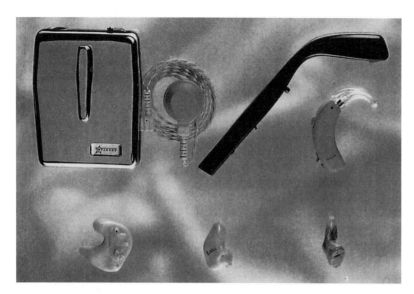

Figure 1–4 Examples of the six basic styles of modern hearing aids. Clockwise from upper left corner: body aid with external receiver, eyeglass hearing aid, BTE aid, CIC aid, ITC aid, and ITE aid. (Courtesy of Starkey Laboratories.)

The electroacoustic performance of eyeglass aids was very similar to the BTE aids of the day, with 2-cc gain ranging up to 60- to 70-dB (peak), and OSPL90 up to about 132-to 134-dB SPL (peak). Early models located the microphones in the paddle portion of the temple with the microphone opening facing to the rear, but in time, microphones were gradually moved to a forward-mounted position, usually on the underside of the temple. The eyeglass hearing aid presented a challenge to hearing aid designers and assemblers because, for the first time, the microphone and receiver were contained in the same housing. This proximity of input (microphone) and output transducer (receiver) caused acoustical and mechanical feedback problems. The result of an ear-level microphone location in eyeglass hearing aids was that the body baffle effect was eliminated so that not only was the low-frequency emphasis obviated but the high frequencies were also well maintained by comparison. This fact, coupled with its cosmetic advantages, contributed to the huge popularity that the eyeglass style continued to enjoy the next 15 or 20 years.

PEARL

It is hard to imagine today how popular the eyeglass aid was at the time. Hearing Aid Industry Conference (HAIC) sales figures for 1959 showed that eyeglass aids constituted nearly 65% of the market, far ahead of BTE aids and body aids, each of which were responsible for only 12% of the sales, respectively (Skafte, 1990).

Eyeglass aids began to be discontinued in the late 1970s because of the rapid growth in popularity of custom ITE instruments and for other reasons. Because of their slender shape and construction, they were somewhat more fragile than BTE or custom aids. Frames having the proper type of hinge for connection to the temples became harder to find. The ability to adjust eyeglass frames for a comfortable nonslip

fit, at one time a necessary skill for the dispenser, became nearly a lost art. When the eyeglass aid needed repair, the patient had to have a spare set of glasses because when the aid was removed, so were the glasses. However, a few previous users to this day still insist on being fitted with this style, a testimony to the strength of the desire to camouflage the presence of hearing aids. A few models are available primarily from European manufacturers, but they have disappeared almost entirely from the catalogs of most North American suppliers. Some manufacturers provide BTE aids that can be directly connected to slim, relatively attractive temples with specially designed adapters for holding the BTE aid in place behind the ear. Finally, a few eyeglass bone conduction aids are available for the relatively few patients with air-bone gaps (and cochlear reserve within normal limits) that cannot benefit from air conduction amplification.

Behind-the-Ear

The BTE style, although first introduced in the 1950s, did not actually rise to prominence until the late 1960s. BTE hearing aids are configured so that the transducers, battery, electronics, and controls are contained within a curved plastic chassis that fits behind the pinna. Amplified sound is transmitted to the ear through an earhook, translucent polyvinyl tubing, and an external earmold. Today, these versatile instruments provide the widest range of gain and output available in ear level aids, with up to as much as 80 dB peak gain in 2-cc and 140 dB SPL peak OSPL90.

In the same way as eyeglass aids the first models were extremely large and clumsy, with rear-facing microphones and few frequency-response adjustment options. The first BTE instruments had their microphones facing toward the rear at the bottom of the case. Later, studies of the effect of head diffraction on the input signal to the microphone revealed that this location had an unfavorable polar directivity pattern (Lybarger & Barron, 1965) (i.e., more signal was received from the rear direction behind the wearer than from the frontal direction). Early production models were beset with internal feedback problems; the magnetic microphones and receivers of the day were extremely susceptible to shock and constituted one of the main causes of breakdown. The microphone had to be distanced as far as possible from the receiver; early attempts to position the microphone at the front of the aid in a forward-facing direction next to the receiver exacerbated feedback problems. This was because the magnetic receivers and microphones, even when mounted at right angles to each other to minimize electromagnetic induction, produced high levels of feedback in all but low and moderate gain instruments.

Introduction of ceramic microphones, and later the modern, lightweight electret condenser microphone in the 1970s greatly reduced feedback problems and provided very broad bandwidth capability (see Fig. 1–5). In 1962, 4 years after eyeglass aids accounted for most annual sales, BTE aids had surpassed them in total volume (Bolstein, 1977). By the mid 1970s, BTE sales had increased to nearly 70% of the total sold in North America. The rapid rise of the BTE style was directly related to the refinement and miniaturization of circuitry, transducers, and controls (Fig. 1–6), and the superior performance that was afforded by the microphone mounted on the head closer to the natural opening of the ear. In addition, greater attention began to be paid to the performance of the instruments on the patient; the introduction of KEMAR (Burkhard & Sachs, 1975) and subminiature microphone assemblies (Knowles, 1975) for performing measurements in the earcanal made possible the first reliable studies of the effects of earmolds and microphone position on the performance of hearing aids.

The BTE style affords the audiologist many optional and desirable features. These include a telecoil, two-position and three-position patient-operated switches that may be used to control direct-audio and frequency modulated (FM) signal input alternatives, extensive response and performance manipulation by means of wide range trimmer controls, optional

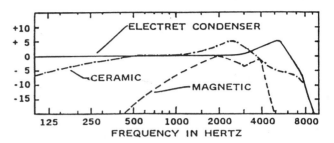

Figure 1–5 Representative response curves of three types of hearing aid microphones, showing the extension of the frequency response provided by the ceramic and the electret microphones compared with the magnetic type. (From Berger [1984], with permission.)

remote controls, and directional and nondirectional microphone switching capabilities. For children, the advent of BTE aids leads to improved performance by eliminating the body baffle effect. Furthermore, the number of binaural as opposed to monaural or Y-cord* fittings that were once customary has increased as has the acceptance of amplification by children and parents alike. Some contemporary BTE hearing aids

---

*Y-cord fittings were a popular alternative for fitting body aids, especially for children. Instead of having a single cord connecting the body aid to one receiver (and one ear), a special branched cord that terminated in two receivers was substituted, one for each ear, to provide a pseudobinaural fitting. Both ears were stimulated, but the arrangement could only be used when both ears appeared to have approximately the same hearing loss; the signal delivered to each ear was essentially identical and monaural in nature. Y-cord fittings dropped virtually out of sight when ear-level aids permitting true binaural amplification became available.

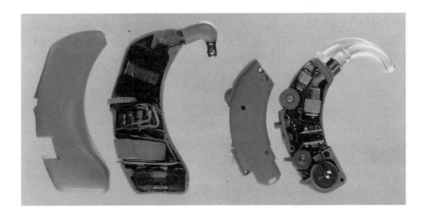

Figure 1–6 Progress in miniaturization and construction of BTE aids over four decades. The larger instrument from the 1960s on the left provided about 40 dB of gain; note the size of the bottom-mounted microphone, the lack of controls or switches, the discrete component amplifier, and the use of bulky rubber cushions to isolate the transducers to prevent feedback oscillation. By contrast, the modern programmable compression instrument on the right provides more than 70 dB of gain with broad bandwidth, and both transducers together are smaller in size than either the microphone or the receiver in the older aid. In addition, the modern instrument provides a three-memory selection switch, a telecoil, and a three-position off-telephone-microphone switch for performance adjustments; its amplifier is a monolithic integrated circuit that incorporates both CMOS and bipolar circuitry. (Courtesy of Starkey Laboratories.)

incorporate an FM receiver and antenna to facilitate listening through RF classroom amplification systems. These designs are intended to supplement more conventional arrangements (e.g., where BTE aids are directly coupled to body-worn FM receivers by means of a cord or BTE aids that receive the FM signal through a telecoil/neck loop arrangement). Other chapters in this text elaborate on assistive listening devices (ALDS) and sound field amplification techniques that are used to augment conventional ear-level amplification in the home, at work, and in the classroom.

When ear-level aids were introduced in the late 1950s and 1960s, it was universally believed by audiologists that the conservative and appropriate course was to continue to recommend body aids because of their superiority in rugged construction and electroacoustic performance compared with BTEs. Within a decade that had begun to change, and the BTE aid eventually became the instrument of choice. In the same way, all new styles, especially the custom-made styles, ITE, ITC, and CIC, when they were first introduced met with a certain amount of rejection. Objections to their small size, early limits on available gain and OSPL90, and assumptions about the instruments' ability to withstand the exigencies of day-to-day handling by patients were among the reasons for audiologists' reluctance to embrace them. Today, however, the custom aid in its various forms has assumed paramount importance in North America, and significant resistance to its use has completely disappeared.

PEARL

Historically, BTE aids were usually the first style to incorporate the most recent and sophisticated technological advantages because of the space for parts they provided, but modern improvements in integrated circuitry and component miniaturization no longer make this true. Now, it is not uncommon to see the latest advances in performance and features introduced to the market not only within BTE aids but also in the custom ITE, ITC, and CIC styles as well.

Custom In-the-Ear, In-the-Canal, and Completely In-the-Canal

By the mid 1950s several separate entrepreneurs independently began to experimentally build aids completely within custom ear shells (Skafte, 1990). Two manufacturers, Earmaster and Goldentone, subsequently dedicated themselves to the manufacture of custom instruments. Both eventually failed because the transducers and circuits of the time were oversized, venting was difficult to accomplish, and production problems were formidable. When reintroduced to the market in the early 1970s, these problems had been largely overcome, and custom aids in all variations rapidly grew to capture almost the entire marketplace and continue to dominate it up to the present, accounting for about 80% of the sales in North America (Kirkwood, 1998).

Besides the fact that custom aids were comfortable and easy to use, three other factors accounted for their astonishing growth. First, in the 1970s, advertising for leads by the

manufacturers for new customers and prospects, then a necessary component of industry sales, had diminished markedly because the advertising practices of the industry had come under serious scrutiny by the Federal Trade Commission (FTC) and the Food and Drug Administration (FDA). Hearing aid dealers' sales had slowed to a standstill as a result. The advent of improved custom aids gave the dealers a chance to recontact and sell their existing file of customers a totally new product, one that promised better hearing and enhanced cosmetic appearance. Most importantly, expensive, questionable advertising was not required.

Second, the leading custom aid manufacturer, Starkey, instituted a policy of a 90-day money-back return privilege in 1973 (Austin, personal communication, 1998), a revolutionary concept at the time that dealers passed on to their customers in the form of a free 30-day trial. This trial was used effectively by the dealers to persuade their existing customers to try the new aids.

Third, the ITE instruments afforded several acoustic advantages over the existing BTE, body, and eyeglass instruments. The first custom aids were essentially simple BTE circuits with their transducers, repackaged. The most used receiver at the time was the Knowles BK series, which when used in BTE aids provided a response that had three characteristic peaks. The first peak was caused by the length of the earhook and the plastic tubing that followed the receiver; this tubing-related resonance occurred at about 1000 Hz. The second and third peaks were related to the mechanical resonance of the receiver itself, which occurred at 2000 Hz and 4000 Hz.

However, when the BK receiver was installed in a custom ITE aid instead of a BTE, the tubing-related resonance at 1000 Hz disappeared because the receiver was now contained within the earshell, close to its medial tip, and only a very short length of tubing was needed (Madaffari & Stanley, 1996; Knowles Electronics, 1976). This constituted a considerable improvement in the response of the aids for the many patients who had better hearing in the low and mid frequencies and greater loss in the high frequencies. These patients could now receive better high-frequency amplification because the absence of the 1000 Hz peak allowed him or her to turn the volume control higher. (Byrne et al, 1981). Furthermore, studies showed that compared with BTE aids with identical performance and components (Griffing & Preves, 1976), the position of the microphone caused an enhancement of the high frequencies by approximately 4- to 6-dB, a very desirable outcome (Fig. 1–2). Finally, by moving the receiver closer to the tympanic membrane, less gain was required to provide appropriate correction for a given hearing loss compared with an equivalent BTE aid, which in turn resulted in reduced current drain and prolonged battery life.

These benefits for patients resulted in extraordinary sales growth and were strong enough to overcome the objections of those who considered the ITE an overpublicized novelty rather than a genuine advance. The ITE's success is an excellent example of a promising concept that with refinement and continuing improvement culminated in advancing the state of the art. Today ITE hearing aids are the instruments of choice for a wide variety and range of hearing losses, from mild to very severe. Featuring peak gain up to 65 dB and peak SSPL90 up to 125 dB SPL, they are easily fitted to very small ears and routinely incorporate two and three, and sometimes up to four, wide-range trimmer controls. At one time ITE telecoils were inadequate in power, but modern telecoils afford the patient with excellent amplification, including those with severe hearing losses. The reader is referred to the section later in this chapter on induction coils. Adaptable to CROS-BICROS* configuration, some manufacturers also provide adapters and cord for connection to FM auditory training systems.

In one form or another a two-piece modular version of the ITE has been in the marketplace since the mid 1960s (Bozarth & Tischbein, 1980; Major, 1971; Stegman, 1966.) A very small chassis with built-in electronics and controls is snapped into or connected to a separate custom-made earmold. The theoretical advantages of the modular version are the lack of need for fabrication of a custom shell, large batch rather than individual unit manufacturing processes, predictable product performance, and immediate ability to replace instruments in the field. Although a very appealing concept, the modular ITE has never been a substantive factor in the North American market, although it has been more successful in Europe and other countries (Clasen et al, 1987). Problems fitting the aids to a wide variety of shapes and sizes of ears, problems with feedback and venting in any but low-powered aids, and less acceptable cosmetic appearance are some of the reasons for its lack of success in North America.

In the early 1980s, President Ronald Reagan was fitted with one of the first custom ITC aids, which were essentially refinements of ITE aids made possible by advances in component miniaturization, especially by the introduction of the Knowles ED receiver. The ED was substantially smaller compared with previous receivers (e.g., the BK) and had a considerably broader bandwidth. The resulting publicity increased industry sales dramatically. The first versions of the ITC had multiple shortcomings, including high incidence of feedback because of undamped, high-frequency response peaks in the ED receiver, lack of appropriate venting, and consequent problems with the occlusion effect. The instruments were considerably smaller than ITE aids and were initially considered useful only for mild losses. Because most persons with mild losses have good hearing in the low frequencies, the incidence of occlusion effect[†] complaints rose considerably, resulting in a high percentage of repairs and returns. In addition, some previous wearers of ITE instruments became dissatisfied with the noticeably enhanced high-frequency quality of the ITC aids, which was due to the markedly wider bandwidth provided by the newer ED receiver. Manufacturers soon learned how to resolve these problems by using advanced venting techniques and frequency-response shaping, resulting in fewer patient complaints and product returns.

---

* The CROS and BICROS hearing aid styles are special adaptations for providing amplification to persons with unilateral and other types of hearing loss. They are more fully described in a subsequent portion of this chapter.

† The occlusion effect is the perception by a patient that his or her own voice sounds hollow or "in a barrel" when he or she is speaking. It is caused by particle vibrations in the cartilaginous portion of the external auditory meatus, which occur when speaking but normally escape to the outside in the unoccluded condition. However, when an earmold terminates in the cartilaginous portion, the particle vibrations, which are essentially low frequency in nature, are blocked from escaping and are transmitted instead directly through the middle ear to the cochlea. If a person has essentially good hearing in the low frequencies, he or she is more liable to be affected.

Measurements showed that the position of the microphone, located closer to the concha-meatal junction, afforded an additional 2- to 4-dB in the high frequencies compared with ITE aids (Bentler & Pavlovic, 1989) (see Fig. 1–2). In his studies, Sullivan (1989a,b) found that when both an ITE and a mini-ITC aid were fabricated from the same impression and had identical electroacoustic performance in a 2-cc coupler, the mini-ITC aid delivered higher SPLs in the residual volume cavity of the earcanal. Part, but not all, of the SPL increase was due to the differences in microphone placement. In addition, he suggested that because the mini-ITC had less retention properties, it slid slightly further down into the ear further reducing the residual cavity volume. Batteries of smaller size and volume, and consequently less expected life, are required for mini-ITC and CIC aids. But as the residual cavity into which instruments deliver their output becomes smaller, the SPL increases, and less electrical gain and current drain are actually required. This has made the downsizing of battery size and performance less of a problem than might be expected. Initially thought to be only useful with mild losses, ITC instruments can now provide 2-cc coupler peak gains up to 45- to 50-dB and peak OSPL90 in the range of 115- to 120-dB SPL, suitable for moderately severe and severe losses. Two trimmer controls are often routinely available, but usually telecoils are only available on a space-available basis.

At present, the ultimate, but certainly not the final, expression of instrument miniaturization is the CIC instrument introduced in the early 1990s. First versions (termed "peritympanic") were developed by Phillips in Holland and involved obtaining two impressions of the complete earcanal down to and including the tympanic membrane (Staab, 1992, 1997). With time it became apparent that deep impressions that extended only beyond the second bend of the external auditory meatus were sufficient. At the time of this writing the CIC style accounts for approximately 10% of sales in North America (Kirkwood, 1998).

The CIC offers three advantageous benefits not achievable with other styles. First, the position of the microphone at or inside the concha-meatal junction provides an additional 3 to 4 dB advantage compared with the ITE style in the higher frequencies (Cornelisse & Seewald, 1997), and because the instrument terminates deep within the earcanal, it produces very high levels of sound pressure within the substantially reduced residual space. Second, the proximity of the receiver to the tympanic membrane reduces the difference in source and load impedance, with the result that high frequencies are more efficiently transmitted. Third, the termination of the medial tip beyond the second bend within the bony portion of the canal results in a significant diminution of the occlusion effect (Bryant et al, 1991; Killion et al, 1988).

Thus for any given hearing loss, to achieve a given output in the earcanal, less amplifier gain is required for CIC aids than is required for any other style of hearing aids. Table 1–1 (Seewald et al, 1997) provides values that can be added to a 2-cc coupler frequency response to obtain an average estimate of the REAR for CIC aids. This transform for estimating real-ear output (TEREO) (Seewald et al, 1997) combines the effects of the microphone position at the concha-meatal junction and the deep insertion of the medial tip of the aid. Table 1–1 illustrates the substantial output SPL (especially in the high frequencies) that is provided by a CIC.

TABLE 1–1   The transform for estimating real-ear output (TEREO) for CIC hearing aids at two azimuths

Azimuth (degrees)	Frequency (kHz)										
	.25	.5	.75	.1	1.5	2	3	4	6	8	
0	6.7	8.6	10.1	11.5	14.2	17.2	23.4	28.2	27.1	17.7	dB
45	9.2	11.4	13.2	14.7	17.5	20.4	26.9	32.7	35.1	23.4	dB

The values in the table can be added to the 2-cc coupler full on gain to obtain an estimate of the real-ear–aided response (REAR) in the patient's ear. (From Seewald et al [1977], with permission.)

Taken together, the CIC often becomes the instrument of choice for persons with high-frequency losses, because it overcomes the biggest problems facing this type of fitting (feedback and occlusion effect), while providing desirable high-frequency amplification.

Typically, CICs are made available either without a volume control or with a screw set volume control, and until recently offered only very small vents and no trimmer controls or telecoils. Some manufacturers have developed external devices for manipulating the gain, and in the case of some digital and programmable CICs, remote controls are provided to adjust gain, change memories, and program the aids. For such small instruments the 2-cc gain and OSPL90 levels that are available are surprisingly high, up to 45- to 50-dB peak gain and 117- to 120-dB SPL peak OSPL90. Despite their favorable advantages, CICs typically are high-maintenance products and are usually recommended only for those patients who can maintain a relatively high level of product hygiene and care, especially with regard to cerumen buildup.

Contralateral Routing of Signals (CROS) Amplification

The contralateral routing of signals (CROS) concept was popularized in North America in a series of papers by Harford and associates at Northwestern University in the 1960s (Dodds & Harford, 1968; Harford, 1966, 1967; Harford & Barry, 1965; Harford & Dodds, 1974; Harford & Fox, 1978). The CROS articles described an eyeglass hearing aid that was divided between two temples. One part of the aid was contained in one temple and connected by a wire installed in the front of the eyeglasses to the other temple. Early versions situated the microphone on the side of the unilaterally impaired ear, and the sound was delivered to the better or normal ear through an unoccluded earmold. Very soon after, it became common practice to use only tubing, without an earmold connected to it, to carry the sound into the earcanal The result of this innovative coupling system was that the low frequencies were markedly reduced, whereas mainly the high frequencies were amplified. This became the impetus for an exhilarating period of progress and discovery because the value of open earcanal, very large vented fittings began to be realized, and an appreciation of the contribution of high frequencies to the intelligibility of the amplified signal was rekindled.

To gain a better understanding of the full impact of CROS, consider the state of the art at the time. Most fittings routinely used full earmolds with no more than small or medium-sized vents at most. Although the acoustic modifier earmold (McGee, 1962), a shortened wide-bore mold with rather large

vents, had been introduced a few years previously, most dispensers and audiologists were relatively ignorant of the effects of a large vent on the frequency response of the earmold; it was viewed by them primarily as a perfect recipe for causing feedback. Body aids were still being fitted with regularity, and most of the literature available about earmolds was based on the external receiver configuration. Most ear-level aids featured relatively broad frequency responses, with insufficient low-frequency reduction capability. Wide-range trimmer controls for changing the low-frequency response of the aids simply did not exist. The consequence was that the most difficult patients to fit were those with good hearing in the low frequencies and poor hearing in the high frequencies. In fact, this lack of ability to modify the frequency response to fit high-frequency losses was one root reason for the dictum that patients with nerve losses could not be helped with hearing aids.

The CROS aid was initially introduced as a method for fitting unilateral losses; the unoccluding earmold or tubing was used to prevent overamplification in the good ear. But Harford and Barry (1965) also suggested that when the better ear had a high-frequency loss rather than normal-hearing, the acceptance of CROS fittings improved. This observation eventually led to the recommendation of CROS amplification for persons who had bilateral high-frequency losses. The separation between the receiver and the microphone was such that substantial amplification could be accomplished before feedback oscillation (Fig. 1–7). The open earcanal allowed low frequencies to enter unimpeded, and the tubing (open earmold) fitting delivered substantial high-frequency amplification. The resultant blend of the two signal sources was highly effective, resulting in at least one ear that could be maximally fitted. Although the CROS aid provided essentially monaural amplification, fitting with one aid was the rule at that time anyway.

Attempts to fit high-frequency losses binaurally by installing two CROS aids operating in opposite directions (CRISS-CROS, DOUBLE-CROS) (Pollack, 1975) failed because the signal introduced into one ear leaked out of that ear and entered the microphone of the other aid. Then it was subsequently amplified and transmitted to the other open ear where it was picked up by the first aid's microphone and transmitted back to the original ear, causing feedback. Audiologists and dealers soon realized they could fit bilateral high-frequency losses with two BTE or eyeglass aids with some form of open earmolds such as tubing only, CROS molds, free field molds, acoustic modifier molds, and so forth (Green, 1969). Incredibly, this type of fitting was termed IROS, for ipsilateral routing of signals, or binaurally, BIROS, for binaural routing of signals (Rowlin, 1972). These tortured acronyms are an indication of

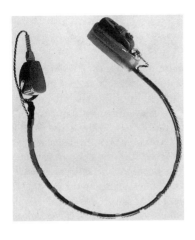 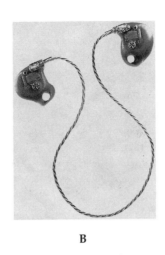 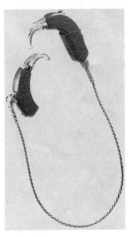

A   B   C

Figure 1–7 Examples of **(A)** a bone conduction CROS aid mounted on a head band, **(B)** an ITE CROS-BICROS aid, and **(C)** a BTE CROS-BICROS aid. (Courtesy of Starkey Laboratories.)

how much the CROS/open earmold idea affected the thinking of the time.

Other forms of CROS became popular, notably Bilateral CROS (BICROS) (Fowler, 1960; Harford & Barry, 1965), which consisted of one complete hearing aid in one temple and an additional microphone located in the other that was wired into the complete hearing aid side. The BICROS was intended for patients with a presumed unaidable hearing loss in one ear, and with a moderate to severe aidable hearing loss in the better ear. A fully occluding earmold instead of an open tubing or earmold was used to deliver the amplified signal to the aidable ear to eliminate feedback. Today the BICROS is a second choice for patients with this kind of loss; usually two complete aids are preferred to provide the benefits of binaural amplification. Hable et al (1990), however, have reported success with an enhanced binaural arrangement called a BICROS-Plus, where a BICROS aid delivers sound to the better ear and a separate power ITE or eyeglass aid is fitted to the poorer ear.

Another useful arrangement, the Power CROS, is sometimes indicated in cases of bilateral, very severe, or profound loss. Here the receiver is crossed to the chosen ear to allow maximum amplification without feedback; it may be an external button type or an internal receiver contained within a custom shell or an earmold. Many subsequent CROS arrangements were discussed in the literature (e.g., Harford & Dodds, 1974; Pollack, 1980), but most were discarded in time, usually because better amplification could be provided with standard BTE or custom aids having the proper coupling configuration.

Although not a true CROS configuration as originally conceived, Sullivan (1988) recommended using a "transcranial" CROS for fitting unilateral losses, where a very powerful ITE or ITC with a long canal is fitted to the "dead" ear. The power aid delivers a signal by means of bone-conducted crossover from the "dead" ear to the better ear, which must have good cochlear reserve in order to perceive the crossed over signal.

As eyeglass hearing aids began to disappear, so did a convenient method for installing CROS. Both BTE and custom ITE aids can be wired for CROS but are not as popular because the wire connecting both sides can be fairly conspicuous. One company (Telex), sensing a need, has developed radio

frequency (RF) CROS and BICROS aids. Instead of signals being transmitted by wire across the head, an RF transmitter on one side broadcasts the signal to a receiver on the opposite side.

CONTROVERSIAL POINT

At that time it was assumed that the best word recognition score that could be obtained by a patient was when tested under audiometric earphones and that an aided word recognition score rarely would exceed that obtained under earphones. In other words, the score under phones represented a maximum performance score that could usually not be improved on, especially with hearing aids (Hirsch, 1952). However, audiologists began to find that word recognition scores obtained by CROS-aided patients in a sound field routinely exceeded those obtained under earphones, and some long-held assumptions began to be examined. Studies of the time (e.g., Green & Ross, 1968; Hodgson & Murdock, 1970; Jetty & Rintelmann, 1970; McClellan, 1967) confirmed that word recognition scores indeed improved as the conditions of coupling were altered appropriately. Later, Harford and Fox (1978) published a study showing improved word recognition performance by patients with flat losses when they were fitted with open, large-vented rather than full, closed molds. Both of these events focused attention on the role that high-frequency amplification played in contributing to word recognition and laid the foundation for today's modern approach to hearing aid fitting.

HEARING AID COMPONENTS

As an acoustic signal enters and travels through the hearing aid, it is processed by successive components/stages during its passage through the instrument. It first encounters the microphone, which converts the incoming acoustic signals to electrical signals; these signals pass to the amplifier, within which three separate stages can be identified: the preamplifier stage, the signal processing stage, and the output stage. The amplifier amplifies and selectively processes the electrical output of the microphone. From the amplifier, the signal is delivered to the receiver (or speaker) and the earmold with its associated tubing (Fig. 1–8). The receiver converts the processed electrical signals from the amplifier output back to acoustic signals. Finally, the battery provides the power needed for operation of all of the preceding components.

All these component parts play an important role in the final performance of the hearing aids. The functions of each interact significantly in determining the characteristics of the hearing aid they are used in and directly affect the ultimate form the amplified signal will take. Poor performance of any of these major components may cause an inadequate fitting and ultimate rejection of the hearing aid by the wearer.

The sequence of the stages of processing and amplification noted previously and shown in Figure 1–8 provide a convenient road map to follow in examining the operation of the hearing aid; we will follow this map and treat each stage in the order given previously in the following sections of this chapter.

Of course, other components in hearing aids, including volume controls, trimmers, and switches, have been exhaustively treated by Agnew (1996b), to which the interested reader is referred; earmolds are covered in Chapter 2 in this volume.

Microphones

Carbon Microphones

Hearing aid microphones are one of the two types of energy transducers used in hearing aids (the other is the receiver). They sense acoustical input signals and convert them to electrical energy. The earliest hearing aid microphones were of the carbon type and dated back to the early 1900s (Fig. 1–9A). A direct current (DC) voltage was applied across a pocket of carbon granules packed tightly behind a diaphragm in an enclosed area. An electrical bias current running through the carbon granules resulted, calculated by Ohms law as current I = Applied voltage/Resistance of carbon granules. The more tightly packed the carbon granules, the smaller the resistance across them. When sound impinged on the diaphragm, the resulting diaphragm movement changed the position of some of the carbon granules relative to each other, causing the resistance across the granules to vary in proportion to the intensity and frequency of the acoustic input. This resistance variation caused a proportional modulation of the bias current, hence converting (transducing) the acoustic signal to an electrical signal. Amplification was restricted to the mid frequencies. The performance of carbon hearing aids was not outstanding because of a crackling or static noise when the position of the granules shifted as the wearer moved, the jagged frequency response, the distortion of the signal transduction (from the carbon granules sticking unevenly together in clumps), and the narrow amplification bandwidth (Berger, 1984; Carver, 1978).

Crystal Microphones

In the mid 1930s the crystal microphone (Fig. 1–9B) came into common use in vacuum tube applications. When pressure is applied to certain crystals, they are deformed and generate an electrical signal, which is then transmitted to the amplifier. Early crystal microphones were extremely sensitive to variations in heat and humidity; they had limited bandwidth and were relatively large. Their high impedance made them quite useful in vacuum tube applications, but they were eventually discontinued when transistor aids became available, which required low-impedance microphones.

Magnetic Microphones

Electromagnetic (also called dynamic) hearing aid microphones were used with vacuum tube hearing aids beginning in the 1920s. Because of their size, low impedance, and excellent energy efficiency, electromagnetic microphones became

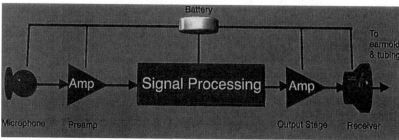

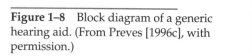

Figure 1–8   Block diagram of a generic hearing aid. (From Preves [1996c], with permission.)

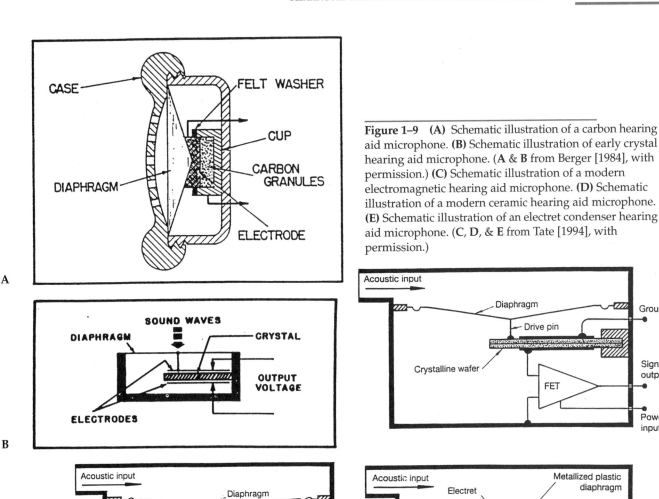

Figure 1–9 **(A)** Schematic illustration of a carbon hearing aid microphone. **(B)** Schematic illustration of early crystal hearing aid microphone. (**A** & **B** from Berger [1984], with permission.) **(C)** Schematic illustration of a modern electromagnetic hearing aid microphone. **(D)** Schematic illustration of a modern ceramic hearing aid microphone. **(E)** Schematic illustration of an electret condenser hearing aid microphone. (**C**, **D**, & **E** from Tate [1994], with permission.)

common when the earliest transistor hearing aids were introduced. The basis of operation for electromagnetic microphones is a magnetic path, formed by metal pole pieces, an air gap, an armature, and a magnet (Fig. 1–9C). A coil is wound around one end of the armature, and the other end of the armature protrudes into the air gap. The armature is connected to the microphone diaphragm by a connecting pin. As incoming sound comes through the microphone port (a hole in the microphone housing), it moves the diaphragm, resulting in one end of the armature moving proportionally within the air gap. The magnetic current changes following the movement of the diaphragm, causing a varying current to flow in the coil by inductive transduction, hence converting the acoustic signal to an electrical signal.

The output of magnetic microphones was relatively low and had to be amplified considerably by the hearing aid amplifier. By the time the signal was amplified sufficiently, feedback problems often resulted from acoustic and mechanical

feedback paths created unintentionally through the inside of the hearing aid and through the hearing aid case, respectively. Also, electromagnetic microphones were sensitive to shock and were easily damaged if the hearing aid was dropped. Their propensity for mechanical feedback and shock damage resulted in hearing aid engineers encasing the microphones in rubber cushions for vibration isolation and increased resistance to shock damage, a practice not common with today's modern microphones. Electromagnetic microphones in the mid 1950s were used mostly in body-worn hearing aids and occupied 3 cm^3 in volume (Killion, 1997).

Ceramic Microphones

A modern version of the crystal microphone, the ceramic (piezoelectric) microphone, was developed in the late 1960s and was considerably more stable and resistant to shock than the electromagnetic microphone (Madaffari & Stanley, 1996). Operation of the ceramic microphone is based on sound moving a diaphragm, which is connected to the piezoelectric material by a strut or pin (Fig. 1–9D). Movement of the diaphragm causes the connecting pin to deform the (ceramic) piezoelectric material, resulting in a varying voltage being produced across it. Ceramic microphones had internal preamplifiers for boosting the microphone output signal and for providing a low output impedance, necessary conditions for their use with transistor amplifiers. Because of the internal preamplifier, the ceramic microphone output signal was typically 15- to 20-dB higher than that from a dynamic microphone. This additional amplification made possible the introduction of more powerful head-worn hearing aids in the 1960s. Also, the ceramic microphone had a much flatter low-frequency response than the magnetic microphone. As a result of the higher output SPL produced, mechanical feedback oscillation often occurred because the high-sensitivity ceramic microphone picked up vibrations from the receiver that were conducted through the hearing aid housing.

Electret Microphones

The problem of oscillation from mechanical feedback in head-worn hearing aids was reduced considerably in the early 1970s with the introduction of the electret microphone (Fig. 1–9E). An electret microphone maintains a permanent charge across its diaphragm; the diaphragm is a thin film of metalized foil that moves in synchrony with the varying pressures that impinge on it. A thin air gap exists between the diaphragm and a backplate, forming a capacitor; as the diaphragm vibrates, the distance between it and the backplate changes according to the amplitude fluctuations of the incoming signal, altering the microphone's capacitance. The resulting capacitance variations, replications of the signal's amplitude fluctuations, produce tiny voltage fluctuations that are transmitted to the preamplifier and thus to subsequent amplifier stages (Olsen, 1986).

The electret condenser microphone, compared with the ceramic microphone, has about the same output amplitude (sensitivity), but because of a low-mass diaphragm construction, is about 20 dB less sensitive to mechanical vibration. As a result, electret microphones do not sense as much mechanical vibration conducted through the hearing aid housing, allowing high gain headworn hearing aids to be produced with fewer internal feedback problems. Electret microphones also have a much higher resistance to shock damage and are able to withstand the hearing aid being dropped. Their low resistance to mechanical vibration, in combination with better resistance to shock, allows them to be used without rubber isolation cushions. Today's smallest electret hearing aid microphones occupy only 0.02-cm^3, a reduction in volume of 150 times compared with hearing aid microphones of 50 years ago (Killion, 1997). The electret microphone is currently used in practically all hearing aids manufactured worldwide. They are available in various frequency responses as shown in Figure 1–10; in most custom aids the frequency response of the aid below 1000 Hz is primarily determined by which microphone is selected by the circuit designer.

Silicone Microphones

Hearing aid microphone development is currently undergoing an important new technological advance: microphones may be formed in the same semiconductor material that is normally used for hearing aid amplifiers, a process that has been referred to as micromachining. Silicone microphones are part of the emerging acoustic silicone sensor technology (Sessler, 1996). The advantages of silicone microphones for hearing aids are (1) their extremely small size (diaphragm areas of about 1 mm^2 compared with about 5 mm^2 for the smallest conventional microphones); (2) extremely low-vibration sensitivity because their diaphragms are so thin (typically < 1 millionth of a meter thick); and (3) a hearing aid microphone may be produced on the same chip as the hearing aid amplifier. This would produce a significant

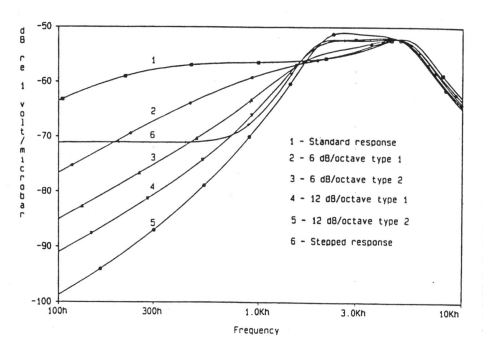

Figure 1–10 Representative frequency responses of microphones available for use in hearing aids. The frequency response below about 2000 Hz, especially in custom aids, is produced by selection of the appropriate microphone slope. (From Madaffari & Stanley [1996], with permission.)

reduction in hearing aid component size and reduce the internal wiring required by eliminating the separate microphone housing. Both electret and piezoelectric silicone microphones have been made. One problem that has delayed the use of silicone microphones in hearing aids has been their relatively high internal noise levels.

For more information on hearing aid microphones, refer to Madafarri and Stanley (1996).

Directional Microphones

Microphones can also be categorized by how much directionality they provide. We have seen that as the diaphragm of a microphone moves back and forth in response to changes in air pressure across it, the energy transducer converts this movement to a proportional output voltage. In an omnidirectional microphone, air is trapped in back of the diaphragm because the rear of the microphone is closed except for a small air leak (Fig. 1–11A). This type of microphone has equal sensitivity to sounds incident from all directions. At present, most hearing aids use omnidirectional microphones.

The earliest directional microphones were bidirectional (Olsen, 1932). A bidirectional microphone is normally made by creating an opening or rear port in the rear cavity behind the diaphragm in an omnidirectional microphone. Bidirectional microphones have equally high output for sounds incident from the front and rear (0 degrees and 180 degrees) and minimum output for sounds incident from the sides (90 degrees and 270 degrees). The first unidirectional microphones (currently called directional microphones) were made by summing the outputs of an omnidirectional microphone element and a bidirectional microphone element (Harry, 1940). For sounds originating from the front, or 0 degrees, the

output voltages of the omnidirectional and bidirectional microphone elements were in phase and added. For sounds coming from the rear, or 180 degrees, the phase of the bidirectional element output was opposite to that of the omnidirectional element and the output voltages canceled. Thus a greater microphone output resulted for sounds incident from the front than from the sides and rear.

Early on, microphone inventors discovered that a bidirectional microphone can be converted to a unidirectional microphone (hereafter called a directional microphone) by covering the rear cavity opening with an acoustic resistance such as a fine mesh screen (Bauer, 1987). The acoustic resistance of the screen acts in combination with the compliance formed by the volume of air in the rear cavity of the microphone to produce a phase shift for sounds entering the rear port of the microphone (Fig. 1–11B). The result of this phase shift is an acoustic delay for sounds entering the rear port of the microphone. The acoustic resistance of the screen is selected such that sounds incident from the rear of the hearing aid wearer are delayed so that they arrive at the back of the diaphragm simultaneously with their arrival at the front of the diaphragm. Typical delays for ITE hearing aid applications depend on the distance between microphone ports and are in the order of 25 to 50 μs. Equal sound pressure arriving on opposite sides of the microphone diaphragm simultaneously results in cancellation of sound from the rear because the diaphragm cannot move. This type of directional microphone is called a *first-order pressure-gradient microphone* because of the directional effect produced by the differential air pressure (gradient) across a single microphone diaphragm.

As discussed later, first-order pressure-gradient directional microphone systems may also be made by combining the outputs of two omnidirectional microphones.

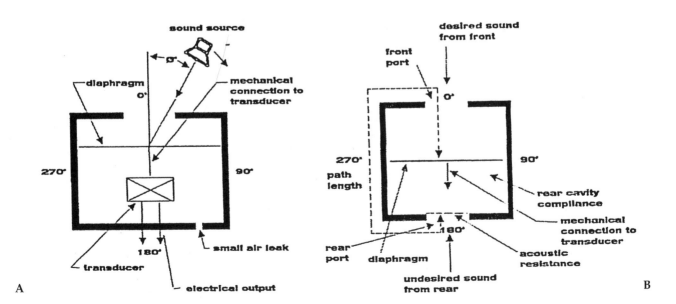

Figure 1–11   Schematic illustrations of **(A)** an omnidirectional microphone and **(B)** a directional microphone. (From Preves [1997], with permission.)

First-order pressure-gradient directional microphones were first used in hearing aids in the early 1970s. Since then, it has been shown that the use of such directional microphones is one of the few methods available for increasing signal-to-noise ratio (SNR) in hearing aid fittings (e.g., Mueller et al, 1983; Valente et al, 1995). The first hearing aids with first-order gradient directional microphones were BTE and eyeglass types. Early prototypes used horse hair and camel hair to create the acoustic resistance that covered the opening in the rear of the microphone housing. These materials did not produce a stable and repeatable acoustic resistance. Later, fine metal mesh screens were used for the acoustic resistance. Hearing aids incorporating first-order pressure-gradient directional microphones have two microphone inlets, one connecting to the air cavity in front of the microphone diaphragm and one connecting to the air cavity in back of the diaphragm (Fig. 1–11B).

During the development of the first directional microphones 50 years ago, acoustical engineers formulated several methods of rating the amount of directivity. Among these were the following:

- *Directivity Factor:* The ratio of microphone output from sounds incident at 0 degrees to that from random sounds incident from all around an imaginary sphere centered on the microphone.
- *Distance Factor:* The square root of the Directivity Factor; indicates how much farther a directional microphone may be from a sound source than an omnidirectional microphone, in the presence of noise incident from all around, for a specific SNR. For example, if a 6 dB SNR was present at a listener with an omnidirectional hearing aid 10 feet from the sound source, the distance could be increased theoretically to 20 feet with a hypercardioid directional microphone without a decrease in SNR.
- *Directivity Index (DI):* The Directivity Factor converted to decibels. The DI simulates the performance of a directional microphone in diffused sound field environments. Some investigators have advocated a DI weighted with the articulation index (AI) (Killion et al, 1998). The AI-DI is derived by multiplying the DI at each frequency by the importance weighting function for that frequency, then performing a root-mean-square (rms) sum on the resulting products.
- *Unidirectional Index (UDI):* The UDI is the ratio of the microphone output from sounds incident on an imaginary front hemisphere (from 270 degrees to 90 degrees, including 0 degrees) to that from sounds incident on an imaginary rear hemisphere (from 90 degrees to 270 degrees, including 180 degrees).
- *Polar directivity pattern:* A graphical plot of the microphone (or hearing instrument) output as a function of angle of sound incidence (see Fig. 1–12). In practice, a polar directivity pattern is obtained by recording the microphone (or hearing instrument) output level (or attenuation relative to that at 0 degrees) at discrete angles as it is turned in circles relative to a loudspeaker in an anechoic chamber. (An anechoic chamber is a room that has wedges on its inside surfaces that almost completely absorb reflective sound.) The concentric reference lines emanating from the center of the polar plot are graduated in decibels. The shapes of polar patterns show in detail how the gain or output SPL of a hearing aid with and without a directional microphone

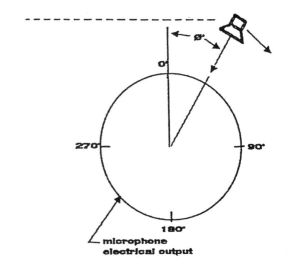

POLAR DIRECTIVITY PATTERNS   **A**

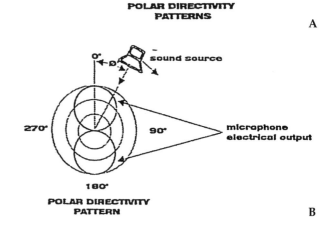

POLAR DIRECTIVITY PATTERN   **B**

Figure 1–12 Theoretical polar directivity of microphones in isolation. **(A)** Omnidirectional and **(B)** bidirectional. (From Preves [1997], with permission.)

varies as the location of the sound source changes. The polar pattern should be thought of as three-dimensional, and the numerical metrics listed above for rating directionality (DI, UDI, etc.) are designed to take into account the noise-suppressing capabilities of a microphone in three dimensions. However, because of the relative difficulty of turning a hearing aid in a vertical arc, polar pattern data are frequently taken only in the horizontal plane and symmetry is assumed in the vertical plane (i.e., the polar pattern in the vertical plane is assumed to be the same as that in the horizontal plane). The Directivity Factor, DI, and UDI are derived from the polar directivity pattern. If symmetry is assumed between the horizontal and vertical planes, these directivity calculations are made in only two dimensions after performing horizontal plane rotation. The type of directionality provided by a hearing instrument is reflected by its polar directivity pattern. An omnidirectional microphone has a perfectly circular polar pattern when tested by itself in an anechoic chamber. Figure 1–12 shows examples of omnidirectional and bidirectional polar directivity patterns.

In any directional hearing instrument the axis of directionality (normally the 0-degree to 180-degree axis in the polar pattern when the hearing aid is not on a wearer) is defined by drawing a line through the two microphone inlet holes. For best results, this axis should be horizontal when the hearing aid is worn. Some manufacturers of directional ITE hearing aids request a line drawn on the ear impression to indicate what the axis of directionality should be when the hearing aid is in place. For directional eyeglass hearing instruments of the 1970s, the axis of directionality passes through two openings on the bottom of the eyeglass temple. For BTE instruments, the axis of directionality passes through front and rear openings near the top of the case (Fig. 1–13A). For a directional microphone in an ITE hearing instrument, the axis of directionality is defined by a line drawn through the two microphone openings in the faceplate (Fig. 1–13B).

Unless compensated for, a directional microphone usually has less low-frequency gain for sounds at 0 degrees incidence than the same microphone with an omnidirectional polar pattern. This reduction in low-frequency gain (Fig. 1–14A) results from the amplitude and phase of the sound pressure condensations and rarefactions being more similar at the two microphone ports for low-frequency waveforms than for high-frequency waveforms (Schulein, personal communication). This effectively produces the same magnitude and phase signals at the two microphone ports for low-frequency sounds. By boosting overall gain and reducing high-frequency gain, this loss of low-frequency gain can be compensated for (Fig. 1–14B).

Figure 1–15 shows examples of cardioid, supercardioid, and hypercardioid polar directivity patterns. At first glance, the supercardioid and hypercardioid polar patterns appear to have less directivity than the cardioid pattern because they have lobes at 180 degrees, whereas the cardioid has a null. However, the supercardioid polar pattern actually has about

---

PEARL

Compensating for loss of low-frequency gain in a switched directional/omnidirectional hearing aid may be advantageous for minimizing the change needed in volume control setting the wearer would have to make in order to equalize loudness between the two operating modes.

---

one half the area (output) of the cardioid for sounds incident on an imaginary rear hemisphere (i.e., twice as much rejection of unwanted sounds from the rear).

CONTROVERSIAL POINT

A "front/back ratio" measurement in an anechoic chamber was used to express the amount of directionality for the first directional hearing aids about 25 years ago (Fig. 1–16). This measurement was contrived by hearing aid manufacturers expressly for directional hearing aids with cardioid microphones. Such a measurement on a coupler shows a cardioid microphone at its best because there is maximum sensitivity for sounds from the front and minimum sensitivity in the null of the cardioid for sounds from 180 degrees. The front-to-back ratio is not a very good measurement for hearing aids with supercardioid or hypercardioid polar patterns, both of which have lobes at 180 degrees, but a higher DI than the cardioid.

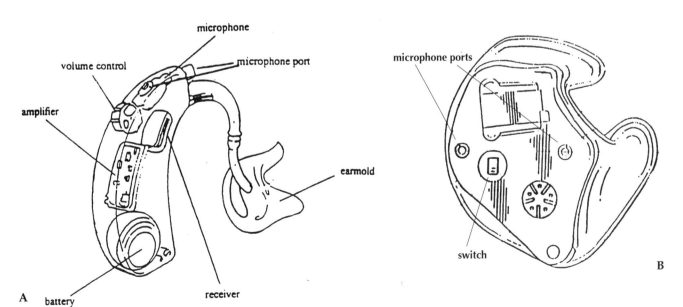

Figure 1–13 **(A)** Schematic illustration of a BTE hearing aid with directional microphone. (From McCracken & Laoide-Kemp [1997], with permission.) **(B)** Schematic illustration of a directional ITE hearing aid. Switch enables wearer to select omnidirectional or directional modes. (From Preves et al [1998], with permission.)

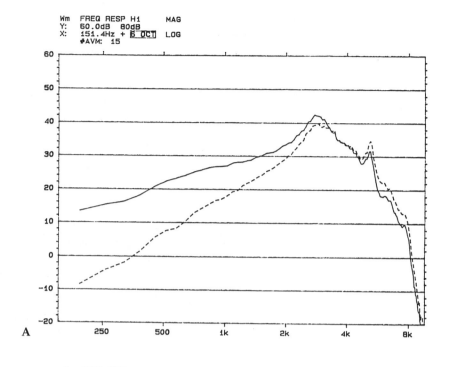

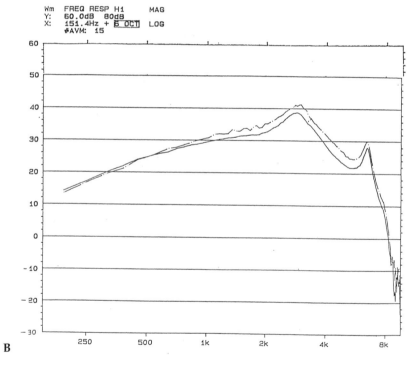

Figure 1–14 Example of **(A)** loss of low-frequency gain produced by a switched ITE directional (*dashed line*)/omnidirectional (*solid line*) hearing aid. **(B)** Same hearing aid with responses equalized.

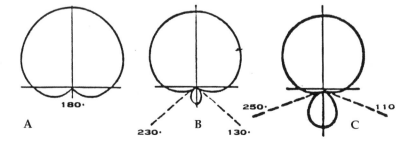

Figure 1–15 Schematized theoretical polar directivity patterns of directional microphones in isolation. **(A)** Cardioid, **(B)** super-cardioid, and **(C)** hypercardioid. (From Preves [1997], with permission.)

TABLE 1–2 Theoretical values for directivity parameters in a free field for microphones having various polar patterns

		Directional		
Parameter	Omnidirectional	Cardioid	Supercardioid	Hypercardioid
Directivity factor	1.0	3.0	3.7	4.0
Directivity index (dB)	0	4.8	5.7	6.0
Unidirectional index (dB)	0	8.4	11.5	8.4
Distance factor	1	1.7	1.9	2

From Preves (1997), with permission.

Table 1–2 gives the theoretical values for the various directivity measures in a free field for microphones having various polar patterns as calculated by several of the early directional microphone inventors (e.g., Glover, 1940). For example, in theory, a supercardioid polar pattern has 3.1 dB more or about twice the unidirectional index of a cardioid polar pattern. The hypercardioid polar pattern also has a DI 0.3 dB higher than the supercardioid in free space, which, in turn has a DI 0.9 dB higher than the cardioid. The microphone designers (e.g., Harry, 1940) reported that directional microphones with hypercardioid polar patterns could produce up to 8 dB more output signal before the onset of acoustical feedback oscillation than those with cardioid polar patterns. In addition, because these directional microphones reduced the amount of transduced low-frequency reverberant energy, perception of desired signals was enhanced in public address applications.

Use of a directional microphone in a hearing instrument is based on two assumptions: (1) The wearer will turn his or her head toward the direction of the desired signal (thus making the axis of directionality adaptive) and (2) Undesired signals are to the back and sides of the wearer. Furthermore, sound diffraction produced by the head of a directional hearing aid wearer alters the theoretical polar patterns shown in Figure 1–15. Even hearing aids with omnidirectional microphones have a noncircular polar pattern when on a hearing aid wearer.

The type of polar pattern provided by hearing instruments with a pressure-gradient directional microphone is determined

CONTROVERSIAL POINT

Contrary to certain trade journal advertising there is no ideal port spacing. The earliest directional microphones required at least a 12 mm separation between the port openings. However, recently, directional hearing aids have been made with excellent directivity with as little as 6 mm separation between port openings by reducing the amount of acoustic delay for sounds entering the rear inlet in the directional microphone.

by the relationship between the time delay created by the acoustic resistor placed over the rear port and the delay caused by the spacing between the two microphone port openings (Madafarri, 1983). The earliest directional hearing instruments were in BTE and eyeglass styles and had cardioid polar directivity patterns (e.g., Preves, 1974, 1975b). Some of the early ITE directional instruments from 20 years ago had supercardioid directivity patterns (e.g, Preves 1976).

A first-order pressure-gradient directional microphone system may also be made by combining the outputs of two omnidirectional microphones (Preves et al, 1998). These systems utilize a switch to use both microphone outputs for directional

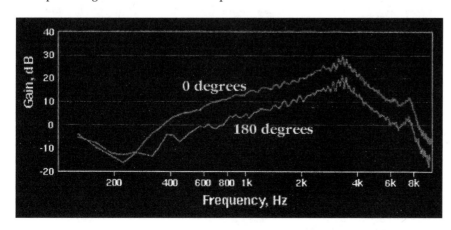

Figure 1–16 Example of frequency responses used as a "front-to-back" directivity measurement. (From Yanz [1997], with permission.)

mode and only one microphone output for omnidirectional mode (Figs. 1–13B and 1–17). An electrical network at the output of the rear microphone contains magnitude-adjusting and phase-shifting circuitry that makes the combination of the two omnidirectional microphones perform like a single first-order gradient directional microphone (Phonak, 1995).

Assessment of directional microphone performance in conventional hearing aid test boxes is problematic because of the sound reflected from the walls inside the test chambers (Preves, 1975a). The use of an anechoic chamber (or a simulated anechoic chamber made by selective time gating) is the one sure way to determine the directional performance of a hearing aid with sound coming from only one direction at a time. Roberts and Schulein (1997) present an overview of technical considerations in measuring the performance of directional microphones with various levels of reverberation in the test environment.

The amount of directivity actually achieved by a wearer of hearing aids with directional microphones depends on the degree of reverberation in the listening environment. Investigators discovered almost immediately that a moderate amount of reverberation can degrade the amount of directionality (Lentz, 1974). Investigators of the performance of hearing aids with directional microphones should be

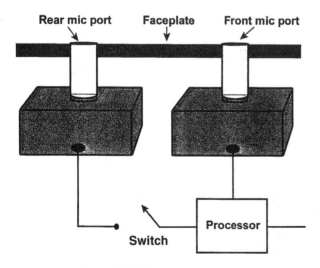

Figure 1–17 Schematic diagram showing combining the outputs of two omnidirectional microphones to form one directional microphone. (From Yanz [1997], with permission.)

cognizant of the critical distance in the test environment (Hawkins & Yacullo, 1984). The critical distance is the distance from the sound source at which the level of direct sound is equal to the level of reverberant sound. At source-test point distances less than the critical distance, sometimes called the near field, the level of direct sound exceeds the level of reverberant sound. At distances greater than the critical distance, sometimes called the far field, the performance of directional microphones in hearing aids is degraded because the level of reverberant sound exceeds the level of the direct sound. For more information on the effect of the critical distance on directionality, readers are referred to Leeuw and Dreschler (1991).

Directional microphones were used many years ago in ITE hearing instruments (e.g. Preves, 1976; Rumoshovsky, 1977). However, since their introduction more than 20 years ago, directional ITE hearing instruments had virtually disappeared from the marketplace until reintroduced recently.

One way of investigating how the directivity of a hearing instrument with a directional microphone is affected by the wearer's body is to determine how the directivity caused by head diffraction interacts with that provided by the directional microphone. This determination can be made by comparing polar directivity patterns and the DIs of an open ear and the same ear with an omnidirectional and directional ITE hearing instruments (Preves, 1997). Preves (1997) compared the DI of a switched ITE hearing aid with directional and omnidirectional operating modes to that of the KEMAR open right ear. At 500 and 1000 Hz, the DIs provided by the open ear were comparable to those provided by the omnidirectional mode of the ITE hearing aid, but the DIs produced in the directional mode were 2- to 3-dB greater than that from the open ear at these frequencies (Table 1–3). At a higher frequency (2000 Hz), the open ear had 0.8 dB and 1.5 dB higher DI than the ITE hearing aid in directional and omnidirectional modes, respectively. Figure 1–18A from this study shows polar directivity patterns at 1000 Hz for these three conditions. In conclusion, a directional ITE hearing aid is viable for improving low-frequency SNR re: unaided.

Few recent behavioral evaluations exist of hearing aids with directional microphones. Killion et al (1998) compared the expected improvement to the actual improvement achieved for an ITE hearing aid with a directional microphone, compared with the same hearing aid with an omnidirectional microphone, on a word recognition in noise task using the Speech In Noise (SIN) test in four real-world

TABLE 1–3 Directivity Index at three frequences obtained for an ITE hearing aid switched between omnidirectional mode and directional mode on KEMAR right ear compared with values for KEMAR open right ear and directional mode in 2-cc coupler

Frequency	0.5 kHz	1 kHz	2 kHz
Open KEMAR ear D.I.	2.3 dB	1.7 dB	5.3 dB
Omnidirectional on KEMAR	2.6	1.2	3.8
Directional on KEMAR	4.3	4.9	4.5
Directional on 2-cc coupler in anechoic chamber	5.8	6.1	5.5

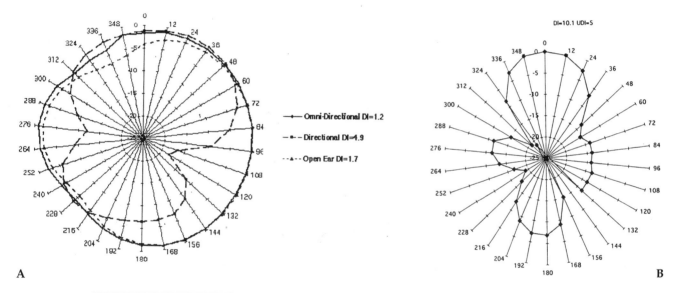

A   B

Figure 1–18   **(A)** Polar directivity patterns at 1000 Hz of KEMAR open right ear *(dotted line)* and an AGC-O ITE hearing aid on KEMAR right ear in omnidirectional mode *(solid line)* and directional mode *(dashed line)*. (From Preves [1997], with permission.) **(B)** 1000-Hz polar directivity pattern on a 2-cc coupler of an ITE BICROS hearing aid with directional microphones on each side. DI = 10.1 dB.

listening situations. They found an actual range of 20% to 60% improvement in word recognition scores was achieved for the directional mode relative to the omnidirectional mode, the exact improvement depending on the combination of hearing loss configuration and the real-world listening situation.

Preves et al (1997) compared the performance of a switched omnidirectional/directional ITE hearing aid fitted binaurally on 10 persons who had never worn hearing aids previously. The study consisted of the Hearing In Noise Test (HINT) (Nillson et al, 1994), Abbreviated Profile of Hearing Aid Benefit (APHAB) (Cox & Alexander, 1995), and subjective preference evaluations performed on the subjects in a first experiment with the frequency responses unequalized between omnidirectional and directional modes and in a second experiment with them equalized. HINT results for both experiments showed a statistically significant 2.4- to 2.8-dB SNR advantage for the directional mode compared with the omnidirectional mode. APHAB results showed statistically

significant advantages for the directional mode on the reverberation subscale and on the background noise and reverberation subscales for frequency responses unequalized and equalized, respectively. Overall, after the second experiment, 7 of 10 subjects preferred the directional mode, 1 preferred the omnidirectional mode, and 2 liked both modes equally well. In both experiments most subjects reported that they would rather not give up the directional-omnidirectional switch option because a variety of listening situations existed in which being able to select omnidirectional or directional operation was an important benefit.

Higher Order Directional Systems and Beamformers

Higher order directional systems can be made by combining the outputs of two or more directional microphones or more than two omnidirectional microphones. Such microphone arrays are called beamformers and have DIs several decibels higher than first-order gradient directional microphones. An example of the polar pattern resulting from combining two-directional microphones in an ITE BICROS hearing aid, each side having a directional microphone with supercardioid polar pattern, is shown in Figure 1–18B. The DI for this system was 10.1 dB on a 2-cc coupler in an anechoic chamber with the two ITE earpieces placed 8.5″ apart. The subject for whom this instrument was made achieved a 6 dB SNR improvement on the HINT test with a 65 dBA competing noise level. Beamformers have the ability to emphasize desired signals while filtering or nulling out one or more noise sources. Some beamforming arrays have nulls (a much reduced output) at fixed locations in their polar directivity patterns that do not change with time. Other beamformers sense the directions of undesirable noises as they move and automatically place their nulls at the locations of these noises in their polar directivity patterns. These directional arrays are called *adaptive beamformers*. Adapting the locations of the nulls is accomplished by using an adaptive filter to "steer" the array. In general, a beamformer can produce up to "*n-1*" nulls in its polar directivity pattern, where "*n*" is the number of microphones used. For example, for the three-microphone array shown in Figure 1–19, 3−1=2 nulls are produced in the polar pattern.

Higher order directional systems with fixed polar patterns can produce excellent performance when used in hearing aid applications because the wearer's head normally turns in the direction of the desired signal, thus making even a fixed beamformer somewhat adaptive. Fixed pattern beamformers have the advantage in hearing aid applications of less hardware size and power consumption because minimal electronics are required. Soede et al (1993a,b) implemented two configurations of fixed-pattern beamformers on an eyeglass hearing aid. Five directional microphones with cardioid polar pattern were placed either in a *broadside array* across the front of the eyeglasses or in an *endfire array* on the right eyeglass

bow. The microphone outputs for the broadside array were simply summed because sounds from the front are incident at the same time for all microphones. For the endfire array, sounds from the front impinge first at the microphone farthest to the front of the wearer's head. Consequently, endfire arrays *use delay and sum beamforming*, meaning that the microphone outputs are delayed by successively smaller amounts going from the front to the back of the wearer's head before they are summed. For example, the output of the microphone farthest to the front of the wearer's head is delayed the most by an amount that makes it arrive at the summing node at the same time as the undelayed output of the microphone farthest to the rear of the wearer's head. In such arrays using omnidirectional microphones, the amount of high-frequency directivity provided depends on the spacing between microphones, and the amount of low-frequency directivity provided depends on the total length of the microphone array. For hearing aid applications in which limited space exists because of cosmetic considerations, the total length of the array limits the amount of directivity provided at low frequencies by the array. That is why it is good to use directional microphones in the array to provide good low-frequency directionality as Soede et al (1993a,b) did. Figure 1–20 shows the comparatively narrow free field polar directivity patterns obtained by Soede et al (1993a) with the broadside microphone array at 4000 Hz. Broadside refers to all microphones in the array receiving sound from straight ahead at the same time. The figure shows that the DI resulting from these patterns was 7.6 dB. In a diffused noise produced by eight loudspeakers, this broadside microphone array produced a mean improvement in the speech reception threshold in noise of 7 dB for 26 subjects relative to that achieved with an omnidirectional microphone.

In another example of a fixed beamformer, Starkey Labs has introduced a chest-worn necklacelike device supported by a neckloop that incorporates six spatially separated microphones made into a directional array (Lehr & Widrow, 1998).

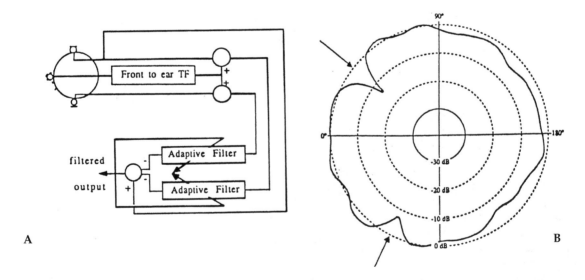

Figure 1–19   Block diagram of a three-microphone beamformer **(A)** and directivity pattern **(B)** achieved showing two nulls within response to uncorrelated noises at 40 degrees and at −60 degrees. (From Preves [1994c], with permission.)

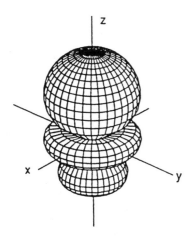

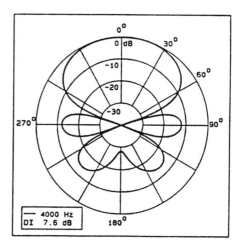

Figure 1–20   Polar directivity patterns at 4000 Hz of five-microphone endfire beamformer; three-dimensional representation *(left)* and two-dimensional representation *(right)*. (From Soede et al [1993a], with permission.)

Output from the array is transmitted by induction (as a wireless link) to any hearing instrument that incorporates a telecoil. The array can be used as a hearing aid in conjunction with a telecoil in a CIC module or BTE hearing aid and can be directly linked to ALDs. The directional signal processing provided by the array improves the SNR available to the wearer by emphasizing sounds in the forward direction by 10- to 20-dB relative to sounds from the sides and rear. The processed frequency range of the array is divided into 12 frequency bands from 0.02 to 6.1 kHz, each with adjustable gain.

Adaptive Directional Systems

One well-known adaptive noise suppression device is the Adaptive Noise Canceller (ANC) (Widrow et al, 1975). The ANC contains an adaptive filter, which changes its characteristics as the amplitude relationships between desired signal and undesired noise change. Referring to Figure 1–21, the signal (S) is the desired input and the signal N is the undesired noise. The two microphones are termed primary and secondary microphones, respectively. The secondary microphone output is used as a reference signal for the adaptive filter. The adaptive filter is adjusted periodically by means of a least mean squares algorithm to minimize the difference between the noise signals in the primary and secondary microphones. The output of the adaptive filter is an estimate of the noise in the primary microphone. The outputs of the primary microphone and adaptive filter are summed (actually subtracted) with the intent of canceling the noise in the primary microphone. Ideally, the summing junction inputs are speech and noise from the primary microphone and an estimate of correlated noise in the primary microphone from the adaptive filter. In the real world, however, reverberation and mismatches in the array allow some of the desired signal to get into the reference microphone, thus canceling part of the desired signal and decreasing the SNR. In hearing aids ANC would be implemented using two microphones, possibly on the same side of the head or with one microphone on each side of the head at each ear in a binaural fitting. In the latter case the microphone outputs need to be processed relative to each

other by the hearing aid circuitry, implying that either a wire between the left and right hearing aids is used or some type of wireless transmission occurs. In such a system with the microphones on opposite sides of the head, an important question arises: What output should be provided to each ear after the two microphone signals are processed? Ideally, the signal from the primary microphone at each ear would be considered the desired signal and the signal from the microphone on the other side of the head would be the reference signal. In a true binaural fitting this would be the case for each ear, implying that two microphones are required on each side of the head.

In theory, only the primary microphone senses the desired signal, and both microphones would have the same noise signal or at least correlated noise signals, conditions not generally achievable with hearing aid fittings. In practice, it is impossible to prevent some primary signal from being picked up by the reference microphone. For more information on the problem of desired signal cancellation in adaptive beamformers, refer to Greenberg and Zurek (1992).

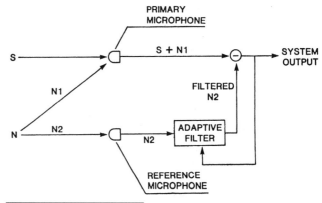

Figure 1–21   Block diagram of adaptive noise canceller (ANC). S, Desired signal; N1, noise in the primary microphone; N2, noise in the reference microphone. (From Preves [1994c], with permission.)

Some investigators have reported results for beamformers with an intelligibility-weighted gain metric (e.g., Greenberg et al, 1993; Stadler & Rabinowitz, 1993). This metric is based on modifications of the articulation index and the speech transmission index. It predicts performance in terms of an intelligibility-weighted SNR for speech (rather than intelligibility) that is not restricted to a minimum or maximum SNR in a given frequency band. The following summarizes results of several fairly recent studies of beamforming for hearing aids. Link and Buckley (1993) theorized that the low frequencies are more important for good speech recognition according to the AI theory, based on equal bandwidths. In their simulations by prewhitening the input to the spacial filter, they improved cancellation of high-frequency interferers that produced improved signal-to-interferer ratio and improved intelligibility averaged gain. Results have been mixed with adaptive beamformers. The main problem has been that when the environment becomes too reverberant, performance with adaptive beamformers degrades because the desired signal may be canceled. Peterson (1987) showed that the 30 dB increase in SNR provided by a two-microphone beamformer of the ANC type in a simulated anechoic chamber is degraded by reverberation to no improvement in a simulated conference room environment. Similar results were achieved by Greenberg and Zurek (1992). Hoffman and Buckley (1995) evaluated a constrained adaptive beamformer in a seven-element, head-worn microphone array for which the amount of cancellation of the desired signal was limited. They evaluated both the effects of mis-steering the microphone array and microphone location variation with an interfering babble noise signal, while simulating head shadow and room reverberation effects. No more than 3 dB cancellation of the desired signal was allowed. Their results showed a substantial improvement in SNR as a function of direct to reverberant energy ratio.

The discouraging results in reverberant environments with adaptive beamformers have led investigators to use fixed beamformers in high levels of reverberation. A *fixed beamformer* has time-invariant processing that produces a fixed polar pattern. Kates and Weiss (1996) compared the performance of several directional systems: (1) a *delay and sum fixed beamformer* (Sydow, 1994) using five nondirectional microphones in an endfire configuration, (2) two types of *superdirective arrays,* and (3) two types of adaptive arrays. A superdirective array has a fixed polar pattern over time and can be implemented by using greater delays in the delay and sum network than those produced by the physical space between the microphones in the array. The spacing between microphones in a superdirective array is less than half of the wavelength of sound (Stadler & Rabinowitz, 1993). The parameters for a superdirective array are set up from the assumed characteristics of the noise to be canceled. Kates and Weiss (1996) evaluated the different systems in an office and a conference room with a male talker located at 0 degrees and uncorrelated multi-talker babble incident from five azimuths. They found that the number of microphones is not an important factor at low frequencies but is important at high frequencies. They recommended using an adaptive array at low-input SNR conditions but to convert to a superdirective array at high-input SNR conditions. Stadler and Rabinowitz (1993) evaluated a fixed microphone array and achieved a DI of more than 7 dB with only two directional microphones in

a broadside array. They stated that beyond the critical distance, a multimicrophone array cannot change the relative levels of the target and background noise, and no gain in intelligibility would be expected to occur. They suggested that the speech transmission index (Houtgast & Steeneken, 1985) be used to calculate performance in such circumstances.

In acknowledgment of the deterioration in performance of adaptive beamformers in high levels of reverberation, investigators have also combined fixed and adaptive beamformers. These arrays normally operate adaptively; however, in high levels of reverberation and in high levels of SNR, the amount of adaptability is considerably reduced and the array essentially becomes a fixed-pattern beamformer. For example, in Kates and Weiss (1996), the adaptive array converges to a superdirective array in a diffuse field.

Amplifiers

The type and quality of the signal processing produced by the hearing aid amplifier is very important in determining how well a person with impaired hearing will function with hearing aids. The hearing aid amplifier selectively processes and amplifies the output signal from the microphone. As discussed previously, the earliest wearable electric hearing aids in the 1920s and 1930s used a carbon microphone that produced an output current whose magnitude was determined, in part, by the applied battery voltage. In essence the microphone (more properly called the transmitter) served as the amplifier of the hearing aid. The variations in current that were produced by the movements of the carbon granules in the transmitter were powered by the battery; the amplified waveform then caused the diaphragm in the earphone to vibrate. If a designer wished to produce greater amplification, a number of methods were used. As many as two, three, or four microphones could be added in series, or the transmitter case could be designed to resonate at desirable frequencies, or the battery voltage could be increased by adding more batteries. Later models incorporated a carbon "booster" for greater gain, but the price was increased distortion. Early wearable carbon aids provided about a 15- to 20-dB peak gain (equivalent in a 2-cc coupler). Later models were able to produce from 25- to 45-dB coupler equivalent peak gain, but essentially, carbon hearing aids were only appropriate for those with mild to moderate hearing loss.

Although primitive vacuum tube hearing aids were introduced in the 1920s, they did not gain substantive popularity until the mid 1930s, when the first wearable models were invented. In fact, carbon aids remained in use well into the early 1940s, because they were stable and fairly rugged compared with the earlier vacuum tube models (Watson & Tolan, 1949). Starting with only one or two vacuum tubes, by 1950, as vacuum tubes began to diminish in size, amplifier designs using up to five or six tubes were introduced. Essentially, the vacuum tube amplifiers of the time were single-ended, class A circuits. Battery sizes also diminished, making possible the monopack hearing aid, where all components were contained in one chassis.

The incorporation of the transistor into hearing aid amplifiers in the 1950s led to the development of smaller headworn hearing aids. The first transistorized hearing aids used point-contact transistors and had circuit noise static problems.

Soon after, performance was improved when the junction transistor began to be used. By 1954, almost all newly developed hearing aid amplifiers used transistor amplifiers (Carver, 1978). Hearing aids with monolithic integrated circuit amplifiers began appearing in the mid 1960s. A monolithic integrated circuit is a semiconductor chip that has many transistors "grown" in it. Modern-day hearing aids are composed of miniature hybrid integrated circuits that package one or more monolithic integrated circuits.

With the advent of programmable and digital hearing aids, both bipolar and complementary metal-oxide semiconductor (CMOS) technology (circuitry developed for use in computers), have been incorporated into hearing aid amplifiers, sometimes on the same chip, to provide the circuitry necessary to provide signal processing that controls the performance of the hearing aid. Frequently, but not always, the signal processing/control portions of the amplifier consist of CMOS technology, whereas the amplification stages are made from bipolar circuitry. Bipolar technology is a semiconductor technology that is the basis for the electronic circuitry that is used in almost all modern electronic appliances and instruments, including radio, television, and stereos. This technology is well understood because it dates back to the invention of the first transistors, is quiet, and continues to be used in most modern hearing aid amplifiers to provide signal amplification. CMOS semiconductor technology was introduced beginning in the early 1980s primarily for digital manipulation of information. It is somewhat noisier than bipolar, but is extraordinarily compact. It is used in more and more hearing aid circuits to facilitate digital operations. Some of the most recently introduced hearing aids use only CMOS circuitry; others combine both types of circuitry: bipolar to provide low noise amplification and CMOS to provide digital control and signal processing of incoming signals.

As mentioned previously, the generic hearing aid amplifier is usually made up of three parts: the preamplifier stage, the signal processing stage and the output stage (Fig. 1–8). The *preamplifier stage* provides enough gain to amplify incoming signals to a level above the circuit noise of the amplifier. The *signal processing stage* manipulates the signal to enhance or extract the information it contains (Kates, 1986). The *output stage* amplifies the output of the signal processing stage and drives the hearing aid receiver. The discussion within the next sections will follow this sequence of components as shown in the block diagram of the hearing aid amplifier in Figure 1–8.

Preamplifier Stage

The first stage of the hearing aid amplifier is a preamplifier, which provides a boost to the microphone (and telecoil) output signals. Sometimes the preamplifier stage is packaged within the microphone (over and above the field-effect transistor normally present). In some hearing aids it also incorporates a signal processing stage.

"Linear" Peak Clipping
Signal Processing Amplifiers

The first hearing aid amplifiers were called "linear" because they had no intentional signal processing such as compression. The definition of a linear system is that a specified

Peak Clipping

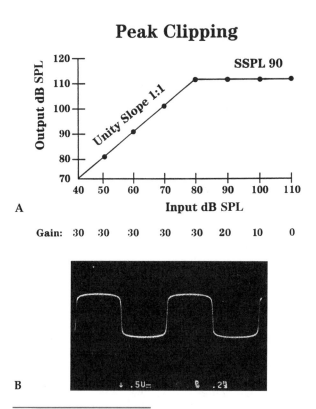

A

Gain: 30   30   30   30   30   20   10   0

B

Figure 1–22 **(A)** Input-output function for a "linear" (PC) hearing aid. **(B)** Example of a pure tone that has been peak clipped. (From Anderson et al [1996], with permission.)

change in input level produces the same change in the output level. The 1:1 relationship between the input signal and the output signal is shown in Figure 1–22A, in which a "unity" (1:1) slope input-output characteristic is depicted. However, in a linear hearing aid, as with any linear audio amplifier, a maximum signal handling capability exists that defines the upper boundary of linear performance. Above that limit, performance is nonlinear because signals are peak clipped due to inadequate headroom, causing saturation. An example of a pure tone signal that has been peak clipped is shown in Figure 1–22B. Limitations in maximum signal handling capability are especially a problem in hearing aids because of the small amount of current they are designed to consume from the tiny, low-voltage batteries used.

PEARL

What is not linear has to be nonlinear. Thus "linear" (PC) hearing aids are actually nonlinear devices at higher input levels because of the distortion produced from saturation. Although saturation is normally associated with the operation of the amplifier output stage and/or receiver, it can occur anywhere in the hearing aid circuitry, i.e., the hearing aid preamplifier or signal-processing sections can saturate at lower input levels than the onset of saturation in the output stage/receiver combination.

The literature uses many terms to describe the various types of amplifiers that are used in hearing aids, and as a result, some confusion exists as to what is meant. The use of the term *linear* to describe PC hearing aids has caused considerable confusion because an important form of compression amplification, discussed in a later section, called *compression limiting* (CL) (Kuk, 1996a; Mueller & Killion, 1996), also has a 1:1 "linear" input/output function below a high-compression threshold (see Figs. 1–22A and 1–23A). Both types of instruments essentially share the same input/output function, yet compression limiting does not result in PC the output signal (up to the level that the compressor continues to function). In point of fact, a compression-limiting amplifier is designed specifically to reduce distortion in the output signal.

Saturation-induced PC was used in early hearing aid designs (and still continues to be used) to limit the maximum output SPL of the hearing aid, defined in ANSI Standard S3.22-1996 as the output SPL with a 90 dB input SPL (OSPL90). In fact, the PC control on linear PC hearing aids, which is sometimes called the output-limiting control, simply allows the onset of saturation to be increased or decreased by the dispenser to prevent output levels from exceeding the loudness discomfort level of the hearing aid wearer. Reducing the OSPL90 in this manner increases distortion caused by PC, which results in a smaller range of linear performance and poorer amplified sound quality at higher input levels. More recent linear (PC) amplifiers (class D) have considerably improved headroom and, consequently, better sound quality at higher input levels compared with older designs (class A).

Nonlinear Distortion Produced in Linear (PC) Hearing Aids

Two types of PC are available for controlling the OSPL90 of a linear (PC) hearing aid: (1) *symmetrical PC*, one that is usually deliberately produced, and (2) *asymmetrical PC*, one that is generally produced by the unmodified characteristics of the hearing aid as it goes into saturation. Symmetrical PC predominantly produces odd harmonics, whereas asymmetrical PC produces a combination of even and odd harmonics. The literature suggests that the sound quality of signals with even harmonics is usually less desirable than a signal with odd harmonics (Agnew, 1998).

A simple test for nonlinear distortion (e.g., harmonic and intermodulation distortion) is to determine whether the hearing aid output contains energy at frequencies that are not present in the input signal (Anderson et al, 1996). For example, if the input signal is 1000 Hz and energy at harmonic frequencies is detected in the output signal, nonlinear distortion is present. Nonlinear distortion in hearing aids is caused by poor headroom. For our purposes, headroom at a particular instant in time can be defined simply as the difference between the OSPL90 and the hearing aid output SPL. Hearing aid output SPL at any moment in time is the sum of input level + gain.

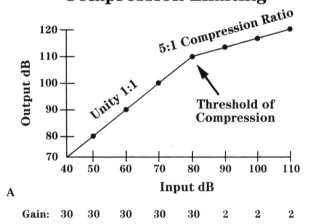

A

Gain: 30   30   30   30   30   2   2   2

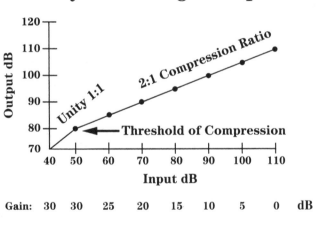

B

Gain: 30   30   25   20   15   10   5   0   dB

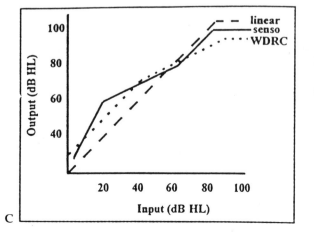

C

Figure 1–23 **(A)** Input-output function of a compression limiting (CL) hearing aid with a 5:1 compression ratio at levels above the compression threshold (CT). **(B)** Input-output function of a wide dynamic range compression (WDRC) hearing aid with a 2:1 compression ratio at levels above the compression threshold. **(C)** Input-output function of a contemporary slow-acting automatic control hearing aid (Widex Senso) compared with that for linear and WDRC hearing instruments. (From Kuk [1998], with permission.)

For example, at a particular frequency, if OSPL90 = 110 dB SPL for a linear hearing aid that has 40 dB gain, an input level component of 75 dB SPL at that frequency will attempt to produce an output SPL of 75 dB SPL + 40 dB = 115 dB SPL. These conditions result in a headroom of negative 5 dB at that frequency, indicating that the linear (PC) hearing aid is trying to produce 5 dB higher output SPL than it can. (In reality, saturation begins to occur at a level a few decibels lower than OSPL90, at the level at which nonlinear distortion begins to increase markedly as the input level increases, resulting in even less headroom.) This negative headroom condition results in nonlinear distortion. Although PC can be used to hold the OSPL90 below the wearer's loudness discomfort level (LDL), the undesirable quality of the amplified signal created by the nonlinear distortion produced by the PC is often quite detrimental to hearing aid performance. Saturation-induced distortion is believed to be undesirable because it may lower the *aided* loudness discomfort level of the hearing aid wearer (Fortune & Preves, 1992). Sound quality may be so poor that in high-noise listening environments, the hearing aid wearer may turn down the gain control or turn the hearing aid off to avoid listening discomfort.

An indication of nonlinear distortion produced in a hearing aid, including circuit noise, may be obtained by performing a coherence or signal-to-distortion ratio measurement (Preves, 1996b). For more information on hearing aid distortion, interested readers are referred to Kuk (1996b) and Agnew (1998).

Compression (Nonlinear) Amplification

Unlike the undesirable nonlinearity caused by PC in linear (PC) hearing aids, hearing aid amplifiers can be deliberately made nonlinear by introducing compression, a type of *automatic gain control (AGC)*. Every type of compressor has a level sensor somewhere in the amplifier that monitors the signal level. The compression circuitry compares the signal level in the amplifier to a preset compression threshold level. Signal level monitoring by the AGC detector may be done with the peaks of the signal or by computing a running average or rms value of the signal. Regardless of the AGC detector type, if the monitored signal level exceeds the compression threshold, compression occurs and the gain of the hearing aid is automatically reduced.

Significant parameters of compression hearing aids are the compression ratio, the compression threshold (kneepoint), and the attack and release times. The compression ratio is the ratio of the change in input SPL to the change in output SPL at a specified input level (ANSI, 1996). For example, if the output from a compression hearing aid changes 10 dB for a 20 dB change in input level, the compression ratio is 2:1. ANSI standard S3.22 (1996) does not include a definition of compression threshold because of a lack of consensus among the working group members for a definition that would apply to all known compressor designs. However, for our purposes, the simplified definition in the IEC 60118-2 standard can suffice: the level at which the input-output characteristic departs from linear by more than 2 dB. This is the lowest signal level at which compression is activated. Attack time is defined in ANSI S3.22 (1996) standard as the elapsed time from an abrupt change in input level of 55- to 90-dB SPL to the time at which the output level settles to within 3 dB of its final value.

This measurement gives an indication of how long a compression hearing aid takes to react to and compress high-level sounds. Release time is defined in the ANSI S3.22 (1996) standard as the elapsed time from an abrupt change in input level of 90- to 55-dB SPL to the time at which the output level settles to within 4 dB of its final value. Release time gives an indication of how long a compression circuit takes to increase its gain after termination of a high-level sound.

Three main types of compression are of interest in hearing aids and will be discussed in the forthcoming section: compression limiting (CL), wide dynamic range compression (WDRC; also called syllabic compression), and slow acting automatic volume control (AVC) (Braida et al, 1979; Dillon, 1996; Kuk, 1996a; Mueller & Killion, 1996; Walker & Dillon 1983).

Compression Limiting

As discussed previously, another type of amplifier with a "linear" (1:1, unity slope) amplification characteristic is the CL amplifier (sometimes called high-level compression (Agnew, 1996a). In 1947 CL amplifiers were described in the Harvard Report (Davis et al, 1947) as a recommended alternative to PC circuits but did not become widespread in use until the 1960s. CL amplifiers usually have a high compression threshold (CT [kneepoint] ≥ 70 dB SPL), a high compression ratio (CR ≥ 4:1) above the compression threshold, and an intermediate release time (150 ms < RT < 350 ms.) (Fortune, 1996). In a CL device, the threshold of compression is set high enough so that average speech signal levels do not exceed the compression threshold (Hickson, 1994), thus ensuring that the number of times the compression threshold is exceeded is not excessive. Consequently, operation of a CL amplifier is essentially "linear" (or 1:1) for input signal levels *less than* the compression threshold or for all except the highest input signal levels. Above the compression threshold, input signals may be severely compressed by a high compression ratio, typically ranging from about 4:1 to more than 10:1, depending on the circuit design (see Fig. 1–23A). Among the studies that have compared behavioral results for linear PC to linear CL, Crain and Van Tasell (1994) found higher speech reception thresholds (SRTs) for greater than 18- to 24-dB peak clipping as compared to SRTs with CL. Onset of SRT elevation coincided with the clipping level at which speech quality was judged unacceptable. Hawkins and Naidoo (1993) found that hearing-impaired subjects preferred the sound quality of compression speech to the quality of asymmetric peak clipped speech.

CL amplifiers may be designed as *either input-dependent compression (AGC-I)* or *output-dependent compression (AGC-O)*. The two types are frequently differentiated by how they perform with changes in gain (volume) control setting (Dillon, 1988). For example, as the gain control setting changes, AGC-I amplifiers keep the dynamic range of the output signal constant, shifting it up and down. The level detector in an AGC-I instrument monitors the signal level in the amplifier before the volume control. That is, as the volume control is rotated up or down, the gain and OSPL90 of the instrument change simultaneously; the two are locked together. As the gain is raised and lowered, so is the OSPL90 (Fig. 1–24A). However, the compression threshold (kneepoint) remains at exactly the same input level no matter where the volume control is set.

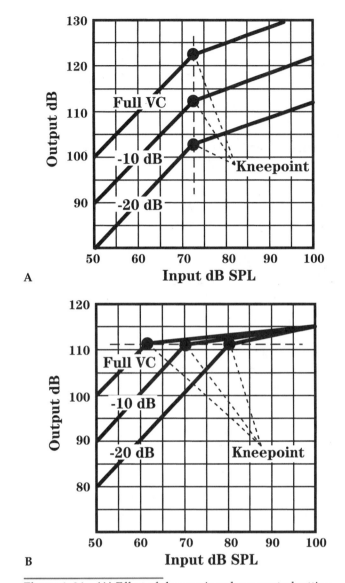

Figure 1–24 **(A)** Effect of changes in volume control setting on the input-output function for an input dependent (AGC-I) compression hearing aid. **(B)** Effect of changes in volume control setting on the input-output function for an output dependent (AGC-O) compression hearing aid. (After Starkey [1995], with permission.)

By contrast, as the gain control setting changes, AGC-O compressors change the dynamic range of the output signal without changing the OSPL90 of the hearing aid. The level detector monitors the signal level in the amplifier after the volume control. Rotation of the volume control does not affect the OSPL90 of the hearing aid (Fig. 1–24B); only the gain changes, so the two parameters are considered to be independent. The compression threshold (referred to input signal level) increases as the volume control reduces gain; as the volume control raises gain, the compression threshold (referred to input signal level) decreases. However, for AGC-O hearing aids, the compression threshold is also frequently defined in terms of the output signal level and thus, in effect, remains relatively fixed.

AGC-O CL hearing aids were in use long before AGC-I CL instruments became available, and the AGC-O type continues to be used as an effective fitting tool even though AGC-I CL instruments have become very popular recently. AGC-O CL aids in which the gain and OSPL90 may be independently adjusted are usually preferred for greater hearing losses. AGC-I CL designs are not usually appropriate for high-power aids because the gain and OSPL90 are locked together. In instances in which high gain is required, the OSPL90 may be too high and might exceed the patient's LDL at the required gain setting.

PEARL

CL circuitry has also been called *output limiting compression* (OLC) in the literature; this terminology has produced some amount of confusion because it suggests that the circuit is of the AGC-O type. As discussed previously, CL amplifiers can be designed either as AGC-I or AGC-O dependent.

Wide Dynamic Range Compression
WDRC amplifiers were first introduced in the early 1970s, (Goldberg, 1972) but were not successful in the marketplace. The reason for their lack of acceptance may be that the compression threshold was too low (i.e., less than about 30 dB SPL) and the compression ratio too high, causing audible pumping artifacts as the circuit went into and out of compression. WDRC instruments were reintroduced, appearing again in the 1980s, and have enjoyed considerable acceptance since then. WDRC amplifiers are characterized by a low compression threshold (i.e., an input level ≤ 55 dB SPL), a low compression ratio (≤ 3:1), and short attack (≤ 10 ms) and release times (≤ 100 to 150 ms) and are designed as AGC-I amplifiers to maintain the necessary low compression threshold irrespective of the volume control setting (Fig. 1–23B).

Restoring normal loudness growth to persons with significantly restricted dynamic range is often cited as a fitting rationale for WDRC amplifiers (Armstrong & Shaver, 1996; Kates, 1993). Studies suggest that the outer hair cells provide mechanical or electrical amplification to low-level acoustic signals in normal auditory systems (Berlin et al, 1996). Thus a nonlinear compression function exists within the auditory system for normal-hearing individuals. Hearing loss up to about 60- to 65-dB HL are associated with loss of outer hair cells (Patuzzi et al, 1989) and thus loss of the compression function. The rationale suggests that use of a WDRC amplifier with the proper compression threshold and compression ratio may replace the lost compression function caused by outer hair cell damage (Killion et al, 1996). Furthermore, because WDRC hearing aids provide greater amplification for soft sounds than for more intense signals, they have the potential to make a wider range of signals audible than instruments having a linear (1:1) input-output function. However, few studies have shown that speech recognition in noise improves with WDRC hearing aids over PC or other forms of compression processing (Dillon, 1996; Killion & Villchur, 1993; Kuk, 1996b).

Differentiating between CL and WDRC circuits may be difficult because, depending on the intentions of the circuit designer, some hearing aids may incorporate atypical relationships between compression threshold, compression ratio, and release time. For example, a given hearing aid may have a compression threshold of 50- or 55-dB SPL, a compression ratio of 10:1 above the kneepoint, and a short release time. Another hearing aid could have a compression threshold of 70- to 75-dB SPL, a compression ratio of 2:1 above the kneepoint, and a long release time. These instruments are neither clearly WDRC or CL circuits but fall somewhere in between. The applicability of such instruments in compensating for hearing loss may depend on other considerations, such as their frequency response or the types of loss for which they are intended by the designers.

Slow-Acting Automatic Volume Control

This third type of compression circuit has not been widely used in our field until recently with the advent of digital amplification (Kuk, 1998). Although slow-acting AVC signal processing is widely used in the audio and broadcast industries, few examples of it exist in hearing aids. Of all the types of compression, slow-acting AVC processing is the most free of audible artifacts because the attack and release times are very long, often in the order of several seconds. Therefore the circuit does not make large changes quickly. Because of its long attack and release times, however, a slow-acting AGC hearing aid may not be able to map faster signal level variations into the reduced dynamic range of a listener with impaired hearing. However, a well-fitted slow-acting AVC hearing aid can bring varying input levels to a most comfortable listening range for a hearing aid wearer. An example of the input-output function for a modern slow-acting AVC instrument is shown in Figure 1–23C by the line denoted "Senso" in the input-output function (refers to the Senso DSP hearing aid manufactured by Widex). Traditionally, for this type of processing, the compression threshold is relatively low and the compression ratio is fairly high (Dillon, 1996; Kuk, 1996a; Walker & Dillon, 1982). For more details, the reader is referred to King and Martin (1984), Dillon (1996), and Kuk (1996a).

Interactions of Compression Parameters

Interactions of compression ratio, compression threshold, and release time can make a dramatic impact on the sound quality of a compression instrument and thus can make or break the success of a fitting. General design guidelines to promote good sound quality are the following combinations of these variables:

1. If a high compression ratio is used (i.e., ≥ 4:1), compression threshold should be kept relatively high (i.e., > 70 dB SPL input level) and release time should not be too short (i.e., > 150 ms). This is the case with CL amplifiers.

2. If a low compression threshold is used (i.e., < 60 dB SPL), compression ratio should be kept relatively low (i.e., < 4:1) and release time should be kept relatively short (i.e., ≤ 150 ms). This is the case with WDRC amplifiers.

Classifying Hearing Aid Amplifier Signal Processing by the Number of Channels (or Bands)

Prior to the last few years, most hearing aids used amplifiers with a single signal path. In single-channel hearing aids the audio signal is processed through a single circuit path.

CONTROVERSIAL POINT

These devices have been called single-channel and single-band amplifiers. Strong feelings exist within our hearing healthcare field that support the appropriateness of both terms. For our purposes, a band is defined simply as a segment of frequencies and a channel is a band with one type of signal processing from input to output. Therefore, a channel may contain several bands.

We have been referring to the block diagram of a generic, single-channel hearing aid shown in Figure 1–8. The variation in frequency response in single channel amplifiers is provided by low-frequency and high-frequency tone controls. Before the use of "active" tone controls having steeper filter slopes that could provide greater attenuation over a smaller frequency range, these amplifiers used "passive" tone controls with less steep filtering that affected a broad frequency range to provide only a relatively small amount of change in gain at extreme low and high frequencies (Sammeth et al, 1993).

Many different types of single-channel amplifiers are implemented with some type of compression circuit. Although compression helps to prevent saturation-induced distortion, two problems are inherent in single-channel compression circuits. The first problem is that a low-frequency environmental noise can reduce gain across all frequencies (i.e., reduce the high-frequency gain and the low-frequency gain). This phenomenon has been illustrated by Schum (1996). In his hypothetical example a high-intensity vowel caused enough compression or gain reduction of the second, third, and fourth formants of speech to render them inaudible. It is not desirable to unnecessarily reduce high-frequency gain. Low-level, information-bearing high-frequency components of speech must be audible for good word recognition. The second disadvantage of some older single-channel compressors with low compression thresholds and high compression ratios is that they may have annoying audible artifacts or "breathing" caused by the activation and deactivation of compression as the signal alternately exceeds and falls below the compression threshold.

The first problem of single-band compressors may be alleviated by using a compression amplifier with a frequency-dependent compression threshold (Curran & Ely, 1979; Sammeth & Ochs, 1991). Such an amplifier may be implemented by reducing low-frequency amplification before the compression detector, thus rendering the compression threshold higher for low-frequency sounds than for high-frequency sounds. The result is that only very intense low-frequency sounds will cause overall gain reduction, and yet the lower compression threshold in the higher frequency region will still protect the listener from aversive high-frequency sounds. The first problem may also be addressed by having independently controlled compression circuits in more than one channel (multichannel). A block diagram of a generic multichannel amplifier is shown in Figure 1–25. As in a single channel amplifier, the preamplifier amplifies the microphone output signal. The preamplifier output, however, then splits into a

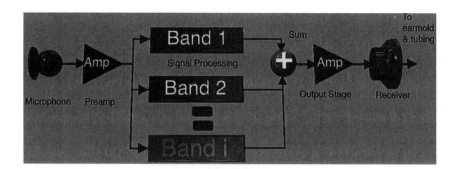

Figure 1–25   Block diagram of a generic multichannel hearing aid. (From Preves [1996c], with permission.)

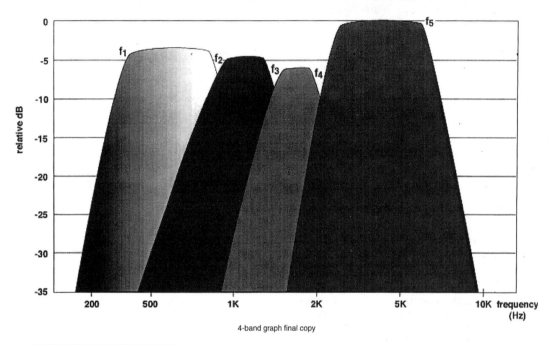

4-band graph final copy

Figure 1–26   Schematic illustration of how a frequency response is formed with a four-channel hearing aid. Crossover frequencies shown are f_2, f_3, and f_4.

number of channels. Each channel in the amplifier performs some type of signal processing, which, for example, may be linear (PC), WDRC, or CL. Thereafter, the outputs of the signal processors in each channel are combined by a summing junction indicated in the block diagram by a "+" sign. The frequency at which two adjacent channels overlap in a multichannel hearing aid is called a *crossover frequency*. In general a multichannel hearing aid has one less crossover frequency than the number of channels it has. For example, a four-channel hearing aid has three crossover frequencies (Fig. 1–26). An amplifier with independent compressors in more than one channel has a theoretical advantage if the slope of the band-splitting filters is steep enough that a low-frequency sound will not cause reduction of high-frequency gain (Goldberg, 1982). Another important advantage of multichannel amplifiers is that they permit finer tuning to match prescriptive target gain requirements (Sammeth et al, 1993). Even a two-band compression system can retain good separation of low- and high-frequency compression processing (Schum, 1996).

Some multichannel amplifiers have compression only in one channel, with linear processing in the other channel(s). Others

may have one compression circuit shared across two or more channels, in which, for instance, both channels share the same compression threshold control. Unfortunately, such hearing aids are sometimes advertised as "multichannel compression" devices. In such quasi-multichannel compression instruments, a low-frequency background noise can still cause compression in the high frequencies like in a single-channel compressor.

The second problem with single-channel compressors noted earlier may be alleviated also by having compression in more than one channel of the hearing aid amplifier. Then, the audible sounds created when a compression amplifier goes into and out of compression will be reduced because compression would theoretically occur across a smaller range of frequencies. Plomp (1988) and his coworkers state that a high number of channels is not desirable, particularly when an independent compression circuit is used in each channel. With more than two or three channels having independent compression circuits, the spectral contrasts in speech may be altered so much that speech recognition may be degraded. This theory is not supported by Crain and Yund (1995) and by Yund and Buckles (1995), who found, respectively, no negative effects on vowel or voiced stop-consonant recognition for up to 31 channels and improved speech recognition in noise with a multichannel compression system having between 8 and 16 independent compressors.

Another approach to reducing audible artifacts of compression processing was taken from the audio industry (Hotvet, 1988; Teder, 1993). The sounds produced by compression activating and deactivating are made less audible by varying the release time of the compression circuit. An adaptive time constant design makes the release time dependent on the length of the high-level portion of the input signal being compressed. For shorter, transient, high-level sounds, the release time is made short so that compression immediately ceases after cessation of a high-level part of the input signal. For longer, more steady-state high-level sounds, the release time is made long so that compression is maintained longer after a high-level part of the input signal ceases. A binary adaptive time constant compression system has been advocated by Moore and Glasberg (1986) and by Moore et al (1991). In this "dual front end" system, there are two sets of attack and release time rather than a continuously variable set. Attack and release times are normally slow until the occurrence of a high-level transient sound, which causes them to be faster.

Studies of the Effect of Release Time on Speech Recognition
Few studies have investigated the effect of release time on speech recognition and whether an optimal release time exists (e.g., Jervall & Lindblad, 1978). The release time should be dependent on the function performed by the compressor (i.e., WDRC or CL). In a multichannel compressor, a longer release time in the low-frequency bands, in which the duration of signals is longer, makes sense so as to avoid compressing (and thus distorting) portions of the low-frequency components of the signal. Likewise, it makes sense to have a shorter release time in the high-frequency bands, in which the duration of the signals is generally shorter and the intensity is generally weaker, so as not to have compression attenuate trailing consonants. In a very early study, Schweitzer and Causey (1977) found that a release time of about 90 ms (compared with 7, 15, 35, 70, 150, and 350 ms) was the most desirable for correct recognition by normal-hearing and hearing-impaired subjects of W-22 lists using a constant attack time of 10 ms. Bentler and Nelson (1997) studied the effect of varying release times in the high and low bands of a two-band compression hearing aid with magnitude estimations of speech intelligibility and found no release time to be superior to any other. However, Jerger

et al (1989) found some benefit for a hearing aid with an adaptive release time for experienced subjects with greater hearing loss.

Behavioral Results Achieved with Compression Hearing Aids
Early studies examined the idea that compression can improve speech recognition in noise (Kretzinger & Young, 1960.) However, in general, this hypothesis has turned out to not be the case, even for multichannel compression. In general, results with linear (CL) devices in comparison to linear (PC) instruments in noisy environments are positive (e.g., Hawkins & Naidoo, 1993). However, Souza and Turner (1996) found no significant benefit of a computer-generated single-channel input compression algorithm with a 60 dB SPL compression threshold and a 5:1 compression ratio, compared with linear processing (to greater than 100 dB SPL input level), with nonsense syllable audibility equalized between conditions. Peterson et al (1990) found greater benefit generally with an AGC-I CL hearing aid than with a PC hearing aid, using a nonsense syllable task in quiet, but better performance with PC than with CL with competing noise at +12 dB SNR.

In contrast, although results have been positive, considerable controversy exists about whether WDRC devices provide any benefit in noise (e.g., Dreschler, 1988, 1989; Tyler & Kuk, 1989). Hickson et al (1994) found no differences in consonant perception in a quiet background for a WDRC system with compression ratios of 1.3:1 and 1.8:1 compared with linear processing (all implemented with a K-AMP circuit). (The K-AMP is named after Mead Killion, its inventor. Further details on the K-AMP are found in a later section in this chapter about TILL signal processing.) In a competing babble condition, consonant perception in the linear condition was significantly better than that for both WDRC configurations. Using the same hearing aid, Hickson and Byrne (1995) studied the effects on consonant-to-vowel ratio (CVR) of linear versus compression (WDRC) amplification using the Nonsense Syllable Test. They found an increased CVR for 17 of 27 syllables with compression amplification compared with linear amplification that was due to increased consonant energy and decreased vowel energy. More information on behavioral evaluations of compression hearing aids is available for the interested reader in Hickson (1994).

In general, results from behavioral studies about the effects of multichannel compression amplifiers have also been mixed. In fact, the best that some studies have been able to say is that multichannel compression does not degrade word recognition (e.g., Barfod, 1978; Crain & Yund, 1995; van Harten-de Bruihn et al, 1997). Moore and Glasberg (1986) found that adding two-channel syllabic compression to slow-acting AVC produced lower SRT in noise and higher questionnaire ratings for sounds encountered in daily life than slow-acting AVC alone. In one of the few studies using real hearing aids, Moore et al (1992) found lower (improved) SRT in noise for 20 subjects with moderate hearing loss with a two-channel compression hearing relative to the same hearing aid (ReSound) in linear compression limiting mode. However, Souza and Turner (1998) stated that the equivocal results for multichannel compression in past studies was due to allowing the subjects to adjust their volume controls, thereby introducing differences in audibility between conditions. They found that two-channel compression produced no improvement in word recognition over that for linear amplification (to a 115 dB SPL input level) if the audibility of speech was maximized for both types of processing. The interested reader is referred to Dillon (1996) and Kuk (1996a) for more information on compression.

Level-Dependent and Fixed-Frequency Response Amplifiers

Another way of categorizing the type of processing performed by linear PC, CL, WDRC, and slow-acting AVC hearing aids is to separate them into *level-dependent* or *fixed-frequency response processing* (Killion et al, 1990). In a fixed-frequency response amplifier, frequency responses do not change as input level changes. With a level-dependent amplifier, the frequency responses continually change as the input level changes. Linear PC instruments and linear single-channel CL amplifiers perform fixed-frequency response processing, whereas multichannel amplifiers are likely to perform level-dependent processing if any compression is present.

Two types of level-dependent processing are *Bass Increases at Low Levels (BILL)* and *Treble Increases at Low Levels (TILL)*. In a BILL amplifier the rationale is to provide good sound quality in quiet environments by providing maximum low-frequency gain. In noisy environments, low-frequency gain is reduced automatically at high-input levels (Kates, 1986). The assumption is that most steady-state, bothersome noises have greater low-frequency energy than high-frequency energy and consequently have the potential to mask high-frequency signals. An example of the effects of BILL processing on frequency response is shown in Figure 1–27. As the input level of a speech-shaped noise is raised in 10 dB steps from 50- to 90-dB SPL, low-frequency gain is reduced. In a PC hearing aid evidence exists that adding BILL processing helps to prevent PC distortion in noisy environments by keeping the amplifier out of saturation (Preves & Newton, 1989). In a simulation of multichannel compression, Van Dijkhuizen (1991) found that, on average for both normal and listeners with impaired hearing, frequency-selective compression that approximated BILL processing compared with wideband compression, provided

lower SRT in a background of broadband noise with the level of the noise raised by 20 dB in the same octave as the frequency-selective compression was applied. Rankovic (1998) performed a similar experiment with frequency-selective compression in the same octave bands as intense noise was produced, but without the broadband noise background, on seven persons with impaired hearing. She concluded that the resulting increases in consonant recognition scores were due to release from masking and that any decreases in consonant recognition scores were due to too much frequency-selective compression. The rationale for BILL processing is based on pathological auditory systems being generally more susceptible to upward spread of masking than are normal auditory systems (Stelmachowicz et al, 1985; Trees & Turner, 1986). Proponents of BILL processing have suggested that it may help to reduce the upward spread of masking (Kates, 1987; Leijon, 1990; Rankovic, 1998; Rankovic et al, 1992; Van Dijkhuizen et al, 1991; Van Tasell & Crain, 1992).

Some investigators have theorized that BILL processing can improve SNR and hence word recognition in noise relative to linear (PC) processing. Some studies support this notion (e.g, Dempsey, 1987; Schum, 1990; Sigelman & Preves, 1987; Stach et al, 1987), whereas other studies do not support this assertion (Cook et al, 1997; Fabry & Van Tasell, 1990; Humes et al, 1997; Tyler & Kuk, 1989). Still other studies support improved word recognition in noise with BILL processing only with a continuous low-frequency-dominated noise (Chiasson & Davis, 1991; Stein et al, 1989; Van Tasell et al, 1988). An excellent overview on this topic is provided by Sammeth and Ochs (1991). Critics of BILL processing have pointed out correctly that if the level of noise is reduced in a particular frequency region, the level of speech is reduced in that region as well, thus rendering SNR unchanged (Fabry & Van Tasell, 1990).

Some studies purporting to evaluate the effects of BILL processing on word recognition in noise have used fixed low-frequency reduction (i.e, a nonvarying low-cut filter) (e.g., Horowitz et al, 1991). However, it is important to realize that BILL processing produces a constantly changing frequency

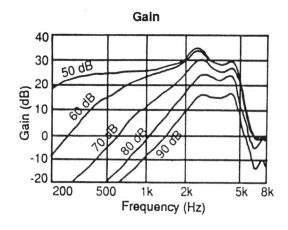

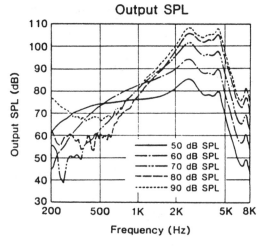

Figure 1–27 Typical effect of BILL processing on family of frequency responses of an ITE hearing aid with speech-weighted noise input levels of 50- to 90-dB SPL. Results are shown for both gain *(left)* and for output SPL *(right)*.

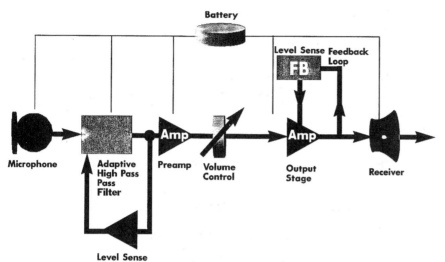

Figure 1–28 Block diagram of a combination BILL and AGC-O signal processor.

response as a result of a constantly changing input level. Thus evaluating a fixed amount of low-frequency reduction simulates the effects of a low-frequency tone control, but not BILL processing. It is also important to realize that not all BILL circuits provide the same amount of automatic low-frequency attenuation. For example, some BILL circuits use voltage-controlled high-pass filters with 12 dB/octave roll-off, and others have 24 dB/octave roll-off. Obviously, much greater low-frequency attenuation results with filters having 24 dB/octave roll-off. Still other BILL circuits use multichannel circuits with compression in the low-frequency band(s). Thus some of the mixed word recognition in noise results with BILL processing could be due to differences in design and/or the BILL processing not attenuating the noise equally in all cases.

Functionally, BILL processing may be accomplished with a voltage-controlled high-pass filter or with a two-channel hearing aid having compression in the lower band. Figure 1–28 is a block diagram of BILL processing combined with an AGC-0 circuit. Because the BILL circuit attenuates high-level, low-frequency-dominated environmental noise, this type of processing does not have the disadvantage of single-band

compression systems in which high-frequency gain is reduced by low-frequency noise.

In a TILL amplifier, high-frequency gain is reduced at high-input levels. A family of frequency responses for a TILL amplifier is shown in Figure 1–29. As the input level of a speech-shaped noise is raised in 10 dB steps from 40- to 80-dB SPL, mid and particularly high-frequency gain is reduced. The rationale for TILL processing involves maximizing gain for low-level high-frequency sounds to make them audible for persons with mild-to-moderate high-frequency hearing loss (Killion, 1979). As mentioned previously, this rationale applies particularly to those with missing outer hair cells that subserve the high frequencies. At those levels, proponents of WDRC/TILL processing maintain that a hearing aid is not needed for persons with mild-to-moderate high-frequency hearing loss because at high-input levels, the loudness growth function of impaired ears approximates that of normal ears. Advocates of WDRC/TILL processing state that hearing aids should not try to filter out background noise. If the hearing aid filters out noise, it also reduces the level of speech. Rather, hearing aids should make all sounds audible and let the brain decide what

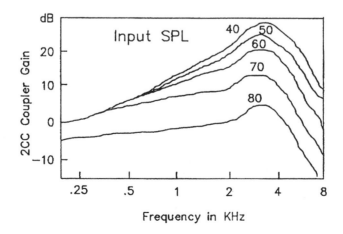

Figure 1–29 Typical effect of TILL processing on estimated family of real-ear insertion frequency response curves (REIR) for input levels of 40-, 50-, 60-, 70-, and 80-dB SPL with a K-AMP circuit (From Etymotic Research, with permission.)

is noise and what is desired signal (Killion, 1993; Villchur, 1993). Because WDRC/TILL hearing aids provide an extra boost to soft high-frequency sounds, a better chance exists that this type of processing will provide audibility across all frequencies compared with hearing aids that do not have WDRC/TILL processing. Only a few studies have evaluated the benefits of nonlaboratory hardware using actual hearing aids with TILL processing. Killion and Villchur (1993) demonstrated improved speech recognition in noise with K-AMP hearing aids compared with unaided and linear PC processing using the SIN test. (At that time, the K-AMP was a TILL processor that had a fixed 2:1 compression ratio and a low compression threshold.) Knight (1992) performed a comparative subjective preference study of K-AMP against their own linear instruments. She found that 55% preferred the K-AMP hearing aids, whereas 27.5% preferred their own instruments, and 17.5% had no preference. Nilsson et al (1997) found no significant differences between those preferring linear class A PC processing to K-AMP class D processing in a double-blind study on 45 experienced hearing-aid wearers. Painton's (1993) results with ITC hearing aids suggested that there would be a more pleasant sound quality for wearers of K-AMP circuitry when listening to their own voices compared with linear and noise reduction circuits. Surr et al (1997) had 18 experienced hearing aid wearers compare and select between a linear PC class D hearing aid with a K-AMP class D for a 30-day trial period. They found no significant difference in the number that chose one or the other or in Profile of Hearing Aid Benefit (PHAB) scores between the two circuits.

Evidence exists that some hearing-impaired-persons perform well with BILL processing and not with TILL processing, some perform well with TILL processing and not with BILL processing, and some can perform well with either BILL or TILL processing (Preves et al, 1997b). Additionally, it is difficult to predict apriori what type of signal processing each hearing-impaired person will perform best with. In recognition of this lack of predictability, some hearing aid amplifiers can be configured to perform either BILL or TILL or simultaneous BILL/TILL processing, the amount of each being adjustable by trimmers or programmable parameters (e.g., Micro-Tech, 1997).

Programmable Hearing Aid Amplifiers

A programmable hearing aid has the parameter settings stored in digital memory rather than by trimmer potentiometer settings. At the time of this writing, most, but not all, programmable hearing aids have analog electronics for their signal processing circuitry with digital storage of the parameter settings. Control of which parameter settings are used is performed digitally. Such devices are termed digitally programmable analog hearing aids. A few programmable hearing aids use digital circuitry for their signal processing in addition to their parameter storage and control functions. These are referred to as DSP (digital signal processing) programmable hearing aids. For a thorough treatment of programmable hearing aids, the interested reader is referred to the programmable hearing aid text by Sandlin (1994) and to Valente et al (1996).

Hearing Aid Amplifier Output Stages

The output stage amplifies the output of the signal processing stage and sends it to the hearing aid receiver. The main types of amplifier output stage are the class A, class B, and class D (Fig. 1–30). Up to the late 1980s, hearing aid output stages were either class A or class B (actually class AB). Thereafter class D or

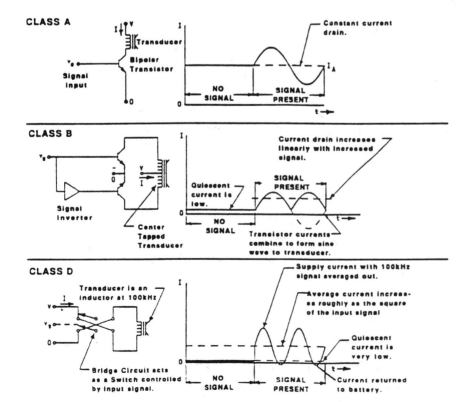

Figure 1–30 Schematic illustrations of output stage configurations and waveforms they produce: class A *(top)*, class B *(middle)*, and class D *(bottom)*. (From Dittardt [1990], with permission.)

pulse width modulation output stages were introduced into hearing aid designs, initially by integrating them into the hearing aid receiver (Carlson, 1988; Killion, 1986), then by making them part of the amplifier itself (Callias et al, 1989). Carlson (1988) estimated that the class D output stage offers a 50% advantage in battery life over a class B output stage with comparable performance, with the differences occurring mainly at high signal levels near saturation. For our purposes, power efficiency of an output stage may be defined as the ratio of usable power it produces to the power it consumes. The efficiency of class A output stages is about 35% to 40% (Lenk, 1971). Various estimates of power efficiency of the class B range from 68% (Watson, 1989) to 78% (Longwell & Gawinski, 1992). Killion, in Johnson and Killion (1994), reported that class D amplifiers are 30% to 40% more efficient than class B amplifiers.

A class A output stage, also called a single-ended design because only a single output drive terminal is used, draws constant current no matter what the input signal level and volume control setting are. Class B output stages, which are traditionally used for higher gain applications, are also called *push-pull* because two output drive terminals are used that operate alternately; when one drive terminal is active, the other is turned off. In a class B output stage, current drawn from the battery varies with the level of the output signal (determined by input signal level and volume control setting). True class B operation implies no idle current is present when no input signal is present. However, true class B operation also produces crossover distortion, a discontinuity in the output signal (Carlson, 1988), when operation is passed from one side of the output stage to the other (Fig. 1–31). For this reason, class AB rather than class B operation is used because crossover distortion is minimized by running a small amount of idle current even when no signal is present. The efficiency of class AB output stages is 50% to 60% (Lenk, 1971).

There are two extremes in comparing class D and class A output stages: for the same amount of current drain, the OSPL90 of a hearing aid with a class D output stage is typically 10- to 12-dB higher than that of a hearing aid with a class A output stage having the same gain. Alternately, for the same OSPL90, the current drain of a hearing aid with a class D output stage is typically one-fourth to one-half that of a hearing aid with a class A output stage having the same gain.

Kochkin and Ballad (1991) reported that sound quality ratings of 110 hearing aid dispensers in listening tests at a convention for ITE and BTE hearing aids with a class D output stage were higher than those for instruments with class A and class B output stages. However, the electroacoustic characteristics of the two types of instruments were not reported so it is not clear what the differences they found were due to. Further investigation revealed that compact discs were used rather than microphones, the devices were line powered rather than battery powered, and the frequency response of the class A device was considerably different from the frequency responses of the class D and class B devices, which were similar to each other (Longwell, personal communication, 1994). Palmer et al (1995) found higher sound quality ratings by normal-hearing and hearing-impaired subjects for hearing aids with class D than with class A output stages having current drains typically found for class A hearing aids. They noted that when the current drain for the class A hearing aid was raised to 3 mA, no difference was found between the sound quality of the class A and class D instruments.

Agnew et al (1997) found that a class D output stage produces 3 dB greater headroom than a class A output stage. They evaluated the sound quality of a test hearing aid amplifier with both a class A and a class D output stage. In their study, when the OSPL90 for the class A and class D operating modes were the same, the class A hearing aid produced greater distortion than the class D hearing aid for the same high-level input signal. When the amount of headroom was matched (OSPL90 of the class A was 4 dB higher than that of the class D), the class D hearing aid had higher distortion than the class A for the same high-level input signal. A general sound quality preference was noted for the hearing aid with the greatest headroom.

Perreault (1994) found that when output level cues were removed, 11 normal-hearing subjects could not hear audible differences between class B and class D output stages. Johnson and Killion (1994) concluded that the sound quality is virtually indistinguishable between well-designed class A, class B, and class D hearing aids. The interested reader may find much more detail about class D amplifiers in Ditthardt (1990).

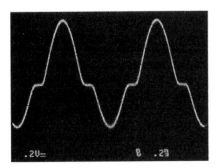

Figure 1–31 Example of crossover distortion produced by a push-pull output stage. (From Anderson et al [1996], with permission.)

PEARL

The reader should note that the hearing aid output stage/function is distinct from the hearing aid signal processing stage/function (Fig. 1–8). Thus a hearing aid with a class A output stage can be designed with either PC or some form of compression signal processing. Similarly, a hearing aid with a class D and push-pull output stages can be designed with either PC or some form of compression signal processing.

Another variation of hearing aid amplifier output stage design is the class H (Gennum, 1996). Class H is similar to class A topologically, but it reduces current consumption by adjusting its bias current adaptively as a function of the signal level. That is, a class H output stage draws significant current in proportion to the level of the signal, and only when a signal is present. The result is essentially class A operation but with somewhat longer battery life. For further information on hearing aid amplifier output stages, the reader is referred to Barry (1998).

Digital Signal Processing (DSP) Hearing Aid Amplifiers

The power of DSP has only been used recently in hearing aids. As in DSP audio applications, in DSP hearing aids the continuous analog incoming signal from the microphone output is first converted by an analog-to-digital converter (ADC) to a binary stream of ones and zeros representing the amplitude of the signal as a function of time.

Early DSP hearing aid efforts were laboratory models designed to show the viability of DSP for hearing aids (e.g., Morely et al, 1988; Nunley et al, 1983). These devices were housed in relatively large boxes and were not generally suitable for use by hearing aid wearers in their own listening environments.

One of the first commercial efforts that was not successful was the Project Phoenix body worn device that connected by means of a cord to a BTE case (Heide, 1994; Roeser & Taylor, 1988). Four batteries were used, three of which were in the body-worn device to boost the supply voltage up to a level sufficient to power the digital circuitry; the fourth battery was in the BTE case. The device had three wearer-operated switches for selecting different noise reduction algorithms. A redesign effort to package the instrument in a self-contained BTE instrument was fairly far along when financial support was withdrawn, rendering the product and miniaturization project essentially dead.

A second early effort involving use of DSP was a feedback reduction algorithm in a self-contained BTE hearing aid (Danavox DFS) intended for persons with severe hearing loss. This device uses only a single 675 battery and has remained in limited use in the hearing aid marketplace (Dyrlund & Bisgaard, 1991).

The issue of *open versus closed platforms* is an important consideration for fitters of DSP hearing aids. The first DSP hearing aids had *fixed algorithms*, and thus had variability of performance parameters for only one algorithm. Examples of these devices were the Oticon DigiFocus (Arlinger et al, 1997; Schum, 1997) and the Widex Senso instruments (Hall & Sandlin, 1997; Kuk, 1997, 1998). In contrast, some DSP instruments can execute several different algorithms that are loaded by means of software into the hearing aid at the time of algorithm selection by the hearing aid fitter. In such an open system the algorithms are software-based, so that the hardware in the same hearing aid does not have to be altered as in analog instrument to run different algorithms. Examples of these devices were introduced jointly by Philips and Micro-Tech (Edmonds et al, 1997). At the time of this writing, several hearing aid manufacturers are tooling up more general purpose DSP platforms that will make future DSP hearing aids even more software controllable. For more information on the use of DSP in hearing aids, the interested reader is referred to Agnew (1997) and Schweitzer (1997).

Future Uses of Digital Signal Processing in Hearing Aids

As DSP is used more and more in hearing aid amplifiers, the number of bands having independent signal processing is likely to increase. In addition to facilitating extreme flexibility in frequency response shaping, DSP technology for hearing aids has been advocated in laboratories for speech enhancement (Preves, 1994b). DSP has also been applied for automatic environmental noise reduction. The noise reduction algorithms involve use of both a single microphone (e.g., spectral subtraction and adaptive Wiener filtering) and beamforming with multimicrophones.

Active noise reduction (ANR) is another approach to noise cancellation that uses DSP but does not use directional microphones or arrays. This idea was first described by Lueg in a 1936 patent. ANR systems have been used to cancel noise in air condition ducts, automobile mufflers, and aircraft cabins. The object is to sense, in a closed cavity, the magnitude and phase of the noise signal that is to be canceled and sum it with an equal but opposite signal formulated by the ANR system. Generally, ANR systems consist of a feedback control microphone, amplifier, filter, and loudspeaker (Fig. 1–32). Briefly explained, the microphone picks up the signal to be canceled in the closed volume (e.g., the external auditory meatus [EAM]) and sends it to an adaptive filter whose parameters are continuously modified as the noise characteristics vary. The processed output from the filter is sent back to the enclosed cavity through the loudspeaker (hearing aid receiver) to be summed acoustically with the residual noise signal. The result is an acoustical "zone of quiet" at a point in space (EAM). The filter parameters are iteratively modified until no noise is present in the microphone output signal. The

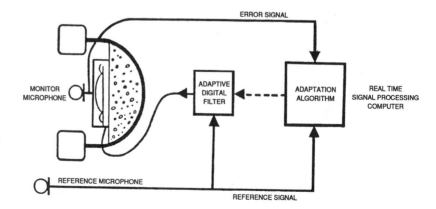

Figure 1–32   Block diagram of an adaptive digital noise reduction system for an Air Force flight helmet. Filter adapts until the error signal (residual noise) is minimized. (From Preves [1994c], with permission.)

adaptation must be accurate to within ± 0.6 dB in amplitude and ± 5 degrees in phase to achieve a 20 dB reduction of a pure tone signal (Elliot & Nelson, 1993). In larger physical volumes, ANR can suppress energy at only very low frequencies.

For smaller dimension applications like communications or noise-canceling headsets and hearing aids, components are much smaller. For example, Rafaely and Furst (1996) described an audiometric probe with ANR consisting of a microphone in the earcanal sealed by a foam plug. The system used a subminiature speaker and two microphones in the foam plug. One microphone picked up error signals in the earcanal and the second or reference microphone picked up ambient noise outside the earcanal. The foam earplug provided passive attenuation. More than 30 dB attenuation of a 500 Hz tone was achieved in four human earcanals during audiometric testing. In this application, the "zone of quiet "was the residual volume behind the foam plug in the earcanal. The system was also able to reduce broad-band noise by 30 dB in an enlarged mechanical model of the ear but was not practical as a broad-band noise reducer for human ears because of excessive group delay in the speaker. In a hearing aid application, slit leaks and vents create a leakage signal that would degrade the algorithm. However, an estimation may be made of these feedback paths to minimize their effects. Whether this technique will become useful for hearing aid applications remains to be seen. A potential problem is that speech may be canceled along with the undesired noise.

DSP processing has been used for suppressing acoustic feedback oscillation problems in hearing aids. For further information on the application of DSP for minimizing acoustic feedback problems, the interested reader is referred to Agnew (1996d) and Preves (1994b).

Hearing Aid Receivers

The receiver is the other energy transducer in hearing aids, converting the processed electrical signal from the hearing aid amplifier back to acoustic energy. Thus the receiver is essentially a loudspeaker in miniature. Some think that calling a subminiature loudspeaker a receiver makes little sense because it would seem that the microphone is receiving the

acoustic energy. However, the term receiver comes from the telephone industry in which the speaker in the handpiece was termed receiver because it received the signal from the telephone line.

In the most simple sense the receiver may be thought of as a microphone used in reverse. In fact, some electromagnetic microphones have been used in reverse as receivers. The first electromagnetic receivers, dating back to the early 1900s, were held in the hand or placed on a flat surface and used with carbon hearing aids. Functionally, alternating current from the amplifier is sent through the coil that is wound around the armature of an electromagnetic receiver. The current variations in the coil are inductively coupled to produce variations in the magnetic current flowing through the armature and magnet pole pieces (Fig. 1–33). This causes proportional armature movement that is transmitted to the diaphragm by means of a connecting pin. The diaphragm moves back and forth, producing compressions and rarefactions having amplitude and frequency proportional to the variations in electrical current from the amplifier. In this manner the receiver converts electrical energy to acoustic energy.

The transfer function of a hearing aid receiver is not without problems. Its phase changes rapidly with frequency, and its frequency response is peaky, unless controlled by damping. These problems lead to an acoustic feedback oscillation problem in hearing aids.

For extremely high gain applications, two receivers have been used"back to back" to cancel mechanical feedback. The two receivers are mounted tightly together, side by side, but with their orientations flipped so that their diaphragms move in opposite directions. The receivers are wired together to the same amplifier output terminals. As stated previously, in a hearing aid receiver, large movements of the diaphragm cause the metal canister the receiver is housed in to vibrate as high SPLs are produced. These movements are conducted through the hearing aid casing and through the air inside the hearing aid and may be sensed by the hearing aid microphone. The result is a feedback path that eventually drives the receiver with an enlarged version of the undesired feedback signal. With dual receivers, such feedback problems are reduced for high-level output signals because when the diaphragm of one receiver moves in one direction, the diaphragm of the other receiver moves in the opposite direction.

Different types of receivers are required for different types of output amplifiers. For example, for a hearing aid with a class A output stage, a "single-ended" two-leaded receiver is normally used that requires a bias current to center the armature in the air gap between the pole pieces in the receiver. Frequently, push-pull amplifiers are used for high-power hearing aids. For a hearing aid with push-pull output stage, the receiver has a coil that is divided in half by attaching a lead wire to the center of the coil. Each side of the push-pull output stage alternately drives one half, then the other half of the "center-tapped" coil inside the receiver. The center of the receiver coil is connected to the positive battery terminal. This arrangement, in effect, forms two coils, each with the same number of turns, connected back to back. For a hearing aid with class D output stage, a "zero-bias" two-leaded receiver is used because no bias current is required to center the armature in the air gap. By adding the cost and size of an extra resistor and capacitor, zero bias receivers may also be

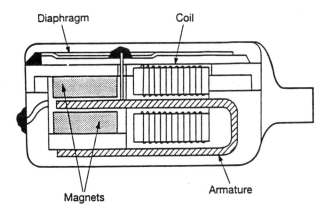

Figure 1–33 Schematic illustration of a hearing aid receiver. (From Tate [1994], with permission.)

used with class A output stages. Some of the first class D output stages for hearing aids were packaged by Knowles Electronics Corp. inside the receiver rather than with the rest of the hearing aid amplifier. This "integrated" class D receiver continues to be widely used today.

Crystal receivers required a large voltage to operate and consequently were well suited for use with vacuum tube amplifiers. Functionally, crystal receivers worked in reverse to the crystal or piezoelectric microphone. Although theoretically interesting and possible to implement, piezoelectric receivers have not been used in modern hearing aids because of the large voltage they require to produce high enough SPLs.

For more information on hearing aid transducers, the interested reader is referred to Killion (1997), Madafarri and Stanley (1996), Berger (1984), and Watson and Tolan (1949).

Hearing Aid Batteries

Batteries are the unsung heroes in hearing aids, providing power to the microphone, amplifier, and sometimes the receiver of the hearing aid. Before the late 1970s, many hearing aids used silver oxide or "silver" batteries. The silver cell system is characterized by a high open circuit voltage—approximately 1.55 volts. This higher voltage was especially important in some voltage-starved high-gain/high-output amplifier designs. When the price of silver rose dramatically in the late 1970s, the silver battery became too expensive and was essentially eliminated from use in all but a few high-power hearing aids. Many hearing aids were re-engineered quickly to permit use of the lower voltage mercuric oxide (mercury) battery. Before the last 10 years, most hearing aids used mercuric oxide or mercury batteries, which were introduced in the 1940s. Mercury system cells are characterized by an open circuit voltage of about 1.4 volts. In the 1990s, after the zinc air battery had been available for some time, ecological considerations mandated against the use of mercury in batteries of all types. In some countries and within certain states in the United States, mercury was banned in the early 1990s from use in batteries. The zinc air system is characterized by an open circuit voltage of about 1.3 volts. In the most recent years, the zinc air battery has taken over as the dominant battery type.

The power delivered by a battery at any point of time is expressed in milliwatts and is the product of the operating voltage and the current supplied. The energy delivered by a battery is the product of power and time and is expressed in milliwatt-hours. For hearing aid–size cells, the zinc air system provides the greatest energy density (in watt-hours per liter), followed by the lithium system (Dopp, 1996).

Battery capacity is rated in milliampere-hours, the product of the number of hours a battery can deliver a particular current. Battery companies have continued to increase the capacity of zinc air hearing aid batteries without increasing their size by downsizing internal parts of the battery to allow room for more zinc. The instantaneous current a zinc air battery can provide is limited by the number and size of its air holes.

As do the other components of the hearing aid, batteries must operate under widely varying climates, from the coldest winter day in Minnesota to the hottest and driest summer day in Arizona to the most humid summer day in Florida. The zinc air battery combines air from the environment with zinc inside the battery. Before use, the air intake hole(s) in zinc air batteries are covered to prevent the chemical reactions in the battery from starting while the batteries are on the shelf. Once the tape tab is removed, the voltage rises quickly to nominally 1.3 volts, and the expected life of the battery is typically about 6 weeks in many climates (Dopp-1996). Zinc air batteries are sensitive to the amount of humidity in the environment. In dry climates or when it is not being used, a zinc air battery may stop working when it experiences a "dry-out" phenomenon as water evaporates from the cell. In humid climates a zinc air battery may stop working when water evaporates inside the cell.

In actual use of the battery, open circuit voltage (battery voltage with no load) is less important than the operating voltage of the battery while it is being used. The operating voltage of a battery fluctuates in class B and class D amplifiers and is determined by its open circuit voltage, the current being drawn by the hearing aid at a particular instant of time, and the output impedance of the battery:

Instantaneous operating voltage = Open circuit voltage −
(Instantaneous current) × (Battery output impedance)

Zinc air batteries have extremely low output impedance. Unlike silver and mercury batteries, the output impedance of zinc air batteries stays quite low throughout the life of the battery. Output impedance of the battery is critical in some hearing aid circuits because of the pulsed inputs hearing aids are required to process. For example, the speech signals produced by hearing aid wearers are high-level, pulsing input signals, in the range of 75- to 80-dB SPL at the microphone inlet (Olsen, 1991). In class B and class D linear hearing aid amplifiers, the current drain in the amplifier output stage rises and falls as the input signal level to the hearing aid rises and falls. The higher the input signal, the greater the peak current the amplifier must draw. If the battery cannot supply enough current to the amplifier during peaks of the input signal, distortion results. Figure 1–34 shows an example of the operating voltage of a hearing aid battery during a pulsed signal. Note that the voltage is significantly decreased during the peaks in the signal.

Two limitations in the battery might prevent the amplifier from drawing the peak currents required to produce an undistorted signal: (1) for zinc air batteries, the minuscule

---

CONTROVERSIAL POINT

At the time of this writing, widespread controversy among battery companies exists over what constitutes an end-of-life voltage of a hearing aid battery. Some believe that it should be 1.0 v or even 0.9 v. The ultimate decision affects what the battery manufacturers can state for their battery capacities in mAH. However, a recent poll among the ANSI working group on hearing aids (S3/WG48) revealed that most members believed it should be 1.1 v. This voltage was deemed the minimum sufficient to allow voltage regulators to continue to operate.

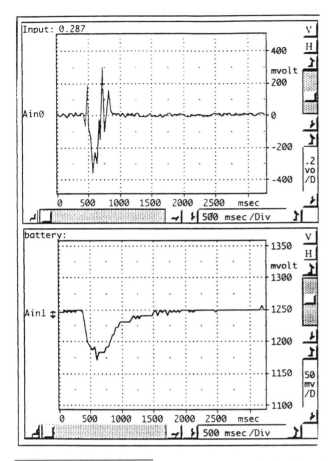

Figure 1–34 Effect on loaded battery voltage of a high-level speech input to a hearing aid. Input signal *(upper)* is /pa/ with an 88 dB peak SPL; loaded battery voltage *(lower)* has up to a 60 mv dip during the speech segment.

hole(s) in the battery may prevent enough oxygen from entering rapidly enough during input signal peaks and (2) the output impedance of the battery causes a significant voltage drop that reduces the operating voltage to the receiver and amplifier during input signal peaks (Fig. 1–34). The amplifier voltage regulator, the part of the circuit that keeps the power supply voltage constant, could "drop out" (cease to function) because of insufficient *loaded* battery voltage. With respect to this problem, it is also important to note how the internal battery impedance varies throughout the life of the battery. Some zinc air batteries start their discharge life with a low-frequency impedance that is much higher than that during the rest of their life, which may cause instability or other performance problems in some hearing aid amplifiers.

At the time of this writing, the most popular battery sizes are the 675, 13, 312, 10A/230, and 5A.

Induction Coils

When using the telephone, placing the telephone handset near the microphone inlet of a custom hearing aid may cause acoustic feedback oscillation, the squealing sound produced when the hearing aid output goes back to the microphone and is reamplified again and again. Also, hearing aid wearers frequently have difficulty understanding telephone conversations in high levels of environmental noise.

Although microphones are used most of the time in hearing aids to pick up acoustical sounds, an induction coil pickup is available to alleviate these two problems (Fig. 1–35). Development of the induction pickup coil for hearing aid aids began in 1947 when Samuel Lybarger, then chief engineer with the Radioear hearing aid company, discovered that magnetic energy leaked out from the receiver in the telephone handset. He also found that this magnetic leakage could be quite useful for hearing-impaired persons if it was sensed with a small induction coil in the hearing aid and then amplified (Lybarger, 1947). Because the pickup is inductive rather than acoustic, the acoustic feedback path created by the telephone receiver will not be sensed by the hearing aid microphone. Also, if only magnetic leakage from the telephone is picked up, environmental sounds will not be heard. As a result of Lybarger's work more than 50 years ago, induction coils (also called telecoils) are now routinely used in hearing aids as an alternate to the microphone for amplifying sounds not only from the telephone but also from audio loops in auditoriums and meeting rooms and from other assisted listening devices.

Unlike the microphone, up until the last few years, the induction coil had no built-in preamplifier, being simply a long coil of wire wound around a piece of metal (Fig. 1–36). Consequently, unless induction coil signals are fed to an external preamplifier, the hearing aid output for signals picked up by an induction coil are much weaker than those transduced by the microphone. Some, but not every, monolithic integrated circuit amplifier chips contain an induction coil preamplifier. If the induction coil preamplifier was not included on the

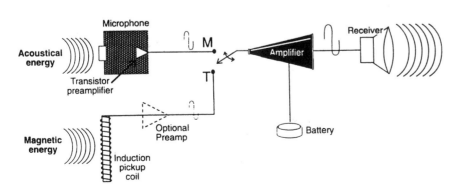

Figure 1–35 Schematic illustration showing switch-selectable microphone and induction coil inputs to a hearing aid amplifier.

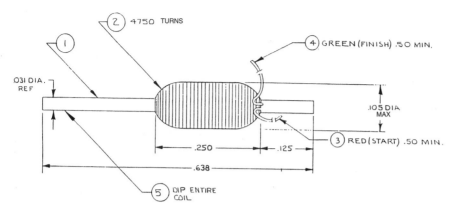

Figure 1–36 Engineering drawing of an induction coil showing turns of wire on a rod.

amplifier integrated circuit, one of two scenarios usually resulted: (1) either no preamplifier was used, rendering the induction coil performance nearly useless to the hearing aid wearer. (To equalize the output signal to that produced by the microphone, the volume control had to be turned up by as much as 15- to 20-dB, an amount of reserve gain frequently not available.); or (2) a separate external preamplifier had to be constructed, often a formidable packaging challenge for those assembling small custom hearing aids. Fortunately, the most recent versions of induction coils include an on-board preamplifier mounted on a hybrid integrated circuit. In addition, to help ensure that preamplifiers will be used, the ANSI (1996) hearing aid performance measurement standard recommends a procedure to determine how different the hearing aid outputs are between microphone and induction coil modes. This measurement is called the Simulated Telephone Sensitivity, which if equal to 0 dB, indicates that the microphone and induction coil should produce about the same hearing aid output SPL at a given volume setting.

Another important consideration is that the induction coil is sensitive to the direction from which the magnetic energy emanates. Some hearing aid wearers are painfully aware of

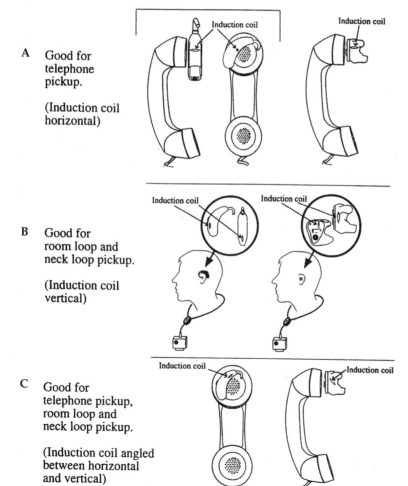

A **Good for telephone pickup.**

(Induction coil horizontal)

B **Good for room loop and neck loop pickup.**

(Induction coil vertical)

C **Good for telephone pickup, room loop and neck loop pickup.**

(Induction coil angled between horizontal and vertical)

Figure 1–37 Illustration showing that directional sensitivity of magnetic pickup depends on the orientation of the induction coil in a hearing aid. Recommended telecoil orientation for good inductive pickup of telephones (**A**), room loops and neck loops (**B**), and both telephones and room loops (**C**). (From Compton [1994], with permission.)

this when they use induction pickup for the telephone because they frequently have to move the telephone handset around the hearing aid case until they get the loudest signal. Sometimes, they have to hold the telephone handset at an odd angle relative to normal telephone handset position to get the maximum signal output. Hearing aid designers can alleviate this situation by orienting the induction coil in the hearing aid for the application(s) of most importance to the hearing aid wearer, (e.g., telephone, audio room loops, or neck loops). Some hearing aids have their induction coils oriented horizontally to pick up sounds from telephones well (Fig. 1–37A) but not sounds from audio room loops or neck loops. Other hearing aids have induction coils oriented vertically so they pick up sounds well from audio room loops and neck loops (Fig. 1–37B) but not sounds from telephones. As a compromise, some hearing aids have their induction coils oriented on an angle so they can pick up sounds well from all three types of magnetic sources (Fig. 1–37C). It is important for those dispensing hearing aids to know how well a particular instrument will work in induction mode for the application(s) most appropriate by the prospective wearer. To aid in this determination, the ANSI (1996) hearing aid performance measurement standard recommends a procedure to determine whether the hearing aid picks up magnetic energy best from telephones or loops. (See the section in this chapter on changes in induction coil measurements in the 1996 version of the ANSI S3.22 standard.) For more information on induction coils for hearing aids, refer to Madafarri and Stanley (1996).

Unfortunately, besides picking up the desired signal, an induction coil may also transduce undesirable magnetic energy from sources such as power lines, computer monitors, transformers, fluorescent lights, and digital wireless telephones (Agnew, 1996b; Preves, 1996b). If strong enough, these magnetic interference signals can make use of the induction coil very difficult because of the high-level continuous hum or buzzing sounds produced in the hearing aids.

Considerable attention has been given to the interference signal generated in hearing aids by digital cordless telephones. The signal consists of an electrical field component and a magnetic field component. As of this writing, hearing aid engineers are working together with telephone company engineers in the ANSI C63 working group to formulate a standard that provides procedures to rate hearing aids for amount of immunity to electromagnetic interference and to rate telephones for amount of electromagnetic radiation. Considerable effort has been made by hearing aid design engineers to reject the magnetic component of the radiated interference signals, but the task is difficult because of the similarity of the desired and undesired signals for hearing aids with induction coil, which must still function effectively for their intended application. As of this writing, engineers have concluded that the magnetic audio frequency component of the interference signal is the problem of the telephone companies.

Other Components in Hearing Aids

Other components in hearing aids include volume controls, trimmers and switches, and the earmold and its associated tubing. For information on these components, the interested reader is referred to Agnew (1996b), Valente et al (1996), and Chapter 2 in this volume.

STANDARDS FOR ELECTROACOUSTIC MEASUREMENTS ON HEARING AIDS

Standard electroacoustic measurements on hearing aids provide those working with hearing aids an indication of how much gain and maximum output SPL (OSPL90) a hearing aid provides and what its frequency response is. They also show how much internal circuit noise and distortion a hearing aid has and how much current it draws from the battery. It is important for those making and using these measurements to understand what their purpose is, under what conditions they are valid, and what their limitations are. The existence of such measurements implies that a consensus has been reached by those involved in the standardization process. In the development of an ANSI standard, all persons likely to be affected are notified so they can participate in the formulation process. The American National Standards Institute (ANSI) has defined the process to be followed for formulating standards and has organized the participants into committees and working groups.

International Electrotechnical Commission (IEC) Standards

The IEC also has standardized hearing aid measurements in its 60118 series of documents. In the 1980s IEC working groups formulated standardized measurements that differed from ANSI procedures that were already in place since the 1970s. These differences result in a hardship for hearing aid companies that export their products internationally. Because of the procedural differences between ANSI and IEC hearing aid standards, manufacturers must provide two sets of data, one set in accordance with ANSI S3.22 for use in the United States and Canada, and the other set for use in countries requiring the IEC 60118 series of hearing aid standards. However, since the early 1990s, a new spirit of cooperation exists between IEC and ANSI working groups in an effort to "harmonize" the standards so that differences will be minimized. At present, the entire series of IEC 60118 hearing aid standards is undergoing major revisions that may make them more compatible with ANSI standards. For example, in revising IEC 60118-7, the hearing aid quality control standard, the IEC hearing aid standards working group, TC29/13, is considering use of a three-frequency average as is used in ANSI standard S3.22.

The Standardization Process

Standardization is a living, ongoing process. Once an ANSI standard exists, every 5 years a decision is required by ANSI from the working group that formulated it to reaffirm it, modify it, or make it obsolete. Changes in ANSI standards are not made arbitrarily because their implementation may require considerable expenditure by hearing aid manufacturers and dispensers to modify test equipment. Recommended changes in standard measurement procedures must be proven viable. Frequently, round-robin testing on the same hearing aids is conducted at several different laboratories to try newly proposed procedures. Procedures recommended in ANSI standards are voluntary unless they are mandated by a regulatory agency. Such is the case with the measurements specified originally in ANSI standard S3.22 (1976), which were adopted by the Food and Drug Administration (FDA) as a set of product testing requirements for hearing aid manufacturers.

"The" ANSI Standard for Characterizing Hearing Aid Performance

Measurements included in ANSI standard S3.22 (1996) have, from the first publication of this document in 1976, been intended mainly for quality control as mandated by the FDA. They are not necessarily representative of the performance of hearing aids in real world listening environments. Because this standard was adopted by the FDA, its measurements are required rather than voluntary. Due to the resulting high visibility of this standard, some people refer to this document as "the hearing aid standard" even though there are several other standards associated with hearing aids. Among the tests in ANSI S3.22 (1996) standard are frequency response, maximum output SPL as a function frequency, bandwidth of a hearing aid, harmonic distortion, internal noise produced by a hearing aid, compression characteristics, and current drain.

At the request of the FDA, the ANSI S3.22 standard included tolerances for the allowable variation in the parameters being measured. Measurements in ANSI standard S3.22 (1996) are performed with couplers. Couplers consist of a metal assembly to couple the output of a hearing aid to a laboratory-quality microphone that converts the acoustic output of a hearing aid to an electrical signal. Coupler measurements are noted for their repeatability, both at the same laboratory and between laboratories. Hence, they are very useful for comparing electroacoustic data for the same hearing aid on hearing aid analyzers at different facilities. In the United States the 2-cc coupler is used as the coupler of choice for specifying hearing aid characteristics in accordance with ANSI standard S3.22 (1996). The 2-cc coupler was thusly named because the static volume behind the microphone is approximately 2-cc (ANSI, 1995). Although this volume of air is fairly representative of the impedance of a normal human ear at low frequencies, it is too large a volume at higher frequencies at which the impedance of the middle ear falls significantly (Burkhard, 1977). This lack of accurate representation should not be taken as a fault because couplers were not designed to represent the earcanal. Such devices as the modified Zwislocki occluded ear simulator and IEC 711 occluded ear simulator are used to fulfill this goal (ANSI, 1979; IEC, 1983).

A typical data sheet showing the electroacoustic performance of a linear custom ITE hearing aid in accordance with ANSI S3.22-1987 is reproduced in Figure 1–38. The FDA requires these data accompany all new custom hearing aids shipped from hearing aid manufacturers. The frequency response with a 60 dB SPL input level with the volume control set at *reference test position* (heavier curve) and saturation SPL with a 90 dB SPL input level *(SSPL90-lighter curve)* curve are both provided in the top graph. The reference test position of the volume control for a linear hearing aid is obtained by setting the high-frequency average (HFA) output SPL with a 60 dB input SPL to a level 17 dB below the HFA SSPL90. If the hearing aid does not have enough gain to reach a level 17 dB below the HFA SSPL90, the volume control is left full-on. The labeling along the left ordinate for the frequency response (lower, bold curve) is in units of decibels of gain (dB). The labeling along the right ordinate for SSPL90 (upper, lighter curve) is in decibels of output sound pressure level (dB SPL). Reference test position for a linear hearing aid is determined in several steps: (1) set the controls on the hearing aid or program the hearing so that it has the widest frequency response bandwidth and the highest SSPL90 and full-on gain; (2) calculate the HFA of the SSPL90 at 1000 Hz , 1600 Hz, and 2000 Hz (or the special purpose average [SPA] of the SSPL90 at three other preferred one-third octave frequencies that are separated by another one-third octave frequency); and (3) lower the volume control setting, if required, until the average output SPL from the hearing aid at the same frequencies with a 60 dB input SPL is 17 dB less than the HFA or SPA SSPL90. The *reference test gain* is the HFA or SPA SSPL90 minus 77 dB or the HFA full-on gain if the volume control is left full-on. SPA frequencies are used for extreme high-pass or low-pass hearing aids (Preves, 1988). An example of a set of SPA frequencies is 2000, 3150, and 5000 Hz.

Below the frequency response and SSPL90 graph are several numerical specifications for the hearing aid. These include Peak SSPL90, the maximum on the SSPL90 curve; HFA SSPL90, the above-referenced three-frequency average; Peak full-on gain, the maximum on the gain curve with the volume control set to maximum gain; HFA full-on gain, the three-frequency average of the output SPL with a 50- or 60-dB input SPL and full-on gain setting minus the 50- or 60-dB input level; Reference Test Gain, the gain at the reference test position of the volume control; Equivalent Input Noise, the output SPL with no input minus the Reference Test Gain; Battery Current, the amount of current drawn by the hearing aid with a 65 dB 1000 Hz pure tone input and the volume control set to Reference Test Position; Low Response Limit F_1, the low-frequency intersection of a horizontal line 20 dB lower than the HFA full-on gain and the frequency response curve with the volume control at Reference Test Position; High Response Limit F_2, the high-frequency intersection of a horizontal line 20 dB lower than the HFA full-on gain and the frequency response curve with the volume control at Reference Test Position; Telecoil Sensitivity, the output of a hearing aid with telecoil activated (if present) at full-on volume control setting for a 1000 Hz magnetic field input with 10 mA/meter field strength; Total Harmonic Distortion (THD) produced by the hearing aid at 500, 800, and 1600 Hz (or at one-half the SPA frequencies) with the volume control at Reference Test Position with input level at 70-, 70-, and 65-dB SPL, respectively. In the figure, HFA full-on gain (18.6 dB) + 60 dB SPL = 78.6 dB SPL, which is less than the HFA SSPL90 (106.2 dB SPL) − 17 dB = 89.2 dB SPL. Therefore the volume control is left at full-on for reference test position, and reference test gain = HFA full-on gain. If this hearing aid had higher gain so that HFA full-on gain + 60 dB SPL >89.2 dB SPL, the volume control would have been turned down for reference test position.

The graph at the bottom of Figure 1–38 is the predicted insertion gain of this hearing aid on the Knowles Electronics Manikin for Acoustic Research (KEMAR), obtained by adding

Custom Designed for:

Date: SEP 18 98 11:55:43   Ear: Right
Model: Full Shell ITE   Circuit: Linear Class D
Serial Number: 98370326   Matrix: 113/30/35 - Variable Vent
Warranty Expiration Date: OCT 20 1999   Options: Variable High Cut
Battery Type: 13

Frequency Response and SSPL90 Curves

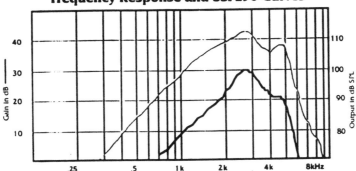

ANSI Specifications

Peak SSPL90 (dB SPL) @ 2600 Hz	113.0
HFA SSPL90 (dB SPL)	106.2
Peak Full-On Gain (dB)	30.0
HFA Full-On Gain (dB)	18.6
Reference Test Gain (dB)	18.5
Equivalent Input Noise (dB SPL)	26.2
Battery Current (mA)	0.8
Low Response Limit (F1 in Hz)	585
High Response Limit (F2 in Hz)	6500
Telecoil Sensitivity @ 1 kHz (dB SPL)	N/A

THD	Frequency	Source
0.0 %	500 Hz	70 dB SPL
0.0 %	800 Hz	70 dB SPL
0.6 %	1600 Hz	65 dB SPL

Predicted Insertion Gain
(per Burnett & Beck, 1987)

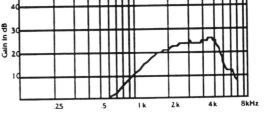

Test Conditions

ANSI S3.22-1987
Aid Type: Linear

Figure 1–38 Typical data sheet in accordance with ANSI S3.22-1987 for a linear custom ITE hearing aid. (Courtesy of Micro-Tech Hearing Instruments.)

correction values determined by Burnett and Beck (1987) to the frequency response.

Figure 1–39 depicts a typical printout of specifications obtained in accordance with ANSI S3.22-1987 for a half-shell hearing aid with an AGC circuit. All the measurements denoted earlier for a linear hearing aid are also required for an AGC hearing aid. For AGC hearing aids, the volume control is left at full-on for reference test position. However,

several measurements are added to report the performance of the compression circuitry. The graph to the right of the frequency response and SSPL90 is the input-output characteristic, plotted for a 2000 Hz pure tone input whose SPL is varied from 50- to 90-dB SPL in 5 dB steps. The ordinate shows the hearing aid output in dB SPL resulting from the input levels denoted by the abscissa. As mentioned previously in this chapter, linear hearing aids become nonlinear at levels above

Custom Designed for:

Date: SEP 18 98 11:30:48   Ear: Left

Model: Half Shell Canal   Circuit: Octiva

Serial Number: 98370147   Matrix: 105/34/22 - Variable Vent

Warranty Expiration Date: OCT 18 2000   Options: Class D AFR Trimmer Compression
                                                 Ratio Control Extended Receiver
Battery Type: 312   Tube Wax Guard Wind Hood

Frequency Response and SSPL90 Curves

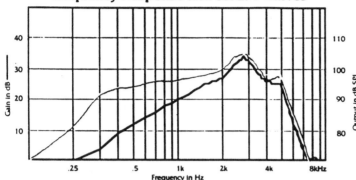

Input/Output Curve @ 2kHz

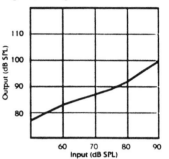

ANSI Specifications

Peak SSPL90 (dB SPL) @ 2700 Hz 105.0

HFA SSPL90 (dB SPL)............................ 99.6

Peak Full-On Gain (dB)............................ 34.0

HFA Full-On Gain (dB) 25.8

Reference Test Gain (dB) 25.8

Equivalent Input Noise (dB SPL).............. 22.4

Battery Current (mA) 0.6

Low Response Limit (F1 in Hz)................. 342

High Response Limit (F2 in Hz) 6700

Telecoil Sensitivity @ 1 kHz (dB SPL)........ N/A

THD	Frequency	Source
1.0 %	500 Hz	70 dB SPL
0.6 %	800 Hz	70 dB SPL
0.9 %	1600 Hz	65 dB SPL

Attack Time (ms) 16

Release Time (ms) 536

Compression Ratio........... 2.4:1

Threshold Knee (dB SPL).... 50

Predicted Insertion Gain
(per Burnett & Beck, 1987)

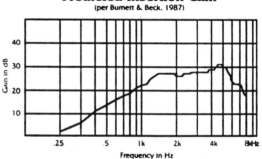

Test Conditions

ANSI S3.22-1987

Aid Type: AGC with EIN test

Figure 1–39 Typical data sheet in accordance with ANSI S3.22-1987 for a half-shell custom hearing aid with a compression circuit. (Courtesy of Micro-Tech Hearing Instruments.)

which peak clipping begins to occur. An input-output characteristic is not usually reported for a linear hearing aid because there would be equal changes in output SPL produced by any change in input level, resulting in a straight line angled upward at 45 degrees. For example, with an input level changing by 10 dB from 60- to 70-dB SPL, the output SPL changes from 85- to 95-dB SPL, so the hearing aid is operating linearly in this input level range. For compression hearing aids, the input-output characteristic becomes nonlinear at input levels above the *compression threshold*. At this time, compression threshold has no official definition in any ANSI standards but is defined in IEC standard 60118-2 (1983a) as the input level at which the input-output characteristic departs from linear by 2 dB. In Figure 1–39, the printout states that the compression threshold occurs at 50 dB input SPL (Threshold Knee). The printout also calculates the *compression ratio* (2.4:1) at input levels above the compression threshold. Compression ratio is defined as the difference in input levels, divided by the difference in output levels, at a specified reference input level. In Figure 1–39, as the input level changes by 10 dB between 60- and 70-dB SPL, the resulting output level changes only from 83-dB to 87.2-dB SPL. Thus the compression ratio is [10/(87.2 − 83)] = 2.4:1.

The attack time and release time are also reported for this hearing aid. The attack time is defined as the length of time taken for the output signal to settle to within 3 dB of the final value as a result of the 2000 Hz input level changing from 55-dB to 90-dB SPL. The release time is defined as the length of time taken for the output signal to settle to within 4 dB of the final value as a result of the 2000 Hz input level changing from 90-dB to 55-dB SPL. Attack and release times provide an indication of how long it will take the circuit to react to fast transient signals.

> ## PITFALL
>
> **Frequent mistakes encountered in making tests in accordance with the 1987 revision of the ANSI S3.22 standard include not closing the vent of a custom hearing aid or earmold, not placing the hearing aid microphone near enough to the location of the reference microphone in the text box, and not orienting the hearing aid for maximum induction coil sensitivity.**

The ANSI S3.22 standard was last updated in 1996. Because this revision contained some major changes, it took 9 years to achieve consensus within the working group, to get the approval of the supervisory Acoustical Society committee and individual experts, and to publish it. The main areas in which this revision of the S3.22 standard departs from the last revision in the 1987 document are the following:

Terminology for Maximum Output SPL

Change terminology from SSPL90 to OSPL90 to be consistent with IEC terminology and in recognition that a 90 dB input SPL will not always cause saturation.

Tests for AGC Hearings Aids

a. Will be tested with the volume control set back to the reference test position using the same calculation procedure as for linear hearing aids rather than at full-on volume.

b. Input level abruptly changes from 55- to 90- to 55-dB SPL for attack and release time measurements rather than from 55- to 80- to 55-dB SPL.

c. *Settling level* is ±3 dB for attack time and ±4 dB for release time measurements rather than ±2 dB for each.

Induction Coil Sensitivity Tests

a. The method used in the 1987 version of the standard (moving the hearing aid adjacent to a coil that radiates magnetic energy until a maximum sensitivity at 1000 Hz is obtained) is moved to an annex.

b. Use *the Telephone Magnetic Field Simulator (TMFS)* instead of an arbitrary size radiating coil.

c. Calculate the *Simulated Telephone Sensitivity (STS)* as a figure of merit for how much the volume control will have to be moved when switching from microphone to telephone on a hearing aid when using it for telephone pickup.

d. Calculate the *Test Loop Sensitivity (TLS)* for a figure of merit for how much the volume control will have to be moved when switching from microphone to telephone on a hearing aid when using it for room or neck loop pickup.

Annexes

A new annex for measuring the circuit noise of the hearing aid in one-third octave bands consistent with IEC procedures.

Moving some tests from ANSI S3.3-1971 to new annexes. Included are how to measure:

- The compression ratio of an AGC hearing aid
- The characteristic of the volume control (gain as a function of rotation)
- Battery current as a function of quiescent current and maximum current
- The effect of a tone control on frequency response
- The effect of an output limiting control on 0SPL90 and frequency response
- The effect of power supply impedance variation on the gain and 0SPL90

At the time of this writing, the FDA has begun the process to adopt the 1996 revision of the S3.22 standard. Thus manufacturers may perform and report measurements as specified in either the 1987 or 1996 versions of the standard.

> ## PEARL
>
> **The reader should be aware that tests specified in annexes of an ANSI standard are for additional information and are not really part of that standard. Thus tests specified in annexes such as the TLS and circuit noise measured in one-third octave bands are optional and would not be required measurements when (if) the FDA adopts the 1996 version of the standard.**

For more detailed information about the rationale and methods for these changes in the ANSI S3.22-1996 standard, the reader is referred to Preves (1996a).

Other ANSI Standards for Hearing Aid Measurements

Coupler Calibration of Earphones (ANSI Standard S3.7-1995)

ANSI S3.7-1995, Method for Coupler Calibration of Earphones, provides specifications for couplers and their use in

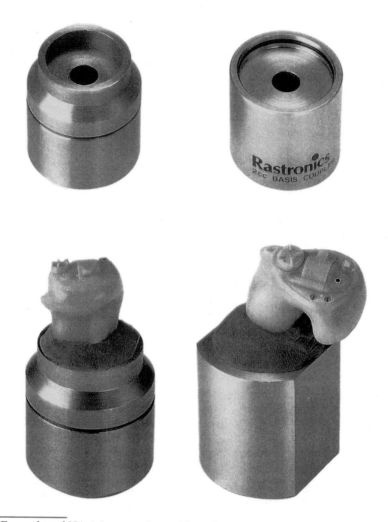

Figure 1–40 Examples of HA-1 2-cc couplers with and without custom hearing aids mounted on them. (Courtesy of Starkey Laboratories.)

calibrating hearing aid and audiometric earphones. (NOTE: A hearing aid earphone pertains to the receiver.) All the HA series couplers except the HA-1 type incorporate an internal earmold simulator. Among the 2-cc couplers used for hearing aid testing are the following:

HA-1 Coupler

This coupler allows direct coupling of an earmold of a postauricular hearing aid, a molded insert with an internal earphone, or a shell of an ITE hearing aid. Clay or putty is used to seal the earmold or shell into the coupler. The S3.22 standard recommends testing with the vent in the hearing aid closed. Examples of custom hearing aids mounted on HA-1 couplers are shown in Figure 1–40.

HA-2 Coupler

This coupler is used for earphones with nubs such as an external receiver of a body aid. The HA-2 coupler is sometimes used with an external tubing to connect an earphone in a hearing aid to an earmold or to an ear insert. For high volume testing, the external tubing may be rigid for longer wear. Unless otherwise stated, the connecting tubing outside of the coupler has a length of 25 mm and an inner diameter of 1.93 mm (No.

13 tubing). This length and diameter may be specified by the manufacturer and simulates the actual tubing used in practice. The earmold simulator in the HA-2 coupler has a 3-mm bore diameter, which may produce a high-frequency boost compared with an actual earmold with 2-mm bore diameter tubing (Lybarger, 1985). An illustration of a BTE hearing aid mounted on an HA-2 coupler is shown in Figure 1–41.

HA-3 Coupler

This coupler is intended for testing modular ITE hearing aids and earphones and insert type receivers that do not have nubs. The entrance tubing may be either flexible or rigid and, unless otherwise stated by the manufacturer, has a length of 10 mm and a diameter of 1.93 mm (i.e., No. 13 tubing). An illustration of an HA-3 coupler is shown in Figure 1–42.

HA-4 Coupler

The HA-4 coupler is a modification of the HA-2 coupler using entrance tubing. It is used for testing postauricular or eyeglass hearing aids in conjunction with a constant sound path bore from the hearing aid output through the earmold of 1.93-mm diameter. An illustration of an HA-4 coupler is shown in Figure 1–43. (The interested reader is referred to Lybarger [1985] for further information on couplers.)

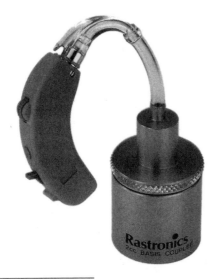

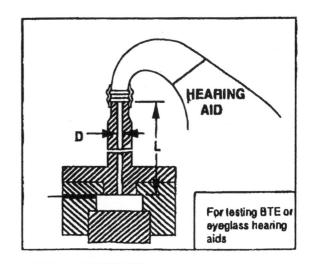

Figure 1–41 Example of a BTE hearing aid mounted on an HA-2 2-cc coupler. (Courtesy of Starkey Laboratories.)

Figure 1–43 Schematic illustration of an HA-4 2-cc coupler. (From Staab & Lybarger [1994] with permission.)

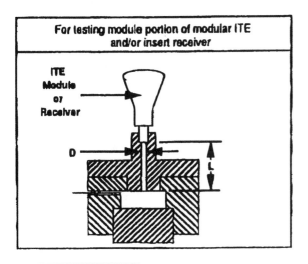

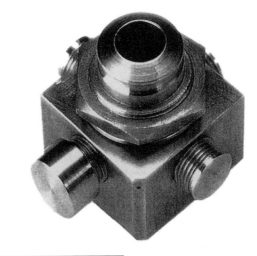

Figure 1–42 Schematic illustration of an HA-3 2-cc coupler. (From Staab & Lybarger [1994], with permission.)

Figure 1–44 Knowles Electronics modified Zwislocki occluded ear simulator. (Courtesy of Starkey Laboratories.)

Occluded Ear Simulator
(ANSI Standard S3.25-1989)

Ear simulators have been specifically designed to represent the characteristics of a normal real-ear over a wide frequency range, unlike the various hearing aid couplers discussed earlier. This standard specifies the physical configuration and acoustical characteristics of the four-branch modified Zwislocki ear simulator (Fig. 1–44). This ear simulator is used in the Knowles Electronics Manikin for Acoustic Research or KEMAR (Burkhard & Sachs, 1975). The occluded ear simulator simulates the portion of the earcanal between the tip of an earmold and the eardrum and also the median acoustic impedance at the eardrum for persons with normal middle ears. A photograph of KEMAR is found in Figure 1–45.

The IEC 711 ear simulator conforms to the specifications of the Bruel and Kjaer ear simulator. Because of slight differences in measurement data, the acoustical performance in the IEC 711 ear simulator standard do not quite meet the

specifications of the four-branch modified Zwislocki ear simulator in ANSI S3.25-1989. The formulation of separate ANSI and IEC ear simulator standards is an example of the difficulty ANSI and IEC have had in developing compatible standards for measuring hearing aid performance.

Manikin Measurements
(ANSI Standard S3.35-1985)

ANSI standard S3.35-1985, Methods of Measurement of Performance Characteristics of Hearing Aids Under Simulated in situ Working Conditions provides guidance on how to use KEMAR for estimating hearing aid performance on an average wearer. Measurements in accordance with this standard are to be performed in a acoustical environment with excellent sound absorption and sound attenuation (an anechoic chamber).

The standard includes the acoustic requirements for the test space and a coordinate system to specify loudspeaker

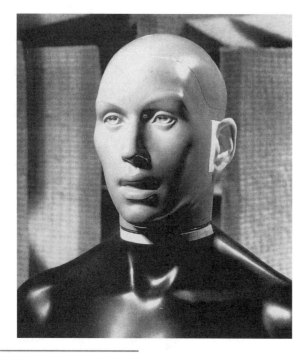

Figure 1–45   Knowles Electronics Manikin for Acoustic Research (KEMAR). (Courtesy of Starkey Laboratories.)

position and direction of sound incidence relative to the manikin. Measurements defined in the standard are as follows:

• Manikin frequency response
• Simulated in situ gain
• Simulated insertion gain frequency response
• Simulated in situ SSPL90 frequency response.

During the formulation of the S3.35 standard, a round robin series of measurements with one postauricular hearing aid was conducted in accordance with the procedures outlined in the S3.35 standard (Teder, 1984). The repeatability of the measurements on the same hearing aid between laboratories was reported in this study. For more information on manikin measurements, consult the Manikin Measurements Conference Proceedings (Burkhard, 1978).

The ANSI manikin standard is very similar to IEC 60118-8, a document that was categorized as a report rather than a standard.

Correction Factors to Convert Between Coupler Gain and Insertion Gain

Correction factors have been used for many years to estimate insertion gain frequency response on KEMAR and on real ears from 2-cc coupler frequency response data. However, as of this writing, correction factors have not been incorporated into a standard. Some hearing aid manufacturers use correction factors to provide estimated insertion gain frequency response, derived from the 2-cc frequency response, on their hearing aid specifications (e.g., Figs. 1–38 and 1–39).

The term CORFIG has been used as shorthand notation for a correction factor. It stands for Coupler Response for Flat Insertion Gain (Killion & Monser, 1980). CORFIG refers to a table of transforms that convert insertion gain frequency

response to a 2-cc coupler frequency response. The inverse of CORFIG converts 2-cc coupler frequency response to insertion gain frequency response and has been termed "GIFROC" (the reverse of CORFIG) by Killion and Revit (1993).

Sam Lybarger calculated the insertion gain that should result from a 2-cc coupler frequency response and from a frequency response on the Zwislocki ear simulator for ITE, BTE, and ITC hearing aids (Lybarger & Teder, 1986). Another "in situ" round robin was created to evaluate these calculations against actual measurements for ITE hearing aids. The round robin consisted of the same six laboratories (that were in the previous round robin reported on by Teder [1984]) making 2-cc coupler and simulated insertion gain frequency response measurements on KEMAR for one ITE hearing aid. The results showed that up to 4000 Hz, the calculated and mean measured inverse CORFIG curves, agreed to within approximately 2 dB.

The Veterans Administration hearing aid distribution program has mandated that manufacturers supplying hearing aids to VA hospitals must also provide either the actual measured insertion gain on KEMAR or an estimated insertion gain. It is difficult to get custom ITE hearing aids having earmolds of various shapes and sizes to fit into the available KEMAR ears. Consequently, an estimate of insertion gain is necessary for a production situation. A set of correction factors to predict insertion gain has been recommended by Burnett and Beck (1987). These correction factors are a result of the S3-48 working group round robin mentioned previously (Lybarger & Teder, 1986). These predicted insertion gain responses serve as a reasonable estimate of the actual insertion gain responses that would be obtained by some but not all hearing aid wearers. The interested reader is referred to Lybarger (1985) for further information on CORFIG.

At the time of this writing, the IEC hearing aid standards working group TC29/13 is considering modifying IEC report 60118-8 to include correction factors to estimate real-ear gain.

ANSI S3/WG48 Directions

In the last few years, the goal of the ANSI hearing aid standards working group, S3/WG48, has been to draft standard measurements that relate to the performance of hearing aids in real-world listening environments. For example, it may be difficult for those persons dispensing hearing aids to determine what type of signal processing a hearing aid amplifier performs because of the proliferation of so many different types of signal processors. For this reason, ANSI standard S3.42-1992 was created as a guide to those making measurements on hearing aids with deliberately designed nonlinear signal processing. S3.42 specifies a speech-shaped broad-band noise for a test signal. With this signal, a family of frequency response curves with different input levels can be obtained on a hearing aid. These frequency responses may be categorized as linear, nonlinear fixed frequency response, or nonlinear level-dependent frequency response. A family of frequency responses for linear (PC) hearing aid have overlaid curves at 50-, 60-, and 70-dB SPL noise input levels. This hearing aid has poor headroom and becomes nonlinear with an 80 dB SPL noise input level (Fig. 1–46A). As the noise input level rises to 90 dB SPL, the gain drops further because of saturation. Figure 1–46B shows a family of frequency responses for a linear (PC) hearing aid with about the same peak gain but with more headroom. This hearing aid has overlaid gain curves at inputs

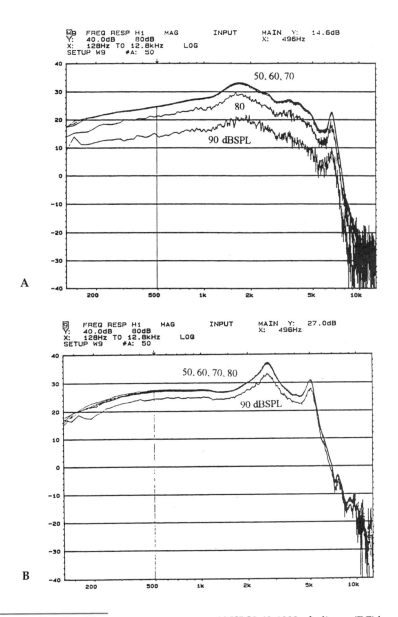

Figure 1–46 Family of frequency responses per ANSI S3.42-1992 of a linear (PC) hearing aid with poor headroom **(A)** and one with better headroom **(B)**. The presence of noticeable irregularities in a sweep frequency response indicates the harmonic and intermodulation distortion.

up to 80 dB SPL. A family of fixed-frequency responses for a compression limiter resemble those of linear instruments: overlaid curves at levels below the compression threshold with the curves becoming parallel at higher input levels (Fig. 1–47).

A family of nonlinear level-dependent frequency responses have parallel curves at levels below the compression threshold with the curves becoming nonparallel in manner at higher input levels to reflect either BILL or TILL or BILL/TILL operation (Fig. 1–48). The previous examples are illustrations of the use of ANSI standard S3.42-1992.

For a more detailed review of electroacoustic measurement standards, the interested reader is referred to Preves (1996b).

The ANSI hearing aid standards working group has recently been considering a number of new measurements with which to characterize more thoroughly the performance

of hearing aids. As mentioned previously, for example, ANSI standard S3.42 (1992), titled *Testing Hearing Aids With a Broad-Band Noise Signal*, was intended to provide a better representation of the real-world performance of nonlinear

---

PEARL

Note that the ordinate scales for the frequency response curves in Figures 1–46A and 1–46B are labeled in gain (dB). This indicates that the spectrum level of the input signal has already been subtracted out. For Figure 1–47, the ordinate is labeled in output SPL (dB), indicating that this is input plus output.

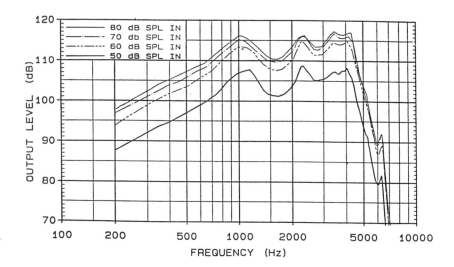

Figure 1–47 Family of frequency responses per ANSI S3.42-1992 of a compression-limiting hearing aid. (From Preves [1996b], with permission.)

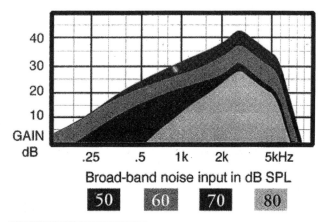

Figure 1–48 Family of frequency responses per ANSI S3.42-1992 for a hearing aid with simultaneous BILL and TILL processing.

hearing aid circuitry than can swept pure tone testing (Preves et al, 1989). In particular, a continuous broad-band noise is appropriate as an input signal to provide additional information about level-dependent signal processing strategies that change frequency response with changes in input level. Early on in the formulation of the ANSI S3.42 standard, the working group recognized that the prediction accuracy of the standard would be somewhat limited because real-world signals are not continuous but are transient in nature. Consequently, the working group has been trying without success for several years to achieve consensus on one or more pulsing signals that would be representative of real-world signals. Such a consensus would advance the level of realism in predicting real-world performance with the measurements specified in the S3.42 standard.

Predicting Whether Hearing Aid Circuit Noise Will Be Audible
Hearing aid circuit noise may be produced at the front end or back end of the hearing aid amplifier (Armstrong, 1995). Traditionally, hearing aid circuit noise has been expressed only

as a single equivalent input noise measurement for quality control purposes. As noted previously, the 1996 draft of the ANSI S3.22 standard included a procedure in an annex for measuring hearing aid noise in one-third octave bands. As an extension to this procedure, Roy Sullivan, a member of the ANSI hearing aid working group, proposed that an audibility prediction for hearing aid circuit noise be accomplished on an individual basis by comparing the hearing aid circuit noise output in one-third octave bands at audiometric frequencies to the hearing thresholds of the hearing aid wearer. Similar techniques to this proposal have been investigated by Macrae and Dillon (1996) and by Agnew (1996c), a member of the ANSI hearing aid standards working group.

At the time of this writing, the working group has been unable to achieve consensus on how to set the volume control, trimmers, and programmable parameters for such measurements.

Effective Compression Ratio
Because the input-output characteristic specified in ANSI S3.22-1996 and ANSI S3.42-1992 have been obtained with steady-state signals, they do not accurately represent the compression ratio of hearing aids with more real-world-like, transient stimuli. Consequently, there has been some interest in specifying the compression ratio for nonlinear hearing aids with pulsatile signals. For example, Stone and Moore (1992) demonstrated that a compressor with release time longer than the repetition rate of the input signal has a lower effective compression ratio than is indicated by the steady-state input-output curve. This may be an important consideration when setting the compression ratio adjustment during fitting of compression hearing aids. Verschuure et al (1996) calculated the effective compression ratio of a compression hearing aid by comparing the temporal modulation depth for a single carrier frequency with a sinusoidal modulating signal at the input to that for the output from the compressor. Although some amount of support seems to exist for using an effective ratio in more closely predicting the real-world performance of compression hearing aids, at the time of this writing, no consensus has been achieved within the working group to standardize this measurement.

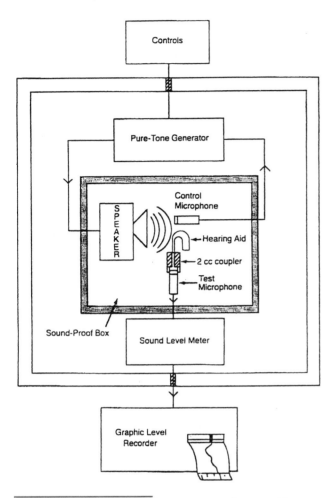

Figure 1–49 Illustration of components of a typical hearing aid analyzer. (From Pascoe [1986], with permission.)

Predicting Hearing Aid Sound Quality
with Electroacoustical Measures

A long-standing quest of the ANSI working group for standardizing hearing aid measurements has been to find electroacoustical measurements that correlate closely to sound quality. As mentioned previously, the harmonic distortion measurements specified in ANSI S3.22 (1996) are for quality control assessment, not for providing an indication of hearing aid sound quality. From a literature review, it appears that the difference frequency distortion measurement, a subtest of

intermodulation distortion, may correlate well to sound quality assessments (Anderson et al, 1996).

Of all of the possibilities considered, recently the working group nearly came to a consensus on an electroacoustical measurement that relates to sound quality—a *signal-to-distortion ratio measurement* (derived from *coherence*) with a broad-band noise input stimulus. Such a distortion measurement would take into account harmonic and intermodulation distortion and internal circuit noise created by a hearing aid.

Equipment Needed to Make Measurements

The hearing aid measurements defined in ANSI standards S3.22, S3.42, and S3.35, for example, and in the IEC 60118 series of standards, can be performed by general purpose spectrum analyzers. The latest of such instruments can be software controlled by means of IEEE488 or RS232 buses to perform the desired measurements in accordance with the preceding standards. Data can be obtained automatically and analyzed off-line with a spreadsheet program. Although this may be expedient for researchers in laboratory settings, it is not convenient for those dispensing hearing aids that wish only to do a quick check on hearing aid performance. Several dedicated hearing aid analyzers are available for such checking (Fig. 1–49). However, such dedicated analyzers may not be flexible enough to perform intermodulation distortion or difference frequency distortion measurements. For more information, the interested reader is referred to Mueller (1998).

CONCLUSIONS

Hearing aid technology has evolved and continues to evolve. Modern hearing aid transducers have improved performance while having experienced considerable miniaturization. Advancements in hearing aid amplifiers have been made possible by innovations in signal processing and dramatic downsizing of semiconductor technology. As a result, hearing aids of the future offer promise for continued technological advances and improved performance for hearing aid wearers. Hearing aid measurement standards evolve in reaction to hearing aid technology evolution.

ACKNOWLEDGMENTS

We are grateful to acknowledge Eric Peterson, Jason Hombach, Earl Harford, Randall Roberts, and Mary MacRae for their assistance in preparing this chapter.

REFERENCES

AGNEW, J. (1996a). Directionality in hearing revisited. *Hearing Review, 3*(8);20–25.

AGNEW, J. (1996b). Hearing aid adjustments through potentiometer and switch options. In: M. Valente (Ed.), *Hearing aids: Standards, options, and limitations* (pp. 210–251). New York: Thieme Medical Publishers.

AGNEW, J. (1996c). The perception of internally-generated noise in hearing amplification. *Journal of the American Academy of Audiology, 7;*296–303.

AGNEW, J. (1996d). Acoustic feedback in hearing aids. *Trends in Amplification, 1*(2);45–82.

AGNEW, J. (1997). An overview of digital signal processing in hearing instruments. *Hearing Review, 4*(7);8–21.

AGNEW, J. (1998). The causes and effects of distortion and internal noise in hearing aids. *Trends in Amplification, 3*(3); 82–118.

AGNEW, J., POTTS, L., & VALENTE, M. (1997). Sound quality judgements in class A and class D hearing aids. *American Journal of Audiology, 6*(2);33–44.

AMERICAN NATIONAL STANDARDS INSTITUTE. (1971). Methods of electroacoustical characteristics of hearing aids (ANSI S3.3–1971). New York: Acoustical Society of America.

AMERICAN NATIONAL STANDARDS INSTITUTE. (1976). Specification of hearing aid characteristics (ANSI S3.22–1976). New York: Acoustical Society of America.

AMERICAN NATIONAL STANDARDS INSTITUTE. (1979). Occluded Ear Simulator (ANSI S3.25–1979). New York: Acoustical Society of America.

AMERICAN NATIONAL STANDARDS INSTITUTE. (1985). Methods of measurement of performance characteristics of hearing aids under simulated *in-situ* working conditions (ANSI S3.35–1985). New York: Acoustical Society of America.

AMERICAN NATIONAL STANDARDS INSTITUTE. (1987). Specification of hearing aid characteristics (ANSI S3.22–1987). New York: Acoustical Society of America.

AMERICAN NATIONAL STANDARDS INSTITUTE. (1989). For an occluded ear simulator (ANSI S3.25–1989). New York: Acoustical Society of America.

AMERICAN NATIONAL STANDARDS INSTITUTE. (1992). Testing hearing aids with a broadband noise signal (ANSI S3.42–1992). New York: Acoustical Society of America.

AMERICAN NATIONAL STANDARDS INSTITUTE. (1995). Method for coupler calibration of earphones (ANSI S3.7–1995). New York: Acoustical Society of America.

AMERICAN NATIONAL STANDARDS INSTITUTE. (1996). Specification of hearing aid characteristics (ANSI S3.22–1996). New York: Acoustical Society of America.

AMERICAN NATIONAL STANDARDS INSTITUTE. (1997). Methods of measurement of real-ear performance characteristics of hearing aids. (ANSI S3.46–1997). New York: Acoustical Society of America.

ANDERSON, B., HAGEN, L., PETERSON, T., PREVES, D., & ROBERTS, R. (1996). Hearing instrument distortion. *Hearing Review, 3*(11);18,22,24,26,69.

ARLINGER, S., BILLERMARK, E., OBERG M., LUNNER, T., & HELLGREN, J. (1997). Clinical trial of a digital hearing aid. *Scandinavian Audiology, 27;*51–61.

ARMSTRONG, S. (1995). Finding and reducing the causes of circuit noise. *Hearing Review, 2*(2);9–11.

ARMSTRONG, S., & SHAVER, D. (1996). Rethinking compression adjustment. *Hearing Review, 3*(8);26–35.

BARFORD, J. (1978). Multichannel compression hearing aids: Experiments and considerations on clinical applicability. *Scandinavian Audiology,* (Suppl. 6);315–340.

BARRY, J. (1998). Review of hearing aid amplification circuits. *Journal of the American Academy of Audiology, 9;*105–111.

BAUER, B. (1987). A century of microphones. *Journal of the Audiological Engineering Society, 35*(4);246–258.

BENTLER, R., & NELSON, J. (1997). Assessing release-time options in a two-channel AGC hearing aid. *American Journal of Audiology, 6*(1);43–50.

BENTLER, R., & PAVLOVIC, C. (1989). Transfer functions and correction factors used in hearing aid evaluation and research. *Ear and Hearing, 10;*58–63.

BERGER, K. (1984). *The hearing aid: Its operation and development* (3rd ed.). Livonia, MI: International Hearing Society.

BERLIN, C., HOOD, L., HURLEY, A., & HAN, W. (1996). Hearing aids: Only for hearing-impaired patients with abnormal otoacoustic emissions. In: C. Berlin (Ed.), *Hair cells and hearing aids* (pp. 99–112). San Diego: Singular Publishing Group.

BOLSTEIN, M. (1977). Thirty years of the hearing aid industry. *Hearing Journal, 31*(2);50–71.

BOZARTH, M., & TISCHBEIN, R. (1980). The evolution of the in-the-ear hearing aid. *Hearing Instruments, 31*(7);16,36.

BRAIDA, L., DURLACH, N., LIPPMAN, R., HICKS, B., RABINOWITZ, W., & REED, C. (1979). Hearing aids—A review of past research on linear amplification, amplitude compression, and frequency lowering. *ASHA Monograph 19,* Rockville, MD.

BRYANT, M., MUELLER, H.G., & NORTHERN, J. (1991). Minimal contact long canal ITE hearing instruments. *Hearing Instruments, 42*(1);12–15,48.

BURKHARD, M. (1977). Measuring the constants of ear simulators. *Journal of the Audiological Engineering Society 25*(12); 1008–1015.

BURKHARD, M. (1978). *Manikin measurements.* Itasca, IL: Knowles Electronics.

BURKHARD, M., & SACHS, R. (1975). Anthropometric manikin for acoustic research *Journal of the Acoustical Society of America, 58*(1);214–222.

BURNETT, E., & BECK, L. (1987). A correction for converting 2-cc coupler responses to insertion responses for custom in-the-ear nondirectional hearing aids. *Ear and Hearing,* (Suppl. 8);89S–94S.

BYRNE, D. (1983). Theoretical prescriptive approaches to selecting the gain and frequency response of a hearing aid. *Monographs of Contemporary Audiology, 4*(1);1–40.

BYRNE, D., CHRISTEN, R., & DILLON, H. (1981). Effects of peaks in hearing aid frequency response curves on comfortable listening levels of normal-hearing subjects. *Australian Journal of Audiology, 3*(2);42–46.

CALLIAS, F., SALCHLI, F., & GIRARD, D. (1989). A set of four IC's in CMOS technology for a programmable hearing aid. *IEEE Journal of Solid-State Circuits, 24*(2);301–312.

CARLSON, E. (1988). An output amplifier whose time has come. *Hearing Instruments, 39*(10);30–32.

CARVER, W. (1978). Hearing aids: A historical and technical review. In: J. Katz (Ed.), *Handbook of clinical audiology* (2nd ed.) (pp. 479–480). Baltimore: Williams & Wilkins.

CHIASSON, C., & DAVIS, R. (1991). Speech recognition in noise for hearing-impaired subjects: Effects of an adaptive filter hearing aid. *Journal of the American Academy of Audiology, 2;*146–150.

CIECHANOWSKI, J., & COOPER, W. (1976) Problems with earphone calibration using a manikin. *Journal of the American Audiological Society, 2*(3);88–94.

CLASEN, T., VESTERAGER, V., & PARVING, A. (1987). In-the-ear hearing aids. *Scandinavian Audiology, 16;*195–200.

COMPTON, C. (1994). Providing effective telecoil performance with in-the-ear hearing instruments. *Hearing Journal, 47*(4);23–33.

COOK, J., BACON, S., & SAMMETH, C. (1997). Effect of low-frequency gain reduction on speech recognition and its relation to upward spread of masking, *Journal of Speech and Hearing Research, 40;*410–422.

CORNELISSE, L., & SEEWALD, R. (1997). Field-to-microphone transfer functions for completely in-the-canal (CIC) instruments. *Ear and Hearing, 18;*342–345.

COX, R., & ALEXANDER, G. (1995). The abbreviated profile of hearing aid benefit. *Ear and Hearing, 16*(2);176–183.

COX, R., & STUDEBAKER, G. (1977). Spectral changes produced by earphone-cushion reproduction of hearing aid-processed signals. *Journal of the American Audiological Society, 3*(1); 26–33.

CRAIN, T., & VAN TASELL, D. (1994). Effect of peak clipping on speech recognition threshold. *Ear and Hearing, 15*(6); 443–453.

CRAIN, T., & YUND, W. (1995). The effect of multichannel compression on vowel and stop-consonant discrimination in normal-hearing and hearing-impaired subjects. *Ear and Hearing, 16*;529–543.

CURRAN, J., & ELY, W. (1979). Input compression by Maico: An achievement from concept to circuit. *Hearing Instruments, 30*(10);24–25.

DAVIS, H., STEVENS, S., NICHOLS, R., HUDGINS, M., PETERSON, G., & ROSS, D. (1947). *Hearing aids: An experimental study of design objectives.* Cambridge, MA: Harvard University Press.

DEMPSEY, J. (1987). Effect of automatic signal-processing amplification on speech recognition in noise for persons with sensorineural hearing loss. *Annals of Otology, Rhinology, and Laryngology, 96*;251–253.

DILLON, H. (1988). Compression in hearing aids. In: R. Sandlin (Ed.), *Handbook of hearing aid amplification* (Vol. 1) (pp. 121–145). Boston: College Hill Press.

DILLON, H. (1996). Compression? Yes, but for low or high frequencies, for low or high intensities, and with what response times? *Ear and Hearing, 17*(4);287–307.

DITTARDT, A. (1990). *Application notes for the Knowles EP integrated receiver.* Itasca, IL: Knowles Electronics.

DODDS, E., & HARFORD, E. (1968). Modified earpieces and CROS for high frequency hearing losses. *Journal of Speech and Hearing Research, 11*(1),204–218.

DOPP, R. (1996) *Zinc air technical introduction.* Rayovac Battery Symposium, Madison, WI.

DRESCHLER, W. (1988). Dynamic range reduction by peak clipping or compression and its effects on phoneme perception in hearing-impaired listeners. *Scandinavian Audiology, 17*;45–51.

DRESCHLER, W. (1989). Phoneme perception via hearing aids with and without compression and the role of temporal resolution. *Audiology, 28*;49–60.

DYRLUND, O., & BISGAARD, N. (1991). Acoustic feedback margin improvements in hearing instruments using a prototype DFS (Digital Feedback Suppression) system. *Scandinavian Audiology, 20*;49–53.

EDMONDS, J., STAAB, W., PREVES, D., & YANZ, J. (1997). "Open" digital hearing aids: A reality today. *Hearing Journal, 50*(10);54.

ELIOT, S., & NELSON, P. (1993). Active noise control. *IEEE Sig Proceedings Magazine 10*(4);12–35.

ERBER, N. (1973). Body-baffle and real-ear effects in the selection of hearing aids for deaf children. *Journal of Speech and Hearing Disorders, 38*;224–231.

FABRY, D., & VAN TASELL, D. (1990). Evaluation of an articulation index-based model for predicting the effects of adaptive frequency response hearing aids. *Journal of Speech and Hearing Research, 33*;676–689.

FORTUNE, T. (1996). Amplifiers and circuit algorithms of contemporary hearing aids. In: M. Valente (Ed.), *Hearing aids: Standards, options and limitations* (pp. 157–209). New York: Thieme Medical Publishers.

FORTUNE, T., & PREVES D. (1992). Hearing aid saturation and aided loudness discomfort. *Journal of Speech and Hearing Research, 35*;175–185.

FOWLER, E. (1960). Bilateral hearing aids for monaural total deafness: A suggestion for better hearing. *Archives of Otolaryngology, 72*;57–58.

GAGNE, J. (1988). Excess masking among listeners with a sensorineural hearing loss. *Journal of the Acoustical Society of America, 83*;2311–2321.

GENNUM (1996). *GS3034 class H CIC hybrid.* Ontario, Canada.

GLOVER, R. (1940). A review of cardioid type unidirectional microphones. *Journal of the Acoustical Society of America, 11*;296–302.

GOLDBERG, H. (1972). Hearing aid compression amplification: Varieties. *National Hearing Aid Journal, 25*(12);9, 32, 46.

GOLDBERG, H. (1982). Signal processors: Application to the hearing-impaired. *Hearing Aid Journal, 35*(4);23–28.

GREEN, D. (1969). Non-occluding earmolds with CROS and IROS hearing aids. *Archives of Otolaryngology, 89*; 512–522.

GREEN, D., & ROSS, M. (1968). The effect of a conventional versus a nonoccluding (CROS type) earmold upon the frequency response of a hearing aid. *Journal of Speech and Hearing Research, 11*;638–647.

GREENBERG, J., PETERSON, P., & ZUREK, P. (1993). Intelligibility-weighted measures of speech-to-interference ratio and speech system performance. *Journal of the Acoustical Society of America, 94*;3009–3010.

GREENBERG, J., & ZUREK, P. (1992). Evaluation of an adaptive beamforming method for hearing aids. *Journal of the Acoustical Society of America, 92*;1662–1676.

GRIFFING, T., & PREVES, D. (1976). In-the-ear aids Part I. *Hearing Instruments, 27*(3);22–24.

HABLE, L., BROWN, K., & GUDMUNDSEN, G. (1990). CROS-plus: A physical CROS system. *Hearing Instruments, 41*(8);27–30,68.

HALL, M., & SANDLIN, R. (1997). The clinical utility of a true DSP hearing instrument. *Hearing Journal, 50*(5);34,37–38.

HARFORD, E. (1966). Bilateral CROS. Two-sided hearing with on hearing aid. *Archives in Otolaryngology, 84*;426–432.

HARFORD, E. (1967). Innovations in the use of the modern hearing aid. *International Audiology, 6*;311–314.

HARFORD, E., & BARRY, J. (1965). A rehabilitative approach to the problem of unilateral hearing impairment: the contralateral routing of signals (CROS). *Journal of Speech and Hearing Disorders, 30*;121–138.

HARFORD, E., & DODDS, E. (1974). Versions of CROS hearing aid. *Archives in Otolaryngology, 100*,50–57.

HARFORD, E., & FOX, J. (1978). The use of high-pass amplification for broad-frequency sensorineural hearing loss. *Audiology, 17*;10–28.

HARRY, W. (1940). Six-way directional microphone. *Bell System Technology Journal, 19*;10–14.

HAWKINS, D., & NAIDOO, S. (1993). Comparison of sound quality and clarity with asymmetrical peak clipping and output limiting compression. *Journal of the American Academy of Audiology, 4*;221–228.

HAWKINS, D. & YACULLO, W. (1984). Signal-to-noise ratio advantage of binaural hearing aids and directional microphones under different levels of reverberation. *Journal of Speech and Hearing Disorders, 49;*278–286.

HEIDE, V. (1994). Project Phoenix, Inc., 1984–1989: The development of a wearable digital signal processing hearing aid. In: R. Sandlin (Ed.), *Understanding digitally programmable hearing aids* (pp. 123–150). Needham Heights, MA: Allyn & Bacon.

HICKSON, L. (1994). Compression amplification in hearing aids. *American Journal of Audiology, 3(3);*51–65.

HICKSON, L., & BYRNE, D. (1995). Acoustic analysis of speech through a hearing aid: Effects of linear vs. compression amplification. *Australian Journal of Audiology, 17(1);*1–13.

HICKSON, L., DODD, B., & BYRNE, D. (1994). Consonant perception with linear and compression amplification. *Scandinavian Audiology, 24;*175–184.

HIRSCH, I. (1952). *The measurement of hearing.* New York: McGraw-Hill

HODGSON, W., & MURDOCK, C. (1970). Effect of the earmold on speech intelligibility in hearing aid use. *Journal of Speech and Hearing Research, 13;*290–297.

HOFFMAN, M., & BUCKLEY, K. (1995). Robust time-domain processing of broadband microphone array data. *IEEE Trans Speech Audio Processing, 3(3);*193–203.

HORWITZ, A., TURNER, C., & FABRY, D. (1991). Effects of different frequency response strategies upon recognition and preference for audible speech stimuli. *Journal of Speech and Hearing Research, 34;*1185–1196.

HOTVET, D. (1988). *Automatic gain control for hearing aid.* U.S. Patent No. 4,718,099.

HOUTGAST, T., & STEENEKEN, H. (1985). A review of the MTF concept in room acoustics and its use for estimating speech intelligibility in auditoria. *Journal of the Acoustical Society of America, 77;*1069–1077

HUMES, L., CHRISTENSEN, L., & BESS, F. (1997). A comparison of the benefit provided by well-fit linear hearing aids and instruments with automatic reduction of low-frequency gain. *Journal of Speech and Hearing Research, 40;*666–685.

INTERNATIONAL ELECTROTECHNICAL COMMISSION. (1981). *Occluded-ear simulator for the measurement of earphones coupled to the ear by ear inserts* (IEC Publication 711). New York: IEC.

INTERNATIONAL ELECTROTECHNICAL COMMISSION. (1983a). *Hearing aids with automatic gain control circuits* (IEC Hearing Aids Publication 60118–2). New York: IEC.

INTERNATIONAL ELECTROTECHNICAL COMMISSION. (1983b). *Measurement of performance characteristics of hearing aids for quality inspection for delivery purposes* (IEC Hearing Aids Publication 60118–7). New York: IEC.

INTERNATIONAL ELECTROTECHNICAL COMMISSION. (1983c). *Measurement of hearing aids under simulated in-situ working conditions* (IEC Hearing Aids Publication 60118–8). New York: IEC.

JERGER, J., JOHNSON, K., & SMITH-FARACH, S. (1989). Signal processing. *Hearing Instruments, 40(11);*12–18.

JERVALL, L., & LINDBLAD, A. (1978). The influence of attack time and release time on speech intelligibility. A study of the effects of AGC on normal-hearing and hearing-impaired subjects. *Scandinavian Audiology, (Suppl. 6);*341–353.

JETTY, A., & RINTELMANN, W. (1970). Acoustic coupler effects on speech audiometric scores using a CROS hearing aid. *Journal of Speech and Hearing Research, 13;*101–114.

JOHNSON, W., & KILLION, M. (1994). Amplification: Is class D better than class B? *American Journal of Audiology, 3(1);* 11–13.

KATES, J. (1986). Signal processing for hearing aids. *Hearing Instruments, 37(2);*19–21.

KATES, J. (1987). Theoretical and practical considerations in signal processing. *Hearing Instruments, 38(8);*23–26, 28.

KATES, J. (1993). Hearing aid design criteria. *Journal of Speech-Language Pathology in Audiology, (Suppl. 1);*18–19.

KATES, J., & WEISS, M. (1996). A comparison of hearing-aid array-processing techniques. *Journal of the Acoustical Society of America, 99(5);*3138–3148.

KILLION, M. (1979). *Design and evaluation of high fidelity hearing aids.* Ph.D. dissertation, Northwestern University, Evanston, IL.

KILLION, M. (1986). *Class D hearing aid amplifier.* U.S. Patent No. 4,592,087.

KILLION, M. (1993). The K-AMP hearing aid: An attempt to present high fidelity for persons with impaired hearing. *American Journal of Audiology, 2;*71–73.

KILLION, M. (1997). Hearing aid transducers. In: M. Crocker (Ed.), *Encyclopedia of acoustics* (pp. 1979–1990). New York: John Wiley & Sons.

KILLION, M., FIKRET-PASA, S., TILLMAN-NIQUETTE, P., & BENTLER, R. (1996). *Required signal-to-noise ratio vs. hearing loss for 4-talker babble SIN test.* Elk Grove Village, IL: Etymotic Research.

KILLION, M., & MONSER, E. (1980). CORFIG: Coupler response for flat insertion gain. In: G. Studebaker, & I. Hochberg (Eds.), *Acoustical factors affecting hearing aid performance* (pp. 149–168). Baltimore: University Park Press.

KILLION, M., & REVIT, L. (1993). CORFIG and GIFROC: Real-ear to coupler and back. In: G. Studebaker, & I. Hochberg (Eds.), *Acoustical factors affecting hearing aid performance* (2d ed.) (pp. 65–85). Boston: Allyn & Bacon.

KILLION, M., SCHULEIN, R., CHRISTENSEN, L., FABRY, D., REVIT, L., NIQUETTE, P., & CHUNG, K. (1998). Real-world performance of an ITE directional microphone. *Hearing Journal, 31(4);*24–38.

KILLION, M., STAAB, W., & PREVES, D. (1990). Classifying automatic signal processors *Hearing Instruments, 41(8);*24.

KILLION, M., & VILLCHUR, E. (1993). Kessler was right—partly: But SIN test shows some aids improve hearing in noise. *Hearing Journal, 46(9);*31–35.

KILLION, M., WILBER, L., & GUDMUNDSEN, G. (1988). Zwislocki was right ... A potential solution to the "hollow voice" problem (the amplified occlusion effect) with deeply sealed earmolds. *Hearing Instruments, 39(1);*14–18.

KING, A., & MARTIN, M. (1984). Is AGC beneficial in hearing aids? *British Journal of Audiology, 18;*31–38.

KIRKWOOD, D. (1998). Hearing aid sales increase 7.5% in 1997: Expansion expected to continue. *Hearing Journal, 51(1);*21–28.

KLEIN, A., MILLS, J., & ADKINS, W. (1990). Upward spread of masking, hearing loss, and speech recognition in young and elderly listeners. *Journal of the Acoustical Society of America, 87;*1266–1271.

KNIGHT, J. (1992). A subjective evaluation of K-AMP vs. linear hearing aids. *Hearing Instruments, 43(10);*8–11.

KNOWLES, H. (1966). Hearing aids are severe test for microphones and receivers. *Hearing Aid Journal, 19(4);*12–14.

KNOWLES ELECTRONICS. (1975). *Information bulletin on XL-9073 probe tube microphone kit-application notes.* Franklin Park, IL: Knowles Electronics.

KNOWLES ELECTRONICS. (1976). *Effects of acoustical termination upon receiver response, Technical Bulletin E-6* (pp 1–8). Itasca, IL: Knowles Electronics.

KOCHKIN, S. (1993). MarkeTrak III: Why 20 million in the U.S. don't use hearing aids for their hearing loss. *Hearing Journal, 46*(1);20–27.

KOCHKIN, S. (1994a). MarkeTrak IV: Impact on purchase intent of cosmetics, stigma, and style of hearing instrument. *Hearing Journal, 47*(9);29–36.

KOCHKIN, S. (1994b). MarkeTrak IV: Will CICs attract a new type of customer and what about price? *Hearing Journal, 47*(11);49–54.

KOCHKIN, S., & BALLAD, W. (1991). Dispenser sound quality perceptions of class D integrated receivers. *Hearing Instruments, 42*(4);25,28.

KRETZINGER, E., & YOUNG, N. (1960). The use of fast limiting to improve the intelligibility of speech in noise. *Speech Monographs, 27*;63–69.

KUK, F. (1996a). Theoretical and practical considerations in compression hearing aids. *Trends in Amplification, 1*(1);1–39.

KUK, F. (1996b). The effects of distortion on user satisfaction with hearing aids In: M. Valente (Ed.), *Hearing aids: Standards, options and limitations* (pp. 327–367). New York: Thieme Medical Publishers.

KUK, F. (1997). Open or closed? Let's weigh the evidence. *Hearing Journal, 50*(10);54.

KUK, F. (1998). Rationale and requirements for a slow-acting compression hearing aid. *Hearing Journal 51*(6); 45–53,79.

LEEUW, A., & DRESCHLER, W. (1991). Advantages of directional hearing aid microphones related to room acoustics. *Audiology, 30*;330–344.

LEHR, M., & WIDROW, B. (1998). *Directional hearing system.* U.S. Patent No. 5,793,875.

LEIJON, A. (1990). Hearing aid gain for loudness-density normalization in cochlear hearing losses with impaired frequency resolutions. *Ear and Hearing, 12*(4);242–250.

LENK, J. (1971). *Handbook of simplified solid-state circuit design.* Englewood Cliffs, NJ: Prentice-Hall.

LENTZ, W. (1974). A summary of research using directional and omnidirectional hearing aids. *Journal of Audiological Technique, 13*;42–46.

LINK, M., & BUCKLEY, K. (1993). Prewhitening for intelligibility gain in hearing aid arrays. *Journal of Acoustical Society of America, 93*(4);2139–2145.

LONGWELL, T., & GAWINSKI, M. (1992). Fitting strategies for the 90s: Class D amplification. *Hearing Journal, 45*(9); 26,28,30–31.

LUEG, P. (1936). *Process of silencing sound oscillations.* U.S. Patent No. 2,043,416.

LYBARGER, S. (1947). Development of a new hearing aid with magnetic microphone. *Electrical Manufacturing*, Nov.

LYBARGER, S. (1985). The physical and electroacoustic characteristics of hearing aids. In: J. Katz (Ed.), *Handbook of audiology* (pp. 849–884). Baltimore: Williams & Wilkins.

LYBARGER, S., & BARRON, S. (1965). Head-baffle effect for different hearing aid microphone locations [Abstract]. *Journal of the Acoustical Society of America, 38*;922.

LYBARGER, S., & TEDER, H. (1986). 2cc coupler curves to insertion gain curves: Calculated and experimental results. *Hearing Instruments, 37*(11);36–40.

MACRAE J., & DILLON, H. (1996). An equivalent input noise level criterion for hearing aids. *Journal of Rehabilitation Research and Development, 33*(4);355–362.

MADAFFARI, P. (1983). *Directional matrix technical bulletin, report 10554-1.* Itasca, IL: Knowles Electronics.

MADAFARRI, P., & STANLEY, W. (1996). Microphone, receiver and telecoil options: Past, present and future. In: M. Valente (Ed.), *Hearing aids: Standards, options and limitations* (pp. 126–156). New York: Thieme Medical Publishers.

MAJOR, M. (1971). All-in-the-ear custom earmolds. *National Hearing Aid Journal, 24*(4);10.

MCCLELLAN, M. (1967). Aided speech discrimination in noise with vented and unvented earmolds. *Journal of Audiology Research, 13*;93–99.

MCCRACKEN, W., & LAOIDE-KEMP, S. (1997). *Audiology in education.* London: Whurr Publishers.

MCGEE, J. (1962). *Acoustic modifier earmold.* U.S. Patent No. 3,126,977.

MICRO-TECH. (1997). *Meridian concept programming manual.* Minneapolis, MN: Micro-Tech.

MOORE, B., & GLASBERG, B. (1986). A comparison of two-channel and single-channel compression aids. *Audiology, 25*;210–226.

MOORE, B., GLASBERG, B., & STONE, M. (1991). Optimization of a slow-acting automatic gain control system for use in hearing aids. *British Journal of Audiology 25*;171–182.

MOORE, B., JOHNSON, J., CLARK, T., & PLUVINAGE, V. (1992). Evaluation of a dual-channel full dynamic range compression system for people with sensorineural hearing loss. *Ear and Hearing, 13*(5);349–370.

MORELY, R., ENGEL, G., SULLIVAN, T., & NATARAJAN, S. (1988). VLSI based design of a battery-operated digital hearing aid. *Proceedings of IEEE ICASSP.*

MUELLER, G. (1998). Probe-microphone measurements: Yesterday, today, and tomorrow. *Hearing Journal, 51*(4);17–22.

MUELLER, G., GRIMES, A., & ERDMAN, S. (1983). Subjective ratings of directional amplification. *Hearing Instruments, 34*(2); 14–16.

MUELLER, G., & KILLION, M. (1996). http://www.compression.edu. *Hearing Journal, 49*(1);10,44–47.

NILSSON, M., SOLI, S., & SULLIVAN, J. (1994). Development of the hearing in noise test for the measurement of speech reception thresholds in quiet and in noise. *Journal of the Acoustical Society of America, 95*(2);1085–1099.

NILSSON, P., VESTERAGER, V., SIBELLE, P., SIECK, L., & CHRISTENSEN, B. (1997). A double-blind cross-over study of a non-linear hearing aid. *Audiology, 36*;325–338.

NUNLEY, J., STAAB, W., STEADMAN, J., WECHSLER, P., & SPENCER, B. (1983). A wearable digital hearing aid. *Hearing Journal, 36*(10);29–35.

OLSEN, H. (1932). Unidirectional ribbon microphone. *Journal of the Acoustical Society of America, 3*;315.

OLSEN, W. (1986). Physical characteristics of hearing aids. In: W. Hodgson (Ed.), *Hearing aid assessment and use in audiologic habilitation* (3rd ed.) (pp. 13–37). Baltimore: Williams & Wilkins.

OLSEN, W. (1991). Clinical assessment of output limiting and speech enhancement techniques. In: G. Studebaker, F. Bess,

& L. Beck (Eds.), *The Vanderbilt hearing-aid report II* (pp. 53–61). Parkton, MD: York Press.

PAINTON, S. (1993). Objective measure of low-frequency amplification reduction in canal hearing aids with adaptive circuitry. *Journal of the American Academy of Audiology, 4;* 152–156.

PALMER, C., KILLION, M., WILBER, L., & BALLAD, W. (1995). Comparison of two hearing aid receiver-amplifier combinations using sound quality judgments. *Ear and Hearing, 16*(6);587–598.

PASCOE, D. (1986). *Hearing aids* (pp. 1–49). Austin, TX: Pro-Ed Studies In Communicative Disorders.

PATUZZI, R., YATES, G., & JOHNSTONE, B. (1989). Outer hair cell receptor current and sensorineural hearing loss. *Hearing Research, 42;*47–72.

PERREAULT, J. (1994). *A comparison of class B and class D hearing aid amplifiers.* Unpublished master's thesis, University of Minnesota, Department of Communication Disorders.

PETERSON, M., FEENEY, P., & YANTIS, P. (1990). The effect of automatic gain control in hearing-impaired listeners with different dynamic ranges. *Ear and Hearing, 11*(3); 185–194.

PETERSON, P. (1987). Using linearly constrained adaptive beamforming to reduce interference in hearing aids from competing talkers in reverberant rooms (pp. 2364–2367). *Proceedings of IEEE ICASSP.*

PHONAK (1995). *Audio zoom-signal processing for improved communication in noise.* Phonak Focus No. 18, Stafa, Switzerland.

PLOMP, R. (1988). The negative effect of amplitude compression in multichannel hearing aids in light of the modulation-transfer function. *Journal of the Acoustical Society of America, 83;*2322–2327.

POLLACK, M. (1980). Special applications of amplification. In: M. Pollack (Ed.), *Amplification for the hearing-impaired* (pp. 243–286). New York: Grune and Stratton.

PREVES, D. (1974). Application of directional microphones in hearing aids. *Hearing Aid Journal, 27*(8);18–19.

PREVES, D. (1975a). Obtaining accurate measurements of directional hearing aid parameters. *Hearing Aid Journal, 28*(4);13,28,34.

PREVES, D. (1975b). Selecting the best directivity pattern for unidirectional noise suppressing hearing aids. *Hearing Instruments, (26)*10;18–19.

PREVES, D. (1976). Directivity of in-the-ear aids with non-directional and directional microphones. *Hearing Journal, 29*(8);7,32–33.

PREVES, D. (1988). Revised ANSI Std. S3.22 for hearing instrument performance measurement. *Hearing Instruments, 39*(3);26–34.

PREVES, D. (1994b). Current and future applications of digital hearing aid technology. In: R. Sandlin (Ed.), *Understanding digitally programmable hearing aids* (pp. 275–313). Needham Heights, MA: Allyn & Bacon.

PREVES, D. (1994c). Future trends in hearing aid technology. In: V. Valente (Ed.), *Strategies for selecting and verifying hearing aid fittings* (pp. 363–396). New York: Thieme Medical Publishers.

PREVES, D. (1996a). Revised ANSI standard for measurement of hearing instrument performance. *Hearing Journal, 49* (10);49–57.

PREVES, D. (1996b). Standardizing hearing aid measurement parameters and electroacoustic performance tests. In: M. Valente (Ed.), *Hearing aids: Standards, options, and limitation* (pp. 1–71). New York: Thieme Medical Publishers.

PREVES, D. (1996c). The role of the hearing instrument amplifier. *Hearing Review, 3*(5);34–35,42–43.

PREVES, D. (1997). Directional microphone use in ITE hearing instruments. *Hearing Review, 4*(7);21–22,24–27.

PREVES, D., BECK, L., BURNETT, E., & TEDER, H. (1989). Input stimuli for obtaining frequency responses of automatic gain control hearing aids. *Journal of Speech and Hearing Research, 32;*189–194.

PREVES, D., LEISSES, M., & WOODRUFF, B. (1997b). Using a hearing instrument manufacturer's database to maximize fitting success. *Hearing Review Supplement 2,* Nov.; 12–18.

PREVES, D., & NEWTON, J. (1989). The headroom problem and hearing aid performance. *Hearing Journal, 42*(10);19–26.

PREVES, D., PETERSON, T., & BREN, M. (1998). *In-the-ear hearing aid with directional microphone system.* U.S. Patent No. 5,757,933.

PREVES, D., SAMMETH, C., & WYNNE, M. (1997a). *Field trial evaluations of a switched directional/omnidirectional ITE hearing instrument.* Poster presentation at NIDCD/VA Hearing Aid Conference, Bethesda, MD.

RAFAELY, B., & FURST, M. (1996). Audiometric earcanal probe with active ambient noise control. *IEEE Trans Speech Audio Processing, 4*(3);224–230.

RANKOVIC, C. (1998). Factors governing speech reception benefits of adaptive linear filtering for listeners with sensorineural hearing loss. *Journal of the Acoustical Society of America, 103*(2);1043–1057.

RANKOVIC, C., FREYMAN, R., & ZUREK, P. (1992). Potential benefits of adaptive frequency-gain characteristics for speech reception in noise. *Journal of the Acoustical Society of America, 91;*354–362.

ROBERTS, M., & SCHULEIN, R. (1997). *Measurement and intelligibility optimization of directional microphones for use in hearing aid devices.* Paper 4515B–3, presented at Audiological Engineering Society Meeting, New York.

ROESER, R., & TAYLOR, K. (1988). Audiometric and field testing with a digital hearing instrument. *Hearing Instruments, 39*(4);14.

ROWLIN, R. (1972). BIROS and tube fittings. *Hearing Journal, 25*(12);13,36,38.

RUMOSHOVSKY, J. (1977). Directional microphones in ITE aids. *Hearing Journal, 30*(6);11,48–50.

SAMMETH, C., & OCHS, M. (1991). A review of current "noise reduction" hearing aids: Rationale, assumptions, and efficacy. *Ear and Hearing, 12*(Suppl. 6);116S–124S.

SAMMETH, C., PREVES, D., BRATT, G., PEEK, B., & BESS, F. (1993). Achieving prescribed gain/frequency responses with advances in hearing aid technology. *Rehabilitation Research and Development, 30*(1);1–7.

SANDLIN, R. (1994). *Understanding digitally programmable hearing aids* Boston: Allyn & Bacon.

SCHUM, D. (1990). Noise reduction strategies for elderly, hearing-impaired listeners. *Journal of the American Academy of Audiology, 1;*31–36.

SCHUM, D. (1996). Speech understanding in background noise. In: M. Valente (Ed.), *Hearing aids: Standards, options, and limitations* (pp. 368–406). New York: Thieme Medical Publishers.

SCHUM, D. (1997). A field evaluation of the ASA fitting rationale. *Hearing Journal, 50*(5);42,44,47,48.

SCHWEITZER, H., & CAUSEY, G. (1977). The relative importance of recovery time in compression hearing aids. *Audiology, 15*;61–72.

SCHWEITZER, H. (1997). Development of digital hearing aids. *Trends in Amplification, 2*(2);41–77.

SEEWALD, R., CORNELISSE, L., RICHERT, F., & BLOCK, M. (1997). Acoustic transform for fitting CIC instruments. In: M. Chasin (Ed.), *CIC handbook* (pp. 83–100). San Diego: Singular Publishing Group.

SESSLER, G. (1996). Silicon microphones. *Journal of the Audiological Engineering Society, 44*(1/2);16–22.

SIGELMAN, J., & PREVES D. (1987). Field trials of a new adaptive signal processor hearing aid circuit. *Hearing Journal, 40*(4);24–28.

SKAFTE, M. (1990). Fifty years of hearing healthcare 1940–1990. *Hearing Instruments, 41*(9);1–130.

SOEDE, W., BERKHOUT, A., & BILSEN, F. (1993a). Development of a directional hearing instrument based on array technology. *Journal of the Acoustical Society of America* (Pt. 1) 94(2); 785–798.

SOEDE, W., BILSEN, F., & BERKHOUT, A. (1993b). Assessment of a directional microphone array for hearing-impaired listeners (Pt. 2). *Journal of the Acoustical Society of America, 94*(2), 799–808.

SOUZA, P., & TURNER, C. (1996). Effect of single-channel compression on temporal speech information. *Journal of Speech-Language-Hearing Research, 39*;901–911.

SOUZA, P., & TURNER, C. (1998). Multichannel compression, temporal cues, and audibility. *Journal of Speech-Language-Hearing Research, 41*;315–326.

STAAB, W. (1992). The peritympanic instrument: fitting rationale and test results. *Hearing Journal, 45,*(10)21–26.

STAAB, W. (1997). Deep canal hearing aids. In: M. Chasin (Ed.), *CIC handbook* (pp. 1–30). San Diego: Singular Publishing Group.

STAAB, W., & LYBARGER, S. (1994). Characteristics and use of hearing aids. In: J. Katz (Ed.), *Handbook of clinical audiology* (4th ed.) (pp. 657–722). Baltimore, MD: Williams & Wilkins.

STACH, B., SPEERSCHNEIDER, J., & JERGER, J. (1987). Evaluating the efficacy of automatic signal processing hearing aids. *Hearing Journal, 40*(3);15–19.

STADLER, R., & RABINOWITZ, W. (1993). On the potential of fixed arrays for hearing aids (Pt. 1). *Journal of the Acoustical Society of America, 94*(3);1332–1342.

STARKEY LABORATORIES (1995). *The compression handbook.* Eden Prairie, MN: Starkey Laboratories.

STEGMAN, H. (1966). Earmold fitting for the new all in-the-ear aids. *Hearing Aid Journal, 19*(9);12–13.

STEIN, L., MCGEE, T., & LEWIS, P. (1989). Speech recognition measures with noise suppression hearing aids using a single-subject experimental design. *Ear and Hearing, 10*(6);375–381.

STELMACHOWICZ, P., JESTEADT, W., GORGA, M., & MOTT. J. (1985). Speech perception ability and psychophysical tuning curves in hearing-impaired listeners. *Journal of the Acoustical Society of America, 2*;620–627.

STONE, M., & MOORE, B. (1992). Syllabic compression: Effective compression ratios for signals modulated at different rates. *British Journal of Audiology, 26*;351–361.

SULLIVAN, R. (1988). Transcranial ITE CROS. *Hearing Instruments, 39*(1);11–12,54.

SULLIVAN, R. (1989a). Custom canal and concha hearing instruments: A real-ear comparison. *Hearing Instruments, 40*(4);23–29,60.

SULLIVAN, R. (1989b). Custom canal and concha hearing instruments: A real-ear comparison. *Hearing Instruments, 40*(7);30–36,58.

SURR, R., CORD, M., & WALDEN, B. (1997). Comparison of linear and K-AMP circuits. *Ear and Hearing, 18*(2);140–146.

SYDOW, C. (1994). Broadband beamforming for a microphone array. *Journal of the Acoustical Society of America, 96*(2); 845–849.

TATE, M. (1994). *Principles of hearing aid audiology.* London: Chapman and Hall.

TEDER, H. (1984). Repeatability of KEMAR insertion gain measurements. *Hearing Instruments, 35*(10);16–22.

TEDER, H. (1993). Compression in the time domain. *American Journal of Audiology, 2*(2);41–46.

TREES, D., & TURNER, C. (1986). Spread of masking in normal and high-frequency hearing loss subjects. *Audiology, 25*;70–83.

TYLER, R., & KUK, F. (1989). The effects of "noise suppression" hearing aids on consonant recognition in speech-babble and low-frequency noise. *Ear and Hearing, 10*(4);243–249.

VALENTE, M., FABRY, D., & POTTS, L. (1995). Recognition of speech in noise with hearing aids using dual microphones. *Journal of the American Academy of Audiology, 6*;440–449.

VALENTE, M., VALENTE, M., & POTTS, L. (1996). Programmable hearing aid systems. In: R. Sandlin (Ed.), *Hearing instrument science and fitting practices* (pp. 647–697). Livonia, MI: National Institute for Hearing Instrument Studies.

VALENTE, M., VALENTE, M., POTTS, L., & LYBARGER, E. (1996). Options: Earhooks, tubing and earmolds. In: M. Valente (Ed.), *Hearing aids: Standards, options and limitations* (pp. 252–356). New York: Thieme Medical Publishers.

VAN DIJKHUIZEN, J. (1991). *Studies on the effectiveness of multichannel automatic gain-control in hearing aids.* Ph.D. dissertation, University of Amsterdam, Holland.

VAN DIJKHUIZEN, J., FESTEN, J., & PLOMP, R. (1991). The effect of frequency-selective attenuation on the speech-reception threshold of sentences in conditions of low-frequency noise. *Journal of the Acoustical Society of America, 90*; 885–894.

VAN HARTEN-DE BRUIJN, H., SIDONNE, C., VAN KREVELD-BOS, G., DRESCHLER, W., & VERSCHUURE, H. (1997). Design of two syllabic nonlinear multichannel signal processors and the results of speech tests in noise. *Ear and Hearing, 18*(1); 26–33.

VAN TASELL, D., & CRAIN, T. (1992). Noise reduction hearing aids: Release from masking and release from distortion. *Ear and Hearing, 13*;114–121.

VAN TASELL, D., LARSEN, S., & FABRY, D. (1988). Effects of adaptive filter hearing aid on speech recognition in noise by hearing-impaired subjects. *Ear and Hearing, 9*(1);15–21.

VERSCHUURE, J., MAAS, A., STIKVOORT, E., DEJONG, R., GOEDEGEBURE, A., & DRESCHLER, W. (1996). Compression and its effect on the speech signal. *Ear and Hearing, 17*(2);162–175.

VILLCHUR E. (1993). A different approach to the noise problem of the hearing-impaired. *American Journal of Audiology, 2*;47–51.

WALKER, G. & DILLON, H. (1982). *Compression in hearing aids: An analysis, a review and some recommendations.* Report No. 90. Sydney, Australia: National Acoustic Laboratories.

WATSON, J. (1989). *Analog and switching circuit design: Using integrated and discrete devices* (2nd ed.). New York: John Wiley and Sons.

WATSON, L. & TOLAN, T. (1949). *Hearing tests and hearing instruments.* Baltimore: Williams & Wilkins.

WIDROW, B., et al. (1975). Adaptive noise cancelling: Principles and applications. *Proceedings IEEE, 63*;1692–1716.

YANZ, J. (1997). *A directional revival.* Micro-Tech Hearing Instruments multi-media presentation.

YUND, W., & BUCKLES, K. (1995). Multichannel compression hearing aids: Effect of number of channels on speech discrimination in noise. *Journal of the Acoustical Society of America, 97*(2);1206–1223.

Chapter 2

Earhooks, Tubing, Earmolds, and Shells

Michael Valente, Maureen Valente, Lisa G. Potts, and Edward H. Lybarger

Outline

The electroacoustic characteristics of hearing aids, measured according to ANSI S3.22–1987 specifications (ANSI, 1987a) in either HA-1 or HA-2 couplers, can be significantly altered by the manner in which the hearing aid is coupled to the ear (de Jonge, 1983). Some alterations of the electroacoustic characteristics (i.e., from head diffraction, concha and earcanal resonances, head shadow and body baffle, residual earcanal volume, and the impedance of the eardrum and middle ear) may be unpredictable and are beyond the control of the audiologist. However, the audiologist can alter, in a fairly predictable way, the electroacoustic characteristics of hearing aids by changes in the transmission line (i.e., earhook, tubing, earmold, and shell) relative to the electroacoustic characteristics originally measured in the coupler.

This chapter will attempt to provide a comprehensive overview of how altering the earhook, tubing, earmold, or shell may affect the electroacoustic characteristics of the delivered signal to the eardrum. The goal of this chapter is to provide the audiologist with the tools necessary to provide a hearing aid fitting that (1) allows aided performance in "quiet" to be significantly better than unaided performance in the same listening situation; (2) allows aided performance in "noise" to be significantly better than unaided performance in the same listening situation. However, it is important for the patient to understand that aided performance in "noise" will not be as satisfactory as aided performance in "quiet." Even normal listeners experience greater difficulty listening in noise compared with listening in quiet! In addition, the hearing aid fitting; (3) allows "soft" input signals to be judged as "soft," but audible, "average" input signals to be judged as "comfortable," and "loud" input signals to be judged as "loud," but not "uncomfortably loud"; (4) provides excellent sound quality and good intelligibility of speech; (5) is relatively distortion free (10% or less) at high input levels; (6) is free of feedback throughout the usable range of the volume control wheel; (7) preserves the balance between the low-frequency and high-frequency regions of the average speech spectrum; (8) when appropriate, extends the high frequency range of the hearing aid; (9) when appropriate, minimizes excessive gain at approximately 1500 Hz; (10) when appropriate, maintains a gently rising frequency response; (11) creates a comfortably fitting earmold or shell; and (12) eliminates the sensation that the patient's head is "at the bottom of the barrel."

As mentioned earlier, the primary goal of this chapter is to provide a comprehensive overview of the transmission line from the earhook to the earmold. Because little has changed over the years regarding the acoustics of the transmission line, we do not feel it necessary to "rewrite" this information.

Audiology: Treatment. Edited by Valente, Hosford-Dunn, and Roeser. Thieme Medical Publishers, Inc., New York © 2000

If the reader is interested in this area, he or she should consult the excellent works of Cox (1979), Egolf (1979a, 1980), Lybarger (1979, 1980), Mynders (1985), Leavitt (1986), and Staab and Lybarger (1994).

DIMENSIONS OF THE TYPICAL TRANSMISSION LINE

The tubing from the receiver encased in the behind-the-ear (BTE), in-the-ear (ITE), or in-the-canal (ITC) hearing aid is typically 8 to 15 mm long and has an internal diameter (ID) of 0.5 to 1.5 mm wide (Cox, 1979; Killion, 1982). The sound bore of the earhook is typically 20 to 30 mm long and 1.2 to 1.8 mm wide (Cox, 1979; Killion, 1982). The tubing from the earhook to the tip of earmold is usually 40 to 45 mm long and 1.93 mm wide (Cox, 1979; Killion, 1982). This latter dimension should be compared with the ANSI S3.22–1989 standard that requires 25 mm of 1.93 mm tubing connected to an HA-2 coupler, which is designed to simulate the average earmold with a bore length of 18 mm and ID of 3 mm. Thus the transmission line of a typical BTE is approximately 75 mm long. In an eyeglass fitting, the transmission line is about 20 to 30 mm shorter because of the absence of an earhook (Staab & Lybarger, 1994). Finally, the dimensions of the typical earcanal from the earmold tip to the eardrum is 13 to 15 mm long and 7.5 mm wide (Cox, 1979; Killion, 1982). Figure 2–1 (Valente, 1984c) provides a schematic drawing of the typical dimensions of the transmission line from the tubing to the eardrum.

EARHOOK

The earhook is a semirigid acoustic connector used to retain the hearing aid over the ear and to conduct sound to tubing that is connected to the earhook. Earhooks are available in a variety of shapes (one-fourth and one-half moon) and materials. The bore diameter of the earhook usually tapers at the tubing end, although some earhooks have minimal tapering (i.e., 2.25 mm at the start and 1.83 mm at the end). Cox (1979) compared the output of a hearing aid–earmold system with a variety of earhooks ranging in length from 20 to 30 mm and with constant diameters of 1.2 to 1.5 mm. She reported 1 to 2 dB greater high-frequency output when using the shorter and wider earhooks.

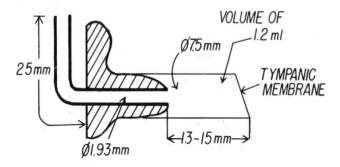

Figure 2–1 Schematic drawing of an earmold coupled to the earcanal.

Some earhooks are delivered with dampers, and others allow the audiologist to add or change the damper. Some earhooks are threaded, and others are of the snap-on type. ANSI S3.37–1987 (ANSI, 1987b) specifies a preferred earhook nozzle thread (5-40 UNC-2A; modified and unmodified) to reduce the number of different earhook styles currently stocked by audiologists in their clinics for replacing damaged earhooks.

Tubing Resonances

As stated earlier, one of the goals for providing a successful fitting is delivering a smooth and gently rising frequency response to the eardrum of the listener. Unfortunately, many hearing aids (particularly, BTE) provide a frequency response that is characterized by numerous sharp resonant peaks that can hamper a successful hearing aid fitting.

As mentioned earlier, the typical length of the transmission line from the receiver to the tip of the earmold is approximately 75 mm, with an ID ranging from 1.0 to 1.93 mm. In a tube open at both ends, a length of 75 mm and a diameter of 1.93 mm will produce one-half wave resonances at approximately 2300, 4600, and 6900 Hz (Cox, 1979). Half-wave resonances will occur at frequencies that are two times the effective wavelength of the tubing. In a hearing aid fitting the tube is closed at the receiver end with relatively low acoustic impedance in the earcanal and eardrum. The presence of the closed tube and the impedance mismatch will create a one-fourth wave resonance where the wavelength of the incoming signal is four times the effective length of the tube. Additional resonances will occur at odd-number intervals of this fundamental frequency. Thus for a 75 mm effective length tube closed at both ends, a one-fourth wave resonance will produce resonances between 1000 to 10,000 Hz at approximately 1100, 3300, and 5500 Hz (Walker, 1979). Figure 2–2 (Valente, 1984c) illustrates the presence of these resonances for a BTE hearing aid when damping was not placed in the earhook (solid line).

Damping
Fused Mesh Dampers

To reduce the sharp resonant peaks in the frequency response to achieve a smooth and gently rising frequency response, several types of damping materials have been introduced in the past. The use of damping allows the user to increase the volume control setting with less probability of feedback and, thus, achieve greater usable gain and output. In addition, the reduction of gain at 1000 Hz will reportedly reduce the upward spread of masking and improve word recognition in noise.

These peaks are undesirable because they reportedly degrade sound quality, introduce transients, and allow the output to exceed the listener's loudness discomfort level. Knowles Electronics introduced fused mesh dampers to reduce the gain and output to acceptable levels and smooth the frequency response (Gastmeirer, 1981; Killion, 1982, 1988a). The fused mesh damper is a finely woven plastic screen held in place by a stainless steel screen and encased in a 2.5 mm long and 2.0 mm wide metal ferrule. The fused mesh damper provides a pure acoustic resistance and negligible reactance and, therefore, does not attenuate the high-frequency region of

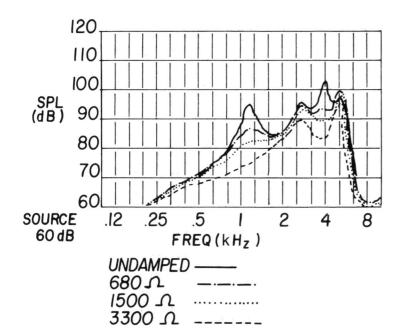

UNDAMPED ——
680 Ω ― · ― · ― ·
1500 Ω ·············
3300 Ω ― ― ― ― ― ―

Figure 2–2 Frequency responses of a hearing aid with an undamped and damped earhook. For the damped conditions, a 680, 1500, and 3300 ohm fused mesh damper was placed at the earhook.

the frequency response; this was one of the problems with previous materials used for damping. They were originally designed to fit snugly inside No. 13 tubing, which has an ID of 1.93 mm. These dampers are available in five discrete resistances of 680, 1500, 2200, 3300, and 4700 Ω, which are color-coded as white, green, red, orange, and yellow, respectively. These dampers allow greater high-frequency output and a smoother frequency response. Figure 2–2 (Valente, 1984c) illustrates the smoothing of the frequency response and increased low-frequency attenuation by adding 680, 1500, or 3300 Ω dampers to the earhook. From Figure 2–2 it can also be seen that the 3300 Ω damper decreased output at 4000 Hz, which may be considered undesirable.

Currently, inserting the damper at the tip of the earhook is the most common position. Inserting the damper further along the transmission line will increase its ability to dampen the peaks, but will increase the probability of the damper becoming clogged with moisture or debris.

The effectiveness of dampers is determined by the density (i.e., resistance in acoustic ohms) of the material and the number and location of the damper(s). Killion (1988a) reported using two fused mesh dampers (one at the tip of the earhook and another at the threaded end) to reduce the gain and output by approximately 15 dB and provide a smoother frequency response. As a cautionary note, if resonances do not appear when electroacoustically analyzing a BTE hearing aid, the manufacturer has probably provided damping; inserting additional dampers will further reduce the gain and output of the hearing aid.

Briskey (1982) reported that a 680 Ω damper reduces average full-on gain and SSPL90 by 3 dB, whereas the remaining four dampers reduce the gain and output by 4-, 5-, 6-, and 9-dB, respectively.

Libby (1979) and Teder (1979) reported that by reducing the peak in the frequency response, the audiologist can increase the "headroom" (i.e., output) of the aid and expand the range of linear amplification. Furthermore, Teder (1979) reported that a peak in the SSPL curve can cause a "volume expansion effect" when high-intensity sounds occur at the peak frequency (i.e., dishes clattering, automobile horns, and typewriters). These sounds are then limited by the output but are higher in intensity than the remainder of the output curve, which is relatively flat.

One of the disadvantages of using dampers, as reported by Chasin (1983a), is that dampers can easily become plugged with moisture or debris. Thus dampers usually need to be changed often and the patient must be counseled regarding this problem and informed of the steps necessary to follow when the aid does not appear to be functioning properly.

PEARL

If a patient reports that a BTE hearing aid is "dead," remove the earhook (after first checking the battery). If the hearing aid begins to produce feedback, the damper in the earhook was clogged. Replace the earhook and damper, and the hearing aid should return to "normal" function.

Other Damping Materials

1. LAMB'S WOOL: This is the earliest damping material. It is usually placed in the earhook or tubing and is typically used on a trial-and-error basis. It is an effective and inexpensive method of damping, but the effect can be very unpredictable.

2. SINTERED STEEL PELLETS: These are small cylinders of stainless steel, welded together in such a manner that their specified resistance in acoustic ohms offers specific amounts of attenuation (Goldstein, 1980; Mynders, 1985). In our clinic we use sintered filters, which are available in different colors

and provide a progressively greater degree of attenuation at 1000 Hz (orange = 3 dB; green = 6 dB; brown = 9 dB; yellow = 12 dB; gray = 15 dB; red = 18 dB). The greatest attenuation occurs at 500 to 1000 Hz, and, as the sintered filter is placed further down the transmission line, it provides even greater attenuation.

3. STAR DAMPER: This is a flexible silicone material that is usually placed in the earhook and does not permit moisture buildup because its design allows drainage of moisture. This damper provides some gain at 2700 Hz to compensate for the loss of the earcanal resonance. The star damper must be cut to different lengths and electroacoustic measures made to ensure that the desired effect has been achieved.

4. DAMPERS IN CUSTOM HEARING AIDS: A variety of dampers are now available in custom hearing aids, which reduce the peak around 2000 Hz. These include, from one manufacturer, a white damper that reduces the output by 3- to 5-dB, a green damper that reduces the output by 7- to 8-dB, and a red damper that reduces the output by 10 dB.

Dampers: Effect on Speech Intelligibility and Clarity

As mentioned earlier, research has suggested that improved speech intelligibility, greater clarity of speech, and increased user satisfaction will result when using dampers (Cox & Gilmore, 1986; van Buuren et al, 1996). However, Decker (1975) reported no significant differences in word recognition scores (W-22) for 10 subjects who listened to the monosyllabic words using broadband and high-frequency emphasis hearing aids with and without the insertion of sintered filters.

Cox and Gilmore (1986) reported that damping could improve speech intelligibility or sound quality by reducing the effects of the upward spread of masking. Suppression of the peaks by damping should reduce these effects and improve the overall fidelity of amplification. They used 10 subjects with sensorineural hearing loss, who evaluated 1½ minutes of male-connected discourse embedded in multi-talker babble presented at 55- and 70-dB Leq using a paired comparison paradigm. In general, they reported that damping the frequency response did not provide improved clarity of speech or a more advantageous preferred listening level. However, they reported that reducing resonant peaks by damping could be useful in reducing feedback.

Special Purpose Earhooks

Killion et al (1984), Killion and Wilson (1985), and Killion (1988c) introduced four special oversized earhooks using open canal fittings or closed earmolds to provide solutions for four hard-to-fit hearing losses (see Fig. 2–3). However, to be useful these earhooks must be coupled to hearing aids using treaded earhooks. These special earhooks include the following:

1. *ER 12-1 (low-pass or K-bass):* Designed for patients with normal-hearing at 2000 to 3000 Hz and hearing loss up to 40- to 65-dB at 250 to 1000 Hz. In the high-frequency region the patient should have hearing thresholds of 0- to 25-dB at 4000 Hz and 0- to 60-dB at 8000 Hz (Killion & Wilson, 1985; Killion et al, 1984). This earhook can be coupled to the earcanal using Lybarger's 1.5 LP open canal reverse horn tube fitting (Lybarger, 1980), which is comprised of No. 15 tubing coupled to 12 mm of No. 20 tubing having an ID of 0.86 mm and extending into the earcanal by at least 16 mm. An alternative tube fitting (Janssen free field) is No. 13 tubing and an 18 mm insert of No. 18 tubing. These tube fittings reduce the gain in the mid-frequency region by 10- to 15-dB and shift the first resonant peak at 1000 Hz downward to 5000 Hz. The ER 12-1 is identified with a silver band with one red stripe at one end that screws onto the hearing aid and has a clear disk in the middle of the earhook (left earhook in Fig. 2–3). The ER 12-1 should be used with power aids having adequate low-frequency gain and a maximum SSPL90 of 130 dB. Killion and Wilson (1985) reported a 76% acceptance rate in 68 fittings.

2. *ER 12-2 (2 kHz notch filter):* This is identified by a silver band with two red stripes and has no clear center disk

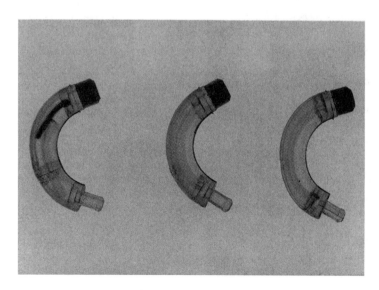

Figure 2–3 Etymotic earhooks. *Left:* ER 12-1; *middle:* ER 12-2; *right:* ER 12-3.

(middle earhook in Fig. 2–3) (Killion & Wilson, 1985). This earhook is used with a conventional earmold and is used for patients with normal or near-normal-hearing at 2000 Hz (10- to 40-dB HL) with hearing loss up to 40- to 60-dB at 500 to 1000 Hz and 3000 to 4000 Hz. The ER 12-2 reduces the gain by 20 dB at 2000 Hz. It produces an acoustic signal that is very similar to the Macrae 2k notch-filter earmold (Macrae, 1981, 1983), which will be discussed in a later section.

3. *ER 12-3 (high pass):* Can be identified with gold band having three red stripes and a small barb at the end (right earhook in Fig. 2–3) (Killion & Wilson, 1985). This earhook is designed to be used with Lybarger's nonoccluding dual diameter earmold (see Fig. 2–4), which uses tubing with an ID of 0.8 mm coupled to 15 mm of No. 13 tubing that should be inserted minimally to obtain maximum high-frequency gain before feedback (i.e., insertion of only 4 to 8 mm). This configuration changes a wideband aid hearing aid into a high-pass aid with reduced output below 3000 Hz to eliminate excessive gain in the frequency region where the patient may have normal-hearing. This combination also provides 12 dB of additional gain at 4000 to 7000 Hz. The ER 12-3 is designed for patients who have hearing thresholds of 25- to 35-dB HL at 500 to 2000 Hz and 50- to 90-dB HL at 4000 to 8000 Hz.

4. *ER 12-4 (cookie bite):* Is the opposite of the ER 12-2 and is designed to be used with patients with reduced hearing at 2000 Hz and better hearing in the frequency regions above and below 2000 Hz. This earhook is used with an open earmold with 1/32-inch tubing coupled to a Lybarger high-pass eartube. It has a silver band on one end that screws onto the hearing aid and has no disk in the center of the earhook.

Finally, Bergenstoff (1983) introduced the "E-Hook" in which a wedge-shaped filter is placed in the earhook. Also, an acoustic resistance element is permanently mounted inside the tubing end of the earhook. Using No. 13 tubing from the end of the earhook to the tip of the earmold, a very smooth real-ear insertion response (REIR) can be obtained when coupled to a hearing aid having a wideband receiver.

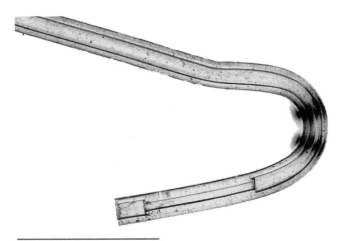

Figure 2–4 Example of a Lybarger high-pass eartube.

TABLE 2–1 Inside diameter (ID) and outside diameter (OD) of tubing sizes as standardized by the national association of earmold labs (NAEL)

Tubing No.	ID		OD	
	Inches	mm	Inches	mm
9	0.094	2.4	0.160	4.1
12	0.085	2.2	0.125	3.2
13 standard	0.076	1.9	0.116	2.9
13 medium	0.076	1.9	0.122	3.2
13 thick wall	0.076	1.9	0.130	3.3
13 double wall	0.076	1.9	0.142	3.6
14	0.066	1.7	0.116	2.9
15	0.059	1.5	0.166	2.9
16 standard	0.053	1.3	0.166	2.9
16 thin	0.053	1.3	0.085	2.2

Tubing
NAEL Sizes

Table 2–1 reports the numerical system used by the National Association of Earmold Laboratories (NAEL) to identify the various tubing sizes. As can be seen, as the number increases, the ID decreases. For example, No. 9 tubing has an ID of 2.4 mm, whereas No. 13 tubing has an ID of 1.93 mm. The outside diameter (OD) can be thin, standard, medium, thick, or double-walled. The thick and double-walled tubing are often used for power BTEs to reduce the probability of feedback and vibration.

Tubing Style

Tubing can be ordered as bulk, preformed, quilled, single-bend, double-bend, or triple-bend. Tubing can also be ordered as clear or tinted or with a cut-tapered end for easier insertion into the earmold sound bore. Tubing is also available as a "dri-tube." This type of tubing is made from a denser and more rubbery material that is reported to eliminate or reduce condensation and is available in the 3 or 4 mm horn, No. 13 medium, and thick walled.

Tubing Adapters

Several variations of adapters are available to connect to tubing. For example, male and female adapters (large and miniature sizes) are available to be used with receiver-type earmolds. These fit onto the tubing to allow direct snap-in connectors to the receiver earmold. In addition, elbows made of hard vinyl with gradual or sharp right angle bends can be ordered that are threaded or cemented into a hole in a Lucite earmold for easier changing of tubing. Another possibility of a tubing adapter is the Bakke horn, which is a hard plastic, stepped-bore permanent elbow that creates an acoustic effect similar to the Libby 4 mm horn, which will be discussed in a later section.

Tubing Cement

Generally, cementing tubing into the bore of an earmold is a relatively simple task when using hard Lucite earmolds. However, for polyvinyl and other soft earmolds, the dispenser should use "sheer" tubing cement. Another solution is to use "tube-lock," "tube-lock plus," and "tubing retention systems" that have recently been introduced. These use a small 14-carat gold-coated brass ring containing a small flange. It is assembled and permanently affixed by the earmold laboratory. With this system, the tubing can never be loosened or pulled out. It is available in two sizes (regular and double walled) and requires a special tool for insertion and removal of tube-lock. The tube-lock can be used with any size tubing and is highly recommended for materials where glue will not easily adhere. More recently, several earmold manufacturers introduced a special tube lock ("EZ Tube") for the JB 1000 and other soft earmolds designed for patients with severe-to-profound hearing loss. This is a permanently installed nozzle in the sound bore of the earmold and the audiologist can remove the old tubing from the nozzle and replace it with new tubing. Another possibility is ordering continuous flow adaptor (CFA) earmolds, which will be explained in greater detail in a later section.

> **PITFALL**
>
> **Never use Super-Glue to glue tubing into the sound bore of an earmold. The use of this product makes it very difficult to replace tubing.**

Tubing Length

Recall that ANSI S3.22–1987 (ANSI, 1987a) required BTE hearing aids to be electroacoustically analyzed using 25 mm of No. 13 tubing coupled to an HA-2 coupler. In reality, changing tubing length is limited because tubing length is related to anatomical dimensions of the head. However, as Figure 2–5 (Valente, 1984c) illustrates, if the length is increased (re: 25 mm), the primary resonant peak will shift downward and the output will increase in the lower frequencies and decrease in the mid and high frequencies. Also, the amplitude of the second and third peaks will be reduced (Egolf, 1980; Lybarger, 1985; Valente, 1984c). If the tubing is shortened (re: 25 mm), the primary and secondary peaks will shift upward in frequency. Also, the output will decrease in the low frequencies and increase in the mid and high frequencies. Table 2–2, Section I, summarizes the effect changing tubing length may have on four regions of the frequency-response curve.

Tubing Diameter

ANSI S3.22–1987 (ANSI, 1987a) also required BTE hearing aids to be electroacoustically analyzed using 25 mm of No. 13 tubing, which has an ID of 1.93 mm. Using tubing with a wider ID (No. 9, No. 11, or No. 12 tubing) will increase the gain between 1000 and 2000 Hz and decrease the gain in the lower frequencies. Using tubing with a narrower ID (No. 14 to No. 16 tubing) will increase the gain in the lower frequencies and decrease the gain in the higher frequencies (Austin et al, 1990c; Lybarger, 1979, 1980, 1985). Table 2–2, Section II, summarizes the effect changing tubing diameter may have on four regions of the frequency-response curve.

Tubing Length and Diameter

Changes in length and diameter are consistent when either length or diameter is varied independently. That is, a

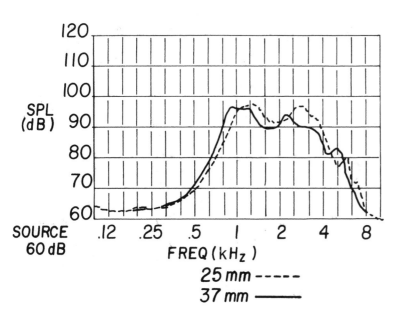

Figure 2–5 Frequency response of a hearing aid coupled to an HA-2 coupler with 25 mm and 37 mm of #13 tubing.

TABLE 2–2   Effect of various modifications upon four regions of the frequency response

Change	Frequency Region (Hz)			
	<750	750–1500	1500–3000	>3000
I. Tubing length				
Short	Slight decrease	Moves peak to higher Hz	Moves peak to higher Hz	Minimal
Long	Slight increase	Moves peak to lower Hz	Moves peak to lower Hz	Decrease
II. Tubing diameter				
Wider	Minimal	Moves peak to higher Hz	Moves peak to higher Hz	Increase
Narrower	May decrease	Moves peak to lower Hz	Reduces height of peak and moves to lower Hz	Decrease
III. Bore length				
Short	Slight decrease	Moves peak to higher Hz	Moves peak to higher Hz	Increase
Long	Slight increase	Moves peak to lower Hz	Moves peak to lower Hz	Decrease
IV. Bore diameter				
Wider	Minimal	Moves peak to higher Hz	Moves peak to higher Hz	Increase
Narrower	Minimal	Moves peak to lower Hz	Moves peak to lower Hz	Decrease
Belling	Minimal	Minimal	Minimal	Increase
V. Tubing insertion				
Medial	Minimal	Minimal	Shift peak to lower Hz	Decrease
Lateral	Minimal	Minimal	Shift peak to higher Hz	Increase
VI. Venting				
Small[1]	Minimal	Minimal	Minimal	Minimal
Medium[2]	Decrease	Increase peak height	Minimal	Minimal
Large[3]	Decrease	Increase peak height	Minimal	Minimal
Parallel	Less attenuation of low-frequency SPL than diagonal venting, but no attenuation of high-frequency SPL			
Diagonal	Greater attenuation of low-frequency SPL than parallel venting, but greater attenuation of high-frequency SPL			

[1]0.8 mm
[2]1.6 mm
[3]2.4 mm
 Adapted from Microsonic, 1994

long tube with a narrow ID will shift the frequency peaks downward. Using a short tube with a wider ID will shift the frequency peaks upward.

Minimal Insertion of Tubing

Up to this point, the discussion has assumed that the audiologist has inserted the tubing to the tip of the earmold. Another strategy is to insert the tubing minimally into the sound bore and create a "dual tube" fitting (Lybarger, 1979, 1985; Valente, 1984b,c). This strategy takes advantage of the fact that when a significant step-up in diameter exists toward the earcanal, a quarter wave open-end resonance in the larger bore section exits into the earcanal. This can result in considerable high-frequency amplification above 2000 Hz.

An example of such a strategy would be inserting No. 13 tubing only 3 mm into the sound bore. Figure 2–6 (Valente, 1984b,c) illustrates 2-cc coupler measures of a BTE hearing aid when No. 13 tubing was inserted 3 mm, 9 mm, and 16 mm (tip) into the sound bore. Notice the improved high-frequency output when the tubing was inserted only 3 mm (solid line) into the sound bore compared with when the tubing was inserted to the tip (dashed line). In this case, 10- to 12-dB greater output at 5000 to 6000 Hz exists than when the tubing was cemented to the tip. Table 2–2, Section V, summarizes the effects insertion of tubing in the sound bore has on four regions of the frequency response curve.

SPECIAL CONSIDERATION

When using the strategy of minimal insertion of tubing into the sound bore, it is very important that a high-quality cement be used to anchor the tubing into the sound bore.

Figure 2–7 (Valente, 1984b, 1984c) reveals that the effect of minimal insertion of the tubing is directly related to the length of the sound bore. That is, as the bore length increases,

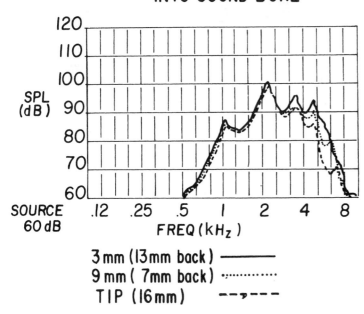

DEPTH OF INSERTION OF TUBING INTO SOUND BORE

3 mm (13 mm back) ———
9 mm (7 mm back) ··············
TIP (16 mm) ‒ ‒ ? ‒ ‒ ‒

Figure 2–6 Change in output when inserting #13 tubing 3 mm, 9 mm, and to the tip of an earmold when the bore length is 16 mm.

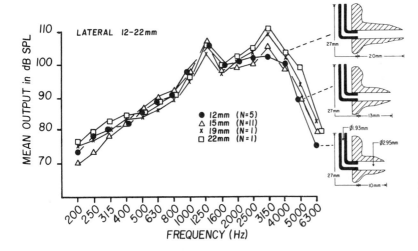

Figure 2–7 Change in output when inserting #13 tubing 2 mm into the sound bore for four earmolds in which bore length is 12 mm, 15 mm, 19 mm, and 22 mm long.

the effect of minimal insertion becomes greater. As bore length is reduced, the advantage of this strategy is diminished. Finally, the magnitude of the effect depends on the length and diameter of the second segment. The longer and wider the second segment, the greater the high-frequency boost (Valente, 1984b, 1984c).

Open Canal Fittings

Tube Fitting

One method of tube fitting is to use a free field mold that is adjusted in varying lengths to create the desired change in the

---

PEARL

If the goal of the hearing aid fitting is to achieve as much high-frequency gain as possible, do not order earmolds with No. 13 tubing cemented to the tip. Instead, order a earmold with a "horn" design or tubing only slightly inserted into the sound bore.

---

frequency response and then cemented in place to a non-occluding earmold (see Fig. 2–8 middle, and Fig. 2–9D). When

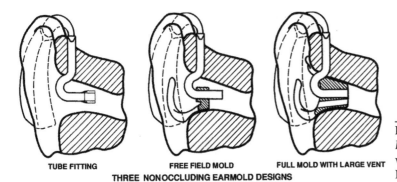

TUBE FITTING   FREE FIELD MOLD   FULL MOLD WITH LARGE VENT

THREE NONOCCLUDING EARMOLD DESIGNS

Figure 2–8 Three nonoccluding earmold designs. *Left*: tube fitting; *middle*: free field; *right*: full mold with a large vent. (Printed with permission from Microsonic, Inc.)

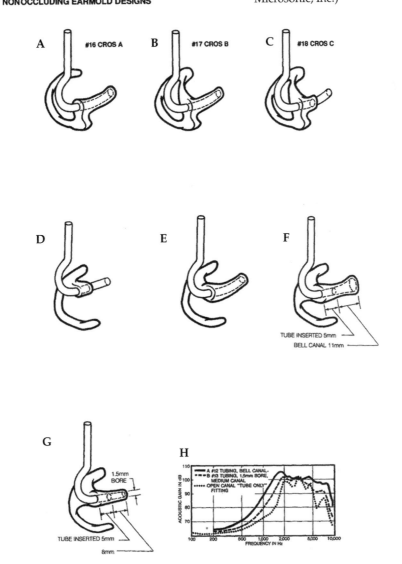

Figure 2–9 Examples of seven nonoccluding earmolds: **(A)** CROS A; **(B)** CROS B; **(C)** CROS C; **(D)** free field; **(E)** Janssen; **(F)** extended range earmold; **(G)** another extended range earmold; and **(H)** frequency response of three nonoccluding earmolds. (Printed with permission from Microsonic, Inc.)

used with a conventional BTE, this would be classified as an (ipsilateral routing of the signal) IROS fitting. Another method is using a tube fitting (Fig. 2–8, *left*) in which the tubing is not cemented (Staab & Nunley, 1982). The rationale is to achieve

maximum high-frequency gain without feedback, obtain maximum low-frequency attenuation (up to 30 dB at 500 Hz), and provide maximum comfort. This type of tube fitting will not occlude the earcanal, which can reduce the transmission of low-frequency sounds by as much as 15- to 30-dB, depending on the magnitude of occlusion by the earmold. This type of tube fitting also takes advantage of the natural resonance of the earcanal, which is around 17 dB at 2800 Hz. For some patients, greater retention of a nonoccluding earmold may be necessary. A design offering the benefits of a nonoccluding earmold, but with greater retention, is illustrated in Figure 2–9C.

Tube fittings should be considered when the patient has a ski-slope audiometric configuration with hearing loss up to 50 dB above 2000 Hz. If the hearing loss is greater than 50 dB, the audiologist should not consider using a tube fitting but, instead, use a conventional earmold with some degree of venting because of acoustic feedback. Also, tube fittings can theoretically eliminate the upward spread of masking by reducing low-frequency amplification and, thus, improve word recognition. Other advantages of this type of fitting may include reduction of harmonic distortion caused by minimal gain below 1000 Hz and providing improved sound quality.

A tube fitting may be considered when an earmold is contraindicated because of middle ear drainage, irritations in the earcanal, allergic reactions to earmold materials, psoriasis, eczema, and scars. It should not be used with a high-frequency emphasis hearing aid but, instead, should be used with a broadband hearing aid. Furthermore, for tube fittings to provide adequate high-frequency gain, insertion of the tubing must be greater than 15 mm beyond the orifice of the earcanal. As the tubing is moved closer to the eardrum, the frequency response below 1500 Hz is shifted downward, producing a broader response. As the tubing is placed further away from the eardrum, low-frequency attenuation is greater. Also, its use in smaller earcanals will produce greater high-frequency gain than in longer canals, with tubing length held constant.

To properly fit tube fittings, it is suggested that the audiologist first use No. 15 tubing (ID, 1.5 mm) and then try tubing with a wider ID (No. 9) to achieve even greater high-frequency emphasis. To achieve maximum comfort, it is necessary to properly bend the tubing to comfortably fit in the earcanal. To do this, it is suggested that isopropyl alcohol be wiped over solid core solder wire whose OD is sufficiently wide enough to fit snugly inside the tubing. The audiologist should then bend the tubing to the desired configuration and add heat by means of an air blower with a heat-directing shield. Cool the tubing in alcohol or water to preserve the configuration and then remove the solder. At this point the tubing will maintain its shape.

Traditional CROS Open Mold

Harford and Barry (1965), Harford and Dodds (1966), Green and Ross (1968), and Green (1969) introduced the contralateral routing of the signal (CROS) (see Figs. 2–9A–2–9C) earmold for unilateral and high-frequency hearing loss. They reported that the CROS mold can improve aided word recognition scores in noise caused by significant low-frequency reduction. Courtois et al (1988) advocated use of CROS molds for patients with mild-to-moderate hearing loss to attenuate low frequencies, thereby reducing both the amplification of ambient noise and the occlusion effect. They measured the sound pressure level (SPL) in closed and open molds and found differences of 30- to 40-dB below 125 Hz, and these differences disappeared at round 2000 Hz. They also report that a

2 mm vent reduces the occlusion effect at 250 to 500 Hz and a 3 mm vent reduces the occlusion effect to 750 Hz.

The CROS mold is similar to a parallel-vented earmold, which has a vent so large that only a small piece of earmold is left to hold the tubing in place (Cox, 1979). Cox (1979) and Lybarger (1979) reported that the acoustic difference between a CROS mold and a tube fit is minimal, providing the earcanal is not so small as to be occluded by the small retention portion of the open mold fitting. If retention does occlude the earcanal, a tube fitting is preferred to obtain the desired acoustic effect. The tube fitting will significantly reduce low-frequency amplification and provide some high-frequency emphasis above the vent-associated resonance. This effect depends on the depth of insertion, the ID of the tubing, and the size of the earcanal. Because insertion depth is closer to the eardrum, less low-frequency energy will escape but, more importantly, greater high-frequency amplification will occur. As tubing diameter is reduced, an overall reduction in output and a shift of the first peak to a lower frequency will occur. If no gain is required below 2000 Hz, the audiologist should use tubing with a narrower ID for greater user satisfaction. However, this strategy will reduce the overall SPL and provide less high-frequency gain. Low-frequency attenuation will be less for a tube fit when fitted to a small earcanal than if the earcanal is of average length.

PEARL

CROS amplification is most effective if the better (aided) ear has a mild-to-moderate high-frequency hearing loss. If the hearing thresholds in the better (aided) ear are within normal limits, the prognosis for success with CROS amplification will be greatly diminished. For these patients, a transcranial CROS should be considered as an option (Valente et al, 1995).

CONTROVERSIAL POINT

Should a hearing aid ever be placed in a "dead" ear? Valente et al (1995) demonstrated that in half of their subjects, a transcranial CROS was viewed by the subjects as providing significant benefit. The authors believe that success with transcranial CROS fittings can occur if (a) the patient has reduced transcranial thresholds, (b) the patient is fitted with a power BTE, and (c) the earmold must be tight fitting and have a long bore and pressure vent. Less success will likely be achieved if the fitting is attempted with a power ITE or CIC.

Libby 3 mm and 4 mm Horns

Libby designed injection-molding techniques to obtain a one-piece 3 mm and 4 mm tapered horn (see Fig. 2–10). The 4 mm design is comprised of 21 mm of No. 13 tubing,

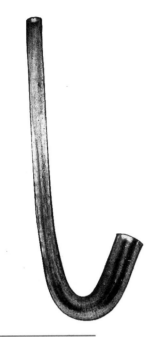

Figure 2–10 Example of a Libby 4 mm horn.

enlarged to 22 mm of tubing 4 mm wide. The 3 mm horn has 21 mm of No. 13 tubing followed by 22 mm of tubing 3 mm wide. The 3 mm horn will provide 5- to 6-dB less gain at 2500

to 3000 Hz compared with the 4 mm horn. Both styles are designed to work best with a 1500 Ω fused mesh damper at the tip of the earhook. Libby advocated that the stepped diameter earmold should be used with a hearing aid having a wide band receiver to obtain high-fidelity sound quality, an extended frequency response, and reduced battery drain. The first two rows in sections A and B in Table 2–3 report the relative changes in the output of a hearing aid produced by the Libby 3 mm and 4 mm designs relative to the output measured in an HA-1 (section A) or HA-2 coupler (section B).

Valente (1983) reported 0.9- to 8.4-dB greater mean functional gain (Fig. 2–11) with an earmold design similar to the Libby 3 mm horn compared with when No. 13 tubing was inserted to the earmold tip. For the same subjects with sensorineural hearing loss, the mean word recognition scores (NU-6) were 8.3% better in quiet and 12.1% better in noise (multitalker babble at a +6dB signal/noise ratio) with the Libby 3 mm horn (Fig. 2–12).

Usually, the Libby 3 mm or 4 mm horn is ordered without a vent. However, Pedersen (1984) reported that a 2 mm diagonal vent intersecting near the end of the earmold did not affect the high-frequency gain provided by the 3 mm or 4 mm horn. The mean difference was less than 1 dB at 6 discrete frequencies between 250 and 4000 Hz. To reduce the likelihood of inducing the occlusion effect, the authors suggest that 3 mm and 4 mm horns be ordered with some degree of venting. We routinely order Select-A-Vent (SAV) or Positive-Venting-Valve (PVV) vent "trees" for all horn fittings. The advantage of this strategy will be presented in a later section.

TABLE 2–3 Changes in gain/output (dB) for several acoustically tuned earmolds relative to the response obtained using an HA-2 coupler or No. 13 tubing to the tip of the earmold measured in an HA-1 coupler

Design	250	500	1000	2000	3000	4000	6000
Earmold Design							
A. Re: #13 Tubing to the Tip (HA-1 Coupler)							
Libby 4 mm	−1	−2	−3	−2	−6	10	6
Libby 3 mm	−1	−2	−2	0	6	8	2
8CR1	−2	−2	−3	0	7	7	2
6R12	−1	−2	−1	−2	1	5	7
6B10	−2	−2	−2	−2	1	7	0
6B5	0	0	2	1	2	4	3
6B0	0	0	0	0	0	0	0
6C5	0	1	0	0	−4	−6	−11
6C10	0	2	−2	−5	−10	−12	−17
B: Re: 3 mm × 18 mm (HA-2 Coupler)							
Libby 4 mm	−1	−1	−2	0	2	3	0
Libby 3 mm	0	0	0	1	3	2	−4
8CR1	−1	−1	−2	0	4	0	−6
6R12	0	0	0	0	0	0	1
6B10	0	0	0	0	0	1	−5
6B5	1	2	3	2	0	−1	−2
6B0	0	1	1	0	−2	−5	−7
6C5	1	2	1	2	−5	−10	−16
6C10	1	3	0	−3	−11	−17	−22

[1]680 ohm damper at earhook tip: dimensions of Libby 4 mm
Dillion, 1985, 1991.

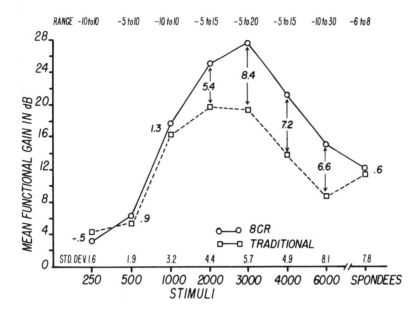

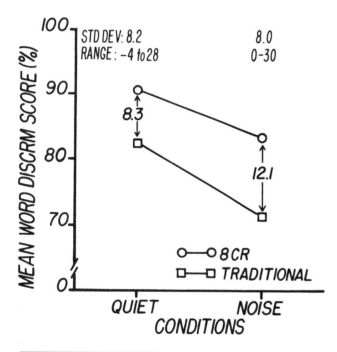

Figure 2–11 Mean functional gain for warble tones and spondee words utilizing conventional and 8CR earmolds. Also provided is the mean difference in warble tone thresholds between the two earmold designs, standard deviation, and range.

Figure 2–12 Mean word recognition in quiet and noise utilizing conventional and 8CR earmolds. Also provided is the mean difference in word recognition scores between the two earmold designs, standard deviation, and range.

Burgess and Brooks (1991) reported that the sound quality from a hearing aid with the Libby horn was rated clearer, more natural, undistorted, and more acoustically comfortable when compared with an earmold where the tubing was cemented to the tip of the earmold. Objectively, real-ear and functional gain measures reported greater gain (mean of 8 dB) in the higher frequencies (1500 to 6000 Hz). They also reported improved recognition of phonemes, especially the fricatives and affricates.

Mueller et al (1981) compared the Libby 3 mm horn with a free field mold for 24 subjects with high-frequency sensorineural hearing loss. Functional gain measures revealed 5- to 10-dB greater functional gain at 3000 Hz with the Libby horn compared with the free field earmold. However, significant differences were found in word recognition scores or subjective ratings between the two earmold designs.

Robinson et al (1989) compared the performance of 21 inexperienced users with the Libby 4 mm horn and an earmold where No. 13 tubing were cemented to the tip of the earmold. Aided scores for speech in noise (+5 dB SNR) using CVC words were, on average, only 2.4% better with the Libby 4 mm horn. However, two thirds of the subjects preferred the sound quality of the 4 mm horn. After a 4-week trial period, the 4 mm horn was preferred by those subjects who had poorer hearing above 2000 Hz. They concluded that improved word recognition could be achieved with a hearing aid providing a smooth rising frequency response in which the response extended the higher frequencies.

Bergenstoff (1983) reported that the real-ear gain above 2000 Hz for a hearing aid coupled to an earmold in which No. 13 tubing is inserted to the tip was as much as 20 dB lower than the gain reported in a 2-cc coupler whose dimensions are 18 mm long and 3 mm wide. When using a 4 mm horn coupled to a hearing aid having a narrow frequency range, the frequency response was extended by almost an octave, the gain was increased by 10- to 15-dB, and the mid-frequency resonant peak was reduced by 4 dB. When the same earmold was coupled to a hearing aid providing a wide-band response, the 4 mm horn extended the frequency response by almost two octaves, increased high-frequency gain by 20 dB, and reduced the mid-frequency resonant peak by 8 dB.

Sung and Sung (1982) compared the performance of the Libby 3 mm and 4 mm horns to a conventional earmold with No. 13 tubing to the tip on 28 subjects with sensorineural hearing loss. Word recognition scores (NU-6 and high-frequency word lists) presented in quiet at 70 dB SPL and noise (SNR of +6 dB) were improved only 0.9 to 4.9%. Functional gain increased by 0.5 dB at 1500 Hz to 6.4 dB at 4000

Hz. For some subjects, the improvement was as large as 15 dB. In addition, 54% of the subjects expressed a preference for the Libby designs.

Fernandes and Cooper (1983) reported on the successful use of an undamped Libby 4 mm horn in nine subjects with severe hearing loss compared with their performance with the same hearing aid coupled to No. 13 tubing to the earmold tip. They reported minimal differences in functional gain below 2000 Hz, but 15 dB greater functional gain at 3150 Hz when using the 4 mm horn. No significant differences were found in speech reception threshold (SRT), most comfortable level (MCL), or loudness discomfort level (LDL). However, an overwhelming preference existed for the 4 mm horn because it reportedly provided better sound quality and clarity.

Lyregaard (1982) reported that the effectiveness of the horn is not diminished significantly if small variations are present in the dimensions of the horn or if different hearing aids with different receivers are used. He reported that the horn effect can improve the high-frequency response by 10 dB. Finally, some audiologists might question the feasibility of the average earcanal being wide enough to accommodate an earmold requiring a 4 mm bore and venting. He concluded that an earmold requiring an ID of 4 mm is feasible for most adult subjects. Clearly, this may be a viable concern when providing services to a pediatric population.

PEARL

If a patient has hearing thresholds no greater than 75- to 80-dB at 2000 to 4000 Hz, use of a 3 or 4 mm Libby horn is essential. It is not in the best interest of the patient to use No. 13 tubing. If the hearing loss is greater than 80 dB, a reversed horn is recommended to reduce the chance of feedback. If feedback occurs, the patient is forced to turn down the volume control wheel that will reduce the gain in the frequency region where hearing thresholds are better.

Bakke Horn

Another method of achieving the acoustic benefits of a 4 mm horn in the transmission line is with a Bakke horn. This is a rigid plastic tube, or horn, which is glued directly into Lucite or soft (Bakke horn-S) earmolds. This horn is designed so that the ID is 2 mm at the tubing end and 3 mm at the earmold end. the Bakke horn is then followed by 4 mm wide and 11 mm long sound bore. These are the same dimensions as the Libby 4 mm horn. However, a major difference exists between the Libby and Bakke horns. With the Bakke horn, it is very efficient and inexpensive to change the tubing from the earhook to the Bakke horn. However, with the Libby horn it is necessary to replace the entire 4 mm tubing. This can be more expensive because the cost for a 3 mm or 4 mm horn is significantly greater than the cost of No. 13 tubing. Finally, when used with a conventional hearing aid, the Bakke horn extends the frequency response by almost one octave and

provides 10- to 15-dB greater high-frequency gain. When used with a wide-band hearing aid, it extends the frequency response by almost two octaves and increases the high-frequency gain by 20 dB.

Reversed Horn

Libby (1990) designed injection molding techniques to obtain a one-piece reverse tapered horn (i.e., the diameter of the tube at the tip is narrower than the diameter of the tube at the earhook) for patients with severe-to-profound hearing loss to reduce the likelihood of feedback for BTE fittings caused by the peaks in the high-frequency region of the frequency response. The reverse horn reduces the gain above 2000 Hz and shifts the energy toward the lower frequencies (8 dB to 10 dB shift in low-frequency gain). This is appropriate for patients who cannot achieve sufficient gain before feedback and must reduce the volume control to eliminate feedback. When feedback is reduced by means of a reversed horn, the subject can achieve sufficient low-frequency gain where their hearing is typically better.

EARMOLDS

Early earmold selection in this country was rather simple. The hearing aid fitter poured plaster of Paris to cast the impression and the completed earmold was fabricated from a black hard rubber material. The only style available was a "regular" earmold and a large button receiver painted in a bright pink and optimistically called "flesh," which was attached to the earmold. An alternative fitting used a flat 2-inch diameter earphone, which covered most of the pinna and was held in place by a 19 mm wide spring steel headband. By World War II, plastic technology grew to include thermosetting acrylic impression materials and methyl methacrylate (Lucite) earmolds.

Today, audiologists have a wide range of material and style options available to them. However, this technology is used in only a quarter of the hearing aid fittings because approximately 75% of hearing aid fittings in the United States incorporate custom hearing aids. This may be unfortunate because when an audiologist sends an impression to a manufacturer, the audiologist has little say in the final configuration of the custom shell. The decision is made by the manufacturer on the basis of accommodation of the circuitry, power supply, and venting. If space is available, the manufacturer can consider patient needs or preferences. In addition, composed with earmolds, shell options are few. Finally, in a large hearing aid manufacturer, a particular shellmaker may never consistently interact with an individual audiologist to get to know the audiologist's needs and impressions.

Earmolds are designed to seal the earcanal, correctly couple the hearing aid to the ear from an acoustical viewpoint, retain the hearing aid on the pinna, be comfortable for an extended period of time, modify the acoustic signal produced by the hearing aid, be able to be easily handled by the patient, and be cosmetically appealing.

Recall that ANSI S3.22–1987 (ANSI, 1987a) specifies the use of a HA-2 2-cc coupler in which the final segment is 18 mm long and 3 mm wide. These dimensions reportedly represent the average length and diameter of an earmold. However, Cox (1979) reported an average length of 14.3 mm for 52 ears. Dalsgaard (1979) reported an average length of 21.9 mm in 100 ears and Valente (1984c) reported an average length of 15.3 mm for 55 ears. Lybarger (1979) and Killion (1981) reported that if earmolds with dimensions of 18 mm by 3 mm were used instead of No. 13 tubing to the tip, they would provide 5- to 7-dB greater high-frequency gain. Table 2–3 reveals

a 2- to 7-dB decrease in output at 3000 to 6000 Hz for the 6BO earmold design (same as No. 13 tubing to the tip of the earmold) compared with an earmold with dimensions of 18 mm by 3 mm. Figure 2–13 (Valente, 1984c) reports the dimensions of a "2-cc earmold," which was manufactured in the clinic by using the appropriate lengths of No. 13 (ID = 1.93 mm) and No. 9 (ID = 3.0 mm) tubing. Figure 2–14 (Valente, 1984c) shows the frequency response of the same BTE hearing aid measured in HA-1 (without the earmold) and HA-2 (with "2-cc earmold") couplers. It can be seen that the two responses are quite similar.

Changing Bore Length

Lybarger (1979, 1985) reported that changing the bore length from minimum to maximum will increase or decrease the overall gain by no more than 2 dB in either direction. However, increasing bore length will increase low-frequency gain and decreasing bore length will increase high-frequency gain. Table 2–2, Section III, summarizes how changing the bore length may affect four regions of the frequency response curve.

Changing Bore Diameter

Lybarger (1979, 1985) reported that the wider the diameter of the bore, the greater the high-frequency emphasis. The narrower the diameter of the bore, the greater the low-frequency emphasis. Table 2–2, Section IV, summarizes how changing the bore diameter may affect four regions of the frequency-response curve.

Changing Length and Diameter

Changes in length and diameter are consistent when either length or diameter is varied independently. That is, a long bore with a narrow ID will shift the frequency response downward. Use of a short bore with a wider ID will shift the frequency response upward.

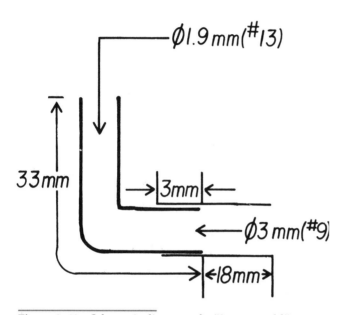

Figure 2–13 Schematic diagram of a "2-cc earmold" stimulating the dimensions of an HA-2 coupler.

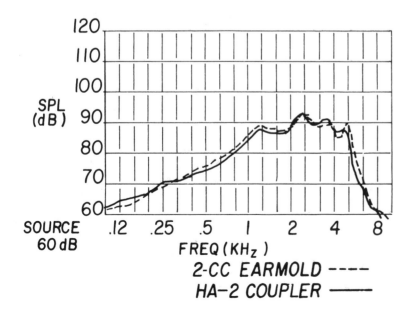

Figure 2–14 Frequency response of a hearing aid measured in HA-2 coupler and the "2-cc earmold" described in Figure 2–13.

Belled Bore

Another method of increasing high-frequency amplification is to drill, or "bell," the last segment of the earmold with a burr to create a wider diameter than at the entrance of the earmold. Cox (1979) and Lybarger (1980) reported that belling the end of the earmold effectively produces a limited horn effect that can increase high-frequency amplification, but its effectiveness depends on the length of the bore. Killion (1980) suggested that a bore length of 17 mm is required for the belling effect to be beneficial. Lybarger (1980) stated a length of 16 to 19 mm is required to obtain maximum benefit when using this strategy. Figure 2–15 (Valente, 1984a) illustrates a belled bore with minimal insertion of tubing and a parallel vent. Figure 2–16 illustrates such an earmold that was prepared for a patient with a gently sloping audiogram. Figure 2–17 (Valente, 1984a) illustrates the performance of a BTE hearing aid measures in a HA-1 2-cc coupler under two conditions. First (*dotted line*), the hearing aid was measured using No. 13 tubing and a 1000 Ω damper at the tip of the earmold. Second, the same hearing aid was measured using a configuration illustrated in Figures 2–15 and 2–16, but with the vent closed with putty. Notice how the belled bore increased high-frequency output and extended the high-frequency response (*dashed line*).

Earmold Impressions

To develop the skills required in taking an acceptable impression of the ear, it is necessary for the audiologist to become familiar with the anatomy of the external ear and have a good knowledge of the vocabulary used to identify key anatomic sites (Fig. 2–18). This is necessary to communicate with the earmold laboratory how the earmold needs to be modified because the earmold/shell is preventing a comfortable and/or appropriate fit. Therefore, it is necessary for the audiologist to become familiar with the terminology used by earmold manufacturers to describe important segments of the earmold in relation to the anatomy of the ear (Fig. 2–19). Recently, Alvord et al (1997) introduced recommendations for the nomenclature that should be used when describing the parts of an earmold. For

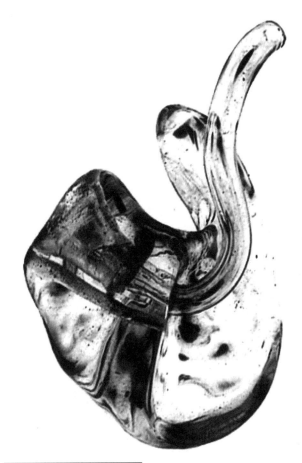

Figure 2–16 Example of an earmold with a belled bore, parallel vent, and minimal insertion of tubing ordered for a patient with a gently sloping audiogram.

example, they suggest using the term *canal stalk* as a replacement for the previous term *canal*. In addition, these authors divide the canal stalk into superior, anterior, inferior, posterior, and medial surfaces. These authors go on to suggest 13 other terms to be used in describing the segments of an earmold.

Examination of the Earcanal

Thoroughly perform an otoscopic observation. For an adult, pull the pinna upward to straighten the earcanal. For a child, pull the pinna downward to straighten the earcanal. Be sure the earcanal is free of cerumen or other foreign objects. Inspect the earcanal to determine whether deformities (i.e., atresia), pathological conditions (warts, moles, tumors), infections (drainage, irritations, redness of the canal wall or eardrum), or abnormalities of the earcanal (stenosis, prolapsed canal, surgically altered canal) are present. If any of the conditions are present, the audiologist should not proceed with the impression and, instead, should refer the patient to an otolaryngologist for consultation.

Selection and Placement of an Otoblock

One of the first decisions made when preparing an earmold impression is to select the appropriate otoblock, which is placed in the earcanal to prevent the impression material from coming into contact with the eardrum. Thread or dental floss

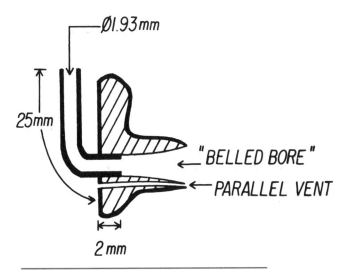

Figure 2–15 Schematic diagram of an earmold with a belled bore, parallel vent, and inserting the tubing 2 mm into the sound bore.

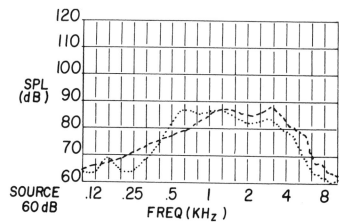

SOURCE 60 dB

BELLED BORE AND 3mm INSERTION OF TUBING
                          WITH 1000 Ω DAMPER ------
#13 TUBING TO TIP OF EARMOLD WITH 1000 Ω DAMPER ....

Figure 2–17   Frequency response using an earmold with a belled bore, 3 mm insertion of tubing and a 1000 Ω damper at the tip of the earhook. Also illustrated is the frequency response generated when using an earmold with #13 tubing to the tip of the earmold and a 1000 Ω damper at the tip of the earhook.

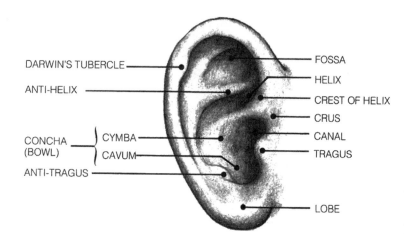

Figure 2–18   Illustration of the anatomical sites of the outer ear. (Printed with permission from Microsonic, Inc.)

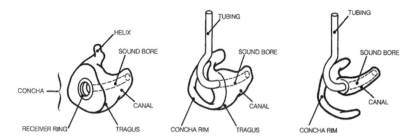

Figure 2–19   Terminology commonly used by earmold laboratories to relate the anatomical sites of the ear with various sections of three common earmolds. (Printed with permission from Microsonic, Inc.)

attached to the otoblock helps in the removal of the impression from the earcanal. However, it is important to remember that the removal of the impression from the earcanal is achieved primarily by pulling back on the impression and not by pulling the thread. This thread should be placed along the floor of the earcanal and draped over the intratragal notch of the pinna.

Morgan (1994) reminded us of the importance of selecting the correct otoblock. An undersized otoblock will allow

impression material past the otoblock or push the otoblock too deep into the earcanal, resulting in an uncomfortable situation for both the patient and audiologist. An oversized otoblock will abnormally expand in the earcanal or prevent the otoblock from being placed sufficiently deep. He suggests that the otoblock be correctly placed with an earlite to beyond the first bend of the earcanal and optimally to at least the second bend. The authors highly recommend deep impressions (i.e., beyond the second bend) for *all* patients regardless of type of fit. This rationale for this suggestion will be presented in greater detail in a later section.

Recently, one earmold manufacturer introduced pressure relief otosystem, (PROS™) which are soft form eardams with a silicone tube running through the center. This reportedly eliminates pressure buildup while injecting impression material into the earcanal and eliminates the sensation of a vacuum reported by many patients when removing the impression.

Impression Materials

The audiologist has a chance of using either powder (polymer) and liquid (monomer) or silicone impression materials. In recent years the advantages and disadvantages of these two impression materials has become a controversial issue for which uniform agreement is not about to occur in the near future. However, agreement exists that for whichever mater-

ial the audiologist chooses to use, it is imperative that he or she carefully follows the instructions provided by the earmold laboratory.

CONTROVERSIAL POINT

Debate continues as to whether powder and liquid or silicone is the best material to use when making impressions of the earcanal. We prefer to use powder and liquid. We believe little difference probably exists in the resulting impression if both were obtained following the instructions of the manufacturer. However, we suspect that most hearing aid manufacturers prefer silicone impressions.

Figure 2–20 illustrates the step-by-step procedure for use of the syringe techniques for taking an earmold impression.

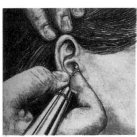

STEP 1
A cotton or foam block is an ABSOLUTE NECESSITY when using the syringe. Set a tight block just past the second bend. Foam blocks MUST be compressed to insure proper results. Be sure to use the correct size foam block even though it may appear to be larger in diameter than the ear canal.

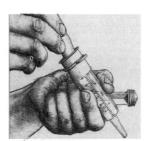

STEP 2
Mix the impression material according to instructions and place in the barrel of the syringe. The quicker you can use the material the better the impression.

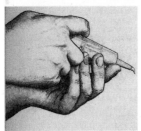

STEP 3
Insert the plunger and gently push the material into the nozzle to remove air pockets.

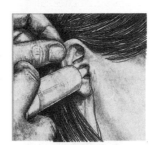

STEP 4
Place the nozzle into the canal and fill the canal.

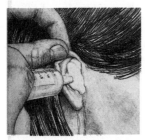

STEP 5
As the material fills the canal, slowly withdraw the syringe and fill the helix and concha areas completely. Then cover the tragus.

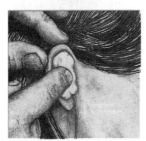

STEP 6
When the external ear has been filled completely, press your finger GENTLY in the concha and helix areas. BE CAREFUL NOT TO PRESS HARD AS IMPRESSION WILL DISTORT.

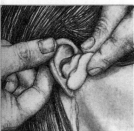

STEP 7
Allow a FULL 10 MINUTES of curing time before removing. The impression can be distorted if removed too soon. To remove, gently press ear away from the impression. Remove helix curl slightly. Bring impression straight out while holding thread. Take your time. Don't strain the impression with a long steady pull.

HELPFUL TIPS FOR BETTER IMPRESSIONS
- If the client wears glasses or dentures, make sure these are in place while taking the impression.
- NEVER flatten or smooth out the finished impression with the palm of your hand while impression material is in the client's ear.
- Ask your client to talk and chew after the impression material is in place. This is to help assure a comfortable fitting custom earmold which will not unseat when the jaw muscles constrict the ear canal.
- Children are sometimes fearful and can be hard to work with. Let the child watch you take an impression of mother's ear to alleviate his fears. Let him play with a piece of the "dough". NOTE: It is difficult to use a block with SOME children. The impression may be better formed without it in these cases.

Figure 2–20 Illustrating the syringe techniques for making an earmold impression. (Printed with permission from Microsonic, Inc.)

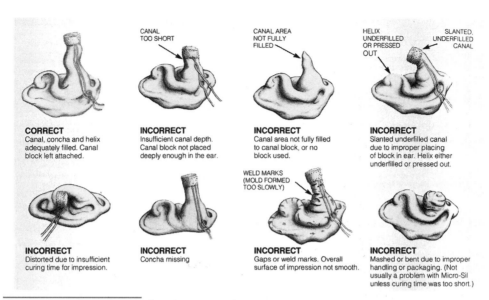

Figure 2–21   Several examples of correct and incorrect earmold impressions. (Printed with permission from Microsonic, Inc.)

With this technique, the impression material is carefully mixed and placed in the syringe and the nozzle of the syringe is placed in the earcanal. Gently press the plunger and gradually withdraw the nozzle as the material fills the earcanal and begins to flow out into the concha. Finally, fill the entire outer ear, especially the helix area. Keep the nozzle submerged in the impression material at all times for better filling of the ear. Do not press the outer surface of the impression because any pressing may lead to distortion of the impression. Allow at least 10 to 15 minutes for the impression to set. Gently break the seal by asking the patient to yawn or use exaggerated facial expressions. Remove the impression by grasping the pinna firmly with one hand and the impression with the other. Rotate the impression slowly with an upward and outward motion. The otoblock should remain on the tip of the impression. Figure 2–21 provides several illustrations of correct and incorrect earmold impressions. Finally, inspect the earcanal with an otoscope to be sure no impression material remains in the earcanal.

> ## CONTROVERSIAL POINT
>
> A general lack of agreement exists as to whether the patient should be allowed to move the jaw (i.e., talk) while an impression of the earcanal is being completed. It is our practice to encourage patients to exercise jaw movement while the impression material is setting up in the earcanal. We find this practice results in less chance of feedback and a greater chance for providing a more comfortable fitting earmold or shell.

Morgan (1994) reported that silicone impression material retains a highly accurate and dimensionally stable impression

of the earcanal from the clinic to the earmold laboratory. Many audiologists are hesitant to use silicone impression material because it is relatively messy in that it requires the proper mixing of two "pastes." One paste is a base material (silano-terminated gum) that is measured in a scoop, and the second paste is an activator agent that is spread over the base material. The two pastes are mixed together by hand for 20 to 30 seconds until an even, consistent color is reached (Fig. 2–22). It is then inserted into a syringe that is specially designed for silicone impressions. Trade names for some silicone impression material across earmold laboratories include Yellow Stuff I and II, XL-80, X-SIL, Otoform A/K, XL-100, XL-200, Micro-SIL, Blue Velvet, Gold Velvet II, Silicone, and Silicast. Prepackaged silicone is available. This material is delivered in prepackaged, self-mixing cartridges and is injected into the earcanal using an injection gun, as illustrated in Figure 2–23.

Staab and Martin (1995) recommend the use of silicone material with a relatively low viscosity rating (20 Shore) for the bony section of earcanal and a higher viscosity rating (40 Shore) for the cartilaginous section of the earcanal. Pirzanski (1996) and Hosford-Dunn (1996) suggest making two impressions. One with the jaw closed and a second with the jaw open. Hosford-Dunn (1996) suggests having the patient insert five tongue depressors between the teeth for the open-jaw impression. At our clinic, we have the patient hold 10 to 15 tongue depressors between their teeth for the open-jaw impression. For patients who cannot accept the 10 to 15 tongue depressors, we will then reduce the number to five tongue depressors. The need for making open *and* closed jaw impressions becomes more critical when the impression is taken for the purpose of manufacturing completely-in-the-canal (CIC) hearing aids.

Although a growing consensus on the advantages of silicone impression material exists, it is our opinion that powder (polymer) and liquid (monomer) impression material can provide an excellent impression if the audiologist uses the proper mix of powder and liquid, and the resulting mixture is

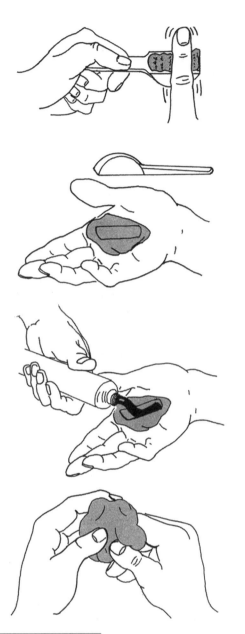

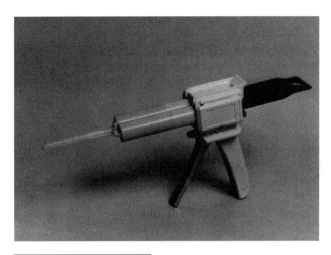

Figure 2–23 Illustration of an impression gun used when making earmold impressions with premixed silicone material.

Figure 2–22 Mixing the "base" material and "activator" agent when making an impression using silicone material. (Printed with permission from Microsonic, Inc.)

correctly syringed into the earcanal in a timely fashion. If the mixture of powder and liquid is incorrect and not properly cured (at least 10 to 15 minutes), the impression can stretch during removal. If the mixture is too dry (too much powder or too little liquid), it will be difficult to push through the syringe and, thus, cause voids. On the other hand, too much liquid makes the impression susceptible to melting.

To reinforce these points, Agnew (1986) reminded us that ethyl methacrylate will shrink if the proportion of the powder and liquid are poorly mixed. The magnitude of shrinkage can be 2% to 3% in 24 hours and 4% to 5% in 48 hours. One key factor for increased shrinkage is increased use of liquid in proportion to the amount of powder. Other reasons may

include not shaking the liquid or powder before use or loss of liquid by evaporation caused by a poorly sealed contained.

Another key factor in providing a good impression of the earcanal is "gel time" or "setup time." This is the time it takes for the mixing of the powder and liquid to become solidified or "cured" in the earcanal. As a general rule, gel time is at least 10 minutes. Gel time decreases with increased temperature and humidity. Thus on a hot and humid summer day, the impression will gel faster than in winter. To retard gel time, some audiologists increase the amount of liquid. To evaluate this strategy, Agnew increased the liquid amounts by 10% and 20% and found that shrinkage increased by 12% and 22%, respectively compared with when the correct mixture ratio was used.

Excessive heat (i.e., impression placed in a mailbox outside) will increase warpage and distortion of the impression. Excessive heat may cause the tip of the impression to distort toward the body by warpage and drooping (1.0 mm) after 5 days. For this reason, it is important to keep the impression in a cool place. Also, it is important not to use excessive force during the impression. This will "balloon" the earcanal, and the resulting earmold will cause the earcanal to become sore.

Morgan (1994) also reminded us to encourage the patient to talk, turn the head in all directions, smile, and chew while the impression material is setting in the earcanal. This will result in a more accurate impression of the dynamics of the earcanal and reduce the probability of feedback when the patient moves the jaw when wearing the hearing aids.

When shipping, it is necessary to glue the powder and liquid impression, but a silicone impression can be shipped loose in the box. Finally, it is important not to allow the order form to come into contact with the impression while in the shipping box because this may result in the order form pressing against the impression and cause distortion.

Earmold Impression on a Surgically Altered Earcanal

Taking an earmold impression on a surgically altered earcanal can present significant challenges to the dispensing audiologist. Figures 2–24A through 2–24C help illustrate the potential problem. Figure 2–24A illustrates a foam dam inserted into the earcanal at the position of the second bend. Medial to the dam is the significantly larger than usual surgically altered earcanal. Figure 2–24B illustrates silicone material injected into the earcanal, stopping at the position of the foam dam. Figure 2–24C illustrates the dam moving because of the force of the injection of the silicone material (silicone material is typically denser than powder and liquid material) combined with the poorer "staying" power of the foam dam and the larger than usual canal size medial to the dam. The movement of the dam now has allowed the impression material to bypass the dam and fill up the earcanal space between the foam dam. When this occurs, removal of the impression material is impossible. If the dispensing audiologist finds any difficulty in removing an impression . . . STOP and immediately seek the assistance of an otologist. Depending on the status of the space beyond the dam, this event can lead to very serious problems and is something all audiologists should avoid. To prevent this from occurring the following precautions should be followed. First, it is highly recommended that *cotton* dams be used instead of foam dams. It has been our experience that properly sized cotton dams are more likely to adhere to the canal wall when material is injected compared with foam dams. *It is often necessary to use numerous cotton dams instead of just one.* Second, powder and liquid material should be used because this material has less viscosity (i.e., less force) and

is less likely to cause the dam to move. Third, when taking an earmold impression of a surgically altered earcanal, it is advised to have an otologist place the dam(s) in the earcanal and have him or her available to assist the audiologist in removing the impression from the earcanal.

Earmold Materials

Earmolds are available in both hard or soft materials, and it is not a simple task to select the appropriate earmold material for a patient. For example, if the pinna is hard, a soft earmold material may be more appropriate. Conversely, if the pinna is soft, a hard earmold material may be more appropriate. If the gain/output requirements of the hearing aids are "high" (usually 70 dB of gain and 125 dB SPL of output), the audiologist might consider ordering a hard Lucite body with a soft canal or a material that softens to the heat of the earcanal, which provides a better seal to prevent feedback. For mild-to-moderate gain aids, a Lucite earmold might be considered. If any indication of an allergic reaction to the earmold material exists, the audiologist might consider polyethylene (hard) or silicone (soft) material. If the patient indicates difficulty with inserting an earmold, a Lucite material may be considered because it is easier to insert earmolds made of hard material. If the audiologist prefers the flexibility of having the ability to make modifications (venting, changing bore length or diameter, and belling), ordering a Lucite material may be better

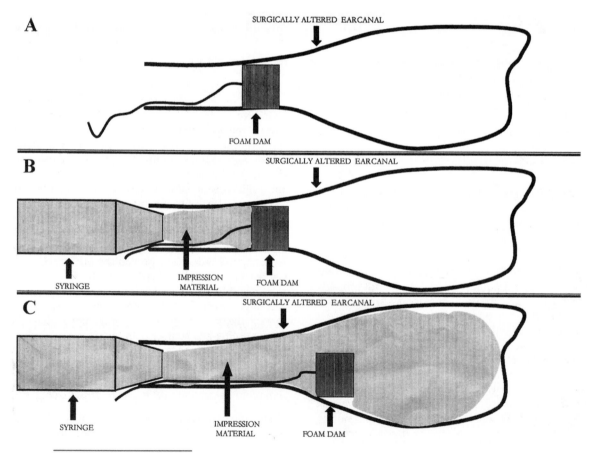

Figure 2–24   (A–C) Earmold impression on a surgically altered earcanal.

because of its greater ease in allowing for such modifications. Finally, the audiologist needs to be familiar with the terminology used by his or her earmold laboratory because quite a variance exists in terminology across earmold laboratories. A description of the various earmold materials provided by one manufacturer is provided in the next section.

1. LUCITE: This is a polymethyl methacrylate dental acrylic. It is a hard material that is easily modified, easy to insert and remove, and is durable. It is available in clear, various tints, and opaque. It is also available as a nontoxic clear or opaque material. The canal portion is rigid and may lead to sound leakage during chewing or other facial movement if applied to a high-gain hearing aid.

2. LUCITE BODY WITH VINYLFLEX CANAL: This earmold combines the body of the earmold made with polymethyl methacrylate (Lucite) material and the canal made by polyethyl methacrylate (Vinylflex) material. This combination of materials is designed for patients who want the comfort and increased sealing capacity of the Vinylflex material when fit with hearing aids having greater gain and output.

3. VINYLFLEX: This is a polyethyl methacrylate material that is a heat-cured semisoft plastic that will soften with body temperature. It is available in clear, beige, and tint. Finally, it is not easy to modify.

4. SEMISOFT: This is a fairly rigid vinyl material that softens at body temperature. This is typically used for additional comfort, while maintaining ease of insertion. It is fairly easy to modify.

5. SOFT VINYL: This is the most common soft material when allergies are not a concern. This material will shrink with

body contact and age and can become discolored over time. Cementing tubing can cause some problems and, therefore, a tube-locking system is recommended.

6. SILICONE: This is a flexible, inert rubber material. It is available in clear, opaque, pink, beige, and brown. It has very little shrinkage and is good for high-power aids; it is not easy to modify. Silicone material will solve most allergy problems. Finally, a tubing lock method is required because cement does not adhere to this material.

7. SOFT SILICONE: This material is recommended for the highest gain requirements. It is most effective when used in a canal or canal-shell earmold design but is not easy to modify. This material also requires an accurate impression to at least the second bend of the earcanal.

8. POLYETHYLENE: This is a hard material that is appropriate for severe cases of allergy, and it is easy to modify. It is only available in opaque white or pink.

9. DISAPPEAR™: This is a new material recently offered by one earmold laboratory where microfibers are embedded in the material so that the earmold has minimal outline and reflection. It is available in hard acrylic or silicone materials.

Recently, E-Compound material was introduced by Emtech Laboratories (Letowski & Burchfield, 1991; Letowski et al, 1992) (see address in Table 2–4). E-Compound is produced by filling a polymeric matrix (Lucite or silicone) with hollow glass microspheres. This new material is reported by the manufacturer to provide better sound quality than conventional materials. Letowski et al (1991) reported the results of 10 normal listeners who provided sound-quality judgments of eight stimuli recorded through KEMAR fitted with

TABLE 2–4 List of several earmold manufacturers

All American Mold Labs 226 S.W. Sixth Street P.O. Box 25751 Oklahoma City, OK 73125 405-232-8144	Mid-States Labs, Inc. P.O. Box 1140 Wichita, KS 67201 800-247-3669
Earmold Designs, Inc. 3424 East Lake Street Minneapolis, MN 55406 800-721-5711	Pacific Coast Labs, Inc. P.O. Box 7981 San Francisco, CA 94120 510-351-2770
Earmold and Research Labs, Inc. P.O. Box 12368 Wichita, KS 67277 316-682-9587	Precision Mold Labs 830 Sunshine Lane Altamonte Springs, FL 32714 800-327-4792
Emtech P.O. Box 12900 Roanoke, VA 24022 800-336-5719	Starkey Labs 6700 Washington Ave, South Eden Prairie, MN 55344 800-328-8602
Microsonic P.O. Box 184 1421 Merchant Street Ambridge, PA 15003 800-523-7672	Westone Labs, Inc. P.O. Box 15100 Colorado Springs, CO 80935 800-525-5071

Lucite and silicone earmolds made with and without E-Compound. Results indicated that only a few of the listeners could detect differences in sound quality between the earmold materials when signals comprised of "noise" were presented. However, they could not detect differences when "non-noise" signals were presented. The authors reported that E-Compound seems to provide better results with silicone material than with Lucite material.

Ridenhour (1988) reported that 76% of 25 subjects wearing ITE hearing aids revealed improved NU-6 word recognition scores, embedded in cafeteria noise at a SNR of +10 dB when wearing E-Compound Lucite shells compared with conventional lucite shells. He reported that the average improvement was 12%, and that 68% of the users preferred the shell made with E-Compound.

Williams and Gutnick (1990) reported the results of 10 listeners who were fitted with conventional Lucite and E-Compound Lucite earmolds. Seventy percent of the patients preferred the E-Compound earmolds, although none of the objective data (functional gain, in situ gain, word recognition scores at 50 dB HL in quiet and noise at +5 and +8 SNR) could reveal statistically different performance between the two materials.

Two-Stage versus One-Stage Impressions

Custom earmolds require two stages. First is the impression of the ear by the audiologist. The impression is then mailed to an earmold laboratory, where it is wax dipped and invested in a matrix medium that is either silicone or plaster. A polymeric material is cured in plaster or silicone and then drilled, tubed, and polished. Many problems may arise that will not allow the finished product to "duplicate the ear." These include poor impression-taking techniques; shrinkage of the impression and/or earmold; incorrect trimming of the impression; and changes in the dimensions of the earcanal between the time of the impression and the fitting.

Single-stage earmolds (i.e., the impression is the earmold) include such commercially available products as Instamold™, Silisoft™, and Otozen™. These earmolds have been used in our clinic as temporary earmolds to allow patients to continue using their hearing aids while waiting for a custom mold to be delivered. We have also used single-stage earmolds instead of stock earmolds for evaluating benefit from amplification during a hearing aid evaluation (HAE).

Some single-stage earmolds have reportedly presented problems such as producing a high degree of heat related to setting reaction that may cause burns to the ear, a high degree of shrinkage, too great a degree of hardness, and poor resistance to tearing, which may lead to difficulties in removal of the earmold (Okpojo, 1992).

Okpojo (1992) reported on a new material for one-stage earmolds that is used in the United Kingdom. This material is reportedly nontoxic and nonirritant, and the setting reaction has a low exothermal release. It is a "polymer power and monomer liquid" mixture that sets in 4 to 7 minutes. Shrinkage is reportedly less than 1% to 2%, and it has suitable mechanical and rheologic properties (elastic, resilient, adequate strength to resist tearing, and comfortable). All these properties led to the development of the soft Otana material.

Custom versus Stock Earmolds

Stock earmolds are available in skeleton, shell, or regular designs and typically are available in a set of five earmolds for each ear. The purpose of these earmolds is to conveniently assess benefit with BTE hearing aids during an HAE, when the patient does not have a custom earmold. Konkle and Bess (1974) reported better performance with custom earmolds compared with stock earmolds. They reported that using stock earmolds presented several problems, which include differences in (a) dimensions between the stock versus custom earmold, (b) vent length and diameter, (c) tubing length and diameter, (d) the size of the residual volume between the tip of the earmold and the eardrum, and (e) sealing capacity. All these differences led the authors to conclude that custom and stock earmolds will deliver different acoustic signals than were evaluated at the time of the HAE with the stock earmold; therefore, the results from the HAE may not be valid. They highly recommended using the custom earmold during the HAE. To punctuate this point, they evaluated 17 patients with sensorineural hearing loss. They compared the performance of six soft and hard acrylic stock earmolds with custom earmolds. They reported no significant differences in functional gain, although mean aided warble tone and speech reception thresholds were lower for the custom earmolds. They also reported that the mean word recognition score was significantly better for the custom earmold.

Disposable Foam Earmolds

Another method of providing a temporary and, in some cases, a permanent earmold is using disposable form earmolds. Smolak et al (1987) reported on seven subjects that used the 3M Comply™ disposable foam earmold. This earmold incorporates retarded recovery foam technology to provide a comfortable fit and eliminate the need for an earmold impression. Venting (four vents) is provided by the use of trench vents in the foam to control the low-frequency response. They reported that differences between a custom earmold and foam earmold was, at its greateset, less than 2 dB. The four vents provided by the disposable foam earmold yielded an average reduction of 3.1- to 6-dB at 250 to 1000 Hz. However, 25% of the ears did not achieve as satisfactory a fit with the disposable foam earmold as they did with their custom earmold. These differences were attributed to the inability of the disposable foam earmold to adequately address earcanals that were unusually narrow or tortuous. These types of earcanals reduced retention and provided inadequate venting. Finally, it was found that the disposable foam earmold was more effective in reducing feedback caused by the adaptive sealing capabilities of the disposable foam and the excellent sealing capability that prevents acoustic signals from re-entering the earcanal by means of a vent or slit leak.

Oliveira et al (1992) reported on results with the Comply disposable foam earmold versus custom earmolds at 15 test sites. They reported significantly better performance of the disposable foam earmold in providing greater comfort and in reducing feedback. However, the disposable foam earmold did present some problems with retention and proper insertion for patients older than 75 years of age.

Another option for a disposable earmold is the ER-13 generic BTE earmold kit, which is delivered with small, medium, and large disposable foam eartips and No. 13 or 3 mm CFA elbows.

EARMOLD STYLES

Sullivan (1985a, 1985b, 1985c) suggested that all hearing aid fittings can be categorized into four classes according to the type of coupling used as follows:

Class I includes earmolds where no loss in transmission of the acoustic signal is present; pinna, concha, and earcanal effects are retained; maximum venting is used; a hermetic seal is not necessary; the volume between the tip of the earmold and the eardrum (V3) is maximum because of the need for a short bore length; maximum in situ gain is 10- to 25-dB and usable in situ output is 75- to 90-dB. Class 1 fittings are appropriate for hearing loss between 15- and 40-dB HL. Examples of Class I fittings would be tube fittings, free field, Janssen, and other nonoccluding designs.

Class II fittings include earmolds where a slight reduction in high-frequency transmission exists; minimal venting is required; the pinna effect is retained, but the concha and earcanal effects are modified; hermetic sealing is not required; there is some reduction in V3 because of the need for a longer bore; maximum in situ gain is 20- to 35-dB; and usable in situ output is 80- to 100-dB. Class II fittings are appropriate for hearing loss between 30- and 55-dB HL and include the use of acoustic modifiers, SAV, Variable-Venting-Valve (VVV), PVV, and fixed venting.

Class III fittings include earmolds where significant loss of high-frequency and mid-frequency transmission exists; the pinna, concha, and earcanal effects are not usable; a limited hermetic seal is required; there is further reduction of V3 because of the need for a longer bore; maximum in situ gain is 30- to 55-dB; and usable in situ output of 95- to 115-dB. Class III fittings are appropriate for hearing loss between 45- and 85-dB HL and include closed molds and use of pressure equalization venting (0.05 mm).

Class IV fittings include earmolds where complete loss of the transmission of the frequency response exists; the pinna, concha, and earcanal effects are not usable; a tight hermetic seal is required; V3 is reduced further because of the need for further increases in bore length; maximum in situ gain is 50 - to 65-dB; and usable in situ output of 110- to 135+-dB. Class IV fittings are appropriate for hearing loss between 70- and 95+-dB HL and include earmolds requiring a closed mold with no venting, tight hermetic seal, and a deep canal fit.

NAEL Earmold Designs

Coogle (1976) reported the nomenclature for earmold designs as agreed to by the National Association of Earmold Laboratories (NAEL). These include the following.

1. *Regular, Receiver, or Standard Earmold* (Fig. 2–25A): This earmold design is typically used for fitting body aids and BTEs. It is usually ordered with a vinyl or metal snap ring that is either 1/4 or 3/16 inch wide. In a body aid fitting the external receiver from a body aid snaps into the snap ring. For BTE fittings, a plastic nub attached to tubing from the earhook snaps into the snap ring or it can be ordered with glued tubing. The plastic nub over which the tubing from the earhook slips onto can be ordered in several sizes (standard, D90, 8080, etc.). An alternative may be a regular earmold with a wire hook for cases where the pinna has little cartilage (i.e., a young child), and this style will hold the weight of the receiver and earmold in place.

   For a regular earmold, bore dimensions of 18 mm by 3 mm will produce a relatively flat frequency response to 3400 Hz. When the bore length is longer and the diameter narrower (23.4 x 2.4 mm), a loss in the high-frequency response occurs. Actually, the use of a long bore may be in the best interest of a patient with a severe hearing loss. This is because attenuating the high-frequency response would reduce the possibility of feedback. In addition, the benefits from high-frequency amplification are questionable in patients with profound high-frequency hearing loss.

   Lybarger (1979) reported that regular earmolds containing a snap ring can reduce the high-frequency gain by 8- to 10-dB above 2800 Hz and increase gain around 1000 Hz by about 4 dB relative to when No. 13 tubing is inserted to the earmold tip. The magnitude of the high-frequency reduction is related to the volume of the cavity in front of the receiver, which has been denoted as V2 by Lybarger (1979). The smaller the V2, the less the reduction of high-frequency gain. Again, as noted earlier, the reduction in high-frequency gain for patients with severe-to-profound hearing loss may be desirable.

2. *Skeleton* (Fig. 2–25B): This is similar to the shell, but the center of the conca section is removed to provide less bulk and greater comfort.

3. *Semi-skeleton* (Fig. 2–25C): This earmold is the same as the skeleton, but the upper portion of the concha ring is removed. It is appropriate for patients who have reduced manual dexterity or hardened ear texture.

4. *Canal* (Fig. 2–25D): This is designed for mild-to-moderate gain hearing aids. It is easy to insert, but retention may be poor and is prone to problems with feedback. This is also available in canal-lock (Fig. 2–25E).

5. *Shell* (Fig. 2–25F): This earmold fills the concha completely. It can be ordered with or without the helix segment. Adding the helix improves retention of the earmold to reduce the possibility of feedback. However, the addition of the helix increases the probability of discomfort in the helix region. It usually selected for high-gain hearing aids.

SPECIAL CONSIDERATION

Should the helix segment be included with the earmold? It is our experience that including the helix will often result in patient discomfort and with greater difficulty in correctly inserting the earmold. At present, we routinely exclude the helix when ordering earmolds.

6. *Half-Shell or Canal Shell* (Fig. 2–25G): The entire helix area is removed, and the earmold covers the bottom half of the concha bowl. It is recommended for patients with reduced manual dexterity.

7. *Nonoccluding Earmolds:* As presented earlier in the sections discussing tubing and earhooks, a variety of nonoccluding earmolds exist. These include tube fitting, free field, CROS, Janssen, Lybarger dual-diameter, Lybarger 1.5LP, and extended range earmolds (see Figs. 2–8 and 2–9).

Non-NAEL Earmold Designs
Acoustically Tuned Earmolds

In the typical BTE fitting, the output from the receiver is transmitted to the earhook by tubing having a length of 10 mm and diameter of 1.0 mm. The earhook typically has a length of 23 mm and diameter of 1.3 mm. The tubing from the earhook to the tip of the earmold is approximately 40 to 45 mm long and 1.93 mm wide. Finally, the signal is delivered to the earcanal, which is typically 13 mm long and 7.5 mm wide (see Fig. 2–1). Thus the typical hearing aid fitting already has a

stepped diameter design. Killion (1980, 1981, 1982, 1984, 1988a, 1988b), Killion and Monser (1980), Killion and Revit (1993), and Libby (1980, 1981) advocated that the stepped diameter design should be extended to the earmold when used with a hearing aid having the newer wideband receiver to obtain maximum high-fidelity sound quality, extended frequency response, and reduced battery drain. Up to that time, receivers had a high-frequency cutoff at 4000 to 4500 Hz. Killion presented 12 new earmold designs that varied in the dimensions of sections of tubing and the placement of damping in either the earhook or tubing. These designs include the 6R12, 6R10, 6K14, 16KLT, 8.5R8, 8CR, 6AM, 6B10, 6B5, 6B0, 6C5, and 6C10; their dimensions have been outlined by Valente and de Jonge (1981). The last seven rows of sections A and B of Table 2–3 report the relative change in output for the 8CR, 6R12, 6R10, 6B5, 6B0, 6C5, and 6C10 earmold designs relative to measures made in HA-1 and HA-2 couplers.

The 6R10, 6R12, and 6K14 earmold designs provide a smooth rising frequency response resulting in 10-, 12-, or 14-dB greater gain at 6000 Hz than at 1000 Hz. The 16KLT provide gain to 16,000 Hz and can only be used if coupled to a receiver whose frequency response extends to 20,000 Hz. The 8.5R8 is a shorter

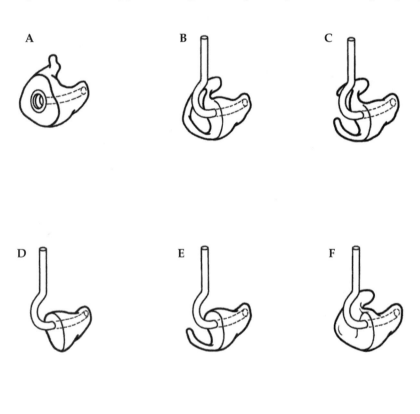

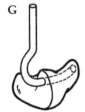

Figure 2–25 Examples of several earmold designs: **(A)** regular; **(B)** skeleton; **(C)** semi-skeleton; **(D)** canal; **(E)** canal-lock; **(F)** shell; **(G)** canal-shell. (Printed with permission from Microsonic, Inc.)

bore design, providing a smooth rising frequency response where the gain is 8 dB greater at 8500 Hz than at 1000 Hz. The 8CR is designed to provide a smooth frequency response, with the greatest gain at 2000 Hz to compensate for the loss of the earcanal resonance, which is eliminated with the introduction of the earmold. It also extends the frequency response to 8000 Hz (see Fig. 2–26; Valente, 1983). The 6AM is an acoustic modifier earmold that extends the frequency response to 6000 Hz. Five additional designs (6B10, 6B5, 6B0, 6C5, and 6C10) either boost (B) or cut (C) the gain at 6000 Hz relative to the gain at 1000 Hz by using either a horn (Boost) or reversed horn (cut) design. As mentioned earlier, the 6B0 is a conventional earmold with No. 13 tubing cemented to the tip of the earmold.

Preves (1980) reported that the advantages of the stepped diameter design could be extended to ITE fittings. He reported that using a stepped bore increased gain by 10 dB at 6000 Hz. In addition, placement of a 2200 Ω damper in the receiver reduced the amplitude of the resonant peak at around 2000 Hz by 4- to 8-dB.

Rezen (1980) evaluated the performance of the 6R12 on 11 subjects with sensorineural hearing loss. She reported functional gain increased from 3.5 dB at 2500 to 4000 Hz to 19.5 dB at 6300 to 10,000 Hz relative to an earmold with No. 13 tubing cemented to the tip. She also reported improved word recognition scores (NU-6, Nonsense Syllable Test, and SPIN) of 8.1% to 15.5% relative to the earmold using No. 13 tubing to the tip of the earmold.

To illustrate the advantages of providing greater high-frequency gain, Schwartz et al (1979) evaluated 12 subjects using conventional high-frequency emphasis amplification versus an experimental high-pass hearing aid that extended the frequency response to 6000 Hz. They reported similar performance between the two hearing aids for word recognition scores in quiet, but the experimental aid provided an average of 9% better word recognition scores in noise. In addition, the experimental aid provided greater functional gain above 4000 Hz and 15- to 20-dB greater high-frequency coupler gain. Finally, eight subjects preferred the sound quality of the experimental aid.

Hartford and Fox (1978) fitted nine subjects having a flat moderate to severe sensorineural hearing loss with a conventional hearing aid and an experimental high-frequency hearing aid that extended the frequency response to 6500 Hz. They reported increased functional gain of 1- to 23-dB at 2000 to 8000 Hz and a mean improvement of 13.5% in word recognition scores (NU-6) embedded in competition. Also, they reported that seven subjects revealed word recognition scores that were 18% or greater than their performance with the conventional aid. Finally, they pointed out that most subjects preferred the performance of the experimental aid in noise, but did not prefer the experimental aid in quiet because it was perceived as "too tinny."

Killion and Tillman (1982) compared the performance of an experimental high-frequency emphasis BTE coupled to an 8CR earmold and ITE hearing aids to high-quality loudspeakers, a pocket radio, a discount stereo, a simulated audiometer, popular headphones, and a monitor loudspeaker. Comparisons were based on six speech samples (nonsense sentences, speech spectrum noise, and four musical passages) recorded through the various listening devices. Subjective fidelity ratings were obtained from three groups of listeners (24 untrained listeners; 5 "golden ears," and 6 trained listeners). Results revealed that ratings for the hearing aids and high-fidelity loudspeaker were equal. Mean fidelity ratings were 82% for the BTE and 91% for ITE. The scores were 63% to 93% for the "low-end" loudspeaker and 89% for high-fidelity loudspeaker. For the 24 untrained listeners, the ITE had a mean subjective fidelity rating of 76%, followed by the BTE, which had a mean rating of 75%. The monitor speakers had a mean rating of 73%, and the popular earphones had a mean rating of 60%. Similar findings were revealed for the "golden ear" and trained listener groups. The results of this study revealed that "high-fidelity" performance was possible with well-designed BTEs and ITEs.

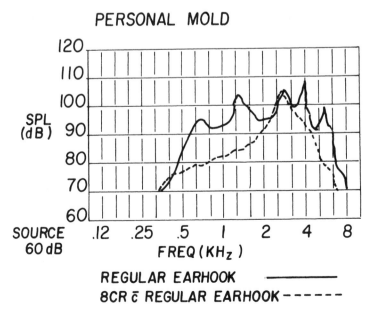

Figure 2–26 Frequency response of a hearing aid coupled to an 8CR earmold and an earmold using #13 tubing cemented to the tip.

Extended Range Earmold

The extended range earmold (ERE) is a specially designed earmold that provides a smooth frequency response between 2000 and 5000 Hz and extends the effective frequency response to 9000 Hz. It is available in two versions from several earmold laboratories. In the first version, No. 13 tubing is inserted to within 5 mm from the lateral end of the earmold, and it is followed by a wide diameter–belled canal that is 11 mm long (Fig. 2–9F). The second version contains a narrower and shorter sound bore that has No. 13 tubing inserted 5 mm into the sound bore followed by a bore length of 8 mm, which is reduced in diameter to 1.5 mm (Fig. 2–9G). This version provides slightly less high-frequency amplification than the first version. Because it is a nonoccluding design, it provides a fair degree of low-frequency attenuation. It is very similar in performance to the Janssen earmold (Fig. 2–9E), which is very similar to a CROS mold except that the canal portion of the mold runs along the top of the earcanal. Figure 2–9H illustrates the improved high-frequency gain with either ERE designs compared with a tub fitting (*dotted line*).

Wide Range Mold

A wide range mold (WRM) is a special resonator earmold that is designed to provide maximum gain at 5000 Hz. It uses No. 13 double-walled tubing inserted 3.2 mm into the sound bore and followed by a short bore 3.4 mm wide. If the audiologist wants a smoother response, the WRM can be ordered with two dampers in the sound bore that are placed between the end of the No. 13 tubing and the beginning of the 3.4 mm sound bore. The WRM also contains a vent, which is 1.35 mm in diameter.

Lybarger Dual Diameter System

The Lybarger dual diameter system is an open canal earmold that is appropriate for patients having normal-hearing from 250 to 2000 Hz followed by a precipitous decrease in hearing above 2000 Hz. This earmold contains a section of tubing with an ID of 0.8 mm, which is cut to the required length and cemented between two sections of No. 13 tubing (see Fig. 2–4). The upper section of the No. 13 tubing is connected to the earhook (containing a 1500 Ω damper), and the lower section of No. 13 tubing is cemented into the nonoccluding earmold and extends between 6.3 to 9.5 mm into the earcanal. The 0.8 mm section of tubing moves the first resonant peak downward, and the open mold provides 20- to 25-dB of attenuation at 500 Hz. The 1500 Ω damper provides a broad and smooth frequency response. Finally, this design provides 12 dB of gain between 4000 to 7000 Hz when used with a wideband receiver (Mynders, 1985).

Frequency Gain Modifier

The frequency gain modifier earmold is available in numerous occluding and nonoccluding designs. Its construction is highlighted by using a stepped-bore, belled canal and a plastic elbow for efficient changing of tubing. Some designs use venting and others do not. This earmold is designed to damp the low-frequency region and amplify the high-frequency region.

Vogel Mold

The Vogel mold is designed for severe-to-profound hearing loss and for patients who illustrate "excessive" mandibular jaw movement. It is comprised of a Lucite base for rigid retention in the outer ear and a soft, flexible silicone section in the earcanal portion that reportedly moves with the earcanal to maintain a constant acoustic seal.

Continuous Flow Adaptors

CFA earmolds are ordered in various numbers (i.e., CFA No. 1, CFA No. 2, etc.) and contain a single snap-in/snap-out elbow that has a constant internal diameter to incorporate the earmold designs of Killion, Libby, and Janssen discussed earlier. The advantages of CFA are the ease of changing tubing and the elimination of damping in the earhook or tubing to smooth the frequency response. Another advantage is the inability of the tubing to become crimped or pinched, which is a common problem when inserting Libby 3 mm or 4 mm tubing inside the sound bore.

It is important for the audiologist to consult his earmold laboratory manual to determine the dimensions and purpose of the various CFA designs because the nomenclature can vary from manufacturer to manufacturer. However, for one manufacturer, CFA No. 1 has a small bore of 1.93 mm that provides high-frequency emphasis at 2000 to 5000 Hz and a smooth frequency response. CFA No. 2 has a belled bore of approximately 4.0 mm, which also provides high-frequency emphasis at 2000 to 5000 Hz and a smooth frequency response. CFA No. 3 has a sound bore between 1.93 and 4.75 mm to provide greater high-frequency emphasis.

CFA No. 4 also contains a large open bore of 4.75 mm to provide even greater high-frequency emphasis. CFA No. 5 is designed for rising configurations and uses venting and a short-wide bore that removes 8 dB to 10 dB of gain at 2000 to 5000 Hz. For all CFA designs it is not necessary to remove the damaged tubing. The audiologist simply needs to pull out the old CFA (with the attached tubing) and snap the new CFA (with the attached tubing) into the seating ring above the sound bore.

Bakke Horn

As previously discussed, the Bakke horn is a hard plastic elbow having a stepped bore design (2 mm at the tubing end and 3 mm at the earmold end), which snaps into the final segment of the earmold having a 4 mm sound bore. It provides an acoustic signal that is very similar to the Libby 4 mm horn.

Macrae 2K Notch Filter

Macrae (1983) reported an earmold designed for hearing losses having an inverted trough configuration (best hearing at 2000 Hz). To accomplish this, the earmold has a Helmholtz resonator that band-rejects the frequency response around 2000 Hz (1400 to 2600 Hz) by 18 dB. His design places a coiled tubing, connected to the sound bore by a T-connector, and recessed into the cavity of the earmold. Then a faceplate was glued over the recess to hide the coiled tube. The reader should be reminded that the Macrae earmold provides the same frequency response as the ER 12-2 earhook that was discussed in an earlier section.

Earmolds Used With Stethoscopes

In our clinic, based in a large medical center, it is common for physicians, nurses, or anesthesiologists to request an earmold that can be used concurrently with their hearing aids or stethoscope because they report difficulties because of their hearing loss or the presence of excessive ambient noise. Mullin et al (1986) described an earmold designed for simultaneous use with a stethoscope and BTE. The earmold (Lucite or soft) accepts the plastic tips (i.e., lug) of stethoscopes. For this earmold design, the rubber tips of the stethoscope are removed and the ends of the stethoscope are inserted into 6.4 mm holes drilled in the earmolds. Peck (1986) described a similar earmold ("stethomold") that does not require the stethoscope's plastic tip to be removed. These earmold designs are available from a number of the earmold laboratories listed in Table 2–4.

Patriot Mold

The Patriot mold was introduced by Emtech Laboratories as a means to control feedback and is available for several earmold laboratories. The Patriot uses E-Compound material and is unique in that the earmold is hollow in the canal area, which reportedly enables it to move with face and jaw movement. The fitting range is reportedly up to 110 dB HL at 250 to 4000 Hz. The manufacturer requests the audiologist use a cotton otoblock, silicone material, and has the patient chew while the ear impression is made.

Other Issues Related to Earmolds

Attenuation or Sealing Capacity of Earmolds

As stated earlier, earmolds are designed to provide (1) an adequate seal, (2) comfort, (3) appropriate gain throughout the entire frequency range, (4) prevention of feedback, and (5) prevention of the sensation that the earmold is "blocking" the ear (i.e., occlusion effect). Macrae (1990, 1991), in a series of studies, reminded us that the seal provided by earmolds and shells has become increasingly important as the microphone has gotten closer to the receiver and for patients with severe-to-profound losses who require greater gain and output.

Sound can propagate through the earmold; vibrate the earmold as a whole; radiate through tissues, cartilage, or bone surrounding the earcanal, and pass through the air pathway between the earmold and the walls of the earcanal by means of unintentional slit leaks. Some of these paths of propagation can cause feedback. The presence of feedback results in the need for the patient to reduce the volume control setting, which results in inadequate amplification. Another outcome of these problems may be unintentional attenuation of low-frequency amplification, which is necessary for patients with severe-to-profound hearing loss, who need as much low-frequency amplification as possible. For these patients, earmolds with minimal pathway for leaks between the sides of the earmold and walls of the earcanal are necessary. The ability to achieve this goal depends on the impression material and technique, as well as the earmold material and style.

To evaluate static pressure seal, Macrae (1990) used an immittance meter attached to the tubing and earmold. With the air pump and manometer connected to the tubing of the earmold, pressure was increased to 200 daPa and maintained for 5 seconds. During this time, the subject was encouraged to talk to determine whether jaw movements broke the seal. If no loss of pressure occurred in 5 seconds, it was concluded that the earmold created an adequate static pressure seal. He evaluated two impression materials (silicone and dental impression) and four earmold materials (hard acrylic, silicone rubber, polyvinyl chloride, and Microlite). For 16 subjects, he found that 12 of the 128 earmold combinations provided an adequate seal, and for those earmolds that did provide an adequate seal, the average length and width of the earcanal was larger. Thus he believed that the dimensions of the earcanal may be a better predictor of maintaining an adequate seal than the impression or earmold materials. He concluded that because only 12 earmolds provided an adequate seal, the chance of sealing the ear with a two-stage earmold process with only a general buildup of the earmold was small. Also, using different impression material or earmold materials did not significantly improve the chances.

In another experiment, Macrae (1991) ordered two earmolds for one impression. He concluded that this method did not improve the chances of maintaining a static seal. In a final experiment, he "patted down" the surface of the impression material after it was syringed into the ear, but before the impression set. He then asked the earmold laboratory to apply a wax buildup to the impression with a hot wax knife. The results of this experiment revealed that "patting down" the impression did not increase the probability of a seal, but the special buildup did increase the probability of maintaining an adequate seal. In fact, in 55% of the cases, a buildup applied to the impression at the earmold laboratory resulted in an adequate seal. He also found that earmolds with round tips are more likely to seal than those with more elliptical tips.

As mentioned earlier, unintentional leaks can occur around the periphery of the earmold. Some estimate that the average leak is equivalent to the presence of a 1.4 mm vent. Lybarger (1979) reported that a vent this wide will have minimal effect on the output of a hearing aid coupled to an unvented earmold. However, when an unintentional leak is presented around an already vented earmold, low-frequency transmission is increased and the effectiveness of the vent is diminished (Cox, 1979).

Frank (1980) compared the performance of Lucite and Vinylflex earmolds (shell and skeleton) with and without the presence of a target lock against the performance of an E-A-R disposable foam earmold. In 20 subjects, he found that the custom earmolds provided approximately 17 dB less attenuation than the E-A-R disposable foam earmold. In addition, he warned against the commonly held belief that an earmold provides adequate hearing protection. The custom earmolds revealed a mean noise reduction rating of 3.3 dB, whereas the E-A-R disposable foam earmold had a mean noise reduction rating of 18.2 dB.

Letowski et al (1991) evaluated the attenuation of silicone and Lucite earmolds on real ears and KEMAR. They reported that silicone earmolds provided greater attenuation than Lucite earmolds, with differences ranging from 13 dB at 500 Hz to 3- to 4-dB at 4000 Hz.

Trychel and Haas (1989) used Bekesy tracking procedures at 250 to 8000 Hz on four subjects in which a hearing aid was coupled to silicone and Lucite earmolds manufactured in several styles (regular, shell, nonoccluding, and skeleton). In 85%

of the comparisons, silicone provided greater attenuation. Also, the regular earmold design provided the greatest attenuation in 63% of comparisons, followed by the shell, skeleton, and nonoccluding earmolds. They cautioned that the audiologist should not overfit a regular or shell earmold because these styles provide greater high-frequency attenuation and theoretically could have a deleterious effect on word recognition in noise.

Parker et al (1992) compared two forms of commercially available silicone impression materials (Amsil™ and Otoform™) to determine differences in accuracy and stability. They used several earmold materials (hard acrylic, soft acrylic, Otoform™, Amsil™, and Molloplast™) on 27 subjects with severe-to-profound hearing loss. They found that Otoform™ provided about 4 dB greater attenuation than Amsil™. They also suggested that using silicone impression material may improve hearing aid fittings by reducing the likelihood of feedback caused by improved attentuation and acoustic seal.

Maximum Real-Ear Gain

For patients with severe-to-profound hearing loss, the audiologist wants to select an earmold that will provide the greatest usable gain before feedback. Madell and Gendel (1984) reminded us that hearing aids, at the time, were available that provided maximum gain in excess of 60 dB and SSPL90, which was greater than 130 dB. For these patients, these authors believe that a soft (vinyl or silicone) earmold used with double-walled tubing is the most suitable because it provides the tightest fit and offers the greatest retention and, therefore, the greatest usable gain.

Kuk (1994) reported on the maximum usable real-ear gain for 10 occluding earmolds (regular with helix lock and No. 13 tubing; shell with helix lock; canal, skeleton without helix lock; skeleton with helix lock; CROS with extended canal; CROS with partial IROS vent; tube mold; and the Oticon E43 earmold designed for patients with hearing loss above 2000 Hz). Kuk reported a tendency among audiologists to believe that a bulkier earmold (regular or shell) will result in greater user gain than those with less bulk (canal or skeleton). His findings revealed that the greatest real-ear gain was achieved by the skeleton and shell earmolds followed by the canal and regular earmold. Furthermore, he reported that the average high-frequency gain was 44 dB for the skeleton and canal earmold, 46 dB for the shell earmold, and 40 dB for the regular earmold. In addition, he reported little advantage of using the helix lock because this addition resulted in increased difficulty in correctly inserting the earmold into the earcanal, increased user discomfort, and increased the possibility of feedback.

Earmold Design and Word Recognition

As mentioned earlier, past research has implied that earmold designs may have an effect on improved word recognition scores. Northern and Hattler (1970) and Hodgson and Murdock (1972) could not demonstrate significant differences in word recognition scores between unvented and vented earmolds in 18 subjects with high-frequency hearing loss. Similar findings were reported by Revoile (1968) using W-22 and CNC word lists at a +6 dB SNR to evaluate four earmold designs (regular with a narrow bore, hollow cavity with a 5.6 mm diameter bore, regular with a diagonal vent of 1.9 mm near the base, and regular with a diagonal vent of 2.2 mm near the base). However, many of the subjects thought the vented earmold provided greater comfort.

If greater gain is desired by the audiologist, the following suggestions may be beneficial.

1. If the pinna is hard, use a softer earmold material.
2. Usable gain can be increased by use of a Lucite body with a soft canal.
3. Consider using one of the "newer" earmold materials where the material expands in response to the heat of the earcanal. Examples include the JB1000, MSL90, Audtex, M2000, or Patriot earmolds, which are available from a number of earmold manufacturers (see Table 2–4).
4. Order an earmold with a long bore that will reduce the likelihood of the occlusion effect and feedback, while at the same time, allow the patient the opportunity to achieve greater usable gain.
5. The earmold design should allow the tip of the earmold to be round and face the eardrum and not the canal wall. If the tip of the earmold faces the canal wall, it will reflect sound back and cause feedback.

Problems with Earmolds

Impressions and the Presence of Perforations

Occasionally, audiologists will observe an eardrum perforation during otoscopic observation while in the process of taking an earmold impression. This should present some concerns for at least two reasons. First, the audiologist clearly needs to select the appropriate otoblock so that the impression material does not pass through the perforation into the middle ear space or expand the width of the perforation. Either event would cause discomfort and increase the possibility of middle ear infection. The second concern is related to the possibility that the presence of the earmold in the earcanal will enhance the probability of creating middle ear infections. Alvord et al (1989) reported that placement of earmolds in the earcanal will increase the risk of infection because the earmold reduces normal ventilation by creating a warm and moist environment for infectious growth. They also stated that bacteria may be introduced by the earmold or the earmold can induce allergic, irritating, or foreign body reactions. They evaluated six subjects with perforations. Four of the six subjects had a regular earmold with no vent, and two subjects had a regular earmold with a 2 mm vent. Their greatest success was with subjects with smaller perforations and vented earmolds. Also, the authors reported that pressure vents of 1 mm or less did not solve the problem and often became plugged. They suggested counseling patients on not using earmolds full time to provide ventilation during times when communication needs are less stressful.

Allergies to Impression and Earmold Materials

Occasionally, patients will report that use of the earmold or shell will cause discomfort to the ear or earcanal. Cockerill (1987) reported on patient allergic reactions to earmold materials. He wanted to determine whether patient complains of allergic reactions to earmolds were related to "true" allergic reactions or were due to irritation caused by a tight fit, surface roughness, lack of hygiene, or simple inflammation caused by constant tissue coverage.

Often, the acrylic resins used in the manufacture of earmolds are in the form of a powder (polymer) and liquid (monomer). Polymerization is the process whereby the monomer is converted into a polymer or the solid end-product. The main component of both the polymer and monomer is methyl methacrylate, with other ingredients including hydroquinine, dibutylphthalate, and benzoyl peroxide acting as inhibitors, activators, and catalysts. nonallergic materials may be vulcanite, silicone rubber, gold, and polyvinyl chloride (PVC), which is usually in the form of a thin coat brushed over the earmold or shell.

Cockerill (1987) evaluated 25 subjects who were subdivided into three subgroups. Group 1 was subjects who reported other skin problems but did not report problems relating to the earmold. Group 2 contained subjects who had or had a history of external otitis or seborrheic dermatitis. Subjects in Group 3 had or encountered otorrhea and had persistent reactions to earmolds. He performed skin patch tests and found reactions to eight substances specifically related to the ingredients used in earmolds. Reactions ranged from dry itchy skin with a slight inflammation of the concha to painful edema of the pinna, cheek, or neck area, which prevented the use of the earmold. Fourteen subjects (55%) showed a reaction to methyl methacrylate. One subject (4%) had a reaction to vulcanite, and two subjects (8%) had a reaction to PVC.

Meding and Ringdahl (1992) reported 22 subjects who had long-standing and severe dermatitis in the earcanal. Patch testing indicated that nine subjects had 15 positive reactions in the standard series. Six patients (27%) had contact allergy to the earmold materials. Four of these six patients had a reaction to methyl methacrylate (sensitizer), and two also had a reaction to ethyleneglycol dimethacrylate and triethyleneglycol dimethacrylate. The diagnosis was allergic contact dermatitis in seven cases and seborrheic dermatitis in six other cases. For the remaining nine subjects, the diagnosis was not obvious, although irritation from occlusion was probable. These authors recommended making another impression using less monomer (liquid) or silicone material. They also recommended consideration for a bone conduction hearing aid and patch testing in cooperation with dermatologists.

When a patient reports an allergic reaction to earmold or shell materials from previous experiences or because of current soreness of the ear, a polyethylene earmold should be ordered in either white or pink opaque colors.

The Elderly

Fitting the elderly can create some special concerns. One of these concerns is manual dexterity and its effect on ease of insertion of the earmold. Meredith and colleagues (1989) evaluated three groups of elderly patients with 20 subjects per group. For each group, they compared ease of handling, comfort, and the general effectiveness of the half shell, skeleton, and skeleton without the tragus notch. Results indicated that the skeleton with the tragus notch removed provided the greatest benefit in all three areas. However, the removal of the

tragus notch did increase the possibility of feedback, and it was suggested that this mold would only be appropriate for low-gain hearing aids. Other generic problems associated with correctly inserting earmolds by the elderly population in this study included (1) placing the tragus notch outside the crus of the tragus rather than underneath; (2) the presence of the concha rim, heel, and helix lock prevented easy insertion into the antitragus and antihelix areas; (3) inserting earmolds back to front or upside down; and (4) incorrect placement of the BTE hearing aid over the ear.

Feedback

In the beginning of the chapter, we stated that a "successful" hearing aid fitting would be one where no feedback was present in the usable range of the volume control wheel.

A number of solutions are available to combat the problem of feedback. Some have been discussed earlier, which may include the sealing ability of the earmold, special earmold designs and materials, dampers, and the depth of insertion of the sound bore. To combat feedback the audiologist might also consider the following:

1. Using antifeedback kits where sleeves (available in four sizes) are snugly fit over the earmold or shell and cemented in place. This strategy has disadvantages because the sleeves are often uncomfortable, develop "ripples," fall off, or cause allergic reactions.

2. Applying a "soft seal" liquid around the surface of the shell or earmold to reduce or eliminate the spaces between the earmold or shell and the canal wall. Other types of "sealing" compounds include (a) soft or hard Addco Addon for a minor buildup or soft or hard earmolds; (b) Adcobuild for a major buildup; (c) Addco Sheen, which is applied over Adcobuild products as a sealer to prevent discoloration.

3. Applying ER-13R E-A-R Ring Seal Kit or "seal rings" around the shell or earmold with tetrahydrofuron (C4H80) in small quantities. They are available in 8 mm, 10 mm, 12 mm, 14 mm, 16 mm, 20 mm, and 22 mm.

4. Using a ER-13MF microphone filter kit, which reportedly reduces gain by 10- to 15-dB at 5000 to 10,000 Hz.

5. Remaking the impression for a new earmold or shell because the original earmold or shell was too loose.

6. Narrowing the diameter of the vent if using any of variable venting schemes, which will be discussed later.

7. Decreasing the overall gain and/or output.

8. Placing a damper along the transmission line or in the vent.

9. Electronically reducing high-frequency gain by means of a high-cut potentiometer, feedback reduction circuit, or feedback notch filter, which are available from a number of ITE and ITC manufacturers. One additional possibility is using digital feedback suppression, which was recently introduced by Danavox, Inc.

10. Making sure the opening from the receiver of the ITE or ITC is not facing the canal wall. This will result in reflection of the amplified sound off the canal wall and induce

feedback. The same can be suggested as a cause for feedback with an earmold in a BTE fitting.

11. Ordering all ITE and ITC hearing aids with receiver extension tube (see Fig. 2–27). This places the output closer to the eardrum and typically results in a lower volume control setting. The lower setting typically results in the patient using less overall gain and, thus, reduces the chances for feedback. In our clinic, receiver extension tubes are ordered on all ITE and ITC hearing aids. An additional benefit of using receiver extension tubing is reducing the possibility that the receiver will be clogged with cerumen because the opening of the tubing is farther away from the receiver.

Occlusion Effect

Again, as stated earlier in this chapter, one of the goals of a "successful" hearing aid fitting is eliminating the sensation that the patient's head is "at the bottom of a barrel," which is commonly referred to as the occlusion effect (OE). Killion (1988d) and Revit (1992) reported that placing an earmold or shell in the earcanal can amplify the patient's own voice by 20- to 30-dB in the lower frequencies. Furthermore, Revit (1992) reminded us that only a 10 dB increase results in a doubling of the perceived loudness of a signal. In this case, inserting the earmold or shell into the earcanal can cause the perceived loudness to be four times as great compared with when the hearing aid is not in the earcanal. This perceived increase in loudness is especially true for the closed vowels /i/ (ee) and /u/ (oo).

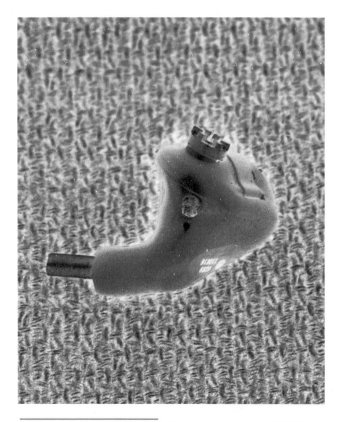

Figure 2–27 Use of extended receiver tube on an ITC hearing aid.

Westermann (1987) measured the OE and reported it was 4- to 10-dB at 200 Hz, 2- to 24-dB at 300 Hz, 11- to 17-dB at 400 Hz, and 1- to 20-dB at 500 Hz. When a 2 mm vent was introduced to the earmold, the trapped sound in the earcanal was "short-circuited" and the subject reported that his voice sounded more natural. Wimmer (1986) reported an overall OE of about 20 dB at 250 to 500 Hz for an occluded earmold on four ears. The mean OE was 22 dB at 250 Hz, 15 dB at 500 Hz, and 6 dB at 1000 Hz. When a 3 mm vent was added, it decreased the OE by 19 dB at 250 Hz, 6 dB at 500 Hz, and 0 dB at 1000 Hz. Staab and Finlay (1991) report that the OE can be 13- to 21-dB for an ITE and 20 dB for a deeply inserted ITC.

In the past, the only tool the audiologist had in dealing with the OE has been subjective reports by the patient because objectively measuring the OE was a challenge. However, Revit (1992) reported on how a real-ear analyzer could perform spectrum analysis of externally generated signals, with and without the hearing aid in place, to objectively measure the OE. First, the patient is asked to vocalize a sustained vowel ("eee" or "on"), which is self-monitored at 70 dB(A) on a sound level meter held 1 m from the lips (see the thicker line in the upper graph of Fig. 2–28). With the hearing aid in place, but turned off, the procedure is repeated (see the thin line in the upper graph of Fig. 2–28). The difference between the two measures, or the OE, is displayed as "insertion gain" in the lower graph of Figure 2–28. For this patient, approximately 15 dB of OE is seen at 800 to 900 Hz. At this point, the audiologist can attempt several steps described below and repeat the measures to determine whether the lower graph can be reduced to as close to 0 dB as possible.

Reducing the Occlusion Effect

One way to reduce or eliminate the OE is to apply venting of the earmold or shell to reduce low-frequency amplification. For example, a 2 mm vent can decrease the measured SPL at 200 Hz by 8.5 dB. Dempsey (1990) reported that venting options to reduce the OE in ITCs are limited as a result of space restrictions and the proximity of the microphone and receiver and the resulting problems of feedback. Usually, vent diameter in ITCs is limited to 2 to 3 mm and, therefore, reducing the OE by means of venting is limited. In this study shells for ITEs and ITCs were manufactured for 10 subjects, and 1.5 to 3 mm vents were introduced. The mean OE was 5.4 dB for the ITEs and 8.6 dB for the ITCs with the vents in place.

Another method for reducing the OE is making a silicone impression and placing a cotton otoblock beyond the second bend of the earcanal in the osseous segment of the earcanal to provide the patient with a deep canal fitting (Killion et al, 1988). In addition, it is important to allow jaw movement during the impression and ask the patient to yawn when removing the impression to reduce the effect of the vacuum created by the deep impression technique. Also, the audiologist should request a parallel pressure vent of 0.05 to 1.5 mm. Revit (1992) reported a 15 dB reduction in the OE at 200 Hz when the patient was fit with a deeply inserted foam tip compared with a medium-length bore that was seated in the cartilaginous portion of the earcanal. Staab and Finlay (1991) reported that a properly seated deep canal fitting where the tip is sealing the earcanal can reduce the OE by 19- to 22-dB at 200 Hz compared with a medium-length fit.

OCCLUSION EFFECT
70 dB(A) OF THE VOWEL "OU"

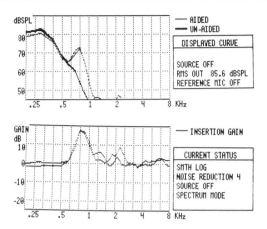

Figure 2–28 Measurement of the occlusion effect using a real-ear analyzer. The upper graph displays the spectrum of an /ou/ sound measured in the earcanal without the hearing aid in place (*dark line*). The light line displays the spectrum of the same sound, but with the hearing aid in place and the volume control turned off. The lower graph displays the resulting occlusion effect.

Completely-in-the-Canal Hearing Aids

A recent development to partly address the issue of reducing the OE has been the CIC hearing aid (Northern et al, 1991; Roesel, 1994). In these hearing aids, the visible end of the hearing aid is 1 to 2 mm inside the opening of the earcanal. On the other hand, as described earlier, a deep canal hearing aid or earmold is simply one in which the tip of the shell or earmold is very close to the eardrum (i.e., past the second bend into the osseous portion of the earcanal). The reported

---

SPECIAL CONSIDERATION

It is very important for the dimensions of the earcanal to be large enough to be an appropriate candidate for a CIC. One manufacturer recommends that the length of the canal section of the impression (i.e., from the tip to the concha bowl) must be *at least* 22 mm. The diameter of the canal section of the impression must be *at least* 5 mm and *greater than* 7 mm if venting is desired. These measurements can easily be achieved by using caliper devices recently introduced by several manufacturers.

---

advantages of the CIC include (a) cosmetic appeal, (b) reduction of the OE, (c) lower requirements for coupler gain and output to achieve the same real-ear gain, and (d) increased gain of 5 dB at the lower frequencies and increased gain of 13 dB at 4000 Hz. Because of the reduced volume of air, the CIC will produce 9 dB greater output than an ITE and 20 dB greater output at the eardrum than is measured in a 2-cc coupler at 4000 Hz. The increased gain occurs because of the deep placement of the shell, whereas the increased output occurs from the increase in gain plus the increased SPL at the

higher frequencies, resulting from the deep concha placement of the microphone. Thus a CIC fitting requires less coupler gain and output to achieve the same level of real-ear performance for an ITE or ITC (Gudmundsen, 1994).

Agnew (1994) also reported that the CIC provides less distortion and better sound quality because of its higher amplifier headroom capabilities. He also reported the elimination of wind noise caused by the deep placement of the microphone and better use of the telephone without feedback. In agreement with past research, Agnew reported that the volume between the shell and the eardrum can be as small as 0.25 cc, which may result in a 12 dB increase in SPL at the eardrum, relative to an ITE fit where the same volume might be 1.0 cc. This may represent as much as a fourfold decrease in volume from an ITE to CIC fitting. Agnew reported that peak gain, as measured in KEMAR, increased from 20 dB to 45 dB as the volume was reduced from 2.0 to 0.12 cc.

Preves (1994) reported that a long bore length (mean of 22.4 mm) provided an average of 6.4 dB greater overall real-ear root mean square (rms) output compared with the rms output measured for five bore lengths that were significantly shorter (mean = 15.2 mm). He reported a 6 dB difference in the higher frequencies and a 3- to 4-dB difference in the lower frequencies. In addition, he found that a 4.4 dB mean overall rms advantage exists for the CIC microphone inlet position compared with the typical ITE microphone inlet position. Finally, he reported that the overall rms output SPL for coupler to real-ear differences (RECD) for the CIC is 25.3 dB, whereas for the ITC it is 17.0 dB and for the ITE it is 11 dB. On average, the CIC provided 8 dB and 14 dB more output SPL than the ITC and ITE, respectively. Thus a CIC fitting would require 14.3 dB less overall gain than an ITE and 8.3 dB less overall gain than an ITC, as measured in a 2-cc coupler.

Minimal Contact Technology

Another method for reducing the OE has been the recent introduction of Minimal Contact Technology (MCT) by

Emtech Laboratories for earmolds and shells. This earmold design reportedly reduces contact between most of the earmold body and the cartilaginous portion of the earcanal. The only point of contact between the body of the earmold and the earcanal wall is the bony portion of the earcanal. The fitting range is reportedly up to 60 dB HL at 250 to 1000 Hz and 90 dB HL at 2000 to 4000 Hz. The earmold is made of E-Compound, which has been described earlier, and the bore length must be between 15 and 20 mm long.

Bryant et al (1991) evaluated eight subjects fit with ITEs manufactured with a conventional shell and a MCT shell. The subjects were asked to wear the aids for 4 weeks and provide their judgments. Real-ear insertion responses were equivalent for both sets of aids with the exception of 4000 Hz, where an average of 12 dB greater gain was reported with the shell made with MCT material. All eight subjects reported that the MCT earmold was initially more difficult to insert and remove. Also, most subjects reported that their voices sounded more natural with the MCT shells. The authors measured OE using real-ear measures while asking the subjects to sustain the /ee/, /um/, /oo/, and /ah/ sounds at a level of 90 dB SPL. They reported that the OE was smaller for the MCT shells for the closed vowels (ee, um, oo), but little difference existed between the shells for the open vowel (ah). The differences in OE varied from 10 dB for the /um/ and 4 dB for the /ee/.

VENTING

It is our belief that virtually every hearing aid fit should have some degree of venting. Dillon (1991) reminded us of the many roles of venting. First, the vent allows some of the low-frequency amplified sound to dissipate outside the earcanal instead of contributing to the SPL buildup at the eardrum. The vent will reduce low-frequency gain and output relative to a closed earmold fitting. Second, the vent allows unamplified signals to enter the earcanal through the vent. This results in less attenuation of the low frequencies and greater attenuation for the higher frequencies. Third, the volume of the vent tube combines with the cavity of the earcanal to produce a Helmholtz resonator to create a vent-associated resonant frequency at 250 to 1000 Hz. At the vent-associated resonant frequency, the vented mold provides greater gain than would have been present if the vent were blocked. Fourth, the vent can reduce or eliminate the occlusion effect. Other advantages of venting include providing pressure release to prevent a sensation of pressure buildup near the eardrum and ventilation to minimize the buildup of moisture in the earcanal.

On a negative note, the presence of a vent can allow the amplified sound in the earcanal to pass back to the hearing aid microphone and lead to suboscillatory (heard by the patient as a "ringing," but not heard by the audiologist) or oscillatory (heard by the audiologist, family members, and, perhaps, the patient) feedback. As vent size increases, the amount of acoustic leakage increases and the probability of feedback heightens. Oscillatory feedback will occur at any frequency when the attenuation along the feedback path is less than the gain of the hearing aid in the earcanal. In BTE fittings, the gain has to be greater or the attenuation along the path less because the length of the path from the earcanal to the microphone of the hearing aid is greater than it is for an ITE or ITC fitting. Even for vents slightly smaller than this critical size, feedback will produce an additional peak in the frequency response and add a "ringing" or transient tone to the sound quality. For many low-gain to medium-gain hearing aids, it is necessary to specify a vent large enough to minimize the OE, but small enough to avoid feedback.

Effect of Vent Diameter

Pressure Equalization

As a general guideline, a pressure vent is approximately 0.06 to 0.8 mm and it will have no measurable effect on the frequency response. Kuk (1994) reported that the pressure vent changed the low-frequency real-ear response by 1- to 6-dB. For a medium length bore (16.6 mm), Lybarger (1977, 1979, 1980) suggested a pressure equalization vent diameter of 0.64 mm (No. 72 drill). Use of a 1.0 mm vent will be too wide because it will change the low-frequency response for earmolds with a short bore length (see Table 2–5). Even "tight" earmolds will provide some degree of "slit leak," which will attenuate the frequency response around 100 Hz by 6 dB and be reduced to 0 dB of attenuation at 250 Hz (Lybarger, 1979).

Low-Frequency Enhancement

Lybarger (1977, 1979) reported that measurements of venting on 2-cc couplers have shown an increase of low-frequency gain as vent diameter increases. However, when the measurements were performed on a Zwislocki coupler, the increase in low-frequency gain was not as apparent (Lybarger, 1979; Studebaker et al, 1978). As seen in Table 2–5, with the same 16.6 mm bore length described above, a 1.0 mm vent will increase gain at 250 to 300 Hz with little effect on the frequency response above 500 Hz. A 2.0 mm vent will increase gain at 250 to 300 Hz with little effect on the frequency response above 500 Hz. A 2.0 mm vent will result in greater low-frequency attenuation below 500 Hz and increased gain between 500 and 700 Hz. A 3.0 mm vent will not provide amplification above the vent-associated resonance but will provide greater attenuation below 550 Hz. Similar low-frequency enhancement is seen for long (22.0 mm) and short (12.2 mm) bore lengths.

Moderate Low-Frequency Reduction

A 2.0 mm vent will provide considerable low-frequency reduction below 500 Hz, depending on the length of the sound bore (see Table 2–5). As the vent size increases, the height of the vent-associated resonance is increased. To reduce or eliminate the undesired peak, Lybarger (1977, 1979, 1980) recommended placing light cloth damping over the lateral end of the vent.

Strong Low-Frequency Reduction

As a general rule, a medium size vent is 1.6 to 2.4 mm wide. A vent this wide will reduce amplification below 500 Hz and result in a vent-associated resonance that will increase

TABLE 2–5 Vent minus unvented response (dB) for simulated earmolds using parallel and diagonal vents (1–3 mm) with bore lengths (L) of 6.0 mm, 12.2 mm, 16.6 mm, and 22 mm and bore diameters (D) of 1.0 mm, 2.0 mm, and 3.0 mm as measured in a DB 100 coupler

Bore L		Parallel Vents											
		6.0			12.2			16.6			22.0		
Vent D	1	2	3	1	2	3	1	2	3	1	2	3
Freq (Hz)													
200	–8	–22	–29	–2	–17	–25	0	–15	–23	2	–14	–22
250	—	—	—	4	–13	–20	6	–11	–19	6	–10	–18
315	—	—	—	7	–8	–16	6	–6	–14	5	–4	–13
400	8	–9	–16	5	–2	–12	4	0	–10	3	3	–8
500	6	–2	–11	3	6	–6	2	9	–4	2	9	–2
630	—	—	—	2	9	1	1	5	5	1	5	6
800	1	5	1	1	3	4	1	2	3	0	1	1
1000	1	4	1	1	3	3	1	3	3	0	2	2
1250	1	3	4	0	2	4	0	2	4	0	1	3
1600	0	2	3	0	1	3	0	1	2	0	1	2

Bore L	Diagonal Vents					
			16.6		22.0	
Vent D			1	2	3	1	2	3
200	–6	–15	–21	–8	–17	–23
250	0	–11	–17	–2	–13	–20
315	6	–4	–11	4	–6	–13
400	6	3	–5	5	1	–7
500	3	6	2	2	4	2
630	1	2	3	0	0	–1
800	0	0	–1	–1	–2	–3
1000	–1	–1	–2	–1	0	–4
1250	–1	–2	–4	–2	–4	–6
1600	–1	–2	–5	–3	–5	–8

For the two diagonal configurations, vent length was 11.9 mm, while the bore length medial to the intersection was 6.3 mm and 11.7 mm, respectively, for the 16.6 mm and 22 mm conditions.
(+) measured SPL is greater.
(–) measured coupler SPL is less.
Lybarger, 1985; Mueller et al, 1992.

amplification at 500 to 1000 Hz. As a general rule, a large size vent is 3.2 to 4.0 mm, which will reduce amplification below 500 Hz, and its vent-associated resonance will increase amplification at 500 to 1000 Hz (see Table 2–5). A wide-short vent will provide strong low-frequency reduction. Extreme low-frequency reduction will occur with an open or nonoccluding earmold. The magnitude of low-frequency reduction will be 25 dB at 250 Hz with a cutoff at 500 Hz. For a long bore (22 mm), there will be an 18 dB reduction at 250 Hz, and the cut-off frequency begins at 800 Hz (Lybarger, 1977, 1979, 1980; Staab & Nunley, 1982).

Extreme Low-Frequency Reduction

For patients with normal-hearing up to 1500 Hz, the use of a tube fitting would be very appropriate because it provides the greatest low-frequency reduction and greatest high-frequency enhancement. For maximum benefit of this strategy, the diameter of the tubing should be wide and the depth of insertion minimal.

Length and Diameter of Vents

The length of the vent is related to the length of the bore and is not really the critical factor in decisions concerning vents. However, as a general rule, as bore length increases, there is less low-frequency attenuation when vent diameter is held constant (see Table 2–5). The crucial decision is usually the diameter of the vent. Chasin (1983b) reported that venting can create a high-frequency antiresonance (notch) that may fall within the frequency range of the hearing aid. All vents have a characteristic vent-associated antiresonance frequency that produces a decrease in gain and whose frequency depends on the length and volume of the vent. The frequency of this vent-associated antiresonance is inversely related to the effective length of the vent. Shortening the effective length of the vent may increase the frequency of the antiresonance until it is above the frequency response of most hearing aids. As a general rule, for each 1.0 mm decrease in vent length, the frequency of the vent-associated antiresonance is increased by 400 Hz. One effective way to eliminate the vent-associated antiresonance is to bell the vent at the medial side of the earmold.

Another issue related to vent diameter is how much gain is available as the diameter is increased before feedback is present. Lybarger (1977) measured the SPL at a point 2.5 cm from the tip of the earmold in which the length of the sound bore was described as "short." He reported that maximum gain before feedback using a 0.8 mm vent was 43 dB, with a reserve gain of 10 dB. For a 3.2 mm vent, maximum gain before feedback was reduced to 36 dB, with a reserve gain of 10 dB.

Finally, as vent length is decreased, a segment of the frequency response exists at which no further reduction in gain is caused by the presence of the vent. This is referred to by some as the high-frequency cutoff. For example, in Table 2–5, when the vent length is 22 mm, the high-frequency cutoff for a 2 mm vent is approximately 315 Hz. However, when the vent is shortened to 6 mm, the high-frequency cutoff is increased to approximately 500 Hz. Also, as the vent length is decreased, attenuation of the low-frequency response is increased (Egolf, 1980; Lybarger, 1985; Mynders, 1985). This latter effect also occurs when the vent is widened.

Types of Venting
Diagonal versus Parallel Venting

Aside from deciding the length or diameter of the vent, the audiologist needs to inform the earmold laboratory if the vent should run parallel (lower example of Fig. 2–29) to the sound bore or if the vent needs to intersect (i.e., diagonal; see upper example in Fig. 2–29) the sound bore at some point between the lateral and medial end. Most research indicates that the primary choice should be a parallel vent because a diagonal vent, relative to a parallel vent, will decrease high-frequency gain by as much as 10 dB and the effect increases as vent diameter increases (see Table 2–5). Most researchers recommend diagonal venting only if space limitation (i.e., narrow earcanal) prevent the use of a parallel vent. If a diagonal vent is the only choice, minimizing high-frequency reduction can

be achieved by ordering a shorter bore length or having the vent intersect the sound bore as close to the medial end possible and then belling the final section of the sound bore Cox, 1979; Egolf, 1980; Studebaker & Cox, 1977; Valente, 1984, 1984c).

> ### PITFALL
>
> **Always order an earmold or shell with a parallel vent. A diagonal vent or intersecting vent will reduce the high-frequency response**

Studebaker and Cox (1977) and Cox (1979) reported the results of measuring the effects of parallel versus diagonal venting on three earmolds measured in a Zwislocki coupler and the real-ear. One earmold had a parallel vent of 16.8 mm. The second earmold had a diagonal vent that was 13.2 mm long and intersected the sound bore 7.6 mm from tip of the earmold. The third earmold had a diagonal vent 8.5 mm long and intersected the sound bore 9.5 mm from the tip of the earmold. Results for the parallel vent showed the expected reduction in low-frequency output below 400 Hz, and a vent-associated resonance as was measured with the parallel vent. However, above the vent-associated resonance there was a 3- to 5-dB attenuation of 3000 Hz. For the second diagonal condition, there was greater low-frequency reduction and a similar vent-associated resonance. However, there was a 10- to 11-dB attenuation in output between 2000 Hz to 3000 Hz. Thus the three venting conditions yielded similar

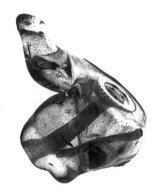

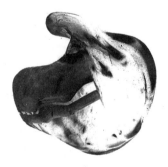

Figure 2–29 Example of diagonal (*upper*) and parallel (*lower*) venting.

low-frequency reduction and vent-associated resonances, but the diagonal vent revealed high-frequency attenuation that increased as the point of intersection moved more laterally in the sound bore. Above the vent-associated resonant frequency, the parallel vent did not reduce high-frequency gain, whereas the diagonal vent did yield greater reduction in high-frequency transmission as the point of diagonal vent did yield greater reduction in high-frequency transmission as the point of intersection was moved more laterally. The magnitude of the high-frequency loss in diagonal vents is related to the diameter of the vent in relation to the diameter of the sound bore. As seen in Table 2–5, reduction in high-frequency gain increases as the vent diameter increases when vent length is held constant. Furthermore, the loss of high-frequency transmission can be as great as 15- to 20-dB if the diagonal vent intersects the main sound bore at a very lateral position and the diameter of the vent is large (3 mm or greater).

Studebaker and Zachman (1970) reported that as the diameter of the diagonal vent increased (0.75 mm, 1.5 mm, and 3.0 mm) there was (1) greater low-frequency attenuation, (2) a shift in the vent-associated resonance to a higher frequency, (3) amplitude of the vent-associated resonance became greater, and (4) greater reduction in high-frequency transmission. During real-ear measures, there was the same low-frequency reduction as was measured in the 2-cc coupler, but the height of the vent-associated resonances was smaller or was not present.

External Venting

Occasionally, the dimensions of the earcanal will be so small that neither parallel nor diagonal venting can be used. In these cases, a "V-shaped groove" can be cut into the bottom surface of the earmold from the outside to the tip. This method of venting is also suggested in cases where the ear may be draining.

PEARL

We routinely order "groove venting" for all CIC fittings. This has significantly reduced the OE in many of our fittings. In addition, it is much easier to remove cerumen from a groove vent than the pressure vent available in most CIC fittings.

Custom Venting

For audiologists who prefer to specify the exact length and diameter of venting, Table 2–6 can be used for ordering vent sizes to specify the vent cutoff frequency at either 250, 500, 750, or 1000 Hz. For example, if the audiologist wants the low-frequency attenuation to extend to 1000 Hz (i.e., greater low-frequency reduction because the patient has normal or near-normal-hearing at 1000 Hz and below), he or she could specify that the bore length should be 8.9 mm and the vent diameter should be 3.0 mm. To achieve the same degree of low-frequency attenuation in an earmold with a shorter bore (i.e., 4.4 mm), the vent diameter would be reduced to 2.1

TABLE 2–6 Custom venting

Frequency (Hz)	Vent Diameter (mm)	Vent Length (mm)
250	1.1	17.8
	0.8	8.9
	0.5	4.4
500	2.2	17.8
	1.5	8.9
	1.1	4.4
750	3.0	17.8
	2.3	8.9
	1.6	4.4
1000	4.3	17.8
	3.0	8.9
	2.1	4.4
	1.5	2.2

Adapted from Microsonic, 1994.

mm. For example, let us assume the patient has some hearing loss in the lower frequencies and the audiologist wants less low-frequency attenuation. In the case of the patient with the longer bore (8.9 mm), the audiologist would order a vent diameter of 0.8 mm. In the case of the patient with the shorter bore length (4.4 mm), the audiologist would order a vent diameter of 0.5 mm.

Adjustable Venting

As mentioned earlier, it is our strong belief that virtually all earmolds/shells should be delivered to the patient with some degree of venting. An issue to consider is should the diameter of the vent be fixed or should the audiologist order a method of adjustable venting to better meet the needs of the patient and the audiologist? The next section will discuss several methods to vary the vent diameter at the time of the hearing aid fitting.

Variable-Venting-Valve

Although not commonly used today, Griffing (1971) and Griffing and Shields (1972) introduced the Variable-Venting-Valve (VVV), which is a gold-plated, brass-tooled threaded valve that is recessed in the earmold in a cavity 4.0 mm deep and 6.4 mm wide. The valve is manipulated by the user to adjust the low-frequency response yielding the most pleasing sound quality for that listening situation. The valve can be rotated 540 degrees from fully open to fully closed. By rotating the valve, the piston is simply moved from a point where it completely seals the 1.5 mm vent to a point where the vent is fully open.

Cooper et al (1975) reported that the VVV was ineffective in reducing low-frequency gain at 400 to 900 Hz in 12 patients, regardless of whether the earmolds had parallel or diagonal vents. These results are not unexpected in view of the fact that the range of adjusting the diameter of the vent is only 1.5 mm from fully open to fully closed.

Select-A-Vent

In the past, audiologists often drilled their own vents on a trial-and-error basis. Table 2–7 provides guidelines for readers who may wish to drill their own vents and the drill size required to accomplish the task. Figure 2–30 illustrates examples of drill sets used in our facility to vent and modify earmolds and shells. Today, however, most audiologists order earmolds or shells with either PVV, SAV, Select-A-Tube (Fig. 2–31), or Mini-SAV changeable venting systems, which eliminate the trial-and-error methods associated with drilling vent holes. For one manufacturer of ITE hearing aids, the ID of the Select-A-Tubes are 1.9 mm, 1.6 mm, 1.3 mm, 0.77 mm, and a plug. Variable venting techniques provide the audiologist with greater flexibility to experiment with different vent diameters and their effect on (a) reducing low-frequency gain, (b) reducing or eliminating the occlusion effect, (c) yielding better sound quality, and (d) reducing or eliminating feedback. This flexibility is permitted by merely inserting different-sized vent plugs (No. 1 to No. 5) or tubes that vary in ID and are inserted in a predrilled vent channel.

The SAV comes with a permanently installed clear styrene seating ring and a removable polythylene venting plug available in a "tree" of five sizes along with a solid plug. The insert channel for the SAV is 4.7 mm deep and 3.6 mm wide. For one

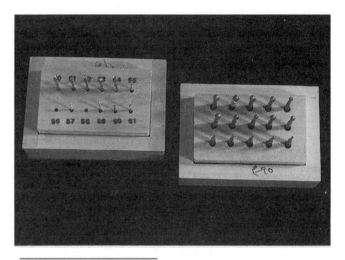

Figure 2–30 Examples of drill and burr sets used to modify earmolds and shells.

manufacturer, the diameters of the SAV inserts are 0.8 mm, 1.6 mm, 2.4 mm, 3.2 mm, and 4.0 mm for inserts No. 1 through No. 5, respectively. There is also a No. 6 insert that is used as a plug to close the vent (see Table 2–8). The SAV is also available from some earmold and hearing aid manufacturers in a mini-SAV format when the sound bore is unusually narrow. For one manufacturer, the diameters of the mini-SAV inserts are 0.5 mm, 0.8 mm, 1.0 mm, 1.6 mm, and 1.9 mm for inserts No. 1 through No. 5, respectively. There is also a No. 6 insert that is used as a plug to close the vent (see Table 2–8). It is important for the reader to understand that the relationship between insert number and the corresponding diameter may be different across manufacturers. In addition, the relationship between insert number and width of the vent may be the reverse from the one described previously. That is, in our clinic, the No. 1 insert has the narrowest diameter and the No. 6 insert plugs the vent. However, for another manufacturer, the No. 1 insert may plug the vent and the No. 6 insert may provide the widest diameter vent.

TABLE 2–7 Common drill sizes and the resulting vent diameter

Drill Size	Vent Diameter (mm)
31	3.17
33	2.93
47	2.00
53	1.57
61	1.00
65	0.89
68	0.79
70	0.72
75	0.54
76	0.51
80	0.35

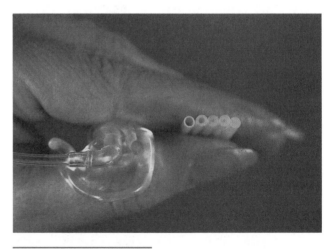

Figure 2–31 Examples of Select-A-Tube venting.

TABLE 2–8 Dimensions of Select-A-Vent (SAV), Mini-SAV, and Positive-Venting-Valve (PVV)

Type	Inches	mm
SAV PLUG		
1	0.031	0.8
2	0.062	1.6
3	0.095	2.4
4	0.125	3.2
5	0.156	4.0
6	closed	closed
MINI SAV PLUG		
1	0.020	0.5
2	0.030	0.8
3	0.040	1.0
4	0.060	1.6
5	0.075	1.9
6	closed	closed
PVV PLUG		
1	0.020	0.5
2	0.030	0.8
3	0.060	1.6
4	0.095	2.4
5	0.125	3.2
6	closed	closed

Adapted from Microsonic, 1994.

Positive-Venting-Valve

The PVV comes with a permanently installed clear styrene seating ring and a removable polythylene venting plug that is available in a "tree" of five sizes along with a solid plug. Compared with the SAV, the PVV has an insert channel that is shorter and wider (2.5 mm deep and 4.0 mm wide). For one manufacturer, the diameters of the PVV inserts are 0.5 mm, 0.8 mm, 1.6 mm, 2.4 mm, and 3.2 mm for inserts No. 1 through No. 5, respectively. There is also a No. 6 insert, which is used as a plug to close the vent (see Table 2–8). Again, the audiologist needs to be careful because earmold laboratories may offer PVV inserts where the order is reversed (i.e., the smallest number insert has the widest vent size and the largest number insert has the narrowest vent size), and the vent diameters may vary slightly from the diameters provided earlier.

SAV versus PVV

For both the PVV and SAV systems there is little change in the low-frequency response between inserts No. 1 to No. 3. However, some differences in low-frequency reduction will occur between inserts No. 4 to No. 5 (Cox, 1979; Killion, 1988a; Lybarger, 1979, 1980, 1985; Mynders, 1985; Valente & de Jonge, 1981). These same researchers favored using the PVV because the PVV uses a shorter and wider insert cup for the vent inserts. These researchers believe that for variable venting systems to work properly, the vent channel must be short and wide so that the vent response will be controlled by the vent hole in the insert rather than the vent channel

itself. If the vent channel is long and narrow (i.e., SAV), changing from one vent insert to another will make little difference in the low-frequency response. It appears that the PVV offers greater low-frequency attenuation because of its shorter and wider insert channel.

Auston et al (1990a,b) reported in separate articles on the differences in real-ear versus 2-cc coupler responses for 47 earmolds with 157 different modifications. They reported that the PW and SAV revealed very small differences in low-frequency reduction between any insert size and the mid-frequency vent-associated resonant peak measured in the coupler was not observed in the real ear. Finally, in agreement with past findings, Austin et al (1990a,b) concluded that the PVV provides greater low-frequency attenuation than the SAV.

Additional Issues Associated with Venting

Intentional versus Unintentional Vents

The level of the signal reaching the eardrum is a result of combing two paths of sound. One path is the "unaided path" where the signal passes through the vent ("intentional vent") and leaks ("unintentional vent") and reaches the eardrum unaided. The second path is the "aided path," where the intensity level of the signal at the eardrum is provided by the hearing aid. Concurrently, these two paths have some of the amplified sound passing to "the outside" through the same vent and leaks to reduce the SPL at the eardrum in a narrow frequency region. At any frequency in which the intensity of one path exceeds the intensity of other path by 20 dB or more, the path with the lesser intensity has an insignificant effect on the total intensity at the eardrum (less than 1 dB). However, at any frequency where the two intensities are within 20 dB of each other, the manner in which the two intensities combine depends on the phase relationship between the two paths. At a frequency where the two paths have equal intensity (often at 250 to 750 Hz), the in phase addition of the two paths will yield an intensity level that is 6 dB higher than the intensity within each path. At frequencies where the two paths are 180 degrees out of phase, there will be a strong attenuation of the signal. The magnitude of the vent effect depends on the dimensions of the vent, the properties of the earcanal and eardrum, and response of the hearing aid. In addition, the presence of vents can sharpen high-frequency resonant peaks so that a rounded response measured in a coupler, with the vent closed, can appear as a sharp peak in the real-ear aided response (Revit, 1994). The degree of "sharpening" of the vent-associated resonant peak from suboscillatory feedback depends on the dimensions of the vent and the earcanal, as well as the impedance of the eardrum. One method to reduce the height of the vent-associated resonant peak is to reduce the diameter of the vent.

Suboscillatory Feedback

Cox (1982) reported that vented earmolds may cause feedback at lower volume control settings than closed molds. This can prevent the user from achieving the desired gain caused by the interference of feedback. In addition, one common practice used by many hearing aid users to adjust the volume control wheel is to rotate the volume control until audible feedback occurs and then "back off" slightly. This strategy may create suboscillatory feedback, which creates a frequency response marked by numerous peaks and troughs. It is clear that the practice of setting the volume control just below the point of audible feedback can have a significant deleterious impact on the frequency response of the hearing aid. If a patient complains that the hearing aid "echoes" or "rings," he or she is probably experiencing suboscillatory feedback.

PITFALL

A common practice is to adjust the volume controls at a position just below where feedback is heard. However, suboscillatory feedback may be present at this setting, which can lead to reduced sound quality and speech intelligibility. It is best to counsel the patient to adjust the volume controls to where speech is comfortably loud.

Acoustic versus Electronic Low-Frequency Attenuation

Audiologists can control the low-frequency response by means of (1) a tone control in combination with a closed mold (electronic tuning) (see Fig. 2–32), (2) use of venting in combination with a hearing aid having a wideband frequency response (acoustical tuning), or (3) combining strategies 1 and 2 where low-frequency output is controlled by the tone control and the vent may or may not provide additional low-frequency attenuation. The first strategy provides a very efficient way to predict low-frequency attenuation. Use of the second strategy is not as strong in predicting low-frequency attenuation. This second method, as mentioned earlier, adds a mid-frequency vent-associated resonant peak and the possibility of altering the frequency response because of audible and suboscillatory feedback, which does not occur with a closed mold.

Cox and Alexander (1983) recorded speech in KEMAR with a hearing aid coupled to closed molds, vented molds, and open molds with the output from KEMAR matched for the different mold conditions. They used a paired comparison paradigm of sound quality and speech intelligibility judgments for connected discourse presented at 65 dB with

signal-to-noise ratios of +5 and +20 dB. They evaluated nine hearing aids, which were divided into three groups, depending on the cutoff frequency (i.e., below 750 Hz, between 750 Hz to 1000, and above 1000 Hz). They evaluated 15 subjects who had normal-hearing in the low frequencies and greater hearing loss in the higher frequencies. Results revealed that the subjects had a slight preference for the electronic modification strategy if the cutoff frequency was less than 750 Hz. However, they had a strong preference for the acoustic tuning strategy (venting) when the cutoff frequency was between 750 to 1000 Hz and an even greater preference for venting when the cutoff frequency was greater than 1000 Hz. These findings were the same for both signal-to-noise ratio conditions and for sound quality or speech intelligibility judgments.

Mackenzie and Browning (1991) evaluated 83 inexperienced subjects with mild-to-moderate severe sensorineural hearing loss. When subjects had normal-hearing to 1000 Hz, they generally preferred combining venting and high-frequency emphasis to achieve the desired balance between low-frequency and high-frequency amplification rather than only relying on the tone control. For subjects having a flatter audiometric configuration from 250 to 4000 Hz, no consistent preferences were present.

Mackenzie and Browning (1989) reported on real-ear measures in 43 ears and found that adjusting the tone control between normal and high-frequency emphasis has less effect in the real-ear than in the 2-cc coupler. Adding a 2 mm vent and returning the tone control to the normal position reduced the output by an average of 8 dB at 750 Hz to 1000 Hz. By turning the tone control to high-frequency emphasis and using an earmold with a 2 mm vent, the low-frequency reduction was extended to 10 dB in the same frequency region.

Perceptual Consequence of Vents

Lundberg et al (1992) evaluated nine subjects with normal-hearing. They reported no difference in sound quality for vented and unvented earmolds while listening to male and female recordings of connected discourse in quiet and noise. Four subjects reported that the unvented earmolds sounded louder than the vented earmolds, and there was an overall tendency of preferring the sound quality produced by the vented condition.

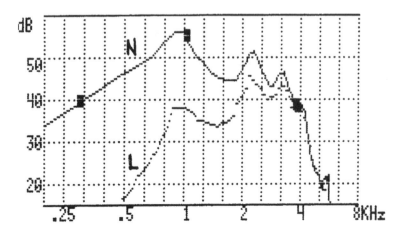

Figure 2–32 Frequency response of a hearing aid when the tone control was rotated for the broadest response (*N*) and the greatest low-frequency attenuation (*L*).

McClellan (1967), Davis and Green (1975), and Kuk (1991) reported higher word recognition scores in noise when venting was introduced to the earmold. However, Revoile (1968), Hodgson and Murdock (1972), and Northern and Hattler (1970) did not report significant improvement in word recognition scores with the introduction of venting. Kuk (1991) evaluated nine subjects with mild-to-moderate severe sensorineural hearing loss using unvented and vented (2.2 mm parallel vent) earmolds. Using a paired comparison strategy and a programmable hearing aid, the subjects shaped their preferred REIR while listening to connected discourse presented at 70 dB SPL. Results indicated that the preferred REIR was similar for the two earmold conditions. However, sound quality for the "clarity" judgment was significantly better for the vented condition. When reading aloud, most subjects preferred the vented condition. No significant differences were found in word recognition scores for W-22 word lists presented at 70 dB SPL. Kuk (1991) concluded that although electronic tuning can be beneficial to ensure that measured REIR matches prescribed REIR, venting is necessary to improve user satisfaction.

Venting in Custom Hearing Aids

Up to this point, the issue of venting has been presented in terms of venting an earmold. Similar decisions need to be made by the audiologist when fitting custom hearing aids. In a custom product, the length of tubing from the output of the receiver to the tip of the shell is typically 10 to 12 mm long and 1 to 2 mm wide (Lybarger, 1985). Preves (1980) described a dual tubing, or stepped bore, arrangement for

an ITE that increased the high-frequency response. In this design, the tubing at the receiver is 6.4 mm long and 1.4 mm wide, which increases to a width of 3.6 mm for the second section. In addition, a 2200 Ω fused mesh damper is placed at the receiver to smooth the frequency response. For short-bore shells, the 3.6 mm segment of tubing is extended beyond the tip of the shell to maintain the desired acoustic effect. Further increases in the high-frequency response can occur as the diameter of the tubing of the second segment is increased (Staab & Lybarger, 1994). To accommodate the damping needs for ITEs, Knowles Electronics has four dampers that fit into cups with outside diameters of 1.12 mm, 1.25 mm, 1.37 mm, and 1.78 mm to fit inside the narrow ID of tubing used in custom hearing aids from the receiver to the tip of the shell. These dampers are available in acoustic resistance of 330 to 3300 Ω for the 1.78 mm diameter cup and 680 or 1500 Ω for the 1.25 mm diameter cup. These dampers have a greater effect on smoothing the second peak instead of the first peak, which is common for BTE fittings (Staab & Lybarger, 1994).

Tecca (1991) believes that most of the research on venting for ITEs carefully eliminated slit-leak effects. In actual use, slit leaks are quite common in ITE fittings. He found that the effect of slit leaks is predominantly at 200 Hz (see Table 2–9). He performed real-ear measures on 10 subjects whose earcanals had an average earcanal length of 22.6 mm and a mean bore length of 8.2 mm. He used vent diameters of 1.3 mm, 2.0 mm, and 3.0 mm. For the 1.3- and 2.0 mm vents, the attenuation was restricted to below 1000 Hz (see Table 2–9).

TABLE 2–9 Mean and standard deviation (in parentheses) of the real-ear vent effects (dB) for three vent diameters (mm) relative to the occluded condition for ITE hearing aids when no sealing (Section A) or sealing (Section B) was placed around the shell of the ITE (Tecca, 1991)

| Diameter | Frequency (Hz) | | | | |
	200	500	1000	1500	2000
A. No Sealing					
1.3 mm	−7.1(3.1)	0.3(2.9)	1.5(0.7)	0.5(0.6)	0.1(0.5)
2.0 mm	−11.1(3.9)	−0.9(3.6)	1.9(0.9)	0.7(0.7)	0.2(0.8)
3.0 mm	−21.9(4.0)	−10.5(3.2)	3.1(2.8)	2.6(1.7)	1.9(0.9)
B. Sealing with E.A.R. Rings					
1.3 mm	−6.8(2.2)	2.8(1.3)	0.8(0.6)	0.3(0.4)	−0.2(0.9)
2.0 mm	−12.1(2.5)	2.2(3.5)	1.7(0.7)	0.6(0.7)	0.3(0.9)
3.0 mm	−25.0(2.6)	−9.8(3.2)	5.1(2.0)	2.9(1.4)	2.0(0.7)
C. Diameter (mm) × Length (mm) (Tecca, 1992)					
0.45 × 22	−4.9(2.6)	0.5(2.0)	0.7(0.8)	0.1(0.9)	0.0(0.8)
0.95 × 22	−9.2(2.0)	2.8(2.5)	1.7(0.7)	0.6(1.1)	0.5(0.7)
1.45 × 22	−12.1(2.1)	1.5(3.9)	2.3(1.0)	1.0(1.1)	0.8(0.7)
2.0 × 22	−13.9(1.7)	0.6(4.0)	2.9(1.3)	1.4(1.1)	1.0(0.7)
2.0 × 16	−15.8(2.3)	−3.7(4.5)	2.5(1.4)	0.9(1.2)	0.3(1.0)
2.0 × 10	−18.9(2.5)	−7.9(3.7)	1.8(1.7)	1.0(1.2)	−0.1(1.5)
2.0 × 4	−22.6(2.9)	−11.4(4.7)	0.7(2.0)	1.5(2.0)	0.3(1.4)
3.0 × 4	−24.6(1.8)	−13.4(3.0)	0.1(2.6)	2.2(2.2)	0.9(1.2)

Section C reports the mean and standard deviation (in parentheses) of the real-ear vent effects (dB) for five vent diameters (mm) and four lengths (mm) (Tecca, 1992).

The attenuation provided by the 3.0 mm vent extended one octave higher (see Table 2–9). When E.A.R. seal rings were used to minimize the effect of slit leak, there was only a slight attenuation of low-frequency gain (see Section B, Table 2–9). In addition, the standard deviation shown in Table 2–9 (0.4- to 4-dB) reveals minimal intersubject variability. Therefore the ability to predict vent effects for a particular individual is rather good. Finally, as reported before, as vent diameter is increased, there is greater low-frequency attenuation, and the vent-associated resonant frequency increases. Table 2–9 indicates that the vent-associated resonance increased for the 1.3 mm and 2.0 mm vent between the sealed and unsealed conditions, but the effect of sealing was minimal for the 3.0 mm vent.

In another study, Tecca (1992) reported that most variable venting systems for custom hearing aids use vent inserts of varying IDs, which are inserted into the lateral end of the vent channel. He evaluated 10 subjects when shells were manufactured having a bore length of 22 mm and vent diameters of 0.45, 0.95, and 1.45 mm. A second condition was where the vent diameter was constant 2.0 mm and vent lengths were 4.0 mm, 10.0 mm, 16.0 mm, and 22.0 mm. A final condition was where there was a vent diameter of 3 mm and vent length of 4 mm. Results revealed (Section C, Table 2–9) that the degree of attenuation at 200 Hz increased as vent diameter increased from 0.45 mm to 1.45 mm and length was held constant at 22 mm. Minimal attenuation occurred above 200 Hz. When vent diameter was held constant at 2.0 mm, attenuation increased as bore length decreased and the vent-associated resonance increased in frequency. Also, differences in the magnitude of low-frequency attenuation

TABLE 2–10   Troubleshooting chart

Problem	Possible Solutions
1. Soreness/discomfort	a. Canal/shell modifications b. New impression c. Hypoallergenic material d. Allergy coating (Verglassen)
2. Allergic reaction	a. Coat shell with hypoallergenic nail polish b. Remake impression for Lucite earmold c. Order hypoallergenic material
3. Too tight	a. Grind/buff areas that may be causing the tightness b. New impression
4. Too loose	a. Buildup shell with Addco Addon (soft or hard) b. New impression
5. Hole/crack in shell	a. Patch with polymer-monomer mix
6. Occlusion effect	a. Wider vent diameter b. Provide a deep canal fit c. Bell the bore d. Reduce low-frequency gain e. Use MCT material f. Increase crossover frequency
7. Tinny or harsh	a. Insert filter in receiver or microphone b. Shift high frequencies with a resonant peak control c. Reduce vent and add filter d. Reduce low-frequency gain e. Reduce crossover frequency f. Reduce high-frequency output g. Increase compression ratio h. Reduce high-frequency gain
8. Too much bass	a. Wider vent b. Reduce low-frequency gain c. Increase crossover frequency
9. Too loud	a. Reduce output with output control b. Reduce gain c. Insert filter in receiver d. Widen the vent e. Reduce compression ratio f. Reduce compression kneepoint

between adjacent vent diameters were 3- to 5-dB at 200 Hz and the effect was predominantly less than 500 Hz. Recall that Cox and Alexander (1983) suggested using electronic tuning instead of acoustic tuning to enhance user satisfaction when the cutoff frequency was less than 750 Hz for venting to result in greater user satisfaction. Finally, Tecca reported that the vent-associated resonance shifted to a higher fre-

quency as vent diameter increased and the mean amplitude varied between 2.0- to 5.1-dB.

Vent diameters for custom hearing aids can also be changed by inserting silicone tubes of different internal diameters into the vent channel (Copeland et al, 1986). This, for example, is the method used by ReSound Corporation for its custom hearing aids. This method of venting has the

TABLE 2–10   (continued)   Troubleshooting chart

Problem	Possible Solutions
10. Too soft	a. Check battery b. Excessive cerumen c. Defective microphone d. Increase overall gain/output e. Increase low-frequency gain f. Increase compression kneepoint g. Decrease compression ratio h. Reduce vent diameter i. Check for excessive battery drain j. Check earcanal for debris k. Check receiver tube for debris l. Clean/replace filter in receiver tube m. Check for moisture
11. Windnoise	a. Use windscreen or windhood b. Place foam in the microphone port c. Decrease high-frequency gain or output
12. Internal feedback	a. Check for loose receiver tube b. Check for hole in vent c. Check for pushed-in receiver tube d. Send for repair
13. External feedback	a. Check for excessive cerumen b. Reduce vent size with SAV, PVV, or REVV (tube vents) c. Buildup or lengthen canal d. Coat shell with non-petroleum-based oil ("soft seal") e. Use receiver extension tubing f. Add damping g. Reduce canal length because tip may be against canal wall h. Reduce high-frequency output/gain i. Remake the earmold/shell j. Use ER-13R ring seals k. Use ER-13MF microphone filter l. Consider receiver extension tube
14. Distortion	a. Increase high-frequency output b. Lengthen high-frequency release time c. Replace microphone d. Circuit repair
15. Intermittent	a. Replace receiver/microphone b. Replace volume control c. Check for moisture buildup and recommend Dri-Aid kit d. Circuit repair
16. Excessive drain	a. Request lower battery drain from manufacturer b. Reduce gain or output c. Circuit repair

Riess and Guthier, 1986.

advantage of knowing that the diameter of the selected vent tube is uniform from the lateral to the medial end of the vent channel.

Problems with Cerumen

One of the most common problems in custom hearing aids is the buildup of cerumen in the tubing from the receiver. The presence of the cerumen will change the electroacoustic characteristics of the hearing aid or attenuate the output so the hearing aid appears "dead." Aside from the need to carefully counsel the patient on this problem and explain preventive measures, several methods have been introduced to help audiologists address this problem.

One recent solution has been the introduction of the Ad-Hear™ wax guards (Oliveira & Rose, 1994). These are easy-to-apply disposable filters that stick onto the shell of the hearing aid and are available in three sizes (ultra-slim, slim, standard, and large). Between the two adhesive strips is a filter that is placed over the tubing opening from the receiver to prevent cerumen from entering the tubing. Reportedly, the Ad-Hear™ wax guards do not change the frequency response of the hearing aid and will last for 1 week before they need to be changed (Oliveira & Rose, 1994). Another solution is a "cerumen filter system." In this case, a small plastic "lid" is pressed into place over the receiver opening. These filters arrive in a pack of 10, and each filter lasts about 1 week.

Audiologists must understand that it is very expensive for manufacturers to replace receivers because of contamination from cerumen. Thus manufacturers have numerous wax guard options available for audiologists to consider. These options include "wax baskets," "spring dampers," or "element dampers," which are placed in the receiver opening to prevent cerumen from reaching the receiver. These devices are reportedly acoustically transparent in that they did not change the frequency response. However, REIR responses at our facility revealed that using a "wax basket" from one manufacturer decreased the real-ear gain around 3000 Hz by nearly 6 dB. Therefore this facility routinely orders translucent receiver tubing and has it extend 3 mm to 4 mm past the tip of the shell (see Fig 2–27). This allows the patient to "see"

the buildup of cerumen and remove it with a "wax loop" before a buildup creates a problem. In addition, the extended receiver tube places the output from the hearing aid slightly closer to the eardrum. This reduces the volume control setting necessary to achieve a comfortable setting and also reduces the likelihood of feedback.

Problems and Solutions

Fitting hearing aids can bring pride and satisfaction for audiologists because of the opportunity to make life more enjoyable and satisfactory for their patients. However, the road to successful fittings will not always be smooth and unchallenging. Table 2–10 lists an array of problems brought to our attention from patients. Also provided are some solutions that have been used successfully to address and correct these problems. Sometimes these solutions eliminate the problem and result in greater user satisfaction. Sometimes these solutions only partially solve the problem, but the degree of improvement is sufficient to make the problem less troublesome. On more occasions than we care to admit, the solutions do not solve the problem, and the patient feels that the problem is sufficiently great enough to discontinue use of amplification. Also, sometimes the solution to one problem can create a previously nonexistent problem. For example, one solution for eliminating the occlusion effect is to widen the vent. It is entirely possible that this solution could result in feedback. As mentioned earlier, the road to successful fittings is not always smooth, but it is challenging.

CONCLUSIONS

It has been stated more than once that fitting hearing aids is an art, as well as a science. It is our belief that greater knowledge of the transmission line's role in shaping the electroacoustic characteristics of hearing aids will help in improving the artistic and dispensing audiologists. It is hoped the information contained within this chapter will provide dispensing audiologists with some of the tools necessary to become better artists and scientists.

REFERENCES

AGNEW, J. (1986). Earmold impression stability *Hearing Instruments, 37*(12);8,11–12.

AGNEW, J. (1994). Acoustic advantages of deep canal hearing aid fittings. *Hearing Instruments, 45*(6);22,24,25.

ALVORD, L.S., DOXEY, G.P. & SMITH, D.S. (1989). Hearing aids worn with tympanic membrane perforations: Complications and solutions. *American Journal of Otolaryngology, 10*(4);277–280.

ALVORD, L.S., MORGAN, R., & CARTWRIGHT, K. (1997). Anatomy of an earmold: A formal terminology. *Journal of the American Academy of Audiology, 8*;100–103.

AMERICAN NATIONAL STANDARDS INSTITUTE. (1987a). *Specifications of hearing aid characteristics (ANSI S3.22–1987).* New York: ANSI

AMERICAN NATIONAL STANDARDS INSTITUTE. (1987b). *Preferred earhook nozzle thread for postauricular hearing aids (ANSI S3.37–1987).* New York: ANSI.

AUSTIN, C.D., KASTEN, R.N., & WILSON, H. (1990a). Real-ear measures of hearing aid plumbing modifications, Part I. *Hearing Instruments, 43*(3);18,20–22.

AUSTIN, C.D., KASTEN, R.N., & WILSON, H. (1990b). Real-ear measures of hearing aid plumbing modifications, Part II.

Hearing Instruments, 43(4);25–30.

AUSTIN, C.D., KASTEN, R.N., & WILSON, H. (1990c). Real-ear measures of hearing aid plumbing modifications, Part III. *Hearing Instruments, 43*(7);30–35.

BERGENSTOFF, H. (1983). Earmold design and its effect on real-ear insertion gain. *Hearing Instruments, 34*(9);46.

BERGER, K., HAGBERG, E., & LANE, R. (1998). *Prescription of hearing aids: Rationale, procedures and results* (5th ed.). Ohio: Herald Publishing House.

BRISKEY, R. J. (1982). Smoothing the frequency response of a hearing aid. *Hearing Aid Journal 3*;12–17.

BRYANT, M.P., MUELLER, H.G., & NORTHERN, J.L. (1991). Minimal contact long canal ITE hearing instruments. *Hearing Instruments, 42*(1);12–15.

BURGESS, N., & BROOKS, D.N. (1991). Earmoulds: Some benefits from horn fitting. *British Journal of Audiology, 25*;309–315.

CHASIN, M. (1983a) Using acoustic resistance in earmold tubing. *Hearing Instruments, 34*(12);18,20,54.

CHASIN, M. (1983b) Vent modification for added high-frequency sound transmission. *Hearing Journal, 6*;16–17.

COCKERILL, D. (1987). Allergies to earmoulds. *British Journal of Audiology, 21*;143–145.

COPELAND, A.B., BURRIS, P.D., & GRIFFING, T.S. (1986). Open fittings for canal and ITE hearing aids. *Hearing Instruments, 37*(4);6,8,11.

COOGIE, K.L. (1976). NAEL's standard terms for earmolds. *Hearing Aid Journal, 3*;5.

COOPER, W.A., FRANKS, J.R., McFALL, R.N., & GOLDSTEIN, D.P. (1975). Variable venting valve for earmolds. *Audiology, 14*; 259–267.

COURTOIS, J., JOHANSEN, P.A., LARSEN, B.V., CHRISTENSEN, P., & BEILIN, J. (1988). Open molds. In: J.H. Jensen (Ed.), *Hearing aid fittings: Theoretical and practical views* (pp. 175–200). 13th Danavox Symposium. Copenhagen: Stougaard Jensen.

COX, R.M. (1979). Acoustic aspects of hearing aid-earcanal coupling systems. *Monographs in Contemporary Audiology, 1*(3);1,44.

COX, R.M. (1982). Combined effects of earmold vents and sub-oscillatory feedback on hearing aid frequency response. *Ear and Hearing, 3*;12–17.

COX, R.M., & ALEXANDER, G.C. (1983). Acoustic versus electronic modifications of hearing aid low-frequency output. *Ear and Hearing, 4*;190–196.

COX, R.M., & GILMORE, C. (1986). Damping the hearing aid frequency response: Effects on speech clarity and preferred listening level. *Journal of Speech and Hearing Research, 29*; 357–365.

Custom Earmold Manual. (1994). Cambridge, PA: Microsonic Earmold Laboratory.

DALSGAARD, S.C. (1975). *Earmolds and Associated Problems.* Seventh Danavox Symposium. Stockholm: The Almqvist & Wiksell Periodical Co.

DAVIS, R., & GREEN, S. (1975). The influence of controlled venting on discrimination ability. *Hearing Aid Journal, 27*(5); 6,34–35.

DECKER, T.N. (1975). The relationship between speech discrimination performance and the use of sintered metal inserts in the hearing aid fitting. *Audecibel* (Summer); 118–123.

DE JONGE, R. (1983). Computer simulation of hearing aid frequency responses. *Hearing Journal, 3*;27–31.

DEMPSEY, J.J. (1990). The occlusion effect created by custom canal hearing aids. *American Journal of Otolaryngology, 11*(1);44–46.

DILLON, H. (1985). Earmolds and high-frequency response modification. *Hearing Instruments, 36*(12);8,11–12.

DILLION, H. (1991). Allowing for real ear venting effects when selecting the coupler gain of hearing aids. *Ear and Hearing, 12*;406–416.

EGOLF, D.P. (1979a). Fundamentals of acoustics and acoustic wave interaction with the human head and ear. In: V.D. Larson, D.P. Egolf, R.L. Kirlin, S.W. Stile, & J.H. Jensen (Eds.), *Auditory and hearing prosthetics research* (pp. 19–37). New York: Grune and Stratton.

EGOLF, D.P. (1979b). Mathematical predictions of electro-acoustic frequency response of in-situ hearing aids. In: V.D. Larson, D.P. Egolf, R.L. Kirlin, S.W. Stile, & J.H. Jensen (Eds.), *Auditory and hearing prosthetics research* (pp. 411–450). New York: Grune and Stratton.

EGOLF, D.P. (1980). Techniques for modeling the hearing aid receiver and associated tubing. In: G.A. Studebaker, & I. Hochberg (Eds.), *Acoustical factors affecting hearing aid performance* (pp. 297–319). Baltimore, MD: University Park Press.

FERNANDES, C.C., & COOPER, K. (1983). Using a horn mold with severe to profound losses. *Hearing Instruments, 34*(12);6,54.

FRANK, T. (1980). Attenuation characteristics of hearing aid earmolds. *Ear and Hearing, 1*;161–166.

GASTMEIRER, W.J. (1981). The acoustically damped earhook. *Hearing Instruments, 32*(10);14–15.

GOLDSTEIN, B.A. (1980). Effects of discriminate and indiscriminate placement of sintered hearing aid filters. *Hearing Aid Journal, 3*;7,30,32,34.

GREEN, D.S. (1969). Non-occluding earmolds with CROS and IROS hearing aids. *Archives of Otolaryngology, 89*;96–106.

GREEN, D.S., & ROSS, M. (1968). The effect of conventional versus a nonoccluding earmold upon the frequency response of a hearing aid. *Journal Speech and Hearing Research, 11*;638–647.

GRIFFING, T.S. (1971). Variable venting of earmolds. *Hearing Dealer, 22*;23.

GRIFFING, T.S., & SHIELDS, J. (1972). Hearing aid performance and the earmold. *Hearing Dealer, 23*;6–9.

GUDMUNDSEN, G.I. (1994). Fitting CIC hearing aids: Some practical pointers. *Hearing Journal, 47*(7);10,45–48.

HARFORD, E.R., & BARRY, J.A. (1965). A rehabilitative approach to the problem of unilateral hearing impairment: The contralateral routing of signals (CROS). *Journal of Speech and Hearing Disorders, 30*;121–138.

HARFORD, E.R., & DODDS, E. (1966). The clinical application of CROS: A hearing aid for unilateral deafness. *Archives of Otolaryngology, 83*;455–464.

HARFORD, E.R., & FOX, J. (1978). The use of high-pass amplification for broad-frequency sensorineural hearing loss. *Audiology, 17*;10–16.

HODGSON, W., & MURDOCK C. (1972). Effect of the earmold on speech intelligibility in hearing aid use. *Journal of Speech and Hearing Research, 13*;290–297.

HOSFORD-DUNN, H. (1996). A basic primer for fitting CICs. *Hearing Review, 3*(1);8,10,12.

KILLION, M.C. (1980). Problems in the application of broadband hearing aid earphones. In: G.A. Studebaker, & J. Hochberg (Eds.), *Acoustical factors affecting hearing aid performance* (1st ed.) (pp. 219–264). Baltimore, MD: University Park Press.

KILLION, M.C. (1981). Earmold options for wideband hearing aids. *Journal of Speech and Hearing Disorders, 46;*10–20.

KILLION, M.C. (1982). Transducers, earmolds and sound quality considerations. In: G.A. Studebaker, & F. Bess (Eds.), *The Vanderbilt hearing aid report* (pp. 104–111). Upper Darby, PA: Monographs in Contemporary Audiology.

KILLION, M.C. (1984). Recent earmolds for wideband OTE and ITE hearing aids. *Hearing Journal, 8;*15–18,20–22.

KILLION, M.C. (1988a). Earmold design: Theory and practice. In: J.H. Jensen (Ed.), *Hearing aid fittings: Theoretical and practical views* (pp. 155–172). 13th Danavox Symposium. Copenhagen: Stougaard Jensen.

KILLION, M.C. (1988b). Principles of high fidelity hearing aid amplification. In: R.E. Sandlin (Ed.), *Handbook of hearing aid amplification* (pp. 45–79). Boston: College-Hill Press.

KILLION, M.C. (1988c). Special fitting problems and open canal solutions. In: J.H. Jensen (Ed.), *Hearing aid fittings: Theoretical and practical views* (pp. 219–228). 13th Danavox Symposium. Copenhagen: Stougaard Jensen.

KILLION, M.C. (1988d). The "hollow voice" occlusion effect. In: J. H. Jensen (Ed.), *Hearing aid fittings: Theoretical and practical views* (pp. 231–242). 13th Danavox Symposium. Copenhagen: Stougaard Jensen.

KILLION, M.C., BERLIN, C.I., & HOOD, L. (1984). A low-frequency emphasis open canal hearing aid. *Hearing Instruments, 35(8);* 30,32,34,66.

KILLION, M.C., & MONSER, E.L. (1980). CORFIG: Coupler response for flat insertion gain. In: G.A. Studebaker, & H. Hochberg (Eds.), *Acoustical factors affecting hearing aid performance* (1st ed.) (pp. 149–168). Baltimore, MD: University Park Press.

KILLION, M.C., & REVIT, L.J. (1993). CORFIG and GIFROC: Real ear to coupler and back. In: G.A. Studebaker, & J. Hochberg (Eds.), *Acoustical factors affecting hearing aid performance* (2nd ed.) (pp. 65–85). Needham Heights, MA: Allyn & Bacon.

KILLION, M.C., & TILLMAN, T.W. (1982). Evaluation of high fidelity hearing aids. *Journal of Speech and Hearing Research, 25;*15–25.

KILLION, M.C., WILBER, L.A., & GUDMUNDSEN, G.I. (1988). Zwislocki was right. . . . *Hearing Instruments, 39(1);*28–30.

KILLION, M.C., & WILSON, D.L. (1985). Response modifying earhooks for special fitting problems. *Audecibel* (Fall); 28–30.

KONKLE, D.F., & BESS, F.H. (1974). Custom-made versus stock earmolds in hearing aid evaluations. *Archives of Otolaryngology, 99;*140–144.

KUK, F.K. (1991). Perceptual consequences of vents in hearing aids. *British Journal of Audiology, 25;*163–169.

KUK, F.K. (1994). Maximum usable real-ear insertion gain with ten earmold designs. *Journal of the American Academy of Audiology 5;*41–51.

LEAVITT, R. (1986). Earmolds: Acoustic and structural considerations. In: W.R. Hodgson (Ed.), *Hearing aid assessment and use in audiologic habilitation* (3rd ed.) (pp. 71–108). Baltimore, MD: Williams & Wilkins.

LETOWSKI, T.R., & BURCHFIELD, S.B. (1991). Study finds greater sound attenuation with silicon than Lucite earmolds. *Hearing Journal, 9;*18, 20–22.

LETOWSKI, T.R., BURCHFIELD, S.B., & HUME, S. (1991). Perceptual differences between earmold materials. *Hearing Instruments, 42(12);*14–16.

LETOWSKI, T.R., RICHARDS, W.D., & BURCHFIELD, S.B. (1992). Transmission of sound, vibration through earmold materials. *Hearing Instruments, 43(12);*11–15.

LIBBY, E.R. (1979). The importance of smoothness in hearing aid frequency response. *Hearing Instruments, 30(4);*20–22.

LIBBY, E.R., (1980). Smooth wideband hearing aid responses—the new frontier. *Hearing Instruments, 30(10);*12–13,15,18,43.

LIBBY, E.R. (1981). Achieving a transparent, smooth, wideband hearing aid response. *Hearing Instruments, 32(10);*9–12.

LIBBY, E.R. (1982). In search of transparent insertion gain hearing aid responses. In: G.A. Studebaker, & F. Bess (Eds.), *The Vanderbilt hearing aid report* (pp. 112–123). Upper Darby, PA: Monographs in Contemporary Audiology.

LIBBY, E.R. (1982). A reverse acoustic horn for severe-to-profound hearing impairments. *Hearing Instruments, 41(12);*29.

LUNDBERG, G., OVEGARD, A., HAGERMAN, B., GABRIELSSON, A., & BRANDSTROM, U. (1992). Perceived sound quality in a hearing aid with vented and closed earmould equalized in frequency response. *Scandinavian Audiology, 21;*87–92.

LYBARGER, S.F. (1977). Sound leakage from vented earmolds. *Hearing Aid Journal, 38;*28,29,40.

LYBARGER, S.F. (1979). Controlling hearing aid performance by earmold design. In: V.D. Larson, D.P. Egolf, R.L. Kirlin, & S.W. Stile (Eds.), *Auditory and hearing prosthetics research* (pp. 101–132). New York: Grune and Stratton.

LYBARGER, S.F. (1980). Earmold venting as an acoustic control factor. In: G.A. Studebaker, & J. Hockberg (Eds.), *Acoustical Factors affecting hearing aid performance* (1st ed.) (pp. 197–217). Baltimore. MD: University Park Press.

LYBARGER, S.F. (1985). Earmolds. In: J. Katz (Ed.), *Handbook of clinical audiology* (3rd ed.) (pp. 885–910). Baltimore, MD: Williams & Wilkins.

LYREGAARD, P.K. (1982). Improvement of the high-frequency performance of BTE hearing aids. *Hearing Instruments, 33(2);*38,40,43,62.

MACKENZIE, K., & BROWNING, G.G. (1989). The real-ear effect of adjusting the tone control and venting a hearing aid system. *British Journal of Audiology, 23;*93–98.

MACKENZIE, K., & BROWNING, G.G. (1991). Randomized cross over study to assess patient preference for an acoustically modified hearing aid system. *Journal of Laryngology, 105;* 405–408.

MACRAE, J. (1981). A new kind of earmold vent—the high cut cavity vent. *Hearing Instruments, 32(10);*18,64.

MACRAE, J. (1983). Acoustic modifications for better hearing aid fittings. *Hearing Instruments, 34(12);*8,11.

MACRAE, J. (1990). Static pressure seal of earmolds. *Journal of Rehabilitation Research and Development, 27;*397–410.

MACRAE, J. (1991). A comparison of the effects of different methods of impression buildup on earmolds. *British Journal of Audiology, 25;*183–199.

MADELL, J.R., & GENDEL, J.M. (1984). Earmolds for patients with severe and profound hearing loss. *Ear and Hearing, 5;*349–351.

McCLELLAN, M.E. (1967). Aided speech discrimination in noise with vented and unvented earmolds. *Journal of Audiology Research, 7;*93–99.

MEDING, B., & RINGDAHL, A. (1992). Allergic contact dermatitis from earmolds of hearing aids. *Ear and Hearing, 13;*122–124.

MEREDITH, R., THOMAS, K.J., CALLAGHAN, D.C., STEPHENS, S.D.G., & RAYMENT, A.J. (1989). A comparison of three types of earmoulds in elderly users of post-aural hearing aids. *British Journal of Audiology, 23;*239–244.

MORGAN, R. (1994). The art of making a good impression. *Hearing Review, 1*(3);10,13–14,24.

MUELLER, H.G., HAWKINS, D.B., & NORTHERN, J.L. (1992). *Probe microphone measurements: Hearing aid selection and assessment.* San Diego, CA: Singular Press.

MUELLER, H.G., SCHWARTZ, D.M., & SURR, R.K. (1981). The use of the exponential acoustic horn in an open mold configuration. *Hearing Instruments, 32*(10);16–17,67.

MULLIN, T.A., GORLIN, B.H., & LASSITER, B. (1986). Stethoscopes and earmolds. *Hearing Instruments, 37*(12);16–17.

MYNDERS, J. (1985). Human acoustic couplers. In: R.E. Sandlin (Ed.), *Hearing instrument science and fitting practices.* (pp. 313–386). Livonia, MI: National Institute for Hearing Instrument Studies.

NORTHERN, J.L., & HATTLER, K.W. (1970). Earmold influence on aided speech identification tasks. *Journal of Speech and Hearing Research, 13;*162–172.

NORTHERN, J.L., KEPLER, L.J., & GABBARD, S.A. (1991). Deep canal fittings and real-ear measurements. *Hearing Instruments, 42*(9);34,35,53.

OKPOJO, A.O. (1992). Advances in earmold technology. *Journal of the American Academy of Audiology, 3;*142–144.

OLIVEIRA, R.J., HAWKINSON, R., & STOCKTON, M. (1992). Instant foam versus traditional BTE earmolds. *Hearing Instruments, 43*(12);22.

OLIVEIRA, R.J., ROSE, D.E. (1994). "Keep your wax guard up." *American Journal of Audiology, 3*(1);7–10.

PARKER, D. J., OKPOJO, A.O., NOLAN, M., COMBE, E.C., & BAMFORD, J.M. (1992). Acoustic evaluation of earmoulds in situ: A comparison of impression and earmold materials. *British Journal of Audiology, 26;*159–166.

PECK, J.E. (1986). The stethomold for hearing aid and stethoscope users. *Hearing Instruments, 37*(12);17–18.

PEDERSEN, B. (1984). Venting of earmoulds with acoustic horn. *Scandinavian Audiology, 13;*205–206.

PIRZANSKI, C.Z. (1996). An alternative impression-taking technique: The open-jaw impression. *Hearing Journal, 49*(11); 30,32,34–35.

PREVES, D.A. (1980). Stepped bore earmolds for custom ITE hearing aids. *Hearing Instruments, 31*(10);24,26.

PREVES, D.A. (1994). Real-ear gain provided by CIC, ITC, and ITE hearing instruments. *Hearing Review, 1*(7);22–24.

REVIT, L.J. (1992). Two techniques for dealing with the occlusion effect. *Hearing Instruments, 43*(12);16–18.

REVIT, L.J. (1994). Using coupler tests in the fitting of hearing aids. In: M. Valente (Ed.), *Strategies for selecting and verifying hearing aid fittings* (pp. 64–87). New York: Thieme Medical Publishers, Inc.

REVOILE, S. (1968). Speech discrimination with ear inserts. *Bulletin of Prosthetic Research Fall;* 198–205.

REZEN, S. (1980). A research application of innovative hearing aid coupling systems. *Hearing Instruments, 31*(9);28,30.

RIDENHOUR, M.W. (1988). The effects of shell material on hearing aid performance. *Hearing Instruments, 39*(9);58–60.

RIESS, R.L., & GUTHIER, J.D. (1986). In-the-ear modification cookbook. *Hearing Instruments, 37*(4);18,21–22,24,54.

ROBINSON, S., CANE, M.A., & LUTMAN, M.E. (1989). Relative benefits of stepped and constant bore earmoulds: A crossover trial. *British Journal of Audiology, 23;*221–228.

ROESEL, G.W. (1994). CIC + WDRC = A logical combination. *Hearing Review, 1*(7);28–27.

SCHWARTZ, D.M., SURR, R.K., MONTGOMERY, A.A., PROSEK, R.A., & WALDEN, B.E. (1979). Performance of high-frequency impaired listeners with conventional and extended high-frequency amplification. *Audiology, 18;*157–174.

SMOLAK, L.H., ISERMAN, B.F., & HAWKINSON, R.W. (1987). Disposable foam earmolds. *Hearing Instruments, 38*(12); 24,27,49.

STAAB, W.J., & FINLAY, B. (1991). A fitting rationale for deep fitting canal hearing instruments. *Hearing Instruments, 42*(1); 6,8–10,48.

STAAB, W.J., & LYBARGER, S.F. (1994). Characteristics and use of hearing aids. In: J. Katz (Ed.), *Handbook of clinical audiology.* (4th ed.) (pp. 657–722). Baltimore, MD: Williams & Wilkins.

STAAB, W.J., & MARTIN, R.L. (1995). Mixed-media impression: A two-layer approach to taking ear impressions. *Hearing Journal, 48*(5);23–24,27.

STAAB, W.J., & NUNLEY, J.A. (1982). A guide to tube fitting of hearing aids. *Hearing Aid Journal, 9;*25–26,28–30,32,34.

STUDEBAKER, G.A., & COX, R.M. (1977). Side branch and parallel vent effects in real-ears and in acoustical and electrical models. *Journal of the American Audiological Society, 3;*108,117.

STUDEBAKER, G.A., COX, R.M., & WARK, D.J. (1978). Earmold modification effect measured by coupler, threshold and probe techniques. *Audiology, 17;*173–186.

STUDEBAKER, G.A., & ZACHMAN, T.A. (1970). Investigation of the acoustics of earmold vents. *Journal of the Acoustical Society of America, 47;*1107–1115.

SULLIVAN, R. (1985a). Part I: An acoustic coupling-based classification system for hearing aid fittings. *Hearing Instruments, 36*(9);25–26,28.

SULLIVAN, R. (1985b). Part II: An acoustic coupling-based classification system for hearing aid fittings. *Hearing Instruments, 36*(12);16,18.

SULLIVAN, R. (1985c). Part III: An acoustic coupling-based classification system for hearing aid fittings. *Hearing Instruments, 36*(12);20–22.

SUNG, G.S., & SUNG, R.J. (1982). The efficacy of hearing aid-earmold coupling systems. *Hearing Instruments, 33*(12); 11–12.

TECCA, J.E. (1991). Real-ear vent effects in ITE hearing instrument fittings. *Hearing Instruments, 42*(12);10–12.

TECCA, J.E. (1992). Further investigation of ITE vent effects. *Hearing Instruments, 43*(12);8–10.

TEDER, H. (1979). Smoothing hearing aid output with filters. *Hearing Instruments, 30*(4);22–23,28.

TRYCHEL, M.R., & HASS, W.H. (1989). Earmold attenuation: The effect on residual hearing. *Hearing Journal, 2;*22,24,27.

VALENTE, M. (1983). *A clinically manufactured stepped diameter earmold for superior aided performance.* Paper presented at the annual meeting of the American-Speech-Language-Hearing Association, Cincinnati, OH.

VALENTE, M. (1984a). *Enhanced aided listening with a belled bore.* Paper presented at the annual meeting of the American-Speech-Language-Hearing Association, San Francisco, CA.

VALENTE, M. (1984b). *Interaction of tubing insertion and bore length upon the frequency response.* Paper presented at the annual meeting of the American-Speech-Language-Hearing Association, San Francisco, CA.

VALENTE, M. (1984c). *Transmission line acoustics.* Unpublished report for the Veterans Administration.

VALENTE, M., & DE JONGE, R. (1981). High-frequency amplification. *Audecibel,* (Fall); 168–177.

VALENTE, M., POTTS, L.G., VALENTE, M., & GOEBEL, J. (1995). Wireless CROS versus transcranial CROS for unilateral hearing loss. *American Journal of Audiology 4;*52–59.

VAN BUUREN, R.A., FESTEN, J.M., & HOUTGAST, T. (1966). Peaks in the frequency response of hearing aids: Evaluation of the effects on speech intelligibility and sound quality. *Journal of Speech and Hearing Research, 39;*239–250.

VASS, W.K., & MIMS, L.A. (1993). Exploring the deep canal fitting advantage. *Hearing Instruments, 44*(12);26,27.

WALKER, G. (1979). Earphone termination and the response of behind-the-ear hearing aids. *British Journal of Audiology, 13;*41–46.

WESTERMANN, S. (1987). The occlusion effect. *Hearing Instruments, 38*(6);43.

WILLIAMS, D.E., & GUTNICK, H.N. (1990). Hearing instrument performance using earmolds with/without a shell additive. *Hearing Instruments, 41*(12);8,10.

WIMMER, V.H. (1986). The occlusion effect from earmolds. *Hearing Instruments, 37*(12);19,57.

PREFERRED PRACTICE GUIDELINES

Professionals Who Perform the Procedure(s)

▼ Audiologists

Expected Outcomes

▼ The hearing aid fitting is free of feedback throughout the useable range of the volume control wheel.

▼ The hearing aid fitting preserves the balance between the low-frequency and high-frequency regions of the frequency response.

▼ The hearing aid fitting, when appropriate, extends the high-frequency range of the hearing aid.

▼ The hearing aid fitting, when appropriate, minimizes excessive gain around 1500 Hz.

▼ The hearing aid fitting, when appropriate, maintains a gently rising REIR with peak gain at approximately 2800 Hz.

▼ The hearing aid fitting provides a comfortable fitting earmold or shell.

▼ The hearing aid fitting is absent of the occlusion effect.

▼ The hearing aid fitting provides appropriate amplification so that low (i.e., <55 dB SPL) input levels are judged as "soft"; average (i.e., ~65 dB SPL) input levels are judged as "comfortable"; and high (i.e., > 80 dB SPL) input levels are judged as "loud, but OK."

Clinical Indications

▼ Hearing aid fitting is conducted for individuals of all ages as a result of an audiologic and hearing aid assessment.

Clinical Process

▼ Electroacoustic evaluation of hearing aids

▼ Selection of earhook, tubing, earmold style and material, shell style and material, and venting based on the audiometric and hearing aid assessment and patient counseling.

▼ Modification of the earhook, tubing, earmold style and material, shell style, and material and venting, if necessary.

▼ Counseling on the care of the earhook, tubing, earmold style and material, shell style and material, and venting.

▼ Patients suspected of having active medical pathological conditions of the auditory system are referred for a medical evaluation before the fitting of the hearing aids.

Documentation

▼ Documentation contains pertinent background information, fitting/orientation results, and specific recommendations.

▼ Documentation includes a record of compliance with state and federal guidelines/laws/regulations for hearing aids.

▼ Documentation includes all information related to the ordering and receiving of the earmold, hearing aid, or shell

▼ Documentation includes all real-ear and behavioral measures.

Chapter 3

Real-Ear Measures

Lawrence J. Revit

Real-ear measures serve two general purposes for audiologists. First, real-ear measures characterize the performance of hearing aids in situ—"in place"—on or in the ear. By knowing

WARNING/DISCLAIMER: The techniques described in this chapter are part of routine clinical practice, and, although they are not dangerous if applied properly, hazards do exist (see later for details). The reader is advised that the author of this chapter makes no warranties as to the safety or effectiveness of the techniques described in this chapter. Also, the author of this chapter is not responsible in any way for injuries sustained as a result of anyone's using these techniques.

the in situ performance of hearing aids, clinicians address the fact that the acoustical properties of individual ears can affect the performance of hearing aids in ways not predicted from published specifications or from tests made in a sound chamber. Second, real-ear measures provide individualized correction factors for maneuvering among the various decibel (dB) measures used in clinical audiology. In the course of a single fitting, a clinician can encounter as many as three different dB systems: Audiometric tests use dB hearing level (HL), manufacturers' hearing aid specification sheets use dB sound-pressure level (SPL) measured in a 2-cc coupler, and verifications of the acoustical aspects of hearing aid fittings use dB SPL measured at the eardrum. Individualized correction factors obtained through real-ear measures permit easy and accurate maneuvering among these three decibel systems. Thus the clinician has two good reasons to become familiar with techniques for obtaining real-ear measures.

BRIEF HISTORY OF REAL-EAR MEASURES

Quoting from Romanow's (1942) article entitled "Methods for Measuring the Performance of Hearing Aids":

> A hearing aid can be considered as a sound transmission system which is interposed in the path between the source of sound and the listener's ear. As such, its performance can be judged by comparing the sound that reaches the ear first through the air path and then through the hearing aid.

Romanow's concept was that observations comparing the sound without and with hearing aids—observations by the *listener*—could give the fitter an idea of the efficacy of the chosen instruments. "Sound that reaches the ear" is the key phrase. Today, clinicians use probe-tube microphone measurements of the sound in the earcanal to gain quantitative, objective comparisons between the unamplified versus the amplified sound that "reaches the ear." Such comparisons are called "real-ear insertion gain" (REIG) measurements.

It is ironic that the article that first introduced this important paradigm for real-ear measures also introduced the 2-cc coupler used in test boxes for standardized electroacoustic measures of hearing aid performance. It is the hearing aid industry's longstanding reliance on the 2-cc coupler, along with the lack of availability of clinical real-ear measurement equipment, that helped steer the focus of hearing aid fitting away from real-ear measures until the mid 1980s, more than 40 years after Romanow's article was published.

105

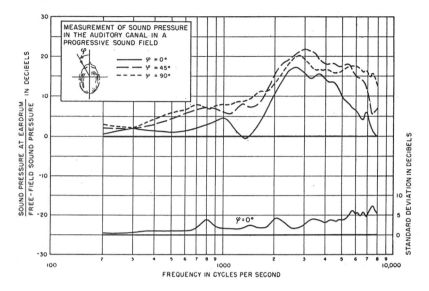

Figure 3–1 Average REUG, re free field, for three azimuths of the sound source in the horizontal plane: 0 degrees *(solid line)*, 45 degrees *(long dashes)*, and 90 degrees *(short dashes)*. (From Wiener and Ross [1946], with permission.)

The first probe-tube microphone measurements of sound in and near the earcanal were reported by Filler et al (1945). In a widely read article discussing those measurements, Wiener and Ross (1946) concluded that "the human ear is . . . an effective 'amplifier,'" referring to the acoustical properties of the outer ear known as "resonances" and "diffraction effects." The earcanal resonance and the diffraction effects of the pinna and the head enhance the SPL of certain frequencies at the eardrum compared with the SPL in the free field (Fig. 3–1). In addition to reporting mean data for sound arriving from three directions (azimuths), Wiener and Ross reported considerable variability among the adult male ears they studied, especially at high frequencies (SD = 5 dB, N = 12).

The combined results of 12 studies of the outer ear "amplifier" appear in a seminal article by Shaw (1974). In this article, Shaw fully described how the transformation of SPL from the free field to the eardrum of unoccluded ears varied as a function of the azimuth of the sound source (Fig. 3–2). Because the primary tube resonance of the earcanal, at about 2700 Hz, does not change with the azimuth of the sound source, the azimuth-dependent effects seen at higher frequencies can be attributed largely to diffraction and resonance effects of the pinna. In later work, Shaw (1975) showed that the pinna causes the sound entering the earcanal to vary as a function of the elevation of the sound source (Fig. 3–3) and of the azimuth of the sound source. In brief summary the SPL at the eardrum of an unoccluded ear is amplified by the diffraction and resonant effects of the outer ear, varying as a function of frequency, varying across individual ears, and varying with the azimuth and elevation of the sound source.

An entirely different system determines the SPL at the eardrum of an *occluded* ear. When sound enters an occluded earcanal through an insert earphone or a hearing aid, the SPL at the eardrum is determined not by the earcanal resonance but by the acoustic impedance "seen" by the sound source, "looking into" the middle ear. Without going into a lengthy discussion of acoustic impedance, this impedance is the same one clinicians measure with an occluding probe as part of an aural acoustic immittance test battery (see Chapter 17 in *Diagnosis*). Of particular importance to clinicians involved in

hearing aid fitting is that the impedance of a 2-cc coupler differs from that of the occluded ear. Addressing the fact that hearing aids occlude the ear and that standardized hearing aid performance is measured in a 2-cc coupler (ANSI, 1996b), Sachs and Burkhard (1972) used real-ear, probe-tube microphone measurements to show how the SPL output of a hearing aid or an insert earphone in a 2-cc coupler differed from that at the eardrum in a nonclinical sample of real-ears (Fig. 3–4). Standard deviations in this measure of the occluded, real-ear-to-coupler difference (RECD) were similar to standard deviations reported by Wiener and Ross (1946) for their measurements of unoccluded ears (approximately 5 dB), again with higher variability at high frequencies (N = 11). Much later, Fikret-Pasa and Revit (1992) measured the RECDs of a clinical population of hearing aid candidates. At high frequencies, standard deviations for RECDs of hearing aid candidates were only slightly higher than those reported for normal ears by Sachs and Burkhard (1972) (Fig. 3–5). However, at low frequencies, standard deviations generally exceeded those of normal ears. Fikret-Pasa and Revit (1992) concluded that the higher standard deviations of the RECDs for their clinical subjects were related to the fact that about half the clinical subjects exhibited some middle ear abnormality, whether by case history or by immittance measurements. Figure 3–6 illustrates examples of RECDs for ears having abnormal (A) and normal (B) middle ears from that study. The "take-home message" was that individual RECDs should be measured whenever 2-cc coupler data are used in context with fittings involving ears having any substantial difference from average adult middle ear function.

In keeping with the early knowledge of unoccluded and occluded outer ear acoustics, Killion and Monser (1980) recognized that the effective frequency response of hearing aids changes markedly, yet systematically, when hearing aids are inserted into ears. In coining the term *CORFIG (coupler response for flat insertion gain)*, Killion and Monser (1980) cautioned audiologists to be aware of the differences between the coupler responses and the REIG responses of hearing aids. Specifically, they described what the HA-2, 2-cc coupler response of behind-the-ear (BTE) hearing aids should look

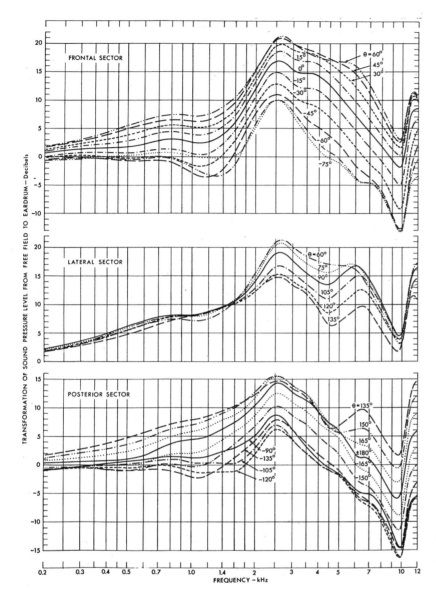

Figure 3–2 Average REUG (12 studies) for various azimuths of the sound source. (From Shaw [1974], with permission.)

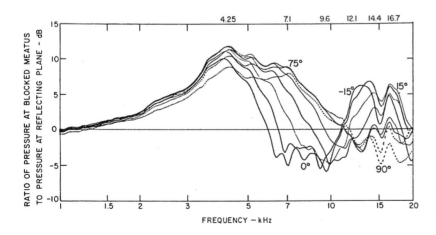

Figure 3–3 Blocked meatus response for various elevations of the sound source at the plane of the earcanal opening. (From Shaw [1975], with permission.)

SPECIAL CONSIDERATION

Very young children have small earcanals. Consequently, the primary resonance of the earcanal begins at about 7000 Hz in newborns, progressing downward to nearly the adult resonant frequency (just less than 3000 Hz) by age 3 (Kruger, 1987). In addition, the RECD in young children far exceeds the amplitudes for the average adult. See Table 3–1A for age-dependent REUG values and Table 3–1B for age-dependent RECD values.

---

like to give a flat, unity-gain* insertion response for a sound source at 0 degrees azimuth and 0 degrees elevation in the average adult ear. Killion et al (1987) expanded the CORFIG data to include in-the-ear (ITE), in-the-canal (ITC), and completely-in-the-canal (CIC) hearing aids[†] in a diffuse sound field. ("Diffuse" means from all directions.) Bentler and Pavlovic (1989) and Killion and Revit (1993) added CORFIGs for a 45-degree azimuth of sound incidence. (See later.)

In discussing average-ear corrections between real-ear and coupler response, Killion and colleagues acknowledged that individual ears can vary substantially in their acoustical properties, and therefore the fitter can make substantial errors in predicting the real-ear responses of hearing aids by relying solely on average-ear correction figures. In addressing this problem Harford (1980) pioneered using real-ear probe-microphone measurements in a clinical setting. He and his staff measured the REIG of hearing aids on approximately 500 adult ears with a miniature microphone (not a probe-*tube* microphone, but a very small microphone housed in a metal case) placed directly in the earcanal between the earmold and the eardrum. They reported that valid measurements could be obtained in all but 10 ears, for which the earcanal was too small to accommodate both the earmold and the microphone. No mention was made of the distribution of male and female subjects in that work.

Along with Harford's early work with miniature microphones, the 1980s brought the widespread availability and use of microcomputers and soft, slender, silicone-rubber tubing that, when affixed to the sound opening of a microphone, could be placed in virtually any earcanal relatively safely and unobtrusively. Steen Rasmussen (Nielsen & Rasmussen, 1984) used these technical advances toward creating the first commercially available, clinical probe-tube microphone, real-ear measurement system, the Rastronics CCI-10. Since that time, significant advances in equipment from various manufacturers have included thinner, more flexible probe tubes; very fast, broadband, real-time digital analysis; and experimental test sequences and displays. On the horizon are new ways of testing the time-varying features of nonlinear hearing aids and how they may provide differing performance in quiet and in noise, ways of testing which better generalize to the real world compared with the "steady-state" tests in common use today.

Another important advance in real-ear measures has been the completion of an ANSI standard for real-ear measures (ANSI, 1997), entitled *American National Standard Methods of Measurement of Real-Ear Performance Characteristics of Hearing Aids*. Whenever the term *standard* is used by itself in this chapter, it refers by default to this standard. It is recommended that every student and practitioner of real-ear measurements obtain a copy of the standard and endeavor to apprehend all of its contents. *Throughout this chapter, numbers in italicized curly brackets refer the reader to section numbers in the standard.* The standard contains definitions of terms and specifications of test conditions and procedures to be used in obtaining real-ear measures. The standard also gives rules and tolerances for test equipment and conditions. This chapter will describe the standardized terms and procedures and other useful methods and properties of real-ear measures. For the most part, where the chapter defines standardized terms, the standard itself contains definitions that are more precise.

THE REAL-EAR MEASURES AND THEIR APPLICATIONS: THE "REs" AND MORE

This section defines and describes the real-ear measures in common use. Almost all these measures are identified by acronyms, which begin with the letters "RE," for "real ear." Most of these are defined in ANSI standard S3.46 (ANSI, 1997), but other measures, not defined in the standard, are also discussed in this chapter.

The reader will see that many of the real-ear measures can be displayed in terms of either "response" or "gain." Response, in this context, is taken to mean an absolute measure of SPL, whereas "gain" is taken to mean a response that is expressed relative to a specified input or reference response. For many real-ear applications, the advantage of observing "gain" is that neither the signal level nor the signal spectrum is apparent in the displayed results, so the observer sees only the effect that the device under test has had on the test signal. For example, the top panel of Figure 3–7 shows the spectrum of a speech-weighted composite signal, as measured by a probe microphone in front of the loudspeaker of a real-ear measurement (REM) system. Note that the speech weighting causes the high frequencies to be increasingly lower in amplitude.[‡] The middle and lower panels are examples of unaided real-ear measures (discussed in detail later) made with this signal, yet with the probe microphone picking up the sound deep in the left earcanal of the author. The center panel is a real-ear unaided gain (REUG) curve made in this manner. The REUG curve shows the gain-versus-frequency effects of the unoccluded outer ear, independently of the signal spectrum. The lower panel is a real-ear unaided response (REUR) curve, showing dB SPL versus frequency. The higher frequencies roll off compared with the REUG because of the superimposed shape of the signal spectrum. As a rule, the choice of viewing gain or SPL depends on the purpose at hand. When prescriptive targets are given in terms of gain, it makes sense to view real-ear measures in terms of

---

*"Unity gain" means no amplification and no attenuation.
[†]Killion et al (1987) used the term *ITC (deep)* for what is now called "CIC."

[‡]The overall (root mean square) amplitude of this signal was 70 dB SPL.

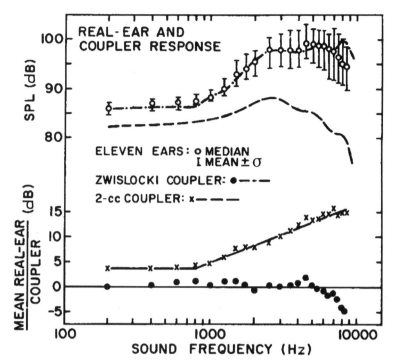

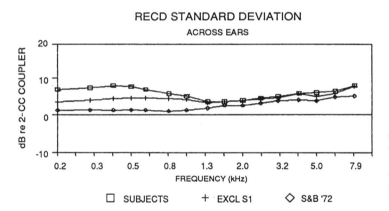

Figure 3–4 Various real-ear and coupler responses of an insert earphone. Data symbols are real-ear data; curves are coupler data as indicated. Solid curve *(through Xs)* is calculated model for RECD on the basis of mean real-ear data. (Adapted from Sachs and Burkhard [1972], with permission.)

Figure 3–5 Standard deviations of RECD for 18 ears *(rectangles)* from Fikret-Pasa and Revit (1992). Crosses are data excluding an ear with a perforated tympanic membrane. *(Diamonds* are data from Sachs and Burkhard [1972], with permission.)

gain. When prescriptive targets are given in terms of earcanal SPL for a given input signal, it makes sense to view real-ear measures in terms of SPL.

REUR/G *{3.4.11/10}*

The REUR is a measure of what the open ear does to sound all by itself—that is, with no hearing aid. It is the SPL at or near the eardrum for a specified sound field outside the ear. When the measure is referred to the sound field outside the ear, it is called the REUG. As described earlier, Figures 3–1 and 3–2 depict average REUGs for various locations of the sound source. The REUR/G serves as a baseline on which amplification must build to obtain an effective "insertion gain" (see later). Because the REUG describes the acoustic transformation from the sound field to the eardrum, it can

also be used in converting unaided sound field thresholds to eardrum SPLs.

> ### SPECIAL CONSIDERATION
>
> **An ear that has a middle-ear pathological condition or an ear that has been surgically treated may present an REUR having an unusual shape. See de Jonge (1996) for a comprehensive discussion, with examples.**

REAR/G *{3.4.6/5}*

The "real-ear aided response" (REAR) is the response of a hearing aid as measured at or near the eardrum for a specified sound field outside the ear. When the measure is referred

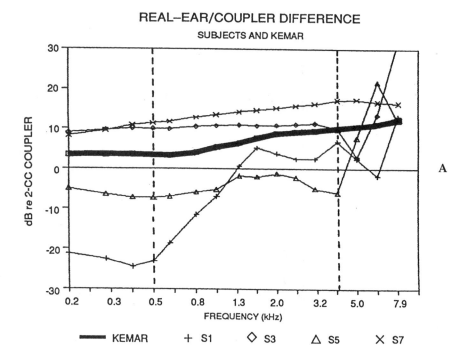

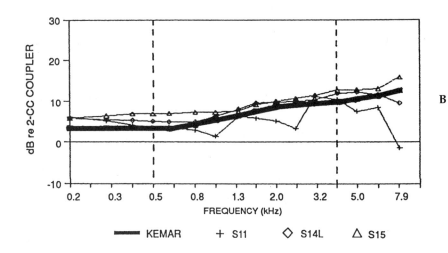

Figure 3–6 Examples of individual RECDs from subjects with abnormal **(A)** and normal **(B)** middle ears. Thick curve is the KEMAR RECD. (From Fikret-Pasa and Revit [1992], with permission.)

TABLE 3–1A   Average, age-dependent values for the REUG (free field reference, 0-degree azimuth and elevation)

	Frequency (Hz)	250	500	750	1000	1500	2000	3000	4000	6000
	<2 mos	−1	−1.4	−1	0	3	4	0	−1	9.5
	2–6 mos	1	1	1.9	2	5	5	4.9	5.8	14
Age:	6 mos–1 yr	0	1	2	2.5	2	1	8	11.8	5.8
	1–2 yr	−2	−2	−2	−1.9	2	9	16.8	15	12
	2–3 yr	0.5	2	2.8	4.5	5	9	16	9	−8
	>3 yr	1	1.8	2.9	2.6	5.3	12	15.3	14.3	7.3

Courtesy Etymonic Design Inc., Dorchester, Ontario, Canada.

TABLE 3–1B Average, age-dependent values for the RECD

	Frequency (Hz)	250	500	750	1000	1500	2000	3000	4000	6000
	<1 yr	7.1	9.4	10.3	11.8	13.2	13.5	17.7	20.7	23.2
	1–2 yrs	9	9.8	10.2	11.4	12.4	13.2	15.3	17.6	16.3
Age:	2–4 yrs	5.7	7.4	9	10.6	11.9	12.2	14.7	15.3	16.2
	4–5 yrs	4.5	7.6	8.8	8.6	10.7	11.7	13.2	14.1	15.6
	>5 yrs	3.9	4.2	4.6	5.1	6.4	7.8	10.4	12.2	14.5

Data courtesy Etymonic Design Inc., Dorchester, Ontario, Canada.

to the sound field outside the ear, it is called the "real-ear aided gain" (REAG). Some prescription strategies (see Chapters 4, 5, 6, 12, and 13 in this volume) are based on one or more target REAR/Gs for a specified input signal or set of input signals.

PITFALL

The presence of the probe tube in the earcanal alongside the earmold or shell can add a "slit leak" to the acoustic picture of a real-ear measurement involving an earmold or shell. A slit leak can add not only unintentional venting but also acoustic damping that is not present without the probe tube. Acoustic damping can reduce the sharpness and amplitude of a Helmholtz resonance caused by an earmold vent (see Chapter 2 in this volume), and therefore the actual REAR may be greater at the peak resonant frequency than what is observed in the probe-tube microphone measure.

REIG {3.4.7}

The REIG is the difference between the REAG and the REUG (or the REAR and the REUR, if both are measured using the same signal amplitude). By subtracting the REUG from the REAG, one observes a measure of the "net" acoustic benefit, in terms of an increase in the SPL at or near the eardrum obtained through the act of inserting a hearing aid. It may seem intuitive to the reader that such a measure of net benefit might be the centerpiece of strategies for prescribing the gain and frequency response of hearing aids, and indeed it is. (See Chapters 4, 5, 6, and 12 in this volume for a thorough discussion of hearing aid fitting strategies.) The reader should note that the REIG was formerly called the "REIR" for "real-ear insertion response." But because the measure is always expressed in terms of gain, S3.46 (ANSI, 1997) changed the term to reflect this fact. Figure 3–8 shows an example of an REIG curve *(upper panel)*, along with the REUG/REAG measurement pair *(lower panel)* that determined the REIG. This set of curves was measured on a KEMAR manikin, with an ITE having a large vent. The target curve *(bold curve, upper panel)* is shown for comparison purposes.

CONTROVERSIAL POINT

Conventional practice (as described in the section on REIG) advocates subtracting the REUR/G from the REAG in verifying that a fitting matches a target REIG and also advocates the use of the REUR/G in formulating a customized 2-cc coupler prescription (e.g., Mueller, 1989). This author advocates *not* using the patient's REUR/G in the preceding applications and instead advocates using average-ear unaided response/gain curves. The rationale for this conclusion can be found in an "open letter" by Revit (1991a). Also, see the "Preferred Practice Guidelines" at the end of the chapter for instructions and worksheets that use these applications.

REOR/G {3.4.9/8}

The "real-ear occluded response" (REOR) is a measure of the SPL at or near the eardrum for a specified sound field, with a hearing aid in place and turned off. When the measure is referred to the sound field outside the ear, it is called the "real-ear occluded gain" (REOG). Mueller (1998) has called the REOR/G the "most misunderstood probe-mic measure." Several authors (e.g., Mueller, 1992; Sullivan, 1985) have studied the REOR and its relation to the REUR, the REAR, and the REIG. But why would the clinician need to know the real-ear performance of a hearing aid that is turned off? One possible use might be as a quick check that the REM system is functioning properly, while the probe tube and hearing aid are already in a patient's ear. If the earpiece of the aid is vented or fits loosely, the REOG should be a low-frequency plateau at 0 dB gain, followed by high-frequency attenuation. If not, something may be wrong with the REM system (H. Dillon, personal communication). An example of such a normal REOG curve is shown in Figure 3–9.

Another possible use of the REOG might be for information purposes, such as in troubleshooting an earmold problem, to be able to observe the part of the sound that gets into the earcanal acoustically, either through the vent or around the earmold or shell. For example, if the REAG has an unwanted resonant peak or dip near 500 Hz (typical with many vented fittings and exemplified by the dip at 630 Hz in

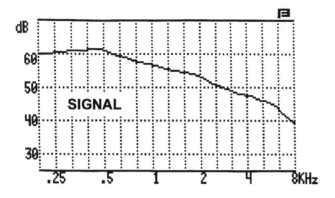

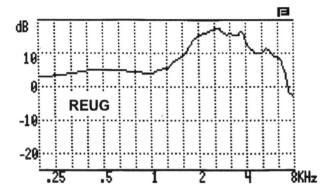

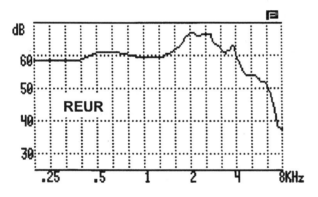

Figure 3–7   Probe-tube microphone responses. Upper curve is spectrum of speech-weighted composite test signal (70 dB SPL rms); middle curve is REUG; lower curve is REUR using signal in upper curve. The REUR rolls off in the high frequencies compared with the REUG because the REUR is the superposition of the REUG and the sloping, speech-weighted signal.

the REAG curve of Fig. 3–8), viewing the REOR can reveal the isolated contribution of the vent resonance to that response anomaly. The dispenser can then make adjustments to the earmold, as desired.

RESR

The "real-ear saturation response" (RESR) is a real-ear measure akin to the test-box measure known as the "output SPL for a 90 dB input SPL" (OSPL-90) (formerly "SSPL-90"). The

RESR is a measure of the real-ear output of a hearing aid that is driven by very loud inputs. Thus it is an estimate of the maximum output of the hearing aid, in terms of the SPL at or near the eardrum. An example of an RESR curve is shown in Figure 3–10.

The term *RESR* is not defined in ANSI S3.46 (ANSI, 1997). One possible reason is that the measure is prone to complexities that make it difficult to standardize. The principal complexity is the name RESR, which itself may be misleading. Many hearing aids do not reach saturation even for the highest signal amplitudes available with REM systems (usually 90 dB SPL, but even less in some cases). Also, the plotted SPLs for an RESR measurement depend heavily on the bandwidth of the test signal. For an overall estimate of maximum real-ear output, using the "root mean square (rms)" output reading with a broadband signal works very well. But for a frequency-by-frequency plot of the maximum real-ear output, using narrowband test signals always gives the best (actually, the worst-case) estimate.

To illustrate the importance of using narrowband signals for the RESR, Figure 3–11 shows two examples of the 2-cc coupler output of a BTE hearing aid using a test signal at 90 dB SPL. The dashed curve was obtained with a broadband (composite) signal, and the curve with filled boxes was obtained with a narrowband (pure tone) signal. The pointy curve is the 2-cc coupler output of the hearing aid in response to the signal of a nearby fax machine. Also shown is the rms (overall) output SPL corresponding to the curve obtained with the broadband signal. The curve obtained with the narrowband signal correctly estimated the possible output of about 110 dB SPL at 800 Hz, which was nearly achieved with the signal from the fax machine. The curve obtained with the broadband signal underestimated the possible output for the fax signal, although the rms output measured using the broadband signal (110 dB SPL) provided a good estimate.

RECD

The RECD is another real-ear measure that is not described in the S3.46 standard (ANSI, 1997). The reasons for the omission are likely that the RECD differs from the other real-ear

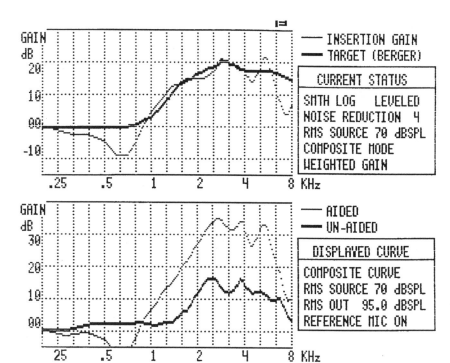

Figure 3–8 REM display for REIG. Lower graph shows the REUG *(thick curve)* and the REAG *(thin curve)*. Upper graph shows the REIG *(thin curve)*, which is the REAG minus the REUG. Thick curve in upper graph is a target curve shown for comparison purposes.

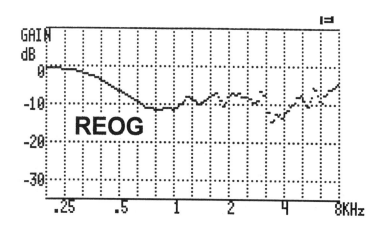

Figure 3–9 Typical REOG curve. The plateau at 0 dB in the low frequencies indicates normal transmission of sound through a pinhole vent or a slit leak. Negative values at higher frequencies indicate attenuation of sounds originating outside the earcanal.

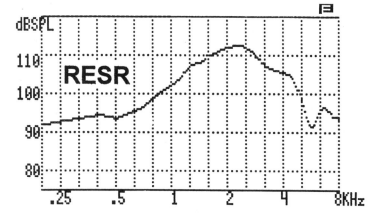

Figure 3–10 Typical RESR curve. The SPL in the earcanal at low frequencies cannot be lower than the signal level (90 dB SPL) because of sound transmission through the earmold vent or slit leak.

measures in form and that the importance of the RECD has only recently become widely known. However, the RECD may, in fact, be the most useful of all the common real-ear measures (Mueller, 1998; Revit, 1993b). Therefore a lot of space in this chapter will be given to describing this measure and its applications.

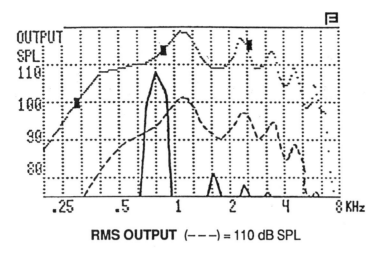

RMS OUTPUT (– – –) = 110 dB SPL

Figure 3–11 2-cc coupler responses of a BTE hearing aid. Pointy, solid curve is the spectrum of a signal from a nearby fax machine recorded through the hearing aid. Upper curve *(filled rectangles)* was obtained using a 90 dB SPL pure tone signal. The pure tone curve correctly indicated the potential hearing aid output at the frequency of the fax signal. The curve plotted using a broadband signal *(dashed curve)* underestimated the potential hearing aid output at the frequency of the fax signal, although the rms output *(indicated below the graph)* provided a reasonable estimate of the potential hearing aid output.

The RECD is the difference between the real-ear response and the 2-cc coupler response of a hearing instrument (i.e., real-ear response minus 2-cc response), using the same stimulus for both component measures. The hearing instrument used in obtaining the RECD can be a hearing aid or an insert earphone. The RECD is not intended to reveal anything about the performance of the instrument used in making the test. It is, however, intended to reveal the difference between the way a hearing instrument will perform in an individual's ear, compared with the way it will perform in a 2-cc coupler. This measure of difference in SPL directly reflects the difference in impedance between the individual ear and the 2-cc coupler. This difference is likely to behave in much the same way for a broad range of hearing instruments, and so it can be used to predict the real-ear response of a range of instruments simply by measuring the 2-cc coupler responses (and vice versa) (Moodie et al, 1994; Revit, 1997). The RECD can also be used in converting hearing-assessment measures, in dB HL, to SPL in the earcanal. More on these applications of the RECD appears in the "Circle of Decibels" section of this chapter.

SPECIAL CONSIDERATION

An ear that has a perforated eardrum will present an RECD having a deep dip or roll-off (10 to 20 dB or greater) in the low frequencies (see Fig. 3–6, *upper panel*, "plus sign" symbols). An ear having a stiffened eardrum, caused, for example, by elevated negative middle ear pressure, will present an RECD having an elevated (by up to about 10 dB) low-frequency to mid-frequency region (see Fig. 3–6, *upper panel*, "X" symbols). See de Jonge (1996) for a comprehensive discussion and examples of the RECD in pathological ears.

REDD

The "real-ear-to-dial difference" (REDD) is somewhat unique among real-ear measures in that its primary purpose does not involve hearing aids. Clinicians use the REDD primarily during audiometry to convert dB HL values to eardrum SPLs or vice versa. Obtaining this measure requires that the REM system and the audiometer be located in the same place. One obtains the REDD by measuring the SPL at or near the eardrum for a set of audiometric tones at a particular setting of the audiometer attenuator dial. One subtracts the dB value of the audiometer attenuator setting from the measured earcanal SPL to arrive at the REDD. More information about applications of the REDD appear in the "Circle of Decibels" section of the chapter.

Measuring the "Occlusion Effect"

"My voice sounds like it's in a barrel." Such is a common complaint of the first-time hearing aid wearer. A hearing aid wearer's own voice can sound "hollow" because low-frequency vocal energy (predominantly in the range of 200 to 500 Hz) enters the earcanals by means of vibration of the cartilaginous portions of the earcanal walls. With unoccluded ears, this vocal sound energy normally exits the earcanals through the earcanal openings. But when hearing aids occlude the ears, such low-frequency vocal energy cannot escape. Thus the spectrum of the hearing aid wearer's own voice in the earcanals becomes excessively bassy, giving one's own voice a "hollow" or "barrellike" sound.

Embodied in the preceding explanation are two clues to ways of alleviating the occlusion effect: (1) the fact that the offending sound energy enters the earcanals through the cartilaginous portions of the earcanals suggests that earmolds or shells having long bores that anchor to the bony portions of the earcanals could effectively block the vibrations of the cartilaginous portions of the earcanals; and (2) the fact that the offending sound energy normally exits through the earcanal openings suggests that increasing vent sizes could let the offending low-frequency energy escape the earcanals more easily. After clinical intervention, aside from simply asking the patient whether the problem has been alleviated, the clinician can use real-ear measurements to document the extent of the occlusion effect objectively, both before and after intervention.

Two REM methods are available to measure the occlusion effect. One method requires special cooperation by the patient; the other frees the patient from active participation. Both methods require using either the "spectrum-analysis" or the "sound-level-meter" mode of operation of the REM system. Both these modes of operation depart from normal REM system operation in that the signal source (loudspeaker) is turned off. Instead, either the patient's own voice or an audiometric bone vibrator provides the test signal.

When the patient's own voice provides the test signal, the patient sustains a vocal "ee" sound while the REM system records the sound level (or spectrum) inside the earcanal. To assist the patient in maintaining a constant vocal level, a separate sound-level meter (SLM) monitors the sound level outside the earcanal, usually from in front of the patient's mouth. The patient strives to maintain a consistent reading on the external SLM under all conditions.

To document the extent of the occlusion effect, measurements can be made with and without the hearing aid in place. The occlusion effect can thus be defined as the difference between the recorded vocal sound level in the earcanal under occluded verses unoccluded conditions for a constant vocal sound level outside the earcanal. Alternately, the vocal sound level in the earcanal can be recorded before and after a change in the earmold or venting to document the change in the occlusion effect under the two conditions. Figure 3–12 shows real-ear spectrum analyses for one subject who sustained an "ee" sound with the test ear unoccluded and with four aided conditions. As can be seen, the highest SPLs in the earcanal were at 300 Hz and less for all conditions. The three venting conditions shown, sealed, 0.6 mm, and 2.0 mm, indicate that as vent size increased, the difference between the unoccluded and the aided SPL for the patient's voice (the occlusion effect) decreased from a maximum of 22 dB to 13 dB. These three venting conditions were for a moderate insertion depth. When a deeply sealed foam eartip was used instead of a conventional earmold, the occlusion effect decreased to only about 5 dB (Revit, 1992).

As previously mentioned, the curves in Figure 3–12 were generated by the patient's own voice. When participation by the patient is not desirable or possible, an audiometric bone vibrator, set to 70 dB HL at either 250 or 500 Hz and placed on the mastoid, can provide a suitable substitute for the patient's own voice. However, the clinician should keep in mind that if the occlusion effect in a given case lies predominantly at a frequency other than the one used, the measurement could fail to show an effect. One way of avoiding this problem in most cases would be to obtain measurements using both 250 and 500 Hz.

INSTRUMENTATION USED IN REAL-EAR MEASURES

What Is a Real-Ear Measurement System?

A REM system is a form of a SLM having its own signal-delivery system. In general, a SLM consists of a microphone and a voltmeter. The microphone responds to sound pressures by generating analogous electrical voltages at its output. The voltmeter measures and displays the voltages generated by the microphone. To display voltage readings in terms of dB SPL, the scale of the voltmeter of a SLM is calibrated in decibels re 20 μPa (microPascals) of sound pressure. That is, the meter will show a reading of 0 dB SPL when the microphone senses a sound pressure of 20 μPa. For a sound pressure of 200 μPa, which is 20 dB greater than 20 μPa, the meter will show a reading of +20 dB SPL, and so forth.

Aside from the basic function of using a probe-tube microphone as the microphone part of a SLM, many REM systems have similar operating features that are dedicated to real-ear measures. Yet each system also has its own unique features. For a brief overview of many of the REM systems available at this writing, see Mueller (1998).

Sound Sources

Because a REM system not only displays SPLs but also the frequencies at which those SPLs occur, a REM system can also be called a "spectrum analyzer." The major difference between a general-purpose spectrum analyzer and a REM system is that a REM system can generate its own, calibrated sound source, usually fed to a loudspeaker but sometimes fed to an insert earphone. "Calibrated" means that the spectrum and amplitude of the sound source are adjusted to known values before the sound is delivered to the ear being tested. This adjustment of the sound source is called "equalization."

Loudspeaker

The most common stimulus for real-ear measures is a test signal generated by the circuitry of the REM system and delivered to the sound field by a loudspeaker. The REUR/G, REAR/G, REIG, and REOR/G all require a sound field loudspeaker as the sound source. The loudspeaker used for these

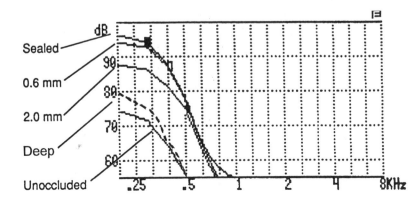

Figure 3–12 Occlusion effect. Real-ear spectrum analyses of sound in earcanal under varied conditions of occlusion. Test signal is subject sustaining an "ee" sound. Increasing vent sizes diminished the occlusion effect. The least occlusion effect was for a foam tip sealed deeply in the bony portion of the earcanal *(dashed curve)*.

real-ear measures should be of a single-radiator or a coaxial-radiator design. Commercially available REM systems generally provide single-element loudspeakers. Single radiator means that the loudspeaker has only one element, or cone, to project all frequencies. Coaxial radiator means that two or more radiators emanate sound along the same axis. A common example would be that a tweeter or a high-frequency horn is positioned at the center of a woofer. If the tweeter and the woofer are separated, signals that emanate from both drivers near the crossover frequency will come from two slightly different directions and may be out-of-phase with each other, causing acoustic interference patterns at the ear.

Insert Earphone

An insert earphone is a good sound source for obtaining the RECD (and also the REDD, if the same insert earphone is used in audiometry). An audiometric insert earphone such as the ER-3A (a.k.a, E-A-RTone-3A) presents a source impedance similar to that of hearing aids. Therefore, when used in obtaining occluded real-ear responses, an insert earphone yields results that relate well to hearing aid performance. Hearing aid venting effects, unfortunately, will not be reflected in insert earphone measures.

Microphones

Reference (Control) Microphone {3.1.8}

Almost all REM systems use a microphone other than the probe-tube microphone for equalizing and calibrating the sound field. This microphone is called the "reference" or "control" microphone. During the equalization process (also called "leveling"), the reference microphone records the spectrum and amplitude of the sound field produced by the loudspeaker. The REM system uses these recordings to adjust the signal source to achieve specified values. The reference microphone is usually placed either just over the pinna (Fig. 3–13), just under the earlobe, or next to the ear. The position of the sound inlet of the reference microphone during equalization is called the "field reference point" {3.1.6}. In measurements of real-ear gain, other than insertion gain, the SPL measured by the reference microphone at the field reference point is subtracted from the earcanal SPL to determine the gain.

Probe-Tube Microphone {3.4.4}

The main measuring microphone of a REM system consists of a slender, flexible tube (often made of silicone rubber) that can be placed unobtrusively in the earcanal, with its sound inlet near the eardrum. The probe tube connects to a small microphone housing placed outside the ear (e.g., as in Fig. 3–13). The frequency response of a probe tube is not flat; it rolls off at high frequencies, typically more than 20 dB at 8000 Hz. Therefore the probe-tube microphone itself requires corrective equalization. Corrective equalization of the probe-tube microphone may be accomplished either acoustically or electronically, or in combination, depending on the specific design of the microphone.

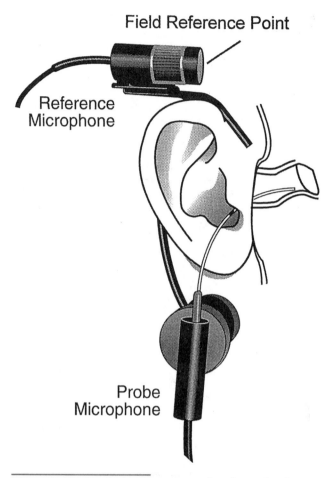

Figure 3–13 Typical arrangement of probe and reference microphones for real-ear measures. Field reference point is the center of the sound opening of the reference microphone. (Courtesy Frye Electronics, Inc.)

Internal Noise {4.3.3}

It is important to recognize that because a probe tube requires more than 20 dB of high-frequency boost to obtain a flat frequency response, this boost also raises the internal noise of a probe-tube microphone at high frequencies. Because of this boost in high-frequency internal noise, the internal noise level of a probe-tube microphone can become a limiting factor in how soft a sound can be measured accurately. ANSI S3.46 (1997) states that the internal noise of the probe microphone must be lower than the lowest SPL to be measured, at a given frequency, by at least 10 dB. For example, if you wish to measure an SPL of 60 dB at 2000 Hz, the equivalent internal noise of the probe microphone (the SPL reading given by the microphone with no signal present) must be no greater than 50 dB SPL at 2000 Hz. This rule of thumb ensures that internal noise does not affect measurements by more than 1 dB.

Cross Talk {3.4.1}

In addition to internal noise, "cross talk" is another potential technical issue the REM operator needs to be aware of. Cross talk is the unwanted "leakage" of a signal from one signal path to another, thus potentially contaminating a measurement. In REMs cross talk can occur between the sound source and the probe microphone {4.3.4} and between the signal paths of the two microphones {4.3.5}. If the sound source is loud enough and if the isolation of the housing of the probe microphone body is insufficient, some sound can bypass the sound inlet of the probe microphone, entering the measuring path directly through the microphone body or through the wall of the probe tube.

With regard to leakage through the probe microphone, ANSI S3.46 calls for an observation of the reading given by the microphone with the sound inlet blocked compared with the reading given with the sound inlet open. In each case, the entire microphone is to be placed in the sound field of interest. The "blocked" reading must be at least 10 dB below that of the "open" reading at each frequency of interest, again ensuring an effect of leakage of less than 1 dB. For cross talk between the main and reference signal paths, ANSI S3.46 (1997) states that the manufacturer of the REM system must report the maximum difference between the signals in the main and reference signal paths as a function of frequency for which cross talk will not affect measurements by 1 dB. This maximum difference usually refers to the maximum acoustic gain of hearing aids that can be measured accurately, although it could also refer to the maximum attenuation of an earplug that can be measured accurately.

Test Signals {4.2.2, Annex A}

Available signals vary considerably across models and manufacturers of REM equipment. Most REM systems have a choice of several test signals. The tester needs to be aware of how a given choice of signal will affect a measurement. For true linear hearing aids, the problem is of little importance: linear hearing aids respond the same way to every test signal. But hearing aids having any sort of adaptive signal processing respond differently to differing signals. Some of the basic variables in test signals are bandwidth, spectrum, crest factor, and so-called temporal properties. With but a few exceptions, most available test signals in REM systems are what is known as "stationary" signals. That is, they do not vary over time; they are of fixed bandwidth, spectrum, crest factor, and temporal properties (all described in the following). Natural signals, such as speech, are not stationary; they constantly vary in the preceding dimensions. Thus no stationary signal can adequately describe hearing aid performance under conditions of natural use.

Much work is ongoing to create signals that better represent natural speech and other real-world signals for the purposes of testing hearing aids. The following descriptions of the properties of test signals are intended to give the clinician questions and answers to aid in the making informed choices of test signal and interpretations of test results.

Bandwidth

Bandwidth refers to the range of frequencies presented by a signal at any given time. Many nonlinear hearing aids perform differently for signals having differing bandwidths. The signal having the narrowest possible bandwidth is a pure tone (or sinusoid). This signal has only one frequency at a time. Two common narrowband signals, whose bandwidths are slightly broader than that of a pure tone, are warble tones

and 1/3-octave bands of noise. An example of a signal having a broad bandwidth is speech-weighted composite noise. This signal presents all the important speech frequencies at once. Natural speech continually varies in bandwidth. But it is almost never as narrow in bandwidth as a pure tone, warble tone, or 1/3-octave band of noise, and it is almost never as wide in bandwidth as a speech-weighted composite noise.

Spectrum

Spectrum refers to the relative amplitudes and phases of the frequencies presented by a signal. Many nonlinear hearing aids perform differently for signals having differing spectral shapes. By manipulating the shape of the amplitude spectrum, one creates what is known as "spectral weighting." In a "speech-weighted" signal, for example, the amplitude spectrum is shaped to conform to that of a long-term sample of speech. Speech-weighted signals can be either narrowband or broadband. By definition, a single pure tone has only one spectral point (has only one frequency) and so can have no spectral shape. However, a succession, or a sweep, of pure tones can be either "iso-amplitude" (the same amplitude at all frequencies) or spectrally weighted such that the collection of tones presented over the course of the sweep follows a spectrally shaped pattern. Sweeps of warble tones or 1/3-octave bands of noise can similarly be either iso-amplitude or spectrally weighted. Broadband signals can also be flat (the same amplitude over frequency) or speech weighted. Broadband speech-weighted signals typically consist of either random noise or deterministic tone composites, also known as pseudorandom noise. The reader is advised to check the manufacturers' specifications to become familiar with the peculiarities of the hearing instrument under test, as related to performance with signals having various spectral shapes.

Crest Factor

Crest factor refers to the decibel ratio of the peak amplitude of a signal versus the rms or long-term effective amplitude of the signal. An example of a signal with a low crest factor—one whose rms level is close to its peak level—is a pure tone or sinusoid. A pure tone has a crest factor of 3 dB; that is, the peak level (as if read on an oscilloscope) is only 3 dB higher than the rms level (as if read on an AC voltmeter). An example of a signal with a high crest factor is a click. If you viewed a click on an oscilloscope, you would see a high peak amplitude that occurs over a very short period of time. If you attempted to measure a click with an AC voltmeter, the signal would begin and end so quickly that the meter would not even have a chance to register. So the ratio of the peak to rms levels (the crest factor) of a click is very high.

Test signals having varying crest factors can result in varying degrees of measured performance (e.g., gain, output, frequency response) for a given hearing aid. It may be important, with certain hearing aids, to use test signals having speechlike crest factors. Natural speech, on average, has a crest factor of about 12 dB, which is higher than that of a sine wave but lower than that of a click. With certain broadband signals, such as digitally generated tone composites, a speech-like crest factor can be achieved (in software) by setting the relative phases of the tonal components of the composite in a certain way (Frye, 1987). With random noise, the peak level can be limited by clipping, which reduces the crest factor but which may alter the signal spectrum.

"Temporal Properties"

A fourth basic quality of test signals is called "temporal properties." What is meant by "temporal properties" is the ways in which a signal varies over time. Natural signals, like speech, are not stationary; they vary in many ways over time. And so hearing aids that adapt with signals that change over time may behave differently with stationary signals compared with the way they behave with natural, temporally varying signals.

Experimental Signals

The stationary test signals mentioned may be the best tools we currently have for real-ear measures,* yet these signals cannot reveal performance that is completely generalizable to the real world. Some experimental signals that address real-world performance are either already available in REM systems or are being tested for future release. Descriptions of some of these follow, including broadband signals with bias tones, roving warble tones, International Collegium of Research Audiologists (ICRA) noise, fluctuating composites, and maximum length sequences.

1. *Broadband signals with bias tones:* With this stimulus, a broadband, speech-weighted signal analyzes the frequency response of hearing aids in the presence of a pure tone or other narrowband "bias" signal. The bias signal simulates the presence of background noise that is constant in amplitude. In automatic gain control (AGC) circuits the bias tone will set the overall gain (as would a constant level of background noise), while the broadband signal reveals the frequency response of the instrument under the "biased" condition. The broadband signal and bias tone can have various relative amplitudes to simulate various signal/noise ratios.

2. *Roving warble tones:* With this stimulus, a sequence of warble tones presents either a predetermined or a random order of frequencies that follow statistically prescribed criteria for duration and amplitude. The notion is to test how hearing aids perform with stimuli that vary somewhat like speech does.

3. *ICRA noise:* The ICRA[†] has created an audio compact disc (CD) containing samples of a novel speech-simulating signal. The signal is a random-type noise that has been modulated by real speech in such a way as to overlay, on the noise, the long-term spectral and short-term temporal qualities of speech. In some digital hearing aids, this signal has been demonstrated to result in performance similar to that achieved with real speech inputs (S. Westermann, personal communication).

4. *Fluctuating composite:* With this signal, a speech-weighted tone composite has been adjusted to fluctuate according to the short-term temporal qualities of real speech. This signal is somewhat similar to ICRA noise, except that it uses a deterministic, pseudorandom source instead of a random source. This signal is currently available in some REM systems, with the feature that the operator has the ability not only to select between the ICRA and S3.42 (ANSI, 1992) long-term spectra but also to add a bias tone to simulate background noise.

5. *Maximum length sequence:* A maximum length sequence (MLS) is a periodic, digitally generated pseudorandom noise. An MLS starts out as a binary sequence that is arranged such that, after conversion to analog form, the amplitudes and phases over the course of the signal are normally distributed, creating a flat spectral shape. The "beauty" of this signal is that, because it is deterministic, a complete frequency response measurement is captured in only one sample; yet its spectral properties resemble those of random white noise, which requires several averaged test samples to get a good reading. Unlike the infinitely high crest factor of random noise (which must be limited by clipping), the crest factor of a maximum length sequence is relatively low.

Room Acoustics {4.1.2}

The validity and repeatability of real-ear measures depend to a large extent on the choice of the test space and on the physical arrangement of the equipment. The following guidelines should be used when deciding where and how to set up a REM system.

Choose as large a room as possible, and one having the least amount of reverberation possible. A rule of thumb to use on room size is that the distance from both the subject and the loudspeaker to any reflective surface (wall, desk, furniture, REM system, etc.) should be at least twice the distance *between* the subject and the loudspeaker.[‡] For example (referring to Fig. 3–14), if the working distance, *WD*, is 18 inches, the minimum distance from both the subject and the loudspeaker to any reflective surface should be 2 x *WD*, or 36 inches. Whenever possible, choose a room large enough to accommodate that criterion. Also, to minimize standing waves and multiple reflections between opposing walls or corners, aim the loudspeaker so it is not pointing directly at a wall or a corner. To minimize reverberation (a form of extraneous noise), cover large reflective surfaces with sound-absorbing materials: The floor should be carpeted (as thickly as is feasible), and the ceiling should be acoustically treated. Drapes on the walls help, too. Audiological test booths, because of their small size, are generally a poor choice for setting up a REM system, even though all surfaces may be "sound treated."

Ambient Noise {4.1.1}

Choose a room that is relatively free of ambient noise. In addition to blatant interference with test signals, excessive

---

*Find a thorough discussion of the interaction of "traditional" test signals with hearing aids in Revit (1994).

[†]For information about ICRA, contact: Dr. W. A. Dreschler, Academisch Medisch Centrum, KNO - Audiologie D2, Meibergdreef 9, 1105 AZ Amsterdam ZO, The Netherlands; or Dr. S. Westermann, Widex Aps, Ny Vestergaardsvej 25, DK 3500, Vaerlose, Denmark.

[‡]The distance between the emanating surface of the loudspeaker and the center of the subject's head is called the "working distance" {3.1.12}, denoted as "*WD*" in Figure 3–14.

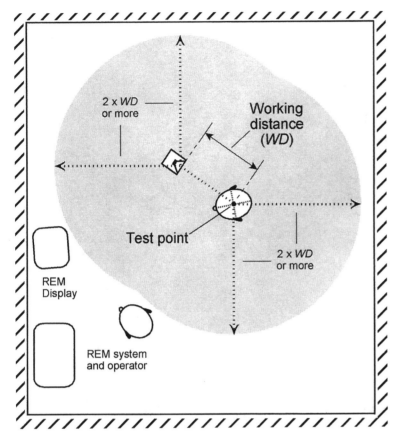

Figure 3–14 Room setup for real-ear measures. The "working distance" is the distance between the center of the subject's head and the emanating surface of the sound source. Ideally, reflective surfaces, such as walls, test equipment, and personnel, should be at least twice the working distance from either the subject or the sound source.

ambient noise can activate AGC action in hearing aids whose compression thresholds are less than the ambient noise level.

Location of the REM Equipment

First of all, remember to apply the rule of thumb given previously regarding the locations of the subject and the loudspeaker. Then, it is important to choose a location for the REM system that lets the clinician operate the equipment conveniently, yet where neither the equipment nor the clinician will be acoustically "in the way." When possible, avoid operating REM equipment from a position near the direct path of sound between the loudspeaker and the patient. The shaded area in Figure 3–14 is the area the operator should avoid. In general, the best place from which to operate the REM system is slightly behind and well to the side of the loudspeaker.

Real-Ear Measures and Clinical Facts of Life

The environment of an audiology clinic presents limitations to obtaining the "perfect" real-ear measures. However, many of these limitations have been minimized by hardware and software processes contained within REM systems. Explanations of some of these limitations and their remedies are given in the following.

Smoothing

Audiological clinicians do not have the luxury of subjects who sit absolutely still and do not wear (acoustically obtrusive) jewelry, stylistic clothing, and coiffures. Also, it is rare to find, in a clinic, a test space large enough or anechoic enough

---

PEARL

Once it is known just where the patients should be during REM testing and where they should face, the video monitor or LCD display of the REM system should be placed where the patient can look at the screen easily when facing the desired direction (see Fig. 3–14). Asking the patient to look at the screen during measurements may help the patient remain still and in the desired position. When a 0-degree azimuth of the loudspeaker (i.e., directly in front of the listener) is used, an orange dot may be placed at the top or bottom of the housing of the loudspeaker for this purpose.

---

to guarantee sound field uniformity and stability (Walker et al, 1984). Because of environmental acoustic anomalies, REMs made under clinical conditions might ordinarily appear so jagged and hard to read as to render a response curve impossible to interpret. This situation can be improved by a common feature of real-ear measures known as "smoothing."

Smoothing is a process by which the resolution (precision) of a measurement is intentionally smeared, across frequency, to bypass many of the effects of environmental acoustic anomalies while maintaining most of the important features of a measurement. An analogy might be a photographer's use

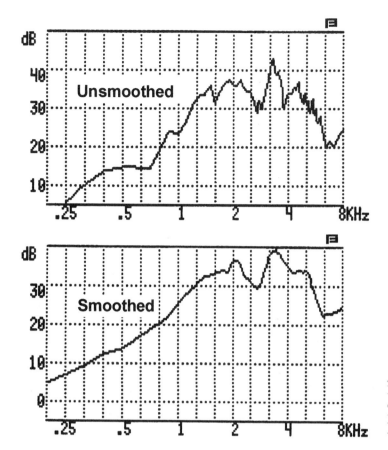

Figure 3–15 Smoothing. Upper curve is an REIG obtained without smoothing. Lower curve is an REIG obtained under the same condition except that post-measurement smoothing was applied.

of a diffusion filter, in portraiture, to obscure the small wrinkles on a face while preserving the important features that define the character behind that face. Figure 3–15 shows an example of an REIG curve whose REAR component was measured with and without smoothing. The important features, such as the amplitudes and frequencies of the primary and secondary resonance peaks, are more clearly visible in the smoothed version *(lower panel)* than in the unsmoothed version *(upper panel)*. However, note that the absolute amplitudes of the peaks are somewhat greater in the unsmoothed version, partly because of the greater precision of the unsmoothed measurement. It is important that the clinician be aware of the compromise on precision from using smoothed curves, yet it is clear that smoothed curves are far more "usable" than unsmoothed ones.

Smoothing can be accomplished by several means, depending on the type of test signal. Each means, however, uses a similar process: Each data point plotted on a frequency response graph, effectively is the average of several data points taken over a range of frequencies. With pure tone stimuli this process is performed mathematically in the software of the REM system. This method is called "post-measurement" smoothing. An example is that a point plotted for 2000 Hz may be the arithmetic average of measurements made at 1800 Hz, 1900 Hz, 2000 Hz, 2100 Hz, and 2200 Hz. The same method would apply for broadband stimuli that are "composites" of many pure tones presented simultaneously. In contrast, with warble tone and 1/3-octave-band noise stimuli, the smoothing process occurs at the same time as the measurement is made. The smoothing is derived from

the intentionally imperfect precision of the signal itself. For example, with a warble tone centered at 2000 Hz, the signal may waver along the frequency range between 1800 Hz and 2200 Hz. Such "frequency modulation" is what makes the tone sound "warbled." The data point plotted for 2000 Hz, in this case, effectively is the average of measurements that were taken over a 400 Hz range centered at 2000 Hz. With 1/3-octave-band noise, each signal spans a 1/3-octave range of frequencies. So a data point plotted for 2000 Hz, again, effectively is the average of measurements taken over the 1/3-octave band centered at 2000 Hz.

Noise Reduction

Another fact of life of clinical real-ear measures is that extraneous noises in the test environment can interfere with the accuracy and repeatability of measurements. REM systems can reduce the effects of extraneous noise without compromising the precision or accuracy of measurements in several ways.

1. *Filtering:* One way to reduce the effects of extraneous noise is to filter the measured signal with a notch-shaped bandpass filter. For example, when measuring the SPL at 2000 Hz, only a narrow band of frequencies centered around 2000 Hz is measured. Other frequencies are filtered out. In this way, noise occurring at frequencies outside the passband of the filter is rejected from the measurement before it is recorded.

2. *Signal averaging:* Some REM systems that operate with deterministic signals use a measurement method known

as "synchronous analysis" {3.4.14}. This method calculates the average of a series of samples of the measured waveform in synchronism with the period of the test signal. Over several synchronized averages, the waveform of the measured signal remains constant in amplitude and phase, whereas the waveform of the extraneous noise randomly fluctuates between positive and negative values across samples. When the samples are averaged, the randomly fluctuating noise cancels out (the average of the positives and negatives approaches zero), but the signal remains intact. The same method is used in brain stem–evoked response measurements to extract specific neural responses from a multitude of neural events, and in otoacoustic emission measurements to extract very weak cochlear signals from the extraneous noises in the test environment.

Sound Field Equalization (Leveling) {3.1.5}

Another clinical fact of life is that the test environment for REMs may be anything but ideal in terms of uniformity of the test sound field. The question of uniformity is: How predictable or repeatable are the level and the spectrum of the test sound field at the field reference point, from one test to another? In almost every clinical test space the answer is that the level and spectrum of the sound field are highly unpredictable, depending on the precise locations of the subject, the person giving the test, the loudspeaker, the reference microphone, and other objects in the room.

The problem of unpredictability of the sound field is solved by correcting the sound field either immediately before or during each measurement. This correction of the sound field is called "leveling" or "equalization" {3.1.5, 6.3}. Equalization of the sound field has the following goal: If the signal source is intended to have a flat spectrum, the signal measured at the field reference point (at the inlet of the control/reference microphone) will also have a flat spectrum. Of course, it follows that if the spectrum of the signal source is shaped in a particular way, the same spectral shaping should appear at the sound field reference point.

In REM systems sound field equalization can occur in two general ways.

1. *Concurrent equalization {3.1.3}:* Also known as "real-time" or "online" equalization, this method adjusts the sound source at the same time as the measurement is made. The REM system continuously adjusts the electrical signal drive to the loudspeaker, such that the intended sound amplitude remains constant at the field reference point (reference microphone) throughout the measurement process. The advantage of this method is that if the subject moves during the measurement, any position-related changes in the sound field will be compensated for.

PITFALL

With concurrent equalization, if the hearing aid is feeding back during measurement, the feedback may enter the reference microphone, and thus influence the control of the test signal.

---

2. *Stored equalization {3.1.9}:* With stored equalization, the REM system records the equalization data at the reference microphone before the measurement is made. With digital REM systems that deliver broadband composite signals, the constant updating of the signal spectrum that would be required by concurrent equalization would be so computationally intensive as to render the measurement process painfully slow. So the fact that the equalization data have already been stored frees the REM system to perform very fast, "real-time" analysis-frequency response measurements that update several times per second.

PITFALL

A potential disadvantage of stored equalization is that if the subject moves between the time of leveling and measurement, resulting changes in the sound field can influence the results. The best way to avoid this pitfall is to level the REM system immediately before each measurement. If it is likely that the subject has moved between leveling and measurement, relevel before making the measurement but be sure any previous measurements that you wish to keep have been properly saved for future use.

Two ways of implementing the preceding equalization methods are the "substitution method of equalization" and the "modified pressure method." Laboratory-controlled real-ear measures often use what is known as the "substitution method of equalization" {3.1.10}. The substitution method is a form of "stored equalization" with which the sound field reference point coincides with the position of center of the subject's head. With the subject absent and with the inlet of the reference microphone at the position in the room where the center of the subject's head will be during testing, the REM system measures and stores the equalization data necessary for leveling the sound field. Later, the subject is positioned at the test point, around which the free-field referred measurements can be made.

For valid, repeatable measurements with the substitution method, the room must exhibit a high degree of acoustic uniformity around the field reference point (Walker et al, 1984). With clinical real-ear measures, such acoustic uniformity is rare, and so an alternate method of equalization becomes the clinical norm. It is called the "modified pressure method of equalization"* {3.1.7}. With this method, the inlet of the reference microphone is placed close to the subject's head, near the test ear, and yet away from the acoustic influence of both the pinna and the hearing aid (exemplified in Fig. 3–13). From this location, the REM system measures the equalization data

---

*Standard test-box measurements of hearing aids use the "pressure method" (ANSI S3.22-1996b). The pressure method calls for the reference microphone to be within a few millimeters of the inlet of the hearing aid microphone. With REMs the reference microphone may be located relatively distantly from the hearing aid microphone; thus the term *modified pressure method* applies.

necessary for leveling the sound field. The modified pressure method can use either concurrent or stored equalization data.

Output Limiting

Perhaps the most important clinical fact of life regarding real-ear measures is the fact that hearing aids can often produce real-ear SPLs that are either uncomfortable or even damaging to the wearer. In fact, the main reason to do real-ear measurements is because one cannot be sure, from coupler measures alone, how a given hearing aid will perform on a given ear. Of special importance is the question: What is the real-ear maximum output? Most clinicians recommend obtaining RESR measures before sending a patient out the door with new hearing aids. The reason is that if the hearing aids are capable of excessive outputs, it is better to find out early, in the clinic, where adjustments can be made, rather than for the patient to find out for oneself later in an intolerably loud real-life situation. Without the proper precautions, such clinical measurements could result in excessive SPLs in the patient's ears.

All REM systems let the clinician specify the maximum SPL permitted at the inlet to the probe microphone. Thus, when the probe microphone is in the earcanal, the REM system effectively limits the maximum real-ear output of the hearing aid. The REM system accomplishes this by reducing the signal drive level the moment the pre-selected SPL is exceeded at the inlet to the probe microphone. Before doing any aided REM on a patient, the clinician must check the setting of the REM system's output limiting to see that the setting is appropriate for that patient.

Preparing to Make Real-Ear Measurements

Otoscopic Inspection

For two purposes, the clinician must inspect the patient's earcanals otoscopically before beginning REM testing (1) to determine that no pathological condition is present that might affect a decision to proceed with testing; and (2) to determine that the earcanal is sufficiently free of cerumen or other obstructions or debris that might interfere with testing. Not only could such obstructions make it difficult to insert the probe tube, but cerumen can easily clog the opening of the probe tube, rendering the probe microphone inoperative. Some REM systems have automatic software that can detect conditions correlating with a blocked probe tube, but it is easy for the clinician to tell when this condition is present just by looking at the measurement results. Figure 3–16 shows an example of two REUG measurements, one *(upper curve)* with a normal probe tube and one *(lower)* with a blocked probe tube. When the probe tube is blocked, the measured output or gain will be unusually low (near the noise floor of the REM system). The same will be true even for an aided response measurement.

Calibration of the Probe-Tube Microphone

The frequency response of a probe-tube microphone is not usually flat without the use of *internal* equalization (distinct from the sound field equalization discussed earlier). The required internal equalization changes somewhat with each type of probe tube. Some REM systems specify the consistent use of a particular model of probe tube, and therefore those systems can store the probe microphone equalization internally. Other REM systems require that the probe-tube microphone be equalized before each use in a simple procedure performed by the operator. The operator places the sound inlet of the probe tube at the center of the sound inlet of the reference microphone, so that each microphone picks up the same signal (see Fig. 3–17). The coincident microphones are then held in front of the loudspeaker while the REM system automatically compares the frequency responses of the two. The REM system then equalizes the probe-microphone response so that it matches the response of the reference microphone. Check the operator's manual of

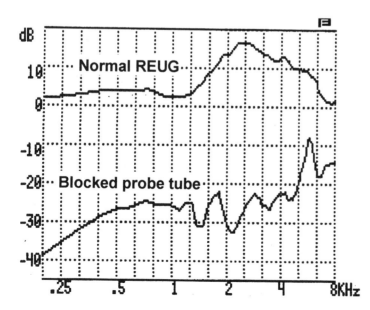

Figure 3–16 Blocked probe tube. Lower curve was an attempt at obtaining an REUG curve, but the probe tube was blocked. Note that all values are well below the 0 dB gain level. Upper REUG curve was measured in the same earcanal after the probe tube was replaced with an unblocked one.

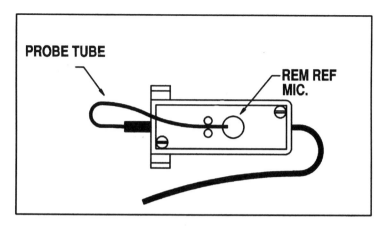

Figure 3–17 Example of housing that combines probe tube and reference microphones. Sound inlet of probe tube is shown in calibration position at sound inlet of reference microphone. (Courtesy Etymonic Design, Inc.)

the REM system to determine what, if any, probe microphone equalization procedure is required.

Placement of the Microphones

The locations of the sound inlets of both the reference and the probe-tube microphones are critical for obtaining of accurate real-ear measures.

Placement of the Reference (Control) Microphone

The location of the sound inlet of the reference microphone determines the field reference point {3.1.6}. The field reference point is the place where the sound field stimulus is calibrated and where the input is determined for real-ear gain calculations.* In some REM systems the reference and probe-tube microphone elements are in the same housing (exemplified in Fig. 3–17). To hold the dual microphone housing in place, these systems generally use a loop placed around the pinna, by which the housing hangs in position either just below the earlobe or else just to the side of the ear.[†] In other REM systems the reference and probe-tube microphone elements are in separate housings (exemplified in Fig. 3–13), and therefore the reference microphone can be placed either above or below the ear, held in place by Velcro-covered fittings. The standard requirement for the location of the reference microphone is only that the operator locate the sound inlet near the head surface, yet out of range of the acoustic influence of either the pinna or the hearing aid.

An additional suggestion might be that the operator chooses a reference microphone location that is precisely repeatable, in case one ever wants to compare current measurements to future or previous ones. The best way to ensure repeatability is to be consistent. For systems using a hanging dual-microphone housing, the clinician should decide on a position relative to the earlobe and always use that position. For over-the-ear reference microphones, the clinician should

decide on a position relative to the apex of the pinna and should always use that position.

Placement of the Probe Tube

The location of the sound inlet of the probe-tube microphone is called the "measurement point" {3.4.3}. The measurement point in the earcanal determines, for high frequencies, how accurately the measured SPL represents the SPL at the eardrum. The REM operator must keep two acoustic conditions in mind. First, at the measurement point in the earcanal, sound reflected from the eardrum can interfere with sound just arriving. Such reflective interference causes sound-pressure nulls at distances from the eardrum equal to one quarter the wavelength of the frequency of interest. Figure 3–18 illustrates this point (Dirks & Kincaid, 1987). Each curve represents the SPL at a given high frequency measured by a probe-tube microphone in the earcanal at varied distances from the eardrum. Note that for relatively lower frequencies (which means longer wavelengths), the pressure nulls occur at greater distances from the eardrum. For frequencies lower than about 2000 Hz, these nulls are not a problem. The take-home message is that for the most accurate estimates of the SPL at the eardrum for high frequencies, one must place the tip of the probe tube as close as possible to the eardrum. However, for clinical purposes, placing the sound inlet of the probe tube within 6 mm (about 1/4 inch) of the eardrum ensures that the measured SPL will agree with the SPL at the eardrum within 2 dB through about 6000 Hz, and within 4 dB through about 8000 Hz. The above, "6 mm" rule of thumb applies to all open-ear and occluded-ear measurements.

A second acoustic consideration for placement of the probe tube applies only for aided REMs. When sound emanates from a small opening into a larger diameter (such as the sound emanating from hearing aids into an earcanal), sound-pressure nulls form at high frequencies in the vicinity of the sound outlet (see Fig. 3–19, Sachs & Burkhard, 1971). These nulls can be explained by the physics of radial waves, which is beyond the scope of this chapter. In simple terms, the greater the distance from the sound outlet, the higher the frequency of the null. Therefore, for accurate estimates of the SPL at the eardrum for high frequencies, the sound inlet of the probe microphone should always be placed well beyond the region of the null at the highest frequency of interest.

---

*"Real-ear gain," in this context, is defined as "output minus input." This definition applies to REAG, REUG, and REOG, but *not* to REIG, which is defined as "REAG minus REUG."

[†]NOTE: When the microphone housing is positioned to the side of the ear, higher than the bottom of the earlobe, the loudspeaker must be placed at 0 degrees azimuth to avoid reflective interference.

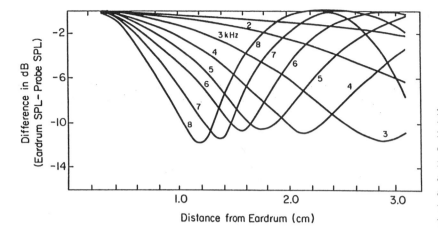

Figure 3–18 Difference between probe microphone SPL and eardrum SPL at varied distances from the eardrum for various frequencies. Sound-pressure nulls occur at distances from the eardrum equal to approximately one-fourth the wavelength of the test tone. (From Dirks & Kincaid [1987], with permission.)

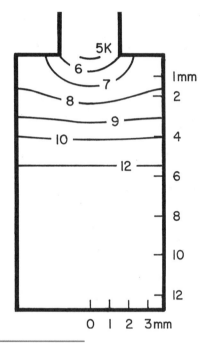

Figure 3–19 Schematic representation of sound entering an occluded earcanal simulator through a 3-mm opening. Contour lines with numbers indicate sound-pressure nulls at indicated frequencies (in kHz). To avoid REM errors caused by these nulls, a rule of thumb is to extend the probe tube at least 5 mm beyond a 3-mm sound outlet. Deeper extension is required for high-frequency accuracy as the diameter of the sound outlet decreases. (From Sachs and Burkhard [1971], with permission.)

For sound outlets of 3 mm or more (for example, a BTE with a 3-mm horn), placing the sound inlet of the probe microphone at least 5 mm medially to the sound outlet of the hearing aid will ensure negligible radial wave interference through about 8000 Hz. For smaller sound outlets (e.g., for No. 13 tubing, which has an internal diameter of 1.93 mm, or for most ITEs, which have a sound outlet diameter of 1.35 mm), a greater distance from the sound outlet is required to avoid interference. None of this, of course, applies to CICs, which are often less than 5 mm from the eardrum to begin with.

PEARL

Because the REIG represents a *difference* between two REMs (REAG minus REUG), the absolute position of the sound inlet of the probe-tube microphone is less important than with other REMs (Hawkins & Mueller, 1986). Any acoustic anomalies related to probe position will be common to both the REAG and the REUG measures and will subtract out of the REIG. What is important is that the measurement point stays in precisely the *same* place for both the REAG and the REUG.

Methods of Positioning the Probe Tube

Researchers and clinicians have developed many methods for determining that the probe tube is in an acceptable position for REMs. This section will present four such methods: the otoscopic method, the acoustic method, the average-length method, and the earmold method.

1. *Otoscopic method:* To many clinicians, viewing the probe tube in the earcanal with an otoscope is the most reliable way to determine, reasonably accurately, that the tip of the probe tube is within 6 mm of the eardrum. First, while looking into the earcanal with an otoscope, visually estimate the length of the earcanal. Then, mark the probe tube at a position you estimate will correspond to the tragus, once the tip of the probe tube lies within 6 mm of the eardrum. On average, the adult earcanal is 24 mm long, so, for an earcanal of average length, the probe tip needs to be positioned at least 18 mm medially to the opening of the earcanal. The distance between the opening of earcanal and the tragus is about another 10 mm. So, for the average-size ear, you would mark the probe tube at 28 mm from the tip. For smaller ears and shorter earcanals, you could use 25 or 26 mm as the starting point; for children's ears, even less. Once you have marked the probe tube, slowly insert it into the earcanal, stopping when the mark lies near the tragus or the intertragal notch. Now look into the ear once more with the otoscope to see how far from the eardrum the tip of the probe tube lies. Carefully adjust the position of the probe tube, if necessary, so that

the tip lies within 6 mm of the eardrum, then confirm the position with the otoscope.

2. *Acoustic method:* Three variations of the acoustic method exist. An acoustic method for positioning the probe tube in REMs was described by Sullivan (1988). Sullivan's method requires that the clinician create a homemade device, with a paper clip used for stabilizing the probe tube at various insertion depths. A 6000 Hz warble tone is introduced into the earcanal at a field reference level of at least 60 dB SPL. The probe tube is slowly inserted until a position is found to produce a minimum SPL. According to Figure 3–18, a null for 6000 Hz corresponds to a distance of about 15 mm from the eardrum. With the probe tube in this position, mark the tube at the tragus or intertragal notch, and then at a point 10 mm lateral to the first mark. Insert the probe tube so that the second mark is now even with the tragus or intertragal notch. The result is a measurement point that is approximately 5 mm from the eardrum.

A variation of this method, using a real-time or repeatedly swept signal, goes as follows: A broadband or repeatedly swept warble tone signal is introduced at a field reference level of 70 dB SPL. While the audiologist watches the real-time readout on the screen, the probe tube is slowly advanced into the earcanal until an SPL minimum at 6000 Hz is observed. The probe tube continues to be advanced slowly, at increments of perhaps 2 mm. The SPL at 6000 Hz will begin to rise out of the null. This is continued until no appreciable additional rise in SPL is seen at 6000 Hz as the tube is advanced the next increment.

3. *Average-length method:* According to various studies (e.g., Zemplenyi et al, 1985; Zwislocki, 1980), the length of the average adult human earcanal is between 23 and 25 mm. The average-length method thus begins by assuming the patient's earcanal is approximately 24 mm long. The pre-REM otoscopic inspection either will support the assumption of an earcanal of average length or will suggest a modification of that assumption. For an earcanal of seemingly average length, the clinician marks the probe tube at perhaps 28 mm from the tip. This distance corresponds to 24 mm for the earcanal, plus 10 mm for the distance between the earcanal opening and the tragus or intertragal notch, minus 6 mm for the target distance from the eardrum. The probe tube is then placed in the earcanal such that the mark is even with the tragus or intertragal notch. Because it is desired to be within 6 mm of the eardrum for all earcanals, the 28-mm rule may be adjusted according to age and sex. The 28-mm mark is often used for adult women, whose earcanals, on average, are at the shorter end of the average adult range. For children's earcanals, or others that on inspection appear to be well shorter than average, the tube is marked closer to the tip (20 to 25 mm for children). For adult men or other longer earcanals, the tube is marked farther from the tip (31 mm for adult men) (Moodie et al, 1994).

4. *Earmold method:* The earmold method is applicable only to insertion-gain measurements, which require only that (a) the probe tube inlet be positioned beyond the influence of radial-wave effects during aided measurements; and (b) the probe tube inlet be at the same position in the earcanal for both the aided and unaided measurements.

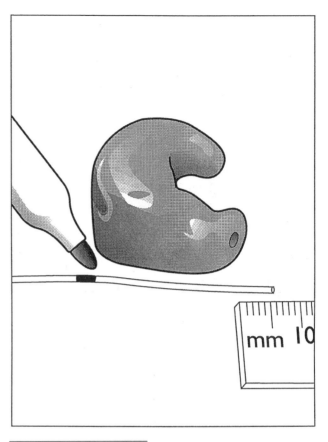

Figure 3–20 Marking of probe tube. Rule of thumb for high-frequency accuracy is that the sound inlet of the probe tube must extend at least 5 mm beyond the sound outlet of the hearing aid for a sound outlet diameter of 3 mm. As the diameter of the sound outlet decreases, greater extension of the probe tube is required for high-frequency accuracy.

1. Align the probe tube along the bottom of the earmold or shell (Fig. 3–20), so that the probe tube inlet lies at least 5 mm beyond the sound outlet of the earmold or shell. A greater distance from the sound outlet to the probe tube inlet is required for sound outlets less than 3 mm in diameter.

2. Mark the probe tube at the point corresponding to the intertragal notch.

3. Place the probe tube in the earcanal such that the mark on the tube is even with the intertragal notch (Fig. 3–13).

PEARL

Once the probe tube is in position in the earcanal, the audiologist may wish to secure it in place by applying surgical tape over the tube and around the earlobe or the helix. Also, when inserting an earmold or shell, the audiologist may wish to hold the probe tube with the finger to prevent the tube from moving.

Positioning the Loudspeaker and Patient

The general locations of the loudspeaker and the patient during REMs have been predetermined by the arrangement of the test room as described and depicted in Figure 3–14. The remaining fine-tuning involves two steps: (1) the precise designation of a "test point" {3.1.11}, which is where the center of the head of the patient will be during testing; and (2) the placement of the loudspeaker relative to the test point. The distance between the emanating surface of the loudspeaker and the test point is called the "working distance" (see Fig. 3–14) {3.1.12}. The greater the working distance, the more that room acoustics can influence the measurement results. The smaller the working distance, the more the patient's head movements can influence the measurement results. Obviously, the clinician must arrive at a compromise. However, with the small loudspeakers normally used in clinical REM systems, a working distance of 30 to 60 cm (1 to 2 feet) usually works well. The horizontal angle of the loudspeaker relative to the "plane of symmetry" directly in front of the patient is called the "azimuth angle" (Fig. 3–21, *upper panel*) {3.1.2}. The vertical angle of the loudspeaker relative to the "horizontal plane" at ear level is called the "elevation angle" (Fig. 3–21, *lower panel*) {3.1.4}. Figures 3–2 and 3–3 show the relative effects of azimuth and elevation for REUR measures. Note in Figure 3–2 that the earcanal SPL generally increases as the azimuth angle increases from 0 to 90 degrees. Also, in Figure 3–3, note that the high-frequency "concha" dip (at about 8000 Hz) moves higher in frequency and becomes more shallow

as the elevation angle increases beyond 0 degrees. (Note that the curves in Figure 3–3 are measurements of the "blocked meatus," not the open earcanal, so the primary canal resonance at 2700 Hz is not seen.)

In real life, people listen from many azimuth angles, and no single azimuth angle will clearly represent most listening positions (see Controversial Point). The question of the best position of the loudspeaker for real-ear testing then becomes which azimuth angle yields the most *reliable* real-ear measures? A 1987 study of insertion-gain repeatability versus loudspeaker location addressed that question (Killion & Revit, 1987). Results showed that placing the loudspeaker at an azimuth angle of 45 degrees toward the test ear produced significantly better repeatability than did placing the loudspeaker at 0 degrees (see Fig. 3–22). These results were independently replicated in a later study (Trede, 1990).

Positioning the Operator

The position of the operator should not influence the sound field during leveling or testing. The shaded area in Figure 3–14 shows where the operator should *not* be. In general terms the operator should be either well behind or well to the side of either the loudspeaker or the patient.

Choosing a Signal Type and Amplitude

The choice of the type and the amplitude of the test signal is, of course, limited to what is available on the REM system.

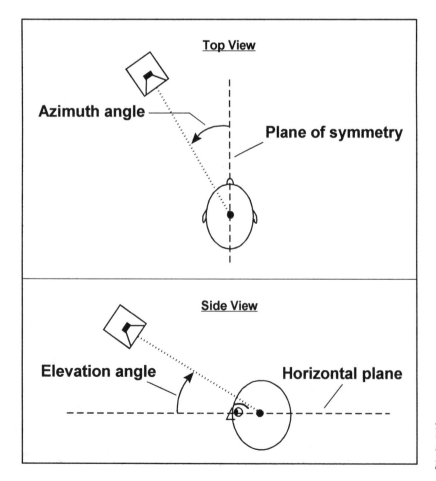

Figure 3–21 Schematic representations of azimuth (*upper panel*) and elevation (*lower panel*) angles.

CONTROVERSIAL POINT

The choice of the azimuth and elevation of the loudspeaker remains in some controversy. Intuitively, it may seem that real-ear testing should be done with the loudspeaker directly in front of the patient. The idea is that, in the real world of conversational speech, the talker and the listener would normally stand or sit facing each other. Yet I observe that people hardly ever face one another directly while conversing; usually, they *partially* face one another, then complete the appropriate eye contact by pointing their eyes toward one another. The reader is asked, sometime soon, to observe a group of two or more diners sitting at adjacent sides of a square table. When the person immediately to a listener's side begins to talk, does the listener turn his or her head as far as is necessary to directly face the talker? Or does the listener turn *partially* toward the talker, and point his eyes in the direction of the talker to complete the appropriate eye contact? If the first case were true, a lot of sore necks would result.

PITFALL

Some portable REM systems have a hinged or built-in loudspeaker, which, when attached to the main unit, sits directly behind a reflective horizontal surface and directly in front of a reflective vertical surface (such as that containing an LCD display). Avoid operating a REM system with the loudspeaker in this configuration because reflective interference from the horizontal and vertical surfaces can confound measurements. In practice, the REM unit itself effectively becomes a nearby reflective floor and wall. With these REM systems, always separate the loudspeaker from the REM unit to avoid interference from the horizontal and vertical surfaces of the unit.

SPECIAL CONSIDERATION

When measuring the RESR, a narrowband signal is used at the highest amplitude possible. If available, use "short bursts" of tones, so that the patient's exposure to loud sounds is minimized. *Before the RESR is tested, the "output-limiting" feature of the REM system should be set properly for patient protection.*

when a linear hearing aid is saturated by a high-amplitude signal, the instrument is no longer operating linearly and is therefore sensitive to the type of signal. For observing the *frequency response* of hearing aids under saturated conditions, a broadband signal is used, if possible. But to see the highest possible case of maximum output (i.e., the RESR), a narrowband signal is used (Revit, 1994).

Compression Hearing Aids
with Single-Channel, Broadband Detectors

To determine the amount of gain to produce for a given circumstance, compression hearing aids have circuits that detect the amplitude of the input signal. Single-channel compression hearing aids (and some multichannel aids, as well) have only one such detector, and it is a broadband one. When the microphones in such hearing aids have flat frequency responses, the measured frequency responses of the instruments will be the same for both broadband and narrowband test signals. But if the response of the hearing aid microphone is sloping, a narrowband signal can yield potentially misleading results for frequency response tests such as those obtained through REMs.

The potential for error arises from the fact that the sloping response of a hearing aid microphone alters the amplitude of the signal entering the detection circuitry of the hearing aid, from one frequency to the next, even though the SPL at the hearing aid microphone may stay constant. Because of the gain-reduction action of wide dynamic-range compression (WDRC), frequencies of relatively low amplitude in the detection circuit will show higher gain than will frequencies of relatively high amplitude. The result is a "blooming" of the frequency-response curve at low frequencies when using iso-amplitude narrowband signals (exemplified in Fig. 3–23). Such blooming of measured low-frequency response would be an accurate portrayal of real-world response for narrowband signals such as whistles and beeps, but not for most speech sounds.

Multichannel Compression Hearing Aids
with Multichannel Detector Circuits

This is a unique class of hearing aids in that, when presented with a broadband signal, the hearing aids themselves narrow the effective bandwidth of the input signal. That is, the circuitry of the hearing aids split the input signal into multiple, comparatively narrow bands, creating multiple channels for both audio processing and level detection. It is possible to have multiple audio channels without having multiple detectors. In such circuits the energy within the range of one frequency band can affect the performance in another frequency band.

Beyond that limitation, the choice depends on what the tester wishes to accomplish.

For real-ear testing of the general performance of hearing aids, the following guidelines may be helpful. In some cases the reader is directed to use a specific signal for a given purpose. In other cases the reader is provided only general information that can help with a decision as to which signal to use.

Linear Hearing Aids

If hearing aids are operating linearly, REM results will be the same regardless of the signal type and amplitude. However,

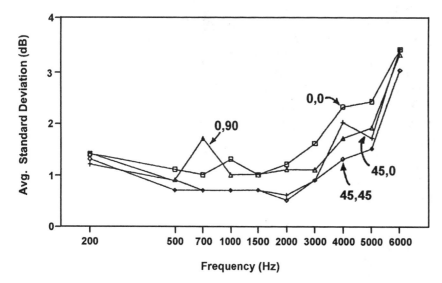

Figure 3–22 Average standard deviations for repeated REIG measurements at various loudspeaker locations. As per convention, each curve label gives the azimuth angle followed by the elevation angle. The best repeatability was obtained using a 45-degree azimuth and a 45-degree elevation. No reference microphone was used in obtaining these measurements. (Adapted from Killion and Revit [1987], with permission.)

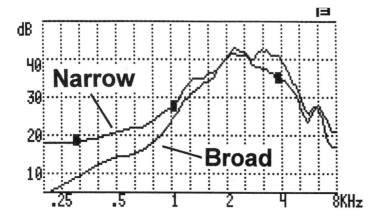

Figure 3–23 REAG measures of a dual-channel, dual-detector hearing aid having WDRC. Curve marked "narrow" *(filled rectangles)* was obtained with a pure tone signal. Curve marked "broad" *(no symbols)* was obtained with a speech-weighted composite signal.

This effect can be seen in the 2-cc coupler curves of Figure 3–24, where changes in the input amplitude of a speech-weighted signal, in which low frequencies predominate, caused changes in the gain at high frequencies. Only one level detector in this circuit controlled the compression in all audio bands.

With multiple detectors, however, each audio channel of the hearing aid behaves independently of the others. In such cases the measured performance depends both on the bandwidth and on the spectral weighting of the signal. When using a broadband signal, measured performance in a particular frequency band will depend on the amplitude of the portion of the signal contained within the band. For example, you might present a speech-weighted noise signal to a two-channel instrument. Speech weighting causes the test signal to have more energy at low frequencies than at high frequencies. With dual-detection two-channel compression, such a signal will produce relatively less gain at low frequencies than at high frequencies compared with a signal having equal spectral weighting in each band. This result can be seen in the REAG curves of Figure 3–23, where a broadband speech-weighted signal in fact produced less low-frequency gain and more high-frequency gain than did an iso-amplitude narrowband sweep.

Choosing Which Tests to Run and When

The choice of which REMs to make depends on the fitting procedure the dispenser is using and also on the patient's

needs. REM-based fitting procedures are covered in detail in Chapters 4, 5, 6, 7, and 12 in this volume. Whatever the fitting method, keep in mind that real-ear measures are but an objective assessment of sound processing. REMs do not replace subjective impressions the patient may offer, nor do they replace appropriate tests of aided speech recognition. In general, confirmatory real-ear measures serve as a jumping-off point in the process of fine-tuning the fit of hearing aids. Always remeasure real-ear performance after making final adjustments. These measures will provide a baseline for future troubleshooting. Also helpful in this regard, the clinician should measure baseline 2-cc coupler responses with the final settings.

Instructions to the Patient

Once seated at the test position, the patient should sit up straight yet comfortably, look straight ahead, and be quiet and still during all the REM procedures. As mentioned earlier, it may be helpful for the patient to have something to look at, directly in front of the patient (as in Fig. 3–14). Doing so may assist the patient in maintaining the desired head position. When testing with high-amplitude signals, the patient should be informed to expect to hear some brief, very loud sounds, but that the REM system is set to shut down automatically or to turn itself down rapidly should excessive

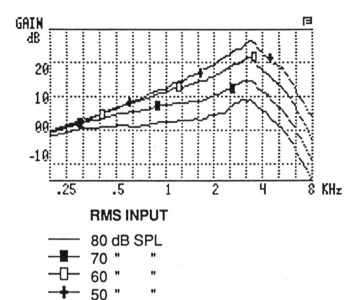

RMS INPUT

—— 80 dB SPL
—■— 70 " "
—□— 60 " "
—+— 50 " "

Figure 3–24 2-cc coupler responses of a single-channel, single-detector WDRC hearing aid having a "treble increases at low levels" (TILL) response characteristic for varied rms input SPLs.

levels be detected in the earcanal. The patient should always be told to let the clinician know immediately if any discomfort is experienced during measurements.

Procedures

Once the appropriate preparations for real-ear measurements have been made, the mechanics of making the actual measurements are relatively simple and easy. The following procedures are given with the assumption that the clinician has completed all the appropriate preparatory steps as summarized in the following.

Summary of Preparations for REMs

NOTE: The precise order of some of the following steps is flexible.

1. Choose which tests to run (e.g., REAG, RESR, etc.).
2. Seat the patient at the test point.
3. Perform an otoscopic inspection of the test ear(s).
4. If required, calibrate the probe-tube microphone.
5. Secure the reference and probe-tube microphones in the appropriate positions.
6. Position the loudspeaker.
7. Choose an appropriate signal type and amplitude.
8. **Check that the output-limiting protection feature of the REM system is set appropriately for the patient.**
9. Assume a position for operating the REM system that is out of the way of acoustic interference.
10. Instruct the patient to sit still and quietly and to face directly forward.

Real-Ear Unaided Response/Or Gain

1. Set the REM system to run an unaided measurement and to display the results as either SPL or gain (as applicable).

2. If applicable, equalize (level) the sound field.
3. Obtain the REUR or REUG.

NOTE: The signal amplitude for the REUR/G is of little consequence because the unaided open ear is a totally passive device that will produce the same relative SPL at the eardrum for any signal amplitude. The only requirement of signal amplitude is that it must exceed the noise floor of the test system (including room noise) by at least 10 dB at all test frequencies.

Real-Ear Aided Response/Gain

1. While taking care that the probe tube does not move appreciably during insertion, insert the earmold or shell of the hearing aid into the test ear.
2. If applicable, equalize (level) the sound field.
3. Turn the hearing aid on and set the volume control or programming to the desired settings.
4. Set the REM system to run an aided measurement and to display the results as either SPL or gain (as applicable).
5. Set the signal type and amplitude as desired.
6. Obtain the REAR or REAG.
7. For nonlinear hearing aids, repeat the REAR/G measurement at several signal amplitudes (e.g., 50-, 65-, and 80-dB SPL) as desired.

PEARL

For insertion-gain measurements, the mark on the probe tube may have to be slightly more medial for the aided measurement than for the unaided measurement to ensure the same position of the tip of the tube for both measurements. This is because of the extra distance the probe tube must cover to get around the shape of the earmold or shell (Revit, 1993a).

SPECIAL CONSIDERATION

FM Systems:

When obtaining real-ear measures of an FM system or other similar assistive listening device, REM procedures must be altered in two ways: (1) The reference microphone used for equalization and calibration must be placed at the location of the transmitting microphone of the FM system. This means that one must be able to separate the reference microphone from the probe microphone if the REM system uses concurrent equalization. (This alteration of procedure applies to all real-ear measures of FM systems, such as the REAR/G and the RESR.) (2) For estimating the REAR/G for real-world speech signals into an FM system, one must use a higher signal level than for hearing aids because the talker is usually very close to the transmitting microphone. Ideally, the amplitude and spectral weighting of the signal should match those of the speech signals generally encountered by the transmitting microphone of an FM system. For a lapel-type transmitting microphone, the nominal level is approximately 85 dB SPL. For a boom microphone, the nominal signal level is very much greater, so the maximum signal level available must be used on the REM system. When possible, a speech-weighted signal and, when applicable, a signal whose speech weighting has been compensated for the location of the transmitting microphone in actual use should be used. NOTE: No consensus has been reached as to the best real-ear procedure to use for fitting FM systems, although the commonly used clinical approach, at this time, is to match the performance of a patient's FM system to that of the patient's hearing aid, assuming the hearing aid has been properly fitted and is working properly.

Real-Ear Insertion Gain

1. Set the REM system for insertion-gain measurement.
2. Obtain the REUR or REUG.*
3. Obtain the REAR or REAG. (NOTE: With REAR measurements for insertion gain, the signal amplitude must be the

---

*For prescriptive insertion-gain applications, the author recommends using a pre-stored, "average-ear" curve for the REUR/G instead of using the individual measure, provided such an average-ear curve is available for the specific system setup you are using. See the Preferred Practice Guidelines at the end of this chapter for details.

same as was used to obtain the REUR or else the REM system must compensate for the level change. This requirement does not apply when working with the REAG and REUG.)

4. The REM system will subtract the REUR/G from the REAR/G, displaying the result as the REIG. For nonlinear hearing aids, the REAR/G should be repeated, thus displaying a new REIG, for several signal levels, as desired (see "Pearl" on wide dynamic-range compression). If working with the REAR for this step, the REIG software should compensate for differences in signal amplitude compared with that used for the REUR.

PEARL

WDRC decreases gain as input level increases above the compression threshold (see Chapter 1 in this volume). Therefore, when fitting WDRC hearing aids, especially when relying on automatic programming schemes or a target REIG strategy, it is a good idea to check the REIG at several input levels. A significant REIG might be observed when using an input SPL of 50 dB, yet the WDRC gain-reduction action could decrease the REIG to zero or less for an input SPL of 70 dB.

Real-Ear Occluded Response/Gain

1. After marking the probe tube and placing it in the ear in the normal way, insert the earmold or shell of the hearing aid into the test ear, taking care not to move the position of the probe tube.
2. The hearing aid should *not* be turned on.
3. Set the REM system to run an aided measurement and to display the results as either SPL or gain (as applicable).
4. Set the signal type and amplitude as desired, but to an amplitude great enough so that the attenuated response measure of sound leaking through the earmold will be more than 10 dB above the noise floor of the REM system for each frequency of interest.
5. If applicable, equalize (level) the sound field.
6. Record REOR or REOG in the same way the REAR or REAG would be recorded.

Real-Ear Saturation Response

1. *Important!* Set the output limiting of the REM system to an appropriate maximum permitted SPL.
2. If applicable, equalize (level) the sound field.
3. Inform the patient to expect a test of maximum possible output of the hearing aid. Tell the patient that he or she will hear very loud sounds, but that those sounds will be very brief and they should not cause discomfort. Explain

that the REM system is set to prevent excessive sound levels, and ask the patient to inform the clinician if any discomfort occurs.

4. Insert the earmold or shell of the hearing aid into the test ear, turn it on, set the volume control and program as desired. (NOTE: For true saturation response, showing the maximum possible output, the volume control should be set to full-on or to the highest possible setting before audible feedback.)

5. Set the REM system to display the output SPL for short tone bursts at the highest possible signal amplitude.

6. Obtain the RESR.

PEARL

For REM systems using stored sound field equalization, it is possible to achieve signal amplitudes higher than the maximum setting on the REM unit. To do this, first level the system in the normal way. Then halve the working distance (move the loudspeaker halfway toward the patient). The signal amplitude will now be 6 dB higher than the setting shows. Halving the working distance again will increase the signal amplitude by another 6 dB.

SPECIAL CONSIDERATION

REMs of CROS and BICROS hearing aids. No standardized methods exist for real-ear testing CROS and BICROS instruments, yet the following special procedures can serve as guidelines.

CROS Head-Shadow Benefit

This procedure can demonstrate how well a CROS instrument overcomes the acoustic shadow of the head for sounds arriving from the "bad-ear" side. (You must be able to place the probe and reference microphones on opposite sides of the head. Some REM systems may require a special accessory.)

1. Referring to Figure 3–25, with the opening of the probe microphone placed in the earcanal of the better ear and with both the loudspeaker and the reference microphone* placed on the "bad-ear" side, obtain and save an unaided measurement (REUR/G).

---

*In Figure 3–25, the reference microphone is shown above the bad ear; the above-the-ear position is only an example. The procedure should use whatever is the normal position of the reference microphone, although at the bad ear.

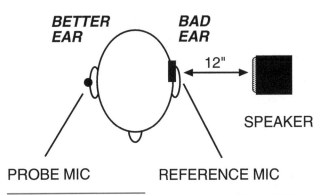

Figure 3–25 Setup for measuring how well a CROS or BICROS hearing aid overcomes the head-shadow effect. (Courtesy Frye Electronics, Inc.)

2. After placing the hearing aid receiver (turned on) into the better ear and the hearing aid microphone at the bad ear, obtain and save an aided measurement (REAR/G).

The difference between the aided and unaided measurements, the REIG, will show the net benefit (to the better ear) for sounds originating from the bad-ear side.

BICROS Head-Shadow Benefit

This procedure is similar to the procedure given previously for CROS aids but with some differences.

1. Referring to Figure 3–25, obtain an aided measurement (REAR/G) with the opening of the probe microphone placed in the earcanal of the better ear and both the loudspeaker and the reference microphone placed on the bad-ear side. For this first measurement, keep the hearing aid microphone on the bad-ear side turned *off* (or unplugged). Save this measurement as if it were an unaided measurement, even though it is actually an aided measurement.

2. Now turn on (or plug in) the hearing aid microphone on the bad-ear side and obtain a second REAR/G, this time saving it as an aided measure.

The curve labeled "insertion gain" (even thought it is not truly an REIG) will show the net benefit to the better ear of adding the microphone on the bad-ear side for sounds arriving from the bad-ear side.

Overall Insertion-Gain Measures for CROS and BICROS Instruments

Follow the normal REIG procedure given earlier, but if you normally use a 45-degree azimuth for the loudspeaker, use exclusively 0 degrees for CROS and BICROS measurements. With BICROS, be sure both hearing aid microphones are turned on.

Real-Ear-to-Coupler Difference

Procedures for obtaining the RECD require changes in the preparation process. The necessary changes will become apparent after studying the procedures. The RECD can be obtained in several ways. Each involves two measurements

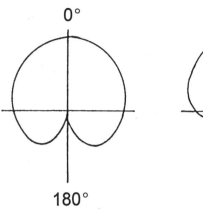

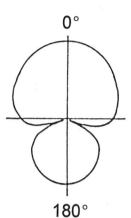

Figure 3–26 Polar plots showing sensitivity as a function of direction for cardioid and hypercardioid directional microphones. Extrapolated to 360-degree space, the cardioid pattern has a single-point null in sensitivity for sounds arriving from 180-degree relative to straight ahead. The hypercardioid has a conical null at about 115 degrees relative to straight ahead. Directional hearing aid microphones having these polar patterns in free space will not have the same patterns when worn on the head.

CONTROVERSIAL POINT

When obtaining REMs of hearing aids having directional microphones, testing with just one direction of the sound source (i.e., from 0 degrees or 45 degrees azimuth) does not provide information regarding the directional performance of these instruments. A possible solution would be to make one measurement from in front of the patient and one from behind. Intuitively, such a comparison would give the tester an idea of how a patient's hearing aids reject "unwanted" signals (from behind) versus "targeted" signals arriving from in front. However, some directional microphones are designed with a "null" (direction of minimum sensitivity) facing directly toward the rear (as with a cardioid pattern), and others have a cone of nulls facing somewhat toward the rear yet slightly off to the side (as with a hypercardioid pattern), as illustrated in Figure 3–26. Theoretical evidence suggests that the latter design may provide better overall rejection of unwanted sounds in real-world conditions, where the listener is immersed in a diffuse, noisy background. However, a front-to-back REM comparison of directional hearing aids having cardioid patterns would indicate superior performance compared with the same test for instruments having hypercardioid patterns, even though the hypercardioid patterns might perform better in real-world conditions. Thus, one is pressed to find a REM protocol that is at least even-handed regarding directional performance. One possible solution might be to make one measurement from in front on each hearing aid and then rotate the patient until a null position is found for each hearing aid (indicated by minimum output). The comparison measurement could then be made from a "customized" null direction in each case. The problem with this procedure is that with WDRC instruments the gain will increase when the signal is at the null position, thus obscuring the directional effects. To date, no REM procedure has been validated to be indicative of real-world performance for directional hearing aids.

---

using the same signal. In general terms: (1) obtain the 2-cc coupler response of an insert earphone or hearing aid, and (2) obtain the real-ear response of the same insert earphone or hearing aid. The procedures following use the "insertion-gain" facility of the REM system to obtain the RECD. Unless the REM system has software dedicated specifically to

obtaining the RECD, it is convenient to use the insertion-gain software for this purpose because, like the REIG, the RECD involves calculating the difference between two measures. If the REM system has dedicated RECD software, the manufacturer's instructions will supersede the procedures following. Check the manufacturer's instructions anyway because each REM system has unique qualities that could alter the RECD procedure—often leading to simplified procedures that may take less of the clinician's time.

If you are using the insertion-gain setup of your REM system, as in the procedures given below, you will use the facility normally used to obtain the REUR/G to instead obtain the 2-cc coupler response of the insert earphone or hearing aid. Then, you will use the facility normally used to obtain the REAR/G, to instead obtain the real-ear response of the insert earphone or hearing aid. The difference between the two measures, what would normally be displayed as the REIG, will instead be the RECD. If you are using the same insert earphone or hearing aid to obtain repeated RECD measurements, you will not need to remeasure the 2-cc coupler response for each RECD. If your REM system has the necessary facility, you can store the 2-cc coupler response in memory and then transfer the data to the REUR/G location of the REM system each time you need it, rather than to measure it each time.

The sound source for the RECD procedure can be a well-damped hearing aid in a sound field, a well-damped hearing aid having a direct audio input (which is, in effect, an insert earphone with active signal processing) or any insert earphone whose source impedance resembles that of a well-damped hearing aid. Three RECD procedures are given in the following. The first procedure uses an ER-3A (a.k.a. E-A-RTone-3A) or other insert earphone as the sound source (Fikret-Pasa & Revit, 1992). Two special features are required of the REM system for this procedure; the operator must be able to (1) disable the reference microphone during measurements, and (2) disconnect the test signal from the loudspeaker and instead connect the signal source to the insert earphone. For REM systems not having these features, an alternative procedure follows, which uses a hearing aid in a sound field instead of the insert earphone (Revit, 1991b). A third RECD procedure is applicable exclusively for use with fitting BTE hearing aids, and therefore is especially applicable to working with young children (Moodie et al, 1994). These procedures are intentionally generic, that is, not directly linked to one REM system or another. Variations will likely be required, depending on the specific features of the REM system you are using.

RECD Procedure Using ER (or EAR-Tone) 3A Insert Earphone

A. **Obtain the HA-1, 2-cc coupler response.**

1. Set the REM system to measure "insertion gain." Also set the REM system to disable the reference microphone during measurements and, if possible, to operate without equalization of the signal source (a condition called "unleveled" with some systems). With some real-ear systems you may have to circumvent the preceding requirement by equalizing the signal drive using the "substitution-method" mode of operation with the loudspeaker still attached.

2. Disconnect the loudspeaker from the signal source of the REM system and instead connect the insert earphone.

3. Using a darning needle, thread a probe tube through the foam eartip of the insert earphone, so that the tip of the probe tube extends 6 mm beyond the sound outlet of the eartip, as shown in Figure 3–27. Always be sure the probe tube extends 6 mm (± 1 mm) with this coupler measurement, even if you will use a different extension of the probe tube for the real-ear measurement in part B. (Doing so results in the tip of the probe tube being placed near the bottom of the 2-cc cavity.)

4. Place a mark on the eartip at the junction between the main tube and the eartip tube, as shown in Figure 3–27. Throughout the procedure, be sure the mark stays aligned in that position, so you know that the probe tube has not changed position relative to the sound outlet of the eartip.

5. As you would an ITE hearing aid, affix the eartip of the insert earphone, which contains the probe tube, to an HA-1, 2-cc coupler (e.g., using putty) as shown in Figure 3–28A. Be sure that the probe tube extends into the coupler. Before proceeding, check to see that the mark on the probe tube is still properly aligned with the junction of the earphone tube and the eartip.

6. Attach the coupler microphone to the 2-cc coupler as if to perform a test-box measurement. The coupler microphone is not actually used in measurement but provides the completion of the normal coupler configuration.

7. Connect the probe tube to the probe microphone of the REM system, taking care not to shift the position of the probe tube relative to the eartip.

8. Using any type of test signal you wish, obtain the 2-cc coupler response of the insert earphone. Use the same equipment operations as you would if you were measuring the REUR. Before capturing the measurement, adjust the signal amplitude to produce approximately 70 dB SPL in the coupler. This will assure that you have an undistorted measurement and that when you measure the real-ear response, the signal will be at a comfortable, yet measurable, level. (NOTE: The signal level in the coupler will not be calibrated to the amplitude setting displayed by the REM system.)

9. Record the measurement as the REUR and, if applicable, store it in permanent memory for future use.

B. **Obtain the real-ear response.**

1. With the probe tube threaded through a foam eartip, as in steps 3 to 4 [A] (Do not yet connect the probe tube to the probe microphone), roll and insert the eartip with the probe tube into the test ear, so that the lateral surface of the eartip aligns with the entrance to the earcanal as shown in Figure 3–28B. Alternately, use the same depth as that which you anticipate the final hearing aid will be inserted. Note that the dimensions shown in Figure 3–27 apply to the real-ear response for the average length of the earcanal of a female patient. For earcanals that are shorter than the female average, you may have to decrease the insertion depth to avoid bumping the eardrum with the probe tube. For earcanals that are longer than the female average, you may have to increase the insertion depth to ensure that you measure close enough to the eardrum. For deep-insertion hearing aids, such as CIC fittings, you will have to use a much shorter protrusion of the probe tube beyond the eartip, as well as a deep insertion of the eartip, unless the REM system has a compensation built into the software. Before proceeding, check to see that the mark on the probe tube is properly aligned with the junction of the earphone tube and the eartip. (Optionally, you do not have to have the probe tube threaded through the eartip for obtaining the real-ear response. You may place the probe tube in the earcanal in the usual way, so that the tip is within 6 mm of the eardrum and then roll and insert the foam tip into the ear, taking care not to shift the position of the probe tube.)

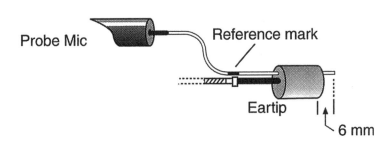

Figure 3–27 Preparation for RECD measurement. Using a darning needle, the probe tube was threaded through the foam eartip of an insert earphone. (Courtesy Frye Electronics, Inc.)

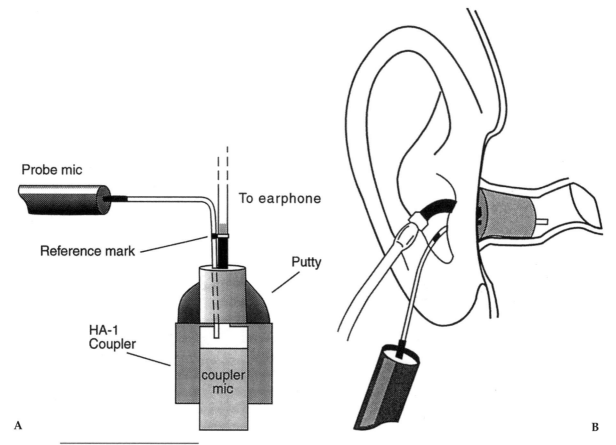

Figure 3–28 **(A)** Coupler part of RECD measurement pair. Response of insert earphone is measured in a 2-cc coupler. (Courtesy Frye Electronics, Inc.) **(B)** Real-ear part of RECD measurement pair. Response of same insert earphone as in **(A)**, using same signal, is measured in the ear. (Courtesy Frye Electronics, Inc.)

2. Using precisely the same signal as used to obtain the 2-cc coupler response, obtain the real-ear response of the insert earphone. Use the same equipment operations as you would if you were obtaining the REAR for an insertion-gain measure.

3. Record the measurement as the REAR. The curve displayed as "insertion gain" is actually the RECD (the real-ear response minus the coupler response).

RECD Procedure Using a Hearing Aid in a Sound Field

A. **Obtain the HA-1, 2-cc coupler response.**

Option #1: If your REM system has a facility by which you can use test-box measurements as REMs, follow these steps for part A:

1. Choose a well-damped "stock" BTE hearing aid having a broad frequency range and relatively low gain.

2. Using the same earmold or stock eartip as you will be using for the real-ear response (part B), affix the hearing aid with the earmold to an HA-1 coupler.

3. In the test box adjust the signal amplitude until you get a coupler SPL of about 70 dB. (This signal level will ensure comfort for the real-ear part B.)

4. Obtain the 2-cc coupler response of the hearing aid. The only differences between this measurement and a standard (ANSI S3.22-1996b) test-box measurement of a BTE hearing aid are that in a standard test-box measurement you would not use the earmold and you would use an HA-2 coupler.

5. Transfer this curve to the "REUR" location of the REM system.

Option #2: If your REM system does not have a facility by which you can use test-box measurements as REMs, use the following steps for part A. The hearing aid will be attached to the 2-cc coupler, and you will hold the coupler and hearing aid at the ear during a sound field measurement.

1. Set the REM system to measure "insertion gain."

2. Choose a well-damped, "stock" BTE hearing aid having a broad frequency range and relatively low gain.

3. Tape the volume control (or set the programming) of the hearing aid so that the gain is very low (perhaps 10 dB of 2-cc coupler gain).

4. Align a probe tube along the bore of the earmold (or stock eartip) such that the tip of the tube extends 6 mm beyond

the sound outlet of the earmold. (Do not yet connect the probe tube to the probe microphone.) Always be sure the probe tube extends 6 mm ($\pm$ 1 mm) with this coupler measurement, even if you will use a different extension of the probe tube for the real-ear measurement in part B. Also, for the coupler measure only, any vent in the earmold must be sealed.

5. Place a reference mark on the probe tube just lateral to the lateral surface of the earmold or eartip or at any convenient place where you will be able to check the position of the probe tube relative to the earmold once they are in the ear.

6. With the tip of the probe tube protruding 6 mm into the coupler and with the reference mark aligned as in the previous step, affix the bore of the earmold or eartip, along with the probe tube, to an HA-1, 2-cc coupler (e.g., using putty). Before proceeding, check to see that the reference mark on the probe tube is still in position.

7. Attach the coupler microphone to the 2-cc coupler as if to perform a test-box measurement.

8. Carefully connect the probe tube to the probe microphone, taking care not to shift the position of the probe tube relative to the earmold.

9. Place the reference microphone in the normal position at the ear. If the reference microphone and probe microphone have the same housing, carefully hold the coupler/hearing aid apparatus at the ear while placing the microphone housing at the ear in the usual way. If the reference and probe microphone have separate housings, place the housing of the probe microphone in its normal place at the ear while holding the coupler/hearing aid apparatus nearby.

10. While holding the coupler/hearing aid apparatus at the ear, place the BTE hearing aid over the ear as it would normally be worn, taking care not to shift the position of the probe tube relative to the earmold.

11. Turn on the hearing aid.

12. While holding the apparatus in place near the ear and with your hand as out of the way of the microphones as possible, level the sound field (if applicable) and measure the coupler response as if you were measuring the REUR. (HINT: You might want to kneel behind the patient during leveling and measurement so as to be as acoustically out of the way as possible.)

13. Record this measurement as the REUR.

B. **Obtain the real-ear response** (this B procedure is used with both options of part A).

1. If not already done, place a reference mark on the probe tube for REMs in the usual way (e.g., corresponding to the intertragal notch).

2. Attach the probe tube to the probe microphone and place the probe tube in the ear such that the tip lies within 6 mm of the eardrum.

3. Insert the earmold or eartip, taking care not to move the probe tube, and place the housing of the hearing aid over the ear.

4. Turn on the hearing aid and be sure the gain is set the same as for the 2-cc coupler measurement.

5. If applicable, equalize (level) the sound field.

6. Using precisely the same signal as used to obtain the 2-cc coupler response, obtain and record the real-ear response of hearing aid (the REAR). The curve now displayed as "insertion gain" is actually the RECD (the real-ear response minus the coupler response).

RECD Procedure for BTEs
(Using HA-2 Coupler and Insert Earphone)*

A. **Obtain the HA-2, 2-cc coupler response.**

1. Set the REM system to measure "insertion gain." Also set the REM system to disable the reference microphone and to operate without equalization of the signal source (a condition called "unleveled" with some systems). With some real-ear systems you may have to circumvent the preceding requirement by equalizing the signal drive using the "substitution-method" mode of operation, with the loudspeaker still attached.

2. Disconnect the loudspeaker from the signal source of the REM system and instead connect the insert earphone.

3. By whatever means available, obtain the HA-2, 2-cc coupler response of the insert earphone. With some REM systems, you can use the normal coupler microphone to obtain this measure, but be sure the system lets you transfer the coupler curve to the REM software. If you are instead using the probe microphone to measure the HA-2 response, you must have a means of positioning the tip of the probe tube inside the coupler, within 3 mm of the bottom of the 2-cc cavity. With some REM systems, you can position the tip of the probe tube inside the coupler by using an adapter that is normally used in calibrating the probe tube. The adapter, which has a channel through which to feed the probe tube, can be fitted to the bottom of the coupler in place of the normal coupler microphone. With other REM systems, the HA-2 coupler has a vent hole large enough to accommodate a probe tube (see Moodie et al, 1994). (With the RECD procedures using the HA-1 coupler, given earlier, the probe tube was threaded through the opening at the top of the coupler. This is not possible with an HA-2 coupler.)

4. Obtain and record the coupler response of the insert earphone as if it were the REUR.

B. **Obtain the real-ear response, using the patient's earmold.**

1. Instead of using the normal eartip, connect the sound outlet (main tube) of the insert earphone to the tubing of the patient's custom earmold.

2. Mark and position the probe tube, as if to obtain the REAR of a hearing aid. But instead of measuring a hearing aid, you will be measuring the real-ear response of the insert earphone, yet delivered through the patient's own earmold.

---

*Some REM systems let you use this procedure in fitting ITEs, ITCs, and CICs, as well as BTEs. With these systems, software-applied corrections compensate for the differences between the HA-2 and the HA-1 couplers and, in the case of CICs, for the assumed deep insertion of the CIC in the earcanal.

3. Obtain and record the real-ear response of the insert earphone, delivered by means of the patient's earmold, as if to record an REAR. The curve displayed as "insertion gain" will actually be the HA-2 RECD (the real-ear response minus the coupler response).

Real-Ear-to-Dial Difference

Obtaining this measure requires that you have your REM system and an audiometer in the same room.

1. Set the REM system so that the probe-tube microphone serves as a SLM (i.e., so that it continuously monitors dB SPL).

2. Mark and place the probe tube in the ear in the normal way.

3. While taking care not to disturb the position of the probe tube, place the audiometric earphone on or in the ear, as applicable. NOTE: When using insert earphones, you can thread the probe tube through the foam eartip, as was described in the first RECD procedure previously.

4. Set the audiometer dial for 70 dB HL.

5. For each audiometric frequency, delivered at 70 dB HL, record the real-ear SPL.

6. Subtract 70 dB from the dB SPL reading from the probe-tube microphone for each frequency. These values constitute the REDD.

THE CIRCLE OF DECIBELS

Aside from providing a means of directly checking the in situ performance of hearing aids (see Chapters 4, 5, 6, 12, and 13 in this volume), real-ear measures can provide individualized conversion factors that let the audiologist transfer patient data from one decibel system to another. In the course of a hearing aid fitting the clinician may encounter three decibel systems. The hearing evaluation is observed in terms of dB HL, the hearing aid prescription is given in terms of dB SPL or gain in a 2-cc coupler, and the acoustic part of the fitting verification is observed in terms of dB SPL or gain at the eardrum of the wearer. Each of these decibel systems has advantages for its intended application. Yet in considering the many phases of hearing aid fittings, clinicians may find it useful to have a means of converting data from one decibel system to another. Computer-driven equipment used in hearing aid fitting (e.g., audiometers, test boxes, and REM systems) often provides such conversions internally to the equipment. Yet even if performed within the software of clinical equipment, the clinician should be aware of the processes and limitations involved in applying those conversions.

The "Circle of Decibels" (Figure 3–29) is a visual aid to understanding how the three decibel systems used in hearing aid fitting are related (Revit, 1997). Eardrum SPL occupies the uppermost position. Ultimately, every acoustic consideration regarding a hearing aid fitting culminates at the eardrum. Connecting "eardrum SPL" with "2cc SPL" and with "dB HL" are two real-ear measures described earlier, the RECD and the REDD. The RECD and REDD are of a special class of measures, called "transforms." They are called "transforms" because, when applied to a set of data, they *transform* the data from one decibel system to another. A third transform, the "2cc/DD," connects "2cc SPL" with "dB HL"

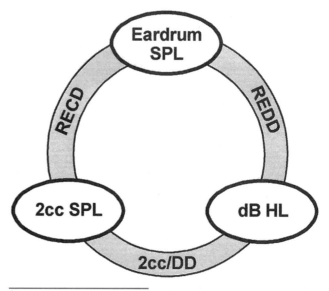

Figure 3–29 The Circle of Decibels. Shows three decibel systems used in hearing aid fittings (*within horizontal ovals*) and the transforms for maneuvering between them (*within circular band*).

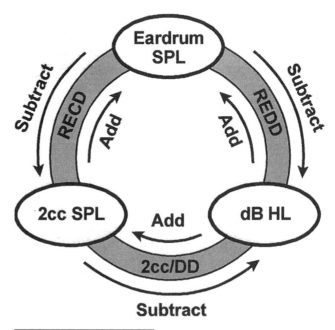

Figure 3–30 The Circle of Decibels, with arrows showing whether to add or subtract a given transform when maneuvering from one decibel system to the next. The rule is to *subtract* when moving *downward* or from *left-to-right* on the circle; *add* when moving *upward* or from *right-to-left* on the circle.

along the bottom of the circle. The "2cc/DD" is not a real-ear measure; it is a known, standard set of values used for calibrating an audiometer for use with insert earphones (e.g., ANSI S3.6-1996a). In ANSI S3.6, these calibration values are called "RETSPLs" for "reference earphone sound pressure levels." Here they are called "2cc/DD" so as to avoid confusing the "RE" of "REMs" with the "RE" of "RETSPLs." Figure 3–30 repeats the circle of decibels, but this time with instructions on how to use the transforms to get from one decibel system to the next. The rules are: When moving from top to bottom or from left to right on the circle, you subtract the transform; when moving from bottom to top or from right to left, you add. For example, to transform data from "dB HL" to "eardrum SPL," you add the REDD to the dB HL values. But you can just as well add the "2cc/DD" and then add the RECD. A study reported by Scollie et al (1998) confirmed that the two alternate paths between "dB HL" and "eardrum SPL" are virtually equivalent. You may, for example, already have a patient's RECD on hand and may not have the REDD. You can therefore use either transformation path interchangeably.

In addition to estimating eardrum SPL from hearing test data in the form of dB HL, another valuable use of the Circle of Decibels is to estimate real-ear performance (eardrum SPL) from 2-cc coupler measurements. After performing just one real-ear measurement, either the RECD or the REDD, the clinician can conveniently do all testing and tuning of the hearing aid in the test box with an accurate eye on real-ear performance.

Table 3–2 summarizes all the possible paths around the Circle of Decibels. The take-home message of Figure 3–30 and Table 3–2 is that as long as you have either the RECD or the REDD, you can transform data from any of the three decibel systems to any other of the three. And you can do so with a high degree of precision because both the RECD and the REDD are individualized real-ear measures. So one real-ear measurement, either the RECD or the REDD, is all that is required to get around the Circle of Decibels.

Coupler Response for Flat Insertion Gain

An older cousin of the Circle of Decibels is CORFIG. CORFIG is the transform used to convert insertion-gain targets to 2-cc

---

PITFALL

When using the Circle of Decibels to estimate eardrum SPL from 2-cc coupler data, the effects of the acoustic coupling of the patient's earmold or shell will not be part of the estimate unless you are fitting a BTE *and* you use the BTE/HA-2 method for obtaining the RECD. Venting effects cannot be predicted using RECDs obtained with insert earphones. Low-frequency venting effects can be included when the RECD is measured using the "sound field" method.

SPECIAL CONSIDERATION

CICS:

When using the RECD to estimate the eardrum SPL of CICs from 2cc SPL, you must account for the fact that the insertion depth of a CIC is much deeper than that of other hearing aids or of audiometric insert earphones. Deeper insertion will increase the relative eardrum SPL, for equal electrical signal drive levels to an insert earphone. Either you must use a deeply inserted earpiece to obtain the patient's RECD data or you must apply an average-ear transform between normal insertion and deep insertion (see Table 3–3). Some REM systems can apply such a transform in software.

TABLE 3–2 Comprehensive instructions for navigating the Circle of Decibels

If You Have	And You Want	Direct Path	Long Way Around
dB HL	Eardrum SPL	Add the REDD	Add the 2cc/DD and add the RECD
dB HL	2cc SPL	Add the 2cc/DD	Add the REDD and subtract the RECD
2cc SPL	Eardrum SPL	Add the RECD	Subtract the 2cc/DD and add the REDD
2cc SPL	dB HL	Subtract the 2cc/DD	Add the RECD and subtract the REDD
Eardrum SPL	2cc SPL	Subtract the RECD	Subtract the REDD and add the 2cc/DD
Eardrum SPL	dB HL	Subtract the REDD	Subtract the RECD and subtract the 2cc/DD

TABLE 3–3 Average 2-cc coupler RECDs for normal and deep (CIC) insertion

Frequency	250	500	750	1000	1500	2000	3000	4000	6000	8000
Avg. RECD normal*:	4	4	4	5	7	8	10	12	15	15
Avg. RECD deep[†]:	6	8	10	11	13	14	17	20	23	23
Correction for CIC:	2	4	6	6	6	6	7	8	8	8

*From Bentler and Pavlovic (1989).
[†]From Seewald et al (1997).

SPECIAL CONSIDERATION

When using the Circle of Decibels to estimate an RESR from an OSPL-90 2-cc coupler measurement, you simply add the RECD to the OSPL-90 to get the estimated RESR. But to estimate an REAR from a 2-cc coupler measure, you must add not only the RECD, but also the presumed acoustic gain seen by the hearing aid microphone because of its location at the ear (see Table 3–8). At low frequencies, these acoustic-gain effects are negligible; and at high frequencies the magnitude of the acoustic gain is generally low, about 3 dB for BTEs (Bentler & Pavlovic, 1989, 1992), increasing to 8 dB for CICs (Cornelisse & Seewald, 1997). However, when observing the REARs of hearing aids that are in compression, you must first divide the microphone-location effects by the compression ratio before adding them to the RECD. So with high-compression ratios (3:1 or greater), microphone-location effects will be minimal.

SPECIAL CONSIDERATION

Young Children:
Using the RECD to estimate the eardrum SPL from 2cc SPL is particularly useful and effective with young children, who do not easily sit quietly and in place even for the brief period of time required for real-ear measures. When fitting BTEs, use the BTE/HA-2 RECD method for the most valid and reliable results (Sinclair et al, 1996). (See Table 3–1B for average RECDs in children of various ages, data that can be used when no individual real-ear measurement is possible.)

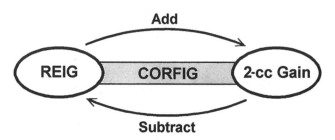

Figure 3–31 CORFIG. Shows whether to add or subtract the appropriate CORFIG when maneuvering between REIG and 2-cc coupler gain.

---

coupler gain prescriptions. Its inverse (sometimes called "GIFROC") is used to estimate REIG performance from 2-cc coupler measures. Figure 3–31 shows how CORFIG is applied. When converting a target REIG to a 2-cc coupler prescription, you add the appropriate CORFIG to the target REIG. To estimate the REIG from 2-cc coupler measures, you subtract the CORFIG from the 2-cc coupler data. Applying a CORFIG to an REIG-based fitting strategy is similar to applying the Circle of Decibels to an REAR-based fitting strategy (see Chapters 4, 5, 6, 12, and 13 in this volume). Both transforms include the RECD and the effects of the location of the hearing aid microphone. Yet because REIG includes both REAG and REUG, CORFIG also includes the REUG. Specifically:

1. CORFIG = REUG − RECD − HA microphone-location effects.
2. Prescribed 2-cc coupler gain = Target REIG + CORFIG.
3. Estimated REIG = 2-cc coupler gain − CORFIG.

The REUG and the effects of the location of the hearing aid microphone are direction-dependent at high frequencies. So CORFIGs will vary with varying locations of the sound source used in obtaining these elemental measures. A "diffuse" sound source has sound coming equally from all directions, and so a diffuse-field CORFIG is essentially the average CORFIG for all possible sound sources. Figure 3–32 shows diffuse-field CORFIGs for the average adult ear from Killion et al (1987). Table 3–4 gives the same data in numerical form and average CORFIG values for 0 degrees and

45 degrees. The Preferred Practice Guidelines at the end of the chapter provide worksheets that can assist with applying CORFIG data to hearing aid fittings on an individualized basis. See Killion and Revit (1993) and Revit (1994) for a broader discussion of CORFIG.

PITFALL

As with the use of the Circle of Decibels to prescribe 2-cc coupler SPL from a target REAR (eardrum SPL), the use of CORFIG to prescribe 2-cc coupler gain from a target REIG will not account for ear- mold coupling effects unless the BTE/HA-2 method is used in obtaining the RECD. Even then, precise, individual estimates of venting effects cannot be made. As a compromise, Table 3–5 provides average venting corrections to use when prescribing 2-cc coupler gain from a target REIG. Add these corrections to the prescribed 2-cc coupler response as applicable. (See Preferred Practice Guidelines at the end of the chapter.)

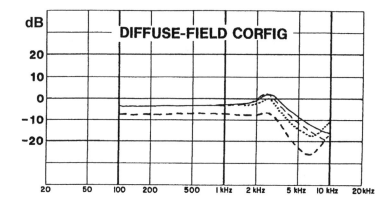

Figure 3–32 Diffuse-field CORFIGs for various hearing aid types: BTE *(solid)*, ITE *(thin dashes)*, ITC *(dots)*, and CIC *(thick dashes)*. (From Killion et al [1987], with permission.)

TABLE 3–4 Average CORFIG values for 0 degrees, 45 degrees, and diffuse incidences of the sound source. For GIFROC values, simply change the sign of each number.

Frequency	250	500	750	1000	1500	2000	3000	4000	6000	8000
0° BTE*:	−4	−4	−3	−3	−3	0	3	−2	−8	−16
45° BTE[†]:	−1	0	−1	−2	−1	4	4	3	−1	−8
Diffuse BTE[‡]:	−3	−3	−3	−3	−2	1	3	−2	−8	−13
0° ITE*:	−4	−4	−4	−4	−1	0	2	−2	−8	−14
45° ITE[†]:	−1	−1	−2	−2	−2	2	3	−2	−6	−10
Diffuse ITE[‡]:	−3	−3	−3	−3	−2	1	2	−4	−10	−15
0° ITC*:	−3	−2	−2	−4	−1	2	1	−4	−10	−11
45°ITC[†]:	−2	−1	−2	−3	−2	1	1	−7	−9	−13
Diffuse ITC[‡]:	−3	−3	−3	−3	−2	1	0	−8	−1	−15
CIC[‡,§]:	−6	−6	−7	−7	−7	−5	−7	−16	−22	−24

(NOTE: The values in the table are rounded to the nearest dB; some values are interpolated.)
*Source: Bentler and Pavlovic (1989) (free field reference).
[†]Source: Killion and Revit (1993) (over-the-ear reference).
[‡]Source: Killion et al (1987) (center-of-head reference).
[§]The diffuse-field CIC values apply for all sound-source angles because the direction-dependent variables cancel in both the CORFIG calculation and the REIG measurement.

TABLE 3–5 Average vent corrections for CORFIG prescriptions of 2-cc gain from a target REIG

Frequency (Hz)	250	500	750	1k	1.5k
Tight seal	—	—	—	—	—
Slit leak	2	2	1	—	—
1 mm	1*	2*	1	—	—
2 mm	7*	1*	—	—	—
Long open	17*	10*	4*	1*	—
Short open	26*	21*	14*	10*	5*

Add these values to the prescribed 2-cc coupler gain to achieve the desired insertion gain. Use starred values only if the prescribed insertion gain is greater than 0 dB at that frequency. Otherwise, use no correction. Blanks indicate use no correction. A slit leak is assumed for all vent conditions except "tight seal." (Derived from Dillon [1991].)

GENERAL CONSIDERATIONS IN REMs

Display Considerations—Interpreting What's on the Screen

Today's REM equipment offers several choices of display environments. Typically, REMs are displayed in either REIG, HL-o-gram, and SPL-o-gram screens.

Figure 3–8 shows a typical REIG screen. The lower graph shows the REAG and REUG curves. The upper graph shows the difference between the two lower curves (the REIG) and a prescriptive REIG target for comparison.

Figure 3–33 shows real-ear data in a different fashion. An audiogram graph displays the patient's thresholds and estimates of aided thresholds on the basis of REAG measurements.* Also shown on this "HL-o-gram" is a "speech banana" and articulation index calculations for unaided and aided conditions. It is also possible to show a target-aided threshold curve based on a prescriptive formula (not in this example).

Figure 3–34 shows yet another form of real-ear display, the "SPL-o-gram." The vertical axis is SPL at the eardrum. In this example the patient's hearing thresholds are indicated with *T*s, and UCLs with *U*s. The thick curve is a target derived for a speech-weighted signal from the NAL fitting formula. The lower curve, labeled with 1s, is the patient's REUR, measured with a speech-weighted composite signal at 65 dB SPL. The curve labeled with 2s is an REAR using the same signal. The 3s indicate the RESR, measured with short tone bursts at 90 dB SPL. According to these results, the gain of the patient's hearing aid is only marginally adequate because the REAR values lie only just above the

thresholds and only at 2000 Hz and less. Also, the RESR values at the high frequencies reach the patient's UCLs, so the maximum output of this hearing aid should be adjusted slightly down in the high frequencies to provide a margin for comfort.

The display in Figure 3–34 and in all the other REM curves presented thus far except for Figure 3–33 are presented in standardized (ANSI, 1996b) aspect ratios. The aspect ratio determines the "look" of a given curve. Specifically, it determines the vertical displacement corresponding to a given horizontal displacement. The aspect ratio for frequency-response graphs is designated in terms of the number of decibels on the vertical axis corresponding to a range of frequency on the horizontal axis. ANSI S3.22 (ANSI, 1996b) recommends an aspect ratio of 50 decibels per decade of frequency when specifying hearing aid performance characteristics. That is, for the length on the frequency scale (*x* axis) corresponding to a 10-fold change in frequency (a decade), that same length on the decibel scale (*y* axis) corresponds to a 50 dB change in amplitude. This is the aspect ratio used in Figure 3–34. For audiograms, ANSI S3.6 (ANSI, 1996a) specifies an aspect ratio of 20 dB per octave of frequency. This is the aspect ratio used in the HL-o-gram of Figure 3–33.

The real-ear performance of a hearing aid can have differing appearances when viewed on displays having differing aspect ratios. In Figure 3–35, the lower graph uses an aspect ratio of 50 dB per decade, whereas the upper graph uses an aspect ratio of about 100 dB per decade. The higher the dB figure in the aspect ratio, the more shallow are the peaks and valleys in a curve. Thus the reduced vertical displacement of the upper graph serves to smooth the peaks and valleys of the REIG compared with the REIG in the lower graph. Smoothing (as described earlier) can either enhance the clarity or "readability" of a curve (as in Fig. 3–15), or it can obscure the impact of amplitude deviations in a measurement. Thus it is important for the clinician to be aware of aspect ratios and other smoothing characteristics when viewing hearing aid performance graphs, both in the clinic and in the literature.

---

*The formula for estimating an aided sound field threshold using REAG measurements is: *Aided sound field threshold = Insert-phone threshold + (Individual RECD$_{2\,cc}$ − Average RECD$_{2\,cc}$) − (REAG − Average REUG).*

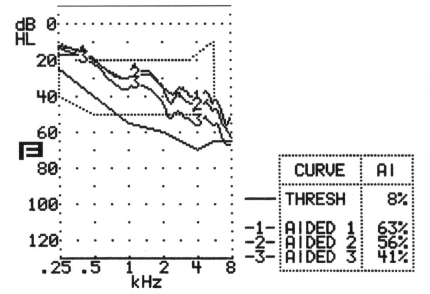

Figure 3–33 HL-o-gram REM display. REM data are presented in terms of HL. Solid curve without numbers is the patient's threshold audiogram. Curves with numbers represent estimated aided thresholds on the basis of REARs for three hearing aid settings or three signal levels. Estimates of the articulation index *(AI)* are given for each curve.

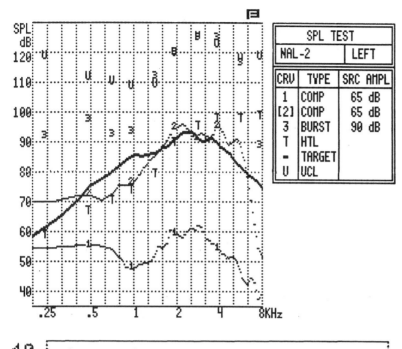

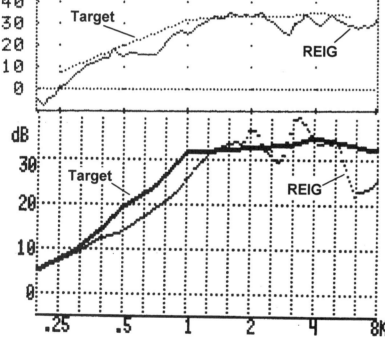

Figure 3–34 SPL-o-gram REM display. REM data are presented in terms of dB SPL at the eardrum. In this example the patient's thresholds are shown as *Ts*, the UCLs as *Us*. A target curve *(bold)* was derived using the NAL formula. Three real-ear measures are shown. Lower thin curve (with *1s*) is the REUR using a speech-weighted composite signal at 65 dB SPL. Upper thin curve (with *2s*) is the REAR using the same signal. 3s indicates the RESR measured with brief tone bursts.

Figure 3–35 Effect of aspect ratio. An REIG was measured twice for the same patient, same hearing aid, using two different REM systems. The data in the lower graph are displayed using conventional (ANSI, 1996b) aspect ratio for hearing aids (50 dB/decade); data in the upper graph are displayed using an aspect ratio of about 100 dB/decade.

Sources of Variability in Real-Ear Measures

Several factors can contribute to within-subject variability in real-ear measures. Table 3–6 lists many of them. However, when real-ear techniques are applied with care, reliable results can be expected. For the techniques described in this chapter, the clinician can expect the variability between test and retest to be on the order of 5 dB through 4000 Hz. This estimate of within-subject variability is based on multiplying the standard deviations shown Figure 3–22 by 2, thus giving the 95% confidence intervals for REIG measures. For a comprehensive discussion of *across*-subject variability in real-ear measures, see de Jonge (1996).

Hazards to the Patient in Clinical Real-Ear Measurements

The hazards to the patient in clinical real-ear measurements are few. Indeed, the risks of *not* obtaining REMs in the course of hearing aid fittings may be greater than the risks of obtaining them. Sending a new hearing aid wearer out the door with hearing aids that are not producing the expected real-ear results can easily lead to rejection of amplification by the patient. Obtaining a quick set of REMs can prevent this result.

In any clinical procedure some hazards are predictable and others are not. The predictable hazards of REMs lie in

TABLE 3–6 Sources of variability in real-ear measures

Source of Variability	Study
Change in placement of the hearing aid across measurements	Killion, 1983
Movement of probe microphone inlet between unaided and aided measurements (for REIG)	Ringdahl & Leijon, 1984
Change in position of probe microphone across measurement pairs	"
Movement of subject's head during or between measurements	"
Room acoustics—reflections, etc.	"
Deformation of probe tube	Dillon & Murray, 1987
Equipment noise	"
Change in level to the hearing aid	Hawkins & Mueller, 1986
Carelessness by the clinician	Hawkins, 1987
Improper seating of earmold or shell	"
Environmental noise in the room	Revit, 1987
Diffraction effects of head ornaments, jewelry, measuring apparatus (housings of probe and reference mics, etc.)	"
Change of insertion depth of eartip, when not a custom earmold	"
Change in density and arrangement of hair in the vicinity of the ear	"
Change in loudspeaker placement	"
Change in hearing aid output/gain	"
Change in body posture	"
Cerumen—change in earcanal impedance and/or blockage of probe tube	"
Noises made by the patient (external and/or internal)	"
Leaks between earmold and probe tube	Tecca et al, 1987
Change in field reference point	Ickes et al, 1991
Varying degrees of slit leak caused by the presence of the probe tube between the earmold and the wall of the earcanal	—

two categories: (1) excessive SPL in the earcanal and (2) contact of the probe tube with the eardrum. Both can cause discomfort and, although unlikely, both can be damaging to the patient.

Excessive SPL in the earcanals can occur either when the amplitude of the input signal is high or when the gain of the hearing aids is high. In particular, the risk of excessive earcanal SPLs is greatest when making RESR measurements with high-gain hearing aids. For example, if the input signal

is 90 dB SPL (typical for obtaining the RESR) and the acoustic gain of the hearing aids is 55 dB, then it is possible to have an SPL of 145 dB in the earcanals during testing. Excessive SPL in the earcanals resulting from signals controlled by REM equipment during measurements can be avoided if, before turning on the signal, the clinician ascertains that the output limiting of the REM system is set to an appropriate amplitude. NOTE: This safeguard works only when the probe microphone is in the earcanal and is active.

The probe tubes used in REM systems are generally very flexible and normally will not cause damage if brought into contact with a healthy eardrum. But if a probe tube comes into contact with a patient's eardrum, it is likely that the patient will be slightly startled or will feel some discomfort. Many patients will not tolerate repeated contact of a probe tube with the eardrum.

Some probe tubes are more flexible than others. Moreover, as the length of the exposed portion of a probe tube decreases, the ability of the tube to bend or buckle decreases, thus making the tube effectively stiffer. For example, when a hearing aid or insert earphone is present along with a probe tube in an earcanal (e.g., Fig. 3–28B), the relatively small length of tubing extending beyond the earpiece is effectively stiffer than when no earpiece is present (e.g., Fig. 3–13). When inserting an earpiece into an earcanal with a probe tube already in place, use care (such as by holding the tube with a finger) to see that the earpiece does not drag the probe tube toward the eardrum as the earpiece is inserted.

SPECIAL CONSIDERATION

When fitting deep-canal (CIC) hearing aids or when fitting hearing aids to small children, small residual earcanal volumes lead to increased earcanal SPLs compared with 2-cc coupler SPLs. Thus the clinician is strongly advised to obtain RESR measures (or to estimate the RESR from the 2-cc coupler OSPL-90 by adding the RECD*) in such cases to prevent excessive earcanal SPLs from occurring once the patient leaves the clinic. For the same reason, extra care must be taken in such cases to avoid excessive earcanal SPLs during clinical RESR procedures.

CONCLUSIONS

With the growing availability of "automatic fitting" software associated with programmable hearing aids, a growing number of fitters are skipping the necessary step of measuring real-ear performance before sending a patient on his or her way (S. Jelonek, personal communication). Although ongoing improvements in hearing aid components and circuitry provide the potential for continued improvements in the auditory lives of hearing aid wearers, audiologists should not overlook the step of verifying, through REIG measures, the simple goal of seeing that a patient's hearing aids amplify conversational speech to levels that exceed the levels provided by the patient's unaided ears.

Toward the future, we look for broader sophistication in real-ear measures. Better test signals, which better represent real-world conditions both in noise free and in noisy backgrounds, should provide better clinical assessments of potential real-world performance. Improved probe microphones that are electrically less noisy and that are mechanically and/or acoustically less obtrusive should provide measurements that are more accurate.

ACKNOWLEDGMENT

Frye Electronics, Inc., Tigard, Oregon, provided funding, REM and hearing aid test equipment, and graphical support for the creation of this chapter.

---

*See the section on the Circle of Decibels and Table 3–2 in this chapter.

REFERENCES

AMERICAN NATIONAL STANDARDS INSTITUTE. (1992). *American National Standard Testing Hearing Aids with a Broad-Band Noise Signal* (ANSI S3.42). Standards Secretariat. New York: Acoustical Society of America.

AMERICAN NATIONAL STANDARDS INSTITUTE. (1996a). *American National Standard Specification for Audiometers* (ANSI S3.6). Standards Secretariat. New York: Acoustical Society of America.

AMERICAN NATIONAL STANDARDS INSTITUTE. (1996b). *American National Standard Specification of Hearing Aid Characteristics* (ANSI S3.22). Standards Secretariat. New York: Acoustical Society of America.

AMERICAN NATIONAL STANDARDS INSTITUTE. (1997). *American National Standard Methods of Measurement of Real-Ear Performance Characteristics of Hearing Aids* (ANSI S3.46). Standards Secretariat. New York: Acoustical Society of America.

BENTLER, R.A., & PAVLOVIC, C.V. (1989). Transfer functions and correction factors used in hearing aid evaluation and research. *Ear and Hearing, 10*(1);58–63.

BENTLER, R.A., & PAVLOVIC, C.V. (1992). Addendum to "Transfer functions and correction factors used in hearing aid evaluation and research." *Ear and Hearing, 13*(4);284–286.

CORNELISSE, L.E., & SEEWALD, R.C. (1997). Field-to-microphone transfer functions for completely-in-the-canal (CIC) instruments. *Ear and Hearing, 18*(4);342–345.

DE JONGE, R. (1996). Real-ear measures: Individual variation and measurement error. In: M. Valente (Ed.), *Hearing aids: Standards, options, and limitations* (pp. 72–125). New York: Thieme Medical Publishers, Inc.

DILLON, H. (1991). Allowing for real-ear venting effects when selecting the coupler gain of hearing aids. *Ear and Hearing, 12*(6);406–416.

DILLON, H., & MURRAY, N. (1987). Accuracy of twelve methods for estimating the real-ear gain of hearing aids. *Ear and Hearing, 8*(1);2–11.

DIRKS, D., & KINCAID, G. (1987). Basic acoustic considerations of earcanal probe measurements. *Ear and Hearing, 8*(Suppl. 5);60S–67S.

FIKRET-PASA, S., & REVIT, L.J. (1992). Individualized correction factors in the preselection of hearing aids. *Journal of Speech and Hearing Research, 35*(2);384–400.

FILLER, A.S., ROSS, D.A., & WIENER, F.M. (1945). *The pressure distribution in the auditory canal in a progressive sound field.* December 1, 1945, Psycho-Acoustic Laboratory, Harvard University Report PNR-5 (available through Publications Board, U.S. Department of Commerce, Washington, D.C.). As cited in Wiener & Ross (1946).

FRYE, G.J. (1987). Crest factor and composite signals for hearing aid testing. *Hearing Journal, 40*(10);15–18.

HARFORD, E.R. (1980). The use of a miniature microphone in the earcanal for the verification of hearing aid performance. *Ear and Hearing, 1*(6);329–337.

HAWKINS, D.B. (1987). Variability in clinical earcanal probe microphone measurements. *Hearing Instruments, 38*(1); 30–32.

HAWKINS, D.B., & MUELLER, H.G. (1986). Some variables affecting the accuracy of probe-tube microphone measures of hearing aid gain. *Hearing Instruments, 37*(1);8–49.

ICKES, M., HAWKINS, D.B., & COOPER, W. (1991). Effect of loudspeaker azimuth and reference microphone location on earcanal probe tube measurements. *Journal of the American Academy of Audiology, 2*;156–163.

KILLION, M.C. (1983). *Individual insertion gain estimates: A comparison of methods.* Paper presented at the meeting of the American Speech-Language-Hearing Association, Toronto, Canada.

KILLION, M.C., BERGER, E.H., & NUSS, R.A. (1987). Diffuse field response of the ear. *Journal of the Acoustical Society of America, 81*(Suppl. 1);S75.

KILLION, M.C., & MONSER, E.L. (1980). CORFIG: Coupler response for flat insertion gain. In: G.A. Studebaker, & I. Hochberg (Eds.), *Acoustical factors affecting hearing aid performance.* (pp. 147–168). Baltimore, MD: University Park Press.

KILLION, M.C., & REVIT, L.J. (1987). Insertion gain repeatability versus loudspeaker location: You want me to put my loudspeaker W-H-E-R-E? *Ear and Hearing, 8*(5 Suppl.); 68S–73S.

KILLION, M.C., & REVIT, L.J. (1993). CORFIG and GIFROC: Real-ear to coupler and back. In: G.A. Studebaker, & I. Hochberg (Eds.), *Acoustical factors affecting hearing aid performance* (2nd ed.), (pp. 65–85). Boston, MA: Allyn and Bacon.

KRUGER, B. (1987). An update on the external ear resonance in infants and young children. *Ear and Hearing, 8*;333–336.

MOODIE, K.S., SEEWALD, R.C., & SINCLAIR, S.T. (1994). Procedure for predicting real-ear and hearing aid performance in young children. *American Journal of Audiology, 3*(1);23–30.

MUELLER, H.G. (1989). Individualizing the ordering of custom hearing aids. *Hearing Instruments, 40*(2);18–22.

MUELLER, H.G. (1992). Terminology and procedures. In: H.G. Mueller, D.B. Hawkins, & J.L. Northern (Eds.), *Probe microphone measurements: Hearing aid selection and assessment.* (pp. 41–66). San Diego, CA: Singular Press.

MUELLER, H.G. (1998). Probe microphone measurements: Yesterday, today, and tomorrow. *Hearing Journal, 51*(4); 17–22.

NIELSEN, H.B., & RASMUSSEN, S.B. (1984). New aspects in hearing aid fittings. *Hearing Instruments,* January;18–20,48.

REVIT, L.J. (1987). *New loudspeaker locations for improved reliability in clinical measures of the insertion gain of hearing aids.* Master's thesis, Northwestern University, Evanston, IL.

REVIT, L.J. (1991a). An open letter: New thinking on the proper application of REMs to prescriptions and fittings. *New Zealand Journal of Audiology, 1*;1–17.

REVIT, L.J. (1991b). Simplified aided-ear customization for target 2-cc FOG prescriptions. *Larry's Corner,* Winter issue, Frye Electronics Inc., Tigard, OR.

REVIT, L.J. (1992). Two methods for dealing with the occlusion effect. *Hearing Instruments, 43*(12);16–18.

REVIT, L.J. (1993a). The tip of the probe—Part 1: Adjusting the probe tube insertion depth. *Larry's Corner,* Winter issue, Frye Electronics Inc., Tigard, OR.

REVIT, L.J. (1993b). The most important real-ear measurement you may ever make. *Larry's Corner,* Spring issue, Frye Electronics Inc., Tigard, OR.

REVIT, L.J. (1994). Using coupler tests in the fitting of hearing aids. In: M. Valente (Ed.), *Strategies for selecting and verifying hearing aid fittings* (pp. 64–87). New York: Thieme Medical Publishers, Inc.

REVIT, L.J. (1996). *Using earphone thresholds and REMs to estimate aided thresholds.* Paper presented at the annual meeting of the American Speech-Language-Hearing Association, Seattle, WA.

REVIT, L. (1997). The circle of decibels: Relating the hearing test, to the hearing aid, to the real-ear response. *Hearing Review, 4*(11);35–38.

RINGDAHL, A., & LEIJON, A. (1984). The reliability of insertion gain measurements using probe microphones in the ear. *Scandinavian Audiology, 13*;173–178.

ROMANOW, F.F. (1942). Methods for measuring the performance of hearing aids. *Journal of the Acoustical Society of America, 13*;194–204.

SACHS, R.M., & BURKHARD, M.D. (1971). *On making pressure measurements in insert earphone couplers and real-ears.* Paper presented at the 82nd Meeting of the Acoustical Society of America, Denver, Colorado, October 19–22. Reprint from Knowles Electronics, Itasca, IL.

SACHS, R.M., & BURKHARD, M.D. (1972). *Earphone pressure response in ears and couplers,* Report No. 20021-2, Knowles Electronics, Itasca, IL.

SCOLLIE, S., SEEWALD, R., CORNELISSE, L., & JENSTEAD, L. (1998). Validity and repeatability of level-independent HL to SPL transforms. *Ear and Hearing, 19*(5);407–413.

SEEWALD, R.C., CORNELISSE, L.E., RICHERT, F.M., & BLOCK, M.G. (1997) Acoustic transforms for fitting CIC instruments. In: M. Chasin (Ed.), *CIC handbook* (pp. 83–100). San Diego, CA: Singular Publishing Group.

SHAW, E.A.G. (1974). Transformation of sound pressure level from the free field to the eardrum in the horizontal plane. *Journal of the Acoustical Society of America, 56*(6);1848–1861.

SHAW, E.A.G. (1975). The external ear: New knowledge. In: S.C. Dalsgaard (Ed.), *Earmolds and associated problems.*

Proceedings of the Seventh Danavox Symposium. *Scandinavian Audiology* (Suppl. 5);24–50. As cited in Shaw, E.A.G. (1980). The acoustics of the external ear. In: G.A. Studebaker, & I. Hochberg (Eds.), *Acoustical factors affecting hearing aid performance* (pp. 109–126). Baltimore, MD: University Park Press.

SINCLAIR, S.T., BEAUCHAINE, K.L., MOODIE, K.S., FEIGIN, J.A., SEEWALD, R.C., & STELMACHOWICZ, P.G. (1996). Repeatability of a real-ear-to-coupler difference measurement as a function of age. *American Journal of Audiology, 5*(3);52–56.

SULLIVAN, R. (1985). An acoustic coupling-based classification system for hearing aid fittings. *Hearing Instruments, 9*;25–28 and *12*;16–22.

SULLIVAN, R. (1988). Probe-tube microphone placement near the tympanic membrane. *Hearing Instruments, 39*(7);43–44,60.

TECCA, J.E., WOODFORD, C.M., & KEE, D.K. (1987). Variability of insertion-gain measurements. *Hearing Journal*, February;18–20.

TREDE, K. (1990). *Real-ear measurements: Issues of loudspeaker angle and room acoustics.* Paper presented at the annual meeting of the American Speech-Language-Hearing Association, Seattle, WA.

WALKER, G., DILLON, H., & BYRNE, D. (1984). Sound field audiometry: Recommended stimuli and procedures. *Ear and Hearing, 5*;13–21.

WIENER, F.M., & ROSS, D.A. (1946). The pressure distribution in the auditory canal in a progressive sound field. *Journal of the Acoustical Society of America, 18*(2);401–408.

ZEMPLENYI, J., GILLMAN, S., & DIRKS, D. (1985). Optical method for measurement of earcanal length. *Journal of the Acoustical Society of America, 78*(6);2146–2148.

ZWISLOCKI, J.J. (1980). An ear simulator for acoustic measurements: Rationale, principles, and limitations. In: G.A. Studebaker, & I. Hochberg (Eds.), *Acoustical factors affecting hearing aid performance* (pp. 127–146). Baltimore, MD: University Park Press.

PREFERRED PRACTICE GUIDELINES— USING REAL-EAR MEASURES TO CUSTOMIZE THE ELECTROACOUSTIC RESPONSE OF HEARING AIDS

Professionals Who Perform the Procedure(s)

▼ People who prescribe and fit hearing aids

Expected Outcomes

▼ The hearing aids are optimized to the prescriptive strategy used.

▼ The hearing aids are optimized to the individual acoustical properties of the patient's ears.

▼ The preceding levels of fitting optimization are possible without the necessity for repeated real-ear measurements.

▼ The manufacturer of custom hearing aids has the best possible information to work with in determining the components and settings of the hearing aids.

▼ The patient can feel better about continuing with amplification by receiving better sounding amplification from the outset.

Clinical Indications

▼ Hearing aid fittings that are based on target REAG, REIG, and/or RESR.

▼ Hearing aid fittings where repeated REMs may be especially troublesome—such as with young children.

Clinical Process

▼ Determine the prescriptive goals in terms of REAG, REIG, and/or RESR.

▼ Measure the patient's RECDs.

▼ If this is a new fitting, use the worksheet provided, entitled "Prescribing Customized 2-cc Coupler Responses," to determine the initial frequency responses required of the patient's hearing aids.

▼ Once you have the hearing aids in hand, ascertain through 2-cc coupler test-box measurements that the hearing aids are set according to the frequency-response requirements determined with the first worksheet (Worksheet 3–1).

▼ Should the patient become available for further REM testing, measure the REAG and calculate the *pseudo* REIG for each hearing aid to verify real-ear performance by use of the worksheet provided, entitled "Verifying the *Pseudo* REIG vs the Target REIG" (Worksheet 3–2). Then make any necessary adjustments and repeat the measurements and calculations.

▼ If this is a check of an existing fitting for which you do not have 2-cc coupler targets, measure the 2-cc coupler responses of the hearing aids and the patient's RECDs, then use the worksheet provided, entitled "Estimating Real-Ear Responses from 2-cc Data," (Worksheet 3–3) for each of the patient's hearing aids.

Documentation

▼ Use the worksheets, entitled "Prescribing Customized 2-cc Coupler Responses," "Verifying the *Pseudo* REIG vs the Target REIG," and "Estimating Real-Ear Responses from 2-cc Data," provided (Worksheets 3–1 through 3–3).

Worksheet 3–1   Prescribing customized 2-cc coupler responses

Frequency	250	500	750	1000	1500	2000	3000	4000	6000	8000
Target REIG:	( )	( )	( )	( )	( )	( )	( )	( )	( )	( )
Add *average* REUG*:	( )	( )	( )	( )	( )	( )	( )	( )	( )	( )
Target REAG or RESR[†]:	( )	( )	( )	( )	( )	( )	( )	( )	( )	( )
Subtract HA mic effects[‡]:	( )	( )	( )	( )	( )	( )	( )	( )	( )	( )
Subtract RECD[§]:	( )	( )	( )	( )	( )	( )	( )	( )	( )	( )
Target 2-cc gain" or OSPL[¶]:	( )	( )	( )	( )	( )	( )	( )	( )	( )	( )
Add desired reserve gain:	( )	( )	( )	( )	( )	( )	( )	( )	( )	( )
Target 2-cc F.O. gain:	( )	( )	( )	( )	( )	( )	( )	( )	( )	( )

*See Table 3–7 for average REUG data for various test conditions. When possible, use data for your particular REM method. Otherwise, use diffuse-field data.

[†] When computing the target OSPL-90, start here, and use target RESR values instead of target REAG values.

[‡] For WDRC hearing aids, divide these values by the compression ratio before subtracting. See Table 3–8 for average microphone effects for various aid types and test conditions. When computing the target OSPL-90, skip this step entirely.

[§] RECD is defined as real-ear response minus coupler response.

"This target does not take venting into account. Add the values in Table 3–5 to correct for average venting effects. Individual venting effects will vary widely.

[¶] Stop here when computing the target OSPL-90 from target RESR values. This line will be the target OSPL-90.

Worksheet 3–2   Verifying the *pseudo* REIG* vs the target REIG

Frequency	250	500	750	1000	1500	2000	3000	4000	6000	8000
Measured REAG:	( )	( )	( )	( )	( )	( )	( )	( )	( )	( )
Subtract *average* REUG[†]:	( )	( )	( )	( )	( )	( )	( )	( )	( )	( )
Pseudo REIG*:	( )	( )	( )	( )	( )	( )	( )	( )	( )	( )
Subtract target REIG:	( )	( )	( )	( )	( )	( )	( )	( )	( )	( )
Fitting error:	( )	( )	( )	( )	( )	( )	( )	( )	( )	( )

*The "*pseudo* REIG" is defined as the REAG minus the *average* REUG (Revit, 1996). Adjusting hearing aid settings to minimize the differences between *pseudo* REIG and target REIG values constitutes the best possible implementation of REIG fitting strategies.

[†] See Table 3–7 for average REUG data for various test conditions. When possible, use data for your particular REM method, that is, data obtained under the same test conditions as used to measure the REAG. Otherwise, use diffuse-field data.

Worksheet 3–3   Estimating real-ear responses from 2-cc data

Frequency	250	500	750	1000	1500	2000	3000	4000	6000	8000
Measured 2-cc gain or OSPL-90:	( )	( )	( )	( )	( )	( )	( )	( )	( )	( )
Add HA mic effects*:	( )	( )	( )	( )	( )	( )	( )	( )	( )	( )
Add RECD[†]:	( )	( )	( )	( )	( )	( )	( )	( )	( )	( )
	—	—	—	—	—	—	—	—	—	—
Estimated REAG[‡] or RESR:	( )	( )	( )	( )	( )	( )	( )	( )	( )	( )
Subtract *average* REUG[§]:	( )	( )	( )	( )	( )	( )	( )	( )	( )	( )
	—	—	—	—	—	—	—	—	—	—
Estimated REIG[‡]:	( )	( )	( )	( )	( )	( )	( )	( )	( )	( )

*For WDRC hearing aids, divide these values by the compression ratio before adding. See Table 3–8 for average microphone effects for various aid types and test conditions. When estimating the RESR from the OSPL-90, skip this step entirely.

[†]RECD is defined as real-ear response minus coupler response.

[‡]These estimates do not take venting into account. Venting will significantly reduce positive, low-frequency, real-ear gain. Subtract the values in Table 3–5 to correct for average venting effects. The minimum estimated real-ear gain value should be 0 dB. Individual venting effects will vary widely.

[§]See Table 3–7 for average REUG data for various test conditions. When possible, use data for your particular REM method. Otherwise, use diffuse-field data.

TABLE 3–7   Average REUG values for various loudspeaker azimuths and field reference points

Frequency	250	500	750	1000	1500	2000	3000	4000	6000	8000
0°, center of head*:	1	2	3	3	5	12	16	14	8	2
45°, over the ear[†]:	2	3	3	3	6	13	14	13	8	4
Diffuse, center of head[‡]:	1	2	3	4	7	11	16	13	9	9

(Values rounded to nearest dB; some values interpolated.)
*Source: Bentler and Pavlovic (1989).
[†]Source: Frye Electronics, Inc., Tigard, OR.
[‡]Source: Killion et al (1987).

TABLE 3–8   Average hearing aid microphone location effects for various loudspeaker azimuths and field reference points

Frequency	250	500	750	1000	1500	2000	3000	4000	6000	8000
0°, center of head:										
BTE*:	1	1	1	0	2	4	3	4	0	3
ITE*:	1	2	2	2	0	4	4	4	2	1
ITC*:	0	0	0	1	−2	2	4	6	2	−2
CIC[†]:	0	0	0	1	2	3	6	8	4	−6
45°, over the ear:										
BTE[‡]:	—	—	—	—	—	—	—	—	—	—
ITE[‡]:	0	1	1	1	1	3	2	5	5	2
ITC[‡]:	0	1	1	1	1	3	3	9	8	5
Diffuse, center of head:										
BTE[§]	1	1	1	2	3	3	3	3	3	3
ITE[§]:	1	1	1	2	2	3	4	5	5	6
ITC[§]:	0	2	2	2	3	4	6	8	8	6
CIC["]	1	1	2	2	3	4	7	10	9	7

*Source: Bentler and Pavlovic (1989).
[†]Source: Cornelisse and Seewald (1997).
[§]Source: Bentler and Pavlovic (1992).
["]Source: Killion et al (1987).
[‡]Source: Frye Electronics, Inc., Tigard, OR.

Chapter 4

Hearing Instrument Selection and Fitting in Children

Dawna E. Lewis

As the title suggests, this chapter will focus on the selection and fitting of amplification in children. One might wonder why this topic is presented in a separate chapter, given that the chapters by Sammeth and Levitt, Kuk, Palmer, Lindley, and Mormer also address amplification. The fact is children are not miniature adults. A number of factors, including physical size, speech and language levels, cognition, and listening environments, must be addressed in the selection and fitting process. The process begins with the selection of instrument and signal processing options. Once these options have been determined, the next step is to select gain and output targets for the hearing instrument. Prescriptive methods that are appropriate for infants and young children are necessary to develop targets. Once it has been determined that the hearing instruments meet prescribed targets, verification of performance is completed. The next step in the process is the validation of auditory function. Any discussion of hearing instruments for the pediatric population would be incomplete without addressing the practical issues involved in use of amplification. Because hearing instruments alone do not provide access to acoustic information in all environments, assistive technology should also be considered. This chapter will address each of these issues in the selection and fitting of amplification in children.

As we begin our discussion of selecting and fitting hearing instruments for children, it is important to remember that amplification is just one aspect of the total (re)habilitation program. A review of hearing loss identification issues and how they relate to the amplification process will help to "set the stage."

IDENTIFICATION OF HEARING LOSS

Recent evidence suggests that children whose hearing loss was identified before 6 months of age had significantly better language development than those whose hearing loss was identified after 6 months of age (Moeller, 1996; Yoshinaga-Itano, 1995; Yoshinaga-Itano et al, 1998). In a review article Ruben (1997) reported on numerous studies that indicate that the critical period for development of phonology is up to 12 months of age. These studies help to confirm the importance of early identification and remediation of hearing loss.

Given the importance of early identification of hearing loss, what are the statistics? Results of a survey by Harrison and Roush (1996) are shown in Table 4–1. The median age of identification ranged from 12 to 22 months. Generally, children with mild to moderate hearing loss who had no known risk factors were identified 9 to 10 months later than those with more significant hearing loss or with known risk factors. For children with known risk factors, the delay between the time that the parents suspected hearing loss and diagnosis of that loss was 4 to 5 months. For children with no known risk factors, the delay was 5 to 7 months, depending on degree of hearing loss. As the results of this survey indicate, the recommendation that all infants with hearing loss be identified and intervention begun by 6 months of age (American Speech-Language-Hearing Association, 1994a) is not being met. As more states implement Universal Newborn Hearing Screening, it is hoped that the age of identification of hearing loss will be lowered significantly.

As the age of identification of hearing loss is lowered, audiologists encounter new challenges when selecting and fitting amplification. The amount of audiological information available varies depending on the age or developmental level of the child. For infants from birth to approximately 6 months of age, the audiologist will be relying primarily on auditory brain stem response (ABR), otoacoustic emission, and immittance test results. After a developmental age of about 6 months of age, behavioral tests can be performed. Depending

Audiology: Treatment. Edited by Valente, Hosford-Dunn, and Roeser. Thieme Medical Publishers, New York © 2000

TABLE 4–1 Median age, in months, for age of suspicion, diagnosis, and hearing instrument fitting for children with and without known risk factors. Also included are lag times between diagnosis and hearing instrument fitting.

Hearing Loss	Children with no known risk factors			
	Suspi-cion	Diagnosis	Hearing instrument fitting	Lag Between diagnosis and fitting
Mild-moderate	15	22	28	6
Severe-profound	8	13	16	3
	Children with known risk factors			
Mild-moderate	8	12	22	10
Severe-profound	7	12	15	3

Adapted from Harrison and Roush (1996). Age of suspicion, identification and intervention for infants and young children with hearing loss: A national study. *Ear and Hearing, 17*(1);55–62. Used with permission.

on factors such as age, developmental status, attention, and/or middle ear dysfunction, these results also can vary from one test session to another. Formal tests of speech recognition generally are not possible with children younger than 3 years of age. For further information on speech perception testing with children, the reader is referred to pertinent references on this topic (Medwetsky, 1994; McCleary & Moeller, 1997; Pediatric Working Group, 1996) and to Chapter 13 in *Diagnosis*.

Once hearing loss has been identified, the next step is to determine whether amplification should be worn. According to The Pediatric Working Group (1996), "thresholds equal to or poorer than 25 dB HL would indicate candidacy for amplification in some form. For children with unilateral hearing loss, rising or high-frequency hearing loss above 2000 Hz, and/or milder degrees of hearing loss (<25 dB HL), need should be based on the audiogram plus additional information including cognitive function, the existence of other disabilities, and the child's performance within the home and

---

CONTROVERSIAL POINT

Many questions remain about the use of amplification for infants and children identified with what is often referred to as auditory neuropathy. No single solution has been found because the individuals who have been identified represent a heterogeneous group. Decisions about the use of amplification should be made on an individual basis with input from a team of individuals, including, but not limited to, family, audiologist, speech-language pathologist, educational, and medical personnel.

---

classroom environment" (p. 54). The following sections will focus on selection, verification, and validation of amplification systems for children.

SELECTION OF AMPLIFICATION SYSTEMS

What Is Different About Fitting Children?

When selecting any amplification system, it is best to define the specific goals and then develop a strategy for achieving those goals. For most degrees of hearing loss, with the possible exception of profound loss, the goal of amplification is to make speech audible, comfortable, and intelligible without allowing sounds to be uncomfortably loud. As stated previously, children are different from adults in a variety of ways. These differences must be considered in the process of achieving these amplification goals. One important difference is that children are learning speech and language. They do not have the same knowledge base that adults have when attempting to make sense of auditory signals that may be distorted, incomplete, or affected by noise (Elliott, 1979; Nittrouer & Boothroyd, 1990). For example, in a study of perception of high and low predictability sentences in noise, Elliott (1979) concluded that lack of knowledge about language rules may have affected the performance of the youngest group tested (9-year-olds). In a study on the effects of context on speech perception in noise, Nittrouer and Boothroyd (1990) reported that young children were unable to use semantic information in the same way as adults.

Research also has shown that infants and young children have poorer thresholds for the detection of speech and tonal stimuli in the presence of background noise than do adults (Allen & Wightman, 1994; Nozza, 1987; Nozza et al, 1990; Nozza et al, 1991). Allen and Wightman (1994), for example, measured the ability of 3- to 5-year-old children to detect tones in the presence of noise. Results indicated that, on average, children's thresholds were 13 dB higher than adults and the slopes of the psychometric functions were shallower. Individual differences across children were large. The authors suggested that the differences in threshold and slope may be related to listening strategies and/or control of selective attention. In a study of infants' speech-sound discrimination in noise, Nozza et al (1990) reported that infants required a greater signal-to-noise ratio (SNR) than adults (approximately 6 dB) for comparable levels of performance.

Another factor that must be taken into account when selecting amplification for children is that they are physically smaller than adults. The small size of infants' and children's earcanals means that the sound pressure level (SPL) delivered to their ears will be greater than measured in adult ears (Feigin et al, 1989; Nelson Barlow et al, 1998; Westwood & Bamford, 1995). The real-ear-to-coupler difference (RECD) is defined as the difference, in decibels, between the SPL measured in a real-ear versus a 2-cc coupler. Feigin et al (1989) measured RECDs in children (ages four weeks to five years) and adults. Results indicated that children's mean RECD values were higher than adults across all frequencies except 250 Hz. The RECD values decreased with increasing age, and the authors predicted that values would fall within 1 standard deviation of the adult mean by approximately 7.7 years of age. Westwood and Bamford (1995) measured RECDs in infants less than 12 months of age. Their findings also revealed higher RECD values than adults. Both reported high intersubject variability.

In addition, the external earcanal resonance peak has been shown to vary as a function of age in children (Bentler, 1989; Dempster & MacKenzie, 1990; Kruger, 1987; Kruger & Ruben, 1987; Westwood & Bamford, 1995). Kruger and Ruben (1987) measured the average external earcanal resonance (also referred to as the real-ear unaided response or REUR) in infants from birth to 37 months of age. Results indicated that the peak resonance frequency decreased as a function of age approaching adult-like values by the second year of life. Bentler (1989) measured REUR for children 3 to 13 years of age. Although results were similar to previously reported data for adults, a large degree of intersubject variability was present. Thus it was recommended that individual values be used whenever possible. Westwood and Bamford (1995) measured REUR over an 18-month period for infants from ≤ 3 to 21 months of age. Their results indicated that the mean peak resonance frequency decreased during the first year of life.

Another difference between children and adults is the amount of information that is available at the time of the hearing instrument fitting. Audiological information for infants and young children may be limited. Delaying amplification until complete audiological information is available may mean that the child is without amplification during critical periods of language development. Thus at the time that hearing instruments are being selected, audiological information might consist of ABR thresholds for clicks and tones or behavioral thresholds (either sound field or for individual ears) at only a few frequencies. In addition, the child's ability to participate in the selection and fitting process may be limited by cognitive and language levels.

Subjective measures of most comfortable level (MCL) and loudness discomfort level (LDL) often are used in adult hearing instrument selection. These measures may not be possible with young children. Kawell et al (1988) tested children (7 to 14 years) and adults using a modification of an LDL procedure reported by Hawkins et al (1987). Results suggested that children with hearing loss who were as young as 7 years could perform the task. The procedure was further modified by Stuart et al (1991). Another LDL procedure was developed by MacPherson et al (1991) using the concept of "too much." After training, children with normal-hearing who had mental ages of 5 years were able to perform the task. No techniques for establishing LDL in younger children have been reported.

Children also will, in general, have less control over their listening environments than adults. Depending on age, the position of the child relative to another talker may vary considerably. Consequently, the level of speech reaching the child's ear also will vary. Stelmachowicz et al (1993) evaluated the effects of distance and postural position on the long-term and short-term characteristics of speech produced by parents of children 2 months to 2½ years. Results indicated that the overall level of the long-term average speech spectrum (LTASS) varied with position and was 10- to 18-dB higher in close conditions (cradle position, hip position) when compared with the reference condition (1 m). In addition, the spectral shape of the LTASS was affected by position. As the child gets older and the distance between talker and listener increases (e.g., on the playground), the expected level reaching the child's ear will be significantly lower. It may not be feasible for the child to change

positions to make speech more audible or to adjust the listening environment to enhance visual cues or reduce noise levels.

Children also may not be able to adjust the volume control settings of their hearing instruments. In noisy or reverberant listening situations, adults often reduce the volume control settings on hearing instruments. Children, on the other hand, often have covers on their volume controls, ensuring that the settings remain fixed regardless of the listening environment. If the hearing instruments use multiple memories to provide different processing for different listening environments, an adult caretaker usually is responsible for selecting the memory that will be used in a particular setting, not the child.

Instrument Options

In general, behind-the-ear (BTE) hearing instruments are the style of choice for infants and young children for many reasons including comfort, safety, and fit because ear size changes over time. The devices should be small enough to fit comfortably on the child's ears. Use of pediatric-sized (also called "kiddie") tone hooks is especially helpful in positioning hearing instruments comfortably on the ears of small children (Fig. 4–1).

Given the lack of audiological information that may be available at the time of the fitting, hearing instruments that have flexible electroacoustical characteristics and that are compatible with a variety of tone hooks are essential. Internal controls to adjust gain, output, and frequency response of hearing instruments allow audiologists to fine tune the devices as more information becomes available about the degree and configuration of the child's hearing loss and his or her auditory responsiveness. Volume controls allow caregivers to increase or decrease the gain of the instruments, within a range specified by the audiologist, on the basis of their observations of the child's auditory responses. For example, if the child reacts negatively to sounds, caregivers may decrease the volume until internal controls can be adjusted by the audiologist. Hearing instruments without volume controls (either on the instruments themselves or on a remote control) prevent caregivers from making those adjustments. Alternately, if hearing-instrument output is tied to the volume control, removing this control will prevent inadvertent changes in output that might result in overamplification or inaudibility.

> ### PEARL
>
> Many earmold manufacturers make soft earmolds in colors that are particularly attractive and may motivate young children to use their hearing instruments consistently.

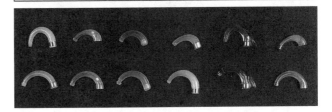

Figure 4–1 Kiddie (*top row*) and adult (*bottom row*) style tone hooks.

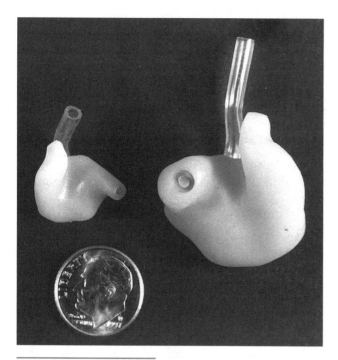

Figure 4–2 Earmold for a 3-month-old infant compared with an earmold for an adult.

Earmolds made of soft material will enhance comfort, retention, and safety. Because children are still growing, their earmolds may need to be replaced more often than adults' earmolds to ensure a good fit. In addition, acoustic modifications such as parallel vents, belled bores, or open molds, which are commonly used in adult hearing instrument fittings, may not be possible with children's molds because of size (Fig. 4–2).

PITFALL

Predicting changes in frequency/gain characteristics of hearing aids on the basis of potential earmold modifications will often be inaccurate for infants and young children. The small size of their earmolds compared with adult earmolds may preclude modifications such as parallel vents, belled bores, or extended canals.

For the safety of younger children, it is important that tamper-resistant battery compartments and volume control covers are available for their hearing instruments. The durability of the device also must be considered given that hearing instruments worn by children may experience greater wear and tear over their lifetimes than those worn by adults. Loss and damage warranties should be recommended, as well as insurance coverage once the manufacturer's warranty expires.

Because children are learning speech and language, it is especially important that they receive auditory signals that are audible, comfortable, not uncomfortably loud, and clear.

PEARL

Products such as Super Seals™ or Moisture Guard™ can be used to protect the battery compartment and/or volume control on hearing instruments without tamper-resistant features. Care should be taken to ensure that the child cannot remove these products because they may be a choking hazard.

Hawkins and Yacullo (1984) reported a significant SNR advantage for binaural over monaural hearing instruments when they evaluated speech recognition in noise and reverberation. In addition, studies of children with unilateral hearing loss indicate poorer performance in noise and reverberation and possible academic difficulties (Bess, 1982; Bess et al, 1986; Culbertson & Gilbert, 1986; Oyler et al, 1988). Because monaural hearing instruments result in a unilateral listener (not to mention that the one ear is impaired), similar problems could be experienced. Binaural hearing instruments are recommended for children unless it can be demonstrated that a particular child performs more poorly with two hearing instruments than with one or if one ear is anacusic.

In many listening environments, hearing instruments alone may not be sufficient to overcome the deleterious effects of noise, distance, and reverberation. Thus hearing instruments should have direct audio input (DAI) and telecoil capabilities that allow them to be compatible with other assistive technology, such as frequency modulated (FM) systems. Assistive listening devices (ALDs) are covered in great detail in Chapter 19 in this volume.

Signal Processing Options

Consideration also must be given to the type of signal processing that will be selected for the child's hearing instruments. At this point in the selection process it may be helpful to refine the goals, making them more specific to the individual child and his or her particular listening environments. Examples of possible goals include the following:

- Make speech audible across a wide range of input levels
- Ensure that speech is undistorted for high level inputs and acoustic conditions
- Increase speech recognition in background noise
- Accommodate a progressive or fluctuating hearing loss
- Amplify an unusual audiometric configuration

Advances in signal processing have resulted in a wide variety of choices for the hearing healthcare professional. Detailed discussion of signal processing options is covered in Chapters 1, 5, 6, and 13 in this volume and will not be repeated here. However, adult findings with different types of signal processing can be helpful when attempting to apply this technology to the pediatric population. Table 4–2

TABLE 4–2   Findings of numerous adult studies of advanced signal processing

Compression

- Wide dynamic range compression (WDRC) processing provides better speech intelligibility over wide range of input levels than does linear processing.

- When hearing instruments are in saturation, quality may be better with compression limiting than with peak clipping. However, some individuals demonstrate preference for peak clipping in these conditions.

- At average conversational levels in quiet, compression limiting does not improve intelligibility.

- Limited objective evidence for improved speech in noise with WDRC circuits.

- For individuals with severe-profound hearing loss, compression systems may not provide sufficient gain and maximum output.

Multimemory

- Studies rely largely on subjective measures.

- Individuals with mild-moderate losses may prefer different amplification schemes in different listening environments.

- Individuals with high-frequency hearing loss greater than 55 dB may be more likely to select different amplification characteristics for different listening environments.

- Hearing instrument should have the ability to vary low-frequency gain by >5 dB in either direction for different memories.

- Individuals who do not demonstrate preferences for different memories in different listening environments may not be candidates.

- Adults tend to use only 2 to 3 memories.

Directional Microphones

- May improve signal-to-noise ratio by 3- to 4-dB with single microphone technology and 5- to 8-dB with dual-microphone technology for adults under optimal conditions.

- Effects increase with binaural hearing instruments.

- Effects decrease in reverberation.

TABLE 4–3   Findings of pediatric studies of advanced signal processing

Compression

- Improved speech recognition in quiet and noise for WDRC and compression compared with peak clipping (PC).

- Little difference in speech recognition between compression limiting and WDRC.

- WDRC provides greater input dynamic range than PC.

- Performance with WDRC significantly better than PC at high input levels.

- Some individuals with hearing loss demonstrate preference for PC over compression limiting at high-input levels.

- For individuals with severe-profound hearing loss compression may result in decreases in performance because of distortion of time/intensity cues.

Multimemory

- Subjective benefit reported with different memories in different listening environments.

- Potential benefit as master hearing instrument.

Directional Microphone

- Improved speech recognition in noise with dual-microphone technology.

FM Systems

- Increase in SNR ratio in FM-only condition compared with HA only.

- SNR ratio advantage decreases when environmental microphone is active.

- Maintains level of talker's voice across distance.

- Response of HA may change when coupled to FM system.

- Improvements in some aspects of language development when FM used as primary amplification.

- Outside interference may affect operation.

summarizes information from numerous studies performed with adults. Studies investigating advanced signal processing options with children are limited. Table 4–3 summarizes information from studies that have been completed with this population. A comprehensive list of readings and references on advanced signal processing, including those used to compile Tables 4–2 and 4–3, is included in Appendix A.

A number of practical issues that must be addressed when selecting a signal processing strategy for a child with hearing loss. As with adults, it is important that the amplified signal children receive be clear and undistorted across a variety of listening environments. As stated previously, children may have more difficulty detecting and understanding auditory signals in the presence of noise than adults. In addition, they cannot use linguistic cues and world knowledge in the same ways as adults to fill in missing information in a message. Given these needs, a number of signal processing options

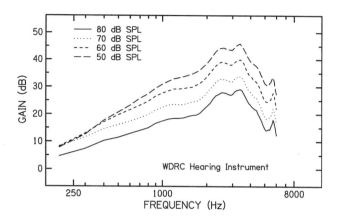

Figure 4–3 Change in gain as a function of input level (50- to 80-dB SPL) for a WDRC hearing instrument.

may be appropriate, including compression circuits, multimemory systems, directional microphones, and FM systems.

Compression Circuits

Wide dynamic range compression (WDRC) circuits apply more gain to less intense signals than to more intense signals (Fig. 4–3). As such, these circuits should provide audibility over a wide range of input levels. On the negative side, the potential for feedback with WDRC circuits is higher because of the increased gain for low input levels. For children, whose ears are smaller and are still growing, feedback may be more of a concern than it would be for an adult. If a WDRC circuit is chosen for a child, it is important that caregivers understand the importance of replacing earmolds when feedback occurs rather than adjusting the volume control to reduce gain of the hearing instrument until their next scheduled visit with the audiologist. If hearing instrument gain is consistently reduced because of feedback, the amplification the child receives may be inadequate and a different circuit may need to be selected.

When considering hearing instruments with input compression circuits, it is important to remember that output is tied to the volume control. That is, as the volume is increased, maximum output also increases. Thus for infants and young children who have been fitted with hearing instruments using input compression, the volume control may need to be fixed to prevent inadvertent changes.

Even compression limiting circuits may not provide enough gain and output to make speech cues and environmental sounds audible for some children with severe to profound hearing loss. Boothroyd et al (1988) used a master hearing instrument with and without amplitude compression to evaluate speech pattern perception for nine children (11 to 16 years) with severe to profound hearing loss. All but one of the children showed small but significant decreases in performance with compression. The authors suggested that distortion of time/intensity cues may have caused the decrement. Dawson et al (1990) measured maximum output for pure tone (90 dB SPL) and speech (86.5 Leq) signals through hearing instruments using peak clipping and compression limiting. Although OSPL90 (measured using pure tone signals) differed

by only 3- to 5-dB, output for speech stimuli differed by 6- to 9-dB, with the compression instruments demonstrating lower output levels. As Dawson et al (1990) report, "undoubtedly this is because such signals have a high crest factor (ratio of instantaneous peak level to Leq), and if the low distortion possible with compression limiting is to be obtained, the aids must be designed so that clipping of the peaks does not occur to a significant degree. This implies that the aid will have a lower long term equivalent output level than would a similar aid employing peak clipping" (p. 4). Such differences in output may render all or parts of the speech signal inaudible for some individuals with severe to profound hearing loss when using compression limiting hearing instruments.

Multimemory Hearing Instruments

Another option that might be considered for children is multimemory hearing instruments. With these systems, different signal processing strategies can be programmed for different listening environments and selected from the memories available in the instrument. Some multimemory hearing instruments use a remote control device to access the various memories, whereas others use switches or push buttons on the hearing instruments. From a practical standpoint, if a caregiver (not the child) will be selecting the memories for various situations, it will be simpler to select a device that uses a remote control. Those in control of selecting the appropriate memory must understand how and when this should be done.

Deciding which memories to program into the hearing instrument and when to use a particular memory raises other issues. It has been suggested that, for very young children, the memories be programmed on the basis of the expected speech inputs to the hearing instrument. Thus one memory might be programmed on the basis of higher input levels when an infant or young child is close to caregivers and a second memory on the basis of lower inputs when the child is farther away from the talker. Another possibility would be to program the first memory with certain frequency/gain characteristics and vary the relative gain in subsequent memories slightly (e.g., a second memory could be set with more gain and a third with less gain than the first). Caretakers would observe the child's responses using the different memories in similar listening situations. Fine tuning of the hearing instruments would be done on the basis of those observations. Once a desired response is achieved in the first memory, other memories could be set for particular situations such as in the car, on the playground, or watching television.

Another important concern when considering multimemory hearing instruments is whether routinely changing the way the hearing instruments operate will be beneficial or detrimental to a child who is learning language. It is possible to argue this point both ways. If selecting different memories makes it easier for the child to hear and understand speech in a greater variety of listening situations, theoretically, at least, multiple memories should provide benefit. On the other hand, if different signal processing is used in different memories, the signal the child receives may sound different, possibly affecting acquisition of speech and language. To date, no tools to determine the efficacy of multiple memories in children are available. Systematic methods of gathering efficacy information, which are sensitive to the possible effects of processing, need to be developed.

Directional Microphones

Hearing instruments with directional microphones also might be considered for children. Single-microphone directional technology has been available for many years. Recently, however, directional microphones using dual-microphone technology have become available. Because hearing instruments in the directional mode of operation attenuate sounds from the sides and rear (i.e., off-axis), a talker directly in front of the listener should be easier to hear. The amount of attenuation provided for off-axis sounds when using a directional microphone can vary across devices and listening situations. With highly directional microphones, it is important that the hearing instrument can be switched from directional to omnidirectional modes of operation. Being able to alter the amount of directionality is important for those instances when, for safety, it is necessary that the user hear sounds from all directions. When the listening situation changes from one main talker (e.g., a lecture) to talkers speaking from a variety of locations (e.g., a classroom discussion), it also is important that the user have the option of changing from directional to omnidirectional mode of operation. For young children who do not understand the rules of communications, directional microphones may hinder interactions that do not take place when the talker and listener are facing one another. In addition, hearing instruments operating in the directional mode may reduce the amount of overhearing a child experiences, hindering learning that takes place incidentally.

SPECIAL CONSIDERATION

Directional microphones should be used with caution for children with visual impairments who need to be aware of sounds from all locations within their environments.

Because adult caregivers may be responsible for determining when the hearing instruments will be used in directional versus omnidirectional mode, it is important that they understand how and when to select the appropriate mode for a given situation. It also is important that the person in charge of the device remember to change modes as the environment changes, such as when a child goes from a single talker situation in a classroom to a game of soccer on the playground.

When signals are degraded by noise, distance, and reverberation, the benefits that can be achieved by even the most advanced hearing instrument technology available today will have limits. In classrooms where children often are learning new information, the effects of noise, distance, and reverberation can be especially detrimental. With the Rapid Speech Transmission Index (RASTI), Leavitt and Flexer (1991) evaluated the integrity of speechlike signals at different locations in a classroom. Perfect reproduction of the transmitted signal would result in a score of 1.0. Results indicated that this score

was achieved only at the location of the reference microphone (6 inches from the loudspeaker). At other distances the scores ranged from 0.83 in the center of the front row to 0.55 in the back row of the class. These findings indicate a decrease in the fidelity of the signal as a function of distance. Thus, even if a hearing instrument were able to perfectly reproduce the signal received at its microphone, distance and interfering noise in the environment would result in an imperfect signal at the listener's ears.

PITFALL

Some individuals incorrectly assume that use of advanced technology in hearing instruments precludes the need for additional assistive technology in educational environments. Often this is based on a comparison of performance between the child's hearing instrument and the environmental microphone of an FM system (which often is linear and may use peak clipping) and not a comparison of FM with hearing instrument performance.

FM Systems

Placing the microphone close to the talker's mouth is a simple, yet effective, way to overcome the effects of noise, distance, and reverberation. FM systems, which have long been used in educational settings, have also been investigated as primary amplification for children at home (Benoit, 1989; Brackett, 1992; Moeller et al, 1996). The signal is sent, by means of FM radio waves, from the transmitter to a receiver worn by the listener. Recent advances in FM technology have produced BTE FM receiver/hearing instrument combinations, and FM receivers in audio boots. The miniaturization of the FM receiver makes FM systems a more practical option as amplification for many children, especially in situations where body-style systems might be considered cumbersome. Despite their small size relative to other FM systems, the BTE FM/hearing instrument combinations typically are housed in a large BTE case that may limit their ability to fit comfortably on very small ears.

In some cases body-style systems may still be the model of choice. For example, if using ear-level environmental microphones results in feedback for children with small ears and/or severe-profound hearing loss, a body-style system with button transducers and environmental microphones on the receiver unit may be a better choice. Also, children with fine motor problems may find the larger controls on body-style units easier to manipulate as they become more independent in the care and maintenance of their devices.

For very young children, the small size of FM receivers in audio boots may pose a choking hazard, and care should be taken if the devices are not tamper proof. Also, the smaller FM receivers do not have "low-battery" and "no FM" lights. Thus they may be more appropriate for use with children who are able to inform caregivers when their systems are not working properly.

PEARL

Young children may have difficulty keeping light-weight headphones worn with FM systems in place or may find them uncomfortable if worn for extended periods. Manufacturers will modify ear-level transducers to reduce output and remove the microphone. When worn with open earmolds, these transducers may fit more comfortably on small heads/ears while producing a response similar to that achieved with lightweight headphones.

If an FM system is to be coupled to a child's personal hearing instrument, it is important to ensure that the instrument selected allows the appropriate coupling (e.g., telecoil, DAI) and that electroacoustical characteristics are maintained. It also is important to ensure that the signal is audible, comfortable, and safe in all modes of operation: FM only, FM plus hearing instrument, and hearing instrument only.

In a longitudinal study of FM use in nonacademic settings, Moeller et al (1996) reported a number of practical problems related to FM use in addition to size and number of components. Concerns about the ability of individuals other than parents to use the systems appropriately even after training by investigators and parents persisted, as well as concerns about appropriate use of the FM system in group situations where there were multiple talkers. FM interference presented problems when the systems were used in different locations. Since the time of that study, additional channels have been allocated for FM system use both in the 72 to 76 MHz frequency region traditionally used by FM systems and in a higher frequency region (216 to 217 MHz) (Federal Communication Commission, 1992). These additional frequencies may help to alleviate some of the interference problems currently plaguing FM users.

Finally, Moeller et al (1996) reported that, despite training, the FM systems often were used inappropriately. Several parents tended to use the FM system as an "intercom" to introduce behavioral control beyond an acceptable range. In addition, the FM transmitter was frequently used in situations where there was not a primary talker. The authors concluded that extensive training regarding proper FM system use and ongoing monitoring would be important to the success of an FM fitting.

An additional factor that must be considered when selecting any amplification system, especially for children, is the cost/benefit ratio. In some areas of the world cost may not be an issue. In others cost may determine whether a family is able to obtain one or two hearing instruments for their child. Cost also may determine whether the family will be able to purchase only hearing instruments or hearing instruments plus additional assistive technology such as FM systems. It is the responsibility of the audiologist to choose devices that will best meet the auditory needs of the child. If expensive technology is chosen, then that expense should be justified

CONTROVERSIAL POINT

With the advent of FM receivers in BTE cases or audio boots, audiologists are more frequently recommending FM amplification for use outside the classroom. When these devices are used in educational settings *and* in other settings, the question of "who pays for what?" begins to arise. Families may argue that the school is responsible because of the need for FM systems for learning. Schools may argue that the family should pay for devices that will be used outside the school, where educational personnel cannot control use, care, and maintenance. As reported by DeConde Johnson et al (1997), "in a Department of Education interpretation (U.S. Department of Education, September 29, 1992) . . . the use of any assistive technology device beyond the school day is permitted provided the need is determined on an individual basis, as required by the student to receive FAPE, and is part of the student's special education services, related services, or supplementary aids and services to meet the goals of his or her IEP" (p. 85). In our experience, even when provision of FM systems outside school is not mandated, many families and school districts work together to cover the expenses (e.g., the school buys the transmitter and the family buys the receiver or the school buys the entire FM system and the family pays for batteries and maintenance). As with all decisions relating to provision of amplification for children with hearing loss, decisions about FM systems must be made on an individual basis, taking into account many factors that are specific to a particular child, his or her family, and the local educational system.

---

by improved ability to meet the amplification goals set for the child. Currently, a critical need exists for efficacy studies of advanced technology with children.

CONTROVERSIAL POINT

Continued debate exists regarding the benefits and limitations of advanced hearing aid technology with children. At our facility, we believe that this should not be an "either/or" debate but that children should be evaluated individually, and the amplification option should be selected that will best meet the needs of the child and his or her family in the listening environments they will encounter.

SELECTING AMPLIFICATION TARGETS

With the information gathered from research with adults and children and the practical considerations that have been discussed thus far, the audiologist is now ready to specify the gain and output characteristics for an individual child's hearing loss. When selecting a prescriptive method for use with young children, it is important to choose one that requires only threshold information because many children initially will be limited in their ability to perform additional measures such as speech recognition, MCL, or LDL. Although many prescriptive methods are available today (e.g., Berger et al, 1989; Byrne & Dillon, 1986; Libby, 1986; Matkin, 1987; McCandless & Lyregaard, 1983), only one has been developed specifically for use with children.

The Desired Sensation Level Approach

Desired sensation level (DSL) is a computer-based formula approach developed by Richard Seewald and colleagues (Cornelisse et al, 1994; Cornelisse et al, 1995; Ross & Seewald, 1988; Seewald, 1991; Seewald, 1994; Seewald & Ross, 1988; Seewald, et al, 1985; Seewald et al, 1987; Seewald et al, 1992; Seewald et al, 1993; Seewald et al, 1997). The DSL procedure was originally designed for children although the most recent versions also can be used for adults. This approach is based on a number of assumptions regarding fitting amplification to children:

1. Children typically wear hearing instruments at fixed settings.
2. Amplification characteristics that are selected are important in speech and language acquisition.
3. Limited audiometric data may be available at the time of hearing instrument selection.
4. A number of factors important for hearing instrument selection will vary with age.

For children, DSL uses the University of Western Ontario speech spectrum (Fig. 4–4) which is a compromise between the average speech levels of adult males, adult females, and children, and the levels of the child's own voice at ear level (Cornelisse et al, 1991). The program allows the clinician to enter thresholds that have been obtained using a range of signal transducers (e.g., TDH earphones, insert earphones, loudspeakers) and appropriate transforms are used to convert all information to dB SPL in the earcanal. The child's own RECD and REUR can be measured individually or the program will use age-appropriate transforms. With the data that are entered and appropriate transforms, the program provides targets for various real-ear and coupler measures. Corrections are made for hearing instrument microphone location (i.e., BTE, in-the-ear [ITE], in-the-canal [ITC], and completely in-the-canal [CIC]), and numerous options for verification are provided. The most recent version of the DSL program, DSL[i/o], provides an algorithm for fitting wide WDRC hearing instruments in addition to linear hearing instruments. Figure 4–5 is a graphic display of target values from DSL[i/o] for a child with a mild to moderate hearing loss. The open squares represent thresholds

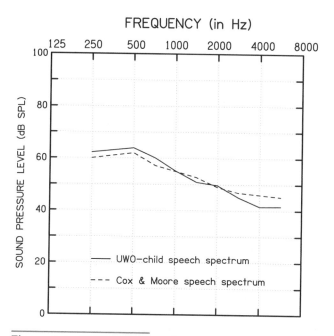

Figure 4–4 UWO-child speech spectrum (*solid line;* Cornelisse, L.E., Gagne, J.P., & Seewald, R.C. [1991]. *Ear and Hearing, 12*(1);47–54.) and adult speech spectrum (*dashed line;* Cox, R.M., & Moore, J.N. [1988]. *Journal of Speech and Hearing Research, 31*;102–107.).

converted to SPL in the earcanal. The dashed lines represent targets for constant level pure tone inputs of 65 (T65) and 90 (T90) dB SPL.

FM System Evaluation

Selecting targets for the FM portion of an FM system varies somewhat from selection of the hearing instrument portion. Although it is beyond the scope of this chapter to discuss these procedures in detail, some important points most be remembered. First, the input level of speech to the FM microphone will, in most instances, be higher than the input level to a hearing instrument microphone. This difference is a result of the proximity of the microphone to the talker's mouth (usually 6 to 8 inches for chest-worn microphones; Fig. 4–6). The input level differences should be taken into account when selecting and verifying FM performance.

SPECIAL CONSIDERATION

Input levels to be used for setting FM systems will vary depending on the location of the FM microphone relative to the talker's mouth (chest level, near the mouth, on a table nearby). Input levels used to set the hearing instrument portion of the system will vary depending on the signal of interest (user's own voice, others not wearing the FM microphone who are close, others not wearing the FM microphone who are farther away).

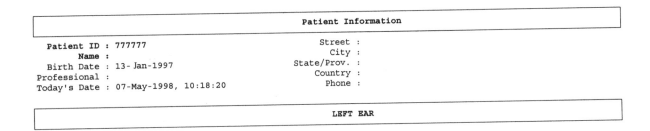

Patient Information	

Patient ID : 777777
Name :
Birth Date : 13-Jan-1997
Professional :
Today's Date : 07-May-1998, 10:18:20

Street :
City :
State/Prov. :
Country :
Phone :

LEFT EAR

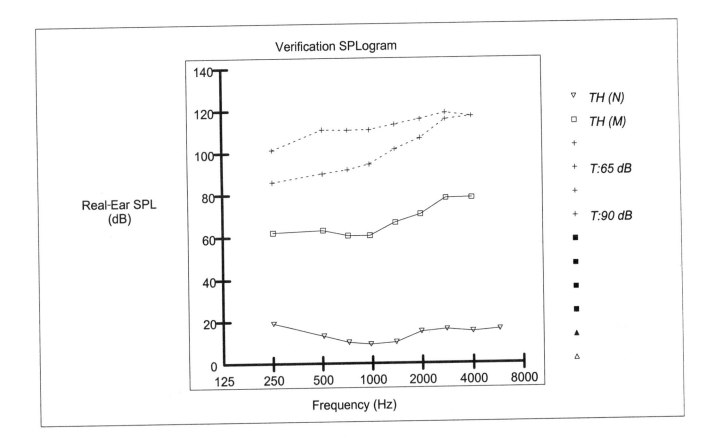

HEARING AID RECOMMENDATION

LEFT EAR
Selection Method : DSL [i/o]

HEARING AID
Style : BTE
Make :
Model :
Serial # :

EARMOLD
Type : NOT SPECIFIED
Tube : NOT SPECIFIED
Bore : NOT SPECIFIED
Vent : NOT SPECIFIED
Material : NOT SPECIFIED

OTHER
Transducer : ER3
HL to SPL : Predicted
HA Style : BTE
Circuit : Linear
RE to 2cc : Predicted

OTHER
Speech : UWO Child

Max. Out : Predicted

	.25	.50	.75	1.0	1.5	2.0	3.0	4.0	6.0
SSPL-90	94	102	101	100	103	106	104	99	
Full-On Gain (Reserve 10 dB)	23	25	26	28	34	39	42	42	
User Gain (Input Speech)	13	15	16	18	24	29	32	32	
Comp. Ratio	1.0	1.0	1.0	1.0	1.0	1.0	1.0	1.0	1.0

Figure 4–5 Graphic display of gain targets for DSL[i/o]. Open squares represent thresholds in earcanal SPL. Dashed lines represent targets for constant level pure tone inputs of 65- and 90-dB SPL.

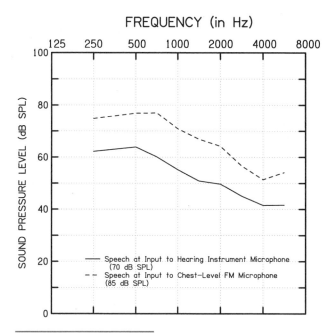

Figure 4–6 Level of speech at a chest-level FM microphone *(solid line)* and a hearing instrument microphone *(dashed line)*.

Second, it is important to remember that, most of the time, the child wearing the FM system will need to hear the talker wearing the FM microphone, others who are not wearing the microphone, and his or her own voice. When setting the system, the goal is to ensure audibility of all three signals while, at the same time, maintaining the SNR advantage for the FM signal. Finally, it is important to always evaluate an FM system in all modes of operation in which it will be used. That is, if the system will be used in FM only and FM plus hearing instrument modes of operation, evaluation should be completed for both. For further information regarding selection and evaluation of FM systems, the reader is referred to relevant texts (ASHA, 1994b; Hawkins, 1987; Hawkins & Mueller, 1992a; Lewis, 1991, 1994, 1998; Lewis et al, 1991; Seewald & Moodie, 1992).

Once amplification targets have been obtained and the hearing instrument has been set to match those targets, the next step is verification. The following section will focus on behavioral and objective methods for verifying hearing instrument performance.

VERIFICATION OF AMPLIFICATION PERFORMANCE

Behavioral Measures

Traditionally, behavioral measures of functional gain have been used to verify aided performance in children. For these measures, a child's sound field thresholds are obtained in both aided and unaided conditions. The difference, in decibels, between these two measures is the functional gain of that particular hearing instrument. Because sound field behavioral testing is familiar to both patients and audiologists and requires only the test equipment that is available in most

audiological settings, it might seem that these measures would be the method of choice for verifying aided performance. However, a number of limitations are associated with functional gain. First, functional gain measures are behavioral and, thus, require both cooperation from the individual being tested and the ability to produce the desired behavioral response. If a child cannot or will not respond behaviorally to the test stimuli or responds inconsistently, little information is obtained. Multiple sessions may be required to complete testing. Because of time constraints, functional gain measures typically provide data only at a few frequencies. This limited sample of frequencies may not give an accurate picture of the performance of the instrument. Functional gain measures also may not provide an accurate estimate of hearing instrument performance under typical use conditions. In regions of normal-hearing functional gain measures may be affected by the noise floor of the hearing instrument and/or noise in the test environment. Thus the gain of the hearing instrument in those regions may be underestimated. Because functional gain measures are made at relatively low input levels to the hearing instrument microphone, they may overestimate the amount of gain available from the hearing instrument for higher level inputs such as normal conversational speech. This discrepancy will occur whenever the hearing instrument is functioning in its nonlinear operating range (e.g., WDRC hearing instruments, linear hearing instruments with low maximum output). Figure 4–7 from Lewis (1997) illustrates this issue. In this figure input/gain curves are shown for three hypothetical hearing instruments. At low input levels (10- to 40-dB) the gain of the instruments is the same. As the input level increases, however, the amount of

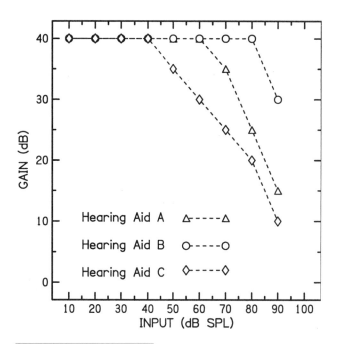

Figure 4–7 Gain (dB) as a function of input (dB SPL) for three different hearing aids. (From Lewis, D. [1997]. In: W. McCracken, & S. Laoide-Kemp (Eds.), *Audiology in education* (pp. 323–347). Manchester: University of Manchester; used with permission.)

gain begins to differ across the three instruments so that at input levels comparable to raised voice (70 dB SPL) the gain is 25-, 35-, and 40-dB for hearing instruments C, B, and A, respectively. If functional gain measures had been used for verification, these devices would have been judged to have similar responses. In real life situations, however, the amplification of speech would be very different. Functional gain measures also will not provide information about the maximum output of the hearing instrument, which is critical when fitting hearing instruments to children.

If functional gain measures are being considered as a means of comparing one hearing instrument to another, it is important to know what differences will be needed to determine that an actual difference in performance exists between the two instruments. Hawkins et al (1987) looked at test-retest variability of aided sound field thresholds. Their results indicated that thresholds would have to differ by greater than 15 dB to be significantly different at the .05 confidence level. Stuart et al (1990) determined the critical difference in aided sound field thresholds for children ages 5 to 9 and 10 to 12 years. They found no statistically significant differences between the two groups and reported that differences in aided thresholds would need to be greater than 10 dB to be statistically significant at the .05 confidence level. One cannot assume that the results of these two studies would hold true for younger children who would be likely to show even greater variability.

Some cases exist where functional gain may be the test method of choice. Stelmachowicz and Lewis (1988) report that functional gain measures may give a more accurate picture of aided performance in cases where unaided thresholds represent vibrotactile rather than auditory responses. Functional gain measures also are the only methods available for verifying aided performance of bone conduction hearing instruments or cochlear implants. Even in these latter cases, it must be remembered that results represent the softest level at which signals can be detected and may not represent performance with higher level input signals.

Objective Measures

Probe microphone measures are a feasible means of assessing the amplification provided by a child's hearing instrument.* Probe microphone measures can be performed with input levels comparable to those that will be encountered in use conditions, providing a more accurate estimate of the audibility of signals. They also provide information about gain in regions of normal-hearing and about maximum output of the hearing instrument. Probe microphone measures are less time consuming and require less cooperation from the child, allowing for more measures than can be obtained in a single session using functional gain measures. They also provide greater frequency resolution than is available with functional gain measures.

Given the benefits of probe microphone measures, one would expect that they would be the verification method of choice for infants and children. However, in a survey of pediatric hearing instrument fitting practices in the United States,

---

*For further information on probe microphone measures, the reader is referred to Chapter 3 in this volume.

SPECIAL CONSIDERATION

When verifying targets using a particular prescriptive method, it is important that the input levels and stimuli that are selected are the ones recommended by the prescriptive method to ensure accurate results.

Hedley-Williams et al (1996) reported that sound field–aided thresholds were used much more frequently than probe microphone measures to verify hearing aid performance.

Let us assume that at least part of the reason probe microphone measures are not used routinely with children is that audiologists are concerned about the difficulties they may experience when attempting these measures. That being the case, how can the ability to obtain real-ear measures with children be improved? It may be helpful if the child is drowsy or asleep during the test procedure. If awake, visual distracters can be used to keep their attention focused without increasing activity levels. If the hearing instrument settings

PEARL

Mirrors, puzzles, and toys used for distraction during testing and even videos without sound can be used to improve cooperation during real-ear probe microphone testing.

have been carefully selected ahead of time with coupler measures, the amount of time needed for real ear testing will be greatly reduced. Probe-tube insertion depths of 10 mm past the earcanal entrance for children less than 5 years of age and 15 mm for older children (not adult sized) may increase comfort during testing. In all cases it is desirable that the probe-tube extend at least 5 mm past the tip of the earmold (Hawkins & Mueller, 1992b).

PEARL

Use of a sealing substance (e.g., Otoform) on the earmold and *f* may prevent the probe from moving during insertion of the earmold and may reduce feedback when testing high-gain hearing aids.

A procedure that can greatly enhance real ear measurements is the RECD procedure developed by Seewald and colleagues (Moodie et al, 1994). In this quick procedure a measurement first is made in a 2-cc coupler. The measurement then is repeated in the child's ear using his or her own earmold. Results of a typical measurement are shown in Figure 4–8. In this graph, the dashed line represents the coupler response and the solid line represents the real-ear response.

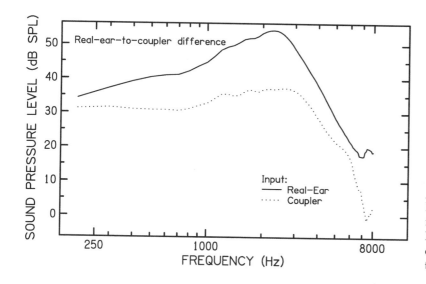

Figure 4–8 RECD measurement. Dotted line represents response in a 2-cc coupler and solid line represents response in the real-ear using the child's custom earmold. The difference between the two curves is the RECD.

The difference between the two curves is the child's RECD. Once the RECD has been measured, subsequent measures can be made in the hearing instrument test box. The RECD is added to the coupler response to predict real-ear aided response (REAR) and real-ear saturation response (RESR).

SPECIAL CONSIDERATION

RECD results will be affected by the size of the child's ear, the earmold being used and the fit of that earmold, and the insertion depth of the probe-tube during measurements. Measurements should be repeated whenever the child receives a new earmold and at least annually.

The validity of the RECD was assessed by Seewald et al (1994). They compared the RECD plus coupler measures and microphone location effects to measurements of REAR and RESR on 15 subjects. Results indicated that REAR and RESR were predicted with a high degree of accuracy using the RECD measures. Sinclair et al (1994) evaluated the repeatability of the RECD for children aged 0 months to 6.9 years of age. Results indicated that the RECD is repeatable as a function of both age and frequency.

When verifying hearing instrument performance using RECD plus coupler measures, several practical issues must be remembered. Because real-ear performance is predicted from measurements made in a coupler, problems with feedback that may prevent use of the instrument at the recommended volume control setting are not addressed. Therefore it is important to try the instrument on the child at use settings, coupled to the personal earmold. If feedback occurs, the hearing instrument and/or earmold may require adjustment. After adjustment, coupler measures should be repeated to provide an estimate of performance at the new settings. It is recommended that RECD measures be repeated whenever the earmold is replaced or at least annually. Adjustments in

hearing instrument settings may be needed on the basis of new RECD values.

The DSL approach allows the user to enter the information obtained during verification measures and will provide a graphic display of the estimated audibility of the speech signal in the aided condition. In the DSL[i/o] version of the software, results for linear gain circuits are displayed for average conversational speech (+12 and −18 dB). Results for WDRC circuits can be displayed for the average long-term speech spectrum (LTASS) of soft (50 dB SPL), average (65 dB SPL), and loud (80 dB SPL) speech. RESR is also displayed for both circuits. Figure 4–9 illustrates results of verification using DSL [i/o]. The open squares represent thresholds for a child with a mild to moderate hearing loss. The dashed lines represent targets for constant level pure tone inputs at 50-, 65-, 85-, and 90-dB SPL (i.e., T50, T65, T80, T90). The filled squares represent verification measurements at the same input levels (i.e., M50, M65, M80, M90).

The ability to evaluate the audibility of different speech levels is helpful because in real life speech does not occur at a single level. Differences in talker-to-listener distances and vocal effort affect the level of speech reaching the hearing instrument microphone. For children who are learning speech and language it is especially important to ensure that speech will be audible to them across many different listening situations. The Situational Hearing Aid Response Profile (SHARP) is a computer program designed to evaluate the audibility and dynamic range of speech over a range of typical listening levels (Stelmachowicz et al, 1994; Stelmachowicz et al, 1996). The user enters audiometric and hearing instrument information into the program, and it calculates unaided and aided LTASS and range of speech, RESR, and an aided audibility index (AAI) for any of 13 different speech spectra (Table 4–4). Results can be used to estimate a hearing instrument's ability to make speech audible across different talker-to-listener distances and vocal efforts to estimate the audibility of the child's own voice and to compare the relative audibility of different signal processing circuits. Figure 4–10 illustrates unaided (A and C) and aided (B and D) speech spectra for average conversational

TABLE 4–4   Thirteen different speech spectrum used in SHARP and their overall RMS levels

Speech Spectrum	Overall RMS level
Average conversational speech at 1 m	60 dB SPL
Raised voice at 1 m	70 dB SPL
Classroom teacher at 1 m	72 dB SPL
Classroom teacher at 2 m	66 dB SPL
Classroom teacher at 3 m	63 dB SPL
Classroom teacher at 4 m	61 dB SPL
Classroom teacher at 7 m	61 dB SPL
Average conversation at 4 m (assumes conversation in a nonreverberant field)	48 dB SPL
Shout	85 dB SPL
Own voice	70 dB SPL
Head shadow at 1 m	60 dB SPL
Cradle position, near ear	68 dB SPL
Hip position, near ear	76 dB SPL

speech (A and B) and the user's own voice (C and D) for a child with a mild to moderate hearing loss. In this figure the X's represent thresholds converted to decibels of sound pressure level in the earcanal. The left column (A and C) shows the unaided condition and the right column (B and D) shows the aided condition. In the left column the solid and dashed lines represent the long-term speech spectrum for average conversational speech (*top*) and own voice (*bottom*). In the right column, the hatched area represents the portion of the speech spectrum that would be audible with a WDRC hearing instrument, and the asterisks represent maximum output of the instrument.

PITFALL

Assuming audibility of speech across a range of input levels on the basis of audibility of speech at a single input level will be inaccurate whenever the hearing instrument is not functioning in its linear operating range.

SHARP was designed for use with single-channel instruments, and, although it can be used for those with multiple channels, different input-output characteristics cannot be entered for the different channels. It also is important to remember that the results provide an estimate of audibility but not intelligibility. In addition, they assume a quiet

listening situation; thus in noisy and/or reverberant backgrounds, audibility of the signal may be poorer.

VALIDATION OF AMPLIFICATION PERFORMANCE

Once the hearing instrument has been selected and set, and testing has verified the performance of the instrument, the next step is validation. According to the Pediatric Working Group (1996), "The purpose of validating aided auditory function is to demonstrate the benefits/limitations of a child's listening abilities for perceiving the speech of others as well as his or her own speech" (p. 56). With infants and children, validation requires input from many sources, including parents/caregivers, educational personnel, audiologists, and other professionals who may be working with the child. Validation will be affected by a variety of factors including the age of the child, the age of onset of the hearing loss, the type and degree of hearing loss, and additional handicapping conditions. Benefits and limitations of amplification also may vary depending on the listening situations and factors related to the hearing instruments being evaluated.

For infants and children, validation is assessed in a variety of ways. *Observable benefit* refers to observed behaviors that suggest the child is responding in some way to the amplified signal provided by the hearing instruments. These might include alerting behaviors, increased vocalizations, or comments from the parents that the child "seems better" when wearing the instruments. *Informal observation* might include situations where the child's auditory responses are observed in a natural environment. Parents/caregivers could be instructed to observe and document the child's behavior in various environments. *Direct measures* of aided auditory function would be used to assess behavioral responses when the hearing instruments are being worn. These might include aided sound field responses (e.g., music, environmental sounds) and speech perception measures. In Appendix B, the Position Statement "Amplification for Infants and Children with Hearing Loss" (Pediatric Working Group, 1996), includes a comprehensive list of speech recognition materials used with children.

Boothroyd (1991) developed a computer-based game (VidSPAC) to evaluate the perception of acoustic contrasts (e.g., vowel height, initial and final consonant voicing) in children. Children as young as 3 to 4 years of age select a colorful character who presents test stimuli. The child responds to changes in a string of stimuli. The program includes animated scenes that are displayed as a reward after a certain number of trials.

Indirect validation measures include functional performance measures. With infants and young children, responses most often are obtained from parents/caregivers and/or educational personnel. One such measure, the Screening Instrument for Targeting Educational Risk or S.I.F.T.E.R. (Anderson, 1989) was developed to identify children at risk for educational problems caused by hearing loss (Appendix C). Teachers are asked to rate the child compared with other students in five areas (academics, attention, communication, classroom participation, and social behavior). On the basis of field testing, "the S.I.F.T.E.R. was felt to be most representative when used

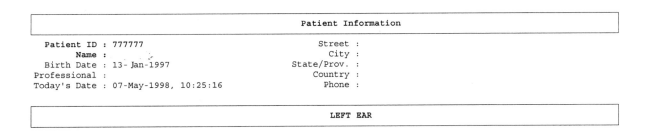

Patient Information

Patient ID : 777777   Street :
      Name :   City :
Birth Date : 13- Jan-1997   State/Prov. :
Professional :   Country :
Today's Date : 07-May-1998, 10:25:16   Phone :

LEFT EAR

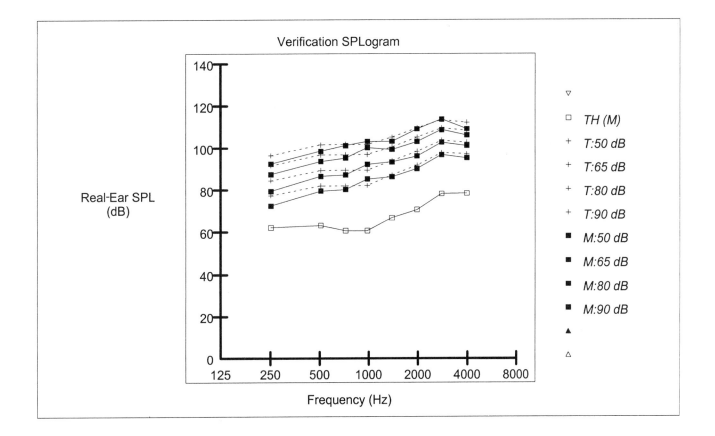

HEARING AID RECOMMENDATION

LEFT EAR
Selection Method : DSL [i/o]

HEARING AID		*EARMOLD*		*OTHER*	*OTHER*
Style : BTE		Type : NOT SPECIFIED	Transducer : ER3	Speech : UWO Child
Make :		Tube : NOT SPECIFIED	HL to SPL : Predicted	Compr. Thresh : IMin
Model :		Bore : NOT SPECIFIED	HA Style : BTE	Loudness : Predicted
Serial # :		Vent : NOT SPECIFIED	Circuit : WDRC (fixed CR)	
		Material : NOT SPECIFIED	RE to 2cc : Predicted	Max. Out : Predicted

	.25	.50	.75	1.0	1.5	2.0	3.0	4.0	6.0
SSPL-90	94	102	101	100	103	106	104	99	
Full-On Gain (Reserve 10 dB)	22	25	24	23	28	32	32	29	
User Gain (Input 65 dB)	12	15	14	13	18	22	22	19	
Comp. Ratio	2.1	2.1	2.0	2.0	2.2	2.2	2.5	2.6	

Figure 4–9 Graphic display of verification using the DSL[i/o]. Open squares represent thresholds in earcanal SPL. Dashed lines represent targets for constant level pure tone inputs at 50-, 65-, 85-, and 90-dB SPL, and filled squares represent verification measurements at the same input levels.

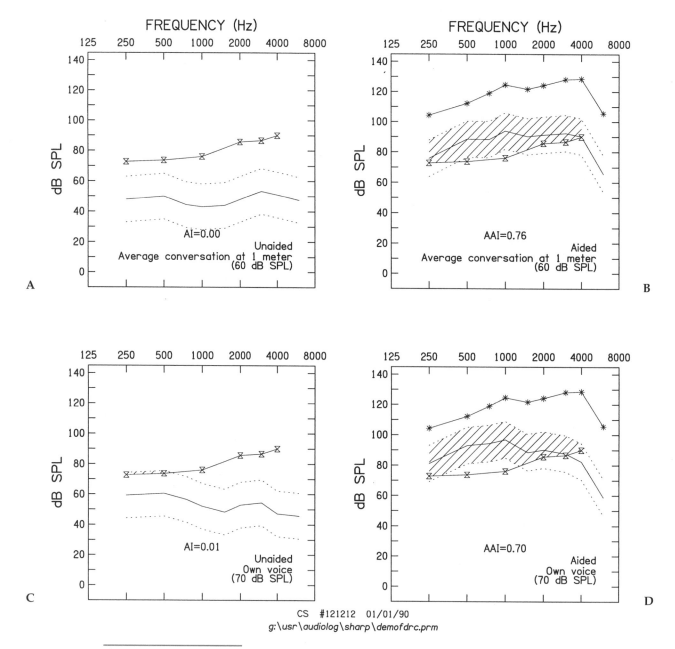

Figure 4–10 Unaided (**A** and **C**) and aided (**B** and **D**) speech spectra for average conversational speech *(top row)* and own voice *(bottom row)* from SHARP. Xs represent thresholds converted to earcanal SPL. Solid and dashed lines represent long-term average speech spectrum. Hatched area represents the portion of the speech spectrum that would be audible in a given condition.

with Caucasian students, grade kindergarten through five, with known hearing loss of faint to moderate degree who are educated in the regular classroom" (Anderson, 1989, p. 2). On the basis of positive feedback from those using the S.I.F.T.E.R., Anderson and Matkin (1996) developed a preschool version of the test (Appendix D). School personnel are asked to rate the child in five areas similar to those used in the original test. From field testing, this version "was felt to have the greatest validity when used with Caucasian students age 3.0 through kindergarten (6.6), with known hearing loss of moderate to profound degree" (Anderson & Matkin, 1996, p. 3).

The Hearing Performance Inventory for Children (HPIC) (Kessler et al, 1990) was developed as a self-assessment tool for children ages 8 to 14 years. The test was designed to assess a child's perceived communication difficulties in various academic environments. In this test students are shown pictures of classroom situations; asked if those situations ever occur in their classes (Fig. 4–11); and if so, how often they experience difficulties (using a 5-point scale from "always" to "never"). Results can be used to help develop individual management programs for students with listening difficulties.

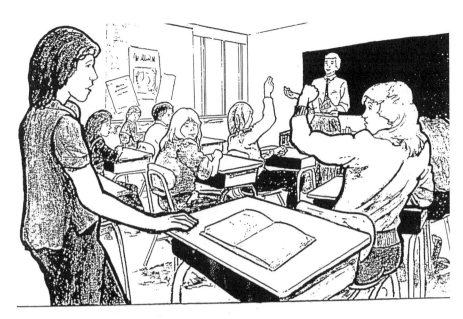

This student is giving an answer in class. The rest of the class is listening. Does that happen in your class? Is it hard for you to hear the other students give answers?

Figure 4–11 Example of one of the picture/classroom situations used in the Hearing Performance Inventory for Children.

The Learning Inventory for Education (LIFE) was developed by Anderson and Smaldino (1997) to determine amplification benefit or effectiveness of an intervention strategy for elementary school students (Appendix E). The LIFE is composed of three inventories. The student inventory uses cartoonlike pictures to identify difficult classroom listening situations. The teacher inventory is used to evaluate the student's attention, classroom participation, and learning. The third inventory, also completed by teachers, uses open-ended questions to gather more information regarding the teacher's observations and opinions. The inventories are intended to be completed before and after classroom intervention such as amplification or acoustic modifications.

Kopun and Stelmachowicz (1998) modified the Abbreviated Profile of Hearing Aid Performance (APHAP) (Cox & Alexander, 1995) for use with children aged 10 to 16 years (Appendix F). The purpose of the CA-APHAP is to allow comparison of aided and unaided performance in a variety of situations. Children with mild to severe hearing loss and their parents were given the test. Results indicated that for children with moderate to severe hearing loss, patterns of responses were similar to aided adult data from Cox and Alexander (1995). Correlations between scores for children and parents were very low, indicating that they did not agree about the communication difficulties the children were experiencing.

The Meaningful Auditory Integration Scale or MAIS (Robbins et al, 1991) was developed for use with children with profound hearing loss. The scale evaluates three aspects of the child's ability to use sound meaningfully in everyday situations (bonding to device, alerting to sound, and deriving meaning from auditory phenomena). An interview format, based on 10 "probes," is used with parents to obtain information about their child's behavior in specific situations.

The Client Oriented Scale of Improvement or COSI (Dillon et al, 1997) was developed as a self-report tool for measuring hearing instrument benefit and satisfaction (Appendix G). With this tool, the individual with hearing loss selects up to five listening situations where they are experiencing hearing difficulty. After rehabilitation, the situations are reviewed relative to improvements. Although the scale was developed using situations encountered by adults, it can be modified to include categories that would be pertinent to infants and children with hearing loss. Examples of categories for young children include the following:

- Changes in behavior (e.g., quiets, smiles in response to sound)
- Increased vocalization
- Requests hearing instrument
- Awareness of loud environmental sounds
- Awareness of soft environmental sounds
- Awareness of voice
- Response to music
- Localization to sound/voice

Parents would complete the form before and after specific rehabilitation such as the introduction of amplification. As the child develops, goals would be changed to reflect developmental changes and expectations.

Professionals at the University of Pittsburgh have developed a set of tools to be used to assess listening needs and evaluate efficacy of intervention (Palmer & Mormer, 1997, 1998). The first tool is the Developmental Index of Audition and Listening (DIAL). The DIAL provides a table of auditory and listening skills that are to be expected at specific ages for children with normal-hearing (Appendix H). The auditory skills of the child with hearing loss are determined as a "starting point" for auditory skill development. The Pediatric Hearing Demand, Ability and Need Profile (HDAN) allows the clinician to assess communication difficulties with and without amplification, current compensations for those difficulties, and recommendations for other solutions (Appendix I). Finally, the information from the DIAL and HDAN are incorporated into the Family Expectation Worksheet (FEW). The FEW is similar to the COSI in that the family, with input from the child when possible, develops goals for (re)habilitation (Appendix J). Using the FEW, the family rates how the child functions currently (before intervention) and how they expect the child to function after intervention. Expectations, based on a variety of factors (e.g., hearing loss, amplification, age) may be adjusted by the audiologist. After intervention the family rates their perception of the child's performance. Thus a goal could be that the child will respond to his or her name. Current levels of success may be "hardly ever" if the child has a severe-profound hearing loss and has not yet been fit with amplification. The family's goal for the child might be that he or she will respond "almost always." The goal might be adjusted to "most of the time" or "half of the time" to account for situations where noise, distance, attention, or the talker's vocal effort would interfere with the child's ability to respond appropriately. If the child is fitted with an ear-level FM system, postintervention success could vary from "most of the time" to "almost always," depending on how and when the FM mode of the system is used.

SPECIAL CONSIDERATION

When children have been followed from a very young age, it is easy to forget to provide them with audiological information that was given to their parents some time previously. It is important that they understand audiological and management issues so that they can participate in and eventually make their own decisions about amplification.

Especially with the youngest children, developing appropriate validation methods may be the most difficult. In addition, a number of questions will remain regardless of the validation tools used to assess performance. For example, how can we assess whether we have achieved optimal performance as opposed to observable improvement? Is "optimal" performance even feasible or is "better" good enough, and if so, how do we quantify? These are questions that do not have easy answers and that will require continued discussion and evaluation as we attempt to develop tools that will demonstrate whether or not intervention strategies are producing desired results.

PRACTICAL ISSUES IN FACILITATING ADJUSTMENT

To achieve goals related to amplification, one of the first issues that must be addressed is consistent use of the hearing instruments. Because with infants and young children caregivers will be in charge of the instruments, it is important that they have a clear understanding of how each device functions,

how to use it correctly, and how to troubleshoot and maintain it. At our facility, families are provided with a "Hearing Instrument Kit" to assist in instrument maintenance. The kit consists of the following items:

- Listening tube
- Battery tester
- Batteries
- Moisture Guard
- Huggie Aids(s) or other retention devices
- Dri-Aid
- Earmold blower

Several hearing instrument manufacturers also produce troubleshooting/maintenance kits for children. In addition, some manufacturers have special programs for children that may include special gifts such as stickers, backpacks, booklets, information for parents and educators, newsletters, and Internet Web sites (Appendix K).

Caregivers are instructed in the care and use of the hearing instruments at the initial fitting. These issues also are discussed at subsequent visits, and families are encouraged to call with any questions or concerns. With children, frequent follow-up is important to monitor hearing, hearing instrument function, and earmold fit, and to allow discussion with families about adjustment, emerging questions, or concerns and changing needs.

Hearing instrument retention is a concern that is often raised by families of infants and children. Retention may be affected by the size of the child's head and ears relative to the hearing instruments or by behavioral issues related to keeping the hearing instrument in place. Pediatric audiologists often must be creative as they assist families with this challenging issue. Because no single strategy works with all children, a variety of options can be tried to select the ones that work best for the individual child and his or her family. Table 4–5 lists a number of strategies to assist in hearing instrument retention and acceptance.

PEARL

When bone conduction hearing instruments are chosen for infants and very young children, it may be difficult to find headbands that will fit well. Alternately, a sweatband, made smaller to fit the child's head, can be used. Both the bone conduction transducer and the hearing instrument are held in place on the band with Velcro.

Hearing instrument adjustment also is enhanced by close communication between the audiologist and educational personnel who work with the child on a regular basis. It is helpful to discuss goals and expectations for amplification (e.g., What is expected to be audible and at what distances?), to review progress and concerns so that modifications can be made when needed, and to provide inservice training regarding use and care of hearing instruments. The child wearing hearing instruments should participate in their care and maintenance

TABLE 4–5 Strategies to assist in hearing and retention and acceptance

Huggie Aids

Fishing line/dental floss and safety pin

Critter Clips

Kiddie tone hooks

Doublestick or toupee tape

Bonnet with hole cut out for hearing instrument microphone

Ribbon with loops for BTE instruments

Eyeglass holders

Sweatbands to hold hearing instruments/earmolds in place

Orthodontic rubber bands to hold BTE instruments to eyeglasses

Vests with pockets for body-worn units

Colored hearing instrument cases

Colored earmolds

Colored beads on earmold tubing

Decorating hearing instruments with stickers

Colored Super Seals

to the extent possible for his or her developmental level. Anderson and Matkin (1998) have developed a counseling tool to assist audiologists when talking with families and schools about a child's hearing loss and educational needs. Counseling pads list 10 degrees of hearing loss along with short discussions of possible effects on understanding of speech and language, possible psychosocial impact, and potential educational accommodations and services (Appendix L).

Even when the hearing instruments selected for a child meet goals and expectations and the child uses them consistently, situations will occur where additional assistive technology is necessary to allow the child to participate more fully in his or her environment. Assistive technology is addressed more fully in Chapter 19 in this volume. The next section will focus, specifically, on selection and use of additional assistive technology with children.

CHOOSING ASSISTIVE TECHNOLOGY FOR CHILDREN

As when choosing hearing instruments, selection of other assistive technology begins with goals. The goals may change over time as the child develops, as needs change, and if hearing loss changes. One of the first goals of assistive technology may be to help the child be aware of auditory events in his or her environment. Children with normal-hearing may learn cause-effect relationships incidentally. For example, the doorbell rings, Mom goes to the door, and someone is there.

After this happens a few times, the child begins to make the association between the doorbell sounding and the presence of someone at the door. Think now of a child with hearing loss who cannot hear the doorbell. The child is playing on the floor; suddenly Mom goes to the door and someone is there. How did she know to go to the door? How will the child learn to understand and interpret these events? By use of a visual alerting device the family can help the child to begin to make associations between the flashing light and the presence of someone at the door.

Another goal of assistive technology is to foster independence. As children get older, it is important for them to be able to do things without assistance from family members. Fostering independence helps prepare the child for the time when they will be living away from their families and to foster self-esteem. One example is helping the child find the most successful method for waking themselves up in the morning. Visual or vibrating alarm clocks or those that ring at higher levels or with different frequencies may be evaluated to select the most appropriate option. When evaluating options, it is important to consider family members with normal-hearing. For example, a sibling sharing the bedroom may tolerate a flashing or vibrating alarm much better than one that uses a more intense auditory signal.

Independence also means increasing degrees of privacy. The ability to have phone conversations without assistance from parents or siblings is especially important as children get older. Use of amplified handsets or telecommunication devices for the deaf (TDDs) used with or without telephone relay services will allow the child to talk to family and peers, make appointments, and even to order pizza. Privacy also extends to the child's own room in the home. For a child with hearing loss, someone knocking at the bedroom door may be inaudible, especially if the child is not wearing his or her hearing instruments. Consequently, family members may get into the habit of entering the room unannounced, an especially distressing event during adolescence. Door knock devices are available that will flash whenever someone knocks on the door. These devices are portable and can be moved around the house as needed.

PITFALL

Making decisions about assistive technology on the basis of audibility of signals when the child is wearing hearing instruments may result in signals that are inaudible without hearing instruments. It is important to know whether the child will be wearing the hearing instrument whenever the device will be used to determine whether the signal should be auditory, visual, or vibrotactile.

As children get older, they also are more likely to be staying home alone or to be caring for other, younger siblings while parents are away. In these cases safety also becomes an issue. It is important that the child with hearing loss be aware when someone is at the door or the phone is ringing, be able to use the phone when needed, and be aware of alarms such as smoke detectors in the home. Again, selecting and evaluating assistive technology before the child is in a situation requiring its use is prudent.

Assistive technology also may be chosen to improve the child's communication skills. Devices for the telephone will enable the child to communicate with a variety of individuals and improve telephone skills. Assistive technology also may help the child communicate in a variety of listening environments where hearing instruments alone are inadequate because of distance, noise, and reverberation. Access to television, radio, tapes and compact discs, and computers also may be enhanced with assistive technology.

PEARL

Remember that assistive technology that is available at home may not be available in other locations. If a child is staying with friends or relatives, it is helpful to have portable assistive devices that the child can take along.

When choosing assistive technology for a child, individual characteristics should be considered. These include the child's age, degree of hearing loss, hearing instruments and their compatibility with assistive technology, any physical limitations, the child's and family's lifestyle, and the family budget. As the child matures, needs will change. For example, a very young child may only need to know that the telephone is ringing. Soon, however, an amplifier or TDD may be needed to allow the child to communicate with family and friends. Later, small portable telephone amplifiers or TDDs, in addition to those on telephones at home, will allow the child to use telephones at friends' homes, at the mall, and so forth.

CONCLUSIONS

Infants and children present a challenge to audiologists during the selection, fitting, and management of amplification. However, it is not an insurmountable challenge, nor is it one that must be met "by hook or by crook." Sources are available that will assist the audiologist in making informed decisions about appropriate amplification from among the myriad of choices that are available today. As the child matures and as available audiological information increases, the process from identification to fitting is a continuous loop: Steps are repeated, goals and fittings are adjusted, and management changes to meet the ever-changing needs of the child and his or her family.

Appendix A
Use of Advanced Signal Processing Hearing Aids with Children
(Adapted from Stelmachowicz, 1997)

Full Dynamic Range
Compression/Compression Limiting

ARMSTRONG, S. (1993). The dynamics of compression: Some key elements explored. *Hearing Journal, 46;*43–47.

BACHLER, H., & BUERKLI-HALEVY, O. (1994). Multi mode limiting: Exploring the endless possibilities. *Hearing Instruments, 45;*26–30.

BOOTHROYD, A., & MEDWETSKY, L. (1986). Effects of compression and spectral equalization on performance/intensity functions. *New Generation Hearing Aids Project (Report #APD15).*

BOOTHROYD, A., SPRINGER, N., SMITH, L., & SCHULMAN, J. (1988). Compression amplification and profound hearing loss. *Journal of Speech and Hearing Research, 31;*362–376.

CORNELISSE, L.E., SEEWALD, R.C., & JAMIESON, D.G. (1994). Fitting wide dynamic range hearing aids: The DSL[i/o] approach. *Hearing Journal, 47;*23–29.

DAWSON, P., DILLON, H., & BATTAGLIA, J. (1991). Output limiting compression for the severe-profoundly deaf. *Australian Journal of Audiology, 13;*1–12.

DeGENNARO, S., BRAIDA, L., & DURLACH, N. (1986). Multichannel syllabic compression for severely impaired listeners. *Journal of Rehabilitation Research and Development, 23;*17–24.

DILLON, H. (1988). Compression in hearing aids. In: R.E. Sandlin (Ed.), *Handbook of hearing aid amplification* (Vol. I) (pp. 121–145). San Diego, CA: College Hill Press.

DILLON, H. (1996). Compression? Yes, but for low or high frequencies, for low or high intensities, and with what response times? *Ear and Hearing, 17;*287–307.

DRESCHLER, W. (1988a). Dynamic-range reduction by peak clipping or compression and its effects on phoneme perception in hearing-impaired subjects. *Scandinavian Audology, 17;*45–51.

DRESCHLER, W. (1988b). The effect of specific compression settings on phoneme identification in hearing-impaired subjects. *Scandinavian Audiology, 17;*35–43.

DRESCHLER, W. (1989). Phoneme perception via hearing aids with and without compression and the role of temporal resolution. *Audiology, 28;*49–60.

DRESCHLER, W.A. (1992). Fitting multichannel-compression hearing aids. *Audiology, 21;*121–131.

DRESCHLER, W., EBERHARDT, D., & MELK, P.W. (1984). The use of single-channel compression for the improvement of speech intelligibility. *Scandinavian Audiology, 13;*231–236.

FABRY, D. (1991). Hearing aid compression. *American Journal of Audiology, 1;*11–13.

FABRY, D.A. (1991) Signal processing hearing aids with the pediatric population. In: J.A. Feigin, & P. G. Stelmachowicz (Eds.), *Pediatric amplification: Proceedings of the 1991 National Conference* (pp. 49–60). Omaha, NE: Boys Town National Research Hospital.

FABRY, D.A., LEEK, M.R., WALDEN, B.E., & CORD, M.A. (1993). Do adaptive frequency response (AFR) hearing aids reduce 'upward spread' of masking? *Journal of Rehabilitation Research and Development, 30*(3);318–325.

HICKSON, L. (1994). Compression amplification in hearing aids. *American Journal of Audiology, 3;*51–65.

HICKSON, L., & BYRNE, D. (1995). Acoustic analysis of speech through a hearing aid: Effects of linear vs. compression amplification. *Australian Journal of Audiology, 17;*1–13.

HICKSON, L., DODD, B., & BYRNE, D. (1995). Consonant perception with linear and compression amplification. *Scandinavian Audiology, 24*(3);175–184.

KIESSLING, J., & STEFFENS, T. (1993). Comparison of a programmable 3-channel compression hearing system with single-channel AGC instruments. *Scandinavian Audiology, (Suppl.), 38;*67–74.

KILLION, M.C. (1993). The K-amp hearing aid: An attempt to present high fidelity for persons with impaired hearing. *American Journal of Audiology, 2;*52–74.

KILLION, M.C. (1995). Talking hair cells: What they have to say about hearing aids. In: C.I. Berlin (Ed.), *Hair cells and hearing aids.* San Diego, CA: Singular Press.

KOLLMEIER, B., PEISSIG, J., & HOHMANN, V. (1993). Real-time multiband dynamic compression and noise reduction for binaural hearing aids. *Journal of Rehabilitation Research and Development, 30;*82–94.

LIPPMAN, R.P., BRAIDA, L.D., & DURLACH, N.I. (1981). Study of multichannel amplitude compression and linear amplification for persons with sensorineural hearing loss. *Journal of the Acoustical Society of America, 69;*524–534.

MOORE, B.C., GLASBERG, B.R., & STONE, M.A. (1993). Effect on the speech reception threshold in noise of the recovery time of the compressor in the high-frequency channel of a two-channel aid. *Scandinavian Audiology (Suppl.), 38;*82–91.

MOORE, B.C.J. (1990). How much do we gain by gain control in hearing aids. *Acta Otolaryngologica (Suppl.), 469;*250–256.

MOORE, B.C.J., LAURENCE, R.F., & WRIGHT, D. (1985). Improvements in speech intelligibility in quiet and in noise produced by two-channel compression hearing aids. *British Journal of Audiology, 19;*175–187.

NABELEK, I.V., & ROBINETTE, L.N. (1977). A comparison of hearing aids with amplitude compression. *Audiology, 16;*73–85.

NEUMAN, A.C., BAKKE, M.H., HELLMAN, S., & LEVITT, H. (1994). Effect of compression ratio in a slow-acting compression hearing aid: Paired-comparison judgments of quality. *Journal of the Acoustical Society of America, 96*(3);1471–1478.

NEUMAN, A.C., BAKKE, M.H., MACKERSIE, C., HELLMAN, S., & LEVITT, H. (1995). Effect of release time in compression hearing aids: Paired-comparison judgments of quality. *Journal of the Acoustical Society of America, 98*(6);3182–3187.

PLOMP, R. (1994). Noise, amplification, and compression: Considerations of three main issues in hearing aid design. *Ear and Hearing, 15;*2–12.

PLUVINAGE, V., & BENSON, D. (1988). New dimensions in diagnosis and fitting. *Hearing Instruments, 39;*28–30.

SEEWALD, R., CORNELISSE, L., JENSTAD, L., MOODIE, S., SHANTZ, J., & PUMFORD, J. (1997). Rationale for WDRC applications in pediatric fittings. *Developments in pediatric audiology: Current issues in assessment and management.* Omaha, NE: Boys Town National Research Hospital.

SMIRGA, D.J. (1993b). Sensorineural hearing loss: A rationale for non-linear circuitry. Part 1: Psychoacoustic and neurophysiologic correlates lead to fitting changes. *Hearing Instruments, 44;*24–28.

SMIRGA, D.J. (1993c). Sensorineural hearing loss: Rationale for non-linear circuitry. Part 2: Formulating problem solving strategies for selecting amplification. *Hearing Instruments, 44;*26–31.

STELMACHOWICZ, P.G., DALZELL, S., PETERSON, D., KOPUN, J., LEWIS, D., & HOOVER, B. (1998). A comparison of threshold-based fitting strategies for non-linear hearing instruments. *Ear and Hearing, 19*(2);131–138.

STELMACHOWICZ, P.G., KALBERER, A., & LEWIS, D.E. (1996). Situational hearing aid response profile (SHARP). In: F. H. Bess, J. Gravel, & A. Tharpe (Eds.), *Amplification for children with auditory deficits.* Nashville, TN: Bill Wilkerson Center Press.

STELMACHOWICZ, P.G., LEWIS, D.E., HOOVER, B.M., & KEEFE, D.H. Subjective effects of peak clipping vs compression limiting in normal and hearing impaired children. *Ear and Hearing* (in press).

STYPULKOWSKI, P., & FRETZ, R.J. (1994). Hearing aid performance: What the test box doesn't tell you. *Hearing Instruments, 45;*11–15.

VERSCHUURE, H., PRINSEN, T.T., DRESCHLER, W.A. (1994). The effects of syllabic compression and frequency shaping on speech intelligibility in hearing-impaired people. *Ear and Hearing, 15;*13–21.

VERSCHUURE, J., DRESCHLER, W.A., DE HAAN, E.H., VAN CAPPELLEN, M., HAMMERSCHLAG, R., MARE, M.J., MAAS, A.J., & HIJMANS, A.C. (1993). Syllabic compression and speech intelligibility in hearing-impaired listeners. *Scandinavian Audiology (Suppl.), 38;*92–100.

WALKER, G., BYRNE, D., & DILLON, H. (1984). The effects of multi-channel compression/expansion on the intelligibility of nonsense syllables in noise. *Journal of the Acoustical Society of America, 76;*746–757.

WALKER, G., & DILLON, H. (1982). *Compression in hearing aids: An analysis, a review and some recommendations (Rep. No. 90).* Sydney, Australia: National Acoustic Laboratories,

YUND, E.W., SIMM, H.J., & EFRON, R. (1987). Speech discrimination with an 8-channel compression hearing aid and conventional aids in a background of speech-band noise. *Journal of Rehabilitation Research and Development, 24;*161–180.

Multimemory Hearing Aids and Related Issues

CHRISTIANSEN, L.A., & THOMAS, T.E. (1997). The use of multiple memory programmable hearing aid technology in children. *Second Biennial Hearing Aid Research and Development Conference,* Bethesda, MD.

FABRY, D.A. (1991). Signal processing hearing aids with the pediatric population. In: J. A. Feigin, & P.G. Stelmachowizc (Eds.), *Pediatric amplification: Proceedings of the 1991 National Conference* (pp. 49–60). Omaha, NE: Boys Town National Research Hospital.

FABRY, D.A., LEEK, M.R., WALDEN, B.E., & CORD, M. (1993). Do adaptive frequency response (AFR) hearing aids reduce 'upward spread' of masking? *Journal of Rehabilitation Research & Development, 30;*318–325.

GOLDSTEIN, D., SHIELDS, A., & SANDLIN, R. (1991). A multiple memory, digitally-controlled hearing instrument. *Hearing Instruments, 42;*20–21.

GRAVEL, J., FAUSEL, N., LISKOW, C., & CHOBOT, J. (1999). Children's speech recognition in noise using dual microphone hearing aid technology. *Ear and Hearing, 20;*1–11.

HORWITZ, A., TURNER, C.W., & FABRY, D.A. (1991). Effects of different frequency response strategies upon recognition and preference for audible speech stimuli. *Journal of Speech and Hearing Research, 34;*1185–1196.

KEIDSER, G. (1995). The relationship between listening conditions and alternative amplification schemes for multiple memory hearing aids. *Ear and Hearing, 16*(6);575–586.

KEIDSER, G., DILLON, H., & BYRNE D. (1995). Candidates for multiple frequency response characteristics. *Ear and Hearing, 16*(6);562–574.

KEIDSER, G., DILLON, H., & BYRNE, D. (1996). Guidelines for fitting multiple memory hearing aids. *Journal of the American Academy of Audiology, 7*(6);406–418.

KUK, F. (1990). Preferred insertion gain of hearing aids in listening and reading-aloud situations. *Journal of Speech and Hearing Research, 33;*520–529.

KUK, F.K. (1992). Evaluation of the efficacy of a multimemory hearing aid. *Journal of the American Academy of Audiology, 3;*338–348.

KUK, F.K. (1993). Clinical considerations in fitting a multimemory hearing aid. *American Journal of Audiology, 2;*23–27.

KUK, F.K., & PAPE, N.M. (1993). Relative satisfaction for frequency responses selected with a simplex procedure in different listening conditions. *Journal of Speech and Hearing Research, 36;*168–177.

MANGOLD, S., ERIKSSON-MANGOLD, M., ISRAELSSON, B., LEIJON, A., & RINGDAHL, A. (1990). Multi-programmable hearing aid. *Acta Otolaryngologica, 469;*70–75.

MANGOLD, S., & LEIJON, A. (1979). A programmable hearing aid with multi-channel compression. *Scandinavian Audiology, 13;*121–126.

RINGDAHL, A. (1994). Listening strategies and benefits when using a programmable hearing instrument with eight programs. *Ear Nose Throat Journal, 73;*192–196.

RINGDAHL, A., ERIKSSON-MANGOLD, M., ISRAELSSON, B., LINDKVIST, A., & MANGOLD, S. (1990). Clinical trials with a programmable hearing aid set for various listening environments. *British Journal of Audiology, 24;235–242.*

STELMACHOWICZ, P.G., LEWIS, D.E., & CARNEY, E. (1994). Preferred hearing-aid frequency responses in simulated listening environments. *Journal of Speech and Hearing Research, 37;712–719.*

TYLER, R.S., & KUK, F.K. (1989). The effects of "noise suppression" hearing aids on consonant recognition in speech-babble and low-frequency noise. *Ear and Hearing, 10;243–249.*

VAN TASELL, D.J., LARSEN, S.Y., & FABRY, D.A. (1988). Effects of an adaptive filter hearing aid on speech recognition in noise by hearing-impaired subjects. *Ear and Hearing, 9;15–21.*

Directional Microphones

BACHLER, H., & VONLANTHEN, A. (1995). Audio zoom-signal processing for improved communication in noise. *Phonak Focus,* No. 18.

BILSEN, F.A., SOEDE, W., & BERKHOUT, A.J. (1993). Development and assessment of two fixed-array microphones for use with hearing aids. *Journal of Rehabilitation Research and Development, 30(1);73–81.*

BUERKLI-HALEVY, O. (1987). The directional microphone advantage. *Hearing Instruments, 38;34–38.*

DEBRUNNER, V.E., & MCKINNEY, E.D. (1995). A directional adaptive least-mean-square acoustic array for hearing aid enhancement. *Journal of the Acoustical Society of America, 98(1);437–444.*

DEMPSEY, J.J. (1985). A functional measure of front-to-back ratio. *Journal of Audiology Research, 25(2);91–100.*

HAWKINS, D.B., & YACULLO, W.S. (1984). Signal-to-noise advantage of binaural hearing aids and directional microphones under different levels of reverberation. *Journal of Speech and Hearing Disorders, 49;278–286.*

HOFFMAN, M.W., & STEWART, R.W. (1996). Simulation of multimicrophone hearing aids in multiple interference environments. *British Journal of Audiology, 30;249–260.*

HOFFMAN, M.W., TRINE, T.D., BUCKLEY, K.M., & VAN TASELL, D.J. (1994). Robust adaptive microphone array processing for hearing aids: Realistic speech enhancement. *Journal of the Acoustical Society of America, 96;759–770.*

LEEUW, A.R., & DRESCHLER, W.A. (1991). Advantages of directional hearing aid microphones related to room acoustics. *Audiology, 30(6);330–344.*

LUDVIGSEN, C., & NIELSON, H.B. (1978). Some experiments with hearing aids with directional microphones. *Scandinavian Audiology, 8;216–222.*

MADISON, T.K., & HAWKINS, D.B. (1983). The signal-to-ratio advantage of directional microphones. *Hearing Instruments, 34;18,49.*

MUELLER, H.G., GRIMES, A.M., & ERDMAN, S.A. (1983). Subjective ratings of directional amplification. *Hearing Instruments, 34;14–16,47–48.*

NIELSON, H.B. (1973). A comparison between hearing aids with directional microphone and hearing aids with conventional microphone. *Scandinavian Audiology, 2;45–58.*

SCHUM, D.J. (1990). Noise reduction strategies for elderly, hearing-impaired listeners. *Journal of the American Academy of Audiology, 1(1);31–36.*

SCHWANDER, T., & LEVITT, H. (1987). Effect of two-microphone noise reduction on speech recognition by normal-hearing

listeners. *Journal of Rehabilitation Research and Develoment, 24(4);87–92.*

SOEDE, W., BERKHOUT, A.J., & BILSEN, F.A. (1993). Development of a directional hearing instrument based on array technology. *Journal of the Acoustical Society of America, 94(2, Pt. 1t);785–798.*

SOEDE, W., BILSEN, F.A., & BERKHOUT, A.J. (1993). Assessment of a directional microphone array for hearing-impaired listeners. *Journal of the Acoustical Society of America, 94(2, Pt. 1);799–808.*

SOEDE, W., BILSEN, F.A., BERKHOUT, A.J., & VERSCHUURE, J. (1993). Directional hearing aid based on array technology. *Scandinavian Audiology (Suppl.), 38;20–27.*

STUDEBAKER, G.A., COX, R., FORMBY, C. (1980). The effect of environment on the directional performance of head-worn hearing aids. In: G.A. Studebaker, & I. Hochberg (Eds.), *Acoustical factors affecting hearing aid performance* (pp. 81–105). Baltimore: University Park.

SUNG, G.S., SUNG, R.J., & ANGELELLI, A. (1975). Directional microphone in hearing aids: effect on speech discrimination in noise. *Archives in Otolaryngology, 101;316–319.*

VALENTE, M., FABRY, D.A., & POTTS, L.G. (1995). Recognition of speech in noise with hearing aids using dual microphones. *Journal of the American Academy of Audiology, 6;440–449.*

WEISS, M. (1987). Use of an adaptive noise canceler as an input preprocessor for a hearing aid. *Journal of Rehabilitation Research and Development, 24(4);93–102.*

Digital Technology

COX, R.M. (1993). On the evaluation of a new generation of hearing aids. *Journal of Rehabilitation Research and Development, 30(3);297–304.*

CUDAHY, E., & LEVITT, H. (1994). Digital hearing aids: A historical perspective. In: R.E. Sandlin (Ed.), *Understanding digitally programmable hearing aids* (pp. 1–13). Boston: Allyn and Bacon.

DEAN, J., & GOLDMAN, E. (1998). *Fitting computer programmed hearing aids on infants and toddlers.* AAA Convention, American Academy of Audiology, Los Angeles, CA: (April, 1998).

HUSSUNG, R.A., & HAMILL, T.A. (1990). Recent advances in hearing aid technology: An introduction to digital terminology and concepts. *Seminar in Hearing, 11;1–15.*

KROKSTAD, A., SVEAN, J., & SORSDAL, S. (1993). Measurement and fitting techniques for digital hearing aids. In: J. Beilin, & G.R. Jensen (Eds.), *Recent developments in hearing instrument technology* (pp. 331–332). Copenhagen: Staugaard Jensen.

LEVITT, H. (1987). Digital hearing aids: A tutorial review. *Journal of Rehabilitation Research and Development, 24(4);7–20.*

LEVITT, H. (1991). Advanced signal processing techniques for hearing aids. In: G.A. Studebaker, F. H. Bess, & L. B. Beck (Eds.), *The Vanderbilt hearing aid report II* (pp. 93–99). Parkton, MD: York Press.

LUNNER, T., HELLGREN, J., ARLINGER, S., & ELBERLING, C. (1997). A digital filterbank hearing aid: Predicting user preference and performance for two signal processing algorithms. *Ear and Hearing, 18;12–25.*

SCHUM, D. (1996). Adaptive speech alignment: A new fitting rationale made possible by DSP. *Hearing Journal, 49;25–29.*

VALENTE, M., FABRY, D., POTTS, L, & SANDLIN, R. (1998). Comparing the performance of the Widex Senso digital hearing aid with analog hearing aids. *Journal of the American Academy of Audiology, 9;*342–360.

VALENTE, M., SWEETOW, R., POTTS, L., & BINJEA, B. (1999). Comparing the performance of the Widex Senso digital hearing aid with directional and omnidirectional microphones with analog hearing aids. *Journal of the American Academy of Audiology, 10;*133–150.

Miscellaneous

CHING, T., NEWALL, P., & WIGNEY, D. (1994). Audio-visual and auditory paired comparison judgments by severely and profoundly hearing impaired children: Reliability and frequency response preferences. *Australian Journal of Audiology, 16;*99–106.

CHING, T., NEWALL, P., & WIGNEY, D. (1995). Reliability and sensitivity of intelligibility judgments by severely and profoundly hearing-impaired children. *Annals of Otology, Rhinology, and Laryngology* (Suppl.), *166* (September);151–153.

EISENBERG, L.S. (1991). Investigation of paired-comparison judgments in normal and hearing-impaired children: Implications in hearing aid selection. In: J.A. Feigin, & P.G. Stelmachowicz (Eds.), *Pediatric amplification: Proceedings of the 1991 National Conference* (pp. 37–48). Omaha, NE: Boys Town National Research Hospital.

EISENBERG, L.S., & DIRKS, D.D. (1995). Reliability and sensitivity of paired comparisons and category rating in children. *Journal of Speech and Hearing Research, 38;*1157–1167.

EISENBERG, L.S., & LEVITT, H. (1991). Paired comparison judgments for hearing aid selection in children. *Ear and Hearing, 12;*417–430.

GIOLAS, T., MAXON, A.B., & KESSLER, A.R. (1995). Hearing Performance Inventory for Children (HPIC), unpublished test instrument.

KAWELL, M., KOPUN, J., & STELMACHOWICZ, P.G. (1988). Loudness discomfort levels in children. *Ear and Hearing, 9;*133–136.

MACPHERSON, B.J., ELFENBEIN, J.L., SCHUM, R.L., & BENTLER, R.A. (1989). A procedure for obtaining thresholds of discomfort in young children. *ASHA, 31;*150.

MACPHERSON, B.J., ELFENBEIN, J.L., SCHUM, R.L., & BENTLER, R.A. (1991). Thresholds of discomfort in young children. *Ear and Hearing, 12(3);*184–190.

SMALDINO, J., & ANDERSON, K. (1997). *Development of the listening inventory for children.* Bethesda, MD: Second Biennial Hearing Aid Research and Development Conference.

STUART, A., DURIEUX-SMITH, A., & STENSTROM, R. (1991). Probe-tube microphone measures of loudness discomfort levels in children. *Ear and Hearing, 12;*140–143.

Appendix B
Amplification for Infants and Children with Hearing Loss

INTRODUCTION

The timely fitting of appropriate amplification to infants and children with hearing loss is one of the more important responsibilities of the pediatric audiologist. Although the importance of providing an audible signal for the development and maintenance of aural/oral communication for formal and informal learning is undisputed, the methods used to select and evaluate personal amplification for infants and children with hearing loss vary widely among facilities. Few audiologists use any systematic approach for selecting and fitting amplification for young children and many do not use current technologies in the fitting process (Hedley-Williams et al, 1996). Because of the improvement in early identification of hearing loss in children (Bess & Paradise, 1994; Stein, 1995), continued changes in technology, and a new array of amplification options available for application to infants and children, there is a critical need for a systematic, quantifiable, and evidence-based approach to providing amplification for the pediatric population. The goal is to ensure that children will receive full-time and consistent audibility of the speech signal at safe and comfortable listening levels.

The audiologist is the professional singularly qualified to select and fit all forms of amplification for children, including personal hearing aids, FM systems, and other assistive listening devices. To perform this function capably, an audiologist must have experience with the assessment and management of infants and children with hearing loss and the commensurate knowledge and test equipment necessary for use with current pediatric hearing assessment methods and hearing aid selection and evaluation procedures. Facilities that lack the expertise or equipment should establish consortial arrangements with those who do.

This statement sets forth guidelines and recommendations associated with the fitting of personal amplification to infants and children with hearing loss. The approach stresses an objective, timely strategy and discourages the traditional comparative approach. We envision the provision of appropriate, reliable, and undistorted amplification as a four-stage process involving assessment, selection, verification, and validation. We herein present a discussion on need, audiologic assessment, preselection of the physical characteristics of hearing aids, selection and verification of the electroacoustic characteristics of hearing aids, and validation of aided auditory function. Because the focus of this position statement is on the fitting process, the topics of counseling and follow-up are discussed but not treated in detail. Readers are referred elsewhere for comprehensive coverage of these important topics (Brackett, 1996; Diefendorf et al, 1996; Edwards, 1996). Finally, we include a question/answer section regarding issues frequently raised by pediatric audiologists.

CRITERIA FOR PROVISION OF PERSONAL AMPLIFICATION

A child needs hearing aids when there is a significant, permanent, bilateral peripheral hearing loss. Some children with variable and/or unilateral losses may also need hearing aids. There are no empirical studies that delineate the specific degree of hearing loss at which need for amplification begins. However, if one considers the acoustic spectrum of speech at normal conversational levels in the 1000–4000 Hz range, hearing thresholds of 25 dB HL or greater can be assumed to impede a child's ability to perceive the acoustic features of speech necessary for optimum aural/oral language development. Hence, thresholds equal to or poorer than 25 dB HL would indicate candidacy for amplification in some form. For children with unilateral hearing loss, rising or high-frequency hearing loss above 2000 Hz, and/or milder degrees of hearing loss (<25 dB HL), need should be based on the audiogram plus additional information including cognitive function, the existence of other disabilities, and the child's performance with the home and classroom.

THE AUDIOLOGIC ASSESSMENT

The efficacy of the hearing aid fitting is predicated on the validity of the audiologic assessment. The ultimate goal of the audiometric evaluation is to obtain ear- and frequency-specific threshold data from the child at the earliest opportunity.

From The Pediatric Working Group of the Conference on Amplification for Children with Auditory Deficits, 1996. Used with permission.
NOTE: This appendix includes the main text of the original document with the exception of the "Questions and Answers" and "Future Directions" sections. For these sections, as well as the Appendices, please refer to the original document.

When testing very young children, however, complete audiologic data are seldom obtained. In the absence of a complete audiogram, and even with one, consistencies among several audiometric measures—behavioral findings, click-evoked and/or tone evoked ABR threshold recordings, aural acoustic immittance measures (reflexes and tympanometry), evoked otoacoustic emissions, and bone-conduction responses (behavioral and/or ABR)—are essential.

For children with a developmental age at or under 6 months, behavioral responses should be confirmed with ABR threshold assessment. When behavioral results are unreliable, such as in the case of children with multiple disabilities, behavioral and ABR assessments should be completed and the findings for both measures should be examined for agreement. However, in the absence of reliable behavioral thresholds, hearing aid fitting should proceed based on frequency-specific ABR results unless neurologic status contraindicates such action. It is not sufficient to base binaural hearing aid fitting only on sound field thresholds, nor is it acceptable to fit hearing aids to infants and young children based solely on a click-ABR threshold. In both such cases critical information is lacking that could affect the efficacy of the fit, or in the worst-case scenario be detrimental to the child's performance. With regard to sound field audiometric assessment, it is inadvisable to assume that both ears have equal hearing loss or hearing loss of the same configuration base on behavioral sound field results alone. Therefore, it is preferable to obtain thresholds using earphones. Insert earphones are recommended because the child's real-ear-to-coupler difference (RECD) (described in the Selection and Verification Section) can then be used to convert threshold measures to real-ear SPL. Other behavioral measures such as speech detection and speech recognition may be useful in determining amplification need. The click-ABR provides insufficient information regarding both the degree and configuration of hearing loss—information that is critical for use with today's prescriptive selection and evaluation procedures. At a minimum, click and 500 Hz tone ABR thresholds should be obtained in order to reflect low- and high-frequency hearing sensitivity (ASHA, 1991). Finally, auditory behaviors should be consistent with parental reports of auditory function as well as more formal, systematic observations of behavioral responses to calibrated acoustic stimuli.

PRESELECTION—PHYSICAL CHARACTERISTICS

Even at a very young age, consideration should be given to the availability of appropriate coupling options on hearing aids, so that the child will have maximum flexibility for accessing the various forms of current assistive device technology. Consequently, hearing aids for most children should include the following features: Direct Audio Input (DAI), telecoil (T), and microphone-telecoil (M-T) switching options. Hearing aids used with young children also require more flexibility in electroacoustic parameters (e.g., tone, gain, output limiting) than for adults, as well as more safety-related features such as battery and volume controls that are tamper resistant.

The physical fit of the hearing aids (in most cases worn behind the pinnae) and the earmolds is important for both comfort and retention. Color of the hearing aids and earmolds needs to be considered across ages, and size of the hearing aids is an especially important cosmetic concern for older children. Earmolds should be constructed of a soft material.

While consideration needs to be given to the aforementioned physical factors, the ultimate goal is the consistency and integrity of the amplified signal that the child receives. Providing the best possible amplified speech signal should not be compromised for cosmetic purposes, particularly in the early years of life when speech-language learning is occurring at a rapid pace.

Binaural amplification should always be provided to young children unless there is a clear contraindication. Even if there is audiometric asymmetry between ears as evidenced by pure tones or speech perception, hearing aids should be fitted binaurally until it is apparent from behavioral evidence that a hearing aid fitted to the poorer ear is detrimental to performance.

In general, behind-the-ear (BTE) hearing aids are the style of choice for most children. However, for children with profound hearing loss, body aids or FM systems may be more appropriate because of acoustic feedback problems limiting sufficient gain to provide audibility of the speech signal in BTE arrangements. Other circumstances that may indicate the need for body-worn amplification include children with restricted motional capacities and those confined by a head restraint. In-the-ear (ITE) hearing aids may be considered appropriate when ear growth has stabilized—at about 8–10 years of age—as long as the flexibility and options available are not markedly restricted by concha and earcanal size.

SELECTION AND VERIFICATION OF ELECTROACOUSTIC CHARACTERISTICS

The use of a systematic approach when selecting the electroacoustic characteristics of hearing aids for children is considered of utmost importance. Sound pressure levels measured in infants' and young children's ears typically exceed adult values (Bratt, 1980; Feigin et al, 1989; Nelson Barlow et al, 1988) and external ear resonance characteristics vary as a function of age (Bentler, 1989; Kruger, 1987). In addition, children may be unable to provide subjective feedback regarding their hearing aid fittings (i.e., comfortable and uncomfortable listening levels). Therefore, probe microphone measurements of real-ear hearing aid performance should be obtained with children whenever possible (Stelmachowicz & Seewald, 1991). If probe measures are used, target values for frequency/gain and frequency/output limiting characteristics should be selected via a systematic approach that seeks to optimize the audibility of speech (e.g., Byrne & Dillon, 1986; Byrne et al, 1991; McCandless & Lyregaard, 1983; Schwartz et al, 1988; Seewald, 1992). Many of these prescriptive approaches were developed for adults and may not be appropriate for children in the process of developing speech and language without some modification. However, such approaches do provide a starting point after which modifications can be made in the verification and validation stages of the process. Some procedures for calculating target gain and output limiting characteristics for children are available in computer-assisted formats (Seewald et al, 1993) although such values can also be calculated manually (Moodie et al, 1994).

Once the preselected hearing aid frequency-gain and output characteristics have been determined theoretically, verification of the selected electroacoustic parameters should be completed. Because large variability in RECDs are expected in young children, custom earmolds should be available at the time hearing aid performance is verified. Prior to the direct evaluation of the hearing aid on the child, the hearing aid gain and maximum output characteristics should be preset in a hearing aid test box using published or preferably measured RECD values (Feigin et al, 1989; Seewald et al, 1993).

Probe microphone measurements are preferable for use in the verification stage. When probe microphone measures of real-ear hearing aid performance are not possible, however, real-ear hearing aid performance can be predicted by applying average RECD values to coupler measures. Average RECD values from adults, however, are not appropriate for use with children due to the differences in adult and children earcanal characteristics (Bentler and Pavlovic, 1989; Hawkins et al, 1990). Thus, transforms designed for use with infants and children should be used to predict hearing aid performance (Moodie et al, 1994; Seewald et al, 1994; Sinclair et al, 1994). No facility should fit hearing aids to children if it lacks the equipment for electroacoustic evaluation.

Verification of Output Limiting

The primary purposes of output limiting are to protect the child from loudness discomfort and to avoid potential damage to the ear from amplified sound. Setting the output-limiting characteristics of hearing aids for children is considered of equal, if not greater, importance as other amplification selection considerations. To this end, the audiologist must know what output levels exist in the earcanal of the child. Coupler-based SSPL targets are insufficient for use with infants and young children in particular unless RECDs are applied (Seewald, 1991; Snik and Stollman, 1995). Recommended options for determining output-limiting levels include direct measurement of the real-ear saturation response (RESR) for each ear or the use of measured or average age-related RECD values added to the tabled response. It is recommended that swept pure tones or swept warble tones should be used when measuring hearing aid output (Revit, 1991; Seewald & Hawkins, 1990; Stelmachowicz, 1991; Stelmachowicz et al, 1990).

Clearly, these approaches are predicated on the availability of frequency-specific threshold data. Thus, in cases where full audiometric information is not available, the clinician must make a "best estimate" of the residual hearing across the frequency range important for speech. The use of formulae may necessitate some extrapolation and interpolation of audiometric information from limited audiometric data, taking into account additional clinical and/or familial information that may be available. In such cases, continued observation and assessment of the child are mandatory.

Although none of the threshold-based selection procedures is guaranteed to ensure that a child will not experience loudness discomfort or that output levels are safe, the

use of a systematic objective approach that incorporates age-dependent variables into the computations is preferred. Finally, frequency-specific loudness discomfort levels should be obtained when children are old enough to provide reliable responses (Gagne et al, 1991; Kawell et al, 1988; Macpherson et al, 1991; Stuart et al, 1991).

Verification of Gain/Frequency Response

The hearing aid should be adjusted to approximate the previously determined target gain values for each ear. Aided sound field threshold measurements are not the preferred procedure for verifying the frequency-gain characteristics of hearing aids in children for several reasons: (a) prolonged cooperation from the child is required, (b) time needed for such testing can be excessive, (c) frequency resolution is poor, and (d) test-retest reliability is frequently poor (Seewald et al, 1996). In addition, misleading information may be obtained in cases of severe to profound hearing loss, minimal/mild loss, or when nonlinear signal processing is used (Macrae, 1982; Schwartz & Larson, 1977; Seewald et al, 1992; Snik et al, 1995; Stelmachowicz & Lewis, 1988).

Gain should be verified using probe microphone measures or 2-cc coupler and RECD (individually measured or age-related average) values. A 60 dB SPL input using swept pure tones or speech weighted-noise should be used with linear hearing aid systems (Stelmachowicz, 1991; Stelmachowicz et al, 1990). When using nonlinear instruments with children, audiologists should be using advanced verification technology such as the use of multiple signal levels and types to obtain a family of response characteristics (Revit, 1994).

VALIDATION OF AIDED AUDITORY FUNCTION

Once the prescriptive procedure is complete and the settings of the hearing aids have been verified, the validation process begins. Validation of aided auditory function is a critical, yet often overlooked, component of the pediatric amplification provision process. The purpose of validating aided auditory function is to demonstrate the benefits/limitations of a child's aided listening abilities for perceiving the speech of others as well as his or her own speech. Validation is accomplished, over time, using information derived through the aural habilitation process, as well as the direct measurement of the child's aided auditory performance.

With input provided by parents, teachers, and speech-language pathologists, the pediatric audiologist determines whether the ultimate goals of the hearing aid fitting process have been achieved. These goals are that the speech signal is audible, comfortable, and clear, and that the child is resistant to noise interference in the vast majority of communication environments in which formal and informal learning takes place. Measurements of aided performance quantify the child's auditory abilities at the time of the initial hearing aid fitting, and, as importantly, serve as a baseline for monitoring the child's incorporation of audible speech cues into his or her communication repertoire. Examples of measures of aided auditory performance include aided sound field responses to various stimuli, including speech measures.

Other functional performance measures include the SIFTER (Anderson, 1989), the Pre-School SIFTER (Anderson & Matkin, 1996), and the Meaningful Auditory Integration Scale (MAIS: Robbins et al, 1991). Measures of aided performance are not to be used for the purpose of changing hearing and settings unless there is an obvious behavioral indicator to the contrary. These include loudness tolerance problems or an inability to perceive particular speech cues that should be audible in the aided condition. It is recommended that performance measures be obtained in a binaural presentation mode unless one's intent is to document asymmetry in aided auditory performance.

It is stressed that the contributions provided by all members of the habilitation team promote an atmosphere of mutual cooperation and respect that ultimately results in more effective management for the child with hearing impairment (Edwards, 1996).

INFORMATION COUNSELING AND FOLLOW-UP

In order to ensure that hearing aids will be used successfully, proper counseling, monitoring, and follow-up are essential. Hearing aid orientation programs should include all family members who will be assisting the child with the hearing aid and any professionals working directly with the child and his or her family (e.g., teachers and therapists). The need for parents, teachers, and therapists to receive inservice training on the routine troubleshooting of the child's hearing instruments and the child's performance using amplification cannot be overemphasized. When appropriate, children should be assisted in understanding the details of their hearing loss; instructed in the use, care and monitoring of their personal hearing aids; and given information on communication strategies under different listening conditions (Edwards, 1996; Elfenbein, 1994; Seewald & Ross, 1988).

It is recommended that young children be seen by an audiologist every 3 months during the first 2 years of using amplification; thereafter children should be seen at least every 6 months if there are no concerns. Reasons for more aggressive monitoring include fluctuating and/or progressive hearing loss (Tharpe, 1996). The follow-up examinations should include audiometric evaluation, electroacoustic evaluation and listening checks of the hearing aid(s), and re-evaluation of the RECD and other probe-microphone measures as appropriate. In addition, the RECD should be measured whenever earmolds are replaced.

Functional measures, as discussed above, should be obtained on a periodic basis to document the development of auditory skills. These measures should include input from family, educators, and other interested professionals regarding communication and educational abilities, and social and behavioral development (Diefendorf et al, 1996). Finally, the audiologist should routinely assess the acoustic conditions in which children use amplification and offer suggestions on ways to optimize the listening environments (Crandell, 1993).

REFERENCES

American Speech-Language Hearing Association. (1991). Guidelines for the audiologic assessment of children from birth to 36 months of age. *ASHA 33* (Suppl. 5); 37–43.

Anderson, K. (1989). *Screening Instrument for Targeting Educational Risk (S.I.F.T.E.R.).* Austin, TX: Pro-ed.

Anderson, K., & Matkin, N.D. (1996). *Screening Instrument for Targeting Educational Risk in Preschool Children (Preschool S.I.F.T.E.R.).* Tampa, FL: Educational Audiology Association.

Bentler, R.A. (1989). External ear resonance characteristics in children. *Journal of Speech and Hearing Disorders* 54;264–268.

Bentler, R.A., & Pavlovic, C.V. (1989). Transfer functions and correction factors used in hearing aid evaluation and research. *Ear and Hearing,* 10;58–63.

Bess, F.H., & Paradise, J.L. (1994). Universal screening for infant hearing impairment: A reply. *Pediatrics,* 94(6);959–963.

Brackett, D. (1996). Developing auditory capabilities in children with severe and profound hearing loss. In: F.H. Bess, J.S. Gravel, & A.M. Tharpe (Eds.), *Amplification for children with auditory deficits* (pp. 369–382). Nashville, TN: Bill Wilkerson Center Press.

Bratt, G.W. (1980). *Hearing aid receiver output in occluded ear canals in children.* Unpublished doctoral dissertation. Nashville, TN: Vanderbilt University.

Byrne, D., & Dillon, H. (1986). The National Acoustic Laboratories (NAL) new procedure for selecting the gain and frequency response of a hearing aid. *Ear and Hearing,* 7;257–265.

Crandell, C.C. (1993). Speech recognition in noise by children with minimal degrees of sensorineural hearing loss. *Ear and Hearing,* 14;210–216.

Diefendorf, A.O., Reitz, P.S., Escobar, M.W., & Wynne, M.K. (1996). Initiating early amplification: Tips for success. In: F.H. Bess, J.S. Gravel, A.M. Tharpe (Eds.), *Amplification for children with auditory deficits* (pp 123–144). Nashville, TN: Bill Wilkerson Center Press.

Edwards, C. (1996). Auditory intervention for children with milder auditory deficits. In: F.H. Bess, J.S. Gravel, & A.M. Tharpe (Eds.), *Amplification for children with auditory deficits.* (pp. 383–398). Nashville, TN: Bill Wilkerson Center Press.

Feigin, J.A., Kopun, J.G., Stelmachowicz, P.G., & Gorga, M.P. (1989). Probe-tube microphone measures of earcanal sound pressure levels in infants and children. *Ear and Hearing,* 10(4);254–258.

Gagne, J.P., Seewald, R.C., Zelisko, D.L., & Hudson, S.P. (1991). Procedure for defining the auditory area of hearing-impaired adolescents with a severe/profound hearing loss II: Loudness discomfort levels. *Journal of Speech Pathology and Audiology,* 15(4);27–32.

Hawkins, D.B., Cooper, W.A., & Thompson, D.J. (1990). Comparison among SPLs in real-ears, 2 cm^3 and 6 cm^3 couplers. *Journal of the American Academy of Audiology,* 1;154–161.

Hedley-Williams, A., Tharpe, A.M., & Bess, F.H. (1996). Fitting hearing aids in children: A survey of practice procedures. In: F.H. Bess, J.S. Gravel, & A.M. Tharpe (Eds.), *Amplification for children with auditory deficits* (pp. 107–122). Nashville, TN: Bill Wilkerson Center Press.

KAWELL, M.E., KOPUN, J.G., & STELMACHOWICZ, P.G. (1988). Loudness discomfort levels in children. *Ear and Hearing, 9*(33);133–136.

KRUGER, B. (1987). An update on the external ear resonance in infants and young children. *Ear and Hearing, 8*(16);333–336.

MACPHERSON, B.J., ELFENBEIN, J.L., SCHUM, R.L., & BENTLER, R. (1991). Thresholds of discomfort in young children. *Ear and Hearing, 12*(3);184–190.

MACRAE. J. (1982). Invalid aided thresholds. *Hearing Instruments, 33*(9);20,22.

McCANDLESS, G., & LYREGAARD, P. (1983). Prescription of gain/output (POGO) for hearing aids. *Hearing Instruments, 34*;16–21.

MOODIE, K.S., SEEWALD, R.C., & SINCLAIR, S.T. (1994). Procedure for predicting real-ear hearing aid performance in young children. *American Journal of Audiology, 3*(1);23–31.

NELSON, BARLOW N.L., AUSLANDER, M.C., RINES, D., & STELMACHOWICZ, P.C. (1988). Probe-tube microphone measures in hearing-impaired children and adults. *Ear and Hearing, 9*(5);243–247.

REVIT, L.J. (1991). New test for signal processing and multi-channel hearing instruments. *Hearing Journal, 44*;20–23.

REVIT, L.J. (1994). Using coupler test in the fitting of hearing aids. In: M. Valente (Ed.), *Strategies for selecting and verifying hearing aid fittings* (pp. 64–87). New York: Thieme Medical Publishers, Inc.

ROBBINS, A.M., RENSHAW, J. & BERRY, S. (1991). Evaluating meaningful auditory integration in profoundly hearing-impaired children. *American Journal of Otology, 12*(Suppl.); 144–150.

SCHWARTZ, D.M., & LARSON, V.D. (1977). A comparison of three hearing aid evaluation procedures for young children. *Archives of Otolaryngology, 103*;401–406.

SCHWARTZ, D.M., LYREGAARD, P., & LUNDH, P. (1988). Hearing aid selection for severe-to-profound hearing loss. *Hearing Journal, 41*;13–17.

SEEWALD, R.C. (1991). Hearing instrument output limiting considerations for children. In: J.A. Feigin, & P.G. Stelmachowicz (Eds.), *Pediatric Amplification: Proceedings of the 1991 National Conference* (pp. 19–35). Omaha, NE: Boys Town National Research Hospital.

SEEWALD, R.C. (1992). The desired sensation level method for fitting children: Version 3.0. *Hearing Journal, 45*(4);36–41.

SEEWALD, R.C., HUDSON, S.P., GAGNE, J-P., & ZELISKO, D.L. (1992). Comparison of 2 procedures for estimating the sensation level of amplified speech. *Ear and Hearing, 13*(3);142–149.

SEEWALD, R.C., RAMJI, K.V., SINCLAIR, S.T., MOODIE, K.S., & JAMIESON, D.G. (1993). *DSL 3.1 user's manual.* London, Ontario: University of Western Ontario.

SEEWALD, R.C., & ROSS, M. (1988). Amplification for young hearing-impaired children. In: M.C. Pollack (Ed.), *Amplification for the hearing-impaired* (3rd Ed.) (pp. 213–27). Orlando: Grune and Stratton.

SEEWALD, R.C., SINCLAIR, S.T., & MOODIE, K.S. (1994). *Predictive accuracy of a procedure for electroacoustic fitting in young children.* American Academy of Audiology, Richmond, VA: (April, 1994).

SINCLAIR, S.T., BEAUCHAINE, K.L., MOODIE, K.S., FEIGIN, J.A., SEEWALD, R.C., & STELMACHOWICZ, P.G. (1994). *Repeatability of a real-ear to coupler difference measurement as a function of age.* American Academy of Audiology, Richmond, VA: (April 1994).

SNIK, A.F.M., & STOLLMAN M.H.P. (1995). Measured and calculated insertion gain in young children. *British Journal of Audiology, 29*;7–11.

STEIN, L.K. (1995). On the real age of identification of congenital hearing loss. *Audiology Today, 7*(1);10–11.

STELMACHOWICZ, P.G. (1991). Clinical issues related to hearing aid maximum output. In: G.A. Studebaker, F.H. Bess, & L.B. Beck (Eds.), *The Vanderbilt/VA hearing aid report* (pp. 141–148.) Parkton: York Press.

STELMACHOWICZ, P.G., & LEWIS, D.E. (1988). Some theoretical considerations concerning the relation between functional gain and insertion gain. *Journal of Speech and Hearing Research, 31*;491–496.

STELMACHOWICZ, P.G., LEWIS, D.E., SEEWALD, R.C., & HAWKINS, D.B. (1990). Complex vs. pure-tone stimuli in the evaluation of hearing aid characteristics. *Journal of Speech and Hearing Research, 33*;380–385.

STELMACHOWICZ, P.G., & SEEWALD, R.C. (1991). Probe-tube microphone measures in children. *Seminars in Hearing, 12*;62–72.

STUART, A., DURIEUX-SMITH, A., AND STENSTROM, R. (1991). Probe-tube microphone measures of loudness discomfort levels in children. *Ear and Hearing, 12*(2);140–143.

THARPE, A.M. (1996). Special considerations for children with fluctuating/progressive hearing loss. In: F.H. Bess, J.S. Gravel, A.M. Tharpe (Eds.), *Amplification for children with auditory deficits* (pp. 335–369). Nashville, TN: Bill Wilkerson Center Press.

Appendix C
Screening Instrument for Targeting Educational Risk

(Anderson, K. [1989]. *Screening Instrument for Targeting Educational Risk [S.I.F.T.E.R.].* Austin, TX: Pro-Ed. Used with permission.)

S.I.F.T.E.R.

SCREENING INSTRUMENT FOR TARGETING EDUCATIONAL RISK

by Karen L. Anderson, Ed.S., CCC-A

STUDENT _____ TEACHER _____ GRADE _____

DATE COMPLETED _____ SCHOOL _____ DISTRICT _____

The above child is suspect for hearing problems which may or may not be affecting his/her school performance. This rating scale has been designed to sift out students who are educationally at risk possibly as a result of hearing problems.

Based on your knowledge from observations of this student, circle the number best representing his/her behavior. After answering the questions, please record any comments about the student in the space provided on the reverse side.

1.	What is your estimate of the student's class standing in comparison of that of his/her classmates?	UPPER 5	4	MIDDLE 3	2	LOWER 1	ACADEMICS	☐
2.	How does the student's achievement compare to your estimation of her/her potential?	EQUAL 5	4	LOWER 3	2	MUCH LOWER 1		
3.	What is the student's reading level, reading ability group or reading readiness group in the classroom (e.g., a student with average reading ability performs in the middle group)?	UPPER 5	4	MIDDLE 3	2	LOWER 1		
4.	How distractible is the student in comparison to his/her classmates?	NOT VERY 5	4	AVERAGE 3	2	VERY 1	ATTENTION	☐
5.	What is the student's attention span in comparison to that of his/her classmates?	LONGER 5	4	AVERAGE 3	2	SHORTER 1		
6.	How often does the student hesitate or become confused when responding to oral directions (e.g., "Turn to page . . .")?	NEVER 5	4	OCCASIONALLY 3	2	FREQUENTLY 1		
7.	How does the student's comprehension compare to the average understanding ability of her/her classmates?	ABOVE 5	4	AVERAGE 3	2	BELOW 1	COMMUNICATION	☐
8.	How does the student's vocabulary and word usage skills compare with those of other students in his/her age group?	ABOVE 5	4	AVERAGE 3	2	BELOW 1		
9.	How proficient is the student at telling a story or relating happenings from home when compared to classmates?	ABOVE 5	4	AVERAGE 3	2	BELOW 1		
10.	How often does the student volunteer information to class discussions or in answer to teacher questions?	FREQUENTLY 5	4	OCCASIONALLY 3	2	NEVER 1	CLASS PARTICIPATION	☐
11.	With what frequency does the student complete his/her class and homework assignments within the time allocated?	ALWAYS 5	4	USUALLY 3	2	SELDOM 1		
12.	After instruction, does the student have difficulty starting to work (looks at other students working or asks for help)?	NEVER 5	4	OCCASIONALLY 3	2	FREQUENTLY 1		
13.	Does the student demonstrate any behaviors that seem unusual or inappropriate when compared to other students?	NEVER 5	4	OCCASIONALLY 3	2	FREQUENTLY 1	SCHOOL BEHAVIOR	☐
14.	Does the student become frustrated easily, sometimes to the point of losing emotional control?	NEVER 5	4	OCCASIONALLY 3	2	FREQUENTLY 1		
15.	In general, how would you rank the student's relationship with peers (ability to get along with others)?	GOOD 5	4	AVERAGE 3	2	POOR 1		

Additional copies of this form are available in pads of 100 each from
The Educational Audiology Association
4319 Ehrlich Road, Tampa, FL 33624
ISBN 0-8134-2845-9

TEACHER COMMENTS

Has this child repeated a grade, had frequent absences or experienced health problems (including ear infections and colds)? Has the student received, or is he/she now receiving, special support services? Does the child have any other health problems that may be pertinent to his/her educational functioning?

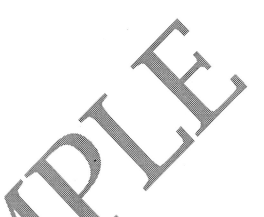

The S.I.F.T.E.R. is a SCREENING TOOL ONLY

Any student failing this screening in a content area as determined on the scoring grid below should be considered for further assessment, depending on his/her individual needs as per school district criteria. For example, failing in the Academics area suggests an educational assessment, in the Communication area a speech-language assessment, and in the School Behavior area an assessment by a psychologist or a social worker. Failing in the Attention and/or Class Participation area in combination with other areas may suggest an evaluation by an educational audiologist. Children placed in the marginal area are at risk for failing and should be monitored or considered for assessment depending upon additional information.

SCORING

Sum the responses to the three questions in each content area and record in the appropriate box on the reverse side and under Total Score below. Place an **X** on the number that corresponds most closely with the content area score (e.g., if a teacher circled 3, 4 and 2 for the questions in the Academics area, an **X** would be placed on the number 9 across from the Academics content area). Connect the **X**'s to make a profile.

CONTENT AREA	TOTAL SCORE	PASS						MARGINAL		FAIL				
ACADEMICS		15	14	13	12	11	10	9	8	7	6	5	4	3
ATTENTION		15	14	13	12	11	10	9	8	7	6	5	4	3
COMMUNICATION		15	14	13		12	11	10	9	8	7	6	5	4	3
CLASS PARTICIPATION		15	14	13	12	11	10	9	8	7	6	5	4	3
SOCIAL BEHAVIOR		15	14	13	12	11	10	9	8	7	6	5	4	3

Appendix D
Pre-School Screening Instrument for Targeting Educational Risk

(ANDERSON, K., & MATKIN, N. [1996]. *Screening Instrument for Targeting Educational Risk in Preschool Children [Preschool S.I.F.T.E.R.].* Tampa, FL: Educational Audiology Association. Used with permission.)

PRESCHOOL S.I.F.T.E.R.

Screening Instrument for Targeting Educational Risk
in Preschool Children (age 3-Kindergarten)

by Karen L. Anderson, Ed.S. & Noel Matkin, Ph.D.

Child _____ Teacher _____ Age _____

Date Completed ____/____/____ School _____ District _____

The above child is suspect for hearing problems which may affect his/her ability to listen, pay attention, develop language, follow teacher instruction and learn normally. This rating scale has been designed to sift out children who are at risk for educational delay and who may need further evaluation. Based on your knowledge of this child, circle the number that best represents his/her behavior. If the child is a member of a class that has students with special needs, comparisons should be made to normal learning classmates or normal developmental milestones. Please share additional comments about the child on the reverse side of this form.

			PRE-ACADEMICS
1. How well does the child understand basic concepts when compared to classmates (e.g., colors, shapes, etc.)?	ABOVE AVERAGE BELOW 5 4 3 2 1		
2. How often is the child able to follow two-part directions?	ALWAYS FREQUENTLY SELDOM 5 4 3 2 1		
3. How well does the child participate in group activities when compared to classmates (e.g., calendar, sharing)?	ABOVE AVERAGE BELOW 5 4 3 2 1		

			ATTENTION
4. How distractible is the child in comparison to his/her classmates during large group activities?	SELDOM OCCASIONAL FREQUENT 5 4 3 2 1		
5. What is the child's attention span in comparison to classmates?	LONGER AVERAGE SHORTER 5 4 3 2 1		
6. How well does the child pay attention during a small group activity or time?	ABOVE AVERAGE BELOW 5 4 3 2 1		

			COMMUNICATION
7. How does the child's vocabulary and word usage skills compare to classmates?	ABOVE AVERAGE BELOW 5 4 3 2 1		
8. How proficient is the child at relating an event when compared to classmates?	ABOVE AVERAGE BELOW 5 4 3 2 1		
9. How does the child's overall speech intelligibility compare to classmates (i.e., production of speech sounds)?	ABOVE AVERAGE BELOW 5 4 3 2 1		

			CLASS PARTICIPATION
10. How often does the child answer questions appropriately (verbal or signed)?	ALMOST ALWAYS FREQUENTLY SELDOM 5 4 3 2 1		
11. How often does the child recall information during group discussions?	ALMOST ALWAYS FREQUENTLY SELDOM 5 4 3 2 1		
12. How often does the child participate with classmates in group activities or group play?	ALMOST ALWAYS FREQUENTLY SELDOM 5 4 3 2 1		

			SOCIAL BEHAVIOR
13. Does the child play in socially acceptable ways (i.e., turn taking, sharing)?	ALMOST ALWAYS FREQUENTLY SELDOM 5 4 3 2 1		
14. How proficient is the child at using verbal language or sign language to communicate effectively with classmates (e.g., asking to play with another child's toy)?	ABOVE AVERAGE BELOW 5 4 3 2 1		
15. How often does the child become frustrated, sometimes to the point of losing emotional control?	NEVER SELDOM FREQUENTLY 5 4 3 2 1		

Additional Copies of this form are available in pads of 100 each from
The Educational Audiology Association 1-800-460-7322
4319 Ehrlich Road, Tampa, FL 33624

TEACHER COMMENTS: (frequent absences, health problems, other problems or handicaps in addition to hearing?)

The Preschool S.I.F.T.E.R. is a SCREENING TOOL ONLY. The primary goal of the Preschool S.I.F.T.E.R. is to identify those children who are at-risk for developmental or educational problems due to hearing problems and who merit further observation and investigation. Analysis has revealed that two factors, expressive communication and socially appropriate behavior, discriminate children who are normal from those who are at-risk. The greater the degree of hearing problem, the greater the impact on these two factors and the higher the validity of this screening measure. If a child is found to be at-risk then the examiner is encouraged to calculate the total score in each of the five content areas. Analysis of the content area score may assist in developing a profile of the child's strengths and special needs. The profile may prove beneficial in determining appropriate areas for evaluation and developing an individual program for the child.

SCORING

There are two steps to the scoring process. First, enter scores for each of the indicated questions in the spaces provided and sum the total of the 6 questions for the expressive communication factor and then the 4 questions for the socially appropriate behavior factor. If the child's scores fall into the At-Risk category for either or both of these factors, then sum the 3 questions in each content area to develop a profile of the child's strengths and potential areas of need.

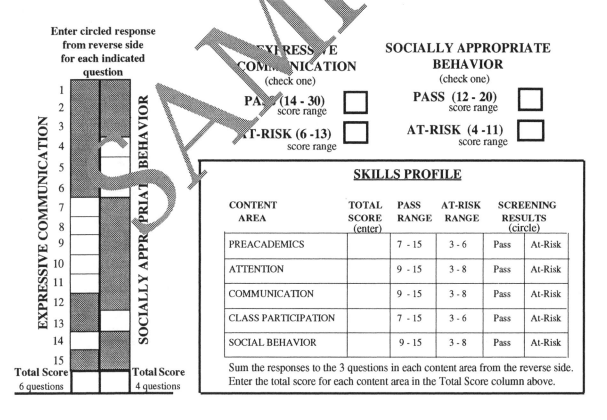

Sum the responses to the 3 questions in each content area from the reverse side.
Enter the total score for each content area in the Total Score column above.

Appendix E
Learning Inventory for Education

(ANDERSON, K., & SMALDINO, J. [1997]. *Learning Inventory for Education [L.I.F.E.]*. Tampa, FL: Educational Audiology Association. Used with permission.)

L.I.F.E.
Listening Inventory For Education
Teacher Appraisal of Listening Difficulty
An Efficacy Tool by Karen L. Anderson, Ed.S. & Joseph J. Smaldino, Ph.D.

Name _____ Grade _____ Date _____
(Complete only for trial periods with individuals)

School _____ Teacher _____

Whole Classroom Sound Field Amplfication Trial Period **Y / N**   Class Trial Period Length___Weeks

Individual Amplification Trial Period **Y / N**   Hearing Aid User **Y / N**   Trial Period Length___Weeks

Type of Hearing Technology Used With Individual: _____

Instructions: Circle the number which best describes student listening and learning behaviors. See reverse for suggestions to aid students in listening and understanding classroom instruction.

The student's:

	AGREE	NO CHANGE	Not Observed	DISAGREE	
1. Focus on instruction has improved (more tuned in to instruction).	(2)	(1)	(0)	(-1)	(-2)
2. Appears to understand class instruction better.	(2)	(1)	(0)	(-1)	(-2)
3. Overall attention span has improved (less fidgety and/or less distracted).	(2)	(1)	(0)	(-1)	(-2)
4. Attention has improved when listening to directions presented to whole class.	(2)	(1)	(0)	(-1)	(-2)
5. Stays on task longer with less need for redirection.	(2)	(1)	(0)	(-1)	(-2)
6. Follows directions more quickly or easily (less hesitation before beginning work).	(2)	(1)	(0)	(-1)	(-2)
7. Answers questions in a more appropriate way or answers appropriately more often.	(2)	(1)	(0)	(-1)	(-2)
8. Improved understanding of instructional videos and/or morning announcements.	(2)	(1)	(0)	(-1)	(-2)
9. More involved in class discussions (volunteer more, follow better).	(2)	(1)	(0)	(-1)	(-2)
10. Improved understanding of answers or comments by peers during discussions.	(2)	(1)	(0)	(-1)	(-2)
11. Improved attention and understanding when noise is present (ventilator fan, transitions).	(2)	(1)	(0)	(-1)	(-2)
12. Improved ability to discriminate similar words or sounds (hat vs back, page 11 vs page 7).	(2)	(1)	(0)	(-1)	(-2)
13. Attention improved when listening in groups (small group/cooperative learning activities).	(2)	(1)	(0)	(-1)	(-2)
14. Socially more confident with other children or more comfortable in peer conversations.	(2)	(1)	(0)	(-1)	(-2)
15. Rate of learning <u>seems</u> to have improved (quicker to comprehend instruction).	(2)	(1)	(0)	(-1)	(-2)
16. Based on my knowledge and observations I believe that the amplification system is beneficial to the student's overall attention, listening and learning in the classroom.	(5)	(2)	(0)	(-2)	(-5)

Comments: (e.g., absences, equipment use problems)

Total Appraisal Score _____

APPRAISAL SUMMARY (circle one)

Highly Successful   26 - 35

Successful   16 - 25

Minimally Successful   5 - 15

Distributed by the Educational Audiology Association
4319 Ehrlich Rd, Tampa FL 33624 1-800-460-7322

LISTENING INVENTORY FOR EDUCATION
SUGGESTIONS FOR ACCOMMODATING STUDENTS WITH AUDITORY DIFFICULTIES

Students with auditory problems face extra challenges learning in a typical classroom setting. Typically, they can hear the teacher talk, but miss parts of speech or do not hear clearly, especially if noise is present. Students usually do not know what they didn't hear because they didn't hear it. They often may not know that they "misheard" a message unless they have already had experience with the language and topic under discussion. Use of amplification, having fluctuating hearing ability, hearing loss in just one ear, permanent hearing loss of any degree or central auditory processing disorders all compromise a student's ability to focus on verbal instruction and comprehend the fragments of speech information that are heard. The following items are suggestions for accomodating these student's special auditory needs and helping them learn their best in your classroom.

1. Seat the student close to where you customarily teach.
Sound weakens as it crosses distance. If a student has any auditory difficulties, how close you are to him/her will make a big difference on how well the student can hear and understand you.
  - Can the student be moved to the front of the room?
  - Can the student be allowed flexible seating so they can move to a better vantage point as classroom activities change? (e.g. move close to TV during movies)
  - If your teaching style causes you to move around the room when you talk, is it possible to stay in close proximity to the student with auditory problems?
  - When giving test directions, can you see the student's face clearly? Are you standing near the student's desk? Is the lighting on your face and not from a window behind you? Be sure the student is watching you.
  - Develop a signal the student can use if he or she does not understand or has missed critical information.

2. Be aware of the benefits and limitations of lipreading.
  - Only about 30-40% of speech sounds are visible on the lips. Lipreading supplements a student's hearing but is most helpful when the topic of conversation and vocabulary are known. New concepts and new vocabulary words have little meaning using lipreading.
  - Is the student seated so they can see your face clearly? Too close and they view your face from a skewed angle, too far and the quick, tiny mouth movements are imperceptible.
  - Lipreading is only possible if you are facing the student. If you use the chalkboard, do not provide verbal instruction while writing or be prepared to summarize or repeat that information for the student.
  - Reading aloud to the class with your face downward makes lipreading very difficult. Hold the book below your chin so your face is easily visualized.
  - Students cannot lipread and take notes at the same time. Classroom notetakers can use carbonized (NCR) paper and share notes easily. The student can use these notes from other students to fill in gaps in understanding.
  - The extra demands of trying to understand using only speech fragments and of constantly trying to lipread can be very fatiguing. Listening breaks are natural, especially after rapid class discussions, lectures or new information.

3. Noise is a barrier to learning.
  - Adults and children with normal hearing usually can tolerate a small amount of background noise without having their speech understanding compromised. Students with auditory problems are already missing fragments of what is said, especially if a message is spoken farther than from 3-6 feet away. Noise covers up word endings and brief words, reverberation smears the word fragments that are perceived.
  - Can the student be allowed flexible seating so they can move away from noise sources? (e.g. lawn mower)
  - Overhead projectors allow the student to clearly view the teacher's face, however, their fan noise interferes with understanding. If the student has a poorer hearing ear, face that one toward the overhead projector (or noisy ventilator, etc.) and seat close, but not next to the projector.
  - If possible, eliminate or dampen unnecessary noise sources. Sometimes apsorbtive material, such as styrofoam or a thick bathtowel placed under an aquarium heater or animal cage will absorb some noise. Seat the student away from animal distractions.
  - Keep your classroom door closed, especially when classes pass in the hall, gym or lunchroom activities are audible.
  - One of the main causes of noise in the classroom is due to the activity of students. Seat away from peers who are very active or habitually noisy. Allow student's time to search their desks so that the noise generated will not occur during verbal instruction. Inform the custodian of especially squeaky desks.

4. Control or allow for distance.
  - During group discussion, students with auditory problems typically can understand the students seated next to them but cannot understand students who are answering from more distant seats.
  - Use a student's name when calling on them to answer a question. This will allow the student with hearing needs a chance to turn to face the answering student and to lipread if at all possible.
  - Summarize key points given by classmates, especially brief messages like numeric answers, yes/no, etc.
  - Allow or assign a student buddy that the student with auditory problems can ask for clarification or cueing.

L.I.F.E.

Listening Inventory For Education
An Efficacy Tool
Student Appraisal of Listening Difficulty

By Karen L. Anderson, Ed.S. & Joseph J. Smaldino, Ph.D.

Name _____ Grade _____ Date _____

School _____ Teacher _____

Hearing Aid User Y / N   Trial Period   Type of Classroom

Trial Period Y / N   Length____Weeks   Hearing Technology_____

Instructions: Circle the item which best describes the student's difficulty listening in the situations shown on picture card items 1-10. Optional items 11-16 can be scored if these situations are encountered in the listening environment. See reverse for intervention suggestions to improve listening and understanding.

Classroom Listening Situations	ALWAYS		SOMETIMES		NEVER
1. Teacher talking in front of room Comments:	(10)	(7)	(5)	(2)	(0)
2. Teacher talking during transition time Comments:	(10)	(7)	(5)	(2)	(0)
3. Teacher talking with back turned Comments:	(10)	(7)	(5)	(2)	(0)
4. Listening with hallway noise present Comments:	(10)	(7)	(5)	(2)	(0)
5. Other students making noise Comments:	(10)	(7)	(5)	(2)	(0)
6. Student answering during discussion Comments:	(10)	(7)	(5)	(2)	(0)
7. Listening with overhead projector fan on Comments:	(10)	(7)	(5)	(2)	(0)
8. Teacher talking while moving Comments:	(10)	(7)	(5)	(2)	(0)
9. Word recognition during a test or directions Comments:	(10)	(77)	(5)	(2)	(0)
10. Watching a video movie in classroom Comments:	(10)	(7)	(5)	(2)	(0)

Additional Listening Situations					
11. Cooperative small group learning	(20)	(15)	(10)	(5)	(0)
12. Listening in gym (inside & outside)	(20)	(15)	(10)	(5)	(0)
13. Listening in school assembly	(20)	(15)	(10)	(5)	(0)
14. Listening to students during lunch	(20)	(15)	(10)	(5)	(0)
15. Students talking while coats are hung up	(20)	(15)	(10)	(5)	(0)

Scoring

		PRE-TEST		POST-TEST
Sum of Items 1 - 10	(100 possible)			
Sum of Items 11-16	(100 possible)	_____	CLASSROOM LISTENING SCORE	_____
Total Score of Items	(200 possible)	_____	ADDITIONAL SITUATIONS SCORE	_____

The LIFE Student Appraisal was inspired by the Hearing Performance Inventory for Children. The authors recognize T. Giolas, A. Brancia Maxon & A. Riordan Kessler for their work in developing the HPIC.

LISTENING INVENTORY FOR EDUCATION
SUGGESTIONS FOR IMPROVING CLASSROOM LISTENING

Mark an X next to each statement that corresponds with the situations indicated on the reverse side in which the student is experiencing any difficulty.

Classroom Difficult Listening Situations

_X_ 1.   Let the teacher know that you cannot understand. Develop a signal system with your teacher.

_X_ 1.   Be sure that you are seated near the teacher. Ask to move if needed.

_____ 2.   Ask a student buddy to explain the directions ("Did she say page 191?).

_____ 2.   Before the teacher hands out a test to the class, ask what kind of test it is and how you take it (fill in all blanks, true/false, multiple choice).

_____ 3.   Have another student or two in your class that will share their class notes with you, the teacher can help to arrange this and provide carbonized paper. It is still your job to listen very carefully as your teacher talks. Notes can help you fill in gaps you may have missed as you study later.

_____ 3.   Be sure that the teacher is aware of how important it is for you to see his/her face. Ask your parent to send a note to the teacher. Ask for the teacher to repeat information, ask a neighbor, use your signal.

_____ 4.   If there is noise in the hall, ask for door to be closed. Arrange with your teacher ahead of time to have permission to get up and close the door whenever it's noisy.

_____ 5.   Let your teacher know that noise from classmates is interfering with your understanding; use your signal system to alert your teacher that it's too noisy.

_____ 6.   Ask your teacher to say student's names when calling on them to answer questions. Watch her face and listen carefully for names so you can quickly turn to face the talking student.

_____ 6.   If you miss information from student answers or discussion: 1) ask answering student to repeat the information, 2) ask the teacher to repeat, 3) ask a neighbor

_____ 7.   If you did not hear all of the announcements, ask the teacher or a neighbor what they were about.

_____ 8.   If you cannot understand what the teacher is saying as he or she talks when the class is getting out books or papers it is important to be sure you are ready and watching the teacher during these times. If you miss a page number or other information be sure to raise your hand and ask - you are probably not the only one who didn't hear the teacher clearly in all the noise of changing activities.

_____ 9.   Spelling tests are easiest if you really know the word list and can tell the difference between similar words (e.g., champion and trampoline have similar sounds but have different endings). Sit close and watch the teacher's face carefully. If you are not sure you clearly heard a word, let the teacher know immediately (you could use your signal).

_____ 10.   Hearing speech clearly in a movie can be hard because of the background music on some videos. Sit close to the TV even if it means sitting in a different seat. If used, ask the teacher to put the FM microphone next to the TV. Have a note taker. Request closed captioned videos be used.

Additional Difficult Listening Situations

_____ 11.   In small group work, be sure to sit close to other students and try to be able to see all of their faces. If used, pass the FM microphone from student to student. Ask students to repeat what you missed. It helps if your group could meet in a quieter spot of the class or in the hall while you work.

_____ 12.   While in the gym, stand close to the teacher for directions and ask other children for directions you may have missed. Ask the teacher to repeat what you missed. Use a signal system to let your teacher know you didn't understand.

_____ 13.   To hear in an assembly it is important to be near the front. If you have a personal FM the person speaking should wear the transmitter.

_____ 14.   Ask your friends to repeat or clarify when something is missed (Did you say tomorrow night?"). Sit where you can easily see their faces and try to sit away from noisier children or noisy areas of your classroom. Remind your friends they may need to tap you to get your attention when it's really noisy and if you are not watching their faces.

_____ 15.   You need to depend on your friends to catch your eye, tap you or for them to wait until they see you looking at them before they talk to you. Ask them to repeat what you have missed (Practice is at what time? You called Suzy when?).

Appendix F
Children's Abbreviated Profile of Hearing Aid Performance (CA-APHAP)

(KOPUN, J.G. & STELMACHOWICZ, P.G. [1998]. Used with permission.)

CHILDREN'S ABBREVIATED PROFILE OF HEARING AID PERFORMANCE (CA-PHAP)

CHILD'S NAME: _____ CHILD'S DATE OF BIRTH: ___/___/___
            Last   First

PARENT NAME: _____ TODAY'S DATE: ___/___/___
            Last   First

TELEPHONE: (home)_____(work)_____

INTERVIEWER_____

INSTRUCTIONS: Please circle the answers that come closest to your everyday experience. Notice that each choice includes a percentage. You can use this to help you decide on your answer. For example, if a statement is true about 75% of the time, circle "C" for that item. If you have not experienced the situation we describe, try to think of a similar situation that you have been in and respond for that situation. If you have no idea, leave that item blank.

A Always (99%)
B Almost Always (87%)
C Most of the time (75%)
D Half-the-time (50%)
E Once in a while (25%)
F Hardly ever(12%)
G Never (1%)

	With Hearing Aid(s)	**Without Hearing Aid(s)**
1. When I am paying for something in a crowded store, I can understand what the cashier is saying	A B C D E F G	A B C D E F G
2. I miss a lot of what the teacher says in my classroom	A B C D E F G	A B C D E F G
3. Sounds that I am not expecting, like smoke detectors or alarms, are uncomfortable	A B C D E F G	A B C D E F G
4. When I am at home with someone from my family, I have difficulty understanding what they are saying	A B C D E F G	A B C D E F G
5. I have trouble understanding what the actors are saying in a movie or play	A B C D E F G	A B C D E F G
6. When I am watching TV and other people are talking, it is hard to hear the person on the TV	A B C D E F G	A B C D E F G
7. I have trouble understanding what one person is saying when I eat dinner with a group of people	A B C D E F G	A B C D E F G
8. Traffic noises are too loud	A B C D E F G	A B C D E F G
9. I understand the words when I am talking with someone across a large, empty room	A B C D E F G	A B C D E F G

NOTE: This questionnaire was adapted from the Abbreviated Profile of Hearing Aid Performance*. It is part of a research project and has not yet been validated.

* Cox and Alexander (1995). The abbreviated profile of hearing aid benefit. *Ear and Hearing, 16*, 176-186.

	With Hearing Aid(s)	Without Hearing Aid(s)

10. When I am asking and answering questions in a small room, it is hard to understand what the other person is saying......A B C D E F G   A B C D E F G

11. Sometimes I go to the theater to watch a movie. I can understand what the movie actors are saying, even when people around me are whispering and rattling papers.........A B C D E F G   A B C D E F G

12. When I talk with a friend in a quiet room, it is hard to understand what he says..A B C D E F G   A B C D E F G

13. The sounds of running water, like a toilet or shower, are too loud..A B C D E F G   A B C D E F G

14. When I am listening to someone talk to a small group of people and everyone is quiet, it is hard to hear the person talking...A B C D E F G   A B C D E F G

15. When I am in a doctor's office, I have trouble understanding what he is saying..A B C D E F G   A B C D E F G

16. I can understand what someone is saying, even when several people are talking....................................A B C D E F G   A B C D E F G

17. The sounds of construction work are too loud.......................A B C D E F G   A B C D E F G

18. When I am in an auditorium or in church, it is hard to understand what the speaker is saying.............................A B C D E F G   A B C D E F G

19. I can understand other people when I am in a crowd.............A B C D E F G   A B C D E F G

20. The sound of a fire engine siren close by is so loud that I want to turn my hearing aid down or off or cover my ears.A B C D E F G   A B C D E F G

21. I can understand the words of the speaker when I'm at church...A B C D E F G   A B C D E F G

22. The sound of squealing tires is too loud................................A B C D E F G   A B C D E F G

23. When I am talking to someone in a quiet room, I have to ask him to repeat what he said...A B C D E F G   A B C D E F G

24. I have trouble understanding others when an air conditioner or fan is on..A B C D E F G   A B C D E F G

Do you use a caption decoder when watching TV?   Yes   No

Age 1st Aided _____

Hearing Aid Fitting:

Monaural_____   Binaural_____

Degree of Hearing Loss:

Right_____ Left_____

A Always (99%)
B Almost Always (87%)
C Most of the time (75%)
D Half-the-time (50%)
E Once in a while (25%l
F Hardly ever (12%)
G Never (1%)

Appendix G
Client Oriented Scale of Improvement

(DILLON, H., JAMES, A., & GINIS, J. [1997]. Used with permission.)

COSI™

The NAL Client Oriented Scale of Improvement

Name: _____

Client Number: _____

oticon

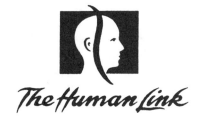

COSI

The NAL Client Oriented Scale of Improvement

Name: _____

Audiologist: _____

Date: 1. Needs established _____

      2. Outcome assessed _____

SPECIFIC NEEDS

Indicate Order of Significance

Degree of Change
"Because of the new hearing instrument, I now hear . . ."

	Worse	No Difference	Slightly Better	Better	Much Better

Final Ability (with hearing instrument)
"I can hear satisfactorily . . . "

	Hardly Ever 10%	Occasionally 25%	Half the Time 50%	Most of Time 75%	Almost Always 95%

The Human link

901 76 311 07/ 01.96

oticon

194

Appendix H
Developmental Index of Audition and Listening

(PALMER, C., & MORMER, E. [1997]. The goals of the hearing aid fitting: Child, parents, and educators. *Remediating pediatric hearing loss through amplification: Taking science into the clinic.* San Antonio, TX: University of Pittsburgh and Oticon, February, 1998. Used with permission.)

Developmental Index of Audition and Listening
(DIAL)

Age Group	Specific Age	Milestone
Infant		
	0-28 days	Startle response; attends to music and voice, soothed by parent's voice; some will synchronize body movements to speech pattern; enjoys time in "en face" position; hears caregiver before being picked up
	1-4 months	Looks for sound source; associates sound with movement; enjoys parent's voice; attends to noise makers; imitates vowel sounds
	4-8 months	Uses toys/objects to make sounds; recognizes words; responds to verbal commands -bye bye; learning to recognize name; plays with noise makers; enjoys music; enjoys rhythm games
	8-12 months	Attends to TV; localizes to sounds/voices; enjoys rhymes and songs; understands NO; enjoys hiding game; responds to vocal games (e.g., So Big!!)
Toddler		
	1 year	Dances to music; sees parent answer telephone/doorbell; answers to name call; attends to books
	2 years	Listens on telephone; dances to music; listens to story in group; goes with parent to answer door; awakens to smoke detector; attends to travel activities and communication
Preschool		
	3 years	Talks and listens on telephone; sings with music; listens to books on tape; smoke detector means danger; enjoys taped books; attends to verbal warnings for safety
	4 years	Telephone play; attends movie theatre; dance/swim lessons; watches TV/videos with family neighborhood play
	5 years	Music lessons; attends to children's service in church; learns to ride bike; plays at playground at a distance from parent
Early School Age		
	6-8 years	Uses telephone meaningfully; enjoys walkman/headphones; uses alarm clock independently; responds to smoke detector independently
Late Elementary		
	8-10 years	Uses television for entertainment & socializing; attends to radio; responds to sirens for street safety; participates in clubs and athletics; enjoys privacy in own room; enjoys computer/audio games; plays team sports
Middle School		
	10-14 years	Uses telephone as social vehicle; attends movies/plays; develops musical tastes; watches movies/TV with friends
Older Adolescent		
	14-18 years	Goes to dances; begins driving (e.g., needs to hear sirens/turn signal); participates in school groups/clubs; employment/ ADA
	18-22 years	Employment/career decisions; travels independently; listens in college lecture halls/classrooms; participates in study groups/extra curricular activities

Appendix I
Pediatric Hearing Demand, Ability, and Need Profile

(PALMER, C., & MORMER, E. [1997]. A systematic program for hearing aid orientation and adjustment. *The Hearing Review, High Performance Hearing Solutions Supplement, 19*;201–210. Used with permission.)

HEARING DEMAND, ABILITY, AND NEED PROFILE

(adapted from Healey, J. (1992) and Palmer, C.(1992))

Name: _____

Age	Description of Communication Milestone/Activity	Communication Problem is Present…. With Hearing Aid: HOME on / off	WORK on / off	TRAVEL	The Problem is Due to…. Hearing	Noise	Distance	Visibility	Current Compensation (describe)
	ALERTING								
	telephone bell								
	doorbell								
	door knock								
	alarm clock								
	smoke alarm								
	siren								
	turn signal								
	personal pager								
	PERSONAL COMMUNICATION								
	telephone								
	tv/stereo/radio								
	one-to-one(planned)								
	one-to-one(unplanned)								
	group								
	large room								
	OTHER ACTIVITIES								
	clubs/games:								
	lessons:								
	sports:								

Further information (e.g., status of hearing aids, telecoil, DAI,communication environment):

Recommendations (Assistive Technology, Communication Strategies, Environmental Manipulation):

Appendix J
Family Expectation Worksheet

(PALMER, C., & MORMER, E. [1997]. A systematic program for hearing aid orientation and adjustment. *The Hearing Review, High Performance Hearing Solutions Supplement, 19*;201–210. Used with permission.)

Family Expectation Worksheet

Child is successful in this situation...

Goal (list in order of priority)	Hardly Ever	Occasionally	Half the Time	Most of the Time	Almost Always
1.					
2.					
3.					
4.					
5.					

C = how the child functions currently (pre-treatment or with current technology/strategies)

E = how the child/family expects to function post intervention(HA, ALD, strategies, etc.)

✓ = level of success that the audiologist realistically targets

I = how the child/family actually perceives level of success post intervention

Appendix K
Partial List of Manufacturers Having Special Programs for Children

Miracle Ear
Miracle Ear Children's Foundation
Phone: 800-255-5049
Web site:
http://www.miracle_ear.com/kid.htm

Phonak
Phonak Pediatric Program
Phone: 800-777-7333
E-mail: email@phonak.com

Oticon
Otikids
Phone: 800-526-3921
Web site:
http://www.oticonus.com/ot4kidssu.htm

Unitron
Unitron Kids Club
Phone: 800-521-5400
Web site:
http://www.sentex.net/
-unitron/pages/cikk.htm#.cikk

Appendix L
Relationship of Hearing Loss to Development and Educational Needs

(ANDERSON, K., & MATKIN, N. [1998]. *Relationship of hearing loss to developmental and educational needs.* Tampa, FL: Educational Audiology Association.)

RELATIONSHIP OF HEARING LOSS TO DEVELOPMENT AND EDUCATIONAL NEEDS

A Counseling Tool for Audiologists & Information for Parents and Schools

by Karen L. Anderson, Ed.S. & Noel D. Matkin, Ph.D

What does the audiogram really mean? Why does my child need to wear hearing aids; he seems to be able to hear me fine at home? Will she need to have special help to learn in school? The school said he was having trouble, could it be because of his hearing loss? Can she hear the teacher okay with her hearing aids?

Families have many questions about how a child's hearing loss will effect their development and learning. The Relationship of Hearing Loss to Development and Educational Needs information pads were developed to aid audiologists as they counsel and work with families after identifying a child with a hearing loss. This information is general and needs to be tailored by the audiologist to the individual characteristics of each child and family and their specific needs and abilities. Explanations are brief and the language level of this information will be too difficult for some parents to fully comprehend and will need further indepth description by the audiologist. This information was also intended to be beneficial to school districts as they plan for the educational needs of the student. A child without effective access to teacher instruction will not receive an appropriate education. A counseling sheet stapled to the audiogram and provided to school districts can encourage communication between the audiologist and school to work together to meet the child's listening and learning needs. Parents can also utilize this information to raise questions about their child's school performance and advocate for appropriate accommodations and programming.

These counseling pads were developed from a handout produced in 1991, called the Relationship of Degree of Longterm Hearing Loss to Psychosocial Impact and Educational Needs. This handout was produced with valuable input from members of the Educational Audiology Association in 1991 and was widely distributed, reprinted and has been in popular use by many clinical and educational audiologists. The enclosed counseling pads were developed out of the desire to provide audiologists with a practical, easy to use format for providing critical development and educational information to families. Information from 1991 was updated and expanded as appropriate to the changes in technology and increased knowledge available from the expansions in educational audiology research which occurred during the 1990's. This information was reviewed and input provided by numerous involved practitioners in the field. We are especially grateful for the input and expertise provided by: Cheryl DeConde Johnson, Casey Morehouse, Barbara Murphy and Michael Pelc.

References: Olsen, W. O., Hawkins, D. B., VanTasseli, D. J. (1987). Representatives of the longterm spectrum of speech. *Ear and Hearing*. Supplement 8, pp. 100-108. Mueller, H. G. & Killion, M. C. (1990). An easy method for calculating the articulation index. *The Hearing Journal*. 43, 9, pp. 14-22. Haenstab, M. S. (1987). *Language Learning and Otitis Media*, College Hill Press, Boston, MA. Bernero, R. J. & Bothwell, H. (1966). Relationship of hearing impairment to educational needs. Illinois Dept. of Public Health & Office of Superintendent of Public Instruction. Crandell, C. C., Smaldino, J. J., Flexer, C. (1995) *Sound-Field FM Amplification: theory and practical applications*. Singular Press, San Diego, CA. Johnson, C. D., Benson, P. V., Seaton, J. B. (1997). *Educational Audiology Handbook*, Singular Press, San Diego, CA.

Reorder Information:

Refills of the counseling pads can be obtained by contacting the Educational Audiology Association at 1-800-460-7322. The 1998 price for refills for each of the 10 pads is $2.50 per pad plus shipping and handling.

CHILD'S NAME
DATE: _____ Average Hearing Loss: R___ L___

MINIMAL HEARING LOSS (16-25 dB)

Possible Effect of Hearing Loss on the Understanding of Language and Speech

Impact of a hearing loss that is approximately 20 dB can be compared to ability to hear when index fingers are placed in your ears. Child may have difficulty hearing faint or distant speech. At 16 dB student can miss up to 10% of speech signal when teacher is at a distance greater than 3 feet. A 20 dB or greater hearing loss in the better ear can result in absent, inconsistent or distorted parts of speech, especially word endings (s, ed) and unemphasized sounds. Percent of speech signal missed will be greater whenever there is background noise in the classroom, especially in the elementary grades where instruction is primarily verbal. Young children have the tendency to watch and copy the movements of other students rather than attending to auditorily fragmented teacher directions.

Possible Psychosocial Impact of Hearing Loss

May be unaware of subtle conversational cues which could cause child to be viewed as inappropriate or awkward. May miss portions of fast-paced peer interactions which could begin to have an impact on socialization and self concept. May have immature behavior. May be more fatigued due to extra effort needed for understanding speech.

Potential Educational Accommodations and Services

Due to noise in typical classroom environments which impede child from having clear access to teacher instruction, will benefit from improved acoustic treatment of classroom and sound-field amplification. Favorable seating necessary. May often have difficulty with sound/letter associations and fine auditory discrimination skills necessary to learn phonics for reading. May need attention to vocabulary or speech, especially when there has been a history of ear problems. Appropriate medical management necessary for conductive losses. Depending on loss configuration, may benefit from low power hearing aid with personal FM system. Inservice on impact of so called "minimal" hearing loss on language development, listening in noise and learning, required for teacher.

Audiologist
Additional Audiologist comments on reverse side.

Developed by Karen L. Anderson, EdS & Noel D. Matkin, PhD ©1998
Available from the Educational Audiology Association 1-800-460-7322

CHILD'S NAME
DATE: _____ Average Hearing Loss: R___ L___

MILD HEARING LOSS (26-40 dB)

Possible Effect of Hearing Loss on the Understanding of Language and Speech

Effect of a hearing loss that is approximately 20 dB can be compared to ability to hear when index fingers are placed in ears. Mild hearing loss causes greater listening difficulties than such a "plugged ear" loss. Child can "hear" but misses fragments leading to misunderstanding. Degree of difficulty experienced in school will depend upon noise level in the classroom, distance from the teacher, and configuration of the hearing loss. At 30 dB can miss 25%-40% of the speech signal; at 35-40 dB may miss 50% or more of class discussions, especially when voices are faint or speaker is not in line of vision. Will miss brief or unemphasized words and consonants, especially when a high frequency hearing loss is present. Often experiences difficulty learning early reading skills such as letter/sound associations. With personal hearing aids alone, child's ability to understand and succeed in the classroom will be substantially diminished by speaker distance and background noise, especially in the elementary grades.

Possible Psychosocial Impact of Hearing Loss

Barriers build with negative impact on self esteem as child is accused of "hearing when he/she wants to," "daydreaming," or "not paying attention." May believe he/she is less capable due to understanding difficulties in class. Child begins to lose ability for selective listening, and has increasing difficulty suppressing background noise causing the learning environment to be more stressful. Child more fatigued due to effort needed to listen.

Potential Educational Accommodations and Services

Noise in typical class will impede child from clear access to teacher instruction. Will benefit from hearing aid(s) and use of a personal FM or sound-field FM system in the classroom. Needs favorable acoustics, seating and lighting. Refer to special education for language/educational evaluation. May need attention to language development, auditory skills, articulation, speechreading and/or support in reading and self esteem. Inservice teacher on impact of so called "mild" hearing loss on listening and learning.

Audiologist
Additional Audiologist comments on reverse side.

Developed by Karen L. Anderson, EdS & Noel D. Matkin, PhD © 1998
Available from the Educational Audiology Association 1-800-460-7322

CHILD'S NAME _____
DATE: _____ Average Hearing Loss: R___ L___

MODERATE HEARING LOSS (41-55 dB)

Possible Effect of Hearing Loss on the Understanding of Language and Speech

Even with hearing aids, child can "hear" but typically misses fragments of what is said. Without amplification, understands conversational speech at a distance of 3-5 feet, only if sentence structure and vocabulary are controlled. The amount of speech signal missed can be 50+% with 40 dB loss and 80+% with 50 dB loss. Child is likely to have delayed or disordered syntax, limited vocabulary, imperfect speech production and flat voice quality. Early consistent use of amplification and language intervention increases the probability that the child's speech, language and learning will develop more normally. Use of a visual communication system to supplement speech may be indicated, especially if large language delays and/or additional disabilities are present. Child will not have clear access to verbal instruction due to typical noise in class. A personal FM system to overcome noise in the classroom and distance from the teacher usually necessary. With personal hearing aids alone, ability to learn effectively in the classroom is at high risk.

Possible Psychosocial Impact of Hearing Loss

Barriers build with negative impact on self esteem as child is accused of "hearing when he/she wants to," "daydreaming," or "not paying attention." Often with this degree of hearing loss, communication can be significantly affected, and socialization with peers can be difficult, especially in noisy settings such as lunch or recess. May be more fatigued than classmates due to effort needed to listen.

Potential Educational Accommodations and Services

Consistent use of amplification (hearing aids/FM) is essential. Needs favorable classroom acoustics, seating and lighting. Program supervision by hearing impairment specialist to coordinate services is essential. Special academic support may be necessary, especially for elementary grades; attention to growth of oral communication, reading, written language skills, auditory skill development, speech therapy, self esteem likely. Teacher inservice required with attention to peer acceptance.

Audiologist
Additional Audiologist comments on reverse side.

Developed by Karen L. Anderson, EdS & Noel D. Matkin, PhD © 1998
Available from the Educational Audiology Association 1-800-460-7322

MODERATE TO SEVERE HEARING LOSS (56-70 dB)

Possible Effect of Hearing Loss on the Understanding of Language and Speech

With hearing aids, child can usually "hear" people talking around him/her, but will miss fragments of what is said resulting in difficulty in situations requiring verbal communication in both one-to-one and groups. Without amplification, conversation must be very loud to be understood; a 55 dB loss can cause a child to miss up to 100% of speech information without working amplification. Delayed spoken language, syntax, reduced speech intelligibility and flat voice quality likely. Reliance on vision to complement hearing to achieve functional access to communication necessary. Age when amplified, consistency of hearing aid use and amount of language intervention strongly tied to development of speech, language and learning. Use of visual communication system often indicated, especially if language delay and/or additional disabilities are present. Use of personal FM system will reduce noise and distance and to allow increased auditory access to verbal instruction. With hearing aids alone, ability to understand in the classroom is greatly impacted by distance and noise.

Possible Psychosocial Impact of Hearing Loss

Often, with this degree of hearing loss, communication is significantly affected, and socialization with peers can be difficult, especially in noisy settings such as lunch or recess. Tendency for poorer self concept and social immaturity will contribute to a sense of rejection; peer inservice helpful.

Potential Educational Accommodations and Services

Full time, consistent use of amplification (hearing aids / FM system) is essential. Depending upon loss configuration, frequency transposition aid may be of benefit. Program supervision by specialist in hearing impairment necessary. May require intense support in language skills, speech, aural habilitation, reading and writing. Sign increasingly useful to access instruction as it becomes more linguistically complex. Note-taking, captioned films and visual aids are needed accommodations. Teacher inservice required.

Audiologist

Additional Audiologist comments on reverse side.
Developed by Karen L. Anderson, EdS & Noel D. Matkin, PhD © 1998
Available from the Educational Audiology Association 1-800-460-7322

UNILATERAL HEARING LOSS
One Normal Ear and One Ear with Permanent Loss

Possible Effect of Hearing Loss on the Understanding of Language and Speech

Child can "hear" but will have difficulty understanding in certain situations, such as hearing faint or distant speech, especially if poor hearing ear is closest to the person speaking. Will usually have difficulty localizing sounds and voices using hearing alone. The unilateral listener will have greater difficulty understanding when environment is noisy and/or reverberant, especially with normal ear towards the overhead projector or other sound source and poor hearing ear towards the teacher. Exhibits difficulty detecting or understanding soft speech from the side of the poor hearing ear, especially in a group discussion.

Possible Psychosocial Impact of Hearing Loss

Child may be accused of selective hearing due to discrepancies in speech understanding in quiet versus noise. Social problems may arise as child experiences difficulty understanding in noisy cooperative learning, lunch or recess situations. May misconstrue peer conversations and feel rejected or ridiculed. Child may be more fatigued in classroom setting due to greater effort needed to listen, especially if class is active or has relatively poor acoustics. May appear inattentive, distractable or frustrated, with behavior or social problems sometimes evident.

Potential Educational Accommodations and Services

Allow child to change seat locations to direct the better ear toward the most effective listening position. Student is at risk for educational difficulties as half of students with unilateral hearing loss experience significant learning problems. Often have difficulty learning sound/letter associations in typically noisy Kdgn and grade 1 settings. Educational monitoring is warranted. Teacher inservice is beneficial. May benefit from a hearing aid on the poorer hearing ear if there is residual hearing or occasionally a CROS aid can be successful. Will benefit from a sound-field FM system in the classroom, especially in lower grades, or a personal FM system with low gain/power.

Audiologist

Additional Audiologist comments on reverse side.
Developed by Karen L. Anderson, EdS & Noel D. Matkin, PhD © 1998
Available from the Educational Audiology Association 1-800-460-7322

MID-FREQUENCY HEARING LOSS or REVERSE SLOPE HEARING LOSS

"Cookie Bite" Loss: Approx. 750 Hz - 3000 Hz
Reverse Slope Loss: Approx. 250 Hz - 2000 Hz

Possible Effect of Hearing Loss on the Understanding of Language and Speech

Child can "hear" whenever speech is present but will have difficulty understanding in certain situations; may have difficulty understanding faint or distant speech, such as a student with a quiet voice from across the classroom. The "cookie bite" or reverse slope listener will have greater difficulty understanding speech when environment is noisy and/or reverberant, such as a typical classroom setting. A mild degree of loss in the low to mid-frequency range may cause the child to miss approximately 30% of speech information, if unamplified; some consonant and vowel sounds may be heard inconsistently, especially when background noise is present. Speech production of these sounds may be affected.

Possible Psychosocial Impact of Hearing Loss

Child may be accused of selective hearing due to discrepancies in speech understanding in quiet versus noise. Social problems may arise as child experiences difficulty understanding in noisy lunch or recess situations. May misconstrue peer conversations. Child may be more fatigued in classroom setting due to greater effort needed to listen. May appear inattentive, distractable or frustrated.

Potential Educational Accommodations and Services

Personal hearing aids important but must be precisely fit to loss. Child likely to benefit from a sound-field FM system, a personal FM system or assistive listening device in the classroom. Student is at risk for educational difficulties. Can experience some difficulty learning sound/letter associations in Kdgn and 1st grade classes. Depending upon degree and configuration of loss, child may experience delayed language development and articulation problems. Annual hearing evaluation to monitor for loss progression is suggested.

Audiologist

Additional Audiologist comments on reverse side.
Developed by Karen L. Anderson, EdS & Noel D. Matkin, PhD © 1998
Available from the Educational Audiology Association 1-800-460-7322

CHILD'S NAME _____
DATE _____ Average Hearing Loss: R _____ L _____

PROFOUND HEARING LOSS (91+ dB)

Possible Effect of Hearing Loss on the Understanding of Language and Speech

Detection of speech sounds is dependent upon the hearing loss configuration and the optimal use of amplification. May be aware of vibrations more than tonal patterns. Degree and configuration of hearing loss, use and appropriateness of amplification, quality of early intervention and individual ability, all combine to influence the degree to which a profoundly deaf child can detect, discriminate, process and understand the sounds of spoken language. If loss is present at birth, speech and language will not develop spontaneously. If loss is of recent onset, speech and language is likely to deteriorate rapidly. Most profoundly deaf children are not able to use hearing by itself for communication and learning, and utilize visual communication systems and languages.

Possible Psychosocial Impact of Hearing Loss

Parents and family members who are fluent in the child's communication mode are essential for the child's feelings of acceptance, self esteem and his/her optimal communication development. Child often more comfortable interacting with deaf or hard of hearing peers due to ease of communication. Relationships with peers and adults who have hearing loss can make positive contributions toward the development of a healthy self-concept and a sense of cultural identity, important tools that can help the child function more effectively in the mainstream. Signing club or class for hearing peers beneficial. Often in the mainstream, child will have greater dependence on adults due to difficulties understanding oral communication. Inservice to hearing peers and teachers is essential to foster acceptance.

Potential Educational Accommodations and Services

There is no one communication system that is right for all hard of hearing or deaf children and their families. Whether a visual communication approach or auditory/oral approach is used, early and extensive language intervention, full-time consistent amplification use, and constant integration of the communication practices into the family will highly increase the probability that the child will become a successful learner. If an auditory/oral approach is used, early training is needed on all auditory skills, speechreading, concept development and speech. Full time, consistent use of amplification (hearing aids/FM) is essential if hearing is to be maximized; older deaf child may decide to discontinue hearing aid use if extremely limited functional benefit. Frequency transposition aid or cochlear implant may be an option if culturally deaf emphasis is used, exposure to deaf, ASL users is vital. Self-contained educational placement with other deaf and hard of hearing students (special school or classes) often a less restrictive option due to access to free-flowing communication with peers and teachers. Specialized supervision, support services and continual appraisal of access to communication is required. Inclusion into regular classes as much as is beneficial to student (with oral or sign interpreter). Note-taking, captioned films and visual aids are necessary accommodations. Training in communication repair strategies helpful.. Inservice of mainstream teachers is essential. School for the Deaf is a social and program consideration.

Audiologist _____
Additional Audiologist comments on reverse side.

Developed by Karen L. Anderson &
Noel D. Matkin, PhD   Available from
the Educational Audiology Association
1-800-460-7322   © 1998

CHILD'S NAME _____
DATE _____ Average Hearing Loss: R _____ L _____

SEVERE HEARING LOSS (71-90 dB)

Possible Effect of Hearing Loss on the Understanding of Language and Speech

Without amplification, may hear loud noises about one foot distant from ear. When amplified optimally, children with hearing ability of 90 dB or better should be able to detect many sounds of speech if presented from close distance or via FM. Individual ability and early intensive intervention will determine the degree that sounds detected will be discriminated and processed into meaningful input. Often unable to perceive higher pitch speech sounds sufficiently loud enough to discriminate them, especially without the use of FM. Reliance on vision to complement hearing to achieve functional access to communication necessary. If loss is present at birth, oral speech and language will likely be severely delayed or not develop spontaneously. Use of visual communication system often indicated. The younger the child wears amplification consistently and intensive language intervention is provided, the greater the probability that speech, language and learning will develop at a more normal rate. Use of child's communication mode by family members is essential. If progressive or recent onset hearing loss, speech will likely deteriorate with quality becoming flat.

Possible Psychosocial Impact of Hearing Loss

Communication is significantly affected, and socialization with hearing peers is often difficult. Child often more comfortable interacting with deaf or hard of hearing peers due to ease of communication. Relationships with peers and adults who have hearing loss can make positive contributions toward the development of a healthy self-concept and a sense of cultural identity. Poorer self concept and greater social immaturity is typical unless child is in a deaf school or within a peer group. Child in mainstream classroom may have greater dependence on adults due to difficulties comprehending oral communication.

Potential Educational Accommodations and Services

There is no one communication system that is right for all hard of hearing or deaf children and their families. Whether a visual communication approach or auditory/oral approach is used, early and extensive language intervention, full-time consistent amplification use and constant integration of the communication practices into the family will highly increase the probability that the child will become a successful learner. Self-contained educational placement with other deaf and hard of hearing students (special school or classes) may be a less restrictive option due to access to free-flowing communication. Specialized supervision, support services and continual appraisal of access to communication is required. Depending on hearing loss, a frequency transposition aid or cochlear implant may be remotely possible options. If an auditory/oral approach is used, early training is needed on all auditory skills, speechreading, concept development and speech. If culturally deaf emphasis is used, frequent exposure to deaf, ASL users is important. Oral or sign interpreter likely necessary in mainstream settings, especially as instruction becomes more linguistically complex. Note-taking, captioned films and visual aids necessary; training in communication repair strategies helpful. Inservice of mainstream teachers is essential.

Audiologist _____
Additional Audiologist comments on reverse side.

Developed by Karen L. Anderson &
Noel D. Matkin, PhD   Available from
the Educational Audiology Association
1-800-460-7322   © 1998

206

HIGH FREQUENCY HEARING LOSS
Approximately 1500 Hz - 8000 Hz

Possible Effect of Hearing Loss on the Understanding of Language and Speech

Child can "hear" but will miss important fragments of speech. Even a mild loss in high frequency hearing may cause the child to miss 20%-30% of vital speech information if unamplified. Consonant sounds t, s, f, th, k,sh, ch likely heard inconsistently, especially in noise. Will have difficulty understanding faint or distant speech, such as a student with a quiet voice from across the classroom and will have much greater difficulty understanding speech when environment is noisy and/or reverberant. Many of the critical sounds for understanding speech are high pitched, quiet sounds, making them difficult to perceive. The words "cat, cap, calf, cast would be perceived as "ca," word endings, possessives, plurals and unstressed brief words are difficult to perceive and understand. Speech production may be affected. Use of amplification often indicated to ease learning.

Possible Psychosocial Impact of Hearing Loss

May be accused of selective hearing due to discrepancies in speech understanding in quiet versus noise. Social problems may arise as child experiences difficulty understanding in noisy lunch or recess situations; may misinterpret peer conversations. Child may be fatigued in classroom due to greater listening effort. May appear inattentive, distractible or frustrated. Could affect self concept.

Potential Educational Accommodations and Services

Student is at risk for educational difficulties. Depending upon onset, degree and configuration of loss, child may experience delayed language and syntax development and articulation problems. Possible difficulty learning some sound/letter associations in Kdgn and 1st grade classes. Early evaluation of speech and language skills is suggested. Educational monitoring and teacher inservice is warranted. Will often benefit from personal hearing aids and use of a sound-field or a personal FM system in the classroom. Use of ear protection in noisy situations is imperative to prevent loss progression from hearing damage.

Audiologist
Additional Audiologist comments on reverse side.

Developed by Karen L. Anderson, EdS & Noel D. Matkin, PhD © 1998
Available from the Educational Audiology Association 1-800-460-7322

FLUCTUATING HEARING LOSS
Conductive Loss Due to Otitis Media with Effusion

Possible Effect of Hearing Loss on the Understanding of Language and Speech

Of greatest concern are children who have experienced hearing fluctuations over many months in early childhood (multiple episodes with fluid lasting three months or longer). Listening with a hearing loss that is approximately 20 dB can be compared to hearing when index fingers are placed in ears; this loss or worse is typical of listening with fluid behind the eardrums. Child can "hear" but misses fragments of what is said. Degree of difficulty experienced in school will depend upon the classroom noise level, the distance from the teacher and the current degree of hearing loss. At 30 dB can miss 25%-40% of the speech signal; child with a 40 dB loss associated with "glue ear" may miss 50% of class discussions, especially when voices are faint, speaker is not in line of vision; will frequently miss unstressed words, consonants and word endings.

Possible Psychosocial Impact of Hearing Loss

Barriers build with negative impact on self esteem as the child is accused of "not hearing when he/she wants to," "daydreaming," or "not paying attention." Child may believe he/she is less capable due to understanding difficulties in class. Typically poor at identifying changes in own hearing ability; with inconsistent hearing, the child learns to "tune out" the speech signal. Children are judged to be immature, have greater attentional problems, insecurity, distractibility and lack self esteem. Tend to be non-participative and distract themselves from classroom tasks.

Potential Educational Accommodations and Services

Primary impact is on attention in class and acquisition of early reading skills, can also delay language development. Screening for language delays necessary starting at a young age. Ongoing hearing monitoring in school with communication between parent and teacher necessary. Educational monitoring is warranted. Will benefit from sound-field FM system or an assistive listening device in class. May need attention to speech/language, reading, self esteem and listening skills development. Inservice teacher beneficial.

Audiologist
Additional Audiologist comments on reverse side.

Developed by Karen L. Anderson, EdS & Noel D. Matkin, PhD © 1998
Available from the Educational Audiology Association 1-800-460-7322

Please Consider in Child's Educational Program:

___ Teacher inservice and seating close to teacher
___ Hearing monitoring at school every ___ mos.
___ Amplification monitoring
___ Contact your school district's audiologist
___ Protect ears from noise to prevent more loss
___ Educational monitoring (e.g. biannual SIFTER)
___ Screening/evaluation of speech and language
___ Educational support services/evaluation
___ Classroom Amplification Trial Period
• ___ Sound-Field amplification system
• ___ Personal FM / Assistive Listening Device
___ Educational consultation/ program supervision by specialist(s) in hearing loss
___ Note-taking, closed captioned films, visual aids
___ Regular contact with other children who are deaf or hard of hearing
___ Use of visual communication system/indicated
___ Specialized program for Deaf/Hard of Hearing

NOTE: All children with hearing loss require periodic audiologic evaluation, rigorous amplification checks, regular monitoring of their access to instruction and the effectiveness of their communication skills. Children with hearing loss (especially conductive) need appropriate medical attention along with educational accommodations and services.

Individual with Disabilities Education Act requires that "hearing aids worn by deaf and hard of hearing children in school are functioning properly." A daily battery/listening check and an electroacoustic evaluation of hearing aid function by an audiologist two or more times per year is important.

Teacher Inservice: All children require access to verbal instruction if they are to succeed in school. **A child without effective access to teacher instruction will not receive an appropriate education.** Distance, noise in classroom and fragmentation caused by hearing loss prevent access. Use of visuals, FM classroom amplification, visual communication systems, notetakers, communication partners, etc. provide access to instruction. Components of good classroom management for a child with hearing loss include: 1) keep in close proximity to the child during instruction, 2) call on students by name during discussions and summarize important points, 3) reduce noise sources, 4) check student comprehension following directions, 5) adapt/modify curriculum for student to experience success 6) utilize classroom amplification daily for all large group instruction, 7) be aware of potential changes in hearing ability and report if suspected, 8) facilitate socialization between the child and peers, 9)keep lighting from windows on teacher's face.

Organization Phone Numbers

Alexander Graham Bell Association
for the Deaf 202-337-5220
American Hearing Research Foundation
312-726-9670
American Society for Deaf Children
800-942-ASDC
American Speech-Language-Hearing
Association 301-897-5700
AT&T National Special Needs Center
800-233-1222
Auditory-Verbal International
703-739-1049
Center for Bicultural Studies
(Bi-Bi) 301-277-3945
Council for Exceptional Children
703-620-3660
Deaftek, USA 508-620-1777
Federation for Children with
Special Needs 617-482-2915
Hear Now 303-695-7797
House Ear Institute 213-483-4431
John Tracey Clinic 213-748-5481
National Association of the Deaf
301-587-1791
National Captioning Institute
703-917-7600
National ued Speech Association
919-828-1218
National Information Center on Deafness
202-651-5051
National Institute on Deafness and Other
Communication Disorders Clearinghouse
800-241-1044
National Parent Network on Disabilities
703-684-6763
National Technical Institute for the Deaf
716-475-6400
EE Center for the Advancement of Deaf
Children 310-430-1467
Self Help for Hard of Hearing People
301-657-2248
Sertoma 816-333-8300
Software to Go, Gallaudet University
202-651-5705
Telecommunications for the Deaf
301-589-3786
World Recreation Association of the Deaf
716-586-4208

Please Consider in Child's Educational Program:

____ Teacher inservice and seating close to teacher
____ Hearing monitoring at school every ____ mos.
____ Amplification monitoring
____ Contact your school district's audiologist
____ Protect ears from noise to prevent more loss
____ Educational monitoring (e.g. biannual SIFTER)
____ Screening/evaluation of speech and language
____ Educational support services/evaluation
____ Classroom Amplification Trial Period
• Sound-Field amplification system
• Personal FM /Assistive Listening Device
____ Educational consultation/ program supervision
by specialist(s) in hearing loss
____ Note-taking, closed captioned films, visual aids
____ Regular contact with other children who are
deaf or hard of hearing
____ Use of visual communication system indicated
____ Specialized program for Deaf/Hard of Hearing

NOTE: All children with hearing loss require periodic audiologic evaluation, rigorous amplification checks, regular monitoring of their access to instruction and the effectiveness of their communication skills. Children with hearing loss (especially conductive) need appropriate medical attention along with educational accommodations and services.

Individual with Disabilities Education Act requires that "hearing aids worn by deaf and hard of hearing children in school are functioning properly." A daily battery/listening check and an electroacoustic evaluation of hearing aid function by an audiologist two or more times per year is important

Teacher Inservice: All children require access to verbal instruction if they are to succeed in school. **A child without effective access to teacher instruction will not receive an appropriate education.** Distance, noise in classroom and fragmentation caused by hearing loss prevent access. Use of visuals, FM classroom amplification, visual communication systems, notetakers, communication partners, etc. provide access to instruction. Components of good classroom management for a child with hearing loss include: 1) keep in close proximity to the child during instruction, 2) call on students by name during discussions and summarize important points, 3) reduce noise sources, 4) check student comprehension following directions, 5) adapt/modify curriculum for student to experience success, 6) utilize classroom amplification daily for all large group instruction, 7) be aware of potential changes in hearing ability and report if suspected, 8) facilitate socialization between the child and peers, 9)keep lighting from windows on teacher's face.

REFERENCES

ALLEN, P., & WIGHTMAN, F. (1994). Psychometric functions for children's detection of tones in noise. *Journal of Speech and Hearing Research, 37*;205–215.

AMERICAN SPEECH-LANGUAGE-HEARING ASSOCIATION. (December, 1994a). Joint Committee on Infant Hearing 1994 Position Statement, *ASHA, 36*;38–41.

AMERICAN SPEECH-LANGUAGE-HEARING ASSOCIATION. (1994b). Guidelines for fitting and monitoring FM systems. *ASHA 36* (Suppl.);1–9.

ANDERSON, K. (1989). *Screening Instrument For Targeting Educational Risk (S.I.F.T.E.R.).* Austin, TX: Pro-Ed.

ANDERSON, K., & MATKIN, N. (1996). *Screening Instrument for Targeting Educational Risk in Preschool Children (Preschool S.I.F.T.E.R.),* Tampa, FL: Educational Audiology Association.

ANDERSON, K., & MATKIN, N. (1998). *Relationship of hearing loss to developmental and educational needs.* Tampa, FL: Educational Audiology Association.

ANDERSON, K., & SMALDINO, J. (1997). *Learning Inventory For Education (L.I.F.E.).* Tampa, FL: Educational Audiology Association.

BENOIT, R. (1989). Home use of FM amplification systems during the early childhood years. *Hearing Instruments, 40*;8–12.

BENTLER, R.A. (1989). External ear resonance characteristics in children. *Journal of Speech and Hearing Disorders, 54*;265–268.

BERGER, K.W., HAGBERG, E.N., & RANE, R.L. (1989). *Prescription of hearing instruments: Rationale, procedures, and results.* Kent, OH: Herald.

BESS, F.H. (1982). Children with unilateral hearing loss. *Journal of the Academy of Rehabilitation Audiology, 25*;131–144.

BESS, F.H., THARPE, A.M., & GIBLER, A.M. (1986). Auditory performance of children with unilateral hearing loss. *Ear and Hearing, 7*(1);21–26.

BOOTHROYD, A. (1991). Assessment of speech perception capacity in profoundly deaf children. *American Journal of Otology, 12*;67–72.

BOOTHROYD, A., SPRINGER, N., SMITH, L., & SCHULMAN, J. (1988). Amplitude compression and profound hearing loss. *Journal of Speech and Hearing Research, 31*;362–376.

BRACKETT, D. (1992). Effects of early FM use on speech perception. In: M. Ross (Ed.), *FM auditory training systems: Characteristics, selection and use* (pp. 175–188). Timonium, MD: York Press.

BYRNE, D., & DILLON, H. (1986). The National Acoustics Laboratories (NAL) procedure for selecting the gain and frequency response of a hearing instrument. *Ear and Hearing, 7*;257–265.

CORNELISSE, L.E., GAGNE, J.-P., & SEEWALD, R.C. (1991). Ear level recordings of the long-term average spectrum of speech. *Ear and Hearing, 12*(1);47–54.

CORNELISSE, L.E., SEEWALD, R.C., JAMIESON, D.G. (1994). Wide dynamic range compression hearing instruments: The DSL[i/o] approach. *Hearing Journal, 47*(10);23–29.

CORNELISSE, L.E., SEEWALD, R.C., & JAMIESON, D.G. (1995). The input/output formula: A theoretical approach to the fitting of personal amplification devices. *Journal of the Acoustical Society of America, 97*;1854–1864.

COX, R.M., & ALEXANDER, G.C. (1995). The abbreviated profile of hearing aid benefit. *Ear and Hearing, 16*(2);176–186.

COX, R.M., & MOORE, J.N. (1988). Composite speech spectrum for hearing aid gain prescriptions. *Journal of Speech and Hearing Research, 31*;102–107.

CULBERTSON, J.L., & GILBERT, L.E. (1986). Children with unilateral sensorineural hearing loss: Cognitive, academic, and social development. *Ear and Hearing, 7*(1);38–42.

DAWSON, P., DILLON, H., & BATTAGLIA, J. (1990). Output limiting compression for the severe-profoundly deaf. *Australian Journal of Audiology, 13*(1);1–12.

DECONDE JOHNSON, C., BENSON, P.V., & SEATON, J.B. (1997). Amplification and classroom hearing technology. *Educational audiology handbook* (pp. 83–106). San Diego: Singular Publishing Group.

DEMPSTER, J.H., & MACKENZIE, K. (1990). The resonance frequency of the external auditory canal in children. *Ear and Hearing, 11*;296–298.

DILLON, H., JAMES, A., & GINIS, J. (1997). Client oriented scale of improvement (COSI) and its relationship to several other measures of benefit and satisfaction provided by hearing instruments. *Journal of the American Academy of Audiology, 8*(1);27–43.

ELLIOT, L.L. (1979). Performance of children aged 9 to 17 years on a test of speech intelligibility in noise using sentence material with controlled word predictability. *Journal of the Acoustical Society of America, 66*(3);651–653.

FEDERAL COMMUNICATION COMMISSION. (1992). Amendment Part 15 (92–163), ET Docket No. 91–150. *Additional frequencies for auditory devices for the hearing-impaired,* April 7.

FEIGIN, J.A., KOPUN, J.K., STELMACHOWICZ, P.G., & GORGA, M.P. (1989). Probe-microphone measures of earcanal sound pressure levels in infants and children. *Ear and Hearing, 10*;254–258.

HARRISON, M., & ROUSH, J. (1996) Age of suspicion, identification and intervention for infants and young children with hearing loss: A national study. *Ear and Hearing, 17*(1);55–62.

HAWKINS, D. (1987). Assessment of FM systems with an earcanal probe-tube microphone system. *Ear and Hearing, 8*;301–303.

HAWKINS, D., & MUELLER, H.G. (1992a). Test protocols for probe-tube microphone measurements. In: H.G. Mueller, D. B. Hawkins, & J. L. Northern (Eds.), *Probe microphone measurements: Hearing instrument selection and assessment* (pp. 269–278). San Diego, CA: Singular Publishing, Inc.

HAWKINS, D., & MUELLER, H.G. (1992b). Procedural considerations in probe-microphone measurements. In: H.G. Mueller, D.B. Hawkins, & J.L. Northern (Eds.), *Probe microphone measurements: Hearing instrument selection and assessment* (pp. 67–89). San Diego, CA: Singular Publishing, Inc.

HAWKINS, D.B., WALDEN, B.E., MONTGOMERY, A., & PROSEK, R.A. (1987). Description and validation of an LDL procedure designed to select SSPL90. *Ear and Hearing, 8*;162–169.

HAWKINS, D.B., & YACULLO, W.S. (1984). Signal-to-noise advantage of binaural hearing instruments and directional microphones under different levels of reverberation. *Journal of Speech and Hearing Disorders, 49*;278–286.

HEDLEY-WILLIAMS, A., THARPE, A.M., & BESS, F.H. (1996). Fitting hearing instruments in the pediatric population: A survey of practice procedures. In: F.H. Bess, J.S. Gravel, & A.M. Tharpe (Eds.), *Amplification for children with auditory deficits* (pp. 107–122). Nashville, TN: Bill Wilkerson Center Press.

Kawell, M.E., Kopun, J.G., & Stelmachowicz, P.G. (1988). Loudness discomfort levels in children. *Ear and Hearing, 9;*133–137.

Kessler, A.R., Giolas, T.G., & Maxon, A.B. (1990). *The hearing performance inventory for children (HPIC): Reliability and validity.* American Speech-Language Hearing Association Convention. Seattle, WA: American Speech-Language-Hearing Association.

Kopun, J.G., & Stelmachowicz, P.G. (1998). Perceived communication difficulties in children with hearing loss. *American Journal of Audiology, 7*(1);30–38.

Kruger, B. (1987). An update on the external ear resonance in infants and young children. *Ear and Hearing, 8;*333–336.

Kruger, B., & Ruben, R.J. (1987). The acoustic properties of the infant ear: A preliminary report. *Acta Otolaryngologica (Stockholm), 103;*578–585.

Leavitt, R., & Flexer, C. (1991). Speech degradation as measured by the rapid speech transmission index (RASTI). *Ear and Hearing, 12;*115–118.

Lewis, D. (1991). FM systems and assistive devices: Selection and evaluation. In: J.A. Feigin, & P.G. Stelmachowicz (Eds.), *Pediatric amplification: Proceedings of the 1991 National Conference* (pp. 115–138). Omaha, NE: Boys Town National Research Hospital.

Lewis, D. (1994). Assistive devices for classroom listening: FM systems. *American Journal of Audiology, 3;*70–83.

Lewis, D. (1997). Selection and assessment of classroom amplification. In: W. McCracken, & S. Laoide-Kemp (Eds.), *Audiology in education* (pp. 323–347). Manchester: University of Manchester.

Lewis, D. (1998). Classroom amplification. In: F.H. Bess (Ed.), *Children with hearing impairment: Contemporary trends.* Nashville, TN: Bill Wilkerson Center Press.

Lewis, D., Feigin, J., Karasek, A., & Stelmachowicz, P. (1991). Evaluation and assessment of FM systems. *Ear and Hearing, 12;*268–280.

Libby, E.R. (1986). The 1/3–2/3 insertion gain hearing instrument selection guide. *Hearing Instruments, 37;*27–28.

MacPherson, B.J., Elfenbein, J.L., Schum, R.L., & Bentler, R.A. (1991). Thresholds of discomfort in children. *Ear and Hearing, 12;*184–190.

Matkin, N.D. (1987). Hearing instruments for children: Premises for selecting and fitting. *Hearing Instruments, 38;*14–16.

McCandless, G.A., & Lyregaard, P.E. (1983). Prescription of gain and output (POGO) for hearing instruments. *Hearing Instruments, 3;*16–21.

McCleary, E., & Moeller, M.P. (1997). Clinical assessment of speech perception skills in children. *1997 Conference on Developments in Pediatric Audiology: Current issues in assessment and management.* Omaha, NE: Boys Town National Research Hospital.

Medwetsky, L. (1994). Educational Audiology. In: J. Katz (Ed.), *Handbook of clinical audiology* (pp. 503–520). Baltimore, MD: Williams & Wilkins.

Moeller, M. (1996). *Efficacy of an early intervention project.* Third International Symposium on Childhood Deafness. Vanderbilt University, Kiawah Island, SC (October, 1996).

Moeller, M.P., Donaghy, K.F., Beauchaine, K.L., Lewis, D.E., & Stelmachowicz, P.G. (1996). Longitudinal study of FM system use in nonacademic settings: Effects on language development. *Ear and Hearing, 17*(1);28–41.

Moodie, K.S., Seewald, R.C., & Sinclair, S.T. (1994). Procedure for predicting real-ear hearing instrument performance in young children. *American Journal of Audiology, 3*(1);23–31.

Nelson Barlow, N.L., Auslander, M.C., Rines, D., & Stelmachowicz, P.G. (1988). Probe-tube microphone measures in hearing impaired children and adults. *Ear and Hearing, 9*(5);243–247.

Nittrouer, S., & Boothroyd, A. (1990). Context effects in phoneme and word recognition by young children and older adults. *Journal of the Acoustical Society of America, 80;*50–57.

Nozza, R.J. (1987). Infant speech-sound discrimination testing: Effects of stimulus intensity and procedural model on measures of performance. *Journal of the Acoustical Society of America, 81;*1928–1939.

Nozza, R.J., Rossman, R.N.F., & Bond, L.C. (1991). Infant-adult differences in unmasked threshold for the discrimination of consonant-vowel syllable pairs. *Audiology, 30;*102–112.

Nozza, R.J., Rossman, R.N.F., Bond, L.C., & Miller, S.L. (1990). Infant speech-sound discrimination in noise. *Journal of the Acoustical Society of America, 87;*339–350.

Oyler, R.F., Oyler, A.L., & Matkin, N.D. (1988). Unilateral hearing loss: Demographics and educational impact. *Language, Speech and Hearing Services in Schools, 19;* 201–210.

Palmer, C., & Mormer, E. (1997). A systematic program for hearing aid orientation and adjustment. *Hearing Review, High Performance Hearing Solutions Supplement, 1;*45–52.

Palmer, C., & Mormer, E. (1998). The goals of the hearing aid fitting: Child, parents, and educators. *Remediating Pediatric Hearing Loss Through Amplification: Taking Science into the Clinic.* University of Pittsburgh and Oticon, San Antonio, TX.

Pediatric Working Group of the Conference on Amplification for Children with Auditory Deficits. (1996). Amplification for infants and children with hearing loss. *American Journal of Audiology, 5*(1);53–68.

Robbins, A.M., Renshaw, J.J., & Berry, S. (1991). Evaluating meaningful auditory integration in profoundly hearing-impaired children. *American Journal of Otology, 12* (Suppl.); 144–150.

Ross, M., & Seewald, R.C. (1988). Hearing instrument selection and evaluation with young children. In: F.H. Bess (Ed.), *Hearing impairment in children* (pp. 190–213). Parkton, MD: York Press.

Ruben, R.J. (1997). A time frame of critical/sensitive periods of language development. *Acta Otolaryngologica (Stockholm), 117;*202–205.

Seewald, R.C. (1988). The desired sensation level approach for children: Selection and verification. *Hearing Instruments, 39;*18–22.

Seewald, R.C. (1991). Hearing instrument output limiting considerations for children. In: J.A. Feigin, & P.G. Stelmachowicz (Ed.), *Pediatric amplification: Proceedings of the 1991 National Conference* (pp. 19–35). Omaha, NE: Boys Town National Research Hospital.

Seewald, R.C. (1994). Fitting children with the DSL method. *Hearing Journal, 47*(9) 10;48–51.

Seewald, R.C., Cornelisse, L.E., Ramji, K.V., Sinclair, S.T., Moodie, K.S., & Jamieson, D.G. (1997). *DSL v 4.1 for Windows: A software implementation of the desired sensation level (DSL[i/o]) method for fitting linear gain and wide-dynamic-range compression hearing instruments.* Hearing Health Care Research Unit.

SEEWALD, R.C., HUDSON, S.P., GAGNE, J.-P., & ZELISKO, D.L. (1992). Comparison of 2 procedures for estimating the sensation level of amplified speech. *Ear and Hearing 13*(3);142–149.

SEEWALD, R.C., & MOODIE, K.S. (1992). Electroacoustic considerations. In: M. Ross (Ed.), *FM auditory training systems: Characteristics, selection and use* (pp. 75–102). Timonium, MD: York Press.

SEEWALD, R.C., RAMJI, K.V., SINCLAIR, S.T., MOODIE, K.S., & JAMIESON, D.G. (1993). *DSL 3.1 User's manual.* London, Ontario: University of Western Ontario.

SEEWALD, R.C., & ROSS, M. (1988). Amplification for young hearing impaired children. In: M.C. Pollack (Ed.), *Amplification for the hearing-impaired* (3rd ed.) (pp. 213–271). Orlando: Grune & Stratton.

SEEWALD, R.C., ROSS, M., & SPIRO, M.K. (1985). Selecting amplification characteristics for young hearing-impaired children. *Ear and Hearing, 6*;48–53.

SEEWALD, R.C., ROSS, M., & STELMACHOWICZ, P.G. (1987). Selecting and verifying hearing instrument performance characteristics for young children. *Journal of the Academy of Rehabilitation Audiology, 20*;25–37.

SEEWALD, R.C., SINCLAIR, S.T., & MOODIE, K.S. (1994). *Predictive accuracy of a procedure for electroacoustic fitting in young children.* American Academy of Audiology Convention. American Academy of Audiology, Richmond, VA (April, 1994).

SINCLAIR, S.T., BEAUCHAINE, K.L., MOODIE, K.S., & FEIGIN, J.A. (1994). *Repeatability of a real-ear to coupler difference measurement as a function of age.* American Academy of Audiology Convention. American Academy of Audiology, Richmond, VA (April, 1994).

STELMACHOWICZ, P.G., KALBERER, A., & LEWIS, D.E. (1996). Situational hearing instrument response profile (SHARP). In: F.M. Bess, J.S. Gravel, & A.M. Tharpe (Eds.), *Amplification for children with auditory deficits* (pp. 193–214). Nashville, TN: Bill Wilkerson Center Press.

STELMACHOWICZ, P.G., & LEWIS, D.E. (1988). Some theoretical considerations concerning the relation between functional gain and insertion gain. *Journal of Speech and Hearing Research, 31*;491–496.

STELMACHOWICZ, P.G., LEWIS, D.E., KALBERER, A., & CREUTZ, T. (1994). *Situational Hearing-Instrument Response Profile (SHARP, version 2.0).* Omaha, NE: Boys Town National Research Hospital.

STELMACHOWICZ, P.G., MACE, A.L., KOPUN, J.G., & CARNEY, E. (1993). Long-term and short-term characteristics of speech: Implications for hearing instrument selection for young children. *Journal of Speech and Hearing Research, 36*(3); 609–620.

STUART, A., DURIEUX-SMITH, A., & STENSTROM, R. (1990). Critical differences in aided sound field thresholds in children. *Journal of Speech and Hearing Research, 33*;612–615.

STUART, A., DURIEUX-SMITH, A., & STENSTROM, R. (1991). Probe-tube microphone measures of loudness discomfort levels in children. *Ear and Hearing, 12*(2);140–143.

WESTWOOD, G.F.S., & BAMFORD, J.M. (1995). Probe-tube microphone measures with very young infants: Real-ear to coupler differences and longitudinal changes in real-ear unaided response. *Ear and Hearing, 16*(3);263–273.

YOSHINAGA-ITANO, C. (1995). Efficacy of early identification and early intervention. *Seminars in Hearing, 16*(2);115–123.

YOSHINAGA-ITANO, C., SEDEY, A., COULTER, D., & MEHL, A. (1998). Language of early- and later-identified children with hearing loss. *Pediatrics, 102*(5);1161–1171.

Chapter 5

Hearing Aid Selection and Fitting in Adults: History and Evolution

Carol A. Sammeth and Harry Levitt

Methods of hearing aid selection depend on the technology of the hearing aids being selected. This technology, in turn, depends on the current state of technological advances in audio signal processing. Because technology is constantly evolving, it is to be expected that methods of hearing aid selection will show a similar pattern of evolution. The underlying principles of acoustic amplification have, for the most part, remained constant despite the substantial technological advances in the implementation of these principles. However, even well-established principles are challenged by technological innovation in some instances. The interplay between technology and hearing aid selection techniques has become increasingly important with the recent introduction of digital hearing aids.

To keep pace with a rapidly changing field and to fit modern hearing aids appropriately, it is essential for the audiologist to understand the theoretical underpinnings of the various methods of hearing aid selection, their relative advantages and shortcomings, and the ways in which these methods are affected by advances in hearing aid technology. An understanding of these issues and the practical constraints imposed on the various methods of hearing aid

selection will not only provide audiologists greater insight with respect to their craft, with concomitant improvements in how hearing aids are fitted, but will also provide them with the ability to deal with ongoing technological developments in hearing aids and associated fitting systems.

This chapter, then, has several purposes: (1) to provide an historical perspective on hearing aids and their selection and fitting in adults; (2) to serve as an overview of the topic in preparation for other chapters in this textbook that provide more detail and practical step-by-step instructions on current practices; and (3) to provide perspective on the current state-of-the-art and the direction of future developments.

HISTORY OF HEARING AIDS

Before the 1900s, persons with hearing loss had to rely on passive sound collection devices such as ear trumpets or hearing tubes. These devices provided relatively little gain with a highly peaked frequency response. For example, ear trumpets commonly used in the late 1800s showed frequency responses with most of the energy concentrated below 1200 Hz and peak gain ranging from 11- to 26-dB (Berger, 1975, p. 3). Therefore, individuals with greater than mild hearing loss were not helped sufficiently. Some of these sound collection devices were quite creative. For example, ear trumpets were built into women's fans or men's hats and even into high-backed chairs to make them less conspicuous. Berger has written a number of excellent reviews of early hearing aids (1970, 1975, 1976, 1978, 1984).

In this century, however, we have seen the development of electric and electronic hearing aids. The hearing aid has evolved from large tabletop electric amplification systems to wearable electronic hearing aids to miniature digital hearing instruments that are small enough to fit in the earcanal. Each major advance in hearing aid development emerged as an offshoot of a significant new invention in communications technology. The key inventions were the telephone, vacuum-tube amplifier, miniature vacuum tubes, the transistor, integrated circuits, and digital audio.

Figure 5–1 illustrates the chronology of each major stage in hearing aid development. Several categories are shown (i.e., type of hearing aid, digital technology, methods of signal processing, and selection and fitting procedure). Also shown on the horizontal axis are the dates of the landmark inventions that engendered the major stages in hearing aid development and selection. The invention of the telephone, and the carbon

Audiology: Treatment. Edited by Valente, Hosford-Dunn, and Roeser. Thieme Medical Publishers, Inc., New York © 2000

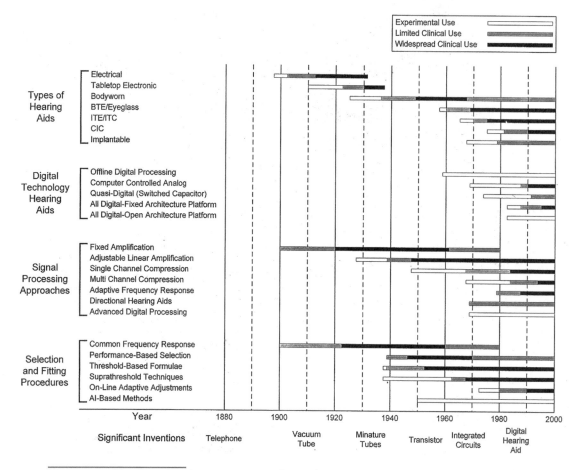

Figure 5–1 Timeline showing approximate dates of major advances in hearing aid technology, signal processing, and fitting approaches. On the horizontal axis are dates of landmark inventions.

microphone in particular, was followed about 20 years later by the invention of the electric hearing aid. The next key invention was the triode vacuum tube, which led to the development of the vacuum tube amplifier and subsequent development of the electronic hearing aid (and the electronic audiometer) about 15 years later. The time between the invention of the transistor and its use in hearing aids was about 5 years. The time taken to reduce new inventions to clinical practice has steadily decreased over the years (with a few exceptions) so that now audiologists are engulfed in a dizzying rate of technological change.

The practical implementation of any new technology necessarily involves an experimental stage and a period of limited use before its general acceptance. The durations of these two stages is not always clear. Thus the timelines shown in Figure 5–1 for the various stages of development should be regarded as no more than approximate, particularly during the early part of the century.

The Electric Era

Carbon Microphone Hearing Aids

The first major era in modern hearing aids began with the introduction of the electric hearing aid after the invention of the telephone by Alexander Graham Bell in 1876 and of the carbon microphone (also known as a carbon transmitter) by

Blake and Hughes in 1878 (Lybarger, 1988). Hutchison received a patent as early as 1899 for an electric hearing aid configured around a carbon microphone. This electric hearing aid became the basis for the "Acousticon" hearing aid, which was introduced commercially in the early 1900s (Berger, 1970).

The electric hearing aid basically consisted of a carbon microphone, battery, and magnetic earphone or eartip, with a sliding resistance volume wheel added around 1912 (Berger, 1975). Electric amplification, unlike earlier passive devices, allowed for several stages of amplification in which the current passes through packs of carbon granules to produce progressively more intense electrical fluctuations. A problem is that each stage of amplification generates noise and distortion in addition to amplifying the noise and distortion of the preceding stage. As a consequence, practical limits on the total amount of amplification can be provided without unacceptably high levels of internally generated noise and distortion. Despite their limitations, early electric hearing aids opened the door to important new concepts, such as amplification by stages and the need to deal with internally generated noise and distortion. An alternative method of increasing the power output of an electric hearing aid was to increase the surface area of the microphone (or to use more than one microphone in parallel) so as to effectively increase the sound power at the input to the electric amplifier (Watson & Tolan, 1949, pp. 272–273). Of course, limitations existed as to how large a microphone or how many microphones could be used in a practical hearing aid.

Although the electric hearing aid provided better amplification than ear trumpets and other nonelectric devices, they were still quite limited in gain and usually had a highly peaked frequency response of limited bandwidth by today's standards. The peak gain of a typical electric hearing aid was about 26 dB, with average gain of 12 dB to 1500 Hz, and a high-frequency response limited to about 3000 Hz (Lybarger, 1988). Electric hearing aids also introduced substantial internal noise and nonlinear distortion.

The Electronic Era

Vacuum-Tube Hearing Aids

The electronic era began with the invention of the triode vacuum tube by DeForest around 1906 and the vacuum-tube amplifier around 1912 (Berger, 1975; Engebretson, 1990; Lybarger, 1988). The vacuum tube was quickly adapted for use in radio applications, but there was a delay before it was applied to hearing aid technology. The first vacuum-tube hearing aid should probably be credited to a patent obtained by Hanson (Berger, 1975) for his 1920 invention of the "Vactuphone" and its release to the market in 1921 (Lybarger, 1988). The earliest vacuum-tube hearing aids were relatively large and expensive, so for a number of years both electric and electronic hearing aids shared the commercial market. Many of these early hearing aids were hybrids in which both electric and electronic amplification were used (Lybarger, 1988). Although some electric hearing aids were wearable, all of the electronic hearing aids of the 1920s were tabletop, nonwearable models.

It was not until the 1930s, after the introduction of the smaller, less expensive, and more stable pentode vacuum tube, that electronic hearing aids reached general popularity (Berger, 1975). Furthermore, the development of practical crystal microphones that used the piezoelectric effect (the generation of an electrical signal with pressure on the crystal) resulted in hearing aids that were smaller with much less noise and distortion than the older electric/electronic hearing aids using carbon microphones. Soon after the introduction of miniature vacuum tubes in the mid 1930s, wearable all-electronic hearing aids were introduced first in England in 1936 and then in the United States in 1937 (Watson & Tolan, 1949, pp. 280–281).

These technological advances coupled with a deeper understanding of electronic circuits, such as between-stage coupling and electronic filtering, led to the first practical attempts at matching the frequency-gain characteristics of hearing aids to the nature of the hearing loss (Hartig & Newhart, 1936; Knudsen, 1939; Littler, 1936). Although the idea that different amounts of gain might be needed for different types of hearing loss originated during the early days of electric amplification (Lybarger, 1988), it was only when advances in technology allowed for these ideas to be implemented in practice that serious consideration was given to the concept of frequency-selective amplification. A related development was that of the electronic audiometer, which provided a means for accurate audiological measurement. With these developments, the stage was set for the new field of audiology (Harford, 1993).

Ongoing advances in electronic miniaturization, including the invention of printed circuits in the 1940s, resulted in

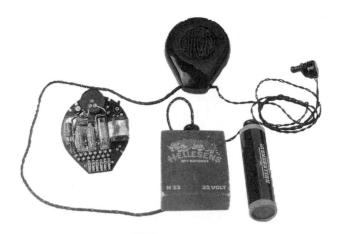

Figure 5–2 Oticon model TA body vacuum-tube hearing aid from 1946 with a vacuum-tube amplifier, a small external receiver with Bakelite earmold, and two batteries. (Photograph courtesy of Oticon.)

smaller, less expensive hearing aids, and pocket-sized hearing aids soon appeared (Engebretson, 1990). The electronic hearing aids of this period were substantially improved in sound quality, frequency response, and power output. The frequency response of a typical 1940s electronic hearing aid extended to about 4000 Hz with a saturation output level as high as 130 dB SPL (Lybarger, 1988). These hearing aids also had considerably less internal noise and distortion than the older hybrid electric/electronic hearing aids. Figure 5–2 shows a vacuum-tube hearing aid from 1946.

Wearable electronic hearing aids had substantially more gain than earlier instruments, resulting in two important developments: the introduction of output limiting to prevent loudness discomfort and possible damage to the ear and the use of high-power hearing aids for severe and profound hearing losses. Many individuals previously labeled as "deaf" had significant amounts of residual hearing and were able to benefit from appropriate acoustic amplification. As a consequence, oral/aural training programs rapidly grew during the 1940s (Berger, 1975). The composition of schools for the deaf also began to change when it was realized that many children with severe hearing loss could be mainstreamed successfully when fitted with appropriate high-gain hearing aids. This development also broadened the field of audiology to include the use of auditory trainers and group hearing aids (Hudgins, 1953; Silverman & Harrison, 1951), and the development of selection and fitting procedures for severe and profound hearing loss.

Transistor Hearing Aids

The invention of the transistor in 1947 by Bardeen, Brattain, and Shockley at Bell Telephone Laboratories and the subsequent development of the germanium junction transistor in 1952 ushered in the era of solid-state electronics. Vacuum-tube hearing aids were soon replaced by smaller and sturdier transistor versions (Berger, 1975; Lybarger, 1988). Transistor hearing aids, in addition to being cosmetically more acceptable because of size reductions, also required almost no warm-up period and, more importantly, had substantially lower power consumption. As a consequence, instead of multiple batteries in a pack, as was needed for even the most modern vacuum-tube hearing aids, the all-transistor hearing aid could function on a single small battery. The reduction in battery power requirements was on the order of 100 to 1 (Lybarger, 1988).

As before, the earliest entrants to the marketplace were hybrid instruments, using a combination of vacuum tubes and transistors (Berger, 1975). This was partly a solution to the problem that the input impedance of early transistor amplifiers was too low for the crystal microphones that were commonly used at that time. The development of low-impedance magnetic microphones (based on the principle of electromagnetic induction) provided a practical solution to this problem. Shortly after the introduction of hybrid versions, all-transistor hearing aids appeared on the market (Lybarger, 1988). Unlike the slower transition from electric to electronic hearing aids, transistorized instruments supplanted vacuum-tube hearing aids within a few years (Berger, 1975). A particularly important development, from an audiological perspective, was that bulky body-worn hearing aids hardwired to an earpiece were soon replaced by one-piece, ear-level instruments.

Transistors, in turn, were replaced by integrated circuits (ICs). IC technology allowed transistors, resistors, capacitors, and their interconnections to be placed on a single small wafer of silicon, thus allowing further significant size reductions. The electronic complexity and signal-processing capabilities of integrated circuits grew rapidly in the 1960s, including the development of the complementary metal-oxide-semiconductor (CMOS) transistor circuit, a type of IC that combined low power and small size (Engebretson, 1990). Eventually these advancements resulted in the introduction in the 1970s of very large scale integrated (VLSI) circuits of enormous complexity and remarkably small size. A modern VLSI microchip can have the equivalent of hundreds of thousands of transistors and other circuit elements.

The economic forces driving the development of VLSI chips were (and are) immense because virtually every industry uses solid-state electronics in some way. The hearing aid industry, like many other small industries, has benefited enormously from the ongoing revolution in solid-state electronics. At the same time, the hearing aid industry has been transformed by this new technology. The cost of developing a new VLSI chip is extremely high, but once a successful chip is developed, the cost of mass producing that chip is extremely low. Because very few hearing aid companies have the resources for their own chip development, the development of solid-state components for hearing aid applications is now concentrated in a small number of companies. Gennum, Inc., for example, produces a substantial proportion of all the chips used in hearing aids worldwide. Similarly, Knowles Electronics, Inc., dominates the market with respect to the manufacture of hearing aid transducers (i.e., microphones and receivers). With respect to hearing aid selection procedures, the trend toward centralization of the component industry has had the important consequence that many of the hearing aids available for clinical use today have similar electroacoustic characteristics because essentially the same components are used by different hearing aid manufacturers.

Improvements in Component Technology

The essential components of a hearing aid are the electronic circuits, input microphone(s), output receiver(s), power supply (battery), and housing (hearing aid case or shell). As is evident from the preceding sections, the electronic circuits in hearing aids have undergone profound changes over the years. The other components of hearing aids have also undergone substantial changes, although not quite as profound. Because Chapter 1 in this volume deals more specifically with hearing aid components, it is the purpose of this section to provide only a brief outline of key historical developments in component technology, with attention to the perspective of hearing aid selection procedures.

Microphones

Microphone technology has evolved dramatically over the years and is perhaps second only to the electronic circuit in terms of the impact that these technological advances have had on hearing aids and hearing aid selection procedures. The early carbon microphones were large (by design, so as to capture as much sound as possible) and generated substantial internal noise and distortion. These were replaced by crystal piezoelectric microphones used with vacuum-tube amplifiers around 1936 that, in turn, were replaced by magnetic microphones used with transistor hearing aids, which were less fragile and more insensitive to temperature and humidity. The miniaturized balanced armature microphone was introduced in hearing aids in 1953 and was the most advanced of the magnetic microphones (Lybarger, 1988).

The invention of the field effect transistor (FET), with its very high input impedance, allowed ceramic microphones to be used in hearing aids. The FET/ceramic microphone, also based on the piezoelectric effect, had a smoother and wider frequency response than did the magnetic microphone, was more rugged, and allowed further miniaturization (Killion & Carlson, 1970). Finally, the electret condenser (electret/FET) microphone was introduced (Killion & Carlson, 1974), which further reduced vibration sensitivity and improved signal-to-noise ratio (SNR) (Staab, 1978, p. 35).

Each stage in the development of microphones for hearing aid use resulted in a microphone that was smaller, more robust, and with superior electroacoustic characteristics to its predecessor. Recent advances in microphone technology indicate that a new era has been reached in which further miniaturization is no longer a primary goal but rather the goal is increasing the role of the microphone in terms of improving the overall performance of hearing aids. For example, a directional microphone not only converts acoustic signals to electrical form, but it also helps reduce background noise by attenuating sounds coming from directions other than that of the signal.

Directional microphones were first used in hearing aids more than 30 years ago (Berger, 1975) but have not been widely used. Early directional microphones provided relatively little directionality and the advantage may not have been obvious. It is possible, however, to increase the directional characteristics of a hearing aid by using two or more microphones. The miniature microphones currently available are well suited for this application, and there is now great interest in directional hearing aids using more than one microphone. This topic is discussed further in the section on signal processing techniques later in the chapter.

Another possible application for a second microphone is to monitor the signal in the earcanal. More effective methods of hearing aid fitting and improved signal control (e.g., for reducing acoustic feedback) can be achieved by this means. Although these developments are still at the experimental stage, the direction of current research indicates that the use of multiple microphones for improved directionality and other features is likely to be an option in hearing aids of the future.

Amplifiers and Receivers

Technological limitations restricted the capability of earlier hearing aids to provide the gain and frequency response required for a patient. Subsequent improvements in amplifier and receiver technology resulted in greater capability to achieve desired electroacoustic characteristics. Older technology included class A amplifier output stages* with narrow-band receivers, and relatively simple low-frequency tone controls that provided only about 6 dB/octave attenuation. Newer technology introduced in the 1980s included class D amplifier output stages (using pulse code modulation techniques) with wide-band receivers, and much steeper rates of attenuation for low-frequency tone controls (e.g., 24 dB/octave). Sammeth et al (1993) demonstrated substantial improvements in fitting prescribed frequency responses with this new technology. An additional advantage of the class D amplifier is that it increases the dynamic range of the output stage, thereby providing greater "headroom" (i.e., additional undistorted gain to better accommodate occasional peaks in the audio signal).

The size of hearing aid receivers underwent significant change over the years from the large supra-aural earphones used in early hearing aids, to the button-type receivers that clipped on to the earmold, to the miniature receivers now being used in hearing aids small enough to fit entirely within the earcanal. As hearing aid receivers became smaller, the maximum acoustic power that could be generated also decreased. At the same time, the closer the receiver could be placed relative to the eardrum, the less the acoustic output power that was needed.

The trend toward smaller hearing aid receivers placed closer to the eardrum created a new problem for hearing aid selection and fitting procedures. Whereas the sound pressure level (SPL) at the eardrum can be predicted reasonably accurately for supra-aural transducers with acoustic coupler measurements, this is not the case for insert receivers or for any sound delivery system in which the acoustic characteristics of the earcanal are altered (e.g., by an earmold or hearing aid shell). A solution to this problem is to measure SPL in the earcanal directly. Clinical probe microphone instrumentation was introduced in the 1980s for this purpose.

Probe microphone techniques for measuring the real-ear gain of a hearing aid, although widely used, are unfortunately also subject to errors of measurement. A probe microphone measures the SPL at the tip of the probe, and the SPL at the eardrum is then inferred from this measurement. Because sound pressure varies with distance along the earcanal as a result of reflections giving rise to standing waves, the accuracy of this type of measurement depends on the distance between the probe tip and the eardrum. The skill of the audiologist in inserting the microphone probe can thus have a significant effect on the accuracy of these measurements (Hawkins & Mueller, 1986). Furthermore, the error can be quite large at frequencies above 2000 Hz because of the magnitude of the standing wave at these higher frequencies. Probe microphone measurements of real-ear gain are covered in great detail in Chapter 3 in this volume.

It is possible to circumvent the above-mentioned problem by measuring acoustic power flow in the earcanal rather than SPL. Acoustic power flow represents the acoustic power that is absorbed by the middle ear. Because it is independent of position in the canal, variations of the position of the microphone probe are not a problem. The measurement of acoustic power flow (or acoustic pressure reflectance, which is directly related to acoustic power flow) is difficult, but modern computer-based techniques have been developed for obtaining these types of measurements (Keefe, 1997; Voss & Allen, 1994). These techniques are still at the experimental stage, but clinical instrumentation using the techniques are currently under development and should be available in the foreseeable future.

Batteries

Battery technology for the power supply of hearing aids has also improved significantly over the years. With carbon and vacuum-tube hearing aids, zinc-oxide batteries were used, which were large, showed gradual reductions in voltage over time, and performed poorly in high temperatures (Berger, 1975). During World War II, the smaller and more robust mercury battery was developed with a more stable discharge characteristic. Even greater energy storage became possible with the introduction of silver-oxide batteries. In 1977 the zinc-air battery was introduced, which is less toxic, does not use relatively scarce materials, has double the capacity of mercury or silver-oxide batteries, and has a much longer shelf life (Lybarger, 1988). Lithium batteries are currently being explored for use with hearing aids, but because of the high energy storage and very low internal impedance of this battery, a short circuit with these batteries can be hazardous.

PEARL

Unlike older mercury batteries, the shelf life of modern zinc-air batteries will not be lengthened by refrigeration.

Hearing Aid Housing/Shells

Hearing aid housing was designed initially to hide the fact that hearing aids were being used. Not much has changed with respect to this cosmetic consideration, although the physical structure of hearing aid housings has undergone vast changes since these early days. Whereas the design

---

*The difference between class A and class D amplifiers is described in Chapter 1 in this volume.

considerations for pocket-worn and behind-the-ear (BTE) style hearing aids were fairly straightforward, the introduction of hearing aids that fit in the concha and/or earcanal has added complex new dimensions to the design and fabrication of appropriate housing for hearing aids. Not only is it necessary to take individual differences in the shape of the earcanal into account, but the electrical, mechanical, and chemical properties of the housing material are of much greater consequence than for body-worn or BTE hearing aids.

The current widely used approach is to take impressions of the earcanals and to create hard shells or earmolds from these impressions. Fabrication of the shells or earmolds is usually done at the hearing aid factory or earmold laboratory. Because a hard substance is used, the shells or earmolds will make contact with the inner walls of the earcanals along a narrow surface rather than making broad surface contact. The acoustic isolation provided by narrow surface contact is limited and can result in unstable acoustic feedback with high-gain hearing aids, particularly given the proximity of microphone and receiver in small instruments. Broad surface contact provides greater acoustic isolation with a concomitant reduction in acoustic feedback, but it is difficult to achieve in practice (Fifield et al, 1977, 1980).

A good fit with substantial surface contact can be obtained with little difficulty by using softer materials with a fair degree of elasticity. Earmolds that use a soft material do not last as long as those using a harder, more durable material. Universal earmolds that fit a wide range of earcanals have been developed using highly compressible materials. These earmolds, however, are not well suited for housing a hearing aid because of the lack of durability. The constraints imposed by these practical considerations have had a significant effect on hearing aid selection and fitting procedures. The issue of shells and earmolds is covered in detail in Chapter 2 in this volume.

Hearing Aid Types

Sizes and Configurations

The size of hearing aids was reduced substantially during both the vacuum-tube and transistor eras. Body aids were supplanted around 1954 by the bulky, but head-worn, eyeglass style of hearing aids with the amplifier and microphone placed in the stem of the eyeglasses (Berger, 1975). Eyeglass hearing aids offered some interesting possibilities with

respect to improving the directional and binaural characteristics of wearable hearing aids but presented difficulties in terms of selection and fitting because of the need to prescribe the eyeglass lenses, as well as the hearing aid.

Fully BTE (also called "postauricular" or "over-the-ear") models of hearing aids were introduced in the late 1950s and replaced body-worn and eyeglass hearing aids within a few years. All in-the-ear (ITE) hearing aids were also introduced initially in the late 1950s but were not practical until the introduction of IC technology in the 1960s. As the sophistication of IC and then VLSI technology increased, the size of hearing aids decreased dramatically. ITE hearing aids showed very rapid miniaturization over time from full shell (filling the entire concha area) to in-the-canal (ITC) models, and ultimately to the completely-in-the-canal (CIC) models introduced in the 1990s. The various styles of hearing aids in common use today are illustrated in Chapter 1 in this volume.

Figure 5–3 illustrates approximate percentages of U.S. hearing aid sales for each major hearing aid style in decades since 1958. A rapid growth occurred in the sale of eyeglass hearing aids as body-worn hearing aid sales declined (note that eyeglass hearing aids saw greater popularity in the United States than in Europe). Similarly, a rapid decline occurred in the sale of eyeglass hearing aids as the popularity of the BTE instruments increased. Body-worn and eyeglass hearing aids were reduced to a negligibly small fraction of the market by the 1970s and are currently limited to special applications only.

BTE hearing aids have lost substantial ground in recent years to ITE (including ITC) hearing aids but have nevertheless maintained a small but significant proportion of the market. Unlike the earlier trend in which smaller hearing aids virtually eliminated their larger predecessors, BTE hearing aids are still being introduced to the market. The reason is due to a change in marketing philosophy. Until the 1990s the thrust in hearing aid development was to produce instruments that were smaller, less noticeable, and hence cosmetically more appealing. With the introduction of small ITC and CIC hearing aids, there was little to gain cosmetically in terms of further reduction in size. Hearing aid manufacturers began, therefore, to focus on improving signal processing capabilities within the space available.

More advanced hearing aids (e.g., programmable hearing aids with multiple memories, multichannel compression hearing aids, and multimicrophone hearing aids) initially require more space than can be accommodated in a CIC shell. As a consequence, new methods of signal processing have

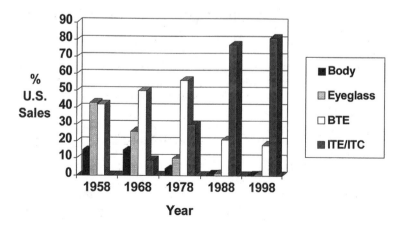

Figure 5–3 Approximate percentages of United States sales for major hearing aid styles in decades from 1958.

usually been first introduced in larger BTE models and later in smaller ITC and CIC instruments. This trend reflects an important change in the forces driving future hearing aid development. The hearing aids of the future are likely to include new forms of signal processing, providing a much wider choice for consumers and more sophisticated methods of hearing aid selection and fitting.

Effects of Ear Level Placement and Miniaturization

It should be noted that, although human vanity was the driving force behind the trend toward smaller, less visible hearing aids, the reduction in size also brought with it other advantages and shortcomings. The transition from body-worn to ear-level hearing aids eliminated body baffle effects and introduced head shadow effects, which are more natural. The term "body baffle effect" refers to the reflection and diffraction of sound around the body. This results in an increase in low-frequency gain when a microphone is placed on the body as it was in early body-worn hearing aids (Erber, 1973).

SPECIAL CONSIDERATION

Although the increase in low-frequency gain produced by the body baffle effect would be undesirable for patients with sloping high-frequency hearing loss, it can be useful for patients with "corner" audiograms (residual hearing only in the lowest audiometric frequencies) who require large amounts of low-frequency gain.

In contrast, when the microphone is placed at ear level, a head shadow effect occurs in which sound is reflected and diffracted around the head. This results in a desirable increase in high-frequency gain, and a reduction in level for sounds coming from the opposite side of the head (e.g., Skinner, 1988, pp. 105–107). The net effect is not only the provision of directional cues but also increased ease of separation of sounds coming from different directions. CIC and some ITC hearing aids may allow for pinna (and concha) resonances that are lost with occlusion by a full-shell or half-shell model. The pinna is not only useful in capturing sound and reflecting it into the earcanal, but these reflections also may increase high-frequency gain and aid in localization (Chasin, 1994).

It has been suggested that deep-canal fitting CICs also may be beneficial for other reasons, including the fact that they can produce greater real-ear output because of the reduced residual earcanal volume. Even with this advantage, however, CIC hearing aids are not powerful enough for severe to profound hearing losses. In addition, a well-fitted CIC hearing aid may reduce the occlusion effect (Mueller, 1994), in which the patient's own voice is perceived as intolerably loud when his or her ear is occluded with a hearing aid.

Hearing aids placed in the canal also open up the possibility of true binaural functioning in which head shadow effects, pinna reflections, and normal interaural differences in amplitude and phase are captured by the hearing aid. A step in this direction is the Cetera hearing aid recently

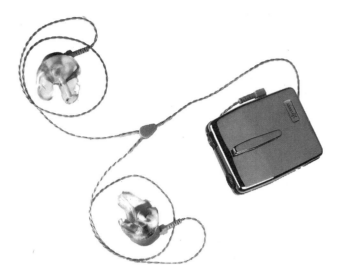

Figure 5–4   Early body hearing aid with a Y-cord for diotic presentation to the ears. (Photograph courtesy of Starkey.)

announced by Starkey Laboratories (Van Tasell, 1998). Binaural listening offers many advantages over monaural listening for normal-hearing listeners. These include summation of energy, important directional cues, the attenuation of unwanted sound that is provided by head shadow effects and pinna reflections, and reduced perceptual interference from noise and reverberation with improved localization ability resulting from binaural processing of sound (see Markides, 1977). These advantages also hold for listeners with hearing loss but to a lesser extent. The older Y-cord format used with body-worn hearing aids, although nominally a "binaural" hearing aid, eliminated important cues needed for true binaural listening. These hearing aids split the output of a single microphone and presented the amplified signal diotically (i.e., the same signal to both ears) as shown in Figure 5–4.

The current practice of using a separate hearing aid on each ear allows for dichotic listening (i.e., different signals to the two ears). The interaural differences obtained in this way can be processed binaurally by the listener, but unless these interaural differences are the same as those for normal listening, this arrangement is still not a "true" binaural hearing aid (although it may have other advantages). It remains to be seen whether a true binaural hearing aid yields performance superior to dichotic listening using two unmatched hearing aids, one on each ear.

SPECIAL CONSIDERATION

Although binaural hearing aid fittings are generally preferred for bilateral hearing losses, patients with a large asymmetry in the hearing loss, particularly one that includes a significant discrepancy in maximum speech recognition scores between the ears, may show degraded performance when a hearing aid is placed on the poorer ear.

The disadvantages of small hearing aids include increased problems with acoustic feedback and cerumen accumulation in the receiver opening, lower power output (although this problem is alleviated to some extent because the transducer is closer to the eardrum), and poorer signal processing capabilities. In addition, the use of a low-voltage battery results in increased nonlinear distortion and a poorer SNR. A remarkable aspect of hearing aid engineering is that audio signals can be amplified with only moderate amounts of nonlinear distortion and reasonably good SNR despite the considerable constraints imposed by the low battery voltage and extremely small size of these instruments.

Special-Purpose Hearing Aids and Components

Telecoils and Telephone Compatibility

A long-standing problem for hearing aid users is that acoustic feedback often occurs when a telephone receiver is held close to the hearing aid. The inductive telephone pickup component, the telecoil or "T-coil", was developed to address this problem. Early telephones used relatively strong electromagnetic (EM) fields to drive the diaphragm in the earpiece. It was found that leakage from this EM field could be used to transmit signals to an electrical coil (the telecoil) mounted inside a hearing aid, thereby bypassing the microphone and eliminating the problem of acoustic feedback when using a telephone.

The first telecoil became available in hearing aid technology in 1936 in an AC-operated desktop vacuum-tube amplifier with a large external coil, but it was not until 1946 that a telecoil was built into a wearable hearing aid (Lybarger, 1988). Telecoils are in relatively common use today and generally accessed by a switch on the hearing aid. For very small ITC or CIC hearing aids, a remotely controlled switch can be used. Remote controls are being used increasingly with hearing aids that are hard to reach by hand.

PEARL

Right-handed patients usually request that the telecoil be placed on the right-ear hearing aid (and vice versa for left-handed patients), but those who frequently need to write information down during a telephone conversation will prefer the telecoil to be placed on the opposite ear from their dominant hand.

The telecoil has proven to be very beneficial for many persons with hearing loss, particularly because the use of high-frequency emphasis and high-power amplification has increased and feedback thus becomes even more of a problem with telephone use. In addition, telecoil use can be very helpful when a patient is listening in high background noise levels or reverberation, for instance at a public pay phone in an airport terminal.

Telecoils became a practical possibility because of the substantial EM leakage in early telephones. Telephone engineers, however, ever concerned with improving the engineering efficiency of telephones, developed new types of handsets that produced very little if any EM leakage. As a consequence, it was not possible to use the telecoil input with these telephones (Gladstone, 1975). Around 1965, the major telephone companies began to introduce these new handsets in coin-operated public telephones (Staab, 1978, pp. 289-291).

Hearing aid users complained that they could no longer use their telecoils with the new telephone handsets and mounted a campaign to reintroduce EM leakage in telephones. As a response, an adapter was introduced in 1974 that could be strapped to the earpiece of the receiver to reintroduce EM leakage for telecoils (Staab, 1978), but it was fairly large and awkward to transport. In the late 1970s, the major telephone companies reintroduced handsets in public telephones with stronger EM fields that were reasonably adequate for telecoil purposes.

A solution to the problem has finally been reached as a result of federal legislation implemented in 1998. Section 255 of the Telecommunications Act requires that all new landline telephones be hearing aid compatible. Wireless (nonlandline) telephones, such as cellular telephones, are exempt from this legislation at the present time but are likely to be subject to the same requirement at some time in the future. To be hearing aid compatible (HAC), a telephone earpiece must generate an EM field that is sufficiently powerful for a hearing aid telecoil.

It is important to realize, however, that hearing aids are not required to be telephone compatible, and there are no requirements on the design of hearing aid telecoils to ensure that they couple effectively with a telephone that meets the requirements of the Telecommunications Act. This is a loophole in the legislation that places an important responsibility on the audiologist. Many hearing aid users do not make use of telecoils because they are either unaware of this capability or because they have great difficulty in coupling the hearing aid's telecoil to the telephone. Audiologists need to know which hearing aids have a telecoil that couples easily and conveniently to a modern landline telephone and to provide this information to their patients, as well as training in the use of the telecoil. In addition, patients should be counseled that some older telephones are not hearing aid compatible.

SPECIAL CONSIDERATION

Many hearing aid users either do not know about telecoils or fail to use them properly. It is an important responsibility of the audiologist to explain to patients the capabilities and limitations of telecoils, their proper use, and which telephones are hearing aid compatible (HAC). NOTE: All modern landline telephones are required to be HAC, but wireless telephones (e.g., cellular telephones) are not as yet subject to this requirement and many of these telephones are not HAC.

It should be noted that the use of telecoils is not restricted to telephones and that other electronic systems for conveying information such as traditional loop systems (for more information, see Chapters 19 and 20 in this volume) and computers can be coupled electromagnetically to hearing aids by means of the telecoil. It is anticipated that as the information revolution progresses, greater use will be made of telecoil coupling.

An emerging problem in this regard is that of "EM pollution" (Levitt, 1997). As increased use is made of EM signal transmission and there is more EM leakage from computer monitors, fluorescent lighting, and other electronic systems, the greater the possibility that audible interference in hearing aids will result from demodulation of the EM fields. The electrical components of hearing aids act as antennae for EM fields. This is particularly true of very high-frequency EM fields such as those produced by cellular telephones. In addition, digital wireless telephones, including the new digital cellular telephone, not only produce relatively strong EM fields, but these fields are modulated at rates within the audible frequency range. If an EM field of this type is picked up by the wiring or other electrical components of a hearing aid (e.g., the microphone) and the hearing aid contains one or more nonlinear components, the EM signal will be demodulated and amplified by the hearing aids. Note that this interference can be picked by any one of a number of electrical components in hearing aids and is not limited to pickup by the telecoil. In many cases the level of interference is so great that the wireless telephone cannot be used with hearing aids. It is also possible for this interference to be audible when a hearing aid user is close to someone else using a digital wireless telephone or some other source of high-frequency EM transmission.

Wireless telephone manufacturers, wireless service providers, and the hearing aid industry, with input from consumer organizations such as Self-Help for the Hard of Hearing (SHHH), are cooperating to find a practical solution to this problem. An American standard is currently being developed (ANSI Working Group PC63.19, of the Accredited Standards Committee on Electromagnetic Compatibility) on how to measure this interference and to establish criteria for acceptable levels of interference. The likely outcome will be two indices, one for wireless telephones and the other for hearing aids. The indices, when added together, will indicate expected levels of interference (e.g., whether the hearing aid/telephone combination will be useable with negligible interference, useable with audible interference, or useable in emergencies only). Audiologists will need to know the meaning of these indices and how to advise their patients with respect to the selection of hearing aids that are likely to be useable with a digital wireless telephone.

> ## PITFALL
>
> **It is a common misconception that electromagnetic (EM) interference is only a problem if a hearing aid has a telecoil. In fact, EM interference is not limited to the telecoil but can be picked up by several hearing aid components, including the microphone.**

Bone-Conduction and Implantable Hearing Aids

Some patients cannot be fitted with standard air-conduction hearing aids because of such conditions as atresia or stenosis of the earcanal, microtia of the pinna, or chronic drainage from middle ear infections. For these patients, bone-conduction

hearing aids have been an alternative, with amplified sound delivered as mechanical stimulation to the mastoid. It is interesting to note that as early as 1879, ear trumpets using bone conduction were developed for patients with conductive hearing loss, with placement either against the mastoid bone, forehead, or teeth (Berger, 1975). Similarly, although most electric hearing aids were designed for use with headphones, some early models used a vibrator and thus were the first electric bone-conduction hearing aids (Berger, 1975). Shown in Figure 5–5, for example, is a 1930 Acousticon body hearing aid that used bone-conduction transmission.

Although bone-conduction hearing aids have improved over time, serious limitations remain with respect to output power, frequency response, and transducer distortion. Figure 5–6 shows one type of conventional bone-conduction hearing aid.

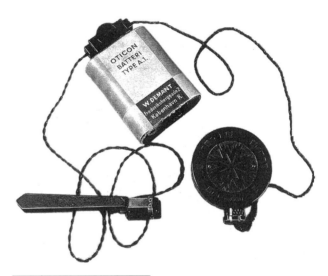

Figure 5–5 Acousticon Model 30 body hearing aid from 1930 using a carbon ball microphone with hand-held bone conductor and battery plugged into an impedance matching unit. (Photograph courtesy of Oticon.)

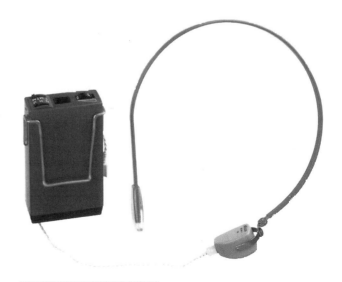

Figure 5–6 Conventional body bone-conduction hearing aid hardwired to a headband for holding the vibrator in place on the mastoid. (Photograph courtesy of Starkey.)

With the vibrator held in place by a headband, it can be difficult to obtain stable placement on the mastoid bone with these hearing aids and they are usually uncomfortable to wear. They also have poor sound quality because of technological constraints in the design of vibrators with good frequency responses. Furthermore, acoustic feedback can occur with large meatuses.

Semi-implantable bone-conduction (bone anchored) devices have also been developed, with implantation in the mastoid portion of the temporal bone (Hakansson et al, 1985; Hough et al, 1986). These devices have the potential to overcome some of the difficulties with conventional bone-conduction hearing aids and appear to be beneficial for those patients with conductive hearing losses who cannot wear air-conduction or conventional bone-conduction hearing aids successfully (Fay, 1991; Hakansson et al, 1990). Researchers have also been experimenting with middle ear implantation, with stimulation directly to the ossicles or cochlear fluids, as a means of obtaining greater power output and higher fidelity amplification in the high frequencies, without acoustic feedback (for reviews see Chasin, 1998; Maniglia, 1995). Although some patients with conductive hearing loss might also be candidates for middle ear implants, the target population is persons with sensorineural hearing loss. Detailed information on both bone anchored and middle ear implantable hearing aids can be found in Chapter 15 in this volume.

A potential problem in fitting the implantable devices (or any other nonconventional method of signal delivery) is that of specifying the sound level generated by the device. One method of specifying equivalent sound levels is to cancel the signal delivered by the implanted hearing aid with a bone-conduction signal using a calibrated bone vibrator. Because of cross-conduction between the ears, two calibrated bone conductors are needed for the cancellation process (Levitt, 1987a). In this way the sound level delivered by the implant can be referenced to an equivalent SPL delivered to a normal ear.

CROS Family of Hearing Aids

Harford and Barry (1965) described a class of special-purpose, air-conduction hearing aids that were particularly popular in the late 1960s and early 1970s. The basic (or "classic") CROS (contralateral routing of signals) hearing aid is intended for use with a patient who has an unaidable unilateral hearing loss, usually by virtue of the extent of the hearing loss (e.g., no measurable hearing or a profound impairment), but sometimes because the impaired ear should not be occluded, as with recurrent otitis media with chronic drainage. These patients, who can only listen with one ear, experience difficulty when the speaker is on the side of their impaired ear because of the head shadow effect. In the CROS hearing aid the signal is simply routed across the head to the normal or near-normal ear with little or no amplification as shown in the top of Figure 5–7.

Early versions of CROS hearing aids were in eyeglass form, so that the signal could be routed by means of wires through the eyeglass frame. With BTE hearing aids, a wire or acoustic routing tube was placed around the back of the patient's neck. Modern CROS hearing aids use wireless FM transmission, typically with a BTE hearing aid containing an FM transmitter on the unaidable ear and an ITE or BTE on the opposite side containing the receiver. Open earmolds or casing are used so

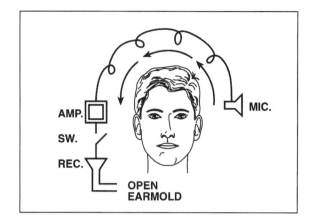

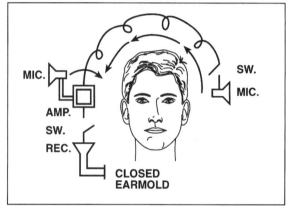

Figure 5–7   Schematic drawings illustrating the functioning of a basic CROS hearing aid *(top)*, and a BICROS hearing aid *(bottom)*.

as to interfere minimally with sound reaching the good ear and also to avoid the negative effects of occlusion.

The bilateral contralateral routing of signals (BICROS) hearing aid is intended for use with patients who have one unaidable ear but who also have aidable hearing loss in the other ear. In these instruments microphones are placed on both ears, with the output of both microphones combined and led to the aidable ear but also with appropriate amplification as shown in the bottom of Figure 5–7. Unlike the open earmold at the receiver ear in the CROS hearing aid, the BICROS hearing aid uses a more closed earmold or casing as appropriate for the hearing loss in the receiver ear.

Unlike the CROS and the BICROS hearing aids in which the purpose was to overcome the head shadow effect, some early CROS-family hearing aids were designed to take advantage of the head shadow effect to allow greater amounts of amplification before feedback. For example, the HI-CROS hearing aid was developed for patients with bilateral hearing loss in the high frequencies only. At that time, conventional hearing aids did not have sharp enough filters with a sufficiently high rate of attenuation so as to attenuate only the high frequencies without overamplifying the low frequencies. Vented earmolds were therefore used to provide additional low-frequency attenuation, which, in turn, produced feedback problems. The HI-CROS hearing aid allowed for the use of an open earmold (or casing) because the microphone and receiver were spatially far apart, thereby avoiding the problem of acoustic feedback. The POWER-CROS hearing aid was developed using a similar rationale; that is, higher gain could be provided without feedback by separating the microphone and receiver. Neither of these CROS-family hearing aids are used today because feedback, although still problematic, is less troublesome with modern hearing aids having filters with sufficiently high rates of attenuation, a smoother frequency response, and new earmold materials that provide a better seal to the ear.

Both CROS and BICROS hearing aids are still used today but less frequently than in the past, partly because fewer hearing losses are unaidable with current hearing aid technology and medical practices. Also, cosmetically conscious patients sometimes reject the notion of wearing a hearing aid on both ears when only one ear is actually receiving amplification. Further, CROS-family hearing aids do not provide binaural cues and benefits because the patient is still listening monaurally.

The newest addition to the CROS family of hearing aids is the transcranial CROS (Sullivan, 1988; Valente, 1995). In this approach, typically a powerful BTE or ITE hearing aid is placed on an ear that is too profoundly impaired for successful aiding, when the other ear has good cochlear reserve function (either normal-hearing, a conductive hearing loss, and/or a mild sensorineural hearing loss). Although the ear on which the hearing aid is placed is not expected to benefit from the power hearing aid, the amplified signal is assumed to cross, by means of bone conduction, to the unimpaired (or minimally impaired) cochlea of the other ear. Pulec (1994) used an implantable bone-anchored hearing aid on the side of a dead ear for the same effect.

CONTROVERSIAL POINT

For a unilateral "dead" ear, should a conventional CROS or a transcranial CROS fitting be tried? According to Valente et al (1995a), conventional CROS amplification may be most effective if the better (aided) ear has at least a mild high-frequency hearing loss, whereas a transcranial CROS may be a better choice if hearing thresholds for the better ear are normal across the audiometric frequencies. A transcranial CROS fitting may also be more acceptable to a patient who, for cosmetic reasons, does not want to wear a hearing aid on both ears.

The Digital Era

The "Computerized" Hearing Aid

Hearing aids from the electric era to those that use transistors all fall under the general umbrella of "analog technology." In analog hearing aids the acoustic waveform, which is a continuous function of time, is transduced by the microphone into an electric waveform with a shape *analogous* to the acoustic waveform and the signal remains a continuous function of time throughout all processing stages. A block diagram of the components of an analog hearing aid is shown in Figure 5–8A.

In the last decade we have seen the introduction of hearing aids that fall under the umbrella of "digital technology," including analog/digital hybrid hearing aids, sampled data hearing aids, and so-called true digital hearing aids. In the hybrid hearing aid, shown in Figure 5–8B, digital techniques are used to control analog components (e.g., amplifiers, filters). Note, however, that the audio signal remains in analog form at all times.

In a sampled data hearing aid, shown in the upper half of Figure 5–9, an analog audio signal is sampled at regular time intervals to produce a sequence of discrete pulses, with the height of each pulse corresponding to the value of the waveform at each sampled instant. These discrete pulses are then processed, usually by means of switched capacitor technology in which the samples are stored as charges in a series of capacitors. These charges are then switched from one set of capacitors to another according to a prescribed algorithm so as to perform the necessary signal processing. After the processing has been completed, the stored electric charges are converted back to an analog waveform.

This is contrasted with a true digital (digital signal processing; DSP) hearing aid, as shown in the lower half of Figure 5–9, in which the audio signal is first sampled and then the magnitude of each sample is converted to binary form and represented by a series of 0s and 1s. This process is performed by an analog-to-digital (A/D) convertor. These binary numbers are then processed using techniques commonly employed in digital computers. After signal processing has been completed, the binary signals are converted back to analog form by a digital-to-analog (D/A) convertor. Low-pass filters are required before the A/D convertor and after the D/A convertor to avoid introducing distortions known as aliasing and imaging errors, respectively. For the interested reader, a number of reviews of the history of digital hearing aids, and the differences between analog and digital hearing aids, are available (see Hussung & Hamill, 1990; Levitt, 1987b, 1988, 1993; Schweitzer, 1997; Sammeth, 1989; Staab, 1985). For a brief nonmathematical tutorial on digital signal processing, see the appendix in Levitt (1987b).

Shown in Figures 5–8C and 5–8D are block diagrams of two forms of digital hearing aids. In Figure 5–8C, a modern digital hearing aid representative of today's technology is illustrated. Hearing aids of this type have a constrained architecture in that processing is limited to multichannel amplification, albeit with tremendous flexibility in controlling amplification characteristics (e.g., filtering, compression) in each channel. In Figure 5–8D, a more sophisticated digital hearing aid is illustrated in which processing is not constrained to a specific form. Digital hearing aids of this latter type are expected to be available in the very near future.

Table 5–1 lists some of the important historical events in the development of digital technology in hearing aids. Digital technology allows many forms of sophisticated processing, but it is not without limitations. Sampling rate and computational speed were initially the major constraints limiting the application of digital technology to the processing of audio signals. Although an experimental system for encoding and processing speech by digital means was developed during World War II (Hodges, 1983), digital processing of audio signals did not become a practical reality until the early 1960s when A/D converters operating at sampling rates fast

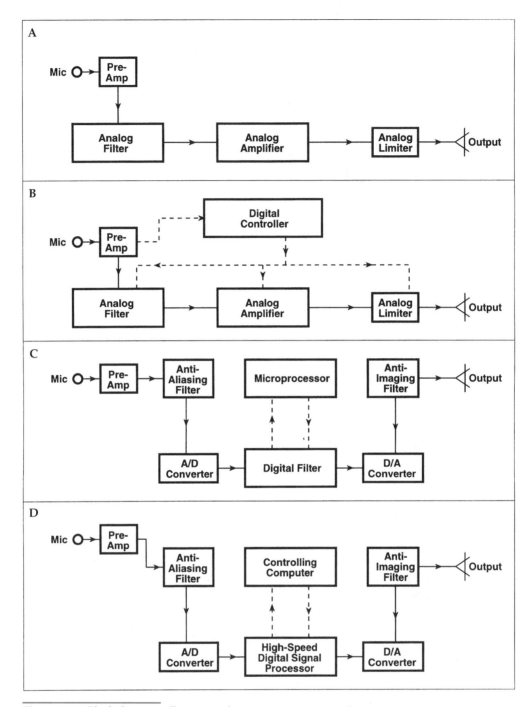

Figure 5–8 Block diagrams illustrating the major components of **(A)** an analog hearing aid, **(B)** an analog/digital hybrid hearing aid, **(C)** a DSP hearing aid with constrained architecture, typically multichannel compression, and **(D)** a DSP hearing aid of the future, with open architecture. Solid lines indicate the amplified signal pathway, and dashed lines indicate information and control signals. (Adapted from Levitt et al [1987a] with permission).

enough and with sufficient precision for audio signals were developed (Bloom, 1985).

Progress in the development of DSP techniques for speech and other audio signals accelerated rapidly once a practical means of digitizing these signals became available. An important milestone during this period was the development of the block diagram compiler (known as BLODI; Kelly et al, 1961). As its name indicates, the input to BLODI consisted simply of a block diagram of the audio system to be simulated, thereby greatly simplifying the task of simulating audio systems on a digital computer. It was possible with this software to simulate a complex audio system, such as an advanced signal

SAMPLED-DATA SYSTEM

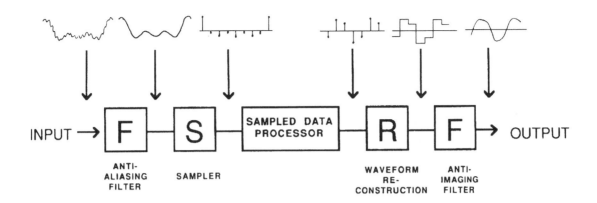

ALL-DIGITAL SYSTEM

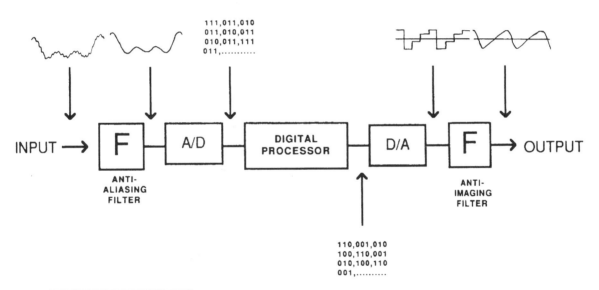

Figure 5–9 The upper block diagram represents an analog sampled–data system. It consists of an anti-aliasing filter, a sampling circuit, a signal processor for operating on sampled-data sequences, a circuit for waveform reconstruction, and an anti-imaging filter. The lower block diagram represents an all-digital or DSP system. It consists of an anti-aliasing filter, an A/D converter containing both a sampler and a circuit for converting the samples to binary form, a digital signal processor, a D/A converter, and an anti-imaging filter. (Reprinted from Levitt [1987b] with permission).

processing multichannel hearing aid, in a minute fraction of the time that it would take for a team of skilled engineers to build such a system.

Despite the substantive advances being made during this period in the digital processing of audio signals, a major limitation still remained and that was the relatively slow computational speed of digital computers. For example, by the end of the 1960s, the time taken for relatively simple forms of signal processing typically exceeded the duration of the signal being processed by more than 100 times (i.e., processing times were more than 100 times *real time*). As a consequence, almost all the work on computer processing of

TABLE 5–1   Some important events in the history of digital technology in hearing aids

	Analog/Digital Hybrid and Quasi-Digital:
1977	Graupe and Causey receive a patent for an analog/digital hybrid adaptive filtering algorithm (Graupe & Causey, 1977).
1979	Mangold and Leijon report experimental multichannel compression hearing instrument using analog/digital hybrid technology (Mangold & Leijon, 1979).
1986	Commercial release of the Intellitech Zeta Noise Blocker microchip for signal processing based on the Graupe-Causey algorithm. It was later withdrawn from the market.
1987	Commercial introduction of a digitally programmable BTE by Audiotone (see D'Amico, 1989).
1988-	Six more digitally programmable hearing aids introduced to the market, including ITE models.
1989	Multiple memory capability, digital remote control, and advanced fitting systems appear. Some of these early models were later withdrawn from the market.
1992	Danavox introduces partially digital power BTE for control of feedback (Dyrlund & Bisgaard, 1991).
1997	Within one decade from the initial introduction, nearly every hearing aid manufacturer offers a line of digitally programmable hearing aids with styles ranging from BTEs to CICs, and sophisticated forms of multichannel signal processing.
	"True" Digital (Digital Signal Processing; DSP):
1967	Researchers at Bell Laboratories simulate digital amplification with a large laboratory computer.
1975	Graupe and Causey report the development of a nonwearable model of a digital hearing aid using an 8080 microprocessor (Graupe & Causey, 1975).
1980	Moser receives a patent for a digital hearing aid (Moser, 1980).
1982	Levitt reports the development of a nonwearable digital hearing aid based on an array processor (Levitt, 1982).
1983	First report in the literature of an experimental body-worn digital hearing aid (Nunley et al, 1983).
1987	First commercial introduction of a DSP hearing aid, with the microphone on a BTE connected via hardwire to a body-worn processor. This hearing aid, the Nicolet Phoenix, was later withdrawn from the market.
1996	Commercial introduction by Oticon and Widex of digital signal processing hearing aids housed entirely in at-the-ear packaging.
1997–1998	Several more "true" digital hearing aids introduced to the market, and DSP hearing aids available even in CIC style.

Adapted from Sammeth (1989) with permission.

speech and other complex audio signals was done off-line (i.e., not in real time). Even with the constraints imposed by off-line processing, substantial progress was made in developing the tools of DSP and methods of computer simulation (see Flanagan, 1965; Levitt, 1987b).

Most of the work during this period focussed on DSP techniques for normal-hearing people. There were, however, a few attempts to apply this technology to help develop sensory aids for people with hearing loss (Guttman & Nelson, 1968; Levitt, 1973). One practical outcome was the development of an improved high-gain telephone handset for hard-of-hearing people. Although the handset itself did not use DSP, digital techniques were used in the development and evaluation of the prototype handset.

Progress in the development and application of DSP techniques for patients with hearing loss was relatively slow at first because of the technological limitations noted previously.

The advent of the laboratory computer allowed for the development of hybrid systems consisting of computer-controlled analog equipment. Experimental amplification systems of this type were used as research tools during this period (Braida et al, 1979; Lippman et al, 1981). At the same time, engineers began working toward digital hearing aids for personal use (Graupe & Causey, 1975; Mangold & Leijon, 1979; 1981). The 3M Corporation eventually marketed an instrument that was based on the work of Mangold and Leijon (1979, 1981). The idea of using a digital computer rather than digitally controlled analog components in a hearing aid was patented by Moser in 1980, but a hearing aid using this concept was not actually built.

The development of the array processor in the mid 1970s opened the door to real-time digital processing of speech signals. The array processor is a special-purpose computer in which whole arrays of numbers are processed simultaneously, rather than one number at a time as is the case in conventional computers. With an array processor it became possible to process speech digitally in real time (i.e., with a negligible delay between input and output). In 1982 a true digital hearing aid was developed configured around a high-speed array processor (Levitt, 1982). The device was not wearable but was used as an experimental master hearing aid in a series of investigations exploring the capabilities of digital hearing aids (Levitt & Neuman, 1991; Levitt et al, 1986a, 1987, 1990, 1993; Neuman et al, 1987). It is interesting to note that this first digital hearing aid actually had an open architecture similar to that shown in Figure 5–8D. Wearable versions of digital hearing aids with an open architecture are expected to be available in the very near future.

Another major advance after the array processor was the development of special-purpose DSP microchips that were designed specifically for high-speed signal processing (such as the TMS320 produced by Texas Instruments). These DSP chips mounted on plug-in boards with supporting software could be used in a personal computer, thereby allowing for the development of relatively inexpensive digital master hearing aids and hearing aid fitting systems (Levitt, 1992; Levitt et al, 1986b; Popelka & Engebretson, 1983; Sullivan et al, 1987). Of greater significance was the fact that the DSP chips were small enough to be housed in a wearable unit. Several experimental body-worn digital hearing aids that used the DSP chips were subsequently developed (Cummins & Hecox, 1987; Engebretson, 1987; Engebretson et al, 1986; Levitt et al, 1988; Nunley et al, 1983).

Early attempts at developing a practical wearable digital hearing aid were not successful, however, because of the relatively large size and power requirements of the DSP chips (compared with the analog microchips being used in hearing aids at that time). The first true digital hearing aid to be marketed, the Nicolet Phoenix, had a body-worn unit with a hardwire connection to a BTE earpiece and multiple batteries with relatively limited battery life (see Hecox & Miller, 1988; Roeser & Taylor, 1988; Sammeth, 1990). Although this instrument embodied many significant advances in hearing aid design, including the development of special-purpose digital circuitry, it was not a commercial success. Schweitzer (1992) also reported the limited introduction overseas of a body hearing aid using DSP by the Japanese company Rion, but it was never released in the United States. Despite the fact that these early products were not successful commercially, they nevertheless demonstrated that wearable, true digital hearing aids were a practical possibility.

At the same time, traditional hearing aid manufacturers and other companies with expertise in digital technology (e.g., 3M Corporation and AT&T, whose hearing aid venture was acquired by ReSound in 1987) began to develop and market analog/digital hybrid hearing aids. Hybrid technology was easier to implement in small size instruments at that time and did not have the large power requirements of DSP. Although these instruments were not true digital hearing aids, they incorporated several important features that were beyond the capability of conventional analog hearing aids; they could be programmed digitally, programs could be stored in memory, and the electroacoustic characteristics of the hearing aid could be changed virtually instantaneously at the touch of a button. The fitting and adjustment of

digitally programmable hearing aids was (and is) accomplished by means of a disconnectable hardwire to a computer or other programming device.

In the 1980s, the first sampled-data hearing aids using switched capacitor technology were marketed, such as the Ensoniq Sound Selector and the Argosy 3-Channel-Clock. The use of sampled-data technology allowed for extremely precise and flexible frequency shaping. The capability of controlling both the amplitude and phase characteristics of a filter with great precision using sampled-data signal processing techniques opened up the possibility of automatic feedback cancellation in a hearing aid. This can be done by establishing an electrical feedback path that is equal in amplitude but opposite in phase to that of the acoustic feedback path in the hearing aid. The acoustic feedback can then be canceled by adding the output of the two feedback paths (Levitt et al, 1988). The Danavox DFS (Digital Feedback Suppression), a power BTE hearing aid introduced in 1992 (Dyrlund & Bisgaard, 1991; Smriga, 1993) uses digital signal processing techniques to accomplish active feedback suppression in this manner.

A signal processing microchip produced by Intellitech Company and known as the "zeta noise blocker" (ZNB, or simply Zeta) also used hybrid technology, but for purposes of adaptive filtering for noise reduction. This chip was incorporated into hearing aids from several manufacturers in the latter part of the 1980s, with processing based on an algorithm developed by Graupe and Causey (1977) using principles of adaptive Wiener filtering (Graupe et al, 1986; 1987). Some clinical benefit from the ZNB was reported (Graupe et al, 1987; Stein & Dempsey-Hart, 1984; Wolinsky, 1986), as well as less than positive experimental results (Van Tasell et al, 1988, 1992). The ZNB was not commercially successful, however, and is no longer manufactured.

Digital technology has continued to advance, and practical, true digital hearing aids have recently been introduced for clinical use. For a period of time in the 1980s a joint collaboration of Danish hearing aid manufacturers (known as "Project Odin") investigated noise reduction for hearing aids using DSP techniques. In 1996 two of these companies introduced true digital hearing aids to the commercial market (the Oticon Digifocus and Widex Senso). Since then, a number of other manufacturers also have marketed true digital hearing aids, and they are now available in BTE, ITE, and CIC versions.

SPECIAL CONSIDERATION

Although digital technology has much to offer, it does not follow that any digital hearing aid will be necessarily superior to any analog hearing aid. Specific devices need to be evaluated on the merit of the signal processing and other capabilities, with respect to the needs, desires, and resources of each individual patient.

Like the programmable hybrid hearing aids, fitting and adjustment of true digital hearing aids is controlled by digital software. When digitally programmable hearing aids first entered the market in the late 1980s, each company produced its own stand-alone programming unit. This was an inefficient approach to the problem and also very expensive for the audiologist to acquire programming units for each brand of hearing aid. An early attempt to create a "universal" programming unit was Siemens's Programmable Multi-Channel (PMC) device, which allowed up to five erasable programmable read-only memory (EPROM) modules to be plugged in for different manufacturers (see Sammeth, 1990). A more cost-effective approach is to use an inexpensive personal computer, now commonly used with a general purpose interface known as a HI-PRO (Hearing Instrument Programmer) box. A special-purpose module and cable connections are needed to access the products of a given manufacturer. The use of these modules protects the proprietary information of each manufacturer while at the same time providing a common hardware platform for controlling the hearing aids of a large number of manufacturers. Shown in Figure 5–10 is a hearing aid connected by means of a HI-PRO box to a modern fitting system.

In addition to the common hardware platform, it is also helpful to have a common software platform. One such platform, known as NOAH, was developed by the Hearing Instrument Manufacturers Software Association (HIMSA) in 1993. The use of NOAH allows audiologists to manage their patient database regardless of which manufacturer's software is used and to automatically transfer information to and from NOAH-compatible measurement and fitting systems.

The economics of solid state circuit development, as previously noted, involve a substantial capital outlay followed by large-scale manufacture and sale of low-cost chips. The larger the market for mass-produced chips, the larger the incentive for more substantial capital investments resulting

in even more advanced solid state chips. Digital microchips using VLSI technology are a direct result of the economics of chip development.

The trend to universal applicability is a key characteristic of digital chips, because these chips can be programmed to perform a very wide variety of functions. The same digital chip can thus be used for an extremely wide range of different applications. As a consequence, digital chips are particularly attractive in terms of the economics of mass production. Furthermore, the versatility of digital circuits combined with their low per-unit cost resulting from large-scale production has created an ever-increasing range of new applications for this technology. The economic forces at work have thus produced self-sustaining growth in that the steps taken to meet the growing demand for digital technology have generated an even greater demand. To be competitive, manufacturers have steadily improved the quality of their products by increasing the computational capabilities of their digital chips, while at the same time reducing their size and power requirements. Because of the economies of scale, these improvements have also been accompanied by reductions in cost. No evidence exists yet that the demand for digital technology is approaching saturation and thus the trend toward smaller, cheaper, and computationally more powerful digital chips is likely to continue for some time to come.

Some engineering compromises have been necessary to achieve the remarkable degree of digital microminiaturization in hearing aids. The true digital hearing aids that are currently available are constrained to a specific architecture (that of a multichannel compression hearing aid as described in the next section), although they have considerably more flexibility in terms of programming their electroacoustic characteristics than was available on the older digitally controlled analog hearing aids. Progress in digital technology is expected to continue unabated. Hearing aids of even greater

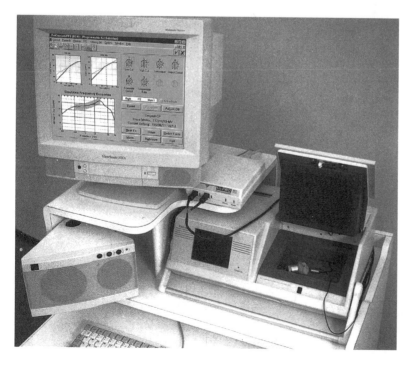

Figure 5–10   A modern hearing aid fitting system with a HI-PRO box and computer for programming of hearing aids. (Photograph courtesy of Starkey.)

flexibility and signal processing capabilities will thus undoubtedly be developed in the years to come. Several companies are already working on digital microchips that will allow for hearing aids to be designed with an open (i.e., relatively unconstrained) architecture. The implications of these developments for future hearing aid development and fitting procedures are immense.

HISTORY OF SIGNAL PROCESSING APPROACHES IN HEARING AIDS

For many years, hearing aids were linear amplifiers (i.e., the output level in dB equaled input level in dB plus gain in dB) so that an increase of x dB in input level produced an identical increase of x dB in output level. It was only at very high input levels that the output of these hearing aids began to saturate (i.e., the hearing aid was no longer linear). Linear amplification over a very wide dynamic range such that saturation was seldom reached was appropriate for most patients in the early days of hearing aid development, because these patients had primarily conductive hearing losses or mixed hearing losses with a mild sensorineural component. These patients typically desire large amounts of gain.

Improvements in the medical/surgical treatment of conductive disorders and the recognition that patients with moderate-to-severe sensorineural hearing losses can be helped with acoustic amplification have altered the demographics of hearing aid prescription. For sensorineural hearing losses, it is important to limit the output of hearing aids at a much lower level than was previously the case. Consequently, modern conventional hearing aids operate linearly over a limited dynamic range. To address the issue of limited dynamic range in sensorineural hearing impairment, new methods of signal processing have been developed, such as multichannel amplitude compression.

In contrast to patients with conductive hearing loss and normal-hearing persons, it is well known that cochlear-impaired patients need a more favorable SNR to achieve their best speech recognition ability in background noise (Cooper & Cutts, 1971; Dirks et al, 1982; Plomp, 1978). How much of the performance deficits are simply caused by the loss of sensitivity itself combined with masking effects of environmental noise, as opposed to nonaudibility factors, is still debated (Humes, 1991). Patients with cochlear hearing loss often have abnormal loudness growth functions (recruitment), and particularly for losses greater than about 60 dB HL (Van Tasell, 1993), suprathreshold deficits in frequency and temporal resolution may be present (e.g., Dreschler & Plomp, 1985; Glasberg & Moore, 1989; Stelmachowicz et al, 1985; see Moore, 1996, for a review). In elderly subjects, often an age-related deterioration of cognitive skills and of central auditory processing ability may also exacerbate problems recognizing speech (i.e., phonemic regression) in noise (van Rooij & Plomp, 1990).

Various forms of nonlinear signal processing have been tried in hearing aids in an attempt to address these problems, and, in particular, to provide greater assistance in adverse listening environments (see Moore, 1996; Preves, 1990; Sammeth & Ochs, 1991; Schweitzer, 1997). To understand the implications of these new methods of signal processing for hearing aid selection and fitting, it is necessary to provide an overview of amplitude compression and methods of nonlinear signal processing for noise reduction and speech enhancement. Further information on signal processing is available in Chapters 1, 6, and 13 in this volume.

Amplitude Compression

The earliest hearing aids consisted of no more than an amplifier with fixed gain and frequency response. The advent of the electronic hearing aid allowed for some limited shaping of the frequency responses of hearing aids, thereby giving rise to the concept of frequency-selective amplification. As the amplification capabilities of electronic hearing aids improved, including the capability of producing amplified signals of high intensity, the need to limit maximum power output for patient comfort and safety became apparent.

A very simple method first used to limit the output power of a linear electronic amplifier was that of peak clipping. In this form of limiting the output voltage is not allowed to exceed a maximum amplitude (i.e., the peaks of the output signal are simply "clipped"). Peak clipping became the preferred method of output limiting early in the electronic era and remained so until the introduction of compression amplification. In fact, output limiting by means of peak clipping is still used, but it is gradually losing ground to more sophisticated methods of controlling the output of hearing aids. The major problem with peak clipping is that it produces significant amounts of harmonic distortion, especially for high-gain instruments. Studies done in the 1960s showed that this distortion was detrimental to speech recognition and long-term success with hearing aids (Jerger et al, 1966a; Kasten & Lotterman, 1967; Kretsinger & Young, 1960; Olson & Wilbur, 1968).

Amplitude compression techniques, which had previously been used for other applications such as loudspeaker systems, were thus introduced for use in hearing aids as an alternative to peak clipping. Amplitude compression produces far less nonlinear distortion than peak clipping, with concommitant improvements in intelligibility (Abramowitz, 1980). Lybarger (1988) reports that the first proposed use of compression for hearing aids was in the vacuum-tube era, but it was not widely used. The current trend toward more sophisticated signal processing in modern hearing aids has resulted in a wide variety of compression techniques being introduced.

The Many Forms of Amplitude Compression

Compression amplification in general refers to the process by which the level of the signal being amplified controls the gain of the amplifier. This process can be implemented in many different ways. In *output compression* the signal level at the output is used to control the gain of the amplifier; in *input compression* the signal level at the input controls amplifier gain. Usually a compression amplifier reduces the range of output signal levels (i.e., an increase in signal level produces a reduction in gain). Note, however, that a compression amplifier can also act as an "expander." In this situation, an increase in signal level produces an increase in gain. Forms of expansion have been explored experimentally in hearing aids (Preves et al, 1991; Sammeth et al, 1996; Walker et al, 1984) but there has been limited commercial application to date. The Widex Senso, a DSP hearing aid currently on the market, uses low-level expansion to reduce the effects of circuit noise.

A common form of compression amplification, known as compression limiting, introduces a substantial reduction in gain when the signal being amplified reaches a critical level. This technique effectively limits the output level of a hearing aid and is used as an alternative to peak clipping to ensure that dangerously loud or uncomfortable levels do not reach the ear of the listener. Limiting only occurs at high input levels (e.g., 80 dB SPL), and the speech signal at lower input levels is still processed linearly.

Another form of compression amplification is known as wide (or "full") dynamic range compression (WDRC), in which compression begins at relatively low input levels. One of the characteristics of cochlear hearing loss, in contrast to conductive hearing loss, is that the threshold of discomfort (the level at which sounds become uncomfortably loud), is often the same or even lower than that of a normal-hearing person because of loudness recruitment. If linear gain is supplied to ensure audibility of soft speech components, louder speech components may be peak clipped or heavily compressed and therefore not available to the patient. In an attempt to "squeeze" the larger dynamic range of environmental sounds into the smaller listening dynamic range found in many patients with cochlear hearing loss, compression has been applied to act at lower input levels. The first attempts at wider range amplitude compression began to compress the signal above about 60 dB SPL. Many modern WDRC hearing aids begin to compress above about 40 dB SPL and thus act on levels over a substantial range.

Static Characteristics

The differences among various compression hearing aids are defined by several key parameters of the compressor amplifier. One of these is the compression ratio (CR), which is equal to the ratio of the change in input level (in dB) to the change in output level (in dB). For example, if an increase in signal level of 30 dB at the input of a compression amplifier results in an increase of only 10 dB at the output of the amplifier, then

$$CR = 30/10 = 3{:}1.$$

Most compression amplifiers also have a parameter known as the compression threshold (also known as the breakpoint or kneepoint), below which the system behaves as a conventional (linear) amplifier and above which compression occurs.

The static characteristics of a compression amplifier are usually represented by a diagram of the input-output function, as shown in Figure 5–11. Three curves are shown. The solid curve shows the input-output relationship for a compression amplifier with a high compression threshold and a high CR. The input stimulus level at the compression threshold in this example is 80 dB SPL, with a corresponding output level of 100 dB SPL (breakpoint A). Thus input signals with levels less than 80 dB SPL are amplified linearly without compression.

The gain of the amplifier below the compression threshold (on the linear portion of the function) is equal to output level minus input level, which is equal to 20 dB for all input signals less than 80 dB SPL. In contrast, for input signal levels above 80 dB SPL, the amplifier gain decreases systematically as the input level goes up. The CR at these levels is 10:1,

meaning that an increase in input level of 10 dB above 80 dB SPL produces an increase in output level of only 1 dB. The output level for an input level of 90 dB SPL is thus 101 dB SPL, which is only marginally higher than the output level at the onset of compression.

Note that at a very high input level of 110 dB SPL, the output level would only be 103 dB (i.e., the output level is actually less than the input level under these conditions). The point at which input level equals output level is known as the zero gain point. For the compression amplifier under consideration, zero gain occurs when the input level is 102 dB SPL. The formula for output level in a compression amplifier is:

(Input level − Input compression threshold)/
CR + Output level at compression threshold

Substituting in the above yields (102 (−) 80)/10 + 100 dB SPL = 102 dB SPL, which is equal to the input level of 102 dB SPL.

The second, dashed curve in Figure 5–11 has two breakpoints (B1, B2), one at an input compression threshold of 50 dB SPL, the second at an input level of 90 dB SPL known as the input saturation threshold. This type of amplifier is often implemented as an input compression circuit, so that the manual gain control also affects the output of the hearing aid. For signal levels below 50 dB, the system acts as a conventional amplifier (i.e., the slope of the input-output curve in this region is 1). Note that the gain over the linear range (output level minus input level) is 30 dB. For signals with levels between 50 dB SPL and 90 dB SPL, which typically includes speech, the system behaves as a compression amplifier with a CR of 2:1 (i.e., slope of input/output curve = 1/2 = 0.5). For input levels above the saturation threshold of 90 dB SPL, the CR is 10:1, yielding a slope of 1/10 = 0.1 for the input/output curve at these high input levels.

The third, dotted curve in Figure 5–11 shows the input/output relationship for a more complex compression system. The curve has no breakpoints identifying well-defined thresholds. Instead, the slope of the curve varies continuously from a slope of greater than one below an input level of 50 dB SPL, to a slope that is approximately one between 50 dB SPL and 65 dB SPL, to a slope that falls well below one at input levels above 90 dB SPL. Thus the characteristics of the compression amplifier represented by the dotted curve are moderate expansion for input signal levels below 50 dB SPL, linear amplification for input signal levels between 50 dB SPL and 65 dB SPL, and substantial compression for input signal levels above 90 dB SPL.

The curves shown in Figure 5–11 are representative of three very different types of compression amplification. The solid curve, in which there is a high compression threshold and a high CR acts as a compression limiter, an alternative to peak clipping to ensure that maximum output levels of the hearing aid are not dangerously or uncomfortably high. The dashed curve, representing a device with a low compression threshold and a low CR is of the WDRC type, proposed for use with patients who have limited listening dynamic ranges (difference between hearing threshold and uncomfortable loudness level). The dotted curve represents an experimental system with curvilinear compression.

Dynamic Characteristics

A compression amplifier is also characterized by its temporal dynamics. Most compression amplifiers require a short period

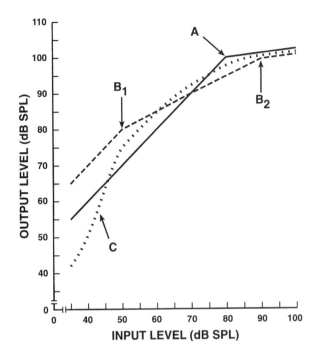

Figure 5–11   Input-output functions illustrating (*A*) compression limiting (*solid line*), with compression threshold A; (*B*) WDRC (*dashed line*), with two compression thresholds B_1 and B_2; and (*C*) experimental curvilinear compression (*dotted line*).

of time to determine the average or peak level of the signal being amplified before adjusting the gain of the amplifier. This time period is known as the attack time. Specifically, it is defined as the time taken for the output of the compression amplifier to come within 3 dB of its steady state level after an abrupt increase in input signal level (ANSI S3.22-1996). The inverse of attack time is release time, which is the time taken for the compression amplifier to come within 4 dB of its new steady state level after an abrupt decrease in input signal level.

The idea of using different time constants for attack and release time in hearing aids was based on the observation that a sudden increase in input sound level could be both uncomfortable and potentially hazardous for the hearing aid user. It was thus considered necessary to reduce the gain for such sounds before the total energy of the amplified sound exceeded an acceptable limit. Attack times of about 50 ms or less are generally considered to be short enough for this application. Very short release times, on the other hand, give rise to an effect known as "pumping" in which low-level background noise is amplified to relatively loud levels during short pauses in the speech. A relatively long release time avoids this problem. Too long a release time, however, creates the phenomenon of "dead time" in which no sound is audible for a short period after a strong transient sound has been compressed.

Hearing aids with more than one release time were introduced by the Telex Corporation in the 1980s (Smriga, 1985), followed by similar releases from other companies. A very short, loud transient (like a door slamming) results in a short release time, whereas an ongoing high-level stimuli (like speech in background noise) produces a longer release time. These adaptive time constant devices provide a practical compromise between the conflicting constraints imposed on the choice of release time.

Some experimental compression amplifiers have a different form of dynamic behavior that is not well specified in terms of attack and release times, such as feed-forward compression

(also called simply forward compression), in which the signal in a given time window is analyzed and a decision made as to how to modify the gain. In this form of compression, the reduction in gain may begin shortly before an increase in signal level.

The term automatic gain (volume) control (AGC or AVC), is used to describe compression amplifiers that have long time constants before effecting a change in gain. AGC was introduced so as to reduce the need to change the gain control setting for varying listening conditions. According to the Swedish Medical Board (Johansson & Lindblad, 1971), hearing aids with release times exceeding 150 ms should be considered AGC hearing aids, whereas Dillon (1988) defines AGC as a release time exceeding 200 ms. Hearing aids with short release times are often referred to as "syllabic compression" hearing aids. The term is not technically correct because these instruments actually provide different amounts of compression for individual speech sounds (phonemes) rather than for whole syllables, as the name implies.

CONTROVERSIAL POINT

No agreement exists at present as to whether syllabic compression is significantly better than automatic gain control with a long release time. The high variability in performance seen across patients suggests a continuing need for research into better candidacy criteria to guide selection of the most benefitial form of compression (or other signal processing) for an individual patient.

The terms "linear amplifier" and "nonlinear amplifier" can also be misleading when they are used to distinguish between peak-clipping and compression amplification. A conventional amplifier with peak clipping to limit the output operates as a linear amplifier for signals below the peak-clipping level, but signals exceeding this level are subjected to substantial nonlinear distortion. Also, an amplifier with compression limiting operates as a linear amplifier for signals below the compression threshold. Signals exceeding the compression-limiting threshold are subject to some nonlinear distortion while the gain is changing, but once the gain has stabilized at a new value, the amplifier operates linearly once again. Furthermore, the amount of nonlinear distortion generated while the gain is changing is quite small in a well-designed compression amplifier. Other forms of signal processing are highly nonlinear, such as spectrum subtraction for noise reduction, so perhaps the term nonlinear amplification should be reserved for hearing aids embodying these highly nonlinear forms of signal processing.

Multichannel Compression

The discussion of compression amplification has, thus far, assumed that only a single channel of amplification is involved. Single-channel compression was used experimentally in the 1950s and saw limited clinical use in the 1970s. Today, single-channel compression hearing aids are common alternatives to linear/peak-clipping instruments. However, one of the criticisms of single-channel amplification is that many speech sounds (and noises) have considerably more acoustic power in the low frequencies, although the weaker high-frequency content of the sound contains important information for identification of the sound. In a single-channel compressor, amplifier gain is determined by overall signal level and, as a result, speech sounds of the above type (or speech in noise) are compressed because of the strong low-frequency components, thereby providing insufficient gain for the weak high-frequency components. In fact, although single-channel instruments may be beneficial for some patients in terms of loudness comfort, much of the early research literature comparing single-channel compression, usually syllabic compression, with linear/peak-clipping hearing aids failed to support compression for speech recognition, showing either no differences or even poorer performance for the compression system (for reviews, see Braida et al, 1979; Walker & Dillon, 1982).

One approach to the problem with single-channel compression is to provide different amounts of compression in different frequency regions. This can be done by means of multichannel compression (Villchur, 1973). In this form of compression the incoming signal is filtered into two or more frequency bands (ranges). Each frequency band is amplified by a separate compression amplifier. When hearing aid technology evolved in the mid 1980s to the point where multiple channels (frequency bands) could be handled differently, compression hearing aids became a viable solution for some patients. The amplification characteristics of each of the separate channels of the hearing aid can be designed to match the spectrotemporal characteristics of the incoming speech signal to that of the impaired auditory system so that, at the output, the various frequency components of the speech signal are amplified appropriately within the patient's available dynamic range.

It was initially recommended that the compressors in the various channels operate independently and that WDRC with short time constants (i.e., syllabic compression) be used (Villchur, 1973). Independent compression in separate channels, however, can destroy important phonetic information, such as overall spectral shape (Haggard et al, 1987; Plomp, 1988). Alternate, experimental methods of multichannel compression have been tried in which compression in different regions of the frequency spectrum operates interdependently (Bustamante & Braida, 1987; Levitt & Neuman, 1991).

Multichannel compression also need not be restricted to WDRC. Many of the multichannel compression hearing aids currently available, for example, use compression limiting. Moore and colleagues (Laurence et al, 1983; Moore & Glasberg, 1986, 1988) have investigated a complex compression system that uses multistage and multichannel processing. In their approach a slow-acting AGC amplifier at the front end of the system is followed by splitting the signal into two channels for subsequent syllabic compression in each channel.

Much controversy exists in the field as to the relative merits of multichannel compression versus single-channel compression. Villchur (1973) in his research on multichannel systems showed significant improvements in speech recognition, but these improvements were obtained against a reference condition that was not the most effective method of single-channel amplification. Subsequent experiments reported conflicting results. For example, Barfod (1979), Abramowitz (1980), Lippman et al (1981), and Walker et al (1984) reported no significant improvements in speech recognition for multichannel compression, whereas Mangold and Leijon (1981), Goldberg (1982), Laurence et al (1983), Yund et al (1987), and Moore and Glasberg (1988) did find significant improvements.

A study by Levitt and Neuman (1991) was revealing regarding the relative merits of different methods of frequency-dependent compression, of which multichannel compression is a special case. The experimental technique used a generalized form of frequency-dependent compression in which the changes to overall spectral shape produced by the compression system were strictly controlled. The optimum compression system within this framework was then obtained for each subject using an adaptive search procedure. The data showed that, for most subjects, single-channel compression yielded speech recognition scores that were as good as those for the most advanced forms of frequency-dependent compression. A few subjects, however, showed a small additional improvement in speech recognition if spectral slope was compressed in addition to overall gain.

Summary

Existing compression amplification systems involve three independent sets of variables. These are (1) the nature of the input/output curve showing the static characteristics of compression threshold and compression ratio, (2) the temporal characteristics of the compression system (i.e., attack time, release time), and (3) the frequency-specific characteristics of the compression system (e.g., multichannel vs. single-channel systems).

The selection and fitting of compression hearing aids is thus a complex problem given the large number of variables involved. The situation is further complicated by ongoing controversies regarding the merits of different forms of compression amplification. The large number of studies showing no significant advantage for multichannel compression indicate that this form of compression is not as effective as initially believed. On the other hand, the positive results that have been reported for certain subjects under certain conditions indicate that specific forms of multichannel compression (or other forms of frequency-dependent compression) may be an appropriate form of signal processing for certain types of hearing loss.

Adaptive Frequency Response Amplifiers

Dynamic control of both the gain and frequency response of an amplifier can provide compression amplification with controlled amounts of spectral shaping. A varying spectral shape across level can also be obtained with other means besides compression, such as with adaptive filtering techniques. Note that programmable hearing aids with multiple memories also can provide the patient with the choice of more than one, albeit fixed, frequency response for different listening situations.

The notion of a dynamically varying frequency response was suggested by various researchers in the 1970s and early 1980s (Goldberg, 1972; Skinner, 1980; Villchur, 1973), based on data illustrating that different frequency responses were needed to produce optimum performance at different listening levels. But it was not until the mid-1980s that such processing was able to be implemented practically in chips small enough to fit into commercial devices. This effect was first achieved in single-channel hearing aids, such as the adaptive high-pass filtering approach used in Argosy's Manhattan circuit (Preves, 1990; Preves & Sigelman, 1986), and hearing aids that incorporated the K-Amplifier (K-Amp) microchip produced by Etymotic Research (Killion, 1990). In addition, many of the multichannel compression hearing aids introduced in the 1980s and 1990s were intentionally designed to produce adaptive frequency responses (AFRs) (Fabry, 1991) for purposes of either reducing the effect of background noise or maintaining comfortable loudness levels across the audible frequency range. These effects were achieved in two-channel instruments by using compression in one channel and conventional amplification in the other channel, or by using a lower compression threshold or a greater CR in one channel than in the other.

Killion et al (1990) categorized amplifiers of this type in terms of how they affect spectral shape as a function of input level. An amplifier that decreases low-frequency gain with increasing signal level (or increases low-frequency gain with decreasing signal level) was given the acronym BILL (base increase at lower levels). Similarly, the acronym TILL (treble increase at lower levels) was used for an amplifier that decreases high-frequency gain with increasing signal level (or increases high-frequency gain with decreasing signal level). Sample families of frequency responses for BILL-type and TILL-type hearing aids can be found in Chapter 1 in this volume.

The rationale for BILL-type and TILL-type processing is different (Sammeth & Ochs, 1991). BILL-type processing appears to be based on several assumptions. The first is that everyday ambient noises have more power in the low frequencies (relative to the high frequencies) than speech. A second assumption is that an unusually high input level indicates the likely presence of ambient noise, thereby requiring a reduction in low-frequency gain. These assumptions are probably true for many, but not all, listening situations. A third assumption is that reducing the gain of the low frequencies as the input level increases will also reduce upward spread of masking. Trees and Turner (1986) and Gagne (1988) have shown that upward spread of masking in cochlear-impaired ears is greater than that in normal ears because of the high SPLs at which they must listen. Some limited support exists for the assumption that reducing low-frequency gain assists in speech recognition in noise (Fabry et al, 1993; Cook et al, 1997), although the degree of upward spread of masking measured in an individual ear does not correspond to the degree of speech recognition benefit seen with reduced low-frequency gain (Cook et al, 1997). Note, however, that these studies used fixed filters for attenuating the low frequencies and not adaptive filters as in BILL-type processing.

> ### SPECIAL CONSIDERATION
>
> **BILL-type hearing aids are typically recommended only for patients who show enough low-frequency hearing loss that significant amounts of low-frequency gain are required (and, thus, can be reduced at higher input levels). An alternate approach is to fit a BILL processor on a patient who has milder low-frequency hearing loss but to provide more low-frequency gain than usual, with the argument that this results in better sound quality for listening in quiet while still preventing excess "base" amplification in high noise levels.**

The TILL approach is intended for use with patients who have mild/moderate sloping hearing losses and loudness recruitment in the high-frequency region. Greater gain is given for lower-level, high-frequency inputs to ensure audibility of speech energy, but less gain is given at higher input levels because of loudness recruitment. In some sense, then, the TILL approach was the first attempt to "normalize" loudness perception in an impaired ear. Variations on the concept of loudness normalization are still debated in fitting and selection practices today, as will be later discussed.

Early studies of AFR hearing aids, which were mostly single-channel analog systems, produced conflicting results (Schum, 1990; Sigelman & Preves, 1987; Stach et al, 1987; Tyler & Kuk, 1989). There appeared to be clear benefits of these types of devices in terms of sound quality, listening comfort, and preventing the hearing aid from going into saturation too often. What was less clear was whether they actually resulted in improved speech recognition in noise. Furthermore, candidacy for each type of approach was also unclear because both BILL and TILL amplification were proposed for patients with similar audiograms.

In a recent study Valente et al (1997) compared performance for subjects with hearing loss who were fitted binaurally with both Oticon MultiFocus BTEs, two-channel analog processors that show BILL-type processing, and the two-channel digitally programmable ReSound BT2-E BTEs, which often produce processing that is similar to TILL-type processing when the manufacturer's fitting algorithm is used. With some exceptions, the results generally suggested that both an audiogram and a level effect were present. Subjects having more severe hearing losses performed better on a speech recognition task in noise with the MultiFocus than with the BT2-E hearing aids for low and moderate input levels but performed better with the BT2-E hearing aids at a very high input level where the MultiFocus likely reached saturation. In contrast, subjects having less severe hearing losses had more comparable speech recognition across both hearing aid sets, but most preferred the sound quality and loudness comfort of the BT2-E hearing aids. Further study is clearly needed to determine appropriate candidacy criteria for different types of signal processing approaches.

Speech Enhancement Approaches

More advanced methods of signal processing are likely on the horizon with the advent of digital techniques and continued microminiaturization of components and chips. In addition to efforts to reduce the effects of background noise, the research literature shows many attempts in laboratory studies to enhance aspects of speech for the cochlear-impaired ear. Included are spectral sharpening or spectral contrast enhancement approaches (Baer et al, 1993; Bunnell, 1990; Bustamante & Braida, 1986; Summerfield et al, 1985), and selective consonant amplification or alteration of the duration of phonemes (Gordon-Salant, 1986, 1987; Kennedy et al, 1998; Montgomery & Edge, 1988).

One phonetically based form of compression amplification that is being investigated experimentally, for example, is that of adjusting the consonant-vowel (C-V) intensity ratio. Most consonantal sounds are weaker than vowels (the exceptions are the nasals, glides, laterals, and voiced /r/, which are vowel-like in terms of their acoustic structure). It has been shown experimentally that increasing the C-V intensity ratio will increase speech recognition for some persons with hearing loss (Gordon-Salant, 1986, 1987; Montgomery & Edge, 1988). The amount by which the C-V ratio needs to be increased for maximizing performance, however, depends on the phonetic environment and on the nature of the hearing loss (Kennedy et al, 1998). Three typical diagrams showing the effect of increasing C-V intensity ratio are shown in Figure 5–12. Figure 5–12A shows a rollover effect in which increasing C-V intensity ratio beyond a critical level produces a reduction in consonant recognition. Figure 5–12B shows a saturation effect in which no further improvement in consonant recognition is obtained. Figure 5–12C shows no change in consonant recognition with increasing C-V intensity ratio because the maximum performance level has already been obtained at the unenhanced C-V intensity ratio.

Methods for implementing adjustments to the C-V intensity ratio in a hearing aid have been investigated (Preves et al, 1991; Sammeth et al, 1996). A simple method is to boost the high frequencies by a combination of frequency filtering and frequency-dependent compression because many of the weaker consonants convey significant information in the high-frequency region. More sophisticated signal processing strategies may be needed, however, to achieve the improvements in speech recognition that are theoretically possible. For example, maximizing performance when rollover occurs (as shown in Figure 5–12A) will require a highly sophisticated method of signal processing that will result in a C-V intensity ratio that is neither too large nor too small. These results and those by Sammeth et al (1998) indicate that optimizing the C-V intensity ratio in an advanced signal processing hearing aid is likely to be difficult. Determining the best form of processing to enhance speech recognition will continue to be a major topic of research in the years to come.

Signal Processing for Noise Reduction

Noise reduction is a problem of general concern and concerted efforts have addressed this problem in many different fields. Methods of signal processing for reducing noise in audio systems are of two basic types: those designed for single-microphone inputs and those designed for multiple-microphone inputs. The single-microphone techniques depend on spectral and/or temporal differences between the signal and noise to either eliminate the noise or reduce its effect on the perception of the signal. Multi-microphone techniques can make use of spatial differences between the signal and noise sources and spectrotemporal differences. Single-microphone techniques are of obvious interest for hearing aid applications because most hearing aids use a single-microphone. The use of more than one microphone in hearing aids is a new development, largely as a result of the less than satisfactory results obtained with single-microphone inputs.

Single-Microphone Techniques

Techniques for improving the intelligibility of speech-in-noise for a single-microphone input have been the subject of considerable research over the years. Lim and Oppenheim (1979) in a review of the many different techniques that had been tried concluded that although SNR could be improved with corresponding improvements in overall sound quality, significant improvements in speech understanding were not obtained. In fact, in many cases the improvement in sound quality was accompanied by a decrease in speech recognition.

The following example illustrates this type of result. Consider speech that is partially masked by high-frequency noise such that recognition is reduced significantly. The speech-plus-noise is now passed through a low-pass filter so as to eliminate all frequency components in the region occupied by the high-frequency noise. The noise is no longer audible, resulting in an improvement in overall sound quality. The process of filtering the speech-plus-noise has increased the SNR because there is no longer any noise in the filtered signal although a significant amount of lower frequency speech remains. However, the high-frequency components of speech have also been eliminated by the filter, and hence the few speech cues that were audible in

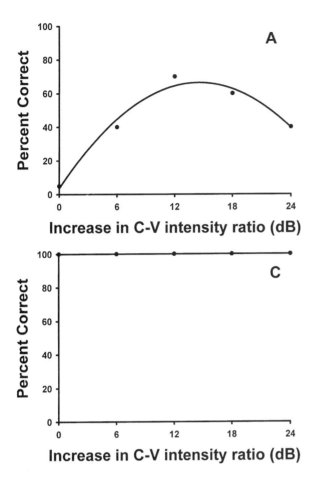

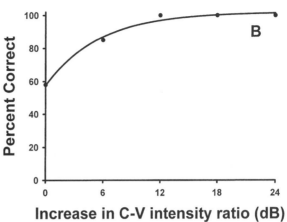

Figure 5–12 **(A-C)** Illustrative performance-intensity (PI) functions for individual nonsense syllables. Data show percent correct as a function of increasing consonant-vowel (*C-V*) intensity ratio. The shape of the PI function depends on the phonetic environment and the characteristics of the hearing loss. (Reprinted from Kennedy [1994] with permission.)

the partially masked high-frequency region are no longer available. This produces a concomitant reduction in speech recognition. In other more advanced forms of noise reduction the reduction in background noise is replaced by subtle distortions of the speech signal and/or low-level processing noise, the effect of which is also to reduce speech recognition.

Although Lim and Oppenheim (1979) considered only signal processing techniques that were developed for and evaluated with normal-hearing listeners, similar results have been reported for listeners with hearing loss using single-microphone systems (Levitt et al, 1990, 1993; Neuman & Schwander, 1987). A few studies, however, have reported small improvements in speech recognition with a single-microphone input under carefully controlled laboratory conditions (Stein & Dempsey-Hart, 1984). As previously noted, when low-frequency amplification produces undesirable upward spread of masking (Gagne, 1988; Trees & Turner, 1986), the effects can be reduced by attenuation of the low frequencies. The improvement in speech recognition obtained in this way is small, however, and if the methods used to attenuate the noise are imperfect, audible components of the speech signal will also be rendered inaudible and speech recognition will be reduced rather than increased. Because of the latter problem, a practical hearing aid has yet to be developed that will selectively reduce the level of high-intensity noise components without at the same time reducing the audibility of speech components in the same frequency region.

There are several ways in which low-frequency noise can be attenuated. The simplest method is to use a fixed frequency response with a low-frequency rolloff. This can be coupled with wide-band AGC so as to maintain a comfortable listening level. A second approach is to use a two-channel hearing aid with compression in the low-frequency channel so as to attenuate the noise, producing BILL-type processing. A third approach is to use a high-pass filter with a cut-off frequency that is increased automatically when the signal intensity in the low frequencies exceeds a level typical of the low-frequency speech spectrum.

In the 1980s some extravagant claims were made in marketing campaigns by some hearing aid manufacturers regarding the noise-reducing (and speech-enhancing) capabilities of their products. Most of the circuits that were being described were variations of the adaptive high-pass filter technique. No experimental data supported the claims that these hearing aids produced substantial improvements in speech understanding in background noise. As a result of legal actions taken by the U.S. Food and Drug Administration (FDA), which regulates medical devices including hearing aids, these types of claims are no longer being made. Rather, most current marketing efforts focus on claims of improved sound quality or listening comfort.

Wiener filtering is a more advanced single-microphone approach to noise reduction that has shown small improvements in speech recognition for at least a few subjects in some noises (Levitt et al, 1993). It is important to understand the strengths and limitations of a Wiener filter. It can be shown mathematically that if the statistical properties of a signal and noise do not vary with time (i.e., both signal and noise are stationary, random processes), the output of the Wiener filter, as derived from the signal and noise spectra, will maximize the SNR. Unfortunately, speech is not a stationary random process and many everyday noises are not stationary processes. It is possible, however, to approximate the speech signal by random processes that are assumed to be stationary over short intervals of time. An adaptive Wiener filter is based on this assumption (i.e., the filter continually adapts to the changes in the short-term spectrum of the speech signal). Because the short-term spectrum of the speech signal is not known in advance, an estimate is used instead so that, in practice, adaptive Wiener filters are only estimates of an approximation to the optimum filter. Of greater consequence is that the derivation of the Wiener filter is based on a mathematical criterion of optimality (minimization of the mean square error). This criteria will not necessarily maximize speech recognition. A filter or other signal-processing strategy that maximizes recognition is more likely to depend on optimizing one or more subjective variables. As previously noted, the ZNB hearing aids of the 1980s used adaptive Weiner filtering. Although several studies (Graupe et al, 1987; Stein & Dempsey-Hart, 1984; Wolinsky, 1986) reported small, but significant improvements on speech tests using the ZNB adaptive Wiener filter, others (Van Tasell et al, 1988–1992) did not.

In contrast, improvements have not been obtained using Weiner filtering for any normal-hearing subjects. A possible explanation of this result is that the auditory filters in a normal ear are relatively narrow in bandwidth, in which case the improvement in SNR that can be obtained with Wiener filtering is negligibly small. On the other hand, the auditory filters are relatively broad in some forms of sensorineural hearing loss, so that it may be possible to take advantage of the increase in SNR provided by a Wiener filter. This hypothesis needs to be tested, but whether or not it is true the fact that substantial individual differences have been reported among listeners with hearing loss with respect to the efficacy of modern signal processing techniques for noise reduction has important implications for selection and fitting of signal processing hearing aids.

In summary, experimental investigations of various advanced methods of noise reduction in single-microphone systems for listeners with hearing loss have, for the most part, shown results similar to those reported by Lim and Oppenheim (1979) for listeners with normal-hearing (i.e., it is possible to improve SNR with concomitant improvements in overall sound quality but without significant improvements in speech recognition on average) (Levitt et al, 1993).

Multi-microphone Techniques

The most promising approach, at present, for improving SNR is the use of multiple microphones. This is not surprising because multi-microphone techniques, in addition to differentiating between sounds coming from different directions, can also incorporate signal processing strategies that have been found to be successful for single-microphone systems. The improvement in going from a single-microphone to a multimicrophone system can be substantial. Several companies have already introduced a dual-microphone hearing aid with a user-selectable option for directional versus omnidirectional

function in BTE or ITE styles. Early studies of these two-microphone hearing aids appear promising (Gravel et al, 1998; Preves et al, 1997; Valente et al, 1995b). Another approach is the D-MIC™, in which the user can select between a directional and omnidirectional microphone. The D-MIC™ has recently been incorporated into a number of ITE models (Killion et al, 1998).

Even greater directionality can be obtained by using arrays of several microphones with appropriate signal processing, sometimes called "beamforming" techniques. The possible use of such arrays at the input stage of hearing aids is currently being evaluated experimentally (e.g., Kates & Weiss, 1995; 1996; Peterson et al, 1987, 1990; Schweitzer & Krishnan, 1996; Schweitzer & Terry, 1995; Soede et al, 1993a,b). A potential problem with multiple microphones is that their placement may be cosmetically unacceptable. Also, the means of connecting the microphones to the hearing aid raises practical problems. Hardwire connections are inconvenient, and the use of radio links can result in high overall power consumption and larger physical size. In one implementation the microphones are placed on the stem and bridge of a pair of eyeglasses (Soede et al, 1993a,b). An alternative, under investigation by Starkey Laboratories, is an array worn around the neck with transmission through an electromagnetic signal to the telecoil of a head-worn hearing aid (Lehr & Widrow, 1998).

Multi-microphone techniques are not only capable of much larger improvements in SNR, but the methods of signal processing also do not typically introduce significant processing noise or distortion. Multi-microphone techniques can be subdivided into two broad classes: directional microphone arrays and adaptive cancellation techniques. These two classes are not mutually exclusive because an adaptive noise-cancellation system may, for example, have directional properties very similar to those of an adaptive directional microphone array. Only a brief description of these techniques will be provided here because detailed information on this topic is available in Chapter 1 in this volume.

The simplest form of directional microphone array is that in which the output of each microphone is delayed and then added to the sum of the other delayed microphone outputs. The delays are chosen to reinforce signals coming from a given direction while attenuating signals coming from other directions (Soede et al, 1993a,b). Greater improvements can be obtained by multiplying the microphone outputs by a set of coefficients that have been optimized for maximum directionality (Kates & Weiss, 1996). Directionality can be increased even further using an adaptive directional array. In this type of microphone array the coefficients are continually updated so as to focus on the signal source (Kates & Weiss, 1996). Adaptive arrays are particularly well suited for situations in which the location of the signal source is not fixed, as in a cocktail party. Directional microphone arrays can effectively separate speech from noise when the signal and noise sources differ substantially in terms of their direction. A directional microphone array is of little value, however, if the signal and noise emanate from the same direction. There is also no advantage to the use of a directional microphone array in a highly reverberant environment because both the signal and noise fields are diffuse (i.e., as a result of the numerous reflections off walls and other surfaces both signal and noise reach the listener from every direction).

It is also possible, using two headworn microphones, to attenuate if not cancel noise coming from a specific direction

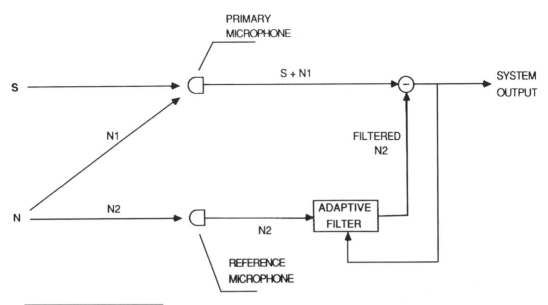

Figure 5–13   Basic adaptive noise canceller. The primary microphone receives the speech signal (S) together with one version of noise signal (*N1*). The reference microphone receives a version of noise signal (*N2*). The adaptive filter adjusts itself until the system output is minimized, which occurs when the filtered N2 noise is approximately the same as N1. In the headworn system the reference microphone picks up some of the speech as well as the noise and when the adaptive filter minimizes the system output, the noise is not cancelled, but there is a substantial improvement in the SNR. (Reprinted from Weiss [1987] with permission.)

by means of advanced signal-processing techniques. Schwander and Levitt (1987), for example, used a technique in which noise picked up by one microphone was used to reduce the noise picked up by the second microphone. This technique, based on the work of Widrow et al (1975), is known as adaptive cancellation and is illustrated in Figure 5–13. The primary microphone points toward the speech source, whereas the reference microphone points away from the speech source. Note that, in this application of adaptive noise cancellation, both microphones can be mounted on the same ear. Adaptive noise cancellation using two microphones can be used to cancel a single noise source, but if more than one noise source is present, additional microphones with additional adaptive filters need to be used. As is the case with directional microphone arrays, adaptive noise cancellation will not work well in a highly reverberant room (Weiss, 1987).

The use of multiple microphones also brings up an issue with respect to binaural listening. The possibility exists that a hearing aid with microphones mounted on each ear and with preprocessing for noise reduction followed by either diotic or dichotic presentation of the signals may yield superior performance in noise and reverberation to conventional hearing aids on each ear. An important finding in this area is that individual differences are large for binaural amplification and the various forms of signal processing that have been tried. This observation has important implications for the selection and fitting of advanced signal-processing hearing aids. For example, a system that works well for one patient may not work well for another, even though the audiograms may be virtually identical.

It remains to be seen whether the movement toward directional hearing aids and/or adaptive noise cancellation with multiple microphones will be commercially successful. The

audiologist needs to be prepared for these developments, however, because the use of multiple microphones (especially those mounted remotely from the hearing aid) will introduce a new dimension to the selection and fitting of hearing aids.

HISTORY OF HEARING AID SELECTION AND FITTING PRACTICES

The principles and practices used to determine hearing aid candidacy and to select and fit hearing aids appropriately have improved substantially over the years. Practices have been modified not only to reflect changes in the hearing aid patient population and technological advances in hearing aids and audiological instrumentation but also in our understanding of sensorineural hearing impairment and its consequences. In the early days when many conductive and mixed hearing losses were not amenable to medical/surgical treatment, hearing aids were thus the intervention of choice for hearing losses of this type and moderate sensorineural hearing losses. For these populations, amplifiers with uniform gain did about as well as any other in compensating for this restricted range of hearing losses. As technology improved, hearing aid candidacy was expanded to include individuals with more substantive cochlear damage, including severe high-frequency hearing losses. A concurrent development was more successful medical/surgical treatment of conductive hearing losses, so that today most candidates for acoustic amplification show primarily sensorineural hearing losses.

As noted by Studebaker (1980), the history of selection and fitting practices can be loosely divided into three overlapping periods. In the earliest period, before about 1946, hearing aid fitting used fairly simple, unvalidated prescriptive techniques. In the second period many hearing aid dispensers used the common-frequency-response approach recommended by the Harvard Report, but the Carhart comparative hearing aid evaluation approach was dominant among practitioners in the new field of clinical audiology. In the third period, beginning in the 1970s, there was a return to the notion of prescriptive fitting, but with much greater refinement of the formulas, better research data to guide their development, and improved techniques to verify accuracy of the fitting.

It should be borne in mind that before the 1980s, linear hearing aids were the norm and thus the major electroacoustic parameters that needed fitting were gain, frequency response, and output limiting. With the introduction of AFRs, multichannel compression, and DSP hearing aids, new fitting methods are in the process of being developed.

Methods of hearing aid selection and fitting can be generally subdivided into five broad categories: (1) the common-frequency-response approach, (2) threshold-based prescriptive formulas, (3) suprathreshold prescriptive techniques, (4) the Carhart selection and evaluation procedure, and (5) on-line adaptive adjustment. These categories are not mutually exclusive. On-line adaptive adjustment, for example, requires a reasonably good initial setting for rapid convergence on the optimum set of electroacoustic characteristics. This initial setting may be arrived at by any of the other selection methods. In addition, some of the suprathreshold prescriptive techniques are essentially modifications of threshold-based prescriptive formulas.

The Common-Frequency-Response Approach and the Harvard/MedResCo Reports

The common-frequency-response approach was developed shortly after World War II when the U.S. government, faced with the problem of large numbers of returning veterans with service-connected hearing losses and cognizant of the dramatic advances in electronics that had been made during the war, commissioned the PsychoAcoustics Laboratory (PAL) of Harvard University to investigate and report on the design requirements of hearing aids that would be maximally effective. The study evaluated patients using a "master" hearing aid, a device in which different frequency-gain characteristics can be selected and performance under each compared (Davis et al, 1946). The now famous report resulting from this investigation, known as the Harvard Report (Davis et al, 1947), suggested that only two frequency responses were needed to produce best performance for all patients: a flat (or "uniform") frequency response for patients with flat or rising audiograms, and a frequency response in which gain increased at approximately 5 or 6 dB/octave for those with downward sloping audiograms.

At about the same time, a similar investigation was commissioned by the British government. The outcome of the British investigation was known as the MedResCo Report (Medical Research Council; Radley et al, 1947). The British report also recommended a limited range of frequency responses for most hearing-aid users, but the range of frequency responses that was recommended was different from that recommended by the Harvard Report.

It is interesting to note that, initially, it was widely believed that the two reports recommended essentially the same

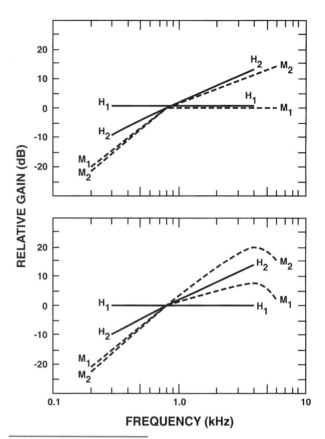

Figure 5–14   The upper diagram illustrates the nominal frequency responses recommended by the World War II era MedResCo Report *(dashed lines M1 to M1, and M2 to M2)* and Harvard Report *(solid lines H1 to H1 and H2 to H2)*. The lower diagram illustrates how the responses differ in the high frequencies when the correction for head diffraction effects that was used by the MedResCo researchers is removed, making calibration procedures comparable across the two studies. (Adapted from Levitt [1978] with permission.)

frequency responses for general use, but after differences in the method of acoustic calibration were taken into account, it was realized that quite different frequency responses were actually being recommended. The upper half of Figure 5–14 shows the nominal frequency responses recommended by the MedResCo and Harvard reports, which appear quite similar. The bottom half of Figure 5–14, however, shows the recommended frequency responses after correcting for differences in the calibration procedures used in the Harvard and MedResCo reports. Significant differences are now apparent in the high frequencies.

It may appear a quandary that two substantive reports recommending a narrow range of frequency response as being the best for the vast majority of hearing aid users should not be recommending essentially the same frequency responses. The answer is that the criterion used for the best response was that of maximizing speech recognition as measured using the traditional monosyllabic PB-word speech recognition tests. Given the relatively poor precision of this measuring instrument, relatively large changes in frequency responses can be tolerated before a significant change in speech recognition score is obtained and therefore the region encompassing the optimum frequency response for general hearing aid use was imprecisely defined. Thus it is not surprising that relatively simple frequency responses (for the chosen method of calibration) were selected as being the optimum responses.

Further evidence in support of the relative insensitivity of traditional speech recognition tests to changes in frequency response was provided by Shore et al (1960), who compared performance across several hearing aids and found no significant differences in speech recognition scores using traditional methods of speech audiometry. More recently, Sullivan et al (1988) also found that scores on traditional speech recognition tests did not differ significantly across four very different frequency responses provided that the subject was allowed to adjust the gain of each to a comfortable overall level.

The common-frequency-response approach to hearing aid fitting had some advantages. The technique was exceedingly simple to administer. Furthermore, the cost of providing acoustic amplification to a large number of patients was low using this method because a wide range of different hearing aids were not needed.

However, the shortcomings of the approach were substantial. At the time the Harvard and MedResCo studies were performed, most individuals who were considered to be candidates for acoustic amplification had either a conductive or a relatively mild sensorineural hearing loss. For these individuals, a flat or mildly sloping frequency response will yield good results, and given the lack of precision in evaluating the quality of the outcome, the prescribed frequency responses appeared to be as good as any. This is no longer the case. Most conductive hearing losses are now treated medically or surgically and most candidates for acoustic amplification today have sensorineural hearing losses. Furthermore, persons with severe sensorineural hearing loss are no longer considered to be untreatable and now form a large and important segment of the population for whom acoustic amplification is the preferred method of intervention. For these individuals, the frequency responses recommended by either the Harvard Report or the MedResCo Report would be a very poor choice. In short, the common-frequency-response-approach to hearing aid fitting was appropriate for the majority of individuals who were considered to be suitable candidates for acoustic amplification at the time that the method was developed, but it is no longer an appropriate approach today.

The Harvard Report also concluded that it was not necessary for the bandwidth of a hearing aid to exceed about 3500 Hz. This was a highly erroneous recommendation based on the observation that telephone speech, which is limited to this bandwidth, is intelligible. Whereas telephone speech is reasonably intelligible for normal-hearing listeners, individuals with hearing loss (particularly those with conductive or mild sensorineural hearing losses) can benefit substantially from a wider bandwidth. Nevertheless, these recommendations of the Harvard Report, coupled with the engineering problems of developing wide bandwidth miniature transducers with high-output power, unfortunately resulted in hearing aids of limited bandwidth being produced for many years.

Prescriptive Approaches

An important advantage of vacuum-tube hearing aids over earlier methods of acoustic amplification was that the frequency-gain characteristics could be adjusted with much greater precision and flexibility than was previously possible. Given this new tool, researchers soon began to investigate the effects of this variable in acoustic amplification and its relationship to hearing loss (Hartig & Newhart, 1936; Knudsen, 1939; Littler, 1936). A related development was the invention of the electronic audiometer, which allowed for the accurate measurement of hearing loss as a function of frequency. These two developments gave birth to the concept of selective amplification in which the electroacoustic characteristics of the hearing aid were selected or adjusted so as to match the characteristics of the hearing loss.

The earliest implementation of selective amplification focused on the frequency-gain characteristics, and formulas were soon developed in which a recommended frequency-gain characteristic was derived based on individual measurements of hearing loss. Prescriptive formulas have since been expanded to include the saturation sound pressure level (SSPL; also called OSPL re: ANSI S3.22-1996) of the hearing aid in addition to the frequency-gain characteristics. Most recently, prescriptive techniques for compression amplification have been developed.

Prescriptive approaches to hearing aid fitting fell out of favor after the Harvard Report was published. A major shift in fitting approaches emerged once again toward the end of the 1960s. As noted by Millin (1975), selective amplification was already being revisited with fitting of specialty hearing aids. For example, the development of CROS aids with the rolloff of low-frequency energy from open-mold fittings had proven to be useful for those with hearing loss only in the high-frequency range. Furthermore, for individuals with profound hearing loss who had residual hearing only at 250 and 500 Hz, extended low-frequency-range hearing aids or those that electronically transposed high frequencies to lower frequencies were being tried (Erber 1971; Ling 1964; Ling & Maretic, 1971). Most importantly, research accomplished in the 1970s and early 1980s, including work by Pascoe, Skinner, and their colleagues at the Central Institute for the Deaf (CID) (Pascoe, 1975, 1978; Skinner, 1980; Skinner et al, 1982), showed that a frequency response could be selected for an individual that would produce the best speech recognition score based on audiological measurements.

A wide variety of prescriptive techniques have been developed over the years. These techniques can be subdivided into two broad groups: threshold-based and suprathreshold prescriptive methods.

Threshold-Based Prescriptive Formulas

Threshold-based prescriptive formulas use information from the pure tone audiogram to select the frequency-gain characteristics of the hearing aid. The earliest prescriptive formulas were based on the belief that by simple "mirroring" of the audiogram (i.e., providing gain equal to the hearing loss at all frequencies), normal-hearing would be restored. This approach actually worked reasonably well with conductive and mild sensorineural hearing losses, which accounts for the use of the approach during the early days of hearing aid fitting when most candidates for amplification had hearing losses of those types. Mirroring the audiogram, however, is contraindicated for more severe sensorineural hearing losses because the high gain predicted by this technique, particularly at high frequencies, would result in sounds of moderate intensity being amplified to exceed the listener's discomfort level by a wide margin.

Rather than mirroring the audiogram, threshold-based formulas that have achieved good results recommend a gain that is proportional, but not equal, to the hearing loss as a function of frequency. One of the earliest and most successful threshold-based prescriptive formulas was developed by Lybarger (1944). It is also one of the simplest, in that the predicted gain is equal to half of the hearing loss at 1000 Hz and higher frequencies. This formula therefore is widely known as the "Half-Gain Rule." At 500 Hz, Lybarger reduced the gain to 1/3 of the hearing loss, and, in fact, most formulas reduce low-frequency gain to avoid overamplifying low-frequency noise and producing excess upward spread of masking.

Many new threshold-based prescriptive formulas were developed in the 1970s and 1980s for calculating frequency-gain characteristics. Some of the more well-known formulas are briefly described in the top section of Table 5–2. This table is not exhaustive of all available formulas nor does it provide information on any means proposed for limiting the maximum output of the hearing aid. Some formulas also have specific calibration and/or measurement procedures, corrections for coupler-to-real-ear differences, and/or for the style of hearing aid and any earmold/shell acoustic modifications. The reader is, therefore, cautioned to consult original article(s) for details on the recommended implementation of any given fitting approach.

SPECIAL CONSIDERATION

It should be kept in mind that prescriptive formulas for selecting hearing aids are based on average data and that the individual patient may differ from the average. In particular, persons with conductive hearing loss typically desire more gain than prescribed by most formulas, whereas some persons with sensorineural hearing loss and loudness recruitment will not tolerate as much gain as prescribed.

It is clear from Table 5–2 that most of the threshold-based formulas are similar to Lybarger's half-gain rule except that different weighting coefficients are used. The prescription of gain output (POGO) approach (McCandless & Lyregaard, 1983), for example, supplies gain that is about 1/2 of the hearing loss (except at the lowest frequencies), whereas Berger et al's (1979, 1988) formula supplies greater than 1/2 gain for middle frequencies and Libby's (1986) approach supplies only 1/3 gain (unless the hearing loss is severe to profound).

In contrast, the NAL formulas involve more than an empirical refinement of a well-established rule. Byrne, Dillon, and others at the National Acoustic Laboratories (NAL) of Australia studied the correlation between threshold and most comfortable listening level (MCL) as a function of frequency. They then came up with a threshold-based formula that, on average, would place the long-term root-mean-square (RMS) speech spectrum at MCL. The original version of this formula (NAL) was published by Byrne and Tonnison (1976) and was subsequently revised (NAL-R) by Byrne and Dillon (1986) to supply greater low-frequency amplification. Essentially the NAL-R approach uses a 1/2-gain rule combined with a 1/3-slope rate, and constants are applied to control for excess gain in cases of severely sloping audiograms. The NAL formulas require more computations than other threshold-based formulas, and many commercial fitting systems include computer programs to calculate the prescribed frequency-gain function. A version of the NAL intended for use with more severe-to-profound losses has also been developed (Byrne et al, 1990), which typically provides more low-frequency emphasis and greater overall gain.

The desired sensation level (DSL) method (Moodie et al, 1994; Seewald, 1992; Seewald & Ross, 1988; Seewald et al, 1993) is intended for use primarily with a pediatric population. The DSL is technically a threshold-based approach because uncomfortable loudness levels (UCLs) used in the calculations are estimated from threshold measurements. Alternately, however, UCLs can be measured directly, in which case the DSL belongs in the suprathreshold techniques category.

Threshold-based prescriptive formulas are well suited for conventional hearing aids (i.e., hearing aids with linear amplification until a limiting output level is reached, at which level the signal is subjected to either peak clipping or output compression limiting). The different prescriptive formulas do, however, result in different frequency-gain functions prescribed for a given audiogram (Byrne, 1987). For example, Figure 5–15A shows a mild-to-moderate sloping audiogram. Figure 5–15B shows the prescribed frequency-gain characteristic for this hypothetical patient using four threshold-based formulas (Berger, Libby, NAL-R, and POGO). Note, however, that the patient is likely to adjust the volume control wheel on the hearing aid. Figure 5–15C shows the effect of adjusting overall gain so that all four frequency-gain characteristics have the same gain at 1000 Hz. Although the differences among the curves are reduced, the Berger formula still provides greater gain at 2000 Hz and less gain at 500 Hz than the other formulas, and POGO prescribes more high-frequency gain than the NAL-R or Libby formulas.

These discrepancies have led to much debate as to which of the threshold-based formulas is the best. In one experimental investigation comparing performance across frequency responses selected using several fitting procedures (including the half-gain rule and the original NAL formula), no significant differences in traditional speech recognition scores were observed once the listeners were allowed to adjust overall gain to comfort (Sullivan et al, 1988). Similarly, Humes and Hackett (1990) found no differences in speech recognition in a comparison of POGO, NAL-R, and a suprathreshold technique.

It should be noted that all the threshold-based prescriptive formulas are based on average data and that some subsequent individualized adjustment may be needed to obtain a good fit. In this respect the use of threshold-based prescriptive formulas, or any prescriptive formula based on average

SPECIAL CONSIDERATION

Although differences exist among prescribed frequency-gain characteristics calculated from different formulas, if the patient is allowed to adjust overall gain to a comfortable listening level, the effect of the differences on performance can be reduced substantially.

PITFALL

With ears having a smaller than average volume, it is important to realize that the output shown in the 2-cc coupler will underestimate the actual SPLs generated in the real ear. Thus real-ear probe microphone measurements are important to preclude the fitting of hearing aids with dangerously high or uncomfortably loud output levels.

data, should probably be regarded as no more than a first estimate of the best frequency-gain characteristic for an individual patient (Bratt & Sammeth, 1991). Furthermore, patients with a conductive component to their loss may require more gain than most formulas prescribe, whereas subjects fitted binaurally may desire slightly less gain than those with a monaural fitting.

Despite these caveats, threshold-based prescriptive formulas are widely used, especially to determine the parameters of ITE-type hearing aids. The reasons are a combination of economics and convenience because the frequency response of conventional hearing aids in a small shell are not easily changed once the circuitry has been mounted in the shell. Because of this constraint, it has become a common practice for audiologists to send to the hearing aid manufacturer a copy of the audiogram with an impression of the earcanal and let the manufacturer select the gain and frequency response. Particularly if potentiometers (trimpots) to allow electroacoustic modifications are not ordered or will not fit into the small shell, the audiologist can do little other than measure the real-ear frequency response once the hearing aid arrives to see if it is grossly appropriate. Given that the formula used by a given manufacturer may not be the best or may not even be known to the audiologist, who is ultimately responsible for selecting the best hearing aids for each patient, this practice of allowing factory technicians to preempt the audiologist's technical expertise with respect to this important stage of the selection process should be discouraged. A better practice is to specify the frequency-gain characteristics by selecting from among the manufacturer's published matrices for a given model. The introduction of programmable hearing aids has returned much of the onus of hearing aid selection to the audiologist, although Byrne (1996) has expressed concern regarding a recent trend toward manufacturer-specific, proprietary fitting systems for some of the more advanced signal processing algorithms, with little or no published validation data.

Beyond determining the gain and frequency response of a hearing aid, the maximum power output, or saturation (SSPL), of a hearing aid must also be determined. Appropriate setting of the maximum output is crucial, not only to avoid acoustic trauma to the ear from excessively high levels of amplified sounds (Macrae, 1991) but also to prevent loudness discomfort from high-level sounds. Yet the output must also be high enough to avoid excess saturation distortion in the hearing aid and to provide an adequately wide listening dynamic range.

Some, but not all, of the threshold-based prescriptive formulas include a means to set the SSPL of the hearing aid.

These formulas typically use predictions of UCLs based on threshold levels (although a few formulas, such as POGO, require individual measurements of UCLs). It is possible to take discomfort into account in this way because, as illustrated in Figure 5–16, UCLs increase, on average, with increasing hearing loss (dB HL). The rate of increase is relatively low for mild-to-moderate hearing losses and fairly high for hearing losses above about 60 dB HL. Notice, however, that substantial individual variation exists about this average relationship. Additional data showing the limited correlation between threshold and loudness levels may be found in Kamm et al (1978), Cox and Bisset (1982), and Sammeth et al (1989).

Dillon and Storey (1998) have recently come up with a threshold-based technique for selecting the SSPL of a hearing aid so as to provide a practical compromise between the conflicting demands of maximizing the dynamic range while minimizing the potential for excess amplification. Experimental evaluation of the procedure (Storey et al, 1998) showed that it provided satisfactory results for about two thirds of the subjects.

Suprathreshold Prescriptive Techniques

Suprathreshold techniques involve, in addition to the audiogram, audiometric measurements at levels well above the threshold of hearing. These techniques can be subdivided into three groups: (1) those that involve the measurement of uncomfortable loudness levels (UCLs) in addition to the audiogram, (2) those that involve the measurement of most comfortable loudness levels (MCLs) and thresholds (and usually also UCLs), and (3) those that measure loudness growth from threshold to UCL level. The middle section of Table 5–2 briefly describes some of the suprathreshold prescriptive techniques that have been introduced in the first two groups as alternatives to the threshold-based prescriptive formulas. Approaches that fall into the third group, measurement of the loudness growth function, are described in the next section on new approaches to fitting WDRC and multichannel compression hearing aids.

The simplest of the suprathreshold prescriptive techniques involves the measurement of UCL for a broadband speech signal. This information is then used to set the SSPL of the hearing aid. The frequency-gain characteristic using this simple approach is determined by a threshold-based formula. In essence, this procedure straddles the boundary between threshold-based and suprathreshold prescriptive procedures.

A more sophisticated use of UCL measurements is to measure UCL levels as a function of frequency and to use this information to determine not only the SSPL of the hearing aid but also its frequency-gain characteristics. One such approach is the bisection method, in which the dynamic range (DR)

TABLE 5–2 Brief descriptions of some of the prescriptive approaches for determining hearing aid frequency-gain characteristics

Threshold-based prescriptive formulas

Lybarger, 1944 (Half-Gain Rule)	Gain = HL × 0.5 ≥ 1000 Hz; HL × 0.33 at 500 Hz.
Berger et al, 1979; 1988	Gain = HL × 0.3 at 500 Hz (0.5 if loss ≥ 50 dB HL), × 0.63 at 1000 Hz, × 0.67 at 2000 Hz, × 0.59 at 3000 Hz, × 0.53 at 4000, × 0.50 at 6000 Hz.
McCandless and Lyregaard, 1983 (POGO)	Gain = HL × 0.5, −10 dB at 250 Hz and −5 dB at 500 Hz
Libby, 1986	Gain = HL × 0.33, −5 dB at 250 Hz and 6000 Hz, and −3 dB at 500 Hz (for patients with more severe to profound hearing loss, a 2/3-gain rule is proposed).
Byrne and Dillon, 1986 (NAL-R)	Gain = HL at each frequency × 0.31 + [0.05 (HL at 500 Hz + HL at 1000 Hz + HL at 2000 Hz)], and with the following correction factors: −17 dB at 250 Hz, −8 at 500 Hz, −1 at 1000 Hz, −1 at 2000 Hz, and −2 at 3000-6000 Hz.
Seewald and Ross, 1988; Seewald, 1992; Seewald et al, 1993; Moodie et al, 1994 (DSL versions 3.0 and 3.1)	Gain = that needed to amplify the average RMS speech spectrum to a level 15-18 dB above threshold at each frequency without exceeding loudness discomfort levels as estimated from thresholds. (NOTE: Can also be a suprathreshold technique if UCLs are measured.)

Suprathreshold prescriptive techniques

Watson and Knudsen, 1940	Mirror MCL curves obtained using tonal stimuli.
Wallenfels, 1967	Bisect listener's DR by amplifying halfway between HL and UCL, with slope of the function dependent on the high-frequency DR.
Bragg, 1977	Bisect DR ≥ 1000 Hz by amplifying halfway between HL and UCL, and amplify to 1/3 of the range at 250 Hz and 500 Hz.
Shapiro, 1976; 1980	Amplify 60 dB SPL input signals to MCL at frequencies ≥ 1000 Hz; Gain at 500 Hz is 10 dB less than the gain at 1000 Hz, and gain at 250 Hz is 15 dB less than the gain at 1000 Hz.
Abramowitz, 1980; modified by Levitt et al, 1987 (UCL-based)	Amplify speech to a level 10 dB less than UCL between 1000 and 6000 Hz, 22 dB below UCL at 250 Hz, and 16 dB below UCL at 500 Hz.
Skinner et al, 1982; Skinner, 1988 (CID)	Amplify long-term average RMS speech spectrum (overall level = 65 dB SPL) to MCL for 500-6000 Hz, with amplification to halfway between threshold and MCL at 250 Hz (1988 modification: also 1/2-way at 6000 Hz).
Cox, 1983; 1985; 1988 (MSU)	Amplify speech spectrum to halfway between threshold and the "upper limit of comfortable loudness" (ULCL; as defined by the procedure). Version 3 also provides a threshold-based procedure in which ULCLs are estimated.

New approaches for WDRC and multichannel hearing aids

Van Vliet et al, 1995 (IHAFF)	Requires loudness growth functions measured at several frequencies; Calculates desired frequency responses for inputs of 50-, 65-, and 80-dB SPL, and suggests compression parameters to achieve these goals.
Killion & Fikret-Pasa, 1993 (FIG6)	Estimates loudness values based on average data; Calculates desired frequency responses for inputs of 40-, 65-, and 90-dB SPL, and suggests compression parameters to achieve these goals.
Cornelisse et al, 1995; Seewald et al, 1996 (DSL [i/o]; also called DSL version 4.0)	Can use estimated or measured loudness values; Calculates desired frequency responses for inputs of 45-, 60-, 75-, and 90-dB SPL, and suggests compression parameters to achieve these goals.

HL, hearing threshold; MCL, most comfortable loudness level; UCL, uncomfortable loudness level; RMS, root-mean-square; DR, dynamic range (UCL minus threshold); WDRC, wide dynamic range compression.

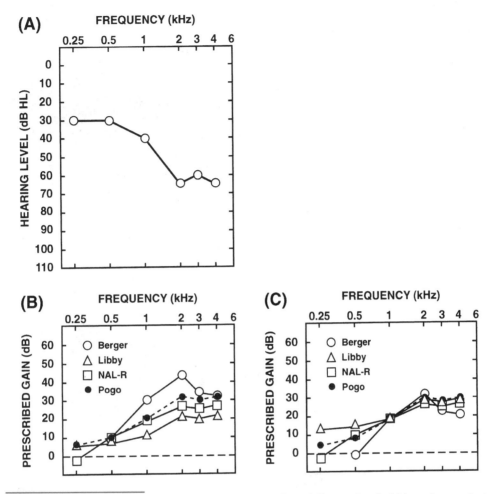

Figure 5–15 Frequency responses calculated under four different threshold-based prescriptive formulas for the audiogram shown in **(A)**. **(B)** is the calculated insertion gain, and **(C)** shows the responses equalized at 1000 Hz, as might occur with volume control adjustment. (Adapted from McCandless [1994] with permission.)

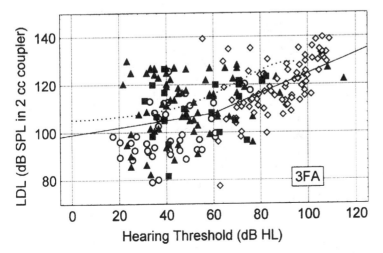

Figure 5–16 Three frequency (500, 1000, 2000 Hz) average (3FA) uncomfortable loudness levels (called "loudness discomfort levels" or LDLs in this figure) versus 3FA hearing threshold levels. Data shown are from Dillon et al (1984, *triangles*), Kamm et al (1978, *crosses*), Storey et al (1998, *circles*), Tonnisson (reported in Dillon and Macrae, 1984, Reference Note 3, *diamonds*), and Shapiro (1979, *squares*). The dotted line is the polynomial fit to Pascoe's (1988) data. (Reprinted from Dillon and Storey [1998] with permission.)

(where DR = UCL minus threshold) is bisected with the goal of positioning speech so that it is approximately halfway between the patient's hearing threshold and the level at which sounds become uncomfortably loud. As early as 1935, Balbi suggested such an approach. Wallenfels (1967) and Bragg (1977) also proposed forms of bisection. Perhaps the most well known of the approaches that involve DR bisection is that developed by Cox (1983, 1985, 1988) at Memphis State University (MSU). In the MSU method, the goal is to position the level of speech so that it is midway between threshold and the "upper limit of comfortable loudness" (ULCL, as defined by the measurement procedure).

Another method, referred to here as the "UCL method," is to specify a frequency-gain characteristic such that the spectrum of speech peaks falls just below the UCL curve. This method maximizes the proportion of the speech signal that is above the threshold of hearing. A problem with this approach is that, because of the high signal levels involved, it is also necessary to take upward spread of masking into account, and individual differences in upward spread of masking for individuals with hearing loss are substantial. Also, because the signals are relatively loud, the subject turns down the overall gain so as to achieve a comfortable listening level, in which case the proportion of the speech signal above the threshold of hearing is no longer maximized. Abramowitz (1980) and Levitt et al (1987 a,b) used this approach with a 6 dB/octave roll-off in the low frequencies to reduce upward spread of masking. Although relatively good results were obtained, speech recognition was not maximized and more accurate and practical means of dealing with upward spread of masking need to be developed. Another problem is that it is not always possible to obtain UCLs without generating signal levels that are potentially dangerous.

Of the various methods of measuring UCL levels, the one most widely used clinically is that of a single measurement with broadband speech. More detailed measurements of UCL levels (e.g., UCL as a function of frequency) have not been widely used to date because the measurements are time consuming and until quite recently most hearing aids did not have the capability for adjusting the shape of the SSPL curve. Modern multichannel programmable hearing aids, however, do allow for some control over SSPL as a function of frequency in that the SSPL can be set independently in each channel.

Figure 5–17 shows UCL data obtained by Dillon and Macrae (1986) for two groups of hearing aid users: 71 children with sensorineural hearing losses and 45 adults with mixed hearing losses. To show the extent to which UCLs vary with frequency, each set of curves has been normalized to a common UCL level at 250 Hz. As can be seen, the range of variation with frequency is on the order of 40 dB for children with sensorineural hearing losses and as much as 60 dB for adults with mixed hearing losses. An important implication of these data is that if a single SSPL value is selected independent of frequency, there will either be a large frequency range over which the dynamic range of the hearing aid is limited unnecessarily or frequency regions in which amplified energy exceeds discomfort level. There is now revived interest in methods of selecting SSPL, and the use of frequency-dependent SSPL settings has potential advantages that need to be further explored.

The second general class of suprathreshold prescriptive procedures is that in which MCLs are measured directly. Knudsen (1939) was the first to suggest use of MCLs in the

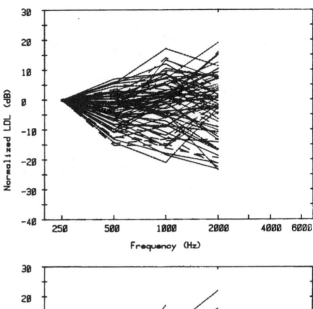

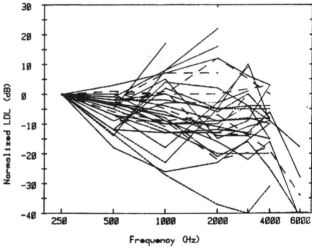

Figure 5–17 Uncomfortable loudness levels (called "loudness discomfort levels" or LDLs in this figure) versus frequency for 71 children with sensorineural hearing losses *(top)* and 45 adults with mixed hearing losses *(bottom)*. All values have been normalized to 0 dB at 250 Hz to illustrate the range of curve shapes encountered. (Reprinted from Dillon and Macrae [1986] with permission.)

prescriptive fitting of hearing aids. In their classic paper Watson and Knudsen (1940) recommended that, instead of mirroring the audiogram (the primary technique used at that time), the MCL curves should be mirrored. Watson and Knudsen (1940), however, measured loudness using tonal stimuli, which can be a difficult task for the typical hearing aid candidate with no previous exposure to psychoacoustic testing. Davis et al (1946) unfortunately discounted the use of loudness measurements in hearing aid prescription, arguing that these techniques are impractical in a clinical setting. As a consequence, the use of loudness measurements in fitting hearing aids remained dormant until Pascoe (1978) and Skinner et al (1982) revived the use of this approach.

Pascoe (1978) used a very simple rating procedure to obtain loudness levels that was easy to use and reliable for listeners with hearing loss who had no previous experience in making loudness judgments. Five rating categories were used, each with an easy-to-understand descriptor: "very soft," "soft," "O.K.," "loud," "too loud." This rating procedure, although less precise than the more sophisticated loudness scaling techniques developed by Stevens (1955), was nevertheless sufficiently accurate for its intended clinical application. The nine-category loudness scale of Hawkins et al (1987) has also seen widespread use. The Pascoe procedure was refined by Allen et al (1990) as part of a joint project between AT&T Bell Laboratories and the Hearing Aid Research Laboratory at the City University of New York (CUNY) in evaluating the AT&T analog/digital hybrid hearing aid (which later became the ReSound hearing aid). The computerized version of the technique, known as LGOB (Loudness Growth in Octave Bands), has been made available commercially by several hearing aid manufacturers for fitting of their instruments.

Skinner et al (1982) used the Pascoe method of loudness scaling to develop her approach to hearing aid fitting, sometimes called the CID (Central Institute for the Deaf) method. The goal is to place the RMS speech spectrum at a comfortable listening level at all frequencies within the bandwidth of the hearing aid, with less amplification at 250 Hz. Shapiro

(1976; 1980) also used MCL measurements as the key parameter in his fitting technique.

Like the threshold-based formulas, suprathreshold techniques can result in different prescribed frequency-gain characteristics. Consider the following example. Figure 5–18A shows the audiogram, ULCL levels, and UCL levels for a hypothetical patient. MCL levels were assumed to be 6 dB less than ULCL levels. Figure 5–18B shows the prescribed frequency-gain characteristics using four suprathreshold techniques (MSU, CID, Shapiro, and the UCL method). The values show some modification of the techniques so that prescribed gain did not amplify the speech spectrum to levels exceeding UCL minus 12 dB (Humes & Halling, 1994). The UCL method prescribes the greatest overall gain, whereas the Shapiro method prescribes the least amount of gain. Note, however, that the patient is likely to adjust the volume control wheel of the hearing aid. Figure 5–18C shows the effect of adjusting overall gain so that all four frequency-gain characteristics have the same gain at 1000 Hz. As can be seen, the differences in the frequency-gain characteristics are substantially smaller.

There are several potential disadvantages to the use of suprathreshold techniques. Additional clinical time is needed

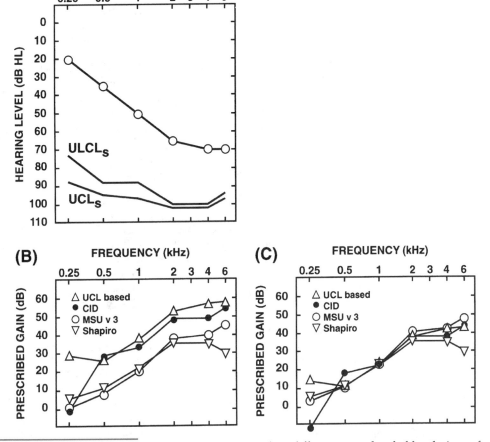

Figure 5–18 Frequency responses calculated using four different suprathreshold techniques for the audiogram shown in **(A)**. **(B)** is the calculated insertion gain, and **(C)** shows the responses equalized at 1000 Hz, as might occur with volume control adjustment. (Adapted from Humes and Halling [1994] with permission.)

to obtain the suprathreshold measurements. Also, as pointed out by the proponents of threshold-based formulas, loudness measurements (MCLs, UCLs) are more variable than threshold measurements (Berger & Soltisz, 1981; Christensen & Byrne, 1980) and can be difficult to obtain accurately in young children or mentally handicapped adults. Furthermore, the issue is not necessarily how well the speech signal can be placed at MCL at all frequencies but rather "how accurately can we specify the frequency-gain characteristics from clinical measurements of thresholds as opposed to clinical measurement of MCL" (Dillon, personal communication, 1998).

The choice between using threshold-based formulas and suprathreshold procedures reduces to two key questions: Do suprathreshold procedures provide improved hearing aid fitting, and if so, does the magnitude of the improvement justify the time and effort required? Whereas definitive answers to these questions have yet to be obtained, the new generation of compression hearing aids will inherently require suprathreshold techniques.

CONTROVERSIAL POINT

Threshold-based techniques have the important advantage of being both practical and time efficient. A well-chosen suprathreshold-based or other more advanced technique requiring additional measurements should in principle, however, provide a better fit. From a cost-effective perspective, is the additional time and effort required by the more detailed approach warranted in terms of improved performance? The answer is likely to be positive for hard-to-fit patients but this may not necessarily be the case for patients who present no difficulties in fitting.

Some experimental fitting procedures have used functional gain measurements. Functional gain is the difference, in dB, between the aided threshold and unaided threshold at a given frequency. The UCL method used by Abramowitz (1980) was modified by Hertzano et al (1979) to obtain frequency-gain characteristics in a form that could be specified in terms of standard coupler measurements. This was done by relating aided UCL measurements in the sound field to standard coupler measurements. Unaided sound field measurements were then obtained to determine the functional gain for UCL levels. In this approach, unlike aided threshold measurements, aided UCL measurements were not affected by the internal noise of the hearing aid. The UCLs could also be used to specify the SSPL of the hearing aid.

Another experimental application of functional gain was called the "Reference Hearing Aid (RHA)" method (Hertzano et al, 1979; Levitt et al, 1987). In this approach, a hearing aid with a relatively flat frequency response (as measured in a standard coupler) and low internal noise is used as a reference. The aided sound field threshold is obtained for the reference hearing aid, followed by measurements of the signal level at which one-third octave bands of conversational speech are comfortably loud. The required gain for each one-third octave band obtained in this way is added to the frequency-gain characteristics of the reference hearing aid as measured in a standard coupler. A hearing aid having this coupler gain, or a close approximation to it, is then selected and fitted to the patient. The RHA method is particularly well suited for fitting programmable hearing aids because there is no need to change hearing aids during the fitting procedure; in this case a relatively flat frequency response is chosen for the reference condition. One of the strengths of this technique is that it bypasses the problem of correcting for coupler-to-real-ear differences.

Approaches for Fitting WDRC and Multichannel Hearing Aids

As more compression and multichannel signal processing hearing aids have entered the commercial market in the last decade, with many audiologist-adjustable compression parameters including crossover frequency(s), compression threshold(s), compression ratio(s), and time constants, prescriptive formulas intended for conventional hearing aids have become largely inadequate. Although it is possible to set the frequency response of multichannel WDRC and/or AFR hearing aids using a linear prescriptive approach and verifying that this is achieved with a moderate-level input (i.e., 60- to 70-dB SPL), the audiologist is left to best-guess what would be most appropriate for parameters such as compression threshold and ratio.

The selection and fitting of compression hearing aids is still at an early stage of development, but suprathreshold techniques are well suited because the very concept of compression involves suprathreshold processing. A number of new approaches have been described, some specifically proposed for multichannel WDRC hearing aids and most with software available for personal computers to ease implementation (see de Jonge, 1996). New methods introduced include the International Hearing Aid Fitting Forum (IHAFF) (Cox, 1995; Valente & Van Vliet, 1997; Van Vliet, 1995), "FIG6" (named after Figure 6 in a publication by Killion and Fikret-Pasa, 1993; also see Gitles & Niquette, 1995), a modified DSL approach called DSL[i/o] (also known as DSL version 4.0; Cornelisse et al, 1995; Seewald et al, 1996), and a modification of the NAL approach that has recently been developed. The stated objective of the latter approach is to maximize speech intelligibility subject to making loudness not greater than normal (NAL Annual Report, 1998). Some of these approaches are briefly described in the bottom section of Table 5–2.

The IHAFF approach incorporates measurements of an individual's loudness growth functions using frequency-specific stimuli (as is also done in manufacturer's fitting approaches that include LGOB measurements). The stated goal of the IHAFF is to compensate for loudness recruitment by determining appropriate compression thresholds and ratios for a two-channel hearing aid so that sounds at soft (50 dB SPL), moderate (65 dB SPL), and loud (80 dB SPL) input levels are perceived at levels comparable to those of a normal ear. This approach, in essence, attempts to "normalize" loudness perception in the impaired ear. The FIG6 procedure calculates desired responses for input levels of 40-, 65-, and 90-dB SPL entirely from threshold data, with estimates of loudness values made from average data. The DSL[i/o] procedure uses measured thresholds and either predicted or measured loudness values to provide compression parameters that will result in a target family of frequency responses for input levels ranging from 45- to 90-dB SPL. These more complex fitting methods intended for use with compression hearing aids are covered in detail in Chapter 6 in this volume.

Important philosophical differences have emerged with respect to both fitting procedures and new methods of signal processing. One philosophical approach is to recreate, as closely as possible, the normal loudness patterns of speech and other complex sounds. Methods that attempt to recreate normal loudness patterns use WDRC with input/output curves that normalize the subject's perception of loudness as a function of frequency. Villchur (1974) demonstrated how abnormal loudness patterns (simulated with expansion amplification in normal ears) might reduce speech recognition and argued that normalization of loudness patterns for cochlear-impaired individuals with abnormal loudness growth functions (i.e., with loudness recruitment) would improve recognition.

Others have argued that insufficient evidence exists that loudness normalization will improve speech recognition over that achieved simply by ensuring that speech is audible but comfortable over a wide frequency range (Byrne, 1996; Van Tasell, 1993). It is very difficult if not impossible to normalize loudness patterns for complex sounds because abnormal loudness growth functions vary not only as a function of frequency but also as a function of signal duration. Whereas it is possible to normalize frequency-dependent loudness growth functions for well-defined psychoacoustic stimuli using multichannel WDRC, it is not clear how to normalize these functions in terms of the time-varying temporal characteristics of speech and the abnormal temporal processing of the ear with sensorineural hearing loss. It is also very difficult to measure and specify how well loudness patterns in speech have been normalized and thus it is not known whether the less-than-ideal results that have been obtained with this approach are due to imperfect loudness normalization (which could be improved with more accurate frequency-dependent compression) or whether the approach is basically flawed. One problem is that different measurement methods and stimuli can result in different loudness growth functions for the same individual, a finding that begs the question of which is the appropriate reference condition (Elberling, 1996).

One of the implications of successful loudness normalization is that a volume control would, in principle, not be necessary because a normal-hearing person does not have the equivalent of a gain control. Hearing aids of this type without a volume control have been introduced but have met with consumer resistance. One interpretation of this result might be that the consumer wants to be "in control" and hence feels uncomfortable without a volume control, or it may be that the normalization was unsuccessful and some sounds were still either too loud or too soft. An alternate explanation, which addresses the core issue, is that additional gain may improve speech intelligibility and that, under certain conditions, abnormally loud but more intelligible speech is preferred over more normal sounding but less intelligible speech. Neuman et al (1995) found that subjects using compression amplification raised overall gain when speech in noise was barely intelligible but lowered gain when the speech was more intelligible (because of a favorable SNR) or was wholly unintelligible because of a very poor SNR.

The second major philosophical approach to fitting compression hearing aids attempts to maximize speech recognition by making as much of the speech signal audible as possible without regard to loudness normalization. Fitting procedures of this type typically provide more gain to low-level speech sounds than would be the case with the loudness normalization approach. As a consequence, weak speech sounds, such as voiceless fricatives, sound louder than in normal speech, but they are also more intelligible.

CONTROVERSIAL POINT

From one perspective, recreating normal loudness functions with compression amplification represents an ideal. Another perspective is that abnormal loudness functions may be a more effective way of improving speech intelligibility. Normal speech heard by normal-hearing listeners is not always fully intelligible and can be made more intelligible by appropriate frequency-dependent and level-dependent gain adjustments.

A method of implementing the preceding approach is to place as much of the speech signal as possible in the residual hearing area. This can be done by selecting a compression system such that at each frequency the peaks of speech fall slightly below the discomfort level (or at the upper bound of the comfort level), whereas the low-level components of speech are amplified to fall above the threshold of hearing. Orthogonal polynomial compression (Levitt & Neuman, 1991) has been used to accomplish this objective. The results showed that intelligibility increased with increased audibility until a point of diminishing returns was reached when further increases in overall audibility (obtained by squeezing more of the speech signal into the residual hearing area) resulted in the destruction of important phonetic cues and a corresponding reduction in performance.

An alternate approach with a strong theoretical basis is that of maximizing the Articulation Index (AI) (Abramowitz, 1980; Radley et al, 1947;* Seewald, 1992; Seewald & Ross, 1988; Seewald et al, 1993). The AI has a value between 0 and 1 that represents the proportion of the speech signal contributing to intelligibility. The AI is derived by dividing the range of speech frequencies into 20 frequency bands that contribute equally to intelligibility. The speech-peak-to-RMS-noise ratio (or speech-peak-to-threshold ratio for noise below the threshold of audibility) is obtained for each frequency band. The maximum and minimum allowable values for each band are 30 dB and 0 dB, respectively. Adjustments are also made for upward spread of masking and other nonlinear effects at high signal or noise levels. The mean speech-peak-to-RMS-noise (or speech-peak-to-threshold) ratio averaged over the 20 bands is then obtained. The AI is equal to this mean speech-to-noise (or speech-to-threshold) ratio divided by 30 for purposes of normalization.

---

*Appendix II of the MedResCo Report, titled "The optimum frequency response characteristics of a hearing aid," used the concept of articulation efficiency, which was a precursor to the Articulation Index.

A problem with the AI approach is that at the high signal levels needed to maximize the index, spread of masking and other nonlinear effects are of critical importance but are not well understood. Individual differences in the magnitude of these effects are also large. Research in this area is progressing (Rankovic, 1991) and a practical method of maximizing the AI for hearing aid users may be developed in the not too distant future.

The objective of maximizing speech recognition is, of course, highly commendable. The problem is that we do not yet know how to process speech to achieve this goal. Fitting approaches in this category and new methods of signal processing have been found to yield some improvement with respect to the primary objective of maximizing intelligibility but less than that hoped for, particularly for the case of speech in background noise (Levitt et al, 1990, 1993). Many different techniques have been found to yield essentially the same intelligibility for speech in noise but with marked differences in overall sound quality. This has led to the introduction of a second criterion, that of maximizing overall sound quality while maintaining speech intelligibility at, or close to, its maximum value.

For the case of speech in noise, overall sound quality can be improved if additional compression is provided in those frequency regions where the noise is likely to exceed the level of the speech peaks. Because most ambient noises have a majority of energy in the low frequencies, a two-channel compression system with additional compression in the low frequencies should improve overall sound quality. The choice of compression threshold(s), CR(s), crossover frequency between the channels, and frequency response before compression, however, depend on the characteristics of the noise, which is not usually known with any degree of precision.

Another area of uncertainty in the selection and fitting of compression hearing aids is the choice of time constants. Relatively good results have been obtained with release times in excess of 500 ms, so that the form of compression amplification is that of AGC (Neuman et al, 1994). From a theoretical perspective, it should be possible to achieve further improvements in speech recognition (in quiet) by the use of short time constants (i.e., by using syllabic compression in addition to AGC). Whereas AGC is very effective in making the overall level of speech comfortably loud, weak sounds may still be inaudible, or barely audible, particularly if masked by a neighboring strong sound. Syllabic compression addresses this problem directly by increasing the audibility of the weaker sounds. As yet, however, no practical methods of fitting syllabic compression systems have been developed that yield significant improvements in speech recognition compared with a well-designed AGC hearing aid that has been fitted properly with an appropriate frequency response. The possibility nevertheless remains that some form of compression may improve speech recognition beyond that which can be obtained using single-channel AGC compression and that appropriate procedures for selecting and fitting such a system will be developed. Research in pursuit of this goal remains active. See, for example, the recent research findings of Kennedy et al (1998).

At present, as in the case of prescriptive formulas developed for linear hearing aids, debate continues about the relative differences and merits of each of the suprathreshold fitting philosophies and approaches for compression hearing aids (see Byrne, 1996). There is little doubt that

existing techniques will continue to be refined and to evolve over time as our knowledge increases and more validation studies are accomplished. Audiologists will need to be vigilant in examining the rationale of and support for new selection and fitting approaches, particularly as more complicated nonlinear signal processing hearing aids enter the market.

The Carhart Method of Hearing Aid Selection

At about the same time as the Harvard and MedResCo Reports, Raymond Carhart of Northwestern University published a series of articles that advocated an empirical method of hearing aid selection on the basis of his experiences fitting large numbers of servicemen and veterans during and after World War II (Carhart, 1946a,b,c; 1950). Carhart's method differed substantially from the prescriptive approaches that have been discussed in that it focused on selecting the best hearing aids for a patient from a set of available instruments. No prescriptive formulas or theoretical justification was used in selecting the appropriate hearing aids (or even in choosing a subset of hearing aids from which the selection was to be made). He was also the first to consider the effects of background noise in developing a fitting technique for hearing aids.

Basically, the approach was to compare the performance of the patient using the hearing aids under consideration, across four dimensions: (1) sensitivity to sound, (2) tolerance limits, (3) efficiency in background noise, and (4) efficiency in distinguishing small sound differences. The hearing aids were evaluated on each of these dimensions using audiological tests including functional gain, aided loudness discomfort and examination of listening dynamic range, and speech recognition tests in quiet and in noise. The hearing aid(s) that best met the needs of the user across these four dimensions was selected. In cases in which hearing aids showed equivalent performance, other criteria were considered such as "convenience, weight and esthetic preferences" (Carhart, 1946c, p. 789).

Carhart's approach was appealing in the 1940s when the merits of individualized prescription versus "one-size-fits-all" frequency responses were being argued. The approach was intended to be part of a multiweek aural rehabilitation program done by those in the emerging audiological profession. The Carhart method was subsequently widely adopted by audiologists, although the method was modified over the years to meet the needs and resources available to various clinics.

Two key elements of the Carhart procedure distinguished it from methods developed by other pioneers in this area. First, performance was evaluated in noise as well as quiet. The inclusion of an evaluation in noise was one of the great strengths of the Carhart method. Many hearing aids have equivalent performance characteristics in quiet but differ significantly in terms of their performance in noise. Because hearing aid users have great difficulty in listening to speech in noise, superior performance on this dimension is particularly important. The second distinguishing characteristic of the Carhart method was that the hearing aids finally selected were instruments actually evaluated on the patient. This is important from a practical perspective. There are cases in which hearing aids prescribed according to a well-established theory or prescriptive formula turn out to be a poor choice because of factors not considered in the prescriptive process, such as internal noise or intermodulation distortion resulting from imperfections in the instrument. It was highly unlikely with the Carhart method that the hearing aids finally selected would have any such hidden flaws because they would be detected in the evaluation stage.

On the negative side, however, there are a number of weaknesses with the Carhart method. First, if the initial choice of hearing aids to be evaluated did not include instruments that were appropriate for the patient, the hearing aids that were finally selected would not be the best choice. Second, the time it took to accomplish all the recommended testing over a group of hearing aids was quite lengthy. Finally, and perhaps most seriously, Carhart used traditional methods of speech audiometry such as phonetically balanced (PB) word lists. These tests have been found to be relatively insensitive to differences among hearing aids (McConnell et al, 1960; Shore et al, 1960). Although there were efforts in the late 1960s and early 1970s to develop more sensitive and reliable speech tests (Campbell, 1965; Jerger et al, 1966b; Margolis & Millin, 1971), this has proven to be a difficult task even today. Thus several researchers began to question the reliability and validity of the Carhart approach (Resnick & Becker, 1963; Shore & Kramer, 1965), and it generally fell out of favor with the revival of interest in threshold-based and suprathreshold prescriptive approaches.

On-Line Adaptive Adjustment

Every method of hearing aid fitting typically ends with some final adjustments to the hearing aids. These final adjustments (or "fine-tuning") are a form of adaptive fitting in that they involve adjustments to previous settings of the hearing aids to improve performance. Often, however, these adjustments are ad hoc in that they depend on the audiologist's skill and intuition in knowing which variable needs to be adjusted and by how much.

Levitt (1978) described an approach in which systematic adaptive adjustment is the primary means of fitting hearing aids and not merely an ad hoc final adjustment. The method begins with an initial estimate of the optimum set of electroacoustic characteristics for the patient. Small adjustments are then made to each variable. If improved performance is obtained, the adjustments are continued in the same direction. If not, adjustments are made in the opposite direction. The process is continued until an optimum condition is reached (i.e., further adjustment of any variable in any direction results in poorer performance).

This adaptive procedure, then, will converge on the best possible settings of the hearing aids for the variables that are being adjusted. If the measure of performance is subject to random errors of measurement, the procedure will converge more slowly on the optimum settings. The final estimate of the optimum settings will also differ from the true optimum by a small statistically insignificant amount, as in any method of statistical estimation.

The advantages of other fitting procedures can be incorporated within the adaptive framework. For example, any reasonable procedure can be used to obtain the initial estimate of the optimum settings. If a very good initial estimate is used, such as that provided by the best available prescriptive formula, the adaptive procedure will converge rapidly on the final estimate. If a poor initial estimate is used, the convergence process will take longer. In either case the final estimate

of the optimum hearing aid settings will result in hearing aid performance that is better than (or at least as good as) that obtained with the best available prescriptive formula.

Another important advantage of the adaptive approach is that any one of a variety of different measures can be used to determine whether performance has improved (i.e., the technique is not constrained to using a single type of testing such as traditional speech recognition tests). It is possible, for example, to use subjective judgments of sound quality and/or clarity using either absolute rating scales or paired-comparison techniques.

In the first experimental implementation of systematic adaptive adjustment, the measures used to examine performance across settings were speech recognition tests administered under conditions representative of actual use (Levitt, 1978). An adjustable, wearable master hearing aid was used for this purpose. Although the adaptive procedure consistently converged on settings that yielded superior performance to the initial estimate of the optimum settings, the time taken to reach this goal was far too long for the technique to be of practical clinical value. Methods of improving the efficiency of the adaptive approach were then investigated, and substantial reductions in the time needed to converge on the optimum settings were obtained by the use of adaptive paired comparison techniques instead of traditional speech recognition tests (Levitt et al, 1987; Neuman et al, 1987).

The availability of computer-controlled programmable hearing aids in the 1980s, combined with the use of paired comparisons (or other time-efficient performance measures), made adaptive on-line adjustment a practical reality. In fact, an on-line adaptive adjustment technique was used to fit the Nicolet Phoenix digital hearing aid upon its initial release. Variations on this type of approach have been suggested for clinical use (Byrne & Cotton, 1988; Kuk, 1994).

Verification and Validation of the Hearing Aid Fitting

Regardless of what selection and fitting approach is used and whether the fitting involves conventional linear hearing aids or multichannel compression, it is necessary to ensure (verify) that the electroacoustic parameters that were selected as best for the patient were in fact accurately matched with the device on the patient's ear. In the early days of fitting hearing aids the differences in decibels between supra-aural headphones calibrated in a 6-cc coupler, hearing aids with 2-cc coupler measurements, and real-ear in situ gain, were not well appreciated. With the widespread adoption in the 1980s of real-ear probe microphone measurement of frequency-gain characteristics, it became easier to verify that a prescription had been met, although technological and manufacturing constraints on the accuracy of obtaining prescribed frequency responses were, and can still be, a problem (Sammeth et al, 1993).

A practical problem in many of the prescriptive fitting procedures is that audiological measurements (thresholds, MCLs, UCLs) obtained with standard earphones need to be corrected for acoustic coupling effects so as to provide accurate predictions of the signal levels reaching the eardrum under conditions of actual hearing aid use. This is not an easy task, varies across earphone type and hearing aid style, and is subject to error. The coupler-to-real-ear corrections that are often used are based on average adult data and can be highly inaccurate for individuals with unusually small ears (especially, the case of young children).

The above problem can be circumvented by using the reference hearing aid technique (Levitt et al, 1987). This technique, however, is not widely used possibly because the earliest implementation of the technique was relatively inconvenient (Hertzano et al, 1979). This technique could be implemented conveniently and efficiently today with modern programmable hearing aids.

PEARL

For ears with unusually large or small volumes, the individual real-ear unaided response (REUR) can be incorporated into the prescribed gain calculation in lieu of the average response to ensure a better fit to target when ordering an ITE hearing aid.

Current clinical practice consists largely of verifying the selected frequency-gain characteristics and SSPL level using real-ear probe microphone measurements. The real-ear saturation response also provides an alternative to measurement of aided UCLs that is easier to obtain in an infant, child, or noncompliant adult. It should be kept in mind, however, that, as previously noted, probe microphone measurements can also be subject to error including inaccuracy in the high frequencies and effects of depth of probe placement (Hawkins & Mueller, 1986).

Before probe microphone instrumentation, one method used to address the problem of determining the gain an individual was receiving was to measure functional gain (difference in dB between the aided and unaided sound field threshold). It can be specified as a single number for broadband speech or as a function of frequency for narrowband stimuli. There are several possible sources of error in the use of functional gain measurements. First, because the value is the difference between two subjective measurements, the threshold-seeking procedure needs to be precise. Second, the internal noise of a hearing aid can produce masking effects during measurements of aided thresholds in regions of less severe hearing loss, thereby underestimating actual functional gain. Third, because these measurements are done in sound field, a better nontest ear must be plugged or muffed adequately during testing. Fourth, errors can occur in ears with sharply sloping audiograms. Noise bands or frequency-modulated signals of finite bandwidth are typically used in measuring unaided thresholds to minimize the effects of standing waves in the test room. In cases of precipitous high-frequency hearing losses, the edge of the finite bandwidth signal can be detected in a neighboring frequency region rather than at the nominal frequency being tested; in other words, off-frequency listening can occur.

Probe microphone measurements are generally preferred over measurement of functional gain because they are faster and provide a view of the entire frequency response rather than only a few selected frequencies. With linear hearing aids, functional gain and real-ear insertion gain (REIG; the difference between the unaided and aided frequency responses obtained with probe microphone measurements) are considered to be comparable, assuming measurement error is negligibly small. However, a few exceptions to this rule exist

(Stelmachowicz & Lewis, 1988). With severe-to-profound hearing loss, functional gain measurement is preferred to REIG because the latter approach may show high levels of gain, but the impaired ear may be unable to use the amplification because of the extensive nature of the hearing loss. Thus REIG may overestimate functional gain in these patients. In contrast, with compression hearing aids, functional gain, which is obtained at threshold levels, will overestimate the gain that the hearing aid supplies to higher speech-level inputs. Thus REIG is the method of choice with compression hearing aids.

As opposed to verification that desired electroacoustics have been achieved, validation refers to measuring whether the patient actually performs well with, and likes, what was prescribed. Validation is important because the hearing aid parameters initially fit may need to be adjusted at follow-up. For some years the use of a prescriptive formula with probe microphone or functional gain verification entailed the entire selection and evaluation process in some clinics. The limitations of this approach are discussed by Ross and Levitt (1997). In contrast to the lengthy rehabilitation program used by Carhart, the use of prescriptive formulas with verification methods sometimes led to limited follow-up with a patient after fitting of the hearing aids.

Awareness has been growing, however, that the original prescription for an individual patient may need to be fine-tuned on the basis of the patients' report of how he is doing with the hearing aids. The prescription may need to be revised for many reasons, including sound quality or comfort factors (e.g., occlusion effect, excessive loudness, perceived "tinniness"), the patients' unique listening environments and personality, and differences in an individual from the average profile on which the prescription was based. Sometimes the audiologist will find that he or she needs to make a tradeoff between the electroacoustic parameters that produce measurably best performance in the clinic and what the patient will tolerate when they wear their hearing aids in the real world. On the other hand, there is reason to encourage a patient to wear the hearing aids long enough to learn to adjust to the new sound, a process that has been called "acclimatization" (Gatehouse, 1992; Turner et al, 1996).

Another reason why validation measures are important is that audiologists, like other health professionals, are under increasing pressure to document to third-party reimbursors that their treatments are, in fact, effective in overcoming the handicap and/or disability imposed by hearing loss. The most commonly used validation approach, beyond informal querying of the patient regarding their everyday performance with the hearing aids, is the use of formalized questionnaires that measure the benefit of the fitting. It is important to note, however, that there are inherent limitations of using questionnaires to validate hearing aid fittings (Ross & Levitt, 1997).

Speech recognition testing can be considered a form of objective validation measure. Another objective measure would be of localization ability, but to date this type of measurement has not been introduced clinically. With the demise of the Carhart comparative procedure, speech recognition testing has largely fallen out of favor. Although some clinicians continue to measure speech recognition unaided and then aided after prescriptive fitting of hearing aids, this practice has dramatically decreased. The problem is that speech recognition testing is not only time consuming but it also rarely results in any change in the choice of hearing aids or their electroacoustic parameters. Rather, the results are typically used only to assist in patient counseling. With the introduction of more complex signal processing approaches, and growing pressure in the health services to document that treatments are effective, the argument may be made for a return to the use of objective validation measurements. New speech recognition tests have been introduced, for example, that appear to have greater potential to differentiate performance across hearing aids, such as the HINT (Hearing In Noise Test; Nillsson et al, 1994), which uses sentence-level materials and an adaptive SNR paradigm. For a comprehensive overview and history of the development of speech recognition tests, a good source is the recent textbook by Mendel and Danhauer (1997).

CONCLUSIONS

The history of hearing aids has shown dramatic technological advances that have revolutionized the field on more than one occasion. These advances have been followed by substantial changes in selection and fitting practices. Furthermore, technological progress has accelerated over the years, with similarly rapid changes in the introduction of new types of hearing aids. The transistor hearing aid, for example, was the first commercial application of the newly invented transistor outside the telephone industry (which nurtured the invention). The hearing aid industry also led the field in developing miniature, low-voltage analog circuits. These rapid technological advances led to the development of the BTE hearing aid, which replaced the older, well-established body-worn hearing aid as the instrument of choice for most hearing aid users within a period of only a few years.

Although each decade of the century-long history of hearing aids has seen major advances in both technology and clinical practice, the most dramatic changes of all have taken place during the most recent decade. These changes have, in essence, brought about the conclusion of one search for the Holy Grail and replaced it with another. For the past century, the driving force in hearing aid development was primarily that of reducing the size of these instruments so as to make them cosmetically acceptable. The 1990s saw the introduction of the CIC hearing aid followed closely by major advances in the development of a fully implantable hearing aid. These instruments represent the culmination of the long quest for an invisible hearing aid. Now that this ultimate cosmetic objective has been reached, the primary focus of hearing aid development has begun to switch to broader objectives. Hearing aids are now designed to do more than simply amplify signals (i.e., some modern hearing aids now incorporate noise reduction techniques, feedback cancellation, signal monitoring, speech enhancement, and other methods of signal processing). The driving force in hearing aid design is thus changing from a focus on miniaturization per se to increasing the signal processing capabilities of hearing aids within the limited space available.

Perhaps the most important development during the past decade has been the introduction of practical digital hearing aids. With digital hearing aids it is necessary to think not only in terms of the hardware of amplification (amplifiers, filters, output limiters) but also in terms of hearing aid software (i.e., programming the hearing aid, storing and transfering

information to and from memory, integrating fitting techniques with other audiological procedures, and computerized methods of record keeping). A digital hearing instrument can be programmed to generate sound and, thus, can also act as an audiometer. The many possibilities of modern digital techniques are almost beyond comprehension.

Today, then, the primary limitation in developing improved hearing instruments is not technological limitations but rather our lack of understanding of how to use the technology to compensate for the effects of sensorineural hearing loss. After many years of research, we have come to a much deeper understanding of the basics of hearing loss and appropriate fitting procedures for conventional hearing aids, but technological advances have outstripped this study rate of increase in our knowledge. The introduction of multichannel hearing aids, each capable of different forms of compression amplification or other means of signal processing, has opened up a Pandora's box of new clinical problems. How does one decide on the most appropriate form of signal processing in a hearing aid for a given patient? How does one fit the many electroacoustic parameters of a modern multichannel compression hearing aid to provide for best performance? These are difficult questions, and the research needed to provide adequate answers may exceed by far the research already completed with respect to the much simpler problem of selecting and fitting conventional hearing aids.

The introduction of new methods of signal processing requires the development of new methods of hearing aid selection and fitting. The techniques developed in the past can serve as useful stepping stones toward the development of new procedures, and we can learn much from both the successes and errors of the past. For example, of the many formulas and techniques for hearing aid fitting that have been developed over the years, the ones that have lasted and yielded the best results are those based on careful experimentation and objective evaluation. If we are to succeed in developing effective fitting procedures for the new methods of signal processing, greater emphasis should be placed on the scientific approach that has succeeded in the past rather than the nonexperimental intuitive approach that has also sometimes been used.

A key concern in this regard is the lack of objective measures for assessing the quality of fit of modern hearing aids. Although consumer satisfaction is an important consideration in hearing aid fitting, it provides an incomplete and sometimes misleading picture of the quality of fit. Patients with low expectations will be satisfied with almost any hearing aid that provides improved hearing (even if poorly fitted) while consumers with unrealistically high expectations are likely to be dissatisfied with even the best hearing aid fitted in the best possible way. Objective measures of performance in combination with unbiased assessments of consumer satisfaction are needed if hearing aid fitting of high quality is to be maintained (and improved systematically over time).

The concept of an "optimum" or "best" fit also needs to be interpreted with caution. Hearing aids are used under a variety of listening conditions (e.g., in quiet, in noise, and under reverberant conditions). It is unlikely that the electroacoustic characteristics that provide optimum performance for one type of listening condition will also be optimum for all other listening conditions. Furthermore, it may be that the optimum set of electroacoustics for one condition (e.g., speech in quiet) is far from optimum for another condition (speech in noise). A better choice is for a set of electroacoustic characteristics that is close to optimum for both listening conditions (i.e., it is better to have a hearing aid that works reasonably well across a broad range of conditions, rather than one that is optimum for one condition only and far from optimum for other commonly occurring conditions). The use of a programmable hearing aid with multiple memories is one approach that attempts to address this problem (i.e., each memory stores the optimum electroacoustic parameters for a different listening condition). Ideally, a "smart" signal processor would be developed that would adapt to the best electroacoustic parameters for any given listening environment, but we are still far from this goal.

Another important issue is the criterion (or set of criteria) used to define optimum performance. Maximizing speech intelligibility is an important criterion, but as noted earlier, it may be possible to maximize intelligibility at the expense of listening comfort (e.g., the amplified signal may be too loud). A possible variation of this criterion is to maximize intelligibility within the range of comfortable listening. An alternative is to maximize overall sound quality while maintaining intelligibility close to the maximum possible value.

Finally, one of the consistent findings in almost all research on advanced methods of signal processing is the extent of individual differences. Several experimental methods of multichannel amplitude compression, for example, have shown significant improvements in speech recognition for some subjects but not for others. Similarly, certain methods of noise reduction have been found to be strongly favored by some subjects, whereas others prefer the unprocessed speech in noise. Individual differences are an important consideration in choosing the appropriate form of signal processing for each patient, but it is often difficult to pinpoint which audiological characteristics and/or personal considerations are most relevant in predicting success with a certain type of amplification. As hearing aids become more advanced in their signal processing capabilities, there will be an increasing number of options to choose from, and much more research is needed to develop candidacy criteria that will assist audiologists in selection of appropriate hearing aids for their patients.

SPECIAL CONSIDERATION

As signal processing capabilities of hearing aids become more sophisticated, large individual differences are to be expected. For example, some patients are likely to favor certain noise reduction strategies more than others. As a consequence, more sophisticated methods of fitting will need to be developed that take these individual differences into account.

In view of how rapidly the field of acoustic amplification is affected by technological advances, it is essential for audiologists to keep abreast of technological change. This is important not only because it will be necessary to anticipate the impact that these changes will have on patient care but also so that audiologists can continue to provide a leading role among hearing healthcare professionals in shaping future directions in the field.

ACKNOWLEDGMENTS

We wish to thank David Kirkwood, editor of *The Hearing Journal* for supplying some of the historical data on U.S. hearing aid sales, Claus Nielsen of Oticon A/S, Preben Brunved of Oticon, Inc., and Jim Curran of Starkey Laboratories for supplying photographs, and Gudrun Carlson of the Roudebush V.A. Medical Center in Indianapolis for drafting some of the figures. Preparation of this chapter was supported in part by Grant No. H133E30015 from the National Institute on Disability and Rehabilitation Research of the Department of Education. The opinions contained in this chapter are those of the grantee and do not necessarily reflect those of the Department of Education.

REFERENCES

ABRAMOWITZ, R. (1980). Frequency shaping and multiband compression in hearing aids. *Journal of Communication Disorders, 13*;485–488.

ALLEN, J.B., HALL, J.L., & JENG, P.S. (1990). Loudness growth in 1/2-octave bands (LGOB) – A procedure for the assessment of loudness. *Journal of the Acoustical Society of America, 88*(2);745–753.

ANSI S3.22-1996. American National Standards Institute. *Specification of hearing aid characteristics.* New York.

ANSI PC63.19-199x Draft Standard. American National Standards Institute/Accredited Standards Committee on Electromagnetic Compatibility. *American national standard for methods of measurement of compatibility between wireless communications devices and hearing aids.* New York.

BAER, T., MOORE, B., & GATEHOUSE, S. (1993). Spectral contrast enhancement of speech in noise for listeners with sensorineural hearing impairment: Effects on intelligibility, quality, and response times. *Journal of Rehabilitation Research and Development, 30*;49–72.

BALBI, C.M. (1935). Adjusted sound amplification. *U.S. Patent #2,003,875* (filed June 1932).

BARFOD, J. (1979). Speech perception processes and fitting of hearing aids. *Audiology, 18*;430–441.

BERGER, K.W. (1970). The first electric hearing aids. *Hearing Dealer, 21*;23–38.

BERGER, K.W. (1975). History and development of hearing aids. In: M. Pollack (Ed.), *Amplification for the hearing-impaired* (pp. 1–20). New York: Grune & Stratton, Inc.

BERGER, K.W. (1976). Early bone conduction hearing aid devices. *Archives of Otolaryngology, 102*(5); 315–318.

BERGER, K.W. (1978). Some ear trumpets of the 1700s and 1800s. *Ear Nose and Throat Journal, 57*(9);387–392.

BERGER, K.W. (1984). *The hearing aid: Its operation and development* (2nd ed.). Livonia, MI: National Hearing Aid Society.

BERGER, K.W., HAGBERG, E.N., & RANE, R.L. (1979). Determining hearing aid gain. *Hearing Instruments, 30;*26–28,44.

BERGER, K.W., HAGBERG, E.N., & RANE, R.L. (1988). *Prescription of hearing aids: Rationales, procedures and results.* Kent, OH: Herald Publishing.

BERGER, K.W., & SOLTISZ, L.L. (1981). Variability of thresholds and MCLs with speech babble. *Australian Journal of Audiology, 3;*1–3.

BLOOM, P. (1985). High-quality digital audio in the entertainment industry: an overview of achievements and challenges. *IEEE ASSP Magazine,* (pp. 2–25).

BRAGG, V. (1977). Toward a more objective hearing aid fitting procedure. *Hearing Instruments, 28*(9);6–9.

BRAIDA, L.D., DURLACH, N.I., LIPPMAN, R.P., HICKS, B.L., RABINOWITZ, W.M., REED, C.M. (1979). Hearing aids: A review of past research on linear amplification, amplitude compression and frequency lowering. *ASHA Monographs,* No. 19.

BRATT, G., & SAMMETH, C. (1991). Clinical implications of prescriptive formulas for hearing aid selection. In: G. Studebaker, F. Bess, & L. Beck (Eds.), *The Vanderbilt/V.A. Hearing Aid Report II* (pp. 23–33). Parkton MD: York Press.

BUNNELL, H. (1990). On enhancement of spectral contrast in speech for hearing-impaired listeners. *Journal of the Acoustical Society of America, 88;*2546–2556.

BUSTAMANTE, D.K., & BRAIDA, L.D. (1986). Wideband compression and spectral sharpening for hearing-impaired listeners. *Journal of the Acoustical Society of America (Suppl.), 80*(1);S12–S13.

BUSTAMANTE, D.K., & BRAIDA, L.D. (1987). Principal-component amplitude compression for the hearing impaired. *Journal of the Acoustical Society of America, 82;*1227–1242.

BYRNE, D. (1987). Hearing aid selection formulae: Same or different? *Hearing Instruments, 38*(1);5–11.

BYRNE, D. (1996). Hearing aid selection for the 1990s: Where to? *Journal of the American Academy of Audiology, 7;*377–395.

BYRNE, D., & COTTON, D. (1988). Evaluation of the National Acoustic Laboratories' new hearing aid selection procedure. *Journal of Speech and Hearing Research, 31;*178–186.

BYRNE, D., & DILLON, H. (1986). New procedure for selecting gain and frequency response of a hearing aid: The National Acoustics Laboratory (NAL) formula. *Ear and Hearing, 7;*257–265.

BYRNE, D., PARKINSON, A., & NEWALL, P. (1990). Hearing aid gain and frequency response requirements for the severely/profoundly hearing impaired. *Ear and Hearing, 11*(1);40–49

BYRNE, D., & TONNISON, W. (1976). Selecting the gain of hearing aids for persons with sensorineural hearing impairments. *Scandinavian Audiology, 5;*51–59.

CAMPBELL, R.A. (1965). Discrimination test word difficulty. *Journal of Speech and Hearing Disorders, 8;*13–22.

CARHART, R. (1946a). Selection of hearing aids. *Archives of Otolaryngology, 44;*1–18.

CARHART, R. (1946b). Volume control adjustment in hearing aid selection. *Laryngoscope, 56;*780–794.

CARHART, R. (1946c). Tests for selection of hearing aids. *Laryngoscope, 56;*780–794.

CARHART, R. (1950). Hearing aid selection by university clinics. *Journal of Speech and Hearing Disorders, 15;*106–113.

CHASIN, M. (1994). The acoustic advantages of CIC hearing aids. *Hearing Journal, 47*(11);13–17.

CHASIN, M. (1998). Current trends in implantable hearing aids. *Trends in Amplification, 2*(3);84–107.

CHRISTENSEN, B., & BYRNE, D. (1980). Variability of MCL measurements: significance for hearing aid selection. *Australian Journal of Audiology, 2;*10–18.

COOK, J.A., BACON, S.P., & SAMMETH, C. (1997). Effect of low–frequency gain reduction on speech recognition and its relation to upward spread of masking. *Journal of Speech Language and Hearing Research, 40;*410–422.

COOPER, J.C., & CUTTS, B.P. (1971). Speech discrimination in noise. *Journal of Speech and Hearing Research, 14;*332–337.

CORNELISSE, L.E., SEEWALD, R.C., & JAMIESON, D.G. (1995). The input/output [i/o] formula: A theoretical approach to the fitting of personal amplification devices. *Journal of the Acoustical Society of America, 97*(3);1854–1864.

COX, R.M. (1983). Using ULCL measures to find frequency/gain and SSPL 90. *Hearing Instruments, 34*(7);17–21, 39.

COX, R.M. (1985). Hearing aids and aural rehabilitation: A structured approach to hearing aid selection. *Ear and Hearing, 6;*226–239.

COX, R.M. (1988). The MSU hearing instrument prescription procedure. *Hearing Instruments, 39*(1);6–10.

COX, R.M. (1995). Using loudness data for hearing aid selection: the IHAFF approach. *Hearing Journal, 48*(2);10,39–44.

COX, R.M, & BISSET, J.D. (1982). Predictions of aided preferred listening levels for hearing aid gain prescription. *Ear and Hearing, 3;*66–71.

CUMMINS, K., HECOX, K. (1987). Ambulatory testing of digital hearing aid algorithm. In: R. Steel, & W. Gerrey (Eds.), *Proceedings of 10th Annual Conference on Rehabilitation Technology* (pp. 398–400). Washington, DC: RESNA – Association for Advancement of Rehabilitation Technology.

D'AMICO, P. (1989). Dispensing options with a programmable system. *Hearing Instruments, 40*(10);13–14.

DAVIS, H., HUDGINS, C.V., MARQUIS, R.J., NICHOLS, R.H., PETERSON, G., ROSS, D.A., & STEVENS, S.S. (1946). The selection of hearing aids. *Laryngoscope, 56;*85–115,135–162.

DAVIS, H., STEVENS, S.S., NICHOLS, R.H., HUDGINS, C.V., PETERSON, G., MARQUIS, R.J., & ROSS, D.A. (1947). *Hearing Aids: An experimental study of design objectives.* Cambridge: Harvard University Press.

deJONGE, R. (1996). Microcomputer applications for hearing aid selection and fitting. *Trends in Amplification, 1*(3); 84–107.

DILLON, H. (1988). Compression in hearing aids. In: R.E. Sandlin (Ed.), *Handbook of hearing aid amplification Vol. I.* (pp. 121–146). Boston, MA: Little, Brown (College-Hill Press).

DILLON, H., & MACRAE, J. (1984). Derivation of design specifications for hearing aids. *NAL Report No. 102.* Sydney: National Acoustics Laboratory.

DILLON, H., & MACRAE, J. (1986). Performance requirements for hearing aids. *Journal of Rehabilitation Research and Development, 23*(1);1–15.

DILLON, H., CHEW, R., & DEANS, M. (1984). Loudness discomfort level measurements and their implications for the design and fitting of hearing aids. *Australian Journal of Audiology, 6;*73–79.

DILLON, H., & STOREY, L. (1998). The National Acoustic Laboratories' procedure for selecting the saturation sound pressure level of hearing aids: theoretical derivation. *Ear and Hearing, 19*(4);255–266.

DIRKS, D.D., MORGAN, D.E., & DUBNO, J.R. (1982). Procedure for quantifying the effects of noise on speech recognition. *Journal of Speech and Hearing Disorders, 47*;114–123.

DRESCHLER, W., & PLOMP, R. (1985). Relation between psychophysical data and speech perception for hearing-impaired subjects II. *Journal of the Acoustical Society of America, 78*;1261–1270.

DYRLUND, O., & BISGAARD, N. (1991). Acoustic feedback margin improvements in hearing instruments using a prototype DFS (digital feedback suppression) system. *Scandinavian Audiology, 20*;49–53.

ELBERLING, C. (1996). *How to integrate knowledge from audiological and acoustical communication with the technological possibilities of tomorrow's hearing aids.* Presented at the conference of the *British Society of Audiology,* Winchester.

ENGEBRETSON, A. (1987). A wearable digital hearing aid. In: R. Steele, & W. Gerrey. (Eds.), *Proceedings of 10th Annual Conference on Rehabilitation Technology* (pp. 392–394). Washington, DC: RESNA – Association for the Advancement of Rehabilitation Technology.

ENGEBRETSON, A. (1990). A brief review of digital audio and the application of digital technology to hearing aids. *Seminars in Hearing, 11*(1);16–27.

ENGEBRETSON, A., MORELY, R., & OCONNELL, M. (1986). A wearable, pocket-sized processor for digital hearing aids and other hearing prosthesis applications. *Proceedings of the International Conference on Acoustics, Speech and Signal Processing (ICASSP)* (pp. 625–628). New York: Institute of Electrical and Electronics Engineers, Inc.

ERBER, N.P. (1971). Evaluation of special hearing aids for deaf children. *Journal of Speech and Hearing Disorders, 36*;527–537.

ERBER, N.P. (1973). Body-baffle and real-ear effects in the selection of hearing aids for deaf children. *Journal of Speech and Hearing Disorders, 38*;224–231.

FABRY, D.A. (1991). Programmable and automatic noise reduction in existing hearing aids. In: G. Studebaker, F. Bess, & L. Beck (Eds.), *The V.A./Vanderbilt Hearing Aid Report II* (pp. 65–78). Parkton, MD: York Press.

FABRY, D.A., LEEK, M.R., WALDEN, E., & CORD, M. (1993). Do adaptive frequency response hearing aids reduce "upward spread" of masking? *Journal of Rehabilitation Research and Development, 30*(3);318–325.

FAY, T. (1991). Implantable auditory systems. In: F. Bess, J. Studebaker, & L. Beck (Eds.), *The V.A./Vanderbilt Hearing Aid Report II* (pp.101–119). Parkton, MD: York Press.

FIFIELD, D.B., EARNSHAW, R., & SMITHER, M.F. (1977). A new ear impression technique. *Hearing Instruments, 28*(12);1–12, 40–41.

FIFIELD, D.B., EARNSHAW, R., SMITHER, M.F. (1980). A new ear impression technique to prevent acoustic feedback with high powered aids. *Volta Review, 82*;33–39.

FLANAGAN, J.L. (1965). *Speech analysis, synthesis and perception.* New York: Academic Press, Springer-Verlag.

GAGNE, J-P. (1988). Excess masking among listeners with a sensorineural hearing loss. *Journal of the Acoustical Society of America, 83*;2311–2321.

GATEHOUSE, S. (1992). The time course and magnitude of perceptual acclimatization to frequency responses: Evidence from monaural fitting of hearing aids. *Journal of the Acoustical Society of America, 92*;1258–1268.

GITLES, T.C., & NIQUETTE, P. (1995). FIG6 in Ten. *Hearing Review, 2*(10);28,30.

GLADSTONE, V.S. (1975). History and status of incompatibility of hearing aids and telephones. *ASHA, 17*(2);103–104.

GLASBERG, B.R., & MOORE, B.C. (1989). Psychoacoustic abilities of subjects with unilateral and bilateral cochlear hearing impairments and their relationship to the ability to understand speech. *Scandinavian Audiology (Suppl.), 32*;1–25.

GOLDBERG, H. (1972). The utopian hearing aid: Current state of the art. *Journal of Auditory Research, 12*;331–335.

GOLDBERG, H. (1982). Signal processors: application to the hearing-impaired. *Hearing Aid Journal, 35*;23–27.

GORDON-SALANT, S. (1986). Recognition of natural and time/intensity altered CV's by young and elderly subjects with normal-hearing. *Journal of the Acoustical Society of America, 77*;664–670.

GORDON-SALANT, S. (1987). Effects of acoustic modification on consonant recognition by elderly hearing-impaired subjects. *Journal of the Acoustical Society of America, 81*(4);1199–1202.

GRAUPE, D., & CAUSEY, G. (1975). Development of a hearing aid system with independently adjustable sub-ranges of its spectrum using microprocessor hardware. *Bulletin of Prosthetic Research 12*;241–242.

GRAUPE, D., & CAUSEY, G. (1977). Method and means for adaptively filtering near-stationary noise from speech. *U.S. Patent #4,025,721,* May.

GRAUPE, D, GROSSPIETSCH, J., & BASSEAS, S. (1987). A single microphone-based self-adaptive filter of noise from speech and its performance evaluation. *Journal of Rehabilitation Research and Development, 24*(4);119–126.

GRAUPE, D., GROSSPIETSCH, J., & TAYLOR, R. (1986). A self adaptive noise filtering system. *Hearing Instruments, 37*(9);29–34.

GRAVEL, J., FAUSEL, N., LISKOW, C., & CHOBOT, J. (1998). Children's speech recognition in noise using dual-microphone hearing aid technology. *Ear and Hearing.* In Press.

GUTTMAN, N., & NELSON, J.R. (1968). An instrument that creates some artificial speech spectra for the severely hard of hearing. *American Annals of the Deaf, 113*;295–302.

HAGGARD, M.P., TRINDER, J.R., FOSTER, J.R., & LINDBLAD, A.C. (1987). Two-state compression of spectral tilt: individual differences and psychoacoustical limitations to the benefit from compression. *Journal of Rehabilitation Research and Development, 24*(4);193–206.

HAKANSSON, B., LIDEN, G., TJELLSTROM, A., RINGDAHL, A., JACOBSSON, M., CARLSSON, P., & ERLANDSON, B. (1990). Ten years of experience with the Swedish bone-anchored hearing system. *Annals of Otology, Rhinology, and Laryngology (Suppl.), 151*;99(10), Part 2.

HAKANSSON, B., TJELLSTRON, A., ROSENHALL, U., & CARLSSON, P. (1985). The bone-anchored hearing aid. *Acta Otolaryngologica (Stockholm), 100*;229–239.

HARFORD, E. (1993). Impact of the hearing aid on the evolution of audiology (1993 Carhart Memorial Lecture). *American Auditory Society Bulletin, 18*(2);7–12,103,108.

HARFORD, E., & BARRY, J. (1965). A rehabilitative approach to the problem of unilateral hearing impairment: the contralateral routing of signals (CROS). *Journal of Speech and Hearing Disorders, 30*;121–138.

HARTIG, H.E., & NEWHART, H. (1936). Performance characteristics of electrical hearing aids for the deaf. *Archives of Otolaryngology, 23*;617–632.

HAWKINS, D., & MUELLER, G. (1986). Some variables affecting the accuracy of probe tube microphone measurements. *Hearing Instruments, 37*(1);8–12, 49.

HAWKINS, D., WALDEN, B., MONTGOMERY, A., & PROSEK, R.A. (1987). Description and validation of an LDL procedure designed to select SSPL90. *Ear and Hearing, 8;*162–169.

HECOX, K., & MILLER, E. (1988). New hearing aid technologies. *Hearing Instruments, 39*(3);38–40.

HERTZANO, T., LEVITT, H., & SLOSBERG, R. (1979). Computer-assisted hearing aid selection. In: J.J. Wolf, & D.H. Klatt (Eds.), *Speech communication papers, 97th Meeting of the Acoustical Society of America* (pp. 627–629). New York: Acoustical Society of America.

HODGES, A. (1983). *Alan Turing: The enigma* (p. 274). New York: Simon and Schuster, Touchstone Books.

HOUGH, J., HIMELICK, T., JOHNSON, B. (1986). Implantable bone conduction hearing device: Audiant™ bone conductor. *Annals of Otology, Rhinology, and Laryngology, 95;*498–504.

HUDGINS, C.V. (1953). The response of profoundly deaf children to auditory training. *Journal of Speech and Hearing Disorders, 18;*273–288.

HUMES, L.E. (1991). Understanding the speech understanding problems of the hearing impaired. *Journal of the American Academy of Audiology, 2;*59–69.

HUMES, L.E., & HACKETT, T. (1990). Comparison of frequency response and aided speech recognition performance for hearing aids selected by three different prescriptive methods. *Journal of the American Academy of Audiology, 1*(2); 101–108.

HUMES, L.E., & HALLING, D.C. (1994). Overview, rationale, and comparison of suprathreshold-based gain prescription methods. In: M. Valente (Ed.), *Strategies for selecting and verifying hearing aid fittings* (pp. 19–37). New York: Thieme Medical Publishers, Inc.

HUSSUNG, R., & HAMILL, T. (1990). Recent advances in hearing aid technology: an introduction to digital terminology and concepts. *Seminars in Hearing, 11*(1);1–15.

JERGER, J., MALMQUIST, C., & SPEAKS, C. (1966a). Comparison of some speech intelligibility tests in the evaluation of hearing aid performance. *Journal of Speech and Hearing Research, 9;*253–258.

JERGER, J., SPEAKS, C., & MALMQUIST, C. (1966b). Hearing aid performance and hearing aid selection. *Journal of Speech and Hearing Research, 9;*136–149.

JOHANSSON, B., & LINDBLAD, A. (1971). The use of compression and frequency-transposition in hearing aids. *Scandinavian Audiology (Suppl.), 1;*68–71.

KAMM, C., DIRKS, D., & MICKEY, R. (1978). Effect of sensorineural hearing loss on loudness discomfort level and most comfortable level judgments. *Journal of Speech and Hearing Research, 21;*668–681.

KASTEN, R.N., & LOTTERMAN, S.H. (1967). A longitudinal examination of harmonic distortion in hearing aids. *Journal of Speech and Hearing Research, 10;*777–781.

KATES, J.M., & WEISS, M.R. (1995). *An adaptive microphone array for hearing aids.* Presented at the 1st biennial NIDCD/V.A. Hearing Aid Research and Development conference, Bethesda, MD.

KATES, J.M., & WEISS, M.R. (1996). A comparison of hearing-aid array-processing techniques. *Journal of the Acoustical Society of America, 99;*3138–3148.

KEEFE, D.H. (1997). Otoreflectance of the cochlea and middle ear. *Journal of the Acoustical Society of America, 102*(5); 2849–2859.

KELLY, L., LOCHBAUM, C., & VYSOTTSKY, V. (1961). A block diagram compiler. *Bell System Technology Journal, 40;*669–676.

KENNEDY, E. (1994). *Consonant/vowel intensity ratio necessary for maximizing consonant recognition for listeners with hearing impairment.* Ph.D. dissertation, City University of New York.

KENNEDY, E., LEVITT, H., NEUMAN, A.C., & WEISS, M. (1998). Consonant-vowel intensity ratios for maximizing consonant recognition by hearing-impaired listeners. *Journal of the Acoustical Society of America, 103*(2);1098–1114.

KILLION, M. (1990). A high fidelity hearing aid. *Hearing Instruments, 41*(8);38–39.

KILLION, M., & CARLSON, E. (1970). A wide-band miniature microphone. *Journal of the Audio Engineering Society, 18;*631–635.

KILLION, M., & CARLSON, E. (1974). A subminiature electret-condenser microphone of new design. *Journal of the Audio Engineering Society, 22;*237–243.

KILLION, M., & FIKRET-PASA, S. (1993). The 2 types of sensorineural hearing loss: Loudness and intelligibility considerations. *Hearing Journal, 46*(11);31–34.

KILLION, M., SCHULEIN, R., CHRISTENSEN, L., FABRY, D.A., REVIT, L., NIQUETTE, P., & CHUNG, K. (1998). Real-world performance of an ITE directional microphone. *Hearing Journal, 51*(4);1–6.

KILLION, M., STAAB, W., & PREVES, P. (1990). Classifying automatic signal processors. *Hearing Instruments, 41*(8);24–26.

KNUDSEN, V.O. (1939). An ear to the future. *Journal of the Acoustical Society of America, 11;*29–36.

KRETSINGER, E.A., & YOUNG, N.B. (1960). The use of peak clipping to improve the intelligibility of speech in noise. *Speech Monographs, 27;*63–69.

KUK, F. (1994). A screening procedure for modified simplex in frequency-gain response selection. *Ear and Hearing, 15;*62–70.

LAURENCE, R., MOORE, B., & GLASBERG, B. (1983). A comparison of behind-the-ear high-fidelity linear hearing aids and two-channel compression aids, in the laboratory and in everyday life. *British Journal of Audiology, 17;*31–48.

LEHR, M.A., & WIDROW, B. (1998). Directional hearing system. *U.S. Patent #5,793,875,* August.

LEVITT H. (1973). Speech processing aids for the deaf: An overview. *IEEE Transactions Audio Electroacoustics,* AU-21;269–273.

LEVITT, H. (1978). Methods for the evaluation of hearing aids. *Scandinavian Audiology (Suppl.), 6;*199–240.

LEVITT, H. (1982). An array-processor, computer hearing aid. [Abstract]. *ASHA, 24;*805.

LEVITT, H. (1987a). A cancellation technique for the amplitude and phase calibration of hearing aids and nonconventional transducers. *Journal of Rehabilitation Research and Development, 24*(4);261–270.

LEVITT, H. (1987b). Digital hearing aids: a tutorial review. *Journal of Rehabilitation Research and Development, 24*(4);7–20.

LEVITT, H. (1988). A brief history of digital hearing aids. *Hearing Journal,* April:15–21.

LEVITT, H. (1992). Adaptive procedures for hearing aid prescription and other audiologic applications. *Journal of the American Academy of Audiology, 3;*119–131.

LEVITT, H. (1993). Digital hearing aids. In: G. Studebaker, & I. Hochberg (Eds.), *Acoustical factors affecting hearing aid performance* (pp. 317–335). Boston: Allyn & Bacon.

LEVITT, H. (1997). New trends – Digital hearing aids: past, present, and future. In: *Practical hearing aid selection and fitting.* Veterans Administration Rehabilitation Research and Development Service, Monograph 001, (pp. xi–xxiii).

LEVITT, H., BAKKE, M., KATES, J., NEUMAN, A., & WEISS, M. (1993). Advanced signal processing hearing aids. *Scandinavian Audiology (Suppl.),* 38;7–19.

LEVITT, H., DUGOT, R., & KOPPER, K.W. (1988). Programmable digital hearing aid system. *U.S. Patent #4,731,850.*

LEVITT, H., & NEUMAN, A. (1991). Evaluation of orthogonal polynomial compression. *Journal of the Acoustical Society of America,* 90(1);241–252.

LEVITT, H., NEUMAN, A., MILLS, R., & SCHWANDER, T. (1986a). A digital master hearing aid. *Journal of the Rehabilitation Research Development,* 23(1);79–87.

LEVITT, H., NEUMAN, A., & SULLIVAN, J. (1990). Studies with digital hearing aids. *Acta Otolaryngologica (Stockholm; Suppl.),* 469;57–69.

LEVITT, H., SULLIVAN, J., & HWANG, J-Y. (1986b). The Chamelion: A computerized hearing aid measurement/simulation system. *Hearing Instruments,* 37(2);16–18.

LEVITT, H., SULLIVAN, J.A., NEUMAN, A.C., & RUBIN-SPITZ, J.A. (1987). Experiments with a programmable master hearing aid. *Journal of Rehabilitation Research and Development,* 24(4);29–54.

LIBBY, E.R. (1986). The 1/3–2/3 insertion gain hearing aid selection guide. *Hearing Instruments,* 37;27–28.

LIM, J.S., & OPPENHEIM, A.V. (1979). Enhancement and bandwidth compression of noisy speech. *Proceedings IEEE,* 67;1586–1604.

LING, D. (1964). Implications of hearing aid amplification below 300 cps. *Volta Review,* 66;723–729.

LING, D., & MARETIC, H. (1971). Frequency transposition in the teaching of speech to deaf children. *Journal of Speech and Hearing Disorders,* 14;37–46.

LIPPMAN, R.P., BRAIDA, L.D., & DURLACH, N.I. (1981). Study of multichannel amplitude compression and linear amplification for persons with sensorineural hearing loss. *Journal of the Acoustical Society of America,* 69;524–531.

LITTLER, T.S. (1936). Hearing aids for the deaf. *Journal of Scientific Instruments,* 13;144–155.

LYBARGER, S. (1944). *U.S. Patent Application SN 532, 278.*

LYBARGER, S. (1988). A historical overview. In: R. Sandlin (Ed.), *Handbook of hearing aid amplification, Vol. I* (pp. 7–29). Boston: College-Hill Press.

MACRAE, J. (1991). Permanent threshold shift associated with overamplification by hearing aids. *Journal of Speech and Hearing Research,* 34(2);403–414.

MANGOLD, S., & LEIJON, A. (1979). Programmable hearing aid with multichannel compression. *Scandinavian Audiology,* 8;121–126.

MANGOLD, S., & LEIJON, A. (1981). Multichannel compression in a portable programmable hearing aid. *Hearing Aid Journal,* 34(6);29–32.

MANIGLIA, A. (Ed.). (1995). Middle and inner ear electronic implantable devices for partial hearing loss. *Otolaryngologic Clinics of North America,* 28(1);1–223.

MARGOLIS, R., & MILLIN, J. (1971). An item-difficulty based speech discrimination test. *Journal of Speech and Hearing Research,* 14;865–873.

MARKIDES, A. (1977). *Binaural hearing aids.* London: Academic Press.

MCCANDLESS, G.A. (1994). Overview and rationale of threshold-based hearing aid selection procedures. In: M. Valente (Ed.), *Strategies for selecting and verifying hearing aid fittings* (pp. 1–18). New York: Thieme Medical Publishers, Inc.

MCCANDLESS, G.A., & LYREGAARD, P.E. (1983). Prescription of gain and output (POGO) for hearing aids. *Hearing Instruments,* 35(1);16–21.

MCCONNELL, F., SILVER, E.F., & MCDONALD, D. (1960). Test-retest consistency of clinical hearing aid tests. *Journal of Speech and Hearing Disorders,* 25;273–280.

MENDEL, L., & DANHAUER, J.L. (1997). *Audiologic evaluation and management, and speech perception assessment.* San Diego: Singular Publishing Group, Inc.

MILLIN, J.P. (1975). Practical and philosophical considerations. In: M. Pollack (Ed.), *Amplification for the hearing-impaired* (pp. 125–126). New York: Grune & Stratton, Inc.

MONTGOMERY, A., & EDGE, R. (1988). Evaluation of two speech enhancement techniques to improve intelligibility for hearing-impaired adults. *Journal of Speech and Hearing Research,* 31;386–393.

MOODIE, K., SEEWALD, R., & SINCLAIR, S. (1994). Procedure for predicting real-ear hearing aid performance in young children. *American Journal of Audiology,* 3;23–31.

MOORE, B. (1996). Perceptual consequences of cochlear hearing loss and their implications for the design of hearing aids. *Ear and Hearing,* 17;133–161.

MOORE, B., & GLASBERG, B. (1986). A comparison of two-channel and single-channel compression aids. *Audiology,* 25;210–226.

MOORE, B, & GLASBERG, B. (1988). A comparison of four methods of implementing automatic gain control (AGC) in hearing aids. *British Journal of Audiology,* 22;93–104.

MOSER, L.M. (1980). Hearing aid with digital processing for correlation of signals from plural microphones, dynamic range control, or filtering using erasable memory. *U.S. Patent #4,187,413,* February.

MUELLER, G. (1994). CIC hearing aids: What is their impact on the occlusion effect? *Hearing Journal,* 47(11);29–30,32,34–35.

NEUMAN, A., BAKKE, M., HELLMAN, S., & LEVITT, H. (1994). The effect of compression ratio in a slow-acting compression hearing aid: paired comparison judgments of quality. *Journal of the Acoustical Society of America,* 96;1471–1478.

NEUMAN, A., BAKKE, M., HELLMAN, S., & LEVITT, H. (1995). Preferred listening levels for linear and slow-acting compression hearing aids. *Ear and Hearing,* 16(4);407–416.

NEUMAN, A., LEVITT, H., MILLS, R., & SCHWANDER, T. (1987). An evaluation of three adaptive hearing aid selection strategies. *Journal of the Acoustical Society of America,* 82(6); 1967–1976.

NEUMAN, A., & SCHWANDER, T. (1987). The effect of filtering on the intelligibility and quality of speech in noise. *Journal of Rehabilitation Research Development,* 24(4);127–134.

NILLSSON, M., & SOLI, S., & SULLIVAN, J. (1994). Development of the Hearing In Noise Test for the measurement of speech reception thresholds in quiet and in noise. *Journal of the Acoustical Society of America,* 95(2);1085–1099.

NUNLEY, J., STAAB, W., STEADMAN, J., WECHSLER, P., & SPENCER, B. (1983). A wearable digital hearing aid. *Hearing Journal,* 10;29–35.

OLSON, W.O., & WILBUR, S.A. (1968). *Hearing aid distortion and speech intelligibility.* Presented at the annual convention of the American Speech and Hearing Association, Denver.

PASCOE, D. (1975). Frequency responses of hearing aids and their effects on speech perception of hearing-impaired subjects. *Annals of Otology, Rhinology, and Laryngology* (Suppl.), 84;1–40.

PASCOE, D. (1978). An approach to hearing aid selection. *Hearing Instruments, 29;*12–16,36.

PASCOE, D. (1988). Clinical measurements of the auditory dynamic range and their relation to formulas for hearing aid gain. In: J. Jensen (Ed.), *Hearing aid fitting, theoretical and practical views* (pp. 129–152). Copenhagen: 13th Danavox Symposium, Stongaard Jensen.

PETERSON, P.M., DURLACH, N.I., RABINOWITZ, W.M., & ZUREK, P.M. (1987). Multimicrophone adaptive beamforming for interference reduction in hearing aids. *Journal of Rehabilitation Research and Development, 24;*103–110.

PETERSON, P.M., WEEI, S., RABINOWITZ, W.M., & ZUREK, P.M. (1990). Robustness of an adaptive beamforming method for hearing aids. *Acta Otolaryngologica (Suppl.), 469;*85–90.

PLOMP, R. (1978). Auditory handicap of hearing impairment and limited benefit of hearing aids. *Journal of the Acoustical Society of America, 65;*533–549.

PLOMP, R. (1988). The negative effect of amplitude compression in multichannel hearing aids in light of the modulation-transfer function. *Journal of the Acoustical Society of America, 83(6);*2322–2327.

POPELKA, G., & ENGEBRETSON, A. (1983). A computer-based system for hearing aid assessment. *Hearing Instruments, 34;*6–9,44.

PREVES, D.A. (1990). Approaches to noise reduction in analog, digital and hybrid hearing aids. *Seminars in Hearing, 11(1);*39–67.

PREVES, D.A., FORTUNE, T., WOODRUFF, B., & NEWTON, J. (1991). Strategies for enhancing the consonant-to-vowel ratio with in-the-ear hearing aids. *Ear and Hearing (Suppl.), 12(6);* 139S–153S.

PREVES, D.A., SAMMETH, C., & WYNNE, M.K. (1997). *Field trial evaluations of a switched directional/omnidirectional ITE hearing instrument.* Presented at the 2nd biennial NIDCD/V.A. Hearing Aid Research and Development Conference, Bethesda, MD.

PREVES, D.A., & SIGELMAN, J.A. (1986). A new signal processor for ITE hearing aid fittings. *Hearing Instruments, 10;*52–60.

PULEC, J.L. (1994). Restoration of binaural hearing with the Audiant implant following acoustic neuroma surgery. *Ear Nose and Throat Journal, 73;*118–123.

RADLEY, W.G., BRAGG, W.L., DADSON, R.S., HALLPIKE, C.S., MCMILLAN, D., POCOCK, L.C., & LITTLER, T.S. (1947). Hearing aids and audiometers. *Report of the Committee on Electroacoustics.* His Majesty's Stationery Office, London.

RANKOVIC, C.M. (1991). An application of the Articulation Index to hearing aid fitting. *Journal of Speech and Hearing Research, 34;*391–402.

RESNICK, D.M., & BECKER, M. (1963). Hearing aid evaluation—a new approach. *ASHA, 5;*695–699.

ROESER, R., & TAYLOR, K. (1988). Audiometric and field testing with a digital hearing instrument. *Hearing Instruments, 39(4);*14.

ROSS, M., & LEVITT, H. (1997). Consumer satisfaction is not enough: hearing aids are still about hearing. *Seminars in Hearing, 18(1);*7–10.

SAMMETH, C. (1989). Hearing instruments: From vacuum tubes to digital microchips. *Hearing Instruments, 40(10);*9–10,12.

SAMMETH, C. (1990). Current availability of digital and hybrid hearing aids. *Seminars in Hearing, 11(1);*91–99.

SAMMETH, C., BIRMAN, M., HECOX, K. (1989). Variability of most comfortable and uncomfortable loudness measurements to speech stimuli in the hearing-impaired. *Ear and Hearing, 10(2);*94–100.

SAMMETH, C., DORMAN, M., & STEARNS, C. (1999). The role of consonant-vowel amplitude ratio in the recognition of voiceless stop consonants by hearing-impaired listeners. *Journal of Speech, Language and Hearing Research, 42(1);*42–55.

SAMMETH, C., & OCHS, M. (1991). A review of current "noise reduction" hearing aids: rationale, assumptions, and efficacy. *Ear and Hearing (Suppl.), 12(6);*116S–124S.

SAMMETH, C., PREVES, D.A., BRATT, G., PEEK, B., & BESS, F. (1993). Achieving prescribed gain/frequency responses with advances in hearing aid technology. *Journal of Rehabilitation Research and Development, 30(1);*1–7.

SAMMETH, C., TETZELI, M., & OCHS, M. (1996). Consonant recognition performance of hearing-impaired listeners using one linear and three nonlinear hearing aids. *Journal of the American Academy of Audiology, 7;*240–250.

SCHUM, D. (1990). Noise reduction strategies for elderly, hearing-impaired listeners. *Journal of the American Academy of Audiology, 1(1);*31–36.

SCHWANDER, T., & LEVITT, H. (1987). Effect of two-microphone noise reduction on speech recognition by normal-hearing listeners. *Journal of Rehabilitation Research and Development, 24(4);*87–92.

SCHWEITZER, C. (1992). Clinical experience with a commercial digital hearing aid. Poster presentation at the *Issues in Advanced Hearing Aid Research* Conference, Lake Arrowhead, CA.

SCHWEITZER, C. (1997). Development of digital hearing aids. *Trends in Amplification, 2(2);*41–77.

SCHWEITZER, C., & KRISHNAN, G. (1996). Binaural beamforming and related digital processing for enhancement of signal-to-noise ratio in hearing aids. *Current Opinions in Otolaryngology Head and Neck Surgery, 4(5);*335–339.

SCHWEITZER, C., & TERRY, M. (1995). *Clinical and experimental results with wearable beamforming digital hearing aids.* Presented at the 1st biennial NIDCD/V.A. Hearing Aid Research and Development Conference, Bethesda, MD.

SEEWALD, R.C. (1992). The desired sensation level method for fitting children: Version 3.0. *Hearing Journal, 45(4);*36–41.

SEEWALD, R., CORNELISSE, L.E., RAMJI, K.V., SINCLAIR, S.T., MOODIE, K.S., & JAMIESON, D.G. (1996). *DSL v4. for Windows: A software implementation of the Desired Sensation Level (DSL [i/o]) method for fitting linear gain and wide-dynamic-range compression hearing instruments.* The Hearing Healthcare Research Unit. The University of Western Ontario, London, Ontario, Canada.

SEEWALD, R.C., RAMJI, K.V., SINCLAIR, S.T., MOODIE, K.S., & JAMIESON, D.G. (1993). *A computer-assisted implementation of the desired sensation level method for electroacoustic selection and fitting in children: DSL 3.1 user's manual.* The Hearing Healthcare Research Unit Technical Report 02. The University of Western Ontario, London, Ontario, Canada.

SEEWALD, R.C., & ROSS, M. (1988). Amplification for young hearing-impaired children. In: M.C. Pollack (Ed.), *Amplification for the hearing-impaired* (pp. 213–267). New York: Grune & Stratton, Inc.

SHAPIRO, I. (1976). Hearing aid fitting by prescription. *Audiology, 15*;63–173.

SHAPIRO, I. (1979). Evaluation of the relationship between hearing threshold and loudness discomfort level in sensorineural hearing loss. *Journal of Speech and Hearing Disorders, 64*;31–36.

SHAPIRO, I. (1980). Comparison of three hearing aid prescription procedures. *Ear and Hearing, 1*;211–214.

SHORE, I., BILGER, R.C., & HIRSH, I.J. (1960). Hearing aid evaluation: Reliability of repeated measurements. *Journal of Speech and Hearing Disorders, 25*;152–170.

SHORE, I., & KRAMER, J. (1965). A comparison of two procedures for hearing aid evaluation. *Journal of Speech and Hearing Disorders, 28*;159–170.

SIGELMAN, J.A., & PREVES, D.A. (1987). Field trials of a new adaptive signal processor hearing aid circuit. *Hearing Journal, 40*(4);24–27.

SILVERMAN, S.R., & HARRISON, C.E. (1951). The National Research Council group hearing aid project. *American Annals of the Deaf, 96*;420–431.

SKINNER, M.W. (1980). Speech intelligibility in noise-induced hearing loss: Effects of high-frequency compensation. *Journal of the Acoustical Society of America, 67*;306–317.

SKINNER, M.W. (1988). *Hearing aid evaluation.* Englewood Cliffs, NJ: Prentice Hall.

SKINNER M.W., PASCOE, D., MILLER, J., & POPELKA, G. (1982). Measurements to determine the optimal placement of speech energy. In: G. Studebaker, & F. Bess (Eds.), *The Vanderbilt hearing aid report* (pp. 161–169). Upper Darby, PA.: Monographs in Contemporary Audiology.

SMRIGA, D. (1985). Modern compression technology. *Hearing Journal, 17*;13–16.

SMRIGA, D. (1993). Digital signal processing to reduce feedback: Technology and test results. *Hearing Journal, 46*(5); 28–33.

SOEDE, W., BERKHOUT, A., & BILSEN, F. (1993a). Development of a directional hearing instrument based on array technology. *Journal of the Acoustical Society of America, 94*; 785–798.

SOEDE, W., BILSEN, F., & BERKHOUT, A. (1993b). Assessment of a directional microphone array for hearing-impaired listeners. *Journal of the Acoustical Society of America, 94*; 799–808.

STAAB, W. (1978). *Hearing aid handbook.* Blue Ridge Summit, PA: Tab Books.

STAAB, W. (1985). Digital hearing aids. *Hearing Instruments, 36*(11);14,16–20,22–24.

STACH, B.A., SPEERSCHNEIDER, J.M., & JERGER, J.F. (1987). Evaluating the efficacy of automatic signal processing hearing aids. *Hearing Journal, 40*;15–19.

STEIN, L., & DEMPSEY-HART, K. (1984). Listener-assessed intelligibility of a hearing aid self-adaptive noise filter. *Ear and Hearing, 6*;199–204.

STELMACHOWICZ, P.G., JESTEADT, W., GORGA, M., & MOTT, J. (1985). Speech perception ability and psychophysical tuning curves in hearing-impaired listeners. *Journal of the Acoustical Society of America, 77*;620–627.

STELMACHOWICZ, P.G., & LEWIS, D.E. (1988). Some theoretical considerations concerning the relation between functional gain and insertion gain. *Journal of Speech and Hearing Research, 31*(3);491–496.

STEVENS, S.S. (1955). The measurement of loudness. *Journal of the Acoustical Society of America, 27*;815–829.

STOREY, L., DILLON, H., YEEND, I., & WIGNEY, D. (1998). The National Acoustics Laboratories procedure for selecting saturation sound pressure level of hearing aids: experimental validation. *Ear and Hearing, 19*;267–279.

STUDEBAKER, G. (1980). Fifty years of hearing aid research: an evaluation of progress. *Ear and Hearing 1*;57–62.

SULLIVAN, J., LEVITT, H., HWANG, J-Y., & HENNESEY, A.M. (1987). Discriminability of frequency irregularities in hearing aids. In: R.D. Steel, & W. Gerrey (Eds.), *Proceedings of 10th Annual Conference on Rehabilitation Technology* (pp. 407–409). Washington, DC: RESNA – Association for Advancement of Rehabilitation Technology,

SULLIVAN, J.A., LEVITT, H., HWANG, J-Y., & HENNESEY, A.M. (1988). An experimental comparison of four hearing aid prescription methods. *Ear and Hearing, 9*(1);22–32.

SULLIVAN, R.F. (1988). Transcranial ITE CROS. *Hearing Instruments, 39*(1);11–12, 54.

SUMMERFIELD, Q., FOSTER, J., & TYLER, R. (1985). Influences of formant bandwidth and auditory frequency selectivity on identification of place of articulation in stop consonants. *Speech Communication, 4*;213–229.

TREES, D.E., & TURNER, C.W. (1986). Spread of masking in normal subjects and in subjects with high-frequency hearing loss. *Audiology, 25*;70–83.

TURNER, C.W., & HUMES, L.E., BENTLER, R.A., & COX, R.M. (1996). A review of past research on changes in hearing aid benefit over time. *Ear and Hearing, 17*(3);14S–28S,90S–98S.

TYLER, R., & KUK, F. (1989). The effects of "noise suppression" hearing aids on consonant recognition in speech-babble and low-frequency noise. *Ear and Hearing, 10*;243–249.

VALENTE, M. (1995). Fitting options for unilateral hearing loss. *Hearing Journal, 48*(4);10, 45–48.

VALENTE, M., FABRY, D.A., & POTTS, L. (1995b). Recognition of speech in noise with hearing aids using dual microphones. *Journal of the American Academy of Audiology, 6*;440–449.

VALENTE, M., POTTS, L.G., VALENTE, M., & GOEBEL, J. (1995a). Wireless CROS versus transcranial CROS for unilateral hearing loss. *American Journal of Audiology, 4*;52–59.

VALENTE, M., SAMMETH, C., POTTS, L., WYNNE, M.K., WAGNER-ESCOBAR, M., & COUGHLIN, M. (1997). Differences in performance between the Oticon Multifocus Compact and the ReSound BT2-E hearing aids. *Journal of the American Academy of Audiology, 8*(4);280–293.

VALENTE, M., & VAN VLIET, D. (1997). The Independent Hearing Aid Fitting Forum (IHAFF) protocol. *Trends in Amplification, 2*(1);6–35.

VAN ROOIJ, J.C., & PLOMP, R. (1990). Auditive and cognitive factors in speech perception by elderly listeners II: Multivariate analyses. *Journal of the Acoustical Society of America, 88*;2611–2624.

VAN TASELL, D.J. (1993). Hearing loss, speech and hearing aids. *Journal of Speech and Hearing Research, 36*;228–244.

VAN TASELL, D.J. (1998). New DSP instrument designed to maximize binaural benefits. *Hearing Journal, 51*;40–49.

VAN TASELL, D.J., LARSEN, S.Y., & FABRY, D.A. (1988). Effects of an adaptive filter hearing aid on speech recognition in noise by hearing-impaired subjects. *Ear and Hearing, 9*;15–21.

VAN TASELL, D.J., THOMAS, R., & CRAIN, M.A. (1992). Noise reduction hearing aids: Release from masking and release from distortion. *Ear and Hearing, 13*;114–121.

VAN VLIET, D. (1995). A comprehensive hearing aid fitting protocol. *Audiology Today, 7*;11–13.

VILLCHUR, E. (1973). Signal processing to improve speech intelligibility in perceptive deafness. *Journal of the Acoustical Society of America, 53*(6);1646–1657.

VILLCHUR, E. (1974). Simulation of the effects of recruitment on loudness relationships in speech. *Journal of the Acoustical Society of America, 56*;1601–1611.

VOSS, S.E., & ALLEN, J.B. (1994). Measurement of acoustic impedance and reflectance in the human earcanal. *Journal of the Acoustical Society of America, 95*(1);372–384.

WALKER, G., BYRNE, D., & DILLON, H. (1984). The effects of multichannel compression/expansion amplification on the intelligibility of nonsense syllables in noise. *Journal of the Acoustical Society of America, 76*(3);746–757.

WALKER, G., & DILLON, H. (1982). Compression in hearing aids: an analysis, a review and some recommendations. *National Acoustics Laboratory Report,* No. 90. Canberra: Australian Government Publishing Service.

WALLENFELS, H.G. (1967). *Hearing aids on prescription.* Springfield, IL: Charles C. Thomas.

WATSON, L.A., & TOLAN, T. (1949). *Hearing tests and hearing instruments.* New York: Hafner Publishing Company (Copyright: Williams & Wilkins, 1967 reprint).

WATSON, N.A., & KNUDSEN, V.D. (1940). Selective amplification in hearing aids. *Journal of the Acoustical Society of America, 11*;406–419.

WEISS, M. (1987). Use of an adaptive noise canceller as an input preprocessor for a hearing aid. *Journal of Rehabilitation Research and Development, 24*(4);93–102.

WIDROW, B., GLOVER, J.R., MCCOOL, J.M., LAUNITZ, J., WILLIAMS, C.S., HEARN, R.H., ZEIDLER, J.R., DONG, E., & GOODLIN, R.C. (1975). Adaptive noise cancelling: Principles and applications. *Proceedings of the IEEE, 63*;1692–1716.

WOLINSKY, S. (1986). Clinical assessment of a self-adaptive noise filtering system. *Hearing Journal, 39*(10);29–32.

YUND, E.W., SIMON, H.J., & EFRON, R. (1987). Speech discrimination with an 8-channel compression hearing aid and conventional aids in a background of speech-band noise. *Journal of Rehabilitation Research and Development, 24*(4);161–180.

Chapter 6

Recent Approaches to Fitting Nonlinear Hearing Aids

Francis K. Kuk

Hearing aids with nonlinear signal processing have been in use for a long time. Braida et al (1979) reported that nonlinear processing, especially the use of compression, can be dated before the 1960s. Some of the ideas prevalent today for compensating for the "abnormal" loudness perception associated with hearing loss have been reflected in the writings of Victoreen (1973). Indeed, the design principles behind the first commercially successful wide dynamic range compression (WDRC) hearing aid can be traced to Villchur (1973), who

argued that a hearing aid should compensate for the equal loudness contour of the hearing-impaired person. Despite such a long history, more than 80% of the hearing aids dispensed in the United States in the late 1980s used linear signal processing and peak clipping as the method for output limiting (Hawkins, cited in Mueller & Killion, 1996). The use of compression in hearing aids grew steadily in the 1990s. It was not until the mid 1990s that almost half of all hearing aids sold in the United States used some form of compression (Mueller & Killion, 1996). This trend that more hearing aids will use compression will likely continue in the future.

This chapter takes the approach that proper fitting of nonlinear hearing aids starts with an understanding of nonlinearity so that the appropriate type of nonlinear hearing aid can be selected at the preselection stage. This minimizes any unnecessary adjustment after the fitting. Thus this chapter will begin with a review of the rationale for nonlinear processing followed by a brief description of the electroacoustic parameters that govern the performance of such devices. On the basis of the available research and clinical experience, a tentative recommendation on the candidates for each type of nonlinear hearing aid will be made. The approaches to fitting these nonlinear hearing aids will be described, followed by a brief section on pertinent issues involved in verification and fine tuning. Validation will be described in greater detail in other chapters within this volume.

WHAT IS LINEAR?

One way to classify hearing aids is by the type of signal processing that they use for typical input levels. Hearing aids that maintain the same magnitude of gain at all input levels (thus preserving the intensity relationship of sounds) until saturation occurs are referred to as linear hearing aids. This is in contrast to nonlinear hearing aids in which gain changes as the input level changes. Figure 6–1A shows the input-output (I-O) curves of three different hearing aids. Hearing aid (i) is linear until an input of 90 dB sound pressure level (SPL). Thereafter the output is limited to about 120 dB SPL. Hearing aid (ii) has kneepoints at 50 dB SPL and 90 dB SPL. Hearing aid (iii) has kneepoints at 20 dB SPL and 60 dB SPL. As is common in all hearing aids, output always increases (or stays the same) as input increases.

The type of processing (linear or nonlinear) becomes clearer if one replots the I-O curves into input-gain (I-G)

Audiology: Treatment. Edited by Valente, Hosford-Dunn, and Roeser. Thieme Medical Publishers, Inc., New York © 2000

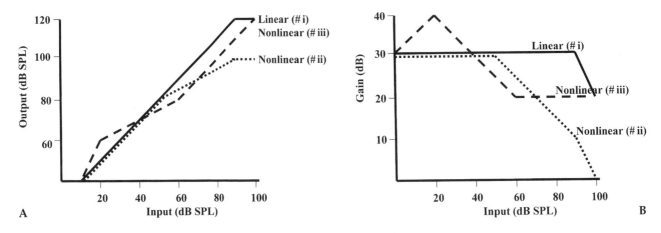

Figure 6–1 **(A)** I-O curves of a linear hearing aid (# *i*) and two nonlinear hearing aids (# *ii* and # *iii*). **(B)** I-G curves for the same linear and nonlinear hearing aids.

curves (Fig. 6–1B). An I-G curve is valuable because it reveals the gain and the type of signal processing at any input range. A linear hearing aid shows a flat straight line (indicating a constant 30 dB gain in this case). Using the definition that linear hearing aids provide the same gain at all input levels, one must agree that the region beyond the input level of 90 dB SPL is nonlinear because gain decreases as input increases. This suggests that even linear hearing aids can behave in a nonlinear manner at high input levels. Obviously, this nonlinearity is saturation distortion and does not reflect the processing of the hearing aids at typical input levels.

In contrast to the flat line seen for the linear hearing aid, the I-G curve for nonlinear hearing aid (ii) shows a flat line below 50 dB SPL. Above that input, gain decreases at a rate of 5 dB gain/10 dB input increase until 90 dB SPL (i.e., a compression ratio [CR] of 2:1). Above that level, gain decreases at a rate of 9 dB gain/10 dB input (i.e., a CR of 10:1). One would describe the hearing aid processing to be linear for inputs up to 50 dB SPL, then nonlinear for input levels greater than 50 dB SPL. Specifically, gain reduction is seen as input increases. This type of nonlinear processing is called *compression*.

Nonlinearity does not always involve gain reduction. The I-O and I-G curves of nonlinear hearing aid (iii) show gain increases as input increases from 0 dB to 20 dB SPL. This region is called *expansion*, and is another form of nonlinear processing used in some digital hearing aids. Expansion is used for the purpose of reaching the desired gain at a particular input level without providing the same amount of amplification to sounds below that input level. Because expansion is not the main form of nonlinear processing in current hearing aids, this topic will not be discussed further in this chapter. Rather, gain reduction nonlinearity (i.e., compression) will be elaborated.

PEARL

Linear hearing aids maintain the same gain at all input levels. Compression reduces gain as input increases. Expansion increases gain as input increases.

WHY NONLINEAR?

Nonlinear processing is used in hearing aids for several reasons. Braida et al (1979), Walker and Dillon (1982), Dillon (1988), Byrne (1996), and Dillon (1996) provided excellent summaries of how compression is used in current hearing aids. All these methods involve gain reduction at some stage of the signal processing so that the output of the hearing aids changes in accordance with the rationale to which compression is applied. A result that is common to all types of compression is that compression reduces the long-term variation in speech and enhances the audibility for soft sounds while providing comfort for loud sounds without the need for adjustment of the volume control (VC) (Dillon, 1996). At present, at least four major uses for compression are recognized.

SPECIAL CONSIDERATION

Gain reduction and enhanced audibility appear to be paradoxical. In reality, when compression is used for better audibility, one purposely assigns more gain to the hearing aid first and then gradually decreases gain as the input level increases so that the range of change in output narrows.

Minimize Saturation Distortion

Compression can be used to prevent the distortion caused by saturation as hearing aids respond to high inputs. With this scenario, the signal processing (linear or nonlinear) is maintained for most of the input levels until a high input level is reached. Beyond that input level, gain reduction (or further gain reduction) occurs as the input increases. The end result is that the output stays minimally increased as the input increases. This use of compression is referred to as *compression limiting* (CL). Because the feedback mechanism (for detection of the need for gain reduction) is located at the output stage of this type of hearing aid, some refer to this type of compression as *output CL, CL,* or *automatic gain control-output*

(AGC-O). Because CL is used only as a means to limit distortion at high input levels, high compression thresholds (>65 dB SPL) and high compression ratios (>5:1) are desirable for such applications. Hawkins and Naidoo (1993) reported that their subjects preferred the sound quality of a CL hearing aid to a peak clipping hearing aid at high input level (greater than 80 dB SPL). Dawson et al (1991) also reached a similar conclusion in a group of subjects with severe hearing loss (pure tone average less than 90 dB HL).

Loudness Normalization

Compression has been used to compensate for the rapid growth of loudness perception associated with sensorineural hearing loss. The desired outcome is that the hearing-impaired ear perceives changes in loudness in the same manner as normal-hearing ears. This goal is different from the goal of linear prescriptive formulas, which is to equalize loudness across different frequency regions so that each is at a comfortable level. Loudness normalization could result in a reduction of the output dynamic range, a reduction of the intensity differences between low-intensity and high-intensity sounds, and perhaps an increase in the proportion of consonantal syllables that are audible (i.e., increases consonant to vowel ratio) (Freyman & Nerbonne, 1989).

Figure 6–2 shows an idealized loudness growth function of a normal-hearing ear and individuals with 40-, 60-, and 75-dB hearing loss (i.e., dashed lines intersecting abscissa at 40-, 60-, and 75-dB HL). A straight line can approximate the loudness-growth function of the normal-hearing ear. The hearing-impaired ears, on the other hand, will not perceive the signal until an input level of 40-, 60-, and 75-dB HL, respectively, is reached. The dynamic range of the listener (or the intensity range between threshold and loudness discomfort) will be 100 dB for the normal, 60 dB for the 40 dB HL case, 40 dB for the 60 dB HL case, and 25 dB for the 75 dB HL case (assuming that the loudness discomfort level [LDL] is 100 dB HL for all cases). A louder perception than the normal ear is reported above the threshold input level (i.e., loudness recruitment). For all degrees of hearing loss, the loudness growth curve of the impaired ear runs parallel to the normal ear above a relatively high input level. This suggests that the impaired ear and the normal ear both process sounds linearly at such input levels (Hellman & Meiselman, 1990).

Theoretically, if one were to design a hearing aid for the listener with the 60 dB HL hearing loss, one would need to provide 60 dB gain at 0 dB HL input to ensure audibility (Cornelisse et al, 1995; Dillon, 1996). Above 0 dB HL, gain reduction should occur to compensate for loudness recruitment (or abnormal growth of loudness perception above threshold). At the high input level, gain should remain at the same reduced level regardless of input. An I-O curve of a linear hearing aid and that of the hypothetical I-O for the three hearing loss cases shown in Figure 6–2A are illustrated in Figure 6–2B. Because gain reduction starts at 0 dB HL, it is possible to map a large range of acoustic inputs onto the reduced dynamic range of the hearing-impaired ear. For this reason, such compression hearing aids are called *wide (or full or whole) dynamic range compression (WDRC)*.

From the preceding description, it is not difficult to conclude that the theoretical compression threshold (CT) should

be close to 0 dB HL for the purpose of restoring normal loudness perception to the impaired ear (Dillon, 1996). Indeed, one nonlinear prescriptive approach (DSL[i/o]) (Cornelisse et al, 1995) prescribes such a low CT level. Unfortunately, commercially available WDRC hearing aids typically have CTs ranging from 40 dB SPL to 65 dB SPL. This is due to technical difficulties with analog techniques in achieving a low CT and the questionable benefit of amplifying sounds at 0 dB SPL. The use of digital technology allows one to choose a lower CT. However, the associated difficulties with amplifying sounds below the CT and the increased likelihood of acoustic feedback still need to be addressed (Dillon, 1996).

CONTROVERSIAL POINT

Although the theoretical CT should be as low as possible, Dillon (1997) showed that adult hearing-impaired people preferred a higher CT. The type of signal processing (linear or nonlinear) below the CT and the number of processing channels in the hearing aid may have resulted in such preference. More research is necessary to determine the optimal CT.

No conclusive evidence supports the assertion that achieving normal loudness guarantees optimal speech intelligibility or sound quality. Indeed, van Buuren et al (1995) showed that a wide variation in speech spectra can still provide the same intelligibility. However, some studies suggest that the use of WDRC enhances speech audibility for soft sounds and maximizes comfort for loud sounds compared with linear hearing aids (e.g., Moore et al, 1992). On the other hand, some suggest that altering the normal loudness relationship may reduce intelligibility (e.g., Festen & Plomp, 1983; Horwitz et al, 1991). More research is needed to clarify this issue.

CONTROVERSIAL POINT

The efficacy of nonlinear signal processing over linear signal processing remains controversial at best. Dillon's (1996) comments on the end result of compression are agreed by most researchers to be the most candid observation on the efficacy of the compression system.

It should be clear that CL and WDRC are independent of each other. CL is a way to limit output and eliminate or reduce distortion. Gain reduction occurs only at a high input level. The signal processing at typical input levels can be either linear or nonlinear (although most CL is used with linear processing). WDRC is a form of signal processing. Gain reduction occurs above low input levels. It can use either CL or peak clipping for output control. Table 6–1 illustrates how signal processing (i.e., linear and nonlinear) can interact with output limiting (peak clipping and CL).

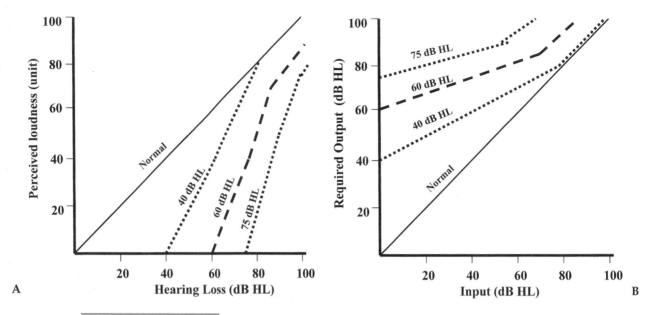

Figure 6–2 **(A)** LGF of a normal-hearing person (*solid line*) and those of three magnitudes of hearing loss: 40 dB HL, 60 dB HL, and 75 dB HL. **(B)** Required I-O curves from a compression hearing aid for the three magnitudes of hearing loss.

TABLE 6–1   Two-by-two matrix showing signal processing and output-limiting combinations

Signal Processing	Output Limiting	
	Peak clipping	Compression limiting
Linear	Most older aids	AGC-O
Nonlinear	AGC-I only	AGC-I and AGC-O

PITFALL

Linear hearing aids receive an unfair assessment when some clinicians assume that linear means peak clipping. Previously this may have been the case when most linear hearing aids used peak clipping for output control. This has changed significantly over the past decade.

Noise Reduction

Compression can be used in specific frequency regions to reduce noise. The assumptions are that "noise" can be isolated to a particular frequency region and that gain reduction of that frequency region will minimize its masking effect on adjacent frequency regions (Sammeth & Ochs, 1991; Tyler & Kuk, 1989). Because typical "noise" is low-frequency weighted (e.g., Keidser et al, 1995), most compression hearing aids adaptively reduce their low-frequency gain as the input level increases (i.e., Bass Increase at Low Level, or BILL processing) (Killion et al, 1990). This action is different from hearing aids that use compression for loudness normalization, where gain reduction occurs in the high-frequency region more than the low-frequency region as input increases (i.e., Treble Increase at Low Level, or TILL) (Killion et al, 1990) or when gain reduction is equal across frequencies.

The effectiveness of compression as a means for noise reduction depends on the properties of the noise signal. When both speech and noise signals have the same spectra, attenuation of the "noise" will invariably attenuate the speech signal. This will not improve the signal-to-noise ratio (SNR) (Tyler & Kuk, 1989). However, when the frequency of the noise source is discrete and different from the spectrum of the desired signal, this method of gain reduction may improve speech intelligibility, sound quality, and overall comfort (Kuk & Tyler, 1990; Kuk et al, 1990; Rankovic et al, 1992).

Another difficulty with the use of compression for noise reduction is that the overall input level determines gain reduction even though the signal may be desirable (i.e., speech). Some method to identify the nature of the input signal before gain reduction may be necessary. The original Zeta Noise Blocker (Graupe et al, 1986) was a good attempt at a difficult issue.

Long-Term Dynamic Range Reduction

Uses for compression hearing aids described previously require the use of short attack (<10 ms) and release time (50 to 100 ms) so that the hearing aid can respond quickly to the required changes in intensity fluctuation. In the process the temporal-intensity relationship between different components of the speech signals may be altered and could be harmful to intelligibility (e.g., Plomp, 1988; Van Tasell, 1993). But if the range of intensity variation (e.g., 30 dB) is less than the residual dynamic range of the hearing-impaired ear, one may not need to use fast-acting compression to retain the range of intensity fluctuation. Rather, one may use a longer attack (e.g., several hundred milliseconds) and release time (e.g., several seconds) so that the short-term intensity difference is maintained and the overall output level of the hearing aids is adjusted to within the person's dynamic range. Pearsons et al (1977) showed that the range of intensity fluctuation within any listening environment is typically less than 30 dB. Pascoe (1988) showed that the average dynamic range for someone with less than 80 dB HL typically exceeds 30 dB. This suggests that the need for hearing aids to respond quickly to intensity changes in a fixed environment is minimal. In other words, compression hearing aids with long attack and release times can be used to preserve the short-term intensity variation of the input signal while reducing the long-term intensity changes without VC adjustment. Compression hearing aids that are used in this manner are called *automatic volume control (AVC) or slow-acting compression* hearing aids. Readers are referred to the following review articles on this topic (Braida et al, 1979; Dillon, 1988, 1996; Kuk, 1996a,b, 1998b; Walker & Dillon, 1982).

CHARACTERIZATION OF A COMPRESSION HEARING AID

The electroacoustic performance of a compression hearing aid can be described by its *static and dynamic* characteristics. The static characteristics refer to the steady-state performance of the hearing aid. An I-O curve derived with a sinusoidal signal (e.g., 2000 Hz) is typically used to represent its static characteristics (ANSI S3.22, 1996). Alternately, an I-G curve, which plots the amount of gain in a compression hearing aid at different input levels, can also convey the same information. Figure 6–3 shows how some of these parameters are defined, first as an I-O curve (A) and as an I-G curve (B).

Static Characteristics

Static characteristics refer to the performance of the compression hearing aid to a steady-state signal, typically a sinusoid. The behavior of the hearing aid with time is not considered. Interactions among frequency components are also not considered.

Compression Threshold

CT represents the input level at which a hearing aid changes its gain. This can be seen as points "A" and "B" on the I-O curve in Figure 6–3. In this case the lower compression threshold occurs at 50 dB SPL, and the upper compression threshold occurs at 90 dB SPL.

The compression thresholds can be easily identified on an I-G curve (Fig. 6–3B). It can be seen that gain stays the same at 40 dB until the input level of 50 dB SPL (i.e., it is linear), thereafter it decreases steadily to 20 dB at an input of 90 dB SPL.

Although the conventional definition of CT is made in reference to the input level at which gain changes, some distinguish CT between an input compression (AGC-I) hearing aid and an output compression (AGC-O) hearing aid (e.g., IHAFF, Valente & Van Vliet, 1997). For an AGC-I system, CT is the input level at which gain reduction occurs. For an AGC-O system, CT is referred as the output level at which gain reduction occurs. Because Figure 6–3A is that of an AGC-I system, the CT is at 50 dB SPL. If Figure 6–3A were the I-O curve of an AGC-O hearing aid, the CT would be 110 dB SPL instead.

Compression hearing aids differ by their compression thresholds. A hearing aid with *CL* typically has a high CT (>65 dB SPL input level). A *WDRC* hearing aid typically has a low CT (between 40 dB SPL and 65 dB SPL), whereas an *AVC* hearing aid has intermediate value (between 55 dB SPL and 75 dB SPL) (Dillon, 1988). Such criteria may be based on the limitations of analog technology in designing today's hearing aids. Digital signal processing may lead to less distinction in classifying hearing aid types on the basis of CT.

SPECIAL CONSIDERATION

One digital hearing aid has a fixed CT at 20 dB HL and a second CT occurring between 50- and 80-dB HL. This hearing aid would not fall neatly into any one of the established categories for compression hearing aid.

Compression Ratio

CR represents the rate of gain reduction. It is computed as the ratio of the change in input level to the corresponding change in output level for the range of intensity at which compression occurs. Hence, the CR shown in Figure 6–3A is (90 to 50)/(110 to 90) or 2:1.

CR in a CL device is necessarily and typically high (>5:1, typically ≥10:1). This is because gain reduction is necessary only when the output level is near saturation or the tolerance limit of the hearing-impaired person (i.e., at high input level). For a WDRC hearing aid, because gain reduction starts early, less gain reduction is necessary over the course of the input range. Typically, the CR on a WDRC hearing aid varies from 1.1:1 to 4:1. The CR on a conventional AVC hearing aid varies between that of a WDRC and a CL hearing aid.

Gain

Whereas gain on a linear hearing aid is constant at all input levels before saturation, gain on a compression hearing aid is level dependent. If one refers to Figure 6–3B, one notices that gain on a compression hearing aid is the greatest at (or below) the compression threshold (maximum gain). Typically, manufacturers report this gain value in all their product specifications. To meaningfully express the gain on a compression hearing aid, it is important to state the input level at which gain is expressed. In this case the gain is 40 dB at 50 dB SPL input, 30 dB at 65 dB SPL input, and 20 dB at 90 dB SPL input. From a practical standpoint, the gain of the hearing aid at the CT (i.e., low or soft input, or G_{soft}), at a normal level (i.e.,

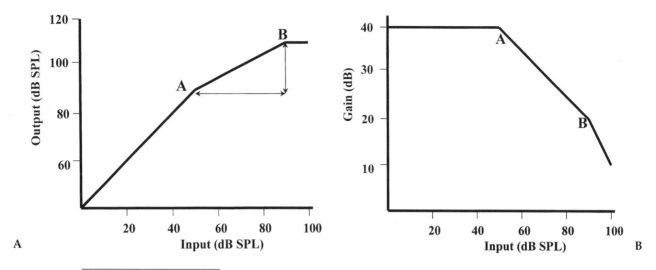

Figure 6–3 **(A)** Static I-O curve for a compression hearing aid. Points A and B are the lower (*A*) and upper (*B*) CTs. **(B)** I-G curve of the compression hearing aid.

around 65 dB SPL, G_{normal}), and at a high (or loud) input level (i.e., 85- to 90-dB SPL, G_{loud}) should be specified. The effect of changing gain at one input level while maintaining gain at another input level will be discussed in the section on fine-tuning.

PITFALL

Knowing the gain at one input and the CR (assuming that it is fixed) allows one to predict gain at the other input levels. Simply knowing the CR is not enough to determine the appropriateness of the compression settings.

Crossover Frequency

A compression hearing aid with multiple channels is called a multichannel compression hearing aid. Each channel processes sounds within a frequency region bounded by its bandwidth, some of which may be adjustable. The frequency at which two channels intersect is the crossover frequency (Fc).

Because the gain within each channel is identical for all frequencies within that bandwidth, one rationale for the choice of Fc is based on the audiometric configuration of the hearing aid wearer. For example, if a patient has a mild hearing loss below 1500 Hz but a severe loss above that frequency, one might agree that the region below 1500 Hz and the region above 1500 Hz receive different gain and compression settings. The optimal Fc should be around 1500 Hz so that separate processing can be applied to each frequency region. Hayes (1994) also showed that hearing aid wearers preferred a Fc that falls near the slope of their audiometric configuration in a two-channel WDRC hearing aid.

Dynamic Characteristics

The dynamic characteristics of a compression hearing aid describe the response of the hearing aid to a stimulus that is changing in level over time. Typically, it is described by the *attack and release times* of the device to a standard stimulus (a sinusoid that goes from 55 dB SPL to 90 dB SPL and back to 55 dB SPL). The most recent ANSI standards (ANSI S3.22-1996) define the attack time as the time it takes the hearing aid to reach within 3 dB of the reduced gain state caused by the 90 dB SPL sinusoid. The release time is the time taken by the hearing aid to return from the reduced gain state to within 4 dB of the linear full-on gain caused by the 55 dB SPL signal.

Attack and Release Time

The attack and release times alter the intensity relationship of different segments of an input signal. Figure 6–4 shows an input signal (B) and its output from a compression hearing aid with a short attack and release time (C) and then a long attack and release time (D) for the same static compression characteristic (A). With a short attack and release time, the gain of the hearing aid changes quickly, and the intensity difference between the more intense sounds and the less intense sounds decreases. This is reflected on the I-O curve (Fig. 6–4C). On the other hand, a longer attack and release time means longer time for the hearing aid to settle to a steady gain state (Fig. 6–4D). This results in a different output than is seen on the static I-O curve and greater intensity difference between the intense and less intense sounds than the case with the short attack and release time.

Recall that the CR is the ratio of the change in input range to the change in output range. If different release times result in different output ranges, one may predict that the CR in real life (i.e., *effective CR*) will be different from the static compression ratio. Indeed, Stone and Moore (1992) and Verschure et al (1996) showed that the effective CR decreases as the release time increases.

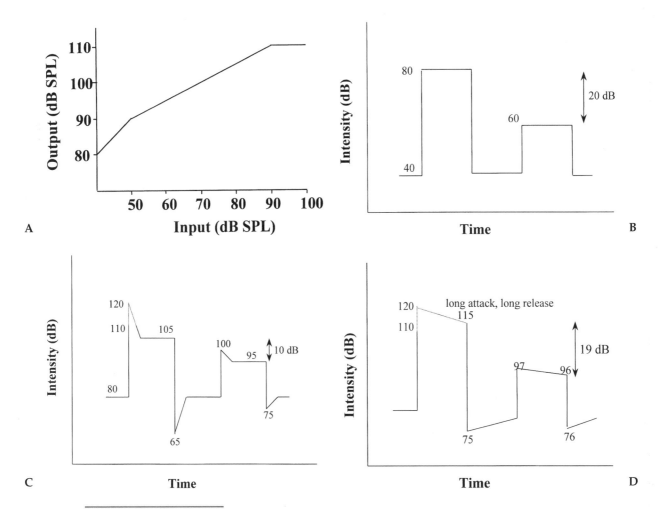

Figure 6–4 Effect of attack and release time on the waveform of a signal. **(A)** Static I-O curve of the WDRC hearing aid. **(B)** Input signal. **(C)** Output from the hearing aid with a fast attack and release time. **(D)** Output from the hearing aid with a long attack and release time.

Compression hearing aids vary in their dynamic characteristics. Because the purpose of a CL hearing aid is to minimize saturation distortion and to protect the wearer from impulse signals, the attack time is usually short (<2 ms) and the release time is usually intermediate in duration (≈100 ms) to minimize artifacts from dramatic gain change. A WDRC hearing aid needs to have relatively short attack and release times for the gain variation to follow the intensity variation seen in the syllabic structures. An attack time of less than 5 ms and a release time of 30 to 50 ms satisfy such requirement. Such a hearing aid has been called a *fast-acting compression* hearing aid. Because the purpose of an AVC hearing aid is to minimize the long-term overall intensity variation while preserving the short-term intensity contrasts, long attack and release times from several hundred milliseconds to several seconds are used. They have also been called *slow-acting compression* hearing aids.

The use of fixed release times, long or short, will have shortcomings in some situations. For example, a fixed short release time may lead to reports of "pumping" "breathiness."

A long release time may lead to inaudibility of low input sounds when they occur after a high input sound. To overcome some of these limitations, adaptive release times are used. Such hearing aids vary their release times on the basis of the intensity and duration of the input signal—short release time for short, intense signal and long release time for longer duration signals. Hearing aids with adaptive release times are available in all types of compression systems—CL, WDRC, or AVC hearing aids.

CANDIDATES FOR DIFFERENT TYPES OF COMPRESSION HEARING AIDS

Compression hearing aids minimize the occurrence of distortion and may enhance audibility for soft sounds and comfort for loud sounds. However, it may alter the intensity relationship among different segments of the speech signal and lead to poor speech intelligibility for some hearing-impaired wearers (Van Tasell, 1993; Verschuure et al, 1996). At present,

PITFALL

Despite the detailed work in specifying the static and dynamic characteristics of compression hearing aids, many clinicians and researchers still only consider the static characteristics of compression hearing aids. In "real life" the output of compression hearing aids is modified greatly by its attack and release time characteristics. Seldom is the static compression ratio achieved in "real life."

a lack of agreement exists among clinicians and researchers as to the type of compression appropriate for each type of hearing loss. However, current research and clinical observations led me to the following general recommendations.

Compression Limiting

Because CL is typically used as a means to avoid saturation distortion at high input levels and not as a means to alter the intensity relationship among sounds, its efficacy should be compared with other types of output limiting approach (i.e., peak clipping).

Dawson et al (1991) compared linear peak clipping and linear CL in a group of subjects with severe-to-profound hearing loss. Forty-three of the 44 subjects with severe hearing loss (pure tone average <90 dB HL) preferred CL, whereas 16 of 32 subjects with profound hearing loss (pure tone average >90 dB HL) preferred peak clipping. The authors attributed the preference for CL to reduced distortion. They hypothesized that the variation in preference seen in subjects with profound hearing loss was attributed to the reduced SPL in the CL hearing aid. The subjects could have responded negatively to the insufficient loudness of the signal, despite the absence of distortion products.

Hawkins and Naidoo (1993) compared the subjective preference between peak clipping and CL by use of subjective judgments of clarity in 12 hearing-impaired subjects with a moderate degree of hearing loss. All the subjects preferred CL over peak clipping when stimuli were presented at high intensity levels (>80 dB SPL).

PEARL

It appears that CL may be more desirable than peak clipping as a means to control for saturation distortion. It should be desirable for all degrees of hearing loss except for the very profound, where the loss of output or distortion products may be viewed negatively by some wearers.

Wide Dynamic Range Compression

A WDRC hearing aid compresses the wide range of acoustic signals into the residual dynamic range of the hearing-impaired ear. The theoretical advantage is higher audibility

for low-input signals and more comfort for high-input signals than linear amplification.

Moore and his colleagues (1992) confirmed this speculation. These authors compared subjects' performance of a commercial two-channel WDRC hearing aid fit linearly and nonlinearly (i.e., WDRC). The hearing aids were adjusted so that conversational speech was comfortable for both hearing aid conditions, and subjects were not allowed to adjust the VC on the hearing aid during the test. Speech recognition scores were obtained at 50 dB SPL, 65 dB SPL and 80 dB SPL in quiet and in babble noise. The results showed significant improvement in speech recognition at the 50 dB SPL level with the WDRC condition over the linear condition. No advantage was seen at the other stimulus conditions. Subjectively, most subjects preferred the WDRC condition to the linear condition. This result can be explained easily in Figure 6–5, which compares the output of a WDRC hearing aid to that of a linear hearing aid when both are matched in output to a conversational input signal (65 dB SPL). More output is seen with the WDRC hearing aid below the 65 dB SPL input level than the linear hearing aid.

A potential drawback of compression is the reduction of intensity contrasts (Plomp, 1988). Van Tasell (1993) commented that such contrasts might disrupt the temporal-intensity cues (e.g., suprasegmental) and affect intelligibility. This may be especially problematic for people with severe-to-profound hearing impairment, who are more reliant on the temporal envelope for speech perception, than those with a milder degree of hearing loss (Boothroyd et al, 1988). Because the width of the auditory filter increases as hearing loss exceeds 40 dB HL (Stone, 1995), a tentative conclusion is that hearing-impaired people with more than a mild degree of hearing loss will more likely experience difficulty with frequency resolution and depend more on temporal resolution. Therefore they may not be good candidates for WDRC. Similarly, Killion and Fikret-Pasa (1993) reported three types of sensorineural hearing loss on the basis of the loudness growth

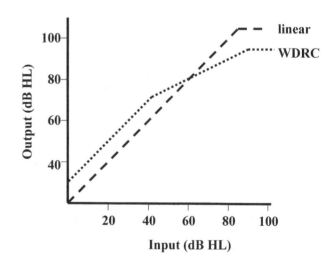

Figure 6–5 Comparison in output between a WDRC hearing aid and a linear hearing aid matched at a conversational input (60 dB SPL). Note the difference in output above and below the 60 dB SPL input level.

function. Type I cases are those with a mild-to-moderate hearing loss with typical loudness growth functions. These are good candidates for WDRC. Type II cases are those with moderate hearing loss and do not show complete recruitment at high input levels. These are also good candidates for WDRC, but they may require greater gain at high inputs. Type III individuals have severe hearing loss, and their maximum speech recognition score occurs at an input level near their uncomfortable listening level (UCL). These patients may benefit from linear processing with CL.

PEARL

A tentative recommendation at this point is that WDRC may be optimal for mild-to-moderate hearing loss when frequency resolution is not a major issue. Its use may be questionable as hearing loss increases because of increased reliance on temporal cues and the potential disruption of temporal cues in a fast-acting WDRC hearing aid.

Slow-Acting Automatic Volume Control

Slow-acting AVC hearing aids are designed to maintain the short-term intensity differences among signals while ensuring long-term audibility and comfort. Furthermore, the chance of saturation distortion is minimized because of gain reduction. From that standpoint, it may overcome some of the limitations of fast-acting WDRC (i.e., reduction of intensity contrast) and linear amplification (i.e., need for VC adjustment for audibility and comfort).

Despite the theoretical advantages and suggestions by some researchers that these hearing aids may be potentially valuable (e.g., Braida et al, 1979; Byrne, 1996; Dillon, 1988, 1996; Walker & Dillon, 1982), such hearing aids are not used commonly. Several reasons may explain such lack of interest. First, earlier studies typically used long release times but short attack times. In those studies a decrease in speech recognition score was seen with prolonged release time (Johansson, 1973; Lynn & Carhart, 1963; Schweitzer & Causey, 1977). This observation is understandable when one realizes that a fast attack time would mean fast gain reduction, but a long release time would mean slow gain recovery. Consequently, the speech signal after compression may not be audible to the hearing aid wearer and thus intelligibility decreased. Interestingly, Neuman et al (1995) found greater subjective preference for a long release time than a short release time. Walker and Dillon (1982), on the basis of Johansson's (1973) findings, suggested that a long release time should be used with a long attack time to minimize gain reduction.

Other reasons may explain the poorer intelligibility with the long release time. The relatively high CT (typically 60- to 70-dB SPL) used in most studies suggests the possibility that these hearing aids may not provide adequate gain for sounds below the CT. A lower CT may be necessary to ensure audibility. Also, the single-channel design in these hearing aids suggests that any gain change will affect all frequency regions. Unless special design considerations are made, the

low-frequency input may put the high-frequency range into gain reduction as well. This may result in poorer audibility. Independent multiple compression channels may be necessary to minimize uniform gain reduction in all frequencies. The conclusion reached in previous studies with slow-acting compression may be modified if these considerations were taken.

Theoretically, candidates for slow-acting AVC hearing aids may include those with a mild-to-severe hearing loss because this type of processing overcomes the limitations of linear (adjusting VC for audibility and comfort) and fast-acting WDRC (potential temporal/spectral smearing) processing. However, insufficient clinical data are available at this time to confirm this speculation. With the advances in hearing aid technology, it is foreseeable that only a well-designed slow-acting compression hearing aid can solve the candidacy question for this type of processing.

PEARL

The listening condition is another consideration for the type of processing. Although fast-acting WDRC is optimal for speech intelligibility in quiet (because of the low CT), most reported studies showed a preference for linear or low CR when listening in noise. A multiple memory hearing aid programmed linearly in one memory and in a WDRC mode in another memory may meet the requirement. Alternately, slow-acting compression may be used instead.

APPROACHES TO FITTING NONLINEAR HEARING AIDS

Compression Limiting

Byrne (1996) recommended high compression parameters in a CL hearing aid because its purpose is to limit saturation distortion. Typically a CT greater than 65 dB SPL is needed. If the CT is specified in output level (i.e., for AGC-O), then the CT should be set to just below the loudness discomfort level (LDL) of the hearing-impaired person. Because gain reduction occurs near the LDL, significant gain reduction (i.e., high CR) is needed to prevent loudness discomfort while avoiding saturation. CRs used in CL hearing aids are generally greater than 5:1, with the typical value at 10:1.

If the CL hearing aid functions linearly at most input levels, the same frequency gain prescription approach for linear hearing aids (e.g., NAL-R) (Byrne & Dillon, 1986) or any other validated approaches (e.g., modified simplex) would also apply. The optimal output sound pressure level at 90 dB input (ANSI S3.22–1996) setting on the hearing aid should be set to just below the UCL or LDL of the wearer (e.g., Hawkins et al, 1987). The reader is referred to Chapters 4, 5, 12, and 13 in this volume on hearing aid selection for details.

Slow-Acting Compression or Automatic Volume Control

At present, no general fitting approach is designed specifically for slow-acting compression hearing aids. A commercial digital hearing aid reportedly has incorporated the effects of attack and release times in its threshold-based fitting formula for its slow-acting compression hearing aid. Consequently, the discussion that follows must be viewed as tentative in nature.

The purpose of an AVC hearing aid is to reduce the long-term fluctuation of the input signal while preserving its short-term level fluctuation. In other words, it must function like a linear hearing aid in the short term (i.e., a dynamic CR of 1:1) and provide gain adjustment in the long term. Because of this, minor variations in the compression settings will probably be inconsequential to the listeners. Indeed, Byrne (1996) suggests that the same compression settings can be used for everyone broadly grouped according to their dynamic ranges. Several considerations are important in choosing an AVC or slow-acting compression hearing aid.

First, audibility must be ensured. One of the reasons for the lack of enthusiasm for past AVC hearing aids is their relatively high CT (60- to 70-dB SPL). This suggests the potential of inadequate gain for sounds less than the 60- to 70-dB SPL, especially when a long release time is used. Thus the first task in fitting AVC hearing aids is to select a low CT (less than 40 dB SPL) to ensure audibility for soft sounds.

Second, the static compression characteristics of the hearing aids (i.e., CR) can be selected broadly based on the ratio of the dynamic range of normal-hearing people to that of the hearing-impaired person. Precise specification is not necessary because the ideal CR of an AVC should be close to 1:1. Third, some means to calculate target gain for conversational input will be necessary so that maximal intelligibility can be ensured. From that standpoint, a linear (e.g., NAL-R) or nonlinear prescriptive target (DSL[i/o]) (Cornelisse et al, 1995) may be used, depending on the clinician's preference. More research is necessary to validate the fitting approach for this type of hearing aid.

Wide Dynamic Range Compression

A stated rationale for WDRC is to restore normal loudness perception in the hearing-impaired ear. Thus it is necessary to examine how loudness is represented and how hearing loss changes this representation. What follows is a general description of the principles behind the loudness compensation approach proposed by Villchur (1973) many years ago.

Equal Loudness Contours

Equal loudness contours (ELC) are a series of lines connecting the SPLs at different frequencies that have the same loudness sensation. Loudness levels are expressed in phons and loudness categories like "soft" and "comfortably loud." Figure 6–6 shows the average ELC for "soft," "normal," and "loud" sounds for normal-hearing listeners (thin lines) and a hearing-impaired listener with a sloping high-frequency sensorineural hearing loss (thick lines).

Let us examine the ELC for the "soft" perception. Below 1250 Hz, no difference exists in the ELC between the normal-

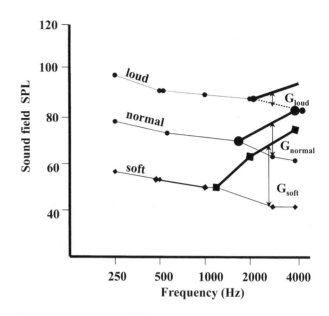

Figure 6–6 Equal loudness contours for "loud," "normal," and "soft" input levels for a normal-hearing listener *(thin line)* and for a patient with a high-frequency hearing loss *(thick line)*. G_{soft} reflects the gain for soft input; G_{normal} reflects the gain for conversational input; and G_{loud} reflects the gain for loud input.

hearing and the hearing-impaired person. Differences between the normal-hearing and the hearing-impaired ELC appear above 1600 Hz. At 3000 Hz, it requires 43 dB SPL for the normal-hearing person and 69 dB SPL for the hearing-impaired person to judge the signal as "soft." The difference in intensity levels for the hearing-impaired person to judge the sound as equally "soft" as the normal-hearing person is the amount of desired gain to restore that ELC. In this case the amount of desired gain (G_{soft}) to restore the "soft" loudness contour is 26 dB at 3000 Hz.

No difference in the ELC is found between the normal-hearing ear and the hearing-impaired ear for the "loud" category below 2000 Hz. At 3000 Hz, the normal ear requires 83 dB SPL and the hearing-impaired ear 91 dB SPL to reach a "loud" judgment (or a gain of 8 dB). It is evident that less gain is required to restore normal loudness for louder sounds than for softer sounds. This is the principle behind Villchur's original design for the WDRC hearing aid.

The last five years had seen a proliferation of approaches targeted at fitting a WDRC hearing aid. Some of these methods involve direct loudness growth measurement, whereas others use a more prescriptive approach with normative data. Both approaches aim to set the compression parameters on the hearing aid so that the loudness perception of the hearing-impaired person matches that of the normal-hearing listeners. Differences between the two approaches reflect the attention paid to individual variation in loudness perception. A description of these approaches follows.

Direct Loudness Measurement

In the direct measurement approach the individual's loudness categories of sounds at different frequencies and intensities are measured. They are used either directly to indicate the amount of necessary gain, or they are compared with the loudness growth function of normal-hearing individuals to derive the optimal compression settings. Direct loudness measurement is justified because it overcomes individual variability in loudness perception (Dillon et al, 1984; Hawkins et al, 1987; Kamm et al, 1978).

Loudness Growth Functions

The ELC gives the clinicians a method of examining loudness information across many frequencies. The loudness growth function (LGF), on the other hand, offers the same information at discrete frequency regions. By definition, a LGF shows how loudness perception changes as the stimulus intensity changes.

One commercial approach to determine the loudness growth information is the loudness growth in octave bands (LGOB) method proposed by Allen et al (1990). In this method one-half octave bands of noise centered at octave intervals from 500 to 4000 Hz are presented through calibrated insert earphones. The patient responds to the loudness of these stimuli by pressing the appropriate buttons on a pad, which are labeled as "too loud," "very loud," "loud," "comfortable," "soft," "very soft," and "did not hear." A practice trial is allowed before actual testing begins. During the actual test, stimulus frequency and intensity are randomized. A LGF is formed when one plots the loudness category on the y axis and the SPL (re: calibrated 2-cc coupler) required for that loudness category on the x-axis.

LGFs can be determined from the ELC. Referring back to Figure 6–6, the normal ear required 43 dB SPL, 62 dB SPL, and 82 dB SPL at 3000 Hz to reach the "soft," "normal," and "loud" loudness categories, respectively. This is drawn as the solid line in Figure 6–7. The hearing-impaired ear, on the other hand, required 69 dB SPL, 78 dB SPL, and 91 dB SPL to reach the same loudness categories. This is drawn as the dotted line in Figure 6–7. The difference between the solid (normal) and the dotted (hearing-impaired) lines represents the amount of gain at each input level (to the normal ear) to bring the impaired ear to the same loudness perception as the nor-

mal ear. In this case 26 dB (69(−)43) of gain (G_{soft}) is required for soft sounds (input level of 43 dB SPL), 16 dB (78(−)62) of gain (G_{normal}) is required for conversational sounds (input level of 62 dB SPL), and 9 dB (91(−)82) of gain (G_{loud}) is required for loud sounds (input level of 82 dB SPL) to reach normal loudness perception.

Calculation of Compression Ratio

The LGF in Figure 6–7 helps determine the required gain from a hearing aid so that it matches the loudness categories of the average normal-hearing listener. If one plots the required output (for the hearing-impaired ear to reach a particular loudness category) against the input (for the normal-hearing ear to reach the same loudness category), one obtains an I-O function similar to the I-O curve of any compression hearing aid.

Figure 6–8 transforms the information from Figure 6–7 into an I-O curve. For example, one reads from Figure 6–7 that it requires 43 dB SPL for the normal ear and 69 dB SPL for the impaired ear to reach a "soft" loudness category at 3000 Hz. Consequently, the (x,y) coordinate on the I-O plane in Figure 6–8 is (43, 69). This point is identified as "soft." At the "normal" level, one reads that 62 dB SPL is required for the normal ear and 78 dB SPL for the impaired ear to reach the "normal" loudness category. Consequently, the (x,y) coordinate on the I-O plane to reach "normal" loudness is (62, 78). This process is repeated for the "loud" loudness category. These three coordinates are connected to create an I-O curve at 3000 Hz. In other words this is the output at 3000 Hz the hearing aid must provide so the hearing-impaired person has the same loudness perception as the average normal-hearing person across intensity levels. Because the CR is defined as the change in input to the change in output (i.e., CR = input change/output change), one can easily calculate the CR at 3000 Hz to be 40/25 or 1.6:1.

Real-Ear Loudness Mapping

The real-ear loudness mapping (RELM) method is similar to the LGOB except that all measurements are calibrated and reflected in the patient's earcanal. Thus in the RELM approach,

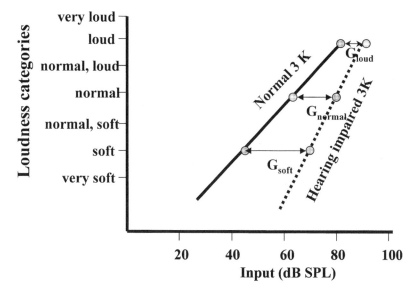

Figure 6–7 Loudness growth function for a normal-hearing and hearing-impaired listener at 3000 Hz. The curves are generated from data in Figure 6–6.

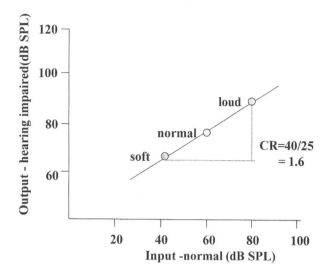

Figure 6–8 Desired I-O characteristics of a compression hearing aid to normalize loudness at 3000 Hz for the hypothetical listener in Figures 6–6 and 6–7.

stimuli (e.g., warble tones) are delivered in the sound field, and the earcanal SPL that corresponds to each loudness perception is directly measured. In performing the task a loudspeaker is placed at about 18 inches and 45 degrees azimuth from the subject. In addition, a probe microphone is placed in the earcanal for SPL measurement. Subjects are instructed and tested in the same manner as in the LGOB test. The earcanal SPL that corresponds to different loudness categories across frequencies is displayed after the whole procedure.

Humes et al (1996) showed that the test-retest variability of the RELM is less than 5 dB across loudness categories and frequencies. To use RELM, Humes et al (1996) recommended that clinicians determine the unaided frequency-specific RELM of the hearing-impaired ear and the real-ear unaided response (REUR) with a 65 dB SPL speech noise. By applying the SPL relationship between the frequency-specific loudness contour and the REUR, the target gain at each input can be specified. This is because for a normal-hearing listener, the REUR for the 65 dB SPL speech noise should follow the "soft" loudness contour for frequency-specific stimuli from 400 to 1000 Hz and about 5- to 10-dB beyond those frequencies. The difference in SPL between the "soft" loudness contour and the REUR at 65 dB SPL defines the target gain that the hearing aid needs to achieve for conversational input. By the same token, one can generate the REUR at 50 dB SPL and 80 dB SPL speech noise and compare that to the subjects' "very soft" and "comfortable" loudness categories for target gain specification at these two input levels. Once the targets are generated, it becomes a matter of adjustment on the hearing aid so that the real-ear aided responses (REAR) at 50 dB SPL, 65 dB SPL, and 80 dB SPL match the corresponding targets.

The RELM method extends beyond the insert earphone LGOB in two ways. First, individual loudness summation across frequencies (from using narrow band signals to approximate broadband loudness) is accounted for. Second, any real-ear modification of the coupler response is directly measured. This increases the precision of fit.

Independent Hearing Aid Fitting Forum

One of the formalized approaches to measure loudness growth for fitting nonlinear hearing aids is proposed by the Independent Hearing Aid Fitting Forum (IHAFF). This is a group of audiologists and hearing scientists who wanted to streamline the fitting of nonlinear hearing aids. The IHAFF group recommended a 10-step hearing aid fitting procedure, from selecting a hearing aid with the desired I-O characteristics to validating the wearer's satisfaction of the hearing aid by use of a standardized questionnaire. Interested readers are referred to the detailed description of the IHAFF protocol by Valente and Van Vliet (1997). Two parts of the IHAFF protocol—the Contour test and the VIOLA test—are especially relevant to the specification of compression settings on a hearing aid. A description of them follows.

Loudness Growth Using the Contour Test

Cox and her colleagues developed the Contour test at the University of Memphis in the early 1990s (Cox et al, 1997) for the purpose of directly measuring loudness growth in the hearing-impaired ear. The test procedure can be conducted automatically by means of software interface with specific audiometers or manually by the clinicians. Warble tones at two frequencies (500 and 3000 Hz) with duration of 200 ms are typically used so that some indication of the dynamic range characteristics in the low-frequency and high-frequency regions can be sampled. However, the clinician may test any frequencies between 250 and 4000 Hz. Typically, five minutes are required to conduct monaural loudness growth at one frequency. Palmer and Lindley (1998) reported good test-retest reliability of the test.

In contrast to the LGOB test that randomizes stimulus presentation, the Contour test uses an ascending approach, with the initial stimulus 5 dB greater than the patient's reported threshold. A step size of 5 dB (2- or 2.5-dB step size for those with dynamic range narrower than 50 dB) is usually followed. Subjects verbally assign a number (1 to 7) to represent the loudness category of the stimulus. A "1" is assigned when the sound is "very soft" and "7" when it is "uncomfortably loud" (Hawkins et al, 1987). Three ascending trials are recommended, and the median intensity level assigned to a particular loudness category is taken to represent its level.

Hearing Aid Selection Using VIOLA

The VIOLA (Visual Input/Output Locator Algorithm) is the part of the IHAFF protocol that helps the clinician to determine the electroacoustic settings on a hearing aid to restore "normal" loudness perception. This algorithm uses the loudness-intensity information determined during the

Contour test to define the residual auditory dynamic range of the hearing-impaired listener. It also identifies the target output SPL level in a HA-1 coupler for three levels of speech input—"soft," "comfortable," and "loud" at the target frequency. The clinician can also enter a set of compression characteristics to determine how close it matches the desired target.

Defining the residual dynamic range

VIOLA takes the results of the Contour test to define the residual dynamic range of the listener. Intensity levels that are assigned the categories of "very soft," "soft," "comfortable, but slightly soft" are assigned the category of "soft." Intensity levels that are assigned the categories of "comfortable, but slightly soft," "comfortable," and "comfortable, but slightly loud" are assigned the category of "comfortable." Intensity levels that are assigned the categories of "comfortable,

but slightly loud," "loud, but ok," and "uncomfortably loud" are assigned the category of "loud." Figure 6–9 shows the VIOLA screen for a 3000 Hz signal. The shaded areas represent the range of SPL for differ ent levels of speech—"soft," "comfortable," and "loud." The dynamic range of the listener is the total area occupied by the shaded areas.

Identifying target output

The loudness growth information obtained during the Contour test was based on perception of frequency-specific, limited-duration auditory stimuli. So that such results can be useful for the perception of broadband stimuli (i.e., speech), Cox (1995) determined from 45 normal-hearing individuals the intensity relationship between speech at different levels (soft, normal, and loud) and the loudness growth data generated during the Contour test. Table 6–2 shows where speech

TABLE 6–2   Relation of speech at different levels to the loudness categories

Frequency (Hz)	Soft	Normal	Loud
250	.01(s)	.50(s)	.87(s)
500	.39(s)	.90(s)	.48(c)
1000	.24(s)	.85(s)	.67(c)
2000	.29(s)	.82(s)	.64(c)
3000	.27(s)	.82(s)	.59(c)
4000	.26(s)	.71(s)	.50(c)

From Cox, R. (1995). *Hearing Journal, 48*(2);10,39–44.

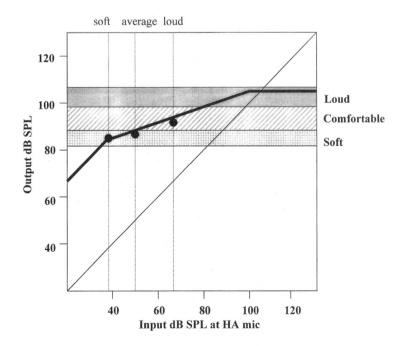

Figure 6–9   Example of a VIOLA screen showing the desired output levels for "soft," "normal," and "loud" speech at 3000 Hz.

at a particular frequency would fall within the dynamic range of that frequency generated using warble tones during the Contour test. It was assumed that soft speech occurs at an overall level of 50 dB SPL, average speech at a level of 65 dB SPL, and loud speech at a level of 85 dB SPL.

For example, average conversational speech at 3000 Hz should be amplified to the top 82% (.82) of the range of intensity that was judged as "soft" (s) using warble tones. Similarly, loud speech at 3000 Hz corresponds to an intensity level that is 59% of the range of intensity that is judged as "comfortable" (c) using warble tones. This conversion is necessary to account for the loudness summation across different critical bands (Scharf & Hellman, 1966; Zwicker et al, 1957) in speech and differences between the crest factor and duration between the frequency-specific stimuli and speech. This relationship found in normal-hearing listeners is then applied to the dynamic range information of the specific hearing-impaired individual to estimate the coupler SPL for "soft," "average," and "loud" speech. This is similar to the approach that Humes et al (1996) took in the RELM test. Note that this conversion does not account for the potential difference in loudness summation between a normal-hearing individual and a hearing-impaired person (Launer, 1995). Furthermore, binaural summation of loudness is not considered in the formulation. This could result in 3- to 5-dB more gain in a binaural fitting than a monaural fitting.

After the desired coupler SPLs for speech at different levels are determined, the input levels for such output is estimated from the data of Pearsons et al (1977). These investigators showed that the SPL at the microphone opening at 3000 Hz was about 38 dB SPL for "soft" speech, 50 dB SPL for "conversational" speech, and 67 dB SPL for "loud" speech. These SPL define the input levels for the desired coupler output levels at the three speech levels. Vertical lines are indicated on the VIOLA screen in Figure 6–9 that correspond to these three input speech levels.

This information allows one to specify the three dots representing the desired hearing aid output at the three input levels of speech. For example, Figure 6–9 shows that at 3000 Hz, soft speech (38 dB SPL) would require an output of 85 dB SPL; average speech (50 dB SPL) an output of 88 dB SPL, and loud speech (67 dB SPL) an output of 90 dB SPL. These computations are performed automatically for the clinician once data from the Contour Test are entered.

Selecting optimal compression characteristics

VIOLA requires the clinicians to join the three dots on the VIOLA screen (Fig. 6–9) to determine the compression settings that match most closely the target I-O curve. They can either examine the target I-O curve and calculate the optimal compression settings or they can enter the available settings from a compression hearing aid to determine whether the entered settings result in an appropriate match.

Comparison of Settings

To help guide the clinicians on the appropriateness of a selected set of compression settings, VIOLA asks that the following information be entered for each test frequency: (1) gain at 40 dB, (2) CT 1, (3) CR 1, (4), CT 2, (5) CR 2, and (6) maximum output. Entries to these six characteristics will allow VIOLA to plot an I-O curve of the comparison hearing

aid and superimpose it onto the VIOLA screen. This allows the clinician to examine whether the I-O curve matches the requirement imposed by the target output (i.e., the three dots). Lindley and Palmer (1997) and Valente and Van Vliet (1997) offered some hints on entering these indices.

Calculation of Settings

The clinicians can also calculate the required compression characteristics. To determine the required optimal gain at 40 dB SPL input (assuming that this is the CT), they can simply draw a vertical line at the 40 dB input point until it intersects with the I-O curve generated from the three dots and note the output level at that point. The difference between the output level and 40 dB SPL is the recommended gain at that input. In this case, the G_{soft} would be about 46 dB.

To determine the compression ratio, one can simply divide the range of input from soft to loud speech to the range of output that corresponds to this range of input. For example, at 3000 Hz, the range of input is 29 dB (or 67 dB SPL to 38 dB SPL), whereas the range of output is 7 dB (or 92 dB SPL to 85 dB SPL). Thus the compression ratio is 29/7 or 4.1:1.

It was indicated earlier that the compression threshold is defined differently by the IHAFF group for input and output compression hearing aids. For input compression, the CT is the lowest input level that signifies gain reduction. Typically, it varies from 40 dB SPL to 65 dB SPL. For the output compression hearing aid, the lowest output level signifies gain reduction. For that reason, VIOLA asks the clinicians to specify the type of compression hearing aid under consideration. An "o" is placed after the numeric entry, (e.g., 100o) to indicate that the CT for this output compression hearing aid is 100 dB SPL.

The maximum output from the hearing aid is simply the outer boundary of the area identified as "loud" in the VIOLA screen. In this case it is 105 dB SPL at 3000 Hz. After these entries are made, VIOLA will generate an I-O curve on the basis of the entries and allow the clinicians to compare their entries with the I-O curves of available hearing aids. The best hearing aid or combination of compression settings is the one with an I-O curve that matches the target curve most closely.

The availability of the IHAFF protocol and, specifically, the Contour Test and the VIOLA procedure is the first systematic attempt at streamlining the fitting of nonlinear hearing aids. It integrates the available information of the time and provides an instructional approach for clinicians to select the most optimal compression hearing aid (or settings). It is the most comprehensive approach to selecting a nonlinear hearing aid.

However, the IHAFF protocol also has several limitations. First, its validity has not been demonstrated. No research has shown that hearing aids selected with the IHAFF protocol are more satisfactory than hearing aids selected with other approaches. Second, the VIOLA generates three points to define the I-O characteristics of the optimal compression hearing aid. This may be superior to predicting the I-O curve simply using threshold and LDL information. It is inadequate, however, for selecting compression systems with a low CT, curvilinear compression, or I-O curves with multiple segments (Dillon, 1996). Third, only the static characteristics of the compression hearing aid (I-O curve) are considered. It is becoming more evident that the attack and release times of the compression hearing aids could alter its static CR (e.g., Stone & Moore, 1992; Verschuure et al, 1996). Similarly, other features of the hearing aid like venting (Fortune, 1997), noise management algorithms, directional microphones, channel interaction, and so forth may also change the static CR and effectiveness of the hearing aid. These considerations could be just as important if not more important than the determination of the static CR.

PRESCRIPTIVE FORMULAS

The stated advantage of direct loudness growth measurement is to account for individual variation in loudness perception. In addition, the test procedure has high test-retest reliability (Humes et al, 1996; Robinson & Gatehouse, 1996). Although good reliability is a prerequisite for an acceptable procedure, several reasons exist that have caused some researchers to propose a prescriptive approach as an alternative to selecting the optimal characteristics on a compression hearing aid. The first reason is the variability in measurement. Olsson et al (1985) showed as much as 20 dB difference between measured real-ear SPL and coupler-specified SPL. Rankovic et al (1992) also showed as much as 35 dB variation between headphone thresholds and real-ear SPL. Fortune (1997) showed that the actual gain (and thus the effective CR) is different between vented and unvented earmolds. In situ loudness measurements (i.e., RELM) can minimize many of these variabilities. However, the extra time and equipment requirement may be a consideration for many.

Second, uncertainty about the loudness perception is being challenged. If loudness is a robust perception, the same loudness growth exponent should be obtained regardless of the method of assessment. This has not been the case. For example, the static CR shown by Hellman and Meiselman (1990) using a *cross-modality matching* task (i.e., matching auditory loudness to visual height) was significantly different from those reported by Kiessling (1995) who used a category rating method (i.e., assigning numbers to loudness categories). Jenstad et al (1997) also showed that the exponents of the individual loudness function vary with the test procedure. Higher exponents are obtained with sequential presentation of stimuli, ascending run, and single tone (without reference) than with random presentation, descending runs, and tones with a reference tone at the start. These findings prompted some to further question the loudness perception that is really being measured during loudness scaling procedures (e.g., Byrne, 1996).

Third, no clinical data support the assertion that compression hearing aids fit using direct loudness scaling can yield higher satisfaction than those fit using a prescriptive approach (Byrne, 1996). Furthermore, it is questionable whether the measured loudness characteristics are even different from the predicted ones. Trine et al (1997) reported on a comparison between the loudness growth exponents determined with direct loudness growth measurement and those predicted on the basis of dynamic range information (threshold and LDL). No difference was found in the outcome of the comparison. This suggests, at least for the average hearing-impaired person, that the actual loudness measurement may not improve the adjustment of a compression hearing aid over that of

prediction. However, Stelmachowicz et al (1998) compared users' gain with the prescription by DSL[i/o], FIG6, and ReSound's LGOB. These investigators found both the DSL[i/o] and FIG6 to prescribe more gain than the wearers used. However, the gain prescribed by ReSound's algorithm was closer to the wearers' daily use than the other two methods. At least for device-specific situations, the prescriptive method may be used efficiently as a first approximation to generate the desired compression characteristics. A summary of several popular prescriptive methods follows.

FIG6

FIG6 (1996) is a computer-aided prescriptive fitting formula that prescribes coupler and real-ear gain for low, medium, and high inputs for a nonlinear hearing aid. In addition, the desired CR can be calculated on the basis of the insertion gain data. This formula is named because the essence of the approach (i.e., gain requirement for different degrees of hearing loss) was reported in Figure 6 of a Killion and Fikret-Pasa (1993) article.

Formulation of FIG6

Killion used a rather eclectic approach to formulate the desired gain at different input levels. Interestingly, the author reported that the recommendation of FIG6 is similar to that of Villchur's (1973) ELC approach.

Gain for Soft Sounds, G_{soft} (<40-dB SPL)

Although normal-hearing individuals have thresholds at or better than 0 dB HL, restoring the aided threshold to 0 dB HL may be counterproductive because of excessive amplification of room noise and the increased likelihood of feedback. Because the softest speech sounds occur at about 20 dB HL, Killion argued that the target-aided threshold should be around 20 dB HL. Consequently, the gain for soft sounds would be the person's threshold minus 20 dB. For example, someone with a 50 dB hearing loss would require 30 dB (or $50 - 20$ dB) gain. Less gain is prescribed for hearing loss greater than 60 dB HL.

Gain for Conversational Sounds, G_{normal} (65 dB SPL)

Killion based the gain requirement for medium level sounds on Pascoe's (1988) data, which showed the relationship among threshold, most comfortable listening (MCL), and LDL in 508 ears. Figure 6–10 shows that the MCL for someone with normal-hearing is at 65 dB HL, whereas it is 77 dB HL for someone with a 40 dB hearing loss. Consequently, the gain requirement would simply be the difference between a hearing-impaired person's MCL and normal MCL (65 dB HL). For patients with more than 60 dB HL, the formula was modified.

Gain for Loud Sounds, G_{loud} (95 dB SPL)

Gain requirement at this input level is estimated by examining the loudness growth curves reported by various researchers, (e.g., Hellman & Meiselman, 1993; Lippman et al, 1977; Lyregaard, 1988). It was shown in Figure 6–2 that patients with different degrees of hearing loss show different degrees of recruitment. For example, a patient with a 40 dB HL shows complete recruitment at high-level sounds, thus no gain is

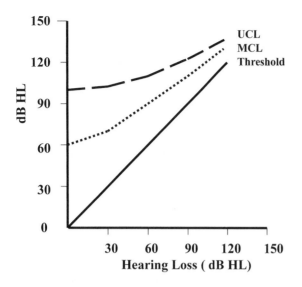

Figure 6–10 Relationship between threshold, MCL, and LDL for 508 ears. (Redrawn from Pascoe, D.P. [1988]. In: J.H. Jensen (Ed.), *Proceedings of the 13th Danavox Symposium.*)

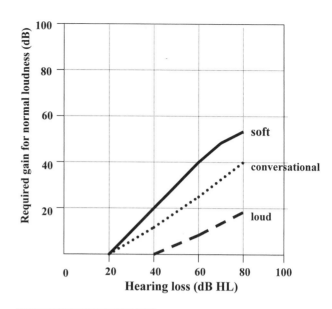

Figure 6–11 FIG6: relationship between hearing loss and desired insertion gain for "soft," "conversational," and "loud" inputs. (From FIG6 [1996], with permission.)

required at high inputs. On the other hand, another patient with a 60 dB HL also shows complete recruitment but at an 8 dB deficit in loudness at high input level. Thus 8 dB of gain is required at high input level for this degree of hearing loss.

Figure 6–11 shows the gain by hearing loss curves (i.e., the original FIG6). To determine the prescribed gain, the clinician simply determines the threshold at each frequency and reads off the corresponding gain for each of the three input values for that hearing loss. For example, a hearing loss of 60 dB HL requires 40 dB gain for soft sounds (G_{soft}), 25 dB gain for conversational sounds (G_{normal}), and 8 dB gain for loud sounds (G_{loud}). The FIG6 manual also included mathematical formulas for calculation of the desired target gain. No gain is prescribed for hearing loss beyond 80 dB HL because Killion recommends a linear hearing aid with CL for hearing loss greater than 75 dB HL (FIG6, 1996). Note that gain prescription is independent of frequency; the same insertion gain is prescribed as long as the frequencies have the same threshold.

Calculation of Compression Ratio

Because CR is simply the change in input to the change in output, the gain recommended at each frequency for low and high level sounds can be used to estimate the CR at such frequency. The recommended CR varies with the input level. Lower CR is recommended for the higher inputs than the low to average input levels above 70 dB HL. Although the optimal CR can be determined for each frequency, the actual CR in a two-channel system will be limited to two values only. In FIG6, the CR for the low band is determined as the average of the CR at 500 and 1000 Hz. For the high band it is the average of the CR at 2000 Hz and 4000 Hz.

The advantage of the FIG6 is its simplicity. Furthermore, it will calculate the desired output for different hearing aid styles (same for IHAFF). Like the IHAFF protocol, its validity has not been demonstrated. Readers can write to Etymotic Research to request a copy of the software.

The Desired Sensation Level (Input/Output)

The DSL[i/o] is a theoretical, device-independent approach formulated by Cornelisse and his colleagues at the University of Western Ontario (Cornelisse et al, 1995). Unlike the other nonlinear approaches, the stated rationale for this approach is not to normalize loudness but to ensure audibility for soft sounds. This formula is to be distinguished from the original DSL formula, which was intended for linear hearing aid fitting in children (Seewald et al, 1985). Despite this difference in origin, Cornelisse et al (1995) indicated that the target defined by the DSL[i/o] for conversational speech is similar to that recommended by the original DSL formula.

The DSL[i/o] approach can be either prescriptive or individualized. To use it in a prescriptive manner, the audiologists enter the patient's audiometric threshold and the type of hearing aids recommended. If no LDL data are entered, the DSL[i/o] will predict this information on the basis of Pascoe's (1988) data. In addition, the software will make the necessary transformations on the basis of average correction factors. To minimize individual variation from the average correction data, the DSL[i/o] recommends entry of the individual's LDL, real-ear-to-coupler difference (RECD), real-ear-to-dial difference (REDD), and REUR so that the individual's threshold data can be converted into real-ear SPL representation. The real-ear threshold and LDL data define the auditory area of the hearing-impaired person and help calculate the target output at each frequency for input levels between 50- and 90-dB SPL.

A unique feature of the DSL[i/o] is that the nature of the compression can be specified. Whereas the IHAFF and FIG6 approaches prescribe a fixed CR for the range of inputs, the DSL[i/o] allows specification of fixed CR (*"linear" compression* in Cornelisse et al's terminology) or variable CRs (i.e., *"curvilinear" compression*). Individual loudness growth data are necessary for the DSL[i/o] to calculate the exponent for the curvilinear compression. The loudness exponent is the ratio of the log of the loudness ratings to the log of the stimulus magnitude. In normal-hearing listeners, it has a value of 0.6. If no loudness growth data are provided, the exponent will be predicted on the basis of the individual thresholds. Furthermore, the DSL[i/o] software allows the entry of real-ear aided response (REAR) so that comparison with the target can be made.

The rationale and steps involved in formulating the DSL[i/o] are detailed in the article written by Cornelisse et al (1995). The following is a summary of the steps involved in its formulation.

Defining the Auditory Area

In contrast to the other approaches, the DSL [i/o] approach presents its recommendation as desired output measured in the wearer's earcanal (dB EC) as a function of input level delivered to the unoccupied sound field (dB SF). Because of this method of presentation, a correction factor, the sound field-to-eardrum transform (SF_t) is added to the input to more accurately reflect the real-ear input level. Figure 6–12 shows all the necessary indices in formulating the recommended compression settings.

PEARL

The derivation of the DSL[i/o] formula appears complex and confusing. This is because of the introduction of the sound field-to-eardrum transforms (SF_t). To simplify its appearance, pretend that SF_t does not exist (i.e., set the SF_t to "0") and the equations will appear to be more straightforward.

Figure 6–12 is an I-O curve of a WDRC hearing aid for a patient with 50 dB hearing loss at 1000 Hz (this will be 60 dB SPL in the earcanal). This figure shows the three regions of WDRC hearing aids defined by Cornelisse et al (1995). Other than the obvious inclusion of the wearer's threshold and LDL information, this I-O curve is similar to typical I-O curves of WDRC hearing aids with a linear region below the compression threshold, a compression region, and a limiting region that is bounded by the upper limit of discomfort of the listener.

A hearing-impaired person's dynamic range is defined by the difference between his threshold (Th_{hi}, e.g., 60 dB) and his upper limit of comfort (UL_{hi}, e.g., 110 dB). Thus the unaided dynamic range is $DR_u = UL_{hi} - TH_{hi}$ (110 − 60 or 50 dB). Because the minimum output from a hearing aid must be greater than the person's threshold and the maximum output of a hearing aid (O_{max}) must be equal to or just below the UL_{hi}, we have:

$$O_{min} = TH_{hi} \text{ or } 60 \text{ dB}$$
$$O_{max} = UL_{hi} \text{ or } 110 \text{ dB}$$

The input level at which maximum output occurs is designated as I_{max} (110 dB). This point should also be the input level, after correction for the sound field-to-eardrum transfer at which loudness discomfort occurs. Thus $I_{max} = UL_{hi} - SF_t$

The minimum input level for compression to activate is the I_{min} (10 dB). This should represent the point of maximum gain of the hearing aid. This point should also be close to the normal-hearing person's threshold so that the hearing-impaired person can have the same audibility as the normal-hearing person. In other words,

$$I_{min} = Th_n - SF_t$$

When a WDRC hearing aid is worn, the aided dynamic range of the wearer should be: $DR_a = UL_{hi} - TH_n$ or 110 − 10 or 100 dB.

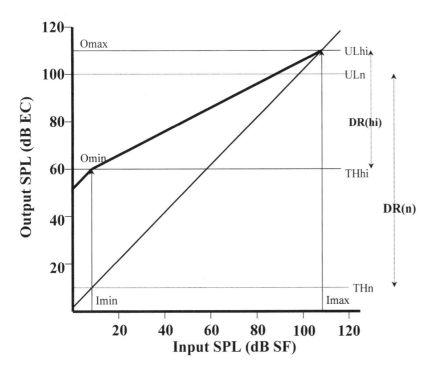

Figure 6–12 Hypothetical I-O function for a 60 dB hearing loss using the DSL[i/o] formula.

Calculating Output and Compression Ratio

The output at different input levels, assuming a "linear" or uniform compression, can be easily calculated.

Region 1: Input less than I_{min}, the output is:
$$\text{Output} = Th_{hi} - [(Th_n - SF_t) - I]$$
For example, if I = 0 dB,
$$\text{Output} = 60 - [(0 + 10) - 0]$$
$$= 50 \text{ dB}$$

Region 2: Input between I_{min} and I_{max} (linear compression), the output is:
$$\text{Output} = \{[(I + SF_t) - TH_n] / [UL_{hi} - TH_n]\}$$
$$\times (UL_{hi} - TH_{hi})\} + TH_{hi}$$
For example, if I = 40 dB
$$\text{Output} = \{\{[(40 - 10) - 10] / [110 - 10]\} \times (110 - 60)\} + 60$$
$$= 70 \text{ dB}$$

Region 3: Input greater than I_{max}:
$$\text{Output} = UL_{hi}$$
For example, if I > 110 dB
$$\text{Output} = 110 \text{ dB}$$

And the CR is:
$$DR_a / DR_u = (UL_{hi} - TH_n) / (UL_{hi} - TH_{hi})$$
$$CR = (110 - 10) / (110 - 60)$$
$$= 2.0$$

Accounting for Curvilinear Compression

The unmodified DSL equation calculates target output from WDRC hearing aids assuming a fixed compression ratio (i.e., same magnitude of gain decrease as input increases). The growth of loudness in some hearing-impaired individuals may not be uniform as described by this equation. Some show rapid loudness growth near threshold and then normal loudness growth, whereas others may show normal loudness growth and then rapid growth afterward. In other words, a linear growth function may not adequately predict the target output in all situations. A curvilinear function can be introduced by including the ratio of the normal and hearing-impaired persons' loudness function exponents in output consideration. Thus for input within the compression range, the output becomes:

$$\text{Output} = \{\{[(I + SF_t) - TH_n] / [UL_{hi} - TH_n]\}^{(En/Ehi)} \times (UL_{hi} - TH_{hi})\} + TH_{hi}$$

where *En* is the exponent of the LGF of normal-hearing listeners and *Ehi* is the loudness growth exponent of a hearing-impaired listener. When the ratio is "1," the LGF of the normal-hearing person is identical to that of the hearing-impaired and "linear" compression results. Otherwise, the function becomes nonlinear. Obviously, loudness growth measurements will need to be taken to determine the ratio of the loudness exponents between the wearer and normal-hearing people. It is not clear which form of compression (i.e., linear or nonlinear) will result in better subject performance.

Similar to the other nonlinear fitting approaches, the DSL[i/o] formula has not been validated.

Modified Linear Prescriptive Method

The implicit assumption of achieving "normal" loudness perception is that the wearers will receive maximum benefit from amplification when the processing is matched to their LGF across frequencies (Cox, 1995). This assumption has been challenged by several researchers and clinicians. In addition to the lack of validation studies to support the efficacy of these approaches and the lack of uniformity of the loudness perception, Byrne (1996) also raised several thought-provoking concerns on the use of loudness normalization. First, he argued that the long-term and short-term spectrum of speech varies considerably among talkers and acoustic conditions. Yet both normal-hearing and hearing-impaired listeners have no problem understanding speech as long as it is audible and comfortably loud. Van Buuren et al (1995) also reached a similar conclusion. This casts doubt on the relative unimportance of loudness relationship.

Second, Byrne (1996) indicated that high-frequency amplification could improve the speech recognition ability even for listeners with normal-hearing. The implication is that normal loudness perception may not always be the best for speech recognition and that restoring normalcy to some aspect of audition (e.g., recruitment compensation) could be counterproductive if other aspects (e.g., frequency resolution) remain abnormal.

Byrne (1996) stressed the importance of an optimal frequency gain response. In a linear fitting using an "equalization" model, the rationale is to maximize audibility for speech by providing differential amplification to each frequency band so that each is equally loud (e.g., Berger et al, 1977; NAL, Byrne & Dillon, 1986; MSU, Cox, 1988; DSL, Seewald et al, 1985). This approach is different from the loudness normalization approach, in which equal amplification is applied to all frequencies of the same degree of hearing loss. At least for the NAL-R formula, Byrne listed the work of Studebaker and Sherbecoe (1992) and Moore and Glasberg (1993), who reported that the frequency gain response recommended by the NAL-R formula yielded the highest audibility in quiet. In addition, the finding that the preferred frequency response and compression settings vary according to the acoustic backgrounds (Keidser et al, 1995; Kuk et al, 1994) further challenges the appropriateness of a loudness normalization model.

In view of these unresolved difficulties and the potential that a compression hearing aid may introduce detrimental consequences to intelligibility and sound quality perception (Boothroyd et al, 1988; Van Tasell, 1993), Byrne (1996) suggested a staged approach to fitting hearing aids. Rather than starting from "scratch" with unproven fitting approaches, this staged approach would recommend optimizing for linear amplification first. If unsuccessful, slow-acting compression, because of the preservation of short-term intensity difference, may be recommended. Syllabic compression will be used only as required.

To extend the application of linear prescriptive formulas into the fitting of nonlinear hearing aids, Byrne (1996) argued that the optimal frequency gain response recommended by a linear prescriptive formula for conversational input should be the same for linear and nonlinear hearing aids. Thus one can use a linear prescriptive formula (e.g., NAL-R) to determine the optimal frequency gain characteristics on a nonlinear hearing aid for the conversational level. Extending beyond Byrne's recommendation, one can use the gain characteristics as a reference and calculate the variation in prescription required at other input levels (e.g., soft and loud) for nonlinear hearing aids. Because this approach involves modification of linear prescriptive formulas, it is named the *modified linear prescriptive (MLP)* method.

Byrne and Dillon (see Chapter 25) will discuss some of their work at the National Acoustics Laboratories (NAL) on the MLP method in this volume. At present, several hearing aid manufacturers are offering this option to specify the gain characteristics on a WDRC hearing aid for different input levels. In this approach the clinician either chooses a particular linear prescriptive target or uses the default linear target recommended by the manufacturer to specify the frequency gain characteristics for conversational speech. Gain at low and high input levels (G_{soft} and G_{loud}) will be calculated automatically if the hearing aid uses a fixed CR. Alternately, the CR can be calculated if the gain requirement at either the low input or the high input is specified. The steps involved in the calculation are found in the following.

Fixed Compression Threshold and Compression Ratio

The goal in adjusting a compression hearing aid with a fixed CT and CR is to set the frequency gain setting (i.e., frequency response and VC) for conversational speech and let the preset compression characteristics determine the gain for low and high input levels. For example, assume that a WDRC hearing aid has a fixed CT at 50 dB SPL and a CR of 2:1. Let us further assume that the NAL-R gain of 30 dB is achieved at a VC setting of 2/4. Thus the required output at an input of 65 dB SPL (assumed conversational speech level) is 95 dB SPL (or 65 + 30). If the hearing aid is in compression from 50 dB SPL to 80 dB SPL, the output at an input level of 50 dB SPL can be calculated as:

$$CR = \text{Change in input/change in output}$$

Therefore

$$2 = (65-50)/(95-X)$$

or

$$X = 87.5 \text{ dB SPL}$$

Thus the gain at 50 dB SPL input is 87.5 − 50 or 37.5 dB. Using the same approach, the gain at an input level of 80 dB SPL is 22.5 dB.

This method ensures that the WDRC hearing aid achieves equal loudness across all frequencies for conversational speech. In contrast to its use on a linear hearing aid, such application on a nonlinear hearing aid also provided 7.5 dB more gain than the NAL-R for soft sounds and 7.5 dB less gain than the NAL-R for loud sounds.

It must be remembered that although the gain for conversational speech is ensured, no guarantee exists that the gain at low and high input levels is optimal because of the fixed CR. This approach may be the least problematic if the fixed CR on the hearing aid approximates the average CR on the basis of a comparison between the wearer's dynamic range to that of the normal-hearing listeners. Killion (in FIG6 manual, 1996) calculated the CR for different degrees of hearing loss. It offers a good estimate on the appropriateness of a WDRC hearing aid (re: CR) for a patient.

Fixed Compression Threshold, but Variable Compression Ratio

To specify the compression characteristics on WDRC hearing aids that allow variable CR is in essence to determine the I-O curve of the hearing aids. If one assumes that the CT is fixed at 50 dB SPL and that the same CR is applied to the whole range of input of interest (i.e., 50- to 80-dB SPL), one could determine the CR if the gain (or output) at two input levels is specified. This is because the minimum requirement for a straight line is to specify two points on the line.

Because the prescribed NAL-R output already represents the output at an input level of 60- to 65-dB SPL (conversational speech), the task is to determine the other point on the I-O curve. This is seen in Figure 6–13, which shows some of the potential I-O curves with the same NAL-R prescribed gain at the typical input level of 65 dB SPL.

One has two options for completing the I-O curve. One can measure the required gain (or output) directly for soft sounds to supply the other point on the I-O curve. Alternately, one can predict the gain requirement at the low input level. For example, the FIG6 procedure (FIG6, 1996) prescribes (HL−20) dB gain for soft sounds, where HL is the audiometric threshold of the hearing aid wearer. In this case a listener with a 50 dB HL hearing loss will require 30 dB (or 50(−)20) of gain. Also, if one assumes that the NAL-R gain is 25 dB, the calculated CR is:

$$CR = \text{Change in input/change in output}$$
$$= (65 - 50)/[(65 + 25) - (50 + 30)]$$
$$= 1.5$$

Thus the calculated CR is 1.5:1. Using this CR, the output at the 80 dB SPL input is calculated to be 100 dB SPL or a gain of (100(−)80) 20 dB is provided by this hearing aid at a high input.

Alternately, one may use the output at a high input level as the second point on the I-O curve. If one assumes that the WDRC hearing aid is fit properly so that the LDL of the hearing aid wearer is not exceeded, the LDL of the wearer could represent the maximum output level of the hearing aid. Thus an estimate of the LDL of the wearer will allow one to specify the other point on the I-O curve. This can be measured directly or predicted. Figure 6–10 reports Pascoe's (1988) data on the relation among threshold, MCL, and LDL of listeners with different degrees of hearing loss. For example, if one assumes that the same hearing-impaired person with the 50 dB hearing loss has an LDL of 100 dB HL, one can calculate the CR to be (80(−)65)/(100(−)90) or 1.5:1. By the same calculation, the gain for soft sounds will be 30 dB. This can be seen in Figure 6–13.

It is possible that the resulting I-O curve from using one estimate may be different from using another estimate (or from the real optimal I-O curve) because the rate of loudness growth may not be uniform at each intensity level (e.g., Hellman & Meiselman, 1990). To increase the precision of fit, gain

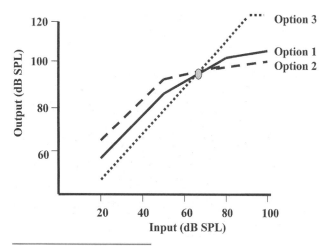

Figure 6–13   Potential I-O curves that have the same CT and output at a 65 dB SPL input.

requirement for low input, conversational input, and high input may need to be available.

The example shown here uses the NAL-R formula to generate targets for conversational speech. The merit of the MLP approach is that any preferred linear prescriptive formulas can be used. This, of course, depends on the preference of the clinician and the experience the patient has with amplification (i.e., how the hearing aid was fitted previously). The NAL-R is chosen because of its extensive validation. Byrne and Cotton (1988) have shown that more than 80% of their subjects selected a frequency-response curve prescribed by the NAL-R when given a choice. Like all the other approaches for a WDRC hearing aid, the potential effects of the attack and release time on the desired gain settings have not been considered. It is foreseeable that the static characteristics determined with this approach might be different from the dynamic characteristics. In addition, loudness summation effects, binaural summation, and so forth are not considered.

WHAT ABOUT OSPL90?

A critical factor in fitting a linear hearing aid is the specification of the *output sound pressure level at 90 dB input (OSPL90)* of the hearing aid so that its maximum output does not exceed the LDL of the hearing-impaired person. This information can be directly measured (e.g., Hawkins et al, 1987) or predicted on the basis of available normative data (e.g., Pascoe, 1988). Recently, several authors have argued that the predicted LDL is as good as the measured LDL in predicting the compression characteristics on WDRC hearing aids (e.g., Dillon, 1997; Trine et al, 1997). In fitting a nonlinear hearing aid, this aspect is frequently not mentioned. In reality the issue of discomfort is somewhat considered when the gain for high input (G_{loud}) is specified. A fundamental difference in circuit design between linear and nonlinear hearing aids gives rise to this difference.

It is important to realize that the maximum output permissible by a hearing aid (assuming that gain is not an issue) is limited by the supply voltage and the receiver output of the hearing aid (Cole, 1993). In most linear hearing aids this maximum output is further regulated by a potentiometer (the OSPL90 or maximum output control) to just below the person's LDL. Figure 6–14A shows the I-O curve of a linear hearing aid as a function of VC position. In addition a hypothetical receiver output limit is indicated on the I-O curve. One can see that the maximum output of the hearing aid is limited by the OSPL90 setting (before it saturates the receiver limit), but independent of the VC position. This means that regardless of the VC position or the input level to the hearing aid, the maximum output of the hearing aid will not exceed the tolerance limit of the wearer.

The typical WDRC hearing aid has AGC-I processing. This means that gain reduction is mediated by the level of the input signal. Figure 6–14B shows the I-O curves as a function of VC position of an AGC-I hearing aid. Clearly, as the VC is adjusted, the output level of the hearing aid is changed. In other words, the maximum output of an AGC-I hearing aid depends on the VC position that is determined when the gain for low (G_{soft}) and high input (G_{loud}) is specified. Because the G_{loud} determines primarily the output at a high input level, this parameter is often called MPO, SSPL90, or UCL setting on nonlinear hearing aids. One must distinguish the use of such terms from linear hearing aids. In a linear hearing aid the output, regardless of VC position, will not exceed the OSPL90 setting. In a nonlinear hearing aid the maximum output of the hearing aid can exceed the so-called MPO setting if sufficiently high input is encountered (> 95-dB SPL) or when the VC is adjusted upward. This is one reason why a VC is not recommended typically on such hearing aids. The output limit of the receiver places the ultimate output limit in such a device.

COMPARISON AMONG VARIOUS FITTING APPROACHES

Although the general goal of nonlinear hearing aid fitting is to provide "normal" loudness sensation to hearing-impaired individuals, these approaches differ in their complexity and their recommendations. Ricketts (1996) compared the results of the VIOLA, the Ricketts and Bentler (RAB), the DSL[i/o], the FIG6, and the NAL-R in fitting a two-channel nonlinear hearing aid. His results showed that the approaches that used direct loudness measurements (i.e., VIOLA, RAB) recommended more gain in the low-frequency and mid-frequency regions than the prescriptive methods (i.e., FIG6, DSL[i/o], NAL-R). In addition, the VIOLA and RAB also provided significantly lower predicted speech intelligibility in noise compared with the measures that assume average loudness growth. However, Lindley and Palmer (1997) reported the opposite findings when comparing the 2-cc target gain. The prescriptive approach actually recommended more gain than the DSL and the IHAFF approaches.

Byrne (1996) compared the recommended frequency gain response between the NAL-R target and the FIG6 target for a flat 50 dB hearing loss at a conversational input. Difference in

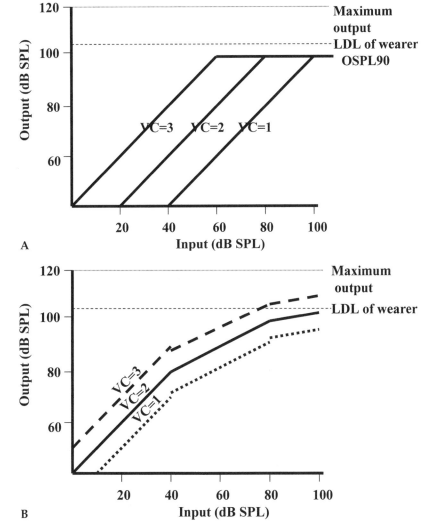

Figure 6–14 **(A)** I-O curves of a linear hearing aid at different VC setting. Note the OSPL90 of the hearing aid is set below the person's LDL. In addition, VC position does not change the OSPL90. **(B)** I-O curves of an AGC-I hearing aid at different VC settings. Note that the maximum output is affected by VC position and the person's LDL is exceeded as VC is increased.

the frequency response was significant even after the curves were matched for overall level. This is especially significant in the mid-frequency region between 750 and 1500 Hz, where the NAL-R target predicted more gain than the FIG6 target. This difference arises as a result of the fitting rationale. The NAL-R is based on equalizing the loudness of various frequency bands. Because the low-frequency region contributes more to the overall loudness than the high-frequency region, less gain is assigned to the low-frequency region than to the high-frequency region for the same degree of hearing loss. This is different from FIG6, which is designed to restore normal loudness without consideration of the loudness contribution by different frequency regions. Killion (FIG6, 1996) also reported similar findings when comparing the FIG6 target to the NAL-R target for different hearing loss configurations.

Stelmachowicz et al (1998) compared wearers' used gain with gain prescribed by the DSL[i/o], FIG6, and predicted LGOB. The DSL[i/o] and FIG6 methods prescribed more gain than the wearer's actual used gain. The gain yielded by the prescriptive LGOB approximated more closely to the user

gain, presumably because the subjects have been wearing hearing aids fit by that approach.

Table 6–3 summarizes the key features of some of the nonlinear fitting approaches discussed in this chapter, including their rationale, the required information, and the recommendations. Procedural differences may also exist among different approaches even though they share the same major features. The choice of a particular approach will be made on the basis of the clinician's rationale, the requirement of the approach, any data supporting the approach, and the time requirement of the approach.

WHICH APPROACHES DO HEARING AID MANUFACTURERS USE?

Many hearing aid manufacturers have adopted various fitting options in their programmable or digital products. Table 6–4 summarizes the approaches that are used by the major hearing aid manufacturers of programmable and digital devices.

TABLE 6–3 Comparison among various nonlinear fitting approaches

	LGOB	IHAFF	FIG6	DSL(i/o)	MLP
Rationale	Loudness normalization	Loudness normalization	Loudness normalization	Loudness normalization	Loudness equalization
Required information	Loudness growth data across frequencies	Loudness growth data at two frequencies	Thresholds across frequencies	Thresholds (minimum) also UCL, RECD, REDD, REUR	Thresholds across frequencies; also formula
Data collection mode	Headphone, inserts, or sound field (RELM)	Headphone, inserts	Headphone, inserts	Headphone, inserts	Headphone, inserts
Hearing loss in dB HL or dB SPL?	Both	Both	dB HL	Both	Both
Use average data?	No, individual loudness data only	No, individual loudness data only	Yes, MCL and LDL	Yes, if LDLs are not entered; no if LDL supplied	Yes-formula, MCL, LDL
Recommendations	Target gain at three inputs	2-cc coupler target gain at three inputs	2-cc coupler target gain and REIG at three inputs	REAR, REAG, 2-cc coupler target at three inputs; aided sound-field target	Coupler or real-ear target at three inputs
Compression parameters?	Yes	No—dispenser calculates	Yes	Yes	Yes
Use with linear hearing aids?	Can be	Can be	Can be	Yes	Yes

Modified from Lindley, G. A., and Palmer, C. U. (1997). *American Journal of Audiology, 6(3);*19–28.

TABLE 6–4 Comparison of fitting approaches used by manufacturers of some programmable and digital hearing aids

Company		Model		LGOB	IHAFF	FIG6	DSL(i/o)	MLP	Special	
Beltone		Composer2000		N	N	N	N	N	Selectafit	
Bernafon-Maico		Dualine		N	N	Y	N	N		
Danavox		DanaSound		Y	N	N	Y	Y	S2000	
									HL-MCL-UCL	
Oticon		Digifocus		N	N	N	N	N	Adaptive speech alignment	
Philips		Digital		N	N	Y	Y	Y	Multiple formulas	
Phonak		PiCS		N	N	N	N	Y	Loud-norm	
Qualitone		Millenium		N	Y	Y	Y	Y		
ReSound		Premium		Y	N	N	N	N		
Siemens		Prisma		Y	N	N	Y	N		
Starkey				Y	Y	Y	Y	Y	Starkey formula	
Unitron		Sound Effect		N	N	Y	Y	N	Adjustment guide	
Widex		Senso		N	N	N	N	N	Loudness mapping MLP in P-series Senso	

One can see a wide range of choices from manufacturers who would only fit their hearing aids with their own proprietary algorithms (e.g., Oticon and Widex) to those who offer a selection of approaches for the clinicians to choose from (e.g., the Starkey Professional Fitting System (PFS) allows the choice of IHAFF, DSL[i/o], FIG6, or the Starkey formula).

Many manufacturers have their own rationales for specific approaches. Although the details of their approaches are proprietary, a description of the general rationale has been available. For example, the *Beltone Selectafit* (Meskan, 1997) uses a variation of the loudness growth test—the comfortable range test—in which the clinician first specifies the patient's thresholds and LDL information. The upper and lower limits of the comfortable range are then determined individually to specify the target gain range.

In the Danavox system, the clinician enters the patient's thresholds, and the S2000 algorithm (Schweitzer, 1997) will predict the target gain for a 55 dB SPL and a 80 dB SPL input signal on the basis of Kiessling's work on loudness scaling (Kiessling, 1995). A unique feature of the fitting software is the *ScalAdapt* test (Kiessling & Dyrlund, 1996), which is a

loudness validation test performed with the patient wearing the hearing aids. ScalAdapt uses the compression settings determined with the S2000 as the starting point and varies the compression settings on the hearing aid in an adaptive manner until the scaled loudness to external stimuli meets the criterion loudness category (e.g., comfortable).

The *adaptive speech alignment* algorithm used by Oticon uses a different compression scheme for its low-frequency and high-frequency channels. In the low-frequency channel, syllabic compression or WDRC with a short attack and release time is used. In the high-frequency channel adaptive gain, or compression with a long attack and release time, is used to preserve the short-term intensity contrasts of the speech signal. Minimally, threshold information is needed to adjust the hearing aid. Schum (1996) provided a discussion on the rationale of this algorithm.

The Philips hearing aid uses different fitting formulas for its four available memories that are designated as the "fidelity," "comfort," "clarity," and "equalizer" programs. The "fidelity" algorithm is designed for sound quality and it uses NAL-R as the target. The FIG6 and DSL[i/o] are recommended for the "comfort" algorithm for use in noisy environments. The

NAL-R is used in the "clarity" algorithm for speech understanding in noise. The "equalizer" recommends the FIG6 and DSL[i/o] algorithms for loudness compensation. The patient presses the memory button on a remote control device to invoke specific processing.

The Widex Senso hearing aid uses slow-acting compression with a much longer attack (10 ms to 2 sec) and release (10 ms to 20 sec) time than most compression hearing aids. A unique feature of the *loudness mapping* algorithm used in the Senso hearing aid is that it considers the effects of attack and release time on its output specification. In fitting this hearing aid the clinician determines the in-situ thresholds of the patient in three frequency channels. This information is used to predict the static loudness growth function on the basis of available psychophysical data (e.g., Hellman & Meiselman 1990, 1993; Pascoe, 1988). In addition, modification of the target gain is made so that the dynamic compression ratio is close to 1:1 (i.e., linear) in any situation. Thus no loudness scaling is performed. Ludvigsen (1997) provided a more detailed description of the rationale behind this device.

Precautions in Verifying the Output of Nonlinear Hearing Aids

A nonlinear hearing aid varies its gain depending on the input level. Consequently, the stimulus input level that is used to evaluate nonlinear hearing aids will affect the outcome of the evaluation. This section discusses some of the issues involved in verification using functional gain and coupler/insertion gain measures.

Functional Gain

Functional gain reflects the threshold difference between aided and unaided condition when the stimulus is presented either in the sound field or under earphones (e.g., for verifying completely in-the-canal hearing aids). Typically, the stimulus is presented in a bracketing manner until the threshold criterion is reached. The measured gain is compared with a linear target to determine the appropriateness of fit. Because a linear hearing aid yields the same gain at all input levels, functional gain reflects the gain for low and high inputs. Because gain on a nonlinear hearing aid depends on the input level and its response time, extra variability in the threshold measurement may be encountered. For example, a high-level stimulus may set the hearing aid into compression so that a lower level stimulus that follows, which is typically audible, may become inaudible because of gain reduction triggered by the preceding stimulus. This could happen because of a high CR, a long release time, or both. The end result is a higher than expected aided threshold (and poorer than expected functional gain). To determine functional gain reliably in nonlinear hearing aids, it is advisable to test in an ascending manner (i.e., from low to high input) when the stimulus is above the compression threshold. The use of small step size (e.g., 5 dB) will limit the amount of gain change, even if the hearing aid is in compression. To minimize the effect of a long release time, ample pauses should be inserted between stimulus presentation so that the hearing aid can recover in gain from compression.

One must be careful in interpreting the results of functional gain measures also. Although functional gain can reflect the gain of a linear hearing aid at conversational level, functional gain for a compression hearing aid only reflects its maximum gain at a low input level. The gain for conversational and loud inputs is not reflected. If two hearing aids, one linear and one nonlinear, are matched in output to a conversational input, the nonlinear hearing aid will likely yield a lower aided threshold (or higher functional gain). If these two hearing aids are matched in their functional gain (meaning same gain for low input), it is likely that the linear hearing aid will provide more output than the nonlinear aid during conversational and loud speech.

Insertion Gain

Insertion gain measure (or real-ear insertion measure) has been used to verify the output of linear hearing aids in the wearer's earcanal. Such a measure can be used to verify whether the output of a nonlinear hearing aid meets the target.

All the nonlinear fitting approaches discussed in this chapter result in a recommended target output/gain level as a function of input levels. Thus verifying that the output of the hearing aid matches the target is simply a matter of presenting the appropriate stimulus at the appropriate input levels. For nonlinear hearing aids, a composite stimulus having energy at all frequencies will yield a more realistic output curve than the use of sweep tones. This is because any potential interactions among frequencies (e.g., intermodulation distortion) can be visualized easily. Furthermore, multiple stimulus levels must be used to document the response of the hearing aid at different input levels. Generally, input levels at 50-, 65-, and 80-dB SPL are recommended to approximate input for soft, conversational, and loud speech.

Many of the current real-ear testing systems also display the result of the measurement in a SPL-O-Gram format. That is, the REARs at different input levels are displayed in relation to the auditory dynamic range of the hearing aid wearer (e.g., Frye 6500 real-ear testing system).

When testing at multiple input levels, one must ensure that the stimulus duration is long enough to fully activate the compression mechanism and that sufficient delay is introduced between presentation so that the hearing aid can completely recover from compression. This is especially critical in testing slow-acting compression hearing aids where the attack and release time of the hearing aid may last several seconds. Consequently, too short a stimulus duration may not yield the steady-state gain of the hearing aid (i.e., no compression tested). The same observation will be true if the delay between presentation is too short. Make sure that the stimulus duration exceeds the longest attack time of the hearing aid and that the delay between presentation exceeds the longest release time of the hearing aid.

A problem with using standard real-ear/coupler systems to verify some of the current digital hearing aids is that these hearing aids have additional signal processing algorithms that may decrease the "real" output. Care must be taken when testing these nonlinear hearing aids so that the appropriate interpretation can be made.

Validating the Performance of Nonlinear Hearing Aids

Subjective Consequence to Parametric Variation

Regardless of the method that one uses to set a compression hearing aid initially, further adjustment or fine tuning of the hearing aid is almost inevitable because of variability in individual preferences and acoustic environments. A nonlinear hearing aid can be adjusted in at least three parameters—the CT, gain for typical sounds (G_{normal}), and gain for high input sounds (G_{loud}). The static I-O curve can help one to understand some of the principles involved in solving a patient's complaints on a compression hearing aid (Kuk, 1998a).

Effect of Compression Threshold—Modification of Gain for Low Inputs

Figure 6–15A shows the effect of adjusting the compression threshold from 40 dB SPL to 65 dB SPL. One notes that the output of the hearing aid remains the same above the 65 dB SPL input, but the output below 65 dB (e.g., 40 dB SPL) has decreased from 80-dB to 70-dB. In this example the effect of increasing the compression threshold is to reduce gain at input levels less than the CT. Because the CT in a WDRC hearing aid varies from 45- to 65-dB SPL, its predominant effect is modifying gain at low to moderately low input level sounds.

The CT may need to be adjusted upward (i.e., reduce gain for soft sounds) to reduce feedback, minimize the perception of ambient sounds, and reduce the "pumping" perception associated with the use of a short release time. On the other hand, the CT can be decreased to increase the audibility of soft sounds like the perception of soft consonants and listening at a distance.

Effect of Typical Gain Setting (G_{normal})—Gain for Soft and Typical Input Levels

Figure 6–15B shows the effect of increasing gain setting on a compression hearing aid. Output from the hearing aid at low and conversational input is increased significantly, but the output of the hearing aid at the high input remains the same. Thus the effect of increasing gain is to increase the CR of the hearing aid and vice versa.

Obviously, the gain on the hearing aid may need to be increased to maximize audibility and loudness for soft and conversational sounds. Complaints like "too soft," "too muffled," and "unclear" are good indications that gain increase may be necessary. On the other hand, too high a gain value will also lead to complaints like "too loud," "unclear," "muffled," and "echoic/hollow."

Effect of Gain at High Input Level (G_{loud})

Various manufacturers allow separate gain adjustment for high input stimulus. These parameters have been called "SSPL90," "UCL," and "Gain$_{80}$" by various manufacturers. Figure 6–15C shows the effect of increasing the gain at high input level (G_{loud}) while keeping G_{normal} constant. As noted, an increase in gain leads to an increase in output above a conversational level and a lowering of the CR. A decrease in high-level gain (G_{loud}) leads to an increase in CR.

Gain for high-level inputs (G_{loud}) may be increased for experienced linear hearing aid wearers who complain that the compression hearing aid is too soft. In addition, it may be increased for music appreciation; for individuals with a conductive or mixed hearing loss, or for those who complained that the amplified sound is "too muffled" or "too unnatural." The gain (G_{loud}) may be decreased for complaints of loudness discomfort.

PEARL

When troubleshooting problems with compression hearing aids, it helps to know the input level at which the patient's complaint is based, so that the proper parameter can be adjusted. Low input complaints involve the CT and/or the G_{soft}, conversational level complaints involve the G_{normal}, and high input level complaints involve the G_{loud}.

Paired Comparison

Paired comparison judgment is a subjective validation technique whereby the subject is presented with two alternative sets of compression settings and is forced to select one that is preferable. The outcome of the comparison will be a combination of compression hearing aid settings that is most preferred by the patient among all the options. This technique can be used as a fine-tuning tool or in selecting the optimal settings on a hearing aid.

Paired comparison can be performed in many ways. They include the round robin, single elimination tournament, double elimination tournament, and adaptive procedure like the modified simplex. Kuk (1994) provided a description of the different tournament strategies and considerations in implementing this technique into clinical use. When this technique is used with today's nonlinear hearing aids, it is important to remember that the duration of the stimulus (e.g., discourse passages) may also affect the outcome. For example, it may take a slow-acting compression hearing aid a few seconds to stabilize to the steady-state level. Consequently, the stimulus must be long enough to allow sufficient time for full activation of the compression hearing aid. This may not be a problem for the linear hearing aid.

Paired comparison technique has been used to validate optimal frequency response (Kuk & Pape, 1993) and preferred compression settings on an AVC hearing aid (Neuman et al, 1994, 1995).

Subjective Questionnaires

The efficacy of a particular nonlinear hearing aid must be documented so that any claims of performance superiority can be substantiated. The subjective questionnaire may also be used in goal setting by identifying the problem areas in which the patient may still have difficulties. Many questionnaires are available today, and interested readers are referred to the excellent article by Weinstein (1997). The two most popular questionnaires—*Abbreviated Profile of Hearing Benefit (APHAB)* and *Client-Oriented Scale of Improvement (COSI)*—will be briefly described.

The *APHAB* was developed by Cox and Alexander (1995) and was included as part of the IHAFF protocol. The patient

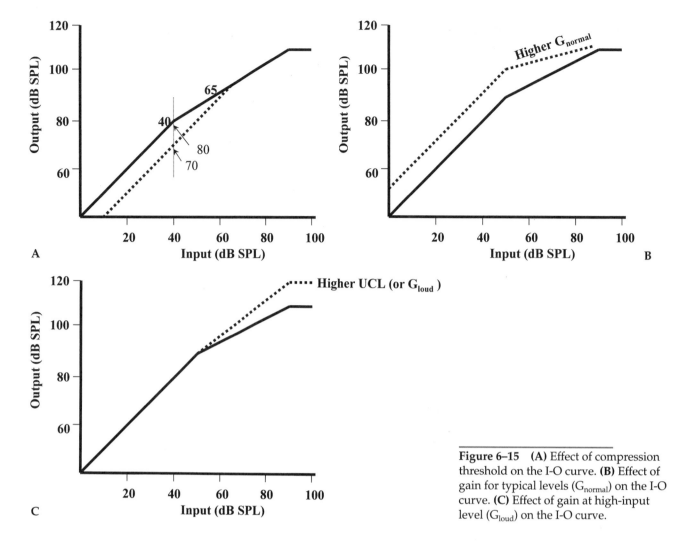

Figure 6–15 **(A)** Effect of compression threshold on the I-O curve. **(B)** Effect of gain for typical levels (G_{normal}) on the I-O curve. **(C)** Effect of gain at high-input level (G_{loud}) on the I-O curve.

indicates the degree of difficulty he or she has in 24 listening situations. These are grouped into four subscales, ease of communication (EC), reverberation (RV), background noise (BN), and aversiveness of sounds (AV). Sampling is done before the hearing aid evaluation and after the hearing aid has been worn for some time. At the end of the trial period the patient is asked again to complete the questionnaire to indicate his or her satisfaction of the chosen settings. The difference between the aided score and the unaided score reflects the benefit that the patient receives from the hearing aid.

The *COSI* was developed by Dillon and his colleagues (Dillon et al, 1997) at the National Acoustic Laboratories (NAL)

as a formalized way to reflect patient benefits with a hearing aid. In this approach the clinician discusses with the patients their areas of hearing difficulties. A list is drawn up with specific goals that are to be achieved with the use of amplification. The clinician and the patients then prioritize the list of goals so that the more important ones are focused on first. The patients indicate their level of functioning on each goal before the hearing aid intervention and at different times after the hearing aids are fit. Proper adjustment of the hearing aid setting or establishment of new goals will take place whenever appropriate.

REFERENCES

ALLEN, J., HALL, J.L., & JENG, P. (1990). Loudness growth in ½ octave bands (LGOB): A procedure for the assessment of loudness. *Journal of the Acoustical Society of America,* 88;745–753.

AMERICAN NATIONAL STANDARDS INSTITUTE. (1996). *American National Standard for Specification of Hearing Aid Characteristics.* ANSI S3.22-1996. (Revision of S3.22-1987). New York: ANSI.

BERGER, K.W., HAGBERG, E.N., & RANE, R.L. (1977). *Prescription of hearing aids: Rationale, procedures, and results.* Kent, OH: Herald.

BOOTHROYD, A., SPRINGER, N., SMITH, L., & SCHULMAN, J. (1988). Amplitude compression and profound hearing loss. *Journal of Speech and Hearing Research, 31*;362–376.

BRAIDA, L.D., DURLACH, N.I., LIPPMAN, R.P., HICKS, B.L., RABINOWITZ, W.M., & REED, C.M. (1979). Hearing aids: A review of past research on linear amplification, amplitude compression and frequency lowering. *ASHA Monograph No. 19.* Rockville, MD: ASLHA.

BYRNE, D. (1996). Hearing aid selection for the 1990s: Where to? *Journal of the American Academy of Audiology, 7*;377–395.

BYRNE, D., & COTTON, S. (1988). Evaluation of the National Acoustic Laboratories' new hearing aid selection procedure. *Journal of Speech and Hearing Research, 31*;178-186.

BYRNE, D., & DILLON, H. (1986). The National Acoustic Laboratories' (NAL) new procedure for selecting the gain and frequency response of a hearing aid. *Ear and Hearing, 7*;257–265.

COLE, W.A. (1993). Current design options and criteria for hearing aids. *Journal of Speech-Language Pathology Audiology Monograph Supplement, 1*;7–14.

CORNELISSE, L.E., SEEWALD, R.C., & JAMIESON, D.G. (1995). The input/output formula: A theoretical approach to the fitting of personal amplification devices. *Journal of the Acoustical Society of America, 97*;1854–1864.

COX, R. (1988). The MSU hearing instrument prescription procedure. *Hearing Instruments, 39*(1);6–10.

COX, R. (1995). Using loudness data for hearing aid selection: The IHAFF approach. *Hearing Journal, 48*(2);10, 39–44.

COX, R., & ALEXANDER, G. (1995). The abbreviated profile of hearing aid benefit (APHAB). *Ear and Hearing, 16*;176–186.

COX, R., ALEXANDER, G., TAYLOR, I., & GRAY, G. (1997). The Contour test of loudness perception. *Ear and Hearing, 18*(5);388–400.

DAWSON, P., DILLON, H., & BATTAGLI, J. (1991). Output limiting compression for the severe-to-profoundly deaf. *Australian Journal of Audiology, 13*;1–12.

DILLON, H. (1988). Compression in hearing aids. In: R.E. Sandlin (Ed.), *Handbook of hearing aid amplification* (Vol. 1) (pp.121–145). Boston: College Hill.

DILLON, H. (1996). Compression? Yes, but for low or high frequencies, for low or high intensities, and with what response times? *Ear and Hearing, 17*;287–307.

DILLON, H. (1997). *Uses of compression in hearing aids.* Presentation at the International Hearing Aid Conference in Iowa City, Iowa. June, 1997.

DILLON, H., CHEW, R., & DEANS, M. (1984). Loudness discomfort level measurements and their implications for the design and fitting of hearing aids. *Australian Journal of Audiology, 6*(2);73–79.

DILLON, H., JAMES, A., & GINIA, J. (1997). Client oriented scale of improvement (COSI) and its relationship to several other measures of benefit and satisfaction provided by hearing aids. *Journal of the American Academy of Audiology, 8*;27–43.

FESTEN, J., & PLOMP, R. (1983). Relations between auditory functions in impaired hearing. *Journal of the Acoustical Society of America, 73*;652–662.

FIG6. (1996). *Hearing aid fitting protocol. Operating manual.* Elk Grove Village, IL: Etymotic Research.

FORTUNE, T. (1997). Real-ear compression ratios: the effects of venting and adaptive release time. *American Journal of Audiology, 6*(2);55–63.

FREYMAN, R., & NERBONNE, G. (1989). The importance of consonant-vowel intensity ratio in the intelligibility of voiceless consonants. *Journal of Speech and Hearing Research, 32*;524–535.

GRAUPE, D., GROSSPIETSCH, J.K., & TAYLOR, R.T. (1986). A self-adaptive noise filtering system. *Hearing Instruments, 37*(9); 29–34.

HAWKINS, D., & NAIDOO, S. (1993). Comparison of sound quality and clarity with asymmetrical peak clipping and output limiting compression. *Journal of the American Academy of Audiology, 4*;221–228.

HAWKINS, D.B., WALDEN, B.E., MONTGOMERY, A., & PROSEK, R.A. (1987). Description and validation of a LDL procedure designed to select SSPL90. *Ear and Hearing, 8*;162–169.

HAYES, D.E. (1994). *Preferred cross over frequencies and compression ratios for a dual channel full range compression hearing aid.* Poster presented at the Convention of the American Academy of Audiology, Dallas, TX.

HELLMAN, R.P., & MEISELMAN, C.H. (1990). Loudness relations for individuals and groups with normal and impaired hearing. *Journal of the Acoustical Society of America, 88*;2596–2606.

HELLMAN, R.P., & MEISELMAN, C.H. (1993). Rate of loudness growth for pure tones in normal and impaired hearing. *Journal of the Acoustical Society of America, 93*;966–975.

HORWITZ, A., TURNER, C., & FABRY, D. (1991). Effects of different frequency response strategies upon recognition and preference for audible speech stimuli. *Journal of Speech and Hearing Research, 34*;1185–1196.

HUMES, L., PAVLOVIC, C., BRAY, V., & BARR, M. (1996). Real-ear measurement of hearing threshold and loudness. *Trends in Amplification, 1*(4);121–135.

JENSTAD, L., CORNELISSE, L., & SEEWALD, R. (1997). Effects of test procedure on individual loudness functions. *Ear and Hearing, 18*(5);401–408.

JOHANSSON, B. (1973). The hearing aid as a technical audiological problem. *Scandinavian Audiology Supplement (3),* T. Lundborg (Ed.), *Symposium on hearing aids* (pp. 55–76).

KAMM, C., DIRKS, D., & MICKEY, M. (1978). Effects of sensorineural hearing loss on loudness discomfort level and most comfortable loudness judgments. *Journal of Speech and Hearing Research, 21*;668–681.

KEIDSER, G., DILLON, H., & BYRNE, D. (1995). Candidates for multiple frequency response characteristics. *Ear and Hearing, 16*;562–574.

KIESSLING, J. (1995). Loudness growth in sensorineural hearing loss—Consequences for hearing aid design and fitting. *Audiological Acoustics, 34*;82–89.

KIESSLING, J., & DYRLUND, O. (1996). Adaptive hearing instrument fitting by loudness scaling (ScalAdapt). *Danavox/Madsen article series* (article number IV of IV).

KILLION, M.C., & FIKRET-PASA, S. (1993). The 3 types of sensorineural hearing loss: loudness and intelligibility considerations. *Hearing Journal, 46*(11);31–36.

KILLION, M.C., STAAB, W.J., & PREVES, D.A. (1990) Classifying automatic signal processors. *Hearing Instruments, 41*(8);6–10.

KUK, F. (1994). Use of paired-comparisons in hearing aid fitting. In: M. Valente (Ed.), *Strategies for selecting and verifying hearing aid fittings* (pp. 108–135). New York: Thieme Medical Publishers, Inc.

KUK, F. (1996a). Theoretical and practical considerations in compression hearing aids. *Trends in Amplification, 1*(1);1–39.

KUK, F. (1996b). Multiple dynamic compression control—Different outputs for different folks? *Hearing Journal, 49*(9); 31–38.

KUK, F. (1998a). Using the I/O curve to help solve subjective complaints with WDRC hearing instruments. *Hearing Review, 5*(1);8–16, 59.

KUK, F. (1998b). Rationale and requirements for a slow acting compression hearing aid. *Hearing Journal, 51*(6);41–53,79.

KUK, F., HARPER, T., & DOUBEK, K. (1994). Preferred real-ear insertion gain for listening in different speech and noise levels. *Journal of the American Academy of Audiology, 5*(2);99–109.

KUK, F., & PAPE, N. (1993). Relative satisfaction for frequency responses selected with a Simplex procedure in different listening conditions. *Journal of Speech and Hearing Research, 36*;168–177.

KUK, F., & TYLER, R. (1990). Relationship between consonant recognition and subjective ratings of hearing aids. *British Journal of Audiology, 24*;171–177.

KUK, F., TYLER, R., & MIMS, L. (1990). Subjective ratings of noise reduction hearing aids. *Scandinavian Audiology, 19*;237–244.

LAUNER, S. (1995). *Loudness perception in listeners with sensorineural hearing impairment*. Ph.D. dissertation. University of Oldenburg, Germany.

LINDLEY, G.A., & PALMER, C.V. (1997). Fitting wide dynamic range compression hearing aids: DSL[i/o], the IHAFF protocol, and FIG6. *American Journal of Audiology, 6*(3);19–28.

LIPPMAN, P.R., BRAIDA, L.D., & DURLACH, N.I. (1977). New results on multiband amplitude compression for the hearing impaired. *Journal of the Acoustical Society of America, 62*;S90(A).

LUDVIGSEN, C. (1997). Basic amplification rationale of a DSP hearing instrument. *Hearing Review, 4*(3);58–67,70.

LYNN, G., & CARHART, R. (1963). Influence of attack and release in compression amplification on understanding speech by hypoacoustics. *Journal of Speech and Hearing Disorders, 28*(2);124–140.

LYREGAARD, P.E. (1988). POGO and the theory behind. In: J. Jensen (Ed.), *Hearing aid fitting: Theoretical and practical views. Proceedings of the 13th Danavox Symposium* (pp. 81–94). Copenhagen.

MESKAN, M. (1997). Understanding differences between nonlinear fitting approaches. *Hearing Review, 4*(4);64–72.

MOORE, B., & GLASBERG, B. (1993). Simulation of the effects of loudness recruitment and threshold elevation on the intelligibility of speech in quiet and in a background noise. *Journal of the Acoustical Society of America, 94*;2050–2062.

MOORE, B., JOHNSON, J., CLARK, T., & PLUVINAGE, V. (1992). Evaluation of a dual channel full dynamic range compression system for people with sensorineural hearing loss. *Ear and Hearing, 13*;349–370.

MUELLER, H.G., & KILLION, M.C. (1996). Page ten: 20 questions—http://www.compression.edu. *Hearing Journal, 49* (1);10,44–45.

NEUMAN, A., BAKKE, M., HELLMAN, S., & LEVITT, H. (1994). Effect of compression ratio in a slow acting compression hearing aid: Paired comparison judgment of quality. *Journal of the Acoustical Society of America, 96*(3);1471–1478.

NEUMAN, A., BAKKE, M., MACKERSIE, C., & HELLMAN, S. (1995). Effect of release time in compression hearing aids: Paired comparison judgments of quality. *Journal of the Acoustical Society of America, 98*(6);3182–3187.

OLSSON, U. (1985). *Hearing aid measurements on occluded-ear simulator compared to simulated in-situ and in-situ measurements*. Report TA 111, Technical Audiology. Stockholm: Karolinska Institute.

PALMER, C., & LINDLEY, G. (1998). Reliability of the Contour test in a population of adults with hearing loss. *Journal of the American Academy of Audiology, 9*;209–215.

PASCOE, D.P. (1988). Clinical measurements of the auditory dynamic range and their relation to formulas for hearing aid gain in presbyacousis and other age related aspects.

In: J.H. Jensen (Ed.), *Proceedings of the 13th Danavox Symposium* (pp. 129–147). Copenhagen.

PEARSONS, K., BENNETT, R., & FIDELL, S. (1977). Speech levels in various noise environments. *EPA report #600/1-77-025.* Washington, DC.

PLOMP, R. (1988). The negative effect of automatic gain control in multichannel hearing aids in the light of modulation transfer function. *Journal of the Acoustical Society of America, 83*;2322–2327.

RANKOVIC, C.M., FREYMAN, R.L., & ZUREK, P.M. (1992). Potential benefits of adaptive frequency gain characteristics for speech reception in noise. *Journal of the Acoustical Society of America, 91*;354–362.

RICKETTS, T. (1996). Fitting hearing aids to individual loudness perception measures. *Ear and Hearing, 17*(2);124–132.

RICKETTS, T., & BENTLER, R. (1996). The effect of test signal type and bandwidth on the categorical scaling of loudness. *Journal of the Acoustical Society of America, 99*;2281–2287.

ROBINSON, K., & GATEHOUSE, S. (1996). Test-retest reliability of loudness scaling. *Ear and Hearing, 17*(2);120–123.

SAMMETH, C., & OCHS, M. (1991). A review of current "noise reduction" hearing aids: A rationale, assumptions, and efficacy. *Ear and Hearing, 12*;116S–124S.

SCHARF, B., & HELLMAN, R.P. (1966). Models of loudness summation applied to impaired ears. *Journal of the Acoustical Society of America, 40*;71–78.

SCHUM, D. (1996). Adaptive speech alignment: A new fitting rationale made possible by DSP. *Hearing Journal, 49*(5);25–30.

SCHWEITZER, C. (1997). New hearing instrument technologies and evolving gain fitting rules: S2000. *Hearing Review, 4*(2);52–56.

SCHWEITZER, H., & CAUSEY, G. (1977). The relative importance of recovery time in compression hearing aids. *Audiology, 16*;61–72.

SEEWALD, R.C., ROSS, M., & SPIRO, M.K. (1985). Selecting amplification characteristics for young hearing-impaired children. *Ear and Hearing, 6*;48–53.

STELMACHOWICZ, P., DALZELL, S., PETERSON, D., KOPUN, J., LEWIS, D., & HOOVER, B. (1998). A comparison of threshold based fitting strategies for nonlinear hearing aids. *Ear and Hearing, 19*;131–138.

STONE, M. (1995). *Spectral enhancement for the hearing-impaired.* Ph.D. Thesis. University of Cambridge, U.K.

STONE, M.A., & MOORE, B.C.J. (1992). Syllabic compression: Effective compression ratios for signals modulated at different rates. *British Journal of Audiology, 26*;351–361.

STUDEBAKER, G.A., & SHERBECOE, R.L. (1992). *LASR3 (SSB): A model for the prediction of average speech recognition performance of normal-hearing and hearing impaired persons.* Laboratory Report 92-02 hearing Sciences Laboratory. Memphis: Memphis State University.

TRINE, T.D., & HORNSBY, B.W.Y. (1997). *Loudness growth measures: Are they worth the time?* Paper presented at the Convention American Academy of Audiology, Fort Lauderdale, FL.

TYLER, R., & KUK, F. (1989). The effects of "noise suppression" hearing aids on consonant recognition in speech babble and low frequency noise. *Ear and Hearing, 10*;243–249.

VALENTE, M., & VAN VLIET, D. (1997). The independent hearing aid fitting forum (IHAFF) protocol. *Trends in Amplification, 2*;6–35.

VAN BUUREN, R.A., FESTEN, J.M., & PLOMP, R. (1995). Evaluation of a wide range of amplitude frequency responses for the hearing impaired. *Journal of Speech and Hearing Research, 38;*211–221.

VAN TASELL, D. (1993). Hearing loss, speech, and hearing aids. *Journal of Speech and Hearing Research, 36;*228–244.

VERSCHUURE, J., MAAS, A.J., STIKVOORT, E., DE JONGE, R.M., GOEDEGEBURE, A., & DRESCHLER, W.A. (1996). Compression and its effect on the speech signal. *Ear and Hearing, 17;*162–175.

VICTOREEN, J.A. (1973). *Basic principles of otometry.* Springfield, IL: Charles C. Thomas Publisher.

VILLCHUR, E. (1973). Signal processing to improve speech intelligibility in perceptive deafness. *Journal of the Acoustical Society of America, 53;*1646–1657.

WALKER, G., & DILLON, H. (1982). Compression in hearing aids: An analysis, a review and some recommendations. *National Acoustic Laboratories of Australia.* Report No. 90.

WEINSTEIN, B. (1997). Outcome measures in the hearing aid fitting/selection process. *Trends in Amplification, 2*(4); 117–137.

ZWICKER, E., FLOTTORP, G., & STEVENS, S.S. (1957). Critical bandwidth in loudness summation. *Journal of the Acoustical Society of America, 29;*548–557.

PREFERRED PRACTICE GUIDELINES

Professionals Who Perform the Selection/Fitting/Evaluation

▼ Audiologists

Indications for Hearing Aid Technology

▼ Fast-acting WDRC: up to a mild-to-moderate (i.e., 50 dB) hearing loss

▼ Slow-acting WDRC: up to severe to severe-profound (i.e., up to 90 to 110 dB) hearing loss

▼ Linear with CL: up to a severe to severe-profound (i.e., up to 90 to 110 dB) hearing loss

▼ Linear with peak clipping: profound loss and only when the other types could not provide adequate output

Clinical Process

▼ Audiologists should have a thorough understanding of the fitting rationale that they follow. This is especially true of the proprietary formulas used by manufacturers.

▼ Use of individual loudness growth measures will minimize individual variability in loudness perception. Thus, if one believes in a loudness normalization model of fitting a compression hearing aid, individual LGF should be generated. If average prediction is used, make sure fine-tuning guidelines are available to correct for individual differences.

▼ If one believes in a loudness equalization model to fitting a nonlinear hearing aid, make sure that the output of the hearing aid matches the target output of the chosen linear prescriptive formula. Fine-tuning guidelines must also be available to correct for individual difference.

▼ Verification of the fitting must be done with real-ear measures at three input levels: 50 dB SPL, 65 dB SPL, and 80 dB SPL. If that is not possible, functional gain measures can be performed with caution on the interpretation.

▼ Validation of the fitting results can be accomplished with the APHAB and/or COSI questionnaires. Other questionnaires may also be appropriate.

Expected Outcomes

▼ The measured output of the selected hearing aid should match as closely as possible the recommended target provided by the chosen fitting approach.

▼ The selected hearing aid provides comfortable and natural listening for conversational speech in quiet (65-dB SPL input). In addition, soft speech (50-dB SPL input) should be audible and loud speech (80-dB SPL) should not be uncomfortably loud.

▼ The selected hearing aid should not produce audible artifacts (e.g., pumping and silence after loud sounds).

▼ The selected hearing aid must decrease the communicative difficulties that the patient reports before wearing the recommended hearing aids.

Documentation

▼ Documentation contains pertinent background information, fitting results on all visits, and specific recommendations.

▼ Documentation should also include a record of compliance with state and federal guidelines for hearing aids. Binaural candidates who opted for a single hearing aid despite the audiologist's recommendation must also be documented.

▼ Documentation on all the pertinent test results, such as speech recognition test, real-ear measures, and questionnaire results, must also be included.

Chapter 7

Counseling for Diagnosis and Management of Auditory Disorders in Infants, Children, and Adults

Jane R. Madell

Outline

NOTE: Part of this chapter is adapted from Madell, J. (1998a). Counseling. In: *Behavioral evaluation of hearing in infants and young children.* New York: Thieme Medical Publishers.

THE ROLE OF THE AUDIOLOGIST AS COUNSELOR

A good audiologist wears many hats. First and foremost he or she needs to be a good diagnostician, but being a good diagnostician is not enough. A good audiologist needs to understand the impact of hearing loss on daily living and needs to be able to identify when additional services are needed and either plan and provide a (re)habilitation program or make appropriate referrals. He or she needs to identify when medical referrals are needed and assist in making educational and vocational recommendations. The good audiologist also needs to provide both educational and supportive counseling. In every aspect of the practice of audiology, the audiologist needs to be a counselor. We can choose to function as specialists who provide technical assistance with little educational or emotional support or we can become partners with our patients and work with them to meet their needs. This usually means more than the basics: more than identifying the degree and type of hearing loss and recommending an amplification system, (re)habilitation, or both. It means providing assistance to the patient and family in accepting the hearing loss, understanding the limitations of amplification, and determining what they can do to make living with a hearing loss easier. To do this, the audiologist needs to be willing to listen and to become involved with the person with hearing loss and his or her family. If we are not willing to do that, we may become good technicians but will not truly be audiologists. The role of counseling in the practice of communicative disorders has been recognized as early as 1962 when Eugene McDonald published *Understand Those Feelings* to assist audiologists and speech-language pathologists in understanding their patients and their behaviors.

PEARL

Evaluation skills are only one part of an audiologist's responsibilities. A successful audiologist will also be a good counselor.

It would appear to be obvious that patients who understand their hearing losses and who know their amplification

Audiology: Treatment. Edited by Valente, Hosford-Dunn, and Roeser. Thieme Medical Publishers, Inc., New York © 2000

and (re)habilitation options will have an easier time dealing with hearing loss. Stephens (1977) demonstrated that hearing aid use increased for patients who received counseling. Brooks (1979) reported that patients who received counseling had greater reductions in perceived hearing handicap than those who did not. Evidence indicates that audiologists are not doing as good a job as they could be doing when it comes to counseling. Fellendorf and Harrow (1970) reported that only half the parents of children with hearing loss were satisfied with the information provided by their audiologists, physicians, or both. Sweetow and Barrager (1980) reported that 20% of parents were uncomfortable asking their audiologist questions, and 35% indicated that the audiologist did not provide them with emotional support in matters related to their child's hearing loss. Adults report similar discomfort with information provided by their audiologists. Despite evidence indicating that we are not providing the counseling services our patients believe we should be providing, Crandell (1997) reports that only 48% of audiology programs offer courses in counseling, and of those that offer courses only 27% require the course. In other words, only 13% of graduate students in audiology are required to take a counseling course. Of the programs that offer courses, 68% were offered within the department rather than by other departments that specialize in counseling such as psychology, human development, or counseling. Although some communicative disorders staff may have had course work and training in counseling, most have not. Even when courses are offered, they are offered by professionals who have probably had minimal training in counseling theory and application. So, is there any question about why our patients are not completely satisfied with our counseling skills?

Listening to our patients and their families is a skill that is infrequently taught in graduate school and certainly not valued. It takes time, time is expensive, and you may hear information that you do not really want to hear. As audiologists, that is difficult for us. What we have been trained to do is "solve the problem." We evaluate hearing and "solve the problem" by providing a device, providing therapy, or making a referral for medical treatment. For many audiologists and patients, hearing aids are viewed as the end of the rehabilitation process, not just one part. That attitude may be the cause of the problem. The devices are not the end, they are only the beginning of a process of learning to function with a hearing loss. Without a doubt, the technical skills in which audiologists excel are to be valued. But are they enough? If we think of how many people have their hearing aids in their dresser drawers and not on their ears, we know that it is not enough. Audiologists who do not feel competent to provide counseling skills have an obligation to their patients to obtain training and improve these skills just as they have an obligation to learn about new technology as it becomes available.

WHAT IS COUNSELING?

Counseling means different things to different people. When most audiologists think about audiological counseling, they think about informational counseling: providing information to patients about hearing loss, amplification, therapy, and so forth. In the field of counseling it is viewed differently. For some it denotes psychotherapy. For others it is supportive assistance and assistance in adjusting to the stresses of daily living. Erdman (1993) and Sanders (1980) talk about two types of counseling in audiology: *informational counseling* and *personal adjustment counseling*. It is sometimes difficult to distinguish between the two. When a family member becomes distressed with the frequent inability of the person with impaired hearing to respond to questions, or when the person with hearing impairment becomes distressed at family members who *"don't speak clearly anymore,"* both informational and supportive counseling are needed. Although parents of newly diagnosed children with hearing impairment need information about the child's hearing loss, they also need help in accepting the hearing loss and dealing with the associated grief.

SPECIAL CONSIDERATION

Two types of counseling are used by audiologists. Informational counseling provides technical information about hearing loss, amplification, and (re)habilitation. Personal adjustment counseling deals with emotional issues related to having a hearing loss, accepting the limitations of hearing loss, and assisting families in dealing with hearing loss.

Approaches to Counseling

Counseling techniques can combine different theories; it may be helpful to review some basic theoretical approaches. Several general counseling approaches exist: the *cognitive* or *rational* approach, the *humanistic or affective approach*, and the *behavioral approach* (Erdman, 1993). Cognitive or rational approaches focus on thought processes and have as their aim an attempt to change the way the person thinks with the goal that if we modify the way the person thinks, the behavior will change. The patient is helped to identify and modify inappropriate assumptions that result in emotional distress or behavior problems. Adler's theory is viewed as an educational experience aimed at increasing self-worth, reducing inferiority feelings, and overcoming discouragement. Inferiority feelings develop when differences exist between the concept of the ideal self and the actual self. This is clinically relevant for clients who are having difficulty accepting their disability (Erdman, 1993).

Humanistic or affective approaches attempt to change the way a person feels to facilitate adjustment. The person is viewed as an agent of change. Carl Rogers' patient-centered therapy (1951) is a well-known affective therapy approach. Rogers views individuals as basically good, realistic and rational, and capable of growth. The intent of therapy is to change the way the person views the world. The counselor is nondirective and encourages the person to determine how to effect change (Erdman, 1993).

Behavioral approaches deal with body and physical actions. Behavioral therapy uses learning theories to change inappropriate behavior and teach appropriate behavior. Pavlov (1927) and Skinner (1953) are the most well-known behavioral theorists. The behavioral technique most familiar to audiologists is visual reinforcement audiometry, which uses behavioral techniques to control behavior and provide information about audition. Wolpe (1982) used behavioral techniques for assertiveness training. This has been successfully used with people with impaired hearing in a number of different settings (DiMichael, 1985; Erdman, 1980). Biofeedback is a behavior therapy that some have found useful in dealing with tinnitus.

Some commonalities exist among counseling approaches regardless of the method (Patterson, 1986). Counseling approaches agree that people are capable of change. They agree that some behaviors are undesirable and result in unhappiness. Counselors expect that the techniques they use can assist patients in making change. Individuals who seek counseling want help. Patients believe change can and will occur. Counselors expect patients to be active participants in making change. Counseling techniques include persuasion, encouragement, advice, support, and instruction. It is clear that all these assumptions have implications for counseling in audiology. The effects of hearing loss can be minimized; communication behavior that is causing problems can be changed. Both audiologists and their patients expect that change will occur, and patients expect and deserve respect and support from their audiologists in effecting change.

The counselor-patient relationship is frequently discussed in the literature and is considered the most powerful variable in counseling. Patterson (1986) reports that warmth, empathy, trust, respect, and unconditional positive regard on the part of the counselor for the patient are the most important variables in the treatment process. Research findings in numerous settings indicate that counselors who communicate warmth, genuineness, and appropriate empathy are more effective in interpersonal relationships.

The model from which individual audiologists function may determine how they view counseling. Audiologists who come from a medical model where patients are passive recipients of care will react differently to the emotional adjustment problems patients experience as a result of hearing loss than those educated in a rehabilitation model that encompasses a helping and co-operative role. Research findings indicate that the more authoritative the counselor is the less compliant the patient is likely to be. Noncompliance issues abound in audiology. Hearing aid use is one of the major issues and has been attributed to cosmetic concerns, denial, and hearing aid limitations. The role of counseling has not been well investigated and may, in fact, play an important role.

COUNSELING THE PATIENT WITH HEARING LOSS

In a review of hearing aid use by the National Health Service hearing aid users in Great Britain, Thomas (1984) determined that people with impaired hearing experienced a high level of psychological disturbance regardless of their degree of hearing loss. If that is the case, then all audiologists need to be prepared to deal with psychological and emotional issues with their patients and to recognize the significant role that counseling will play. Counseling enables individuals to cope effectively with their disabilities. By use of a variety of counseling techniques, the audiologist can significantly effect

change. Although patients may receive appropriate technical care, if they do not receive sufficient psychological care, they are not likely to be satisfied with their treatment (Erdman & Demorest, 1998a,b).

Time constraints are often stated as the reason audiologists cannot listen to patients concerns, but those audiologists who do not listen to their patients are perceived as lacking empathy. When counselors express empathy, when they appear to care and understand, patients are more relaxed and optimistic about treatment outcome. Some patients elicit more empathy from clinicians than others. Managing patients who seem to be difficult or uncooperative is a challenge for all clinicians. It is frequently best accomplished by trying to see things from the patient's perspective. When patients are uncooperative, they are frequently feeling unable to cope with a situation. Patients who are late for appointments, who do not use their hearing aids consistently, parents who come with their children's hearing aids in their pockets or who miss therapy appointments may be expressing their distress and frustration. David Luterman (1996b) talks about "listening with the third ear." He suggests that we need to listen to what the person is telling us and try to understand the underlying message. By doing so we are likely to learn what is really causing the patient to be "noncompliant," which will enable us to help the person resolve the issues that are interfering with compliance. This will, in fact, make our job easier and more successful in the long run.

Many things affect patient-clinician relationships. An important one is the way messages are communicated. Messages communicated in a private area are more likely to be heard than messages communicated in a public space like a hallway or waiting room. A patient who is hesitant or afraid is not likely to be able to reach out to the person standing in the doorway but may, given time, be able to communicate with the clinician who has taken the time to sit down and listen.

COUNSELING ADULT PATIENTS

Determining the Reason for the Visit

Who Initiated the Appointment?

PEARL
It will be easier to work with a patient if you understand the reason for the evaluation appointment. Who initiated the appointment? Does the patient want the evaluation? Is the family pressuring the patient? What does the patient perceive as the problem, and what does he or she hope to gain from the evaluation?

Although it may seem obvious, not everyone spends time trying to find out why the patient came for the visit. Knowing the answer to this basic question will help provide information about what the patient is expecting. Sometimes the person comes because of concerns about hearing and is requesting assistance. When patients request an appointment, they are usually coming first for information, and supportive counseling will be the second concern. The patient may have been sent by a physician with little or no explanation and may have no idea why he or she is there. The person who comes as a result of a referral may have significant concerns about why the referral was made and about the appointment. Some patients come because family members think a problem exists, but the person does not believe anything is wrong. These are the times we frequently hear patients tell us *"I hear what I want to hear,"* or *"The reason I don't understand is because they mumble."* If the patient is coming because family members have insisted on the appointment, a great deal of supportive counseling will be needed for both the patient and the family. The patient will need help in accepting the hearing loss and the necessary rehabilitation. The family will also need assistance in understanding the views of the family member with impaired hearing, including the need to allow the person to make his or her own decisions.

When a patient is being seen as the result of physician referral, it is difficult to determine in advance what kind of counseling will be needed. The patient may know that he or she has a hearing loss and want assistance, may have other medical problems that need evaluation, or may be unprepared to learn about a hearing loss. When a patient is referred from a physician, additional concern exists about who is responsible for counseling—the audiologist or physician. Many physicians choose to counsel their patients and request that audiologists function in a more technical role and not counsel the patient. For many audiologists, this situation is uncomfortable.

What Does the Patient Perceive as the Problem?

The patient's perception of the problem is critical. The first question the audiologist should ask is, *"Why are you here?"* Without that information we can only guess at the reason for the evaluation and provide limited service. If the patient is aware that he or she has a hearing loss and is seeking assistance, our job is relatively easy. If the patient is not aware of the hearing loss, thinks it is minor, or thinks that it is someone else's problem, the audiologist's job will be much different.

When patients seek treatment, it is because they are experiencing disability or handicap rather than hearing impairment. They are concerned about their ability to communicate. As any experienced audiologist knows, an individual's communication and adjustment problems cannot be predicted accurately from the audiometric data. This is another reason why it is critical to determine how the person feels about his or her handicap; to learn as much as possible about the person's communication needs at home, work, school, and so on, and to evaluate the person's communication difficulties to obtain a complete picture.

Expectations for the Evaluation: What Does the Patient Hope to Learn?

Obviously, most patients would prefer to hear that their fears are unfounded and that they do not have a hearing loss. However, most people who come for an evaluation thinking that they have a hearing loss are likely to find that they are correct. They may have ideas already about whether they wish to try hearing aids and, if they do, about which type.

They probably do not have a good idea about what to expect from hearing aids and know little if anything about assistive listening or assistive living systems or other forms of (re)habilitation that may make communication and daily living easier.

Knowing the patient's expectations helps the audiologist in planning the evaluation. If, for example, the patient is certain that he or she does not have a problem and, in fact, he or she does, it will be important for the audiologist to be able to demonstrate that. A standard hearing test with word recognition testing under earphones at comfortably loud levels will not be helpful because the person will not be aware of what he or she is missing in daily conversation.

Counseling About Diagnostic Test Results

Because hearing loss is so familiar to audiologists, it is easy to forget that the people we are counseling do not have as much technical knowledge about hearing loss as we do. We need to keep this in mind when describing test results. How much technical information does the person need at this time? If the person has a hearing loss that is temporary and caused by fluid in the middle ear space, does the person need to understand in detail how to read an audiogram? If a permanent sensorineural hearing loss is causing problems in communication, does the person need to understand how to read an audiogram? Part of the answer to this question is how much the person wants to know. Sometimes, as audiologists, we want to provide information that the patient does not want or is not ready to hear. Patients are entitled to understand everything they want to understand about their hearing. For some patients that means they want to know as much as we know and for other patients it means as little as necessary. Sometimes patients do not want information but may need to hear it anyway.

Audiologists are attached to audiograms, but patients are not. What can we expect a patient to understand when we show an audiogram that indicates a sloping sensorineural hearing loss from 20 dB at 500 Hz to 70 dB at 8000 Hz? Will he or she understand the implications this hearing loss has for communication? That is, of course, the information that needs to be understood. We need to be very careful about the terms we use. We need to provide sufficient technical information so the patient understands but in a way that is not confusing. Telling a patient that he or she has a moderate sloping sensorineural hearing loss is not likely to be helpful. It might be more useful to indicate that testing demonstrates that in the low pitches the person hears normally but has more difficulty hearing in the higher pitches and further explain that with this hearing loss we expect that the person will easily be able to tell when someone is talking and will recognize low-pitched sounds, such as vowels, and low-pitched consonants, such as "b" and "m," but will have more difficulty recognizing high-pitched sounds like "s," "sh," and "f." Some patients may have an easier time understanding men rather than women or adults rather than children. We can then describe what kinds of problems the person might expect to have in the presence of noise. Using the information obtained from word recognition testing will help the person understand the implications of the hearing loss, especially if the word recognition testing includes phoneme scoring, which can help the person recognize some specific problems he or she may be experiencing.

PEARL

A good way to help a person with hearing impairment understand the effect of hearing loss is to demonstrate the effect on daily communication by measuring speech perception at normal and soft conversational levels in quiet and in noise.

Describing the results of special diagnostic tests presents additional problems. In some cases, special diagnostic tests are requested by physicians, and the audiologist functions in a technical capacity. Although the patient wants to know the results, and to be assured that nothing is wrong, the relationship with the physician may prevent the audiologist from discussing them. This is a difficult position for both parties. Even if the audiologist cannot discuss results, he or she can provide comfort and support. We can assure the person that results will quickly be forwarded to the physician for interpretation, check that the patient has an appointment to learn of the test results, and provide the opportunity for the person to vent concerns. This is one of those times when we can provide a good ear.

Counseling About Management Issues

What does the patient really want? Most patients will prefer to have to do as little as possible. For many, using hearing aids is sufficient. The patient may hope to hear well with the hearing aids and will be satisfied with whatever the results are. If the results are less than optimal, some will not be satisfied and will be willing to attend hearing aid orientation, speechreading, or auditory training classes or use assistive listening systems—in other words, do whatever is necessary to be successful. Others are not willing to make the effort. Some who continue to take classes are seeking significant improvement in communication skills, whereas others may have unrealistic expectations about how they will be able to function. The audiologist needs to be optimistic and realistic and assist the person in determining realistic goals. Sometimes low expectations are the audiologist's problem and not the patient's problem.

Years ago when assistive listening systems were less available I had a patient who was unhappy about the quality of hearing he could get from the available amplification and wanted more. Other audiologists and technical staff and I told him that he had unrealistic expectations and *"had to accept his hearing loss."* He was furious. Because no commercially available devices existed that we could recommend, he made one of his own using a stereo amplifier, high-quality earphones, and a microphone that he would pass to whomever was speaking. At the time, my initial reaction was that the idea was ridiculous, but on reflection I realized that this was my prejudice and it was not my place to pass judgment. This person needed to hear better. I would have been a much better audiologist if I had listened to him, if I had heard his

message and helped him solve his problem. Shortly after, he helped me to understand the value of listening to patients. I and others began to explore assistive listening systems and frequency-modulated (FM) systems for people with hearing impairment to use in a variety of different listening situations.

As audiologists, we have a greater responsibility than solving the auditory problem by providing amplification. By inquiring about communication difficulties on the part of the person with hearing impairment and the family members, we can help provide strategies for improving communication skills. We can also help open lines of communication between family members by discussing feelings about hearing loss and the difficulties of living with this loss.

Amplification Counseling

We see few patients who enthusiastically come into our offices requesting amplification and, when fitted, are completely delighted and report no problems or concerns. Almost no one would choose to wear amplification if they had the option. We, unfortunately, live in a culture that does not easily accept differences or disability. In addition, we are not a culture that values aging. Unlike some other cultures that view senior members of the community as people with wisdom who can contribute to the growth of others, we frequently see senior members of our community as people who are losing the capacity to do things and have less value. When an older adult comes in needing hearing aids, he or she is not likely to be enthusiastic. He or she knows that this will make him or her appear to the world to be infirm, incapacitated, and of less value. It should be no surprise, therefore, that the most popular hearing aids are the smallest and least visible.

When most people think about hearing aids, they remember people who had hearing aids that whistled, that they were always adjusting, and that they did not believe helped them to hear well. If they did know people who had good experiences with hearing aids, they frequently do not remember them. As a result, most people come to the hearing aid experience with negative feelings. What most people know about rehabilitation devices comes from eyeglasses. For most people when they put on eyeglasses their vision problems are solved. New hearing aid users expect to experience the same things when they put on hearing aids. Advertising that promises hearing aids that completely eliminate noise or that ensures new digital technology will eliminate all problems contributes to the disappointment experienced by many hearing aid users.

Counseling about amplification is complicated. We need to provide information about amplification options and to provide realistic expectations about benefit. Most people come for amplification assistance after several years of difficulty hearing. Although those tiny hearing aids may work well for some patients, they will not work well for all. Some patients will not be able to hear well with them, some will not have sufficient manual dexterity to manipulate the hearing aids, and some may have visual problems that will prevent them from dealing with the battery door or other controls. For some people the primary concern is cosmetic, and for others it is function. First-time hearing aid users and many experienced users do not know what they can expect from a new aid. They also do not know how to decide between an in-the-ear (ITE), completely in-the-canal (CIC), behind-the-ear (BTE), or programmable hearing aid.

The technical or informational component of counseling requires that the audiologist help the patient understand what to expect from different amplification systems and when the more sophisticated ones will be required. But as important as providing technical information is assisting the patient in having realistic expectations about amplification. The patient needs to know what he or she can expect to be able to hear and in what areas the difficulty can be expected. This is a difficult line to tread. If we play up the problems too much, we may scare the person away from even trying hearing aids, but if we play them down, the person is likely to be disappointed and may be one of those who ends up with hearing aids in the drawer or returned for credit much to the dismay of both the audiologist and the hearing aid manufacturer. (See Chapters 1, 5, 6, 12, and 13 in this volume.) A person who understands the situations in which he or she can expect to have difficulty hearing will be less disappointed than the person who thinks that the hearing aids will solve all problems. The audiologist who spends time helping the patient understand what to expect will have less difficulty with follow-up and will have a patient who more easily accepts amplification.

Communication Training

As any audiologist knows, hearing aids do not solve all communication problems. Many people with impaired hearing would benefit from additional rehabilitation services. Unfortunately, many audiology programs do not offer additional rehabilitation services. The result is that audiologists frequently do not counsel patients about the benefit they might receive from these services. Because no hearing aids completely solve communication problems in difficult listening situations, audiologists need to assist patients in recognizing the situations in which they have difficulty and in recommending additional rehabilitation.

First the audiologist needs to help the patient analyze the listening problems he or she is having to determine whether assistance is needed. Next the audiologist needs to help the person understand the value of taking the time to improve communication skills. This might include speechreading, auditory training, or both. It might include assertiveness training to assist the person in obtaining what he or she needs in communication assistance, including the ability to ask people to modify their communication styles, to turn off the TV when talking, and so on. It may also include providing assistance in managing the auditory environment with technology (FMs and other assistive listening and living systems) and by using such modifications as carpeting and acoustic tiles. (See Chapters 19 and 20 in this volume.)

FAMILY PARTICIPATION

As audiologists, we need to help families understand the effect that poor communication has on family dynamics and to help them develop strategies to improve communication with each other.

Hearing loss is the one disability that puts the onus of the disability on the nondisabled person. A hearing loss affects

---

the entire family. It interferes with the activities of daily living: chatting at the dinner table, talking while you are getting chores done, driving in the car, or discussing a program while watching TV. When listening is a chore for one family member, communication becomes a chore for the whole family, and the joys of casual conversation become difficult. The whole family has to deal with the hearing loss. Many family members have difficulty understanding what the person with impaired hearing can be expected to hear. They frequently assume that he or she could hear more "if he or she paid attention" and almost certainly assume that the hearing aids solve all listening problems.

The audiologist can do a great deal to assist families in understanding about hearing loss. With the permission of the person with impaired hearing, it can be very helpful to invite family members into the test room to help them understand the effects of hearing loss. By testing in sound field, family members will be able to see exactly what the person with impaired hearing can and cannot hear so they can begin to understand why the patient is having difficulty communicating. Word recognition testing in sound field at normal (65 dB SPL) and soft (50 dB SPL) conversational levels in quiet and in the presence of competing noise (+5 dB signal-to-noise ratio [SNR]) will make it clear to family members that the problems are beyond the control of the family member with impaired hearing.

Inviting family members to attend hearing aid orientation classes can also be very helpful. When everyone in the family understands how they can modify the listening environment, family members are more likely to support the person with impaired hearing in making the necessary modifications. Listening to other people with impaired hearing discuss the problems they are having hearing will help make it clear that their family member's problems are not unique and do not indicate that their family member is just being difficult. It also gives them an opportunity to talk with family members of other people with impaired hearing, to share their difficulties communicating, and to provide suggestions for making change.

A good counselor may be able to provide opportunities for family members and the person with impaired hearing to open a dialogue about hearing and communication and help them improve communication and understanding about the difficulties that the hearing loss is causing in the family dynamic.

CULTURAL ISSUES AFFECTING HEARING LOSS

PITFALL

It is important to understand how hearing loss is viewed in the culture of the patient. If disability is viewed negatively, pushing the patient to accept amplification may push the patient and family out of the office. The audiologist must gently help the family work through these issues. Other members of the community or religious leaders may be helpful.

It is important to understand the value system of everyone we deal with if we wish to provide counseling successfully. Different cultural and ethnic groups deal differently with hearing loss and disability. Understanding the value system of the people with whom we are working will help us better meet their needs. For example, in certain cultural groups marriage is arranged or marriage partners are chosen from a very small set of people. Identifying a hearing loss in one or two family members may make it more difficult for other family members to marry. As a result, some families may resist providing amplification for their children with hearing loss for fear that other children in the family will have difficulty finding marriage partners.

Cultures in which family elders are revered may have less need for amplification or assistive listening devices because other family members will be willing to do whatever is necessary to communicate with the elder who has a hearing loss. On the other hand, groups who have difficulty accepting disability may reject family members with hearing loss and attempt to hide them or remove them from the group.

Some groups will require approval from a religious or cultural leader before agreeing to amplification. For other groups amplification will only be used at certain times (e.g., not on Sabbath). For some, the value of hearing for school or work will be high and for others it will be less important. Without knowing who your patient is you are not likely to be able to provide the kind of support needed for a successful adjustment to hearing loss and hearing rehabilitation. As audiologists, it behooves us to learn as much about the cultural mores of the community in which we work to permit us to provide the best possible services to our patients.

COUNSELING PARENTS/CAREGIVERS OF NEONATES

As universal hearing screening becomes more frequent, more and more audiologists will find themselves in a position of needing to counsel families of neonates. Most children who fail neonatal screenings are born into families with no history of hearing loss, so the families we are counseling have little or no information about hearing loss. Parents of most neonates are overwhelmed at the time of the infant's birth. Learning that their neonate has or may have a significant disability can be overwhelming. Luterman (1997) has recently presented an argument against infant hearing screening arguing that families need time to bond with their infants before receiving the diagnosis that the infant has a hearing loss. A survey he conducted indicated that parents were split about this. Although some parents did not want to know about their infant's hearing loss at birth, others did.

In an ideal world it might be possible to delay hearing screening for awhile to let families bond with their infants and still identify hearing loss early enough to provide excellent management. However, at present we do not live in an ideal world, and infants who are not screened in the neonatal nursery will probably not be screened at all. We need to keep this in mind when we counsel families about infant screening.

If possible, we would like to have the opportunity to rescreen infants who failed the initial hearing screening before needing to counsel parents. At least some of the infants who failed the initial screen will pass, and rescreening means that fewer families will need to hear potentially bad news. No matter what the test protocol is, some families will need to be told that their infants failed the screening.

Who Should Provide Screening Test Results?

The first question to be answered is who is responsible for counseling the family. An audiologist is usually responsible for implementing the hearing screening program. An audiologist, aide, or student is responsible for the actual screening. The hospital pediatric staff is responsible for the infant's care while the infant is in the neonatal nursery, and another pediatrician may be responsible for the infant's aftercare. Who is responsible for discussing results with the family? Although the medical staff is most knowledgeable about the infant's health, they are probably not very knowledgeable about hearing loss. It would probably be best if an audiologist was involved in providing information to families.

How Should Test Results Be Reported?

Part of the decision about how test results should be presented will depend on how the program operates. As a rule, counseling should be done in person and not by mail. If families come from a great distance, counseling will need to be done before the infant leaves the hospital. If the family lives nearby and has identified a pediatrician who will follow the neonate after discharge, counseling can be provided by the pediatrician at the first or second checkup. If counseling is not provided while the infant is in the hospital, some system needs to be developed to ensure follow-up contact at a later date.

It is important to remember that screening results are just that—screenings. The results of a hearing screening do not indicate that a child has a hearing loss, only that the child did not respond appropriately. It is important to counsel parents that the test results indicate only that the infant is in need of further testing. It is important, however, to stress the importance of hearing in the development of language and the need for follow-up. The line to toe is a very fine one and requires careful thought and a supportive attitude.

Supporting Parents Through the Diagnostic Process

Infants who fail a hearing screening will need follow-up. When parents return for follow-up a few weeks after hospital discharge, they are likely to be anxious. The audiologist will need to be sensitive to the parents' situation. The best first question probably needs to be an inquiry as to how the parents are doing rather than about the child. If this is the family's first child, they are probably not sufficiently knowledgeable about infant development to feel comfortable stating whether the infant hears. If the family has other children, they will be able to report whether the infant responds to sound the way the others did at the same age. Once the audiologist has assisted the family in getting through the initial diagnostic testing, further evaluations and counseling will be similar to that required of other families who have concern about their infants' hearing.

COUNSELING FAMILIES OF INFANTS AND YOUNG CHILDREN

The Parents' Perspective

SPECIAL CONSIDERATION

Every hearing evaluation is stressful for parents. The audiologist can make it easier for parents by providing a warm, welcoming attitude, and by sitting down prepared to listen to their concerns. Sitting conveys the message that you are there to listen. Standing in the door conveys the message that you are too busy to really listen.

Bringing a child for a hearing evaluation is a very stressful event. It is stressful the first time a child is evaluated and continues to be stressful for many years to come. The first time a child is brought for evaluation it is because someone is concerned about the child's auditory status. Except when the infant is referred as the result of a failed hearing screening, by the time they arrive for a hearing evaluation the parents have probably been worried for some time. From the parents view, however, the problem can never be minor and little could be worse than having something wrong with your child. From their viewpoint, *"Something is wrong with my child."*

Re-evaluations for children already diagnosed with hearing loss are also stressful. Every re-evaluation brings up all the old fears and emotions. It is a reinforced reminder that their child has a hearing loss, and it causes parents to face fears about whether the loss has gotten worse and to assess their child's functioning. *"Is my child doing well enough? Will he or she go to college? Will he or she be able to hold a job?"* These fears and concerns are not different from those experienced by all parents, but they are more intense for parents of a child with a disability. During daily activities parents can usually manage to put them off to the side if not completely out of their minds, but coming for an evaluation will usually bring them all back.

Although middle ear disease usually has less of a long-term effect than a sensorineural hearing loss, it cannot be overlooked, and to some parents it will be very distressful. As audiologists, we need to listen to parents and try and understand their distress and concern.

When Counseling Begins

Counseling begins when we first meet the family in the waiting room. The way we present ourselves tells the families a lot about what they can expect. Do we introduce ourselves very formally, indicating that we are in charge, or more casually, indicating that we are partners in the evaluation experience? Do we talk to the child and try and make both child and parents comfortable? Are we smiling or stern? Do we conduct all our business standing up, indicating that time is limited and that we can only spend a few minutes on this, or do we sit down next to the parents (not behind a desk) and make the parents feel that we will take the time to understand their concerns and answer their questions. How do we begin talking with the family? It may be helpful to start by asking how they are and, if they seem distressed, acknowledge that we understand that this is a difficult time. Acknowledging their distress can make them feel more at ease. It does not eliminate it, but it gives it value.

Who Initiated the Appointment?

Counseling continues as we take the history. During this time we find out why the parents are there, what they are concerned about, and what they may be ready to do. The first thing to find out is who requested the appointment. If the parents were concerned about the child's hearing and requested the appointment themselves, they are more likely to be ready to hear that a problem exists. If parents have come because the infant failed a hearing screening or because the pediatrician or the grandparents wanted the appointment and the parents do not have any concerns of their own, they will have a much more difficult time accepting test results that indicate something is wrong. If this is the child's first evaluation, the parents will not know what to expect. Parents (and the audiologist) may have a guess about what testing may reveal but, as of yet, no test information exists. Sometimes parents have sought out several other opinions before the current evaluation. Sometimes they will share this with the audiologist, and other times they will not.

Sometimes both parents are not in the same place. One parent (frequently the mother who may spend more time with the child) may be concerned and seeking evaluation, whereas the other parent is coming along but really has no concerns. It is not unusual to hear one parent say, *"I think he hears fine but my wife/husband is the nervous type so we came for a hearing test."* When this happens, counseling is difficult because both parents will want and need different things.

It is important that we remember our role. We are here to educate the parents, to provide information, and to help parents make their own decisions. We provide guidance.

Although we may know much more about hearing loss or developmental disabilities than the parent, they know more about their child and family. It is they, and not us, who will have to live with the consequences of any decision that is made.

PITFALL

We need to be careful not to express disapproval of parents' decisions. Our responsibility is to provide information and to assist the family in making decisions that will meet their needs, not ours.

The Parent in the Test Situation

Because parents will, in fact, be making treatment and management decisions, they need to have as much information as we can possibly provide. This means that they need to be involved in all testing and testing decisions. Parents who are in the test room during the evaluation will be in a better position to understand what the child can and cannot hear. If

grandparents are along, they should also be invited in if there is enough room. If not, they may be able to observe testing by sitting with the audiologist and looking through the test room window. Every effort should be made to find a way to have the parent observe, especially if the parent has any question about the presence of hearing loss. If the parent cannot observe, it will be difficult for them to understand test results and make appropriate decisions, making counseling more difficult.

Discussing Test Results

The first step in discussing test results is to explain what happened in the test room. Begin by describing testing and what was observed. Ask the parents what they thought about the testing. Did they think it was a good test? Did they feel the child was cooperative? Let the parents direct the way you proceed. Audiologists are attached to audiograms but most parents are not, and for many parents they are very difficult to understand. If we use an audiogram, we need to describe it in detail, show where we expect children with normal-hearing to respond, and show where their child responded. An audiogram that shows familiar sounds and speech sounds (Fig.

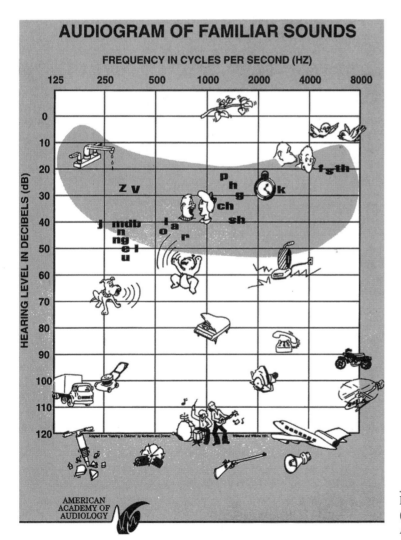

Figure 7–1 Familiar sounds audiogram. (Reprinted with permission of the American Academy of Audiology.)

7–1) can help parents develop a little perspective about what the hearing loss means. As part of counseling, we need to explain what we know and what we do not know. If we did not use earphones, we need to explain that we do not know what hearing is like in each ear. If the child ceased responding after two to three threshold determinations, we need to explain that we need more information to fully understand the child's auditory status and why we need more information.

The audiologist needs to try and determine what the parent can accept. If the parent has normal-hearing and heard sounds the child did not hear, it will be difficult to deny the test results. Parents may question whether children hear at the same levels as adults, whether attention was a factor, or whether the toys were too distracting. We need to be prepared to answer these questions. If a child has a sloping audiogram and responds to some sounds and speech but not to other sounds, we need to explain how this will affect speech, language, and academic development.

If the parents are not ready to accept the results, you cannot proceed. We can only proceed as quickly as the parents can. If the parents need some time to adjust, suggest a re-evaluation as quickly as the parents are ready to proceed. Ask if the parents want another opinion. We need to be clear that we will not be insulted if they seek one. To help parents accept the hearing loss suggests that between this appointment and the re-evaluation the parents observe and record what sounds the child hears when no visual or situational clues are present, what words he or she understands, and what directions he or she can follow without gesture or situational cues. It is important that the parents believe that the audiologist is accepting their opinion and is respectful of their views. If the audiologist does not respect their views, the parents will probably sense the annoyance or disapproval, and it is unlikely that the audiologist will be able to develop a respectful working relationship with the parents.

Once the audiologist tells parents that their child has a hearing loss, it is not likely that the parents will hear or retain much else. No matter how prepared they think they are for the information, it is a shock. If they appear confused, it may be useful to ask if they wish to stop and discuss it later. Offer paper and pen to take notes. Although every parent reacts differently, we can assume that every parent is disappointed and distressed. Whatever they imagined for themselves and their child during the pregnancy and until the time of the diagnosis is now going to change. It does not mean that the child will not be loved and wanted, but their dream of a certain kind of child and their expectations for that child's life and for themselves are lost. We need to recognize this and accept their grief.

Providing Information

Some parents are not capable of taking anything away from the initial evaluation, and we need to accept that. Although we all recognize the value of early identification, nothing terrible will happen if the child waits an additional 2 weeks to get services. When the parent is ready for information, we need to be prepared to provide resources. The basic information that needs to be shared is (1) a description of hearing loss, (2) habilitation/educational options, (3) amplification options, and (4) resources for additional information.

PEARL

It is difficult for parents to hear information after they are told that their child has a hearing loss. Providing written information that they can review at home and can reread and share with family members will be helpful.

We need to provide this information in as objective a fashion as possible. Parents of a child with a severe or profound hearing loss needs to know that differences of opinion exist about educating children with impaired hearing and they need to be encouraged to learn about all of them before making a decision for their child. They need to understand that different amplification options exist, each with positive and negative features. Regardless of the educational option parents select, the child will need amplification, so while parents are learning about educational options they can begin the amplification process.

For many parents, the need to do something immediately is critical. Amplification is a good place to begin. Some parents will want to move quickly and will be prepared to take earmold impressions on the day the hearing loss is diagnosed. Other parents are stunned by the diagnosis and need a little time to adjust before moving on. Others may do better by making an appointment for earmolds in a few days or a week to allow everything to sink in. When they return for earmold impressions, they may be better able to ask questions and hear explanations.

Because it is so difficult for parents to retain information provided at early counseling sessions, it may be helpful to provide written information. It is useful to have a selection of materials that can be provided to parents. These might include the following:

- Basic description of hearing loss
- A description of educational options
- A description of amplification options
- Resources for additional information
- Information and resources on different communication modes
- Financial information for obtaining therapy and amplification
- Contact list of other parents of children with impaired hearing
- Information about parent support groups

The audiologist can select any or all of the information pieces to provide to parents. The material that parents take home can be read over and over until it is understood. It is very likely that parents will have many questions that come to mind after they leave the office. They should be encouraged to get a notebook to write down concerns and questions to discuss at the next visit. If the next visit is a long way off and they feel they cannot wait they should be given permission to call. The audiologist needs to be clear that he or she is there for them. Answering questions as they come up will make life easier for the parents and, by extension, for the audiologist. If parents abuse this and start calling on a daily basis with noncritical issues, they can be asked to write their questions down so they can be discussed at the next visit. Sometimes, when parents call to discuss noncritical issues, the parents really are concerned about other things. It may be helpful for the audiologist to try and find out what those concerns might be (Madell, 1998a).

Providing Emotional Support

Having a child diagnosed with a significant disability is very distressing for any parent. All parents will go through a period of grief or mourning when a disability is diagnosed. Initially they are in shock. As the shock lessens, they begin to feel anger, sadness, and sometimes denial. Parents frequently feel guilt, blame, disappointment, confusion, and helplessness. Eventually, these feelings decrease and parents reach acceptance and recognition, although many parents say the pain never completely disappears. Different people spend different amounts of time in each stage of grief. Many parents move back and forth between stages. They move forward and then when something changes (a change in hearing levels, amplification, school setting, a birthday party), earlier feelings resurface. As audiologists, we need to recognize the stages of grief and be aware of how they are affecting the parent and child. Frequently parents are angry and may react as such with us or other members of the staff. It is usually not us with whom they are really angry, but we are a convenient place to let the anger out. We need to acknowledge their anger and frustration without taking it personally. When a parent repeatedly comes late for appointments, misses appointments, or brings the child without hearing aids or with dead batteries, we know that the parent is angry and possibly in denial. Getting angry at the parent will not help. It may help to acknowledge the situation by saying something like, *"You seem to be having a really difficult time. Having a hearing-impaired child is very difficult."* We have to let the parent know that we accept the problem without passing judgment. Once we have done this we increase the possibility that the parent can accept our assistance.

Some parents will need to deal with their grief before being able to deal with their child's needs. Others will refuse to deal with their emotional needs until their child's needs are met. When parents are ready, it may be helpful to have them speak with other families with hearing-impaired children. The audiologist can give the parents phone numbers of other families or arrange to have another family contact them. If parent support groups are available, they should be invited to attend. Other parents will be able to provide information and support that professional staff cannot provide. They have been there. We have not.

Coping With a Diagnosis

People cope in different ways. Some people are able to recognize the positive things about their child that are not affected by the diagnosis. Some can count their blessings or seek out support from friends or from other families in the same situation. Some people seek spiritual support through their church or temple, through meditation, or through reading. Some seek out support groups. Others learn as much as they can about the disorder through reading, workshops, and conferences. For others, the diagnosis is overwhelming and professional counseling is needed to get through it.

Initially many parents express guilt: *"Why didn't I recognize this sooner?" "Did I do something while I was pregnant that caused this?" "Is this because I drank wine on New Year's Eve?"* Our role is to provide comfort and information to help parents move forward. Parents want to know what caused the hearing loss. It is frequently not possible to find the answer, and this may be very difficult for the parent to accept. They need answers and we do not have them. For some parents this need for information interferes with the ability to move forward. Other parents can provide for their child's needs and work through their grief as they proceed.

Listening To Parents

A good counselor is genuine in caring about the child and family, honest in providing information and expressing feelings, and a good listener. A good counselor can accept parents' feelings without judgment and recognizes that his or her values and the parent's values may be different. The parents and audiologist may come from different cultures and have different expectations about education, behavior limits, and goals for children.

David Luterman (1979, 1996a,b; and Atkins, 1995) says the most important clinical skill we can bring is the ability to listen. We need to be able to listen to parents and hear what they are saying. We need to acknowledge their feelings whatever they are. Feelings are not good or bad. When a parent expresses concern about something he or she may have done during the pregnancy, we need to recognize the underlying message (*"Did I cause this?"*) and respond to that—it is easy to feel guilty when you have a child with a handicap. We need to hear the parents' concerns. Telling the parent not to worry is not a good tactic. It does not make him or her feel better. Their concerns are not minor no matter what they are and we need to acknowledge that.

The best thing we can offer parents are the skills to solve their problems by themselves and assurance of our faith in their ability to do so. Empowering parents is the greatest gift we can provide. Listening to parents rather than "telling" them sends the message that we believe they are capable of making decisions on their own. As Luterman (1979, 1996a,b) reminds us, listening means really listening, not trying to come up with counterarguments while you are listening. It means setting your views aside and trying to understand without judging. It is one of the most challenging tasks we can do. It is also one of the most important.

Who Should Provide Counseling?

The audiologist who is responsible for diagnosis and management of the child's hearing loss has the child as his or her first responsibility. This person provides information to parents and certainly provides support, but other people should be available who have primary responsibility for supporting the parents. This person may be an audiologist, a social worker, a psychologist, or a peer counselor. This person can provide a place where parents can discuss their concerns without judgment and without it interfering with their child's management. If this is not available in the center where the child is receiving services, the child's audiologist should be able to arrange for counseling at another facility.

Dealing with Angry Parents

It is not unusual for parents to be angry with the audiologist. Audiologists are frequently the bearers of bad news. We tell parents things they did not want to hear and assist them in planning for a life they did not choose. On one level the parents know that we are not responsible for the fact that their child is hearing-impaired but making us angry may be less dangerous than alienating family members. In some cases it is the clerical staff who are recipients of the parents' anger. Parents may feel that they do not need something from the clerical staff but will need help from the audiologist so it is safer to express anger at secretaries. Everyone needs to realize that this is misplaced anger and try not to take it personally. When a parent yells at us, we need to say something like, *"You seem very upset. This must be difficult for you."* This gives the parent the opening to talk about what is troubling them.

On the other hand, sometimes their anger is legitimate and we also need to recognize that. If a child has an appointment at 2 PM and we have not yet seen the child an hour later, the parent may really be distressed. The child may be getting fidgety and the parent may be concerned about another child who will arrive home shortly from school. We might have avoided the anger if someone had informed the parent that the audiologist was late, tied up with another patient, and assured the parent that the audiologist will spend as much time with their child as is needed. Although this will not completely solve the problem for the parent, it assures them that they are not being ignored and that we respect their time needs, too.

When a parent frequently arrives late for appointments, audiologists can become distressed. We have other patients scheduled and having a family come late can disrupt the schedule. It is not productive to be angry at the family. Sometimes parents are late for legitimate reasons: the car broke down, a traffic jam, and so on. Sometimes the reasons are not legitimate: something else to do that delayed them or difficulty getting up in the morning. Sometimes parents are used to clinic appointments when everyone is told to arrive early and are taken in turn. When families are late, we have several options. We can start the evaluation and complete as much as time allows or we can reschedule the appointment. Although this may "teach the parent to come on time," the person we are really punishing is the child.

Dealing with other Family Members

In this day and age many different versions of family exist. Some are conventional "nuclear" families, but many are not. In some cases extended family members are a part of the child's life and should be included in our efforts to provide information. If siblings are old enough to understand what is happening, they should be included. The parents will need to lead the way and determine who should be included and when. The audiologist should be available to provide information and counseling to others when needed. If a mother says, *"My mother is driving me nuts. She cries every time she sees Lucy with a hearing aid,"* we need to first acknowledge how difficult this must be for her. Then we need to ask why she

thinks her mother is reacting this way. Maybe it would be helpful if grandma came to the next hearing test or therapy session and learned a little more about hearing loss. It is difficult for parents to accept that the grandparents are going through the same stages of grief they are. This comes at a time in the grandparents' lives when they thought they were done with the difficult aspects of childrearing and expected only the joys of grandparenting. In addition, the grandparents do not have the advantage of doing something proactive to help the child as the parents do. If grandparents can provide support, they can be of great assistance. They can provide respite for parents, can assist with driving to therapy or hearing tests, and, most importantly, they can provide emotional support. If, however, the grandparents cannot provide support, the parents may need to carry on alone.

> ### PITFALL
>
> **Siblings can get neglected when a child is diagnosed with a hearing loss. Families need to be assisted in recognizing the needs of the normal-hearing siblings and in finding ways to meet their needs.**

Siblings will need special support. Because the child with impaired hearing requires a lot of attention, the non-disabled sibling sometimes feels left out. The audiologist can be of assistance by reminding parents that the siblings need to understand what is happening and need some time alone with the parents. As they get older, they may need to talk about their feelings about having a sibling with a hearing loss. They have to deal with their anger at time taken away from them and guilt at being normal-hearing. They need to be given the opportunity to express their feelings and referred for counseling if needed (Roush & Matkin, 1994).

COUNSELING CHILDREN WITH HEARING LOSS

When hearing loss is identified, a great deal of time is spent educating the child's family about hearing loss. By the time a child is 7 or 8 years old, the parents know a lot about hearing loss and counseling, and the hearing testing takes much less time if the hearing loss is stable. However, by this age, hearing-impaired children are ready to understand about hearing loss. The audiologist needs to start to explain the audiogram to the children, show them what they can and cannot hear with hearing aids and with their FM systems, and give them the opportunity to ask questions. The first time I asked an 8-year-old if he had any questions about his hearing loss, he asked when he would be old enough not to need hearing aids anymore. His parents and I were both surprised to realize that he did not understand that his hearing loss was permanent. I recently asked a 12-year-old girl if she had any questions about her hearing loss and she asked why her twin had normal-hearing and she did not. It gave her the opportunity to express her anger about the situation and to cry about it. Her parents were very surprised by the strength of her emotions because she had never expressed them before.

Children with impaired hearing may need to go through the same grieving process as their parents did when the hearing loss was first identified. It frequently comes as a surprise to the parents because they have usually finished grieving when the child is ready to start. It is also difficult for the child because he or she is grieving alone. Support groups for children are valuable; they enable them to express feelings and ask questions of peers—something parents and audiologists cannot provide.

COUNSELING TEENS AND THEIR PARENTS

The teenage years are very difficult ones for children who are developing normally. They are extremely difficult for children who are in any way different from their peers. Wearing hearing aids and having difficulty communicating is definitely stressful. Although very young children may not have difficulty with their peers, hearing-impaired teens may begin to feel isolated. In the attempt to become accepted by their peers, many reject amplification, therapy, resource room, and anything that makes them stand out.

If they do not already do so, teenagers need to be helped to understand hearing loss in general and their hearing loss in particular. They need the basic information about hearing loss, including what causes hearing loss, an explanation of different types of hearing loss, and information about treatment for hearing loss. Then they need the same information about their hearing loss that we have given to their parents and that we provide to adults with hearing loss.

Receiving Amplification for the First Time

Teenagers need to be involved in selecting amplification. Teens who are receiving amplification for the first time are likely to be distressed. They are having hearing loss diagnosed at a time when appearance is critical and now someone who they have no reason to trust is telling them that they need to wear hearing aids. This news is not likely to be well received. Unless the audiologist can demonstrate the benefit that amplification provides and, more importantly, the problems that will result without amplification, little likelihood exists that amplification will be accepted. First, teens must believe that the audiologist is there to support them and that he or she understands the problems involved and is suggesting amplification because that is the only choice. If the audiologist can gain the trust of the teenager, it is possible that the teenager will be willing to at least try amplification.

Selecting Amplification

Amplification cannot be selected *for* a teenager. The teenager needs to be an integral part of the selection process. Any audiologist who works with this population has heard teenagers state that they would no longer wear their hearing aids or their FM systems or would wear them only at school. This is very clearly an expression of the teen's distress and must be addressed that way. Saying, *"This must be awful for you, I'm sure you hate having a hearing loss or wearing hearing aids"* gives

the teen an opportunity to express feelings about hearing loss. Once he or she has expressed feelings, it may be possible to get him or her to consider making some attempt to rectify the situation by trying amplification. The audiologist may need to agree to try amplification that would not necessarily appear to be the most appropriate choice (an ITC hearing aid for a very profound hearing loss) to get the teen to agree.

It is critical that the teenager understand the choice that is being made. He or she needs to understand what will be heard and what will be missed without amplification with the kind he or she is willing to wear and with the kind recommended by the audiologist. Unless we can demonstrate why a particular amplification system is needed, we are not likely to have full cooperation. Speech perception at normal and soft conversational levels and in the presence of competing noise will assist in providing some of the necessary documentation.

Bargaining and contracts are tools frequently used with teens. *"I will give you these less than perfect hearing aids, which you prefer, but you must promise that you will wear them"* or *"You can try going to school without an FM system, but if your grades drop, you need to start using the FM again."*

This kind of bargaining requires constant follow-up and requires that the audiologist continue to work at having a good cooperative relationship with the teen.

Peer Counseling

An effective counseling tool is to arrange for teens to talk to each other. Teens who are mainstreamed may not have sufficient contact with other hearing-impaired teens. Arranging for peer group meetings is helpful. Peers all have similar issues. They will be able to encourage each other and to provide assurance that others are experiencing similar problems. Many of the issues for discussion will be those typical of all teens. Others will be specific to those with impaired hearing.

Assertiveness Training

Teens need help in advocating for themselves as do many people with impaired hearing. Those who have difficulty discussing hearing loss may need the most assistance. Assertiveness training can be helpful in getting teens to remind their peers to face them when they talk, in reminding the teacher to turn on the FM transmitter, and in asking friends to choose a quiet restaurant rather then a noisy one. Assertiveness training is usually well done in groups and can be a part of peer counseling.

SUPPORT GROUPS

Support groups are a useful counseling setting for all people who have hearing loss and for their families. Support groups are made up of people with similar needs so they can provide assistance to each other. Parents can provide each other support in adjusting to hearing loss and in managing the needs of young hearing-impaired children. The group will help them understand how to separate concerns about hearing loss from those of being 2 years old; it will help them develop the skills to fight for school placement and for additional therapies when needed.

Older children and teens will benefit from peer groups to assist them in understanding that they are not alone and in developing skills for coping with peers at school and in social situations. Groups for grandparents and siblings help with issues they may have difficulty expressing to the hearing-impaired child or to parents.

Adult groups help adults with hearing loss and their families work out improved communication strategies, develop assertiveness skills, and provide increased understanding about hearing loss and the communication skills that result.

THE IMPACT OF DIAGNOSING HEARING LOSS ON PROFESSIONAL STAFF

Each time an audiologist diagnoses a child or adult with a hearing loss we, as professionals, may go through a stage of grief that is similar, but less severe, to that experienced by the parents or the person with impaired hearing. The first few times are the worst. If we get the opportunity to diagnose hearing loss frequently, it becomes a little less painful, but the distress never really disappears. That is good because it permits us to become better counselors and to provide better support. If we, as professionals, are seeing many sad families and are not feeling hopeful about the future of our patients, our jobs become depressing and eventually we shut ourselves off from the families. We need to pay attention to how we are feeling. If we are shutting ourselves off, we may need a break from working with this population. Many professionals benefit from a support group to assist in dealing with the grief of hearing loss. It may be as simple as eating lunch together once a week to talk about concerns, or it may require a more structured environment. The more we understand about our feelings the better we will be at doing our job. Again, as with our patients, feelings are not good or bad, they just are. We need to remember this as we deal with our feelings and with our patients' feelings.

REFERENCES

Atkins, D.V. (1995). Beyond the child: Hearing impairment and the family. *Volta Voices, 14*;17,22.

Brooks, D.N. (1979). Counseling and its effect on hearing aid use. *Scandinavian Audiology, 8*;101–107.

Crandell, C.C. (1997). An update on counseling instruction within audiology programs. *Journal of the Academy of Rehabilitative Audiology, 30*;77–86.

DiMichael, S.G. (1985). *Assertiveness training for persons who are hard of hearing.* Rockville, MD: SHHH Publications.

Erdman, S.A. (1980). The use of assertiveness training in adult aural rehabilitation. *Audiology, 5*;12.

Erdman, S.A. (1993). Counseling hearing-impaired adults. In: J.G. Alpiner, & P.A. McCarthy (Eds.), *Rehabilitative audiology: Children and adults* (2nd ed.) (pp. 374–414). Baltimore: Williams & Wilkins.

Erdman, S.A., & Demorest, M.E. (1998a). Adjustment to hearing impairment I: Description of a heterogeneous clinical population. *Journal of Speech, Language and Hearing Research, 41*;107–122.

Erdman, S.A., & Demorest, M.E. (1998b). Adjustment to hearing impairment II: Audiologic and demographic correlates. *Journal of Speech, Language and Hearing Research, 41*;123–136.

Fellendorf, G., & Harrow, I. (1970). Parent counseling 1961–1968. *Volta Reviews, 72*;51–57.

Luterman, D. (1979). *Counseling parents of hearing-impaired children.* Boston: Little Brown & Co.

Luterman, D. (1996a). *Counseling the communicatively disordered and their families.* Austin, TX: Pro-Ed.

Luterman, D. (1996b). Listening with the third ear. *Hearing Instruments, 47*;12.

Luterman, D. (1997). Counseling families of hearing impaired children. Annual Conference of the American Academy of Audiology. Fort Lauderdale, FL.

Madell, J. (1998a). Counseling. In: *Behavioral evaluation of hearing in infants and young children* (pp. 130–141). New York: Thieme Medical Publishers, Inc.

Madell, J. (1998b). Helping adolescents accept amplification. *Hearing Journal, 51*;(5)69.

McDonald, E. (1962). *Understand those feelings.* Pittsburgh: Stanwix House, Inc.

Patterson, C.H. (1986). *Theories of counseling and psychotherapy.* New York: Harper & Row.

Pavlov, I.P. (1927). *Conditioned reflexes.* London: Oxford University Press.

Rogers, C.R. (1951). Client centered therapy. Boston: Houghton-Mifflin.

Roush, J., & Matkin, N.D. (1994). *Infants and toddlers with hearing loss: Family centered assessment and intervention.* Baltimore: York Press.

Sanders, D.A. (1980). Hearing aid orientation and counseling. In: M.C. Pollack (Ed.), *Amplification for the hearing-impaired* (2nd ed.) (pp. 343–392). New York: Grune & Stratton.

Skinner, B.F. (1953). *Science and human behavior.* New York: Macmillian.

Stephens, S.D. (1977). Hearing aid use by adults: A survey of surveys. *Clinics in Otolaryngology, 2*;385–402.

Sweetow, R., & Barrager, D. (1980). Quality of comprehensive audiological care: A survey of parents of hearing-impaired children. *ASHA, 22*(10);841–847.

Thomas, A.J. (1984). *Acquired hearing loss: Psychological and psychosocial implications.* London: Academic Press.

Wolpe, J. (1982). *The practice of behavior therapy* (3rd ed.). New York: Pergamon Press.

PREFERRED PRACTICE GUIDELINES

Professionals Who Perform the Procedure(s)

▼ Audiologists

Expected Outcomes

▼ The audiologist understands the impact of hearing loss on daily living and can communicate this to patients and families.

▼ The audiologist can assist patients in accepting hearing loss and making appropriate management decisions.

▼ The audiologist provides both informational counseling to assist the patient and family in understanding technical information and personal adjustment counseling to deal with emotional issues related to having a hearing loss.

▼ The audiologist understands the value of having families participate in (re)habilitation and includes them in diagnostic and treatment sessions.

▼ Families are comfortable communicating with the audiologist and discussing their concerns.

▼ Families are comfortable making decisions about amplification and management for their children with impaired hearing.

▼ Counseling is a part of every meeting with a patient and/ or family of a patient with hearing loss.

Clinical Indications

▼ Counseling is a part of every meeting with a patient and/ or family of a patient with hearing loss.

Clinical Process

▼ Informational and personal adjustment counseling is available.

▼ Sufficient time is available to provide necessary counseling.

▼ The audiologist understands the patient's view of the problem and expectations for treatment.

▼ Counseling about management is routinely available.

▼ Families routinely participate in evaluation and management.

▼ The audiologist is knowledgeable about cultural issues regarding hearing loss and disability.

▼ The audiologist understands the parents' perspective about having a hearing-impaired child.

▼ Older children and teens are included in counseling.

Documentation

▼ Documentation includes a description of the topics discussed with the patient and the family and their reaction to the information during each audiological encounter.

▼ Documentation includes materials presented to patients and families for informational counseling.

▼ Documentation includes referrals for other supportive counseling, including parent groups and adult support groups.

Chapter 8

National and State Policies Effecting Hearing Aids, Assistive Listening Devices, and Cochlear Implants

Holly S. Kaplan and John W. Hesse, II

Hearing aids have come a long way. This worn cliché truly describes the evolution of hearing aids from the mere cupping of the hand next to the auricle to the recent introduction of digital signal processing. The need for government and national association intervention to protect consumers and professionals involved in dispensing has also evolved over time. The dispensing of hearing aids is regulated at the federal and state levels by a variety of laws and agencies. The consumer and the dispensing audiologist are also protected by ethical codes and practice guidelines written by professional and consumer organizations.

Approximately 14,448 audiologists hold the American Speech-Language-Hearing Association (ASHA) Certificate of Clinical Competence in Audiology (CCC-A) (ASHA, 1997e). Recent surveys reveal more than 50% of audiologists dispense hearing aids (ASHA, 1996b) and more than 70% of audiologists dispense amplification *and* related products (i.e., assistive listening devices) (ASHA, 1993). Today, most hearing aids in the United States are dispensed by audiologists (Lentz, 1991). This is a significant change in the service delivery in hearing healthcare compared with 20 years ago. As late as 1978, almost no audiologists were dispensing hearing aids in the private sector because of constraints against this practice delineated by ASHA's Code of Ethics (Punch & Jarrett, 1994).

The goal of this chapter is to briefly present the history of hearing aid dispensing within the profession of audiology, emphasizing the changes in ASHA's policy in relation to members dispensing amplification. The chapter then focuses on the various national association ethical codes and best practice patterns related to dispensing hearing aids. The various federal and state regulations regarding hearing aid dispensing and consumer rights are also discussed. Finally, the chapter concludes with information on training programs in audiology and national certification programs. Contact information and addresses for the five largest audiology associations dealing with hearing aid dispensing can be found in Table 8–1.

HISTORICAL PERSPECTIVES

Only recently have audiologists dispensed hearing aids. Before the late 1970s, audiologists were prohibited by the Code of Ethics of ASHA to dispense any device recommended to a consumer/patient. Audiologists wrote hearing aid prescriptions on the basis of audiological test results. Hearing aid dispensers then used these prescriptions to dispense the hearing aids. ASHA argued for the practice of writing prescriptions versus direct dispensing because ASHA viewed the latter as a conflict of interest. The audiologist would sell and profit from a device he or she had recommended. Hearing aid dispensing was believed by ASHA to be the purview of salesmen and should not be associated with the medically based profession of audiology.

Audiologists fighting for the right to dispense within the ASHA Code of Ethics pointed to the model of surgeons recommending and performing surgical procedures from which they would profit. Surgeons were not accused of conflict of

Audiology: Treatment. Edited by Valente, Hosford-Dunn, and Roeser. Thieme Medical Publishers, Inc., New York © 2000

TABLE 8–1   Contact information for the major professional associations for audiologists

Name	Address	Telephone/Fax	Web site
American Speech-Language-Hearing Association (ASHA)	10801 Rockville Pike, Rockville, MD 20853	1-800-498-2071 1-301-897-5700 Fax: 1-301-897-7354	www.asha.org
American Academy of Audiology (AAA)	8201 Greensboro Drive, Suite 300, McLean, VA 22102	1-800-222-2336 Fax: 1-703-610-9005	www.audiology.org
Academy of Rehabilitative Audiology (ARA)	Box 26532, Minneapolis, MN 55426	612-920-0196 Fax: 612-920-6098	Ara@incnet.com Web site under construction
Educational Audiology Association (EAA)	4319 Ehrlich Road, Tampa, FL 33624	1-800-460-7322 Fax: 1-813-968-3597	http://pip.ehhs.cmich.edu/eaa/
Academy of Dispensing Audiologists (ADA)	3008 Millwood Ave., Columbia, SC 29205	803-252-5646 Fax: 803-765-0860	www.audiologist.org

interest and were certainly not viewed as "salesmen" in the minds of the public. Consumer need for convenient service and accountability was also promoted as a reason for the audiologist to directly dispense hearing aids. Audiologists complained of a lack of appropriate audiological follow-up to determine whether the hearing aid dispenser correctly applied the prescription. Audiologists also noted the loss of patients and revenue to the hearing aid dispenser.

The pro-dispensing audiologists delineated educational and training differences between audiologists and hearing aid dispensers. Audiologists had to have at least a master's degree, had to have passed a national examination in audiology, and had to meet stringent practicum hour requirements to receive both their degree and Certificates of Clinical Competence in Audiology (CCC-A) through ASHA. Hearing aid dispensers, at best, had minimal professional training and licensure with minimal competency-based requirements. Audiologists argued that audiologists were the professionals best trained to provide total hearing healthcare and therefore should dispense the recommended hearing instrument.

A brief review of the resolutions voted on by the ASHA Legislative Council (LC) during this period reveals policy changes needed to enable audiologists to dispense, while abiding by the ASHA Code of Ethics. In 1971 the LC voted unanimously to permit the ASHA Executive Board to develop "explicit guidelines" related to the dispensing of hearing aids by audiologists as part of a program of auditory rehabilitation (ASHA,1997b). The resolution noted the need for ASHA to enunciate its position on the topic and that ASHA supported the "general intent" of the role of certified audiologists in hearing aid dispensing. The resolution noted that a variety of national and state plans regarding hearing aid dispensing were being considered and that these plans could have a direct bearing on ASHA member audiologists.

However, in 1973 the LC defeated a resolution (LC 42-73) to permit audiologists to dispense hearing aids in commercial settings (ASHA, 1997b). The defeated resolution recognized the relevance of fitting hearing aids to the role of clinical audiologists and noted persons with hearing loss

were obtaining hearing aids without obtaining adequate professional service when fit by hearing aid dispensers. The resolution described the *ASHA Code of Ethics* as a "barrier" between the needs of individuals with hearing loss and direct service provided by audiologists.

Immediate confusion on the part of ASHA member audiologists followed. Some audiologists had been dispensing in "noncommercial" venues, and the ethics of this practice was now in question. The following resolution was passed in 1973 to alleviate this confusion (ASHA, 1997b):

Whereas, the Legislative Council in 1971 endorsed the concept that audiologists should be permitted to dispense hearing aids, and

Whereas, proposed methods of implementation have not been acceptable to the Ethical Practice Board and/or to the Membership, and

Whereas, the sense of the Legislative Council in rejecting Resolution Number 42 (1973) was that this provisions might damage the professional image and standing of the America Speech and Hearing Association and its Members, and

Whereas, under the present Code of Ethics, Members can dispense hearing aids if certain criteria, developed by the Ethical Practice Board, are met; therefore

Resolved, That the Legislative Council reaffirms its enforcement of the concept that audiologist may dispense hearing aids under conditions which are considered ethical by the Ethical Practice Board and endorsed by the Executive Board; and further

Resolved, That the Executive Board disseminate in writing as soon as possible, to the Membership, descriptions of procedures that audiologist may follow to be able to dispense hearing aid without being in violation of the present Code of Ethics; and further

Resolved, That the Executive Board continue urgently to study and develop procedures to implement the dispensing of hearing aids by audiologists.

The profession continued to progress into the arena of full "commercial" hearing aid dispensing. In 1975 the LC recognized a significant number of ASHA member audiologists were dispensing under the ethical provisions of the Code of

Ethics. These individuals needed further professional guidance and policy in the area of amplification in light of concurrent efforts by federal and state regulatory bodies and interest in the development of policies by the hearing aid industry. The LC voted to establish a *Committee on Amplification for the Hearing-Impaired* charged to study and make recommendations regarding amplification. Topics to be studied included the continuation of the role of the audiologist in determining hearing aid candidacy, models for dispensing, continuing education needs, and changes required in the accreditation and certification requirements (ASHA, 1997b).

The ASHA Ethical Practices Board (EPB) recognized the need for audiologists to obtain hearing aid dealer licensure to be in accordance with state laws and unanimously adopted a resolution that audiologists with such licenses were not necessarily in violation of the current Code of Ethics. The LC supported this stand in resolution LC 12-76 (ASHA, 1997b). The resolution reads:

> Resolved, That the American Speech and Hearing Association affirms that a Member is not in violation of the Code of Ethics in obtaining a hearing aid dealer's license, certificate, or registration which may be required for his engagement in dispensing hearing aids within the Association's "Principles Governing the Dispensing of Products to Persons with Communicative Disorders."

Once ASHA fully approved the dispensing of hearing aids by audiologists, a variety of policies were written to support the practice. The LC in 1978 resolved that it would be a policy of ASHA to "foster the legal right of audiologists to dispense hearing aids under that licensing or registration authority which controls their audiological rehabilitation activities." The resolution continues, "(ASHA should) take steps to foster correction of the situation in which audiologists are required by law to be licensed or registered as hearing aid dealers and that assistance be provided to state associations undertaking such corrective action."

CURRENT NATIONAL ASSOCIATION POLICIES ON HEARING AID DISPENSING BY AUDIOLOGISTS

National professional associations serve the profession by providing technical assistance, fostering and sponsoring continuing education programs, and developing and maintaining certification standards for both the profession and educational training programs. Professional associations serve as clearing houses of information for the consumers of audiological services and provide media opportunities for the profession at local and national levels. Volunteer members aid in these efforts and give valuable time in the effort to promote audiology and audiologists as the hearing healthcare professional of choice. A significant part of this effort is the writing of policy documents that define the profession, give guidance regarding ethics and excellence in practice, and serve as record of the stance of audiology on related professional issues. The following is a review of national association policy documents that pertain to hearing aids, assistive listening devices (ALDs), and cochlear implants.

PEARL

Practicing audiologists need to be aware of the legislative, regulatory, and reimbursement issues in their profession. National associations and their state/local chapters are a wonderful source of such information, while also serving the professions well in many other arenas. National associations depend on volunteer member involvement. Join. Volunteer. Participate. Audiology is only as strong as each audiologist.

American Speech-Language-Hearing Association

The American Speech-Language-Hearing Association (ASHA) is the largest national professional association for professionals in communication-related disorders. ASHA is comprised of over 93,000 audiologists, speech-language pathologists, and speech-language-hearing scientists. The ASHA national office is based in Rockville, MD. Publications from ASHA include a *Asha* quarterly magazine, *Asha Leader* a biweekly newspaper, the *Journal of Speech and Hearing Research*, the *American Journal of Audiology*, and *Language, Speech, and Hearing in the Schools*. Information about ASHA can be found at their Web site (www.asha.org). Refer to Table 8–1 for alternate contact information.

Current ASHA policy is clear in its support of the practice of hearing aid and assistive listening devices (ALDs) dispensing by audiologists. ASHA policy documents are written by ad hoc committees of volunteer members selected on the basis of their expertise in the given area of practice. A national office staff member serves as ex officio and an Executive Board member serves as a monitoring officer. The drafts of the ASHA policy documents go through select *and* widespread peer review by association members and are edited and revised on the basis of that review. The revised draft is then presented to the Executive Board and the Legislative Council for a vote at the annual ASHA convention.

Code of Ethics

ASHA policy documents are developed in a hierarchical model with the Code of Ethics serving as the primary guiding document. The *ASHA Code of Ethics* (ASHA, 1994a) is written in an outline format with general ethical statements or principles followed by specific rules under each. The Code of Ethics is periodically reviewed and updated on the basis of changes in standards of practice and changing technologies. An appointed volunteer member board, The ASHA Board of Ethical Practices (formerly EPB) is responsible for adjudicating complaints or concerns regarding the Code and members' possible violations thereof. The current Code of Ethics preamble states, "the preservation of the highest standards of integrity and ethical principle is vital to the responsible discharge of obligations in the professions of speech-language pathology and audiology." (Refer to Table 8–1 for information on how to obtain a copies of association policy documents noted.)

Although the entire code has to be followed by ASHA-member practicing audiologists, several of the delineated principles have specific relevance for dispensing audiologists. Member audiologists should fully inform consumers about the nature and possible effects of products dispensed, and members should evaluate the effectiveness of the products. Members should not guarantee the results of any services, nor should they misrepresent any dispensed product.

Suspected violations of the Code of Ethics are to be reported to the ASHA Board of Ethical Practices. Members can contact the Board at ASHA's national office, 1-800-498-2071. All members are responsible for cooperating with the Board during any investigation of an infraction.

The Scope of Practice in Audiology

The practice of audiology has grown significantly in the past 10 years, and the current revision of the *ASHA Scope of Practice in Audiology* (ASHA, 1996c) reflects this growth by listing 23 practice activities in audiology. The current version of the Scope has several references to hearing aid and ALD dispensing in the definition of an audiologist and the practice of audiology. Specifically, the definition of an audiologist in the Scope states, "Audiologists select, fit, and dispense amplification systems such as hearing aids and related devices."

The Scope of Practice includes the following activities:

- Provision of hearing care by selecting, evaluating, fitting, facilitating adjustment to and dispensing prosthetic devices for hearing loss, including hearing aids, sensory aids, hearing assistive devices, alerting and telecommunication systems, and captioning devices.

- Assessment of candidacy of persons with hearing loss for cochlear implants and provision of fitting, programming, and audiological rehabilitation to optimize device use.

- Assessment and nonmedical management of tinnitus using biofeedback, masking, hearing aids, education, and counseling.

- Consultation to industry on the development of products and instrumentation related to the measurement and management of auditory or balance function.

The Scope of Practice ends with a view to the future, suggesting the real need for treatment outcome and efficacy data be developed for the practice of audiology. Hearing aid dispensing is included in this section. The following are outcomes listed in the Scope that a consumer of audiology services related to amplification might expect:

- Counseling for personal adjustment and discussion of the effects of hearing loss and the potential benefits to be gained from audiological rehabilitation, sensory aids including hearing and tactile aids, hearing assistive devices, cochlear implants, captioning devices, and signal/ warning devices.

- Selection, monitoring, dispensing, and maintenance of hearing aids and large-area amplification devices.

- Development of a culturally appropriate, audiological rehabilitative management plan, including, when appropriate, fitting and dispensing recommendations, and educating the consumer and the family/caregivers in the use of and adjustment to sensory aids, hearing assistive devices, alerting systems, and captioning devices (ASHA, 1996c).

Preferred Practice Patterns for the Profession of Audiology

Several other ASHA documents delineate best practice patterns for the dispensing of hearing aids and other forms of amplification. *The Preferred Practice Patterns for the Profession of Audiology* (ASHA, 1997d) are an attempt to define the universally accepted characteristics of practices directed toward clients, including the basic framework of the practice, duties to be performed, and outcomes intended. The Preferred Practice Patterns are used in conjunction with the Code of Ethics and other policy documents by audiologists, government policymakers, and administrators in defining the practice of audiology. Refer to Table 8–1 for ASHA contact information to obtain copy of the Preferred Practice Patterns for the Profession of Audiology. Specific practice patterns related to amplification include audiological rehabilitation assessment, audiological rehabilitation, hearing aid fitting, product dispensing, product repair/modification, assistive listening system/device selection, and sensory aids assessment.

Other ASHA Documents

Another important ASHA policy document related to amplification and dispensing is the *Guidelines for Hearing Aid Fitting for Adults* (ASHA, 1998a). Copies can be obtained from ASHA (refer to Table 8–1). This guideline was written to address the technical aspects of hearing aid fitting with an emphasis on the hearing aid being only one part of the total audiological rehabilitation plan. Comprehensive audiological assessment, treatment planning, hearing aid selection, verification, hearing aid orientation, and validation are discussed in depth. The Guidelines delineate the following eight components in achieving a successful fitting:

- Hearing aid fitting services should be provided by an ASHA-certified and, where applicable, licensed audiologist or a clinical fellow audiologist under the supervision of an ASHA-certified and, where applicable, licensed audiologist.

- It is essential that the audiologist, client, and family/caregivers combine their efforts to achieve optimum outcome of the hearing aid fitting process.

- The audiologist has sole responsibility for preselection of the appropriate electroacoustic characteristics of the hearing aids.

- Probe microphone measures are the preferred method for verifying the real-ear performance of the hearing aids.

- Thresholds of discomfort should be directly measured with frequency-specific stimuli when possible to accurately assess/adjust the appropriate output and/or compression characteristics of the hearing aids.

- The treatment plan should include assessment and recommendations for ALDs, other assistive technologies, and communication training when appropriate.

- It is essential to assist the client and family/caregivers on what they can realistically expect from amplification, ALDs, and audiological rehabilitation.

- The assessment and validation process should include measures to document the outcome of the intervention.

A schedule exists for periodic review and revision of all ASHA policy documents. Several of the ASHA policy documents related to audiologic rehabilitation are currently under revision by the *ASHA Ad hoc Audiologic Rehabilitation Working Group* and the *Ad Hoc Committee on FM Assistive Listening Devices*. These documents include: *Definitions and Competencies on Aural Rehabilitation* (ASHA, 1984), *Guidelines for Graduate Education in Amplification* (ASHA, 1990), and *Guidelines for Fitting and Monitoring FM Systems* (ASHA, 1994b).

If the LC approves revisions of these documents, the revised documents should be available in 2000. Current amplification-related documents, not under revision include: *Amplification as a Remediation Technique for Children with Normal Peripheral Hearing* (ASHA, 1991a) and *Use of FM Amplification Instruments for Infants and Preschool Children with Hearing Impairment* (ASHA, 1991b).

American Academy of Audiology

The American Academy of Audiology (AAA) was founded in 1988 and celebrated its 10-year anniversary at its national convention in Los Angeles in April 1998. AAA has more than 6000 members. Policy statements from AAA include the *Code of Ethics* (AAA, 1991), *Position Statement: Audiology: Scope of Practice* (AAA, 1996), and *Position Statement: Aged Persons with Hearing Loss* (Task Force on Hearing Impairment in Aged People, 1991). AAA publications include *Audiology Today, Audiology Express*, and the *Journal of the American Academy of Audiology*. Information on AAA is located on their Web site (www.audiology.org) or refer to Table 8–1 for contact information.

Code of Ethics

The *Code of Ethics* (AAA, 1991) is similar in structure to that of the ASHA Code of Ethics with stated principles and a series of rules that pertain to each principle. The Preamble notes the Code, "specifies professional standards that allow for the proper discharge of audiologists' responsibilities to those served, and protect the integrity of the profession."

Principles 4, 5, and 8 specifically deal with issues related to amplification and the dispensing of products. Principle 4 notes that members should only provide services and products that are in the best interest of the consumer. The rules under Principle 4 note that the members should not exploit persons while delivering services, not charge for services not rendered, and not participate in activities that are in conflict of interest.

Principle 5 notes that members should provide accurate information about the communication disorder, service, and products. Rules under this principle note that the information given should be to the extent a reasonable person would need, statements of prognosis should not guarantee results, and the member should document all professional services rendered.

Principle 8 deals with the enforcement of the Code of Ethics. Members should inform the AAA EPB if they believe a violation of the Code has taken place and members should cooperate with the EPB in matters related to the Code.

Scope of Practice

AAA also has defined the practice of audiology through a *Scope of Practice* (AAA, 1996). AAA defines the audience for their Scope of Practice as audiologists, allied professionals, consumers of audiological services, and the general public. AAA emphasizes the document should be viewed as a reference for policymakers and third-party payers rather than a laundry list of services or practices that limit the profession. To emphasize this point, the Scope concludes with the following statement:

> Some audiologists, by virtue of education, experience and personal choice choose to specialize in an area of practice not otherwise defined in this document. Nothing in this document shall be construed to limit individual freedom of choice in this regard provided that the activity is consistent with the *American Academy of Audiology Code of Ethics*. This document will be reviewed, revised, and updated periodically in order to reflect changing clinical demands of audiologists and in order to keep pace with the changing scope of practice reflected by these changes and innovations in this specialty.

The Scope of Practice notes that audiologists through education, training, and experience are the professionals who provide, "the full range of habilitative and rehabilitative services for persons with hearing impairment and disorders of equilibrium." The provision of amplification and hearing aid services is viewed under the umbrella of total audiological rehabilitative management. The document continues, "The audiologist is responsible for the evaluation and fitting of amplification devices, including assistive listening devices. The audiologist determines the appropriateness of amplification systems for persons with hearing impairment, evaluates benefit, and provides counseling and training regarding their use. Audiologists conduct otoscopic examinations, clean earcanals and remove cerumen, take earcanal impressions, fit, sell, and dispense hearing aids and other amplification systems."

The audiologist's role in providing other forms of amplification is further delineated. The AAA Scope of Practice notes the audiologist serves as a member of the cochlear implant team determining candidacy, and provides presurgical and postsurgical assessment, counseling, auditory training, rehabilitation, implant programming. The audiologist also maintains implant hardware and software.

The document also emphasizes the educational and counseling aspects of the profession. Qualifications that health professionals must possess to perform and interpret the pre-purchase comprehensive audiological assessment include: (a) a graduate or post-bachelor's professional degree with emphasis in hearing or hearing-related areas from an accredited university; (b) formal clinical training in the provision of audiological diagnostic and treatment services under the supervision of licensed and/or certified professionals; and (c) passing a standardized national examination.

Position Statement: Aged Persons with Hearing Impairment

The AAA's Task Force on Hearing Impairment in Aged People developed a position statement delineating the roles and responsibilities of the audiologist working with aged persons (Task Force on Hearing Impairment in Aged People, 1991). The position statement describes the changing demographics creating the phenomena of the "aging of America" and gives statistics regarding the prevalence of hearing loss in the aging population. On the basis of this information, the AAA

Task Force notes that the audiologist is the "primary hearing healthcare provider for aged individuals with hearing impairment." The paper also notes that "audiologists are uniquely qualified to provide a full range of auditory rehabilitative service to aged individuals."

AAA recommends five strategies for improving the quality of life of individuals who are aged with hearing loss.

1. AAA advocates the use of screening procedures for identifying persons with hearing loss, with the goal of identifying the greatest number of aged persons with hearing loss.

2. State-of-the-art technology should be used with aged individuals in the evaluation and rehabilitation of hearing loss.

3. AAA promotes funding for research into hearing loss in aged persons.

4. AAA promotes third-party payments from various funding sources for both audiological services and specifically hearing-related devices.

5. AAA promotes public education about hearing loss in aging individuals.

Other Audiology Organizations

Many other professional organizations and foundations have developed over the years to serve the general profession and specific interest groups within the profession. Although too numerous to name all of the organizations, several of the larger associations with specific interest in amplification are noted in Table 8–1.

CONSUMER GROUPS

Consumer organizations related to hearing impairment are made up of members with hearing loss, their families, and professionals. These organizations serve as an important link between audiologists and the individuals who use audiologic services. Consumer organizations serve as sources of practical and clinical information, provide training in self-advocacy, and lobby policy-making bodies on behalf of individuals with hearing loss. The following is a summary of the larger consumer organizations with specific interest and policies related to amplification and cochlear implants.

Self Help for Hard of Hearing People

Self Help for Hard of Hearing People (SHHH) is a national consumer-based organization for individuals with hearing loss and their family/caregivers. SHHH serves as a national advocacy group for individuals with hearing loss, and, as such, SHHH has developed a series of policy documents related to hearing loss, amplification, and education of individuals with hearing loss (Ross, 1994; SHHH, 1995a,b; 1996a,b,c). Information on SHHH policy documents can be found at their Web site, www.shhh.org. A description of the mission of SHHH's can also be found on their Web site. The mission statement notes that SHHH members are catalysts that make mainstream society more accessible to people with hearing loss. The document is written as a series of value statements. The first value noted is education of members,

our families, friends, co-workers, teachers, hearing healthcare providers, industry, government, and others about hearing loss. The mission statement implies that education provides adults and children with tools for self-help; sensitizes the general population about the special needs of people with hearing loss; and promotes understanding of the nature, causes, complications, and remedies of hearing loss. Education about hearing loss also provides members with information on many aspects of hearing loss, from technological and medical advances to coping and parenting strategies. Knowledge regarding hearing loss also provides members with the tools to become informed consumers in making decisions on options available to help make the best decisions on how to deal with hearing loss.

Advocacy is the second value noted in the mission statement. The statement notes SHHH is a leading voice in improving communication access for people with hearing loss through advocacy for communication access in the workplace, hotels, schools, court systems, and medical and entertainment facilities. SHHH also promotes new technology, medical research, and legislation that will alleviate the effects of hearing loss. SHHH encourages research in the areas of hearing aids, ALDs, and other technologies to meet the needs of consumers with hearing loss. Research on understanding the causes of hearing loss and for development of new treatments is also valued. The mission statement also notes the role of SHHH members in testifying and implementing federal, state, and local legislation and regulation regarding hearing loss.

The mission statement notes that the concept of "self-help" is a value of the association. "SHHH believes people with hearing loss can help themselves and one another to participate fully and successfully in society. SHHH promotes self-confidence; empowers individuals with skills to improve their lives; and provides an opportunity for affiliation among people with hearing loss, their friends, families, and professionals. We work to develop options for ourselves and open doors for others."

SHHH's *Position Statements on Hearing Aids* (SHHH, 1995a) delineates the Association's positions on binaural amplification, standards for hearing aid dispensers, and hearing aid return policies. SHHH policy statements reflect the association's belief in the primacy of the individual with the hearing loss to receive optimal care while maintaining control over the care given. SHHH recommends that binaural amplification be viewed as the normative fitting because "two ears normally provide superior listening capabilities than one ear, for all normal-hearing people, and for the majority of those with hearing losses." SHHH recommends that hearing aid evaluations include objective and subjective measures of monaural versus binaural fittings.

In regard to standards for hearing aid dispensers, SHHH emphasizes the preferred training of the dispenser rather than the degree or professional title. The policy states that no one should dispense hearing aids unless he or she can demonstrate mastery of the ever-expanding base of knowledge related to hearing aid technology and hearing aid evaluation procedures. SHHH believes the current state-based licensure system for hearing aid dealers is inefficient and not in the best interests of the consumer. The SHHH document notes, "We recommend that a national and uniform standard be adopted for state licensing of hearing aid dispensers."

SHHH has also gone on record in its statement (SHHH, 1995a) in support of a minimum 60-day trial period for hearing aids. The document notes 30 days is not sufficient time to try hearing aids. SHHH notes consumers should be able to try the fitting for a minimum of 60 days with a money-back trial period (minus earmold costs and a "reasonable" user fee). The document notes the ambiguity of the term "reasonable," however, suggests the upper limit of the fee should not exceed one-tenth the cost of the hearing aids.

The SHHH *Position Statement on Group Hearing Aid Orientation Programs* (SHHH, 1996b) is also consumer centered, but focuses on issues related to counseling during a hearing aid fitting. The position statement notes that inherent limits to one-to-one counseling exist between the dispenser and the client, and SHHH proposes that group hearing aid orientation programs can overcome these limits. SHHH notes these group sessions should supplement the individual counseling sessions and include such topics as types of hearing loss, understanding the audiogram, trouble shooting hearing aids, using ALDs, coping with conversational breakdowns, and the implications of the *Americans with Disabilities Act* (1990) for individuals with hearing loss. The goals of such programs should be to aid hearing aid users in understanding that their experiences are not unique, to share their problems and solutions with others, to provide mutual support, and to provide a foundation for a more positive outlook for the future.

Alexander Graham Bell Association for the Deaf

The Alexander Graham Bell Association for the Deaf (AGB) was founded in 1890 by the inventor of the telephone. Bell's mother and wife were both deaf, and he spent most of his adult life attempting to invent devices to aid individuals with hearing loss and advocate for services for such individuals. AGB is currently a nonprofit organization with the goal of empowering persons who are hearing-impaired to function independently by promoting universal rights and optimal opportunities to learn to use, maintain, and improve all aspects of their verbal communications, including their abilities to speak, speechread, use residual hearing, and process both spoken and written language. AGB is very proactive in its support of the use of residual hearing through technologies, including hearing aids, ALDs, and cochlear implants. AGB can be contacted at their Web site (www.agbell.org).

National Association for the Deaf

The National Association for the Deaf (NAD) founded in 1880 is the oldest and largest association for individuals with disabilities in the United States with more than 22,000 members. NAD monitors and responds to legislation and regulations affecting accessibility and civil rights issues. NAD is a private, nonprofit organization with 51 state association affiliates. NAD can be reached through their Web site (www.nad.org).

CONTROVERSIAL POINT

Do not assume all associations with similar missions to "serve the profession and individuals seeking audiology services" agree on a particular issue. An excellent example is the controversy surrounding the use of cochlear implants with children. The Food and Drug Administration first approved the use of cochlear implants in individuals 2 to 18 years of age in 1990. ASHA and AAA both have the provision of rehabilitation and product fitting in their respective Scopes of Practice. AGB supports the cautious use of cochlear implants for children, SHHH supports their use in children with stated caveats, and NAD has been opposed to their use.

Practicing audiologists need to be aware of the issues and respect the values and cultures of these various constituencies. Parents and other healthcare providers do turn to audiologists for advice—all too often on controversial issues. As a profession, audiologists need to be fair in their presentation of information but realize it is "okay" to support a given professional opinion on the basis of an equitable weighting of clinical experience, education, and personal values.

FEDERAL REGULATION OF HEARING AID DISPENSING

Federal Trade Commission

The Federal Trade Commission (FTC) has responsibility for monitoring business practices, including those of hearing aid dispensers and vendors. The FTC is empowered to take action against companies that attempt to mislead or deceive consumers. Practices under the purview of the FTC include deceptive sales and advertising policies, falsifying hearing loss diagnosis, overrating a hearing aid's performance, lying about refund policies, or warranty coverage. The FTC is also responsible for enforcement of the *Magnuson Moss Warranty Act* (1975). This is legislation that protects consumers with certain regulations regarding warranties. Magnuson Moss requires companies, including hearing aid manufacturers and dispensers offering warranties, to fully disclose all terms and conditions (FTC, 1991).

The FTC also monitors all mail order hearing aid sales. No federal laws exist against mail order sales. However, several states have prohibited mail order hearing aid sales. The FTC requires companies who send the purchase made by mail in the timeframe promised or give customers the option to cancel the order.

The FTC does not enforce individual complaints against companies. The Commission does monitor companies for patterns of business practice. Business patterns that suggest repetitive illegal practices can lead to action against a company by the FTC. Complaints regarding unfair business practices can be reported to the FTC Division of Marketing Practices, Bureau of Consumer Protection at (202) 382-4357 or FTC, CRC-240, Washington, DC, 20580.

A secondary mission of the FTC is to educate the public regarding fair trade practices and the legislation and regulation related to consumer rights. The FTC homepage (www.ftc.gov) has a link to the document entitled, *"Facts for Consumers: Hearing Aids"* (FTC, 1991). This informative document was written in conjunction with the American Association of Retired Persons.

The Food and Drug Administration

The federal government recognizes hearing aids as medical devices. The Food and Drug Administration (FDA) therefore has federal regulatory power over the sale of such devices. The document entitled *Department of Health, Education, and Welfare, Food and Drug Administration Hearing Aid Devices Professional and Patient Labeling and Conditions for Sale* (United States Department of Health, Education and Welfare, Food and Drug Administration, 1977) delineates these regulations and their purpose. The FDA is specific in noting the labeling of a hearing aid must provide the dispenser and the consumer with adequate directions for its safe and effective use. The labeling of the device must be extensive and technical enough to ensure the dispenser can select, fit, and repair the hearing aid as necessary. At present, hearing aid manufacturers must keep adequate records in house to pass FDA review of the provisions.

The 1977 regulations were written in response to a series of hearings held in the United States Senate by the *Subcommittee on Government Regulations of the Select Committee on Small Business* and the *Senate Permanent Subcommittee on Investigations* in 1975 and 1976. Senator Percy of Illinois, chair of the latter subcommittee, recommended the promulgation of hearing aid regulations by the FDA. FDA regulations have the force of federal law. According to the FDA, all dispensers must meet the following conditions before selling a hearing aid:

- Dispensers must obtain a written statement from the patient signed by a licensed physician. It must be dated within the previous 6 months, state that the patient's ears have been medically evaluated, and state that the patient is cleared for fitting with a hearing aid.

- A patient, age 18 or older, can sign a waiver for a medical examination, but dispensers must advise the patient that waiving the examination is not in the patient's best health interest.

- Dispensers must avoid encouraging the patient to waive the medical evaluation requirement.

- Dispensers must advise patients who appear to have a hearing problem to consult promptly with a physician.

- An instructional brochure must be provided with the hearing aid that illustrates and describes its operation, use, and care. The brochure also must list sources for repair and maintenance and include a statement that the use of a hearing aid may be only part of a rehabilitative program.

In response to requests to update the 1977 regulations, the FDA released an *Advanced Notice of Proposed Rulemaking: Medical Devices; Hearing Aid Requirements, Proposals for Revising the Regulations on the Sale, Use and Distribution of Hearing Aids* (Federal Register, November 10, 1993). In response to the issuance of the notice, The Academy of Dispensing Audiologists, The Academy of Rehabilitative Audiologists, The American Academy of Audiology, The American Speech-Language-Hearing Association, and The Educational Audiology Association developed joint testimony (Audiology Coalition, 1994). Refer to Table 8–1 for contact information for these organizations.

The testimony of the audiology organizations was summarized in a letter addressed to David A. Kessler, Commissioner of the FDA dated January 6, 1994. The following are the key points of the letter written to Dr. Kessler:

- All persons interested in obtaining a hearing aid should receive a comprehensive audiological assessment performed and interpreted by a qualified and licensed hearing care professional before obtaining a hearing aid. The minimum components of a comprehensive audiological assessment should include a complete case history, otoscopy and external earcanal management, measures of auditory sensitivity for tones and speech, tympanometry, acoustic reflexes, and other appropriate tests to identify the degree and type of hearing loss, the site of the lesion, and the need for medical and professional referral.

- Neither a medical evaluation nor warning signs are necessary components of the prepurchase hearing evaluation, if an audiologist conducts the comprehensive audiologic assessment. The results of a comprehensive audiologic assessment should remain valid, for the purpose of obtaining a hearing aid for 12 months.

- At a minimum, the qualifications that health professionals must possess to perform and interpret the prepurchase comprehensive audiological assessment include a graduate or post-bachelor's professional degree with emphasis in hearing or hearing-related areas from an accredited institution of higher education.

Until such time as the revised regulations are released, the 1977 regulations remain the federal law. Complaints or concerns about the regulations should be addressed to the FDA *Center for Devices and Radiologic Health* at www.fda.gov.

PEARL

Individual audiologists working in concert with their national professional associations can make a difference. Audiologists recently became concerned with the claims made in advertising for a particular brand of mail order hearing aid. Individual audiologists and national associations reported these possible infractions to the FDA. The FDA investigated and a letter of warning was sent to the company in question (Hartwigsen, 1998).

Federal Communications Commission

The Federal Communications Commission (FCC) is an independent government agency responsible for the development and implementation of regulations for interstate and international communications, including radio, television, telephone, cable, and satellite systems. As such, the FCC has the responsibility to write and enforce regulations for federal legislation specific to hearing aid to telephone compatibility and access by individuals with hearing loss to telecommunications. Two major pieces of legislation under the enforcement purview of the FCC are the *Hearing Aid Compatibility Act of 1989* or *HAC Act* (Compton, 1991) and the *Telecommunications Act of 1996* (1996). Recognizing the importance of disability access issues in regard to the enforcement of these laws, the FCC has established *The Disability Issues Task Force* to serve as a link between citizens with disabilities and the agency. Information about the Task Force and its members can be accessed via the internet at www.fcc.gov.

PEARL

Audiologists can get involved in the regulatory process. The FCC, for example, develops regulations through the "notice and comment" process. A Notice of Inquiry or a Notice of Proposed Rulemaking is issued and citizens are encouraged to study the documents and express any concerns. These documents list deadlines for filing comments or reply comments. Comments and reply comments form the "record" of the proceeding and are given considerable weight by the FCC in decision making.

The *Hearing Aid Compatibility Act of 1988* (HAC Act) (Compton, 1991) was written to ensure federally mandated access to the telephone by individuals with hearing loss. The HAC Act required the FCC to write regulations to ensure that virtually all wire-line telephones would be both electromagnetically (telecoil) compatible and have a volume control. To make telephones accessible to persons with hearing disabilities, the HAC Act required that, after August 16, 1989, virtually all wire-line telephones manufactured or imported for use in the United States be hearing aid compatible. In establishing regulations the FCC was mandated to weigh the economic burden and potential benefits. The resulting initial regulations promulgated by the FCC (1995) gave a deadline of May 1, 1993, for all telephones in establishments of 20 or more employees to be electromagnetically compatible with hearing aids.

This initial deadline was viewed as unrealistic and too expensive by the business community. However, extension of the deadline was vehemently opposed by organizations such as the AGB. The FCC convened a working group of concerned manufacturers and consumer organizations to proceed with negotiated rulemaking. Under negotiated rulemaking, all parties go to the table to discuss the relevant issues and attempt to reach consensus on the regulatory issue (Federal Communications Commission, 1995).

The working group filed a final report with the FCC in August 1995. The report recommended that, in place of the suspended rules, the Commission adopt new rules for the workplace, for confined settings, and for hotels and motels. The group also suggested that business owners could presume, after time, that all of their telephones are hearing aid compatible because of the need to periodically replace such equipment. If a telephone was found to be noncompatible, the owner would be given 15 days to replace it. The report recommended that workplaces with fewer than 15 employees be exempt, although their owners must provide hearing aid–compatible telephones to employees with hearing disabilities. Negotiated rulemaking also led to suggestions regarding technical standards for telecoil, the use of volume controls, and product labeling.

The FCC issued a *Notice of Proposed Rulemaking* in late 1995 to initiate further discussion of the proposals generated during the negotiations (FCC, 1995). The final rule was adopted in June 1996. However, an extension was given to the manufacturers in July 1997. Because of the extensions granted to the telephone manufacturing industry, the law will not be in effect until January 1, 2000.

On February 8, 1996, President Clinton signed into law the *Telecommunications Act of 1996* (1996). Enforcement of the Act was delegated to the FCC. This act was the first serious review/revision of federal telecommunications policy since 1934. Service provision and accessibility of all forms of telecommunication for individuals with disabilities was one of the major goals of the legislation.

Two sections of the law—Section 255 and Section 713—center on access issues and require the FCC to develop enforcement regulations. Section 255 or the *Access by Persons with Disabilities* section requires all manufacturers of telecommunications equipment and providers of telecommunications services to ensure that their products and services are designed and developed to be accessible to and usable by individuals with disabilities. However, Section 255 notes that these design and development changes must only be implemented if readily achievable. The FCC has not yet written regulations for this section.

Section 713 or *Video Programming Accessibility* legislates that video services are accessible to individuals with communication disabilities. The law requires the FCC to examine the level at which video programming is closed captioned and to create a timetable for closed-captioning requirements. The FCC is currently proceeding with the implementation of the legislative requirements.

Several other sections of the *Telecommunications Act of 1996* are of potential interest to audiologists. Section 706 requires the FCC to encourage the use of advanced telecommunications to all Americans, especially children, including children with disabilities in educational settings. The FCC is mandated to determine the level at which advanced telecommunications are available and then, if necessary, push the use of such services by fostering investment in the needed products and services.

Section 254 concerns universal service or the right of all Americans to broad telecommunications services at reasonable rates. The concept of universal service has been expanded from providing telecommunication services to remote areas to include services to include schools, libraries, and healthcare facilities. The FCC and the state governments must work together to further define universal service and determine what rates are reasonable.

Architectural and Transportation Barriers Compliance Board (Access Board)

The *Architectural and Transportation Barriers Compliance Board (Access Board)* is a Federal regulatory agency comprised of a board of 25 members, including 12 federal agency members and 13 members from the public. The president appoints the latter. The Access Board is responsible for writing guidelines for accessibility as part of the *Architectural Barriers Act of 1968* (ABA) (1968) (Public Law 90-480), the *Americans with Disabilities Act* (1990) (Public Law 101-336), and the *Telecommunications Act of 1996* (1996).

The Americans with Disabilities Act (ADA) was signed into law in 1990 by then President George Bush. The legislation and its accompanying regulations are of interest to audiologists for their impact on both service provision and employment. The ADA covers several audiological services and products, including large room acoustics, telephone compatibility to hearing aids, warning alarms and signals, and group amplification systems.

The employment provisions of the ADA also effect audiologists. Audiologists who make hiring decisions cannot discriminate against individuals on the basis of disability, and audiologists as employers must also make reasonable accommodations for employees with disabilities. As small business owners, audiologists need to follow the ADA in relation to accommodating the physical structure of their office, including building appropriate ramps into audiological test suites. Audiologists who provide services to the general public are also responsible for providing interpreters for the deaf when given notice by the client of the need.

The ADA is enforced by the Department of Justice, however the compliance guidelines were written by the Access Board. The ADA is covered in depth in Chapter 19. Information about compliance can be obtained at the Access Board Web site (www.access-board.gov). Information specific to the communication aspects of the ADA can be obtained through ASHA (www.asha.org).

Although as noted previously in this chapter, the FCC enforces the disability sections of the *Telecommunications Act of 1996*, the Access Board was legislated the responsibility of writing guidelines for compliance to these sections. The Access Board opted for a negotiated process and appointed a committee, the *Telephone Access Advisory Committee* (TAAC), which is made up of telecommunications service providers, telecommunications manufacturers, software/hardware manufacturers, organizations from the disability community, and organizations representing audiologists and speech-language pathologists. In writing the guidelines, the Access Board used the TAAC recommendations. Copies of this document are available from the Access Board or via the internet at the Access Board's Web site.

STATE POLICIES AND REGULATIONS REGARDING AMPLIFICATION

State Licensure in Audiology and Hearing Aid Dispensing

Some form of licensure or registration for the practice of audiology is required in 47 states (Lynch & Hesse, 1997). Audiologists are permitted to dispense hearing aids under their audiology license in 23 states. Licensed audiologists in Oklahoma and Utah are permitted to dispense based on an interpretation of the existing statutes by the state attorney general. New York permits audiologists in non-profit settings to dispense without being registered as a hearing aid dealer, audiologists in for-profit settings must carry both licenses. Refer to Table 8–2 for state-specific licensure information. Current contact addresses and continuing education requirements by state can be obtained from ASHA (refer to Table 8–1).

An excellent review of the issues surrounding audiology and hearing aid dispensing licensure can be found in Punch and Jarrett (1994). The authors discuss specific requirements of state hearing aid dispensing licenses, including exemptions for certain medical personnel (audiologists and physicians), candidacy requirements (age, good moral character), reciprocity, and types of examinations. The latter usually includes both a written and practical skills examination.

Punch and Jarrett (1994) discuss several areas that may affect hearing aid dispensing licensure and the need for audiologists to carry hearing aid licensure to dispense. First, is the issue of whether nonaudiologist dispensers and audiologists can work together to write licensure bills versus fighting over turf. Second, the authors note that audiologists have worked against the concept of one license by complaining that graduate programs do not teach the art and science of dispensing. Punch and Jarrett (1994) postulate that improvements in graduate education in the area of amplification and increased political awareness on the part of audiologists will help in the effort to move to one audiology-centered license.

ASHA, in its efforts to lobby for licensure of audiology, has written a model licensure bill (ASHA, 1997c). Audiologists and state professional associations can use the model in their efforts to develop or improve current licensure bills. Recent successful efforts include the state of Washington requiring

TABLE 8–2 Delineation of licensure requirements for audiologists to dispense hearing aids by state (ASHA, 1998b)

Audiology License Only	Hearing Aid Dealer Licensure Only–No state licensure in Audiology	Audiology and Hearing Aid Dealer–Both required
Alabama	Idaho	Arizona
Alaska	Michigan	California
Arkansas	Vermont	Delaware
Colorado	District of Columbia	Hawaii
Connecticut (conditional)		Illinois
Florida		Iowa
Georgia		Kansas
Indiana		Kentucky
Louisiana		Maine
Maryland		Minnesota
Ohio		Mississippi
Rhode Island		Missouri
South Carolina		Montana
South Dakota		Nebraska
Tennessee		Nevada
Texas		New Hampshire
Washington		New Jersey
West Virginia		New Mexico
New York (Non-profit settings)		New York (For-profit settings)
Wisconsin		North Carolina
*Oklahoma		North Dakota
*Utah		Oregon
		Pennsylvania
		Virginia
		Wyoming

*Licensed audiologists are permitted to dispense based on an interpretation by the state attorney general.

state-based certification for audiologists and South Dakota passing a licensure bill. Salient points of the ASHA model bill include definition of the profession of audiology, description of the use of support personnel, rules specific to hearing aid dispensing, and delineation of disciplinary actions.

Consumer Protection Legislation

Consumer protection or "lemon laws" permit consumers to return medical devices for a full refund for various reasons. Lemon laws were originally written in response to numerous consumer complaints against motorized wheelchair or "scooter" manufacturers and distributors. Twelve states have lemon laws with hearing aid provisions, with recent legislation passed in Hawaii, Oregon, and Rhode Island. Legislation with hearing aids included is pending in Illinois, Indiana, Michigan, New Mexico, South Carolina, Tennessee, Texas, and Virginia. The Rhode Island bill was written in direct response to a resident of the state who was dissatisfied with a hearing aid (Hearing Industries Association, 1998). Current information on the status of lemon law legislation in a specific

state can be obtained by contacting the State Policy and Advocacy Group at ASHA (www.asha.org).

Hearing Industries Association (HIA), the national association for hearing aid manufacturers, is opposed to lemon law legislation for hearing aids. HIA notes many lemon laws have exclusions for contact lenses because they are dispensed by medical personnel. HIA argues that hearing aids are also dispensed by medical personnel. Further concerns raised by HIA centers on the excellent warranties provided by manufacturers of hearing aids and the need for clarification as to what constitutes a "lemon." Hearing aids may require several adjustments, necessitating return to the factory. HIA argues that such adjustments should not be viewed as repairs under a lemon law. HIA also notes the expenses associated with lemon laws will be passed on to consumers.

Consumer organizations that are in favor of lemon laws without restrictions note that the user of amplification devices deserves protection under the state codes and regulations. Audiologists need to be aware of their responsibilities under the specific consumer protection laws in the states in which they practice (Hearing Journal, 1997a).

GRADUATE EDUCATION IN AUDIOLOGY

Programs

There are 125 graduate programs in audiology in the United States and Puerto Rico, with 48 offering a doctoral degree. Refer to Table 8–3 for a delineation of audiology programs by state and type of degree awarded. A current complete listing of programs in speech language pathology and audiology with addresses and contact names can be obtained by contacting the *Council on Academic Accreditation* (CAA) at ASHA (www.asha.org).

ASHA's CAA accredits graduate programs in audiology. ASHA has been setting standards for and awarding accreditation for more than 30 years. The CAA came into being in January 1996, replacing the Educational Standards Board (ESB). The current Council is comprised of 11 members, with 5 from each profession and 1 consumer member. Within the professional members, the Council has three practice-based members and seven academic members.

The first directive to the CAA in 1996 was to revise the standards for accreditation. The standards were revised to be more outcomes based in nature with the goal of avoiding prescriptive rules. The new standards became effective in January 1999. Individuals interested in knowing more about academic accreditation should contact CAA at ASHA (www.asha.org).

Audiology Doctorate

Audiology as a profession is moving toward a professional doctorate (Au.D.) as the entry-level degree. The decision by national associations and institutions of higher education in audiology to move toward a clinically based doctorate is based on perceived needs of the consumer of audiology services and extensive research into the knowledge base and clinical skills necessary to practice audiology (ASHA, 1996a). In response to the perceived need and skills validation study, ASHA certification will require the doctoral level for entry into the field in 2012 (refer to the section on ASHA certification). Funding for graduate programs to develop Au.D. programs is being provided by a coalition of audiology organizations and related associations including AAA, ASHA, and the Department of Veterans Affairs (Hearing Journal, 1997b). At present, 6 programs offer the Au.D. degree, including Ball State University, Central Michigan State University, Gallaudet University, NOVA Southeastern University, University of Florida, and the University of Louisville. Baylor College of Medicine has awarded the degree of Au.D., but the program is not currently accepting new applications. Gallaudet, Florida, and Louisville will begin their programs in the fall of 1998. Refer to Table 8–4 to learn more about programs offering the Au.D.

PROFESSIONAL CERTIFICATION

As a method to ensure both minimal and ongoing competence among members of the profession, the national professional associations support audiology professional certification. The ASHA certificate has been offered for more than 35 years and has been used as a model standard for

many state licensure bills. The AAA is now also offering a certification program for their members.

Certificate of Clinical Competence in Audiology

The ASHA certificate of clinical competence in audiology (CCC-A) is awarded to individuals who have completed a specific level and type of course work, participated in a specified amount of clinical practicum as a student, passed a national examination in audiology, and participated in a supervised clinical fellowship year. The CCC-A permits the audiologist to provide independent clinical services and to supervise student trainees, noncertified clinicians, and support personnel.

TABLE 8–3 United States programs in communication sciences and disorders by state with degrees awarded by program noted

State	No. Programs in state	Degrees Offered by Programs in State		
		Masters	Au.D.	Doctoral
AL	4	4		1
AZ	2	2		2
AR	1	1		
CA	7	7		
CO	2	2		1
CT	2	2		1
WDC	3	3	1*	
FL	4	3	2*	2
GA	1	1		1
HI	1	1		
ID	1	1		
IL	6	6		2
IN	3	3	1*	2
IA	2	2		1
KS	2	2		2
KY	1	1	1*	
LA	4	4		1
MD	2	2		1
MA	3	3		2
MI	4	3	1*	2
MN	1	1		1
MS	2	2		1
MO	3	3		1
NE	1	1		1
NJ	1	1		
NM	1	1		
NY	15	12		6
NC	3	3		
ND	1	1		
OH	8	8		4
OK	1	1		1
OR	1	1		
PA	4	4		2
RI	1	1		
SC	1			1
SD	1	1		
TN	4	4		3
TX	6	5	1†	2
UT	3	3		1
VA	3	3		1
WA	3	3		1
WV	1	1		
WI	3	3		1
WY	1	1		
PR	1	1		
TOTALS	**125**	**118**	**7**	**48**

Data from the November 1997 Report from the ASHA Council on Academic Accreditation.
*Gallaudet University, Washington, DC, the University of Florida, and the University of Louisville are accepting students into their Au.D. program beginning in the fall of 1998. Central Michigan, Ball State, and NOVA Southeastern are currently awarding the Au.D. degree.
†Baylor College of Medicine Au.D. program has candidacy standing with the Council on Academic Accreditation as an emerging graduate educational program. Baylor is not currently taking applications into their Au.D. program.

TABLE 8–4   Highlights of programs offering the Au.D.

The Au.D. at Central Michigan State University
- Oldest and largest program, began in August 1994.
- First class of seven graduates May 1998.
- Six PhD faculty and four master's level clinicians.
- Distance and on-campus program for Masters level clinicians begins 1999.

The Gallaudet University, Au.D.
- First class started fall 1998.
- Strong emphasis in audiologic rehabilitation and communication therapy.
- Students will be immersed in deaf culture and American Sign Language.
- Excellent practicum sites, including Walter Reed AMC, Johns Hopkins UMC.

Ball State University—Au.D. Highlights
- Science-oriented preaudiology undergraduate program—parallels predentristry.
- Clinically focused Au.D.
- First students admitted in 1996.
- Final year is spent in clinical residencies.

NOVA Southeastern University—The Distance Au.D.
- Post-master's doctoral program, post-baccalaureate slated for 2000.
- Current students all work full time.
- Program uses home-based desktop videoconferencing to access classes, students and instructors.
- Individualized professional research project.

University of Florida Au.D.—Go Gators
- First class started fall 1998.
- Six Ph.D. faculty, five master's level supervisors.
- Program is in part based out of the UF/Shands Medical Center.
- Classes offered in counseling, gerontology, medical administration.

On the basis of member concerns and the movement toward a doctoral degree in audiology, ASHA's Council on Professional Standards in Speech-Language Pathology and Audiology (Standards Council) has rewritten the standards for clinical certification in audiology. The rewrite was based on a skills validation study, practice literature, feasibility studies, and member input. The 1997 Standards for the Certificate of Clinical Competence in Audiology (ASHA, 1997a) are intended to make the scope and level of professional education in audiology match the actual practice of the profession. The standards will affect individuals who are seeking certification beginning in 2007.

Important features of the new standard include increased number of academic hours of post-baccalaureate study and an increased amount of supervised practicum experience resulting in a doctoral degree after December 31, 2011. The educational program must be begun and completed in a program accredited by the Council of Academic Accreditation in Audiology and Speech-Language Pathology.

American Academy of Audiology Board Certification in Audiology

In response to their membership the American Academy of Audiology has initiated board certification in audiology as of 1998 (American Academy of Audiology, 1997b). Board certification seeks to recognize audiologists whose knowledge and skills meet established standards of practice and who participate in advanced training and other continuing educa-

tion activities. Certification will be administered by the American Board of Audiology, an administratively independent entity of the American Academy of Audiology. Audiology board certification is available to all audiologists regardless of membership in AAA.

Audiologists seeking audiology board certification must complete a post-baccalaureate degree in Audiology from an accredited university. Individuals must also complete a year of professional practice, pass a national examination in audiology, and subscribe to the Board's Code of Ethics. The certification will be good for 3 years, and renewal will depend on participation in various forms of continuing education.

CONCLUSIONS

Audiology as an autonomous profession has come a long way, and the policies of national associations, federal government, and state government reflect the trip. Audiology has come from being viewed as a part of speech pathology to being recognized as its own profession (ASHA, 1997b). Since the early inception of audiology after World War II, audiologists have moved from providing hearing evaluations and therapy to becoming full practitioners of hearing healthcare, including intraoperative monitoring, hearing aid dispensing, occupation hearing conservation, audiological rehabilitation, cochlear implant rehabilitation, and vestibular diagnosis and rehabilitation. National policies and regulations have grown in number and complexity as the scope of practice of the field has grown.

Demographics are also having a major impact on the profession. The "Baby Boomers" are aging, and in our noisy society, with age comes noise-induced hearing loss, presbycusis, and the potential for disorders of balance. Popular publications have noted the potential for growth in audiology (Marable, 1995). Increased numbers of individuals seeking services will change methods of service delivery and payment while also making an impact on the funding for research into improved technologies in amplification. Audiologists need to be aware that increased use of our services may lead to changes in state regulations regarding insurance and licensure, federal regulation in regard to Medicare payments, and national association policy changes regarding practice guidelines and practice patterns.

Other forces also continue to push the need for policies and regulations in audiology. The move to the professional doctorate creates a need for changes in certification and state licensure. These changes will in turn effect revisions in academic training and practice policy. Changes in service delivery, including the use of support personnel in audiology and provision of services by means of telephone and Internet, will create the need for revisions in state laws, insurance policies, and perhaps the ethical codes of national associations.

To remain effective, all types of policy must be fluid and open for revision. Audiologists need to be aware of the policies that affect their ability to practice and the policies that maintain their standing as autonomous professionals. Changes in policy, legislation, or regulation can be positive and move the field toward greater prestige, or changes can be destructive, affecting the very survival of the profession. It is hoped that this chapter will serve as an open invitation for all audiologists to participate in creating positive policies for audiology.

PEARL

Telehealth refers to the burgeoning practice of medicine, nursing, rehabilitation, and counseling being provided by means of telecommunication networks. Audiologists have been using various forms of telehealth for years—follow-up calls to discuss hearing aid orientation concerns are a simple example of telehealth. The possibilities for expansion of this type of service provision are endless and include reprogramming hearing aids by means of telephone lines, group audiological rehabilitation sessions online, and practice-based Web sites where appointments could be scheduled, questions could be answered, and batteries sold.

Telehealth also serves as a policymaker's dream. Is telehealth compatible with current ethical codes? How will best practice patterns change if the client is on the other end of the line instead of across the desk? In which state will the practitioner need to be licensed? Should the federal government become involved because of the possibility of interstate commerce? The questions are being asked and the answers are yet to come.

REFERENCES

ADVANCE FOR SPEECH-LANGUAGE PATHOLOGISTS AND AUDIOLOGISTS. (1998). ASHA files lawsuit against AFA over AuD. *Advance for Speech-Language Pathologists and Audiologists, 8*(30);27.

AMERICAN ACADEMY OF AUDIOLOGY. (1991). Code of ethics. *Audiology Today, 3*(1).

AMERICAN ACADEMY OF AUDIOLOGY. (1996). *American Academy of Audiology position statement: Audiology scope of practice.* Arlington, VA: American Academy of Audiology.

AMERICAN ACADEMY OF AUDIOLOGY. (1997a). AAA President testifies at Indiana Health Professions Bureau. *Audiology Express.*

AMERICAN ACADEMY OF AUDIOLOGY. (1997b). You've asked for it—Here it is coming in 1998 audiology board certification. *Audiology Express.*

AMERICAN SPEECH-LANGUAGE-HEARING ASSOCIATION. (1984). Definition and competencies for aural rehabilitation. *ASHA, 26*(5);37–41.

AMERICAN SPEECH-LANGUAGE-HEARING ASSOCIATION. (1990). Guidelines for graduate training in amplification. *ASHA, 33*(Suppl. 5); 35–36.

AMERICAN SPEECH-LANGUAGE-HEARING ASSOCIATION. (1991a). Amplification as a remediation technique for children with normal peripheral hearing. *ASHA, 33*(Suppl. 3); 22–24.

AMERICAN SPEECH-LANGUAGE-HEARING ASSOCIATION. (1991b). Use of FM-amplification systems for infants and preschool children with hearing impairment. *ASHA 35* (Suppl. 5); 1–2.

AMERICAN SPEECH-LANGUAGE-HEARING ASSOCIATION. (1993). *ASHA omnibus survey.* Unpublished raw data.

AMERICAN SPEECH-LANGUAGE-HEARING ASSOCIATION. (1994a). *Code of Ethics of the American Speech-Language-Hearing Association.* Rockville, MD: American Speech-Language-Hearing Association.

AMERICAN SPEECH-LANGUAGE-HEARING ASSOCIATION. (1994b). Guidelines for fitting and monitoring FM systems. *ASHA, 36*(Suppl. 122); 1–9.

AMERICAN SPEECH-LANGUAGE-HEARING ASSOCIATION. (1996a). *Background information for the standards and implementations for the certificate of clinical competence in audiology.* Rockville, MD: American Speech-Language-Hearing Association.

AMERICAN SPEECH-LANGUAGE-HEARING ASSOCIATION. (1996b). *Membership Update Survey 1996*. Unpublished raw data.

AMERICAN SPEECH-LANGUAGE-HEARING ASSOCIATION. (1996c). *Scope of practice in audiology. ASHA, 38*(Suppl. 16); 12–15.

AMERICAN SPEECH-LANGUAGE-HEARING ASSOCIATION. (1997a). *1997 Standards for the certificate of clinical competence in audiology.* Unpublished manuscript.

AMERICAN SPEECH-LANGUAGE-HEARING ASSOCIATION. (1997b). *American Speech-Language-Hearing Association Legislative Council Resolutions Log.* Unpublished manuscript.

AMERICAN SPEECH-LANGUAGE-HEARING ASSOCIATION. (1997c). Model bill for state licensure of speech-language pathologists and audiologists, relevant paper. In: *ASHA desk reference.* Rockville, MD: American Speech-Language-Hearing Association.

AMERICAN SPEECH-LANGUAGE-HEARING ASSOCIATION. (1997d). *Preferred practice patterns for the profession of audiology.* Rockville, MD: American Speech-Language-Hearing Association.

AMERICAN SPEECH-LANGUAGE-HEARING ASSOCIATION. (1997e). *Semi-annual count of the ASHA membership and affiliation for the period Jan 1–Dec 31, 1997, Table 1.* Unpublished raw data.

AMERICAN SPEECH-LANGUAGE-HEARING ASSOCIATION. (1998a). Guidelines for hearing aid fitting for adults. *American Journal of Audiology, 7;*5–13.

AMERICAN SPEECH-LANGUAGE-HEARING ASSOCIATION. (1998b). *State requirements for audiologists to dispense hearing aids, February 13, 1998.* Unpublished raw data.

AMERICANS WITH DISABILITIES ACT. (1990). Public Law 101–336.

ARCHITECTURAL BARRIERS ACT OF 1968. (1968). Public Law 90–480.

AUDIOLOGY COALITION. (1994). *Response to the advanced notice of proposed rulemaking: Medical devices; hearing aid requirements* (Federal Register, November 10, 1993, 58 FR 59695). Proposals for revising the regulations on the sale, use, and distribution of hearing aids. Testimony prepared by the Audiology Coalition: The Academy of Dispensing Audiologists, The Academy of Rehabilitative Audiology, The American Academy of Audiology, The American Speech-Language-Hearing Association, The Educational Audiology Association.

COMPTON, C. (1991). Clinical management of assistive technology users issues to consider. In: G.A. Bess, F.H. Studebaker, & L.B. Beck (Eds.), *The Vanderbilt hearing aid report II.* Parkton, MD: York Press.

FEDERAL COMMUNICATIONS COMMISSION. (1995). *FCC 95-474, in the matter of access to telecommunications, CC Docket No. 87-124, Equipment and services by persons with disabilities.*

FEDERAL REGISTER. (November 10, 1993). *Advanced notice of proposed rulemaking: Medical devices; hearing aid requirements.* 58 FR 59695.

FEDERAL TRADE COMMISSION. (1991). *Facts for consumers hearing aids. Federal Trade Commission Office of Consumer/Business Education.* Washington, DC: Federal Trade Commission.

HARTWIGSEN, G. (1998). FDA warns Comtrad about Crystal Ear, echoes ASHA concerns. *ASHA Leader*, March 3, 1998, p. 1.

HEARING INDUSTRIES ASSOCIATION. (1998). *State Assistive Device Warranty Legislation.* Unpublished raw data.

HEARING JOURNAL. (1997a). More "lemon laws" introduced. *Hearing Journal, 50*(4);8.

HEARING JOURNAL. (1997b). VA initiative moving ahead. *Hearing Journal, 50*(5);8.

LENTZ, W.E. (1991). A perspective from private practice. *Audiology Today, 3*(5);24–26.

LYNCH, C., & HESSE, J. (1997). *Characteristics of state licensure laws.* Rockville, MD: ASHA.

MAGNUSON-MOSS WARRANTY-FEDERAL TRADE COMMISSION IMPROVEMENT ACT (1975). Public Law 93-637, *15 U.S.C. 2301.*

MARABLE, L.M. (1995). The fifty hottest jobs in America. *Money,* March 1995:115–117.

MOORE, M. (1997). Higher education helps defeat non-earned Au.D. in Indiana. *The ASHA Leader, 2,*(16).

PUNCH, J.L., & JARRETT, A.M. (1994). Hearing aid licensing statutes and the audiologist. *American Journal of Audiology, 3*(1);43–54.

ROSS, M. (1994). Position statement on cochlear implants Self Help for Hard of Hearing People, Inc. *SHHH Journal* (January/February);32–33.

SELF HELP FOR HARD OF HEARING PEOPLE. (1995a). Position statements on hearing aids. *SHHH Journal,* (July/August);18.

SELF HELP FOR HARD OF HEARING PEOPLE. (1995b). Position statement on residual hearing. *SHHH Journal,* (September/October);36.

SELF HELP FOR HARD OF HEARING PEOPLE. (1996a). Position statement: Beyond hearing aids: Other hearing assistance technologies. *Hearing Loss,* (November/December);29–30.

SELF HELP FOR HARD OF HEARING PEOPLE. (1996b). Position statement on group hearing aid orientation programs. *SHHH Journal,* (May/June);29.

SELF HELP FOR HARD OF HEARING PEOPLE. (1996c). Position statement on telecoils. *Hearing Loss,* (September/October);29–30.

TASK FORCE ON HEARING IMPAIRMENT IN AGED PEOPLE. (1991). Position statement on hearing impairment in aged people. *Audiology Today, 3*(6);17–20.

Telecommunications Act of 1996, Public Law 104–104, 110 Stat. 56 (1996).

U.S. DEPARTMENT OF HEALTH, EDUCATION, AND WELFARE. Food and Drug Administration. (1977, February 15). *Hearing aid devices: Professional and patient labeling and conditions for sale.* Table 21. Chapter 1, Sub-Chapter H, Part 801.

Chapter 9

Medical and Surgical Management of Middle Ear Disease

Elizabeth A. Dinces and Richard J. Wiet

Outline

This chapter is not intended to fully discuss all treatments of disease occurring in the middle ear. Instead, we present the more common pathological conditions and some current standard treatments. The surgical treatments outlined here are intended to provide the audiologist with an example of how the middle ear is altered during the most common surgical procedures. We do not mean to imply that they are the only surgical techniques to be used. Understanding the anatomy of the middle ear is critical to understanding how middle ear disease occurs, how middle ear disease becomes chronic or resolves, and how the anatomy of the middle ear is related to the varied pathological conditions.

ANATOMY

The anatomy of the middle ear determines the response of the middle ear to disease. The developments of the middle ear structures are linked together. This helps the reader

323

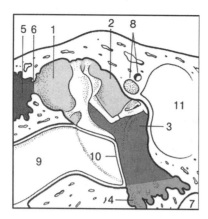

Figure 9–1   Anatomy of the middle ear: 1 and 2, epitympanum or attic; 3, mesotympanum; 4, hypotympanum; 5, mastoid antrum; 6, entrance to the antrum; 7, internal jugular vein; 8, facial nerve narrowing the lower part of the attic (2); 9, EAC; 10, tympanic membrane.

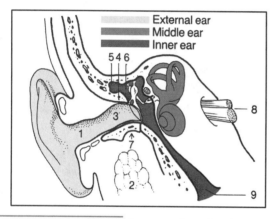

Figure 9–2   Relationship of the external canal and middle ear: 1, cartilagenous EAC; 2, parotid gland; 3, bony EAC; 4, lateral wall of the attic; 5, entrance to the mastoid; 6, attic; 7, temporomandibular joint; 8, internal auditory canal; 9, eustachian tube.

understand how middle ear disease arises, progresses, and responds to treatment (Figs. 9–1 and 9–2).

External Earcanal

The external earcanal (EAC) derives from first branchial groove. Initially this area is solid. At the seventh month, the epithelial core begins to absorb at the medial end, leaving a layer of cells to form the tympanic membrane (TM). The medial aspect of the external canal is formed by the tympanic ring. Malformation of this tympanic ring can lead to a bony atretic plate at the level of the tympanic membrane (Bellucci, 1981). In the infant the tympanic membrane is found just at the medial edge of the cartilaginous EAC. As the mastoid bone develops and is pneumatized, it grows around and lateral to the tympanic ring, thus extending the bony canal and effectively moving the TM medially. Because the external ear and canal form at a different time in fetal development from both the middle ear

and the inner ear, an abnormality may exist in one, with normal structures and function in the other two. Frequently, however, abnormalities of the first branchial pouch (external ear and canal) are accompanied by abnormalities of the first and second branchial arches (ossicles) (Belluci, 1981). Because the stapes footplate develops from the otic capsule, it is usually present and normal in ears with congenital atresia.

Abnormalities of the stapes footplate may be seen in conjunction with aberrant facial nerves. In the human, facial nerves that develop between the embryonic stapes superstructure and the otic capsule can prevent contact between the otic capsule and the stapes superstructure, causing discontinuity of the ossicular chain. This can also lead to failure of development of the oval window (Lambert, 1990).

Tympanic Cavity

The middle ear consists of the tympanic cavity and the eustachian tube (ET). The tympanic cavity is bordered by the TM laterally and the bony labyrinth medially. Superiorly, the tegmen separates the tympanic cavity from the dura of the middle fossa. The inferior boundary is the skull base with a thin layer of bone over the jugular foramen and a variable system of air cells, which may track underneath the bony labyrinth toward the petrous apex. The tympanic portion of the facial nerve and the chorda tympani (both arising from cranial nerve seven) run through the tympanic cavity, along with a network of small blood vessels and nerves.

Two muscles act within the tympanic cavity. The tensor tympani muscle arises from the superior edge of the ET orifice (in the anterosuperior portion of the tympanic cavity). It then courses within its bony semicanal to turn at the cochleariform process and attach to the neck of the malleus. The stapedius muscle enters the tympanic cavity at its posterior edge through a triangular piece of bone called the pyramidal process, and its tendon then extends from this pyramidal process to the head of the stapes.

The chorda tympani enters the tympanic cavity just lateral to the pyramidal process and courses under the malleus to its canal in the anterior wall of the cavity. The facial nerve enters the middle ear just lateral to the cochleariform process and courses laterally within the bony facial canal superior to the oval window toward the mastoid (Fig. 9–3). Any course of the facial nerve over the oval window or through the stapes crura is aberrant and can be seen in atretic ears and in otherwise normal ears. Dehiscences in the tympanic portion of the facial canal have been reported in up to 50% of temporal bones (Moreano et al, 1994). The facial recess is located between the chorda tympani and the pyramidal process. This area is important because disease can be difficult to eradicate from this deep and narrow recess. The scutum is that portion of bone that forms the lateral wall of the epitympanum or attic. The epitympanum is the space above the tympanic cavity. It is separated from the cavity by malleolar and incudal ligaments and contains the head of the malleus and the body of the incus. Both the attic and the scutum can become involved with cholesteatoma, and changes on computed tomographic scanning (CT scan) in these areas can indicate the presence of cholesteatoma.

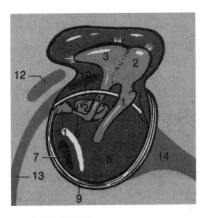

Figure 9–3 View of the medial wall of the middle ear: The facial nerve, (13) enters the middle ear behind the head of the malleus (2) and body of incus (3) superior to the stapes (5) and turns into the mastoid at the lateral semicircular canal (12). It then sends off the chorda tympani (10), which traverses the middle ear between the long processeses of incus (4) and malleus (1) to exit near the ET (14).

Vascular Supply

The blood supply to the middle ear consists of branches of the anterior tympanic and deep auricular arteries, each of which arise from the internal maxillary artery. The anterior tympanic artery supplies the mucosa of the middle ear and has a branch that is the main supply to the incus and malleus. The deep auricular artery supplies the TM. The middle meningeal artery supplies the superficial petrosal artery that sends branches to the geniculate ganglion and facial nerve. From here separate branches are sent to the stapedial tendon, the incudostapedial joint, and the posterior crus of the stapes. The superior tympanic artery supplies the tensor tympani, some of the middle ear mucosa, and joins with the inferior tympanic artery to form a plexus to the anterior stapes. Caroticotympanic arteries arise from the carotid and anastomose with this plexus along with a branch from the ascending pharyngeal artery.

Tympanic Membrane

The TM is conical shaped and is approximately 9 to 10 mm wide and 8 to 9 mm high (Wajnberg, 1987). The TM sits at an oblique angle at the medial end of the external canal, with the posterior edge being the most lateral edge. The normal TM is about 0.1 mm thick and has three layers, an outer layer consisting of squamous epithelium, a middle fibrous layer, and an inner layer of mucosa that is in continuity with the middle ear mucosa. Landmarks seen through a normal TM can include the short process and handle (long process) of the malleus, the lenticular process of the incus, the incudostapedial joint, the round window niche, the ET orifice, and the chorda tympani nerve. The umbo is the end of the handle of the malleus and is the point from which the radial fibers of the middle layer of the tympanic membrane emanate. The umbo also defines the deepest or most medial portion of the TM. The TM has been described as a canternery lever, which is thought to enhance sound transmission.

The TM consists of the pars tensa, which makes up most of the TM and the pars flaccida. The pars flaccida begins at the short process of the malleus and extends superiorly to the uppermost portion of the tympanic ring. This portion of the TM is also known as "Shrapnel's membrane" and is thought to be more compliant because of a difference in the arrangement of the fibrous layer at this portion of the TM. It is from retractions or perforations of the pars flaccida that attic cholestetaomas form.

Middle Ear Mucosa

The mucosa of the middle ear and ET consists largely of ciliated respiratory epithelium and mucous-secreting cells. It also contains some B-cells that secrete immunoglobulins to assist in the body's defense against invading organisms. The cilia beat selectively toward the nasopharynx. They form the "motor" for a mucociliary blanket that is produced by the secretory cells. This blanket of mucous and immune system proteins sits on top of the ciliary layer; as the cilia beat they act to sweep secretions from the middle ear and antrum toward the nasopharynx by way of the ET. A healthy oxygenated environment is needed to maintain the function of the cilia.

Ossicles

The incus and the malleus develop from the cartilages of the first and second branchial arches in the embryo before the sixteenth week of development. These arches develop cartilaginous connections during development. It is from these connections in the roof of the tympanic recess (which will become the tympanic cavity) that the body of the incus and the head of the malleus develop (Hanson et al, 1962). The forming ossicles then develop inferiorly extending processes, which form the long process of the incus and the handle of the malleus. Failure of any of these processes to develop or ossify will result in ossicular abnormalities. The ossicular chain is normally attached directly to the TM along the handle of the malleus. The incus is attached to the malleus and to the stapes by means of joints that are susceptible to the same pathological processes as other similar bony joints in the body. In addition, the ossicles themselves can be affected by systemic and local disease.

The stapes is the third bone in the ossicular chain, and its superstructure is thought to develop from the second branchial arch cartilage. The footplate of the stapes develops and ossifies in conjunction with the otic capsule and thus takes its origin from the otic placode in the embryo. An absent or anomalous superstructure does not rule out a normal and mobile stapes footplate within the oval window. The stapes is shaped like a stirrup, with the arch developing as a result of the stapedial artery coursing through the cartilage as it ossifies. Eventually this artery regresses and may leave a small remnant behind. The head or capitulum of the stapes articulates with the long process of the incus and its articulating surface is covered by cartilage. The tendon of the stapedial muscle extends from the pyramidal process to the posterior crus of the stapes, which is usually thicker and more curved than the anterior crus. Contraction of this muscle helps to dampen loud sounds to help protect the cochlea from noise trauma. The footplate of the stapes sits in the oval window

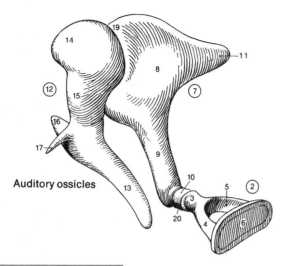

Auditory ossicles

Figure 9–4   The ossicles: View of the articulation and positions of the ossicles from the middle ear looking out. The stapes (2), anterior crus (5), posterior crus (4), footplate (6), capitulum (3). It articulates with the long process of the incus (9) at the incudostapedial joint (10). The incus also has a short process (11), and its body (8) articulates with the head of the mallues (14) at the incudomalleolar joint (19). The malleus (12) has a neck (15), a lateral process (16) (or short process), and an anterior process (17), which usually regresses.

and transmits sounds through this window to the inner ear (Fig. 9–4).

An annular ligament attaches the footplate to the margins of the oval window and enables the stapes to move in a complex fashion within the window. Five other ligaments are found within the tympanic space and act to suspend the ossicular chain within the tympanic space. Three ligaments suspend the malleus: the anterior, lateral, and superior malleolar ligaments. Two other ligaments suspend the incus, the superior incudal ligament, and the ligament of the short process, which is found within the fossa incudis.

Middle Ear Transformer Function

The TM normally acts as a physical barrier between the external earcanal and the middle ear space. The TM and ossicular chain also act as a transformer to enable sound waves traveling through the air to act within the fluid of the inner ear and stimulate the organ of hearing (the organ of Corti within the cochlea). In addition, the middle ear acts as an impedance-matching device, increasing the transmission of sound from air to the higher impedance fluids of the inner ear. Without the middle ear, most sound energy in our environment would not be of sufficient magnitude to vibrate the surface of the cochlear fluid. The transformer function of the middle ear is accomplished through three factors. First, because of the difference in surface area between the TM and the footplate of the stapes, the gain in sound pressure at the stapes footplate has been shown to be about 18:1 (Wever & Lawrence, 1954). Second, the sizes and connections of the ossicles within the ossicular chain enable the chain to act as a lever. The malleus head moves a greater distance than the long process of the incus in response to TM motion; thus, the incus will exert a greater pressure over

the shorter distance in the transmission of that force. The gain based on the ossicular chain lever is about 3:1 (Bekesy, 1960). The third factor is the cone shape of the TM (canternary lever), which enables some areas of the membrane to vibrate at a greater amplitude than others, adding force to the vibrating ossicular chain. Applying these factors, the middle ear transformer adds 25- to 30-dB of sound pressure to the signal that reaches the inner ear. The TM also transmits changes in ambient pressure through its motion and thus can change the effective size of the middle ear space. It is most compliant when the pressure is equal on both sides, and its stiffness increases with positive or negative pressure. Diseases of the TM change its compliance and thus influence the effectiveness of sound transmission. At low frequencies, the entire TM transmits sound as it acts to displace the ossicles. At high frequencies (greater than 1500 Hz) it acts as a baffle directing the sound to the handle of the malleus, which is displaced directly by the sound wave (Tonndorf & Khanna, 1970).

Eustachian Tube

The middle ear is part of a system whose function depends on the anatomy and health of its surroundings. The ET is the corridor by which nasopharynx and middle ear/mastoid systems communicate. Normally the ET is closed, preventing the flow of secretions or infections into the middle ear from the nasopharynx. This also protects the middle ear from the dramatic changes in nasopharyngeal pressure seen commonly with coughing, sniffing, sneezing, and nose blowing. In the infant, the ET lies in a horizontal plane, and its opening into the nasopharynx is a slit parallel to the skull base at rest. This opening is controlled by the tensor veli palatini muscle, which, when contracted, pulls on the lateral edge of the ET cartilage in the nasopharynx to open the ET. The levator veli palatini muscle inserts onto the medial portion of this cartilage and aids the tensor in the opening of the ET in the adult. The entrance of the ET into the middle ear is in the anterosuperior portion of the middle ear and can often be seen through a translucent and intact TM. The ET has three functions: (1) to aid in the removal of secretions from the middle ear space, (2) to aerate the middle ear and to equalize pressure between the nasopharynx and the middle ear, and (3) to prevent nasopharyngeal secretions from entering the middle ear space. The ET achieves these three functions by being passively closed and actively opened. Because the muscles of the nasopharynx and palate control the opening of the ET, diseases or anatomical malformations of the nasopharynx or palate can lead to dysfunction of the ET. The distal two thirds of the ET consists of an incomplete cartilaginous tube, which is flexible enough to collapse and close when the attached muscles are relaxed. Because the mucosa of the ET is in continuity with both the mucosa of the middle ear and the mucosa of the nasopharynx, the pathological processes that may be occurring in either of these two locations affect it. Changes in the mucosal lining of the ET affect how well it performs each of its three functions. The success of the ET in performing its functions can be affected by any pathological condition affecting its neighboring spaces. Because the system is a closed system at rest, resorption of the gases of the middle ear and mastoid results in negative pressure within the middle ear and mastoid. Swallowing opens the ET and air is pulled into the middle ear space from the nasopharynx because of this negative pressure. The proper functioning of the ET depends on the integrity of both the middle ear system, the ET itself, and the nasopharynx. Any change in the anatomy or function of these spaces will affect the ET's ability to perform any or all of its three functions.

SPECIAL CONSIDERATION

- **Because of its course through the temporal bone, the facial nerve is at risk for injury during any otologic procedure.**
- **A stenotic or atretic external earcanal can be associated with normal middle ear structures.**
- **The otoscopic examination can be normal in the presence of middle ear pathosis.**
- **A limited blood supply to the long process of the incus puts it at risk for necrosis when middle ear disease is present.**
- **ET function depends on the anatomy and physiology of the middle ear and the nasopharynx.**

PATHOLOGICAL CONDITIONS OF THE EXTERNAL CANAL

The external canal links the middle ear with the external environment. It directs sound to the middle ear but can also act as a conduit for obstruction of that sound. The canal is lined with skin containing cerumen glands. The canal skin is directly attached to cartilage in the lateral two-thirds of the earcanal and bone in the medial one-third.

General dermatological diseases can affect the skin of the earcanal. The most commonly seen dermatological diseases are local inflammatory reactions; infections, both fungal and bacterial; squamous cell carcinoma; basal cell carcinoma; and melanoma. Autoimmune diseases of the skin affect the earcanal and psoriasis, lupus erythematosus, and scleroderma can all cause lesions within the external canal. The cartilaginous portion of the external canal is susceptible to perichondritis from local infection and systemic causes. Edema and obstruction of the external canal occur with the progression of cartilaginous and dermatological diseases and can cause hearing loss, dysfunction, and discomfort of hearing aids. Cutaneous reactions to shampoos, medications, and foreign material in the earcanal can be severe and require rapid attention to prevent scarring and stenosis of the soft tissues of the external auditory canal.

Some common diseases affect the bony portion of the external canal. Osteomas and exostoses of the bone can cause complete obstruction of the canal and a significant conductive hearing loss. Osteomas are singular benign bony tumors, often with no identifiable cause. Exostoses of the external canal are rounded multiple bony outgrowths that occur as a result of chronic irritation of the external canal. The most common cause of exostoses of the EAC is cold water swimming in childhood. These lesions are usually bilateral and can

continue to grow for many years, even after the patient is no longer swimming. Tumors and obstructing lesions of the external canal require surgical excision with some type of canal reconstruction (called canalplasty). Diagnosis of lesions of the external canal is made on the basis of a careful history and cultures or biopsy when appropriate.

Otitis Externa

Otitis externa is an infection of the external earcanal. It commonly occurs as "swimmer's ear" and often results from contaminated water retained in the external canal after swimming or bathing. Otitis externa can also occur in patients wearing poorly vented hearing aids that prevent the evaporation of perspiration from the earcanal. The retained water macerates the skin and allows organisms to enter and infect the skin. It can also occur after trauma to the canal skin and can be worsened by retained cerumen or other debris within the canal. Fungal infections are often seen in the setting of chronic antibiotic use, both topical and systemic. The most common fungal pathogen found in earcanal infections is *Aspergillus* (Singer et al, 1952).

Initially the patient experiences mild edema and itching. If the infection progresses, edema increases and the TM becomes thickened and less compliant. The canal can narrow as a result of edema, preventing medications from entering and allowing the accumulation of sloughed skin and debris, which acts to encourage infectious growth. The patient can experience conductive hearing loss as a result of canal occlusion and TM thickening. If the infection progresses or spreads, it can involve the cartilage of the external canal, producing severe pain, local swelling, and erythema. Fungal and bacterial pathogens may co-exist. Some patients develop a chronic inflammatory otitis in this situation.

The skin can be chronically irritated by either scratching, local irritation, recurrent low-grade infections or other causes such as systemic disease. Thickening of the canal skin with decreased or absent production of cerumen and associated thickening of the TM with scarring is present. Occasionally, the patient may have an associated serous effusion in the middle ear space, which contributes to the hearing loss. Treatment consists of frequent cleaning of the canal and ear wicks to help carry topical medications to the medial portion of the canal and to help reduce edema. Acetic acid drops help to acidify the canal skin, re-establishing a normal microbial-resistant environment. Antibiotic drops applied topically will help to remove bacteria from the skin crevices, and often a steroid is included in the drops to reduce inflammation. Occasionally, systemic antibiotics are required. Of utmost importance is the instruction of the patient to avoid placing fingers or foreign bodies (like Q-tips or bobby pins) into the earcanal for prevention of future infections and for the avoidance of spread of the current infection.

In uncomplicated otitis externa, treatment with acidification of the EAC, debridement and cleansing of the canal, and topical antibiotics will usually normalize the canal within a few weeks. Avoidance of occluding plugs or hearing aids, as well as keeping the earcanal dry, is necessary. If infection persists despite vigilant care, cultures of the canal skin and occasionally biopsies of any lesions may be warranted. If the infection has caused significant edema such that the EAC is narrowed and the topical medications cannot enter the earcanal, a wick should be placed to help expand the canal. The wick also acts to carry topical medications deep into the canal. With significant edema often the condition of the TM is unknown, and only topical medications that are appropriate for the middle ear are applied to the wick. Topical medications that are fungicidal like gentian violet, clotrimazole lotion, and acetic or boric acid solutions are used when fungal infections are identified. Systemic antibiotics are used in immunocompromised or diabetic patients. They are also used when cellulitis, adenopathy, severe pain, or fever accompany the infection. With prolonged infection, irreversible changes in the skin of the EAC may render it susceptible to recurrent or chronic otitis externa. Consequently, the canal skin becomes thickened and does not produce adequate cerumen. Treatment may require skin excision and grafting.

Malignant otitis externa (also called necrotizing otitis externa) is a potentially fatal form of otitis externa usually caused by *Pseudomonas aeruginosa* infection. This disease is usually seen in diabetic patients, but can also be seen in patients with other immunodeficiencies. This disease originates as an otitis externa in the skin of the EAC but quickly becomes invasive with infection of surrounding soft tissues, cartilage, and eventually bone. The hallmark of malignant otitis externa is granulation tissue in the floor of the external canal and pain out of proportion to the external disease. Once the skull base becomes involved, the patient is at risk for cranial nerve palsies, meningitis, intracranial thrombosis, and brain abscess. The disease progresses rapidly if not treated because diabetic angiopathy predisposes the EAC to inadequate or tenuous blood supply. This poor blood supply to the skin of the EAC can lead to tissue ischemia and enables bacterial infection to progress unchecked. The presence of cranial nerve involvement is associated with a 20 to 60% mortality rate despite treatment (Damiani et al, 1979). Treatment involves antibiotics and strict control of blood glucose. Hyperbaric oxygen and surgical debridement are used for resistant cases as necessary. The antibiotics chosen should be effective against *Pseudomonas* infection because this is the most common pathogen in malignant otitis externa. Infection can involve the TM and middle ear structures, with destruction of the bony canal and ossicles. Infection often extends into the parotid gland and glenoid fossa with local tissue destruction. The facial nerve is at risk in the parotid gland, mastoid process, and at the skull base.

TYMPANIC MEMBRANE DISEASES

Although the TM often remains unaffected by disease in the EAC, the skin of the earcanal is in continuity with the external epithelial layer of the TM. External disease can impinge on the TM's ability to move normally or can invade the TM itself.

Dermatitis of the Canal Skin and TM

Exfoliative dermatitis can cause sloughing of the external canal skin and outer layer of the TM with secondary infection. Both middle ear and external infections can cause thickening of the TM with calcified deposits or scarring that is visible years later and that can potentially affect the sound transmission properties of the TM. A chronically thickened and stiff TM that causes hearing loss may require tympanoplasty (replacement or reconstruction of the middle ear structures) to restore the compliant properties of the TM and improve hearing. Replacement of all or part of the TM with grafted material often results in improvement of the air-bone gap and can be undertaken in conjunction with a reconstruction of the ossicular chain when indicated.

Patients with seborrheic dermatitis of the scalp or other cutaneous areas can also have this condition develop in the skin of the EAC and external surface of the TM. Otitis externa that does not respond to the usual cleansing and topical treatments and that presents as dry scaly skin with itching may be the result of seborrheic dermatitis. Eczema and fungal infections also cause significant pruritus but are also associated with other signs. Weeping of the skin with crusting is seen in eczematous dermatitis, and a grayish membrane and fungal hyphae are seen with fungal infections. The treatment of seborrheic dermatitis of the earcanal is similar to that for the scalp or any other skin involvement. Topical medications and shampoos are tried first. Tar preparations can be applied to a wick placed in the external canal. All wicks placed in the EAC should be removed or changed every 7 to 10 days to avoid superinfection of the canal. Frequent cleanings under microscopic view may be necessary in refractory cases.

Myringitis

Infections of the external canal can involve the TM, causing a myringitis in the absence of otitis media. Acute myringitis can also be the result of middle ear infections because the medial or innermost layer of the TM consists of mucosa in continuity with the middle ear mucosa. Acute myringitis is characterized by thickening of the TM with edema of the involved layer and increased vascularity. An inflammatory reaction with invasion of the layers of the TM by white blood cells is common in the presence of infection. Focal cell death by the pressure of a middle ear effusion or by local invasion of the TM itself by infecting organisms usually leads to TM perforation.

Treatment of myringitis is usually symptomatic, with analgesics and topical drops containing steroids to reduce the inflammation and associated pain. In the presence of middle ear disease and an intact TM, a systemic antibiotic taken orally is usually also prescribed.

Viral Myringitis

Bullae or blisters on the external surface of the TM are the result of acute inflammation often caused by viral disease like that seen with influenza virus. Serum and blood collect between the fibrous and squamous epithelial layers and are often, but not always, painful. The associated viral infection can lead to hearing loss by damaging the inner ear without causing lasting middle ear pathosis. Treatment of viral myringitis is similar to that of bacterial myringitis in that topical medications are often required to make the patient more comfortable. In addition, opening the blisters and relieving pressure can speed recovery. When this is necessary, water precautions and topical antibiotic drops are prescribed until the TM re-epithelializes to help prevent concurrent bacterial infection.

TM Retractions and Middle Ear Atelectasis

Pathological processes affecting the TM most commonly arise from associated middle ear disease. They can lead to healing with scar or chronic perforations. A diseased TM usually causes some degree of hearing loss. Treatment of any underlying problems improves the success of treatment of the TM pathosis.

Obstruction of the ET in the setting of chronic otitis media (COM) or otitis media with effusion (OME) leads to negative pressure in the middle ear and mastoid as gases and fluid are reabsorbed by the middle ear mucosa. This negative pressure pulls the TM inward. In some patients, as the TM is pulled back toward the ET, it slowly yields to this negative pressure causing retraction pockets in areas of increased compliance within the TM. In severe cases complete obliteration of the middle ear space can occur.

In middle ear atelectasis the TM is pulled back onto the ossicles and exerts pressure on them, initially transmitting sound directly, but eventually increasing the stiffness of the ossicular chain and causing a conductive loss. Over time, the pressure of the TM on the ossicles compromises the blood supply to the long processes of the incus and malleus, resulting in erosion and, eventually, ossicular discontinuity. Thinning of the TM, from recurrent episodes of acute otitis media, causes it to become more susceptible to retraction and atelectasis. The TM goes through stages of retraction and atelectasis before it eventually becomes adherent to the bone of the promontory and ossicles with the absence of intervening middle ear mucosa. Once the TM adheres to the bone with no intervening mucosal surfaces, the condition is called adhesive otitis (Sade & Berco, 1976). Treatment of middle ear atelectasis before the adhesive stage is often initiated with myringotomy and tube insertion.

When the negative pressure acts only on areas of increased compliance within the TM (like the pars flaccida or dimeric areas resulting from healed perforations), retraction pockets result. If the negative pressure is allowed to continue acting on these areas, the retractions will be pulled backward toward the mastoid antrum or into anatomical niches like the sinus tympani or ET orifice. Retraction of the TM into tight anatomical spaces leads to the formation of closed cystic spaces where the epithelium of the TM is trapped as it desquamates and eventually develops into a cholesteatoma.

Placement of a ventilating tube has been shown to reverse or arrest the progression of retractions of the TM (Graham & Knight, 1981; Sade et al, 1989). When a ventilating tube is unsuccessful, erosion of the ossicular chain or adhesive otitis is present, then tympanoplasty is an option to recreate an aerated middle ear space with healthy mucosa is indicated. In situations in which the mastoid process has become sclerotic or contracted from chronic otitis media, a mastoidectomy may be indicated to help aerate the middle ear and prevent recurrence of retraction and adhesion.

Tympanostomy Tubes

The placement of tympanostomy tubes has become a frequent therapy for chronic or recurrent otitis media and OME. These tubes act to hold open a surgically created opening in the TM and can sometimes lead to TM and middle ear disease, as well as help to eradicate them. The most common complications of tympanostomy tubes include failure of the TM to close after the tube falls out (or is removed) and chronic drainage from the tubes while they are in place. Drainage occurs either because the middle ear disease is persistent or because the tubes themselves are a source of irritation to the middle ear mucosa.

The choice of tympanostomy tube depends on the disease and the surgeon's preference. Tubes placed for chronic middle ear effusion should have a wide bore to allow drainage and are usually short. They drain fluid well but can easily become plugged by cerumen. Tubes placed for retractions and middle ear ventilation are fairly long and are less susceptible to plugging from cerumen but do not drain effusions as well. Typically tubes last from 6 months to 1 year and are extruded from the TM. Tubes designed to last longer than 1 year have extended flanges that help to prevent extrusion. Occasionally a tube will remain in place longer than the surgeon intended and it will then be removed to allow the TM to heal the perforation. Tubes are removed when they are deemed no longer necessary or when they are causing problems like chronic drainage in the absence of infection (Fig. 9–5).

Tympanic Membrane Perforation

Most TM perforations heal spontaneously regardless of their cause. Infection and trauma are by far the most common causes of TM perforation. Loss of a large portion of the TM or a prolonged or recurrent infection can lead to permanent TM perforations. Perforations are classified as (1) *central perforations*, which occur in the pars tensa and leave at least a rim of TM by the anulus intact; (2) *marginal perforations*, which also occur in the pars tensa and go up to or involve the anulus; and (3) *attic perforations*, which involve the pars flaccida at the superior aspect of the TM. Complications of TM perforations

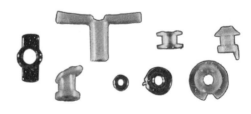

Figure 9–5 Tympanostomy tubes: Examples of tympanostomy tubes. Various types of short-acting and long-acting tympanostomy tubes.

occur when the squamous epithelium of the external layer of the TM grows to cover the edge of the perforation, preventing its closure. In some cases the epithelium grows around the edges of the perforation into the middle ear space, invading the middle ear and inner TM mucosal layers.

Hearing loss from TM perforations varies depending on the size and location of the perforation. Small chronic dry perforations that do not involve the anulus often require surgical repair. Although the risk of ingrowth of squamous epithelium into the middle ear space is less than that of a marginal perforation, this risk is significant. Careful and frequent follow-up of chronic dry central perforations to monitor the middle ear space for the development of cholesteatoma is necessary if the surgical option is initially declined.

The degree of conductive hearing loss from a small TM perforation (in the presence of an otherwise normal middle ear) depends on the location of the perforation and on an individual's specific anatomy. Small anterior perforations and perforations of the pars flaccida often cause little if any conductive loss if they do not interfere significantly with the middle ear transformer mechanism.

Despite little conductive loss, small chronic dry perforations can cause other symptoms that lead a patient to choose surgical repair. A sensation of fullness in an ear with a TM perforation is not uncommon and is uncomfortable for some patients. This can be due to a lack of TM mobility, changes in the middle ear mucosa from exposure to the external environment (e.g., changes in temperature, low humidity). Tinnitus associated with a chronic TM perforation can be seen, even in the absence of conductive hearing loss. Occasionally, patients may complain of intermittent ear pain associated with a chronic dry perforation. Discomfort with temperature extremes, especially cold air, is also reported by our patients. Patients will rarely complain of vertigo when cold air hits the exposed middle ear.

Small dry perforations in the posterior quadrant can enable sound waves to bypass the middle ear transformer and act directly on the incudostapedial joint or the stapes footplate with a resultant conductive hearing loss. Perforations that allow sound waves to directly access the round window can also cause a significant conductive hearing loss.

Medium and large central perforations of the TM usually cause hearing loss. The cause of the perforation will often determine the condition of the ossicular chain and middle ear mucosa. Dry medium or large perforations will usually permit visual inspection of the remainder of the middle ear including the ossicles under microscopic view. The symptoms of fullness, tinnitus, ear pain, and sensitivity to environmental changes can all be seen with medium to large central perforations. In the absence of infection or ingrowth of squamous epithelium, these perforations may also be watched carefully for the development of complications if a patient initially opts not to have a surgical repair.

The most immediate health concern in a patient with a chronic perforation of the TM is repeated or prolonged infection of the middle ear, associated drainage from the perforation, and chronic changes to the remaining TM and middle ear mucosa. Chronic or repeated infections of the middle ear cause damage to the blood supply and tissues of the TM, ossicles, and middle ear mucosa. This can result in an enlarging perforation, ossicular erosion, scarring, and tympanosclerosis, as well as the complications associated with acute otitis

media. Patients with chronic TM perforation must be extremely careful to avoid moisture in the earcanal and to treat the onset of infection or drainage aggressively. The second most immediate health concern is the growth of squamous epithelium around the edges of a perforation and into the middle ear. The presence of squamous epithelium in the middle ear invariably leads to the formation of cholesteatoma, either the creeping, spreading type or the formation of keratin pearls and cysts.

Medical Management of Perforations

The medical management of draining perforations includes topical antibiotic drops. Occasionally acute purulent drainage or pain associated with drainage or water exposure is treated with oral antibiotics. Coverage for *Staphylococcus, Streptococcus,* and *Pseudomonas,* when appropriate, is required in these situations. Acetic acid solutions and sterile irrigations can also be effective in curing an acute infection in the presence of a perforation.

Dry TM perforations can be managed with watchful waiting. In the absence of infection, a perforation requires very little care to avoid complications. Avoidance of water or other substances that many potentially carry infection is strictly enforced by most otologists. Swimming with ear plugs in chlorinated or other disinfected water is allowed by some practitioners, but the patient must be prepared to treat any discomfort or drainage immediately to avoid a serious infection. Long-term observation of perforations is necessary to evaluate for the development of cholesteatoma. Cholesteatoma can develop even in ears with long-standing stable perforations. The conductive hearing loss that often accompanies perforation of the TM can be treated with hearing aids if the patient chooses that option. Discomfort in an ear with a TM perforation exposing middle ear mucosa can be treated with plugging of the meatus to prevent temperature or humidity fluctuations from affecting the middle ear. Tinnitus can often be successfully treated with a hearing aid or other masking device.

Surgical Management of Perforations

Once the patient decides on surgical closure of a chronic TM perforation, the surgeon must decide on the type of procedure and the approach. Options include myringoplasty, tympanoplasties type II to V with and without ossicular reconstruction, tympanoplasty with cartilage graft, and tympanomastoidectomy with or without ossicular reconstruction.

Myringoplasty or patching of a small (less than 5%) chronic perforation can be attempted in the office setting. The TM is anesthetized with topical medication (phenol or topical anesthetic) or alternatively by canal injections of 2% lidocaine with 1:100,000 epinephrine. The edges of the perforation are freshened with silver nitrate cautery. A cigarette paper patch, piece of moist gelatin sponge, or fat from the ear lobe is applied to the perforation. The patient is instructed to avoid Valsalva maneuvers and to adhere to strict water precautions. The TM is followed at regular intervals to assess healing. If this method fails, or the perforation is not amenable to patching (too large), tympanoplasty is considered.

The principle behind tympanoplasty is a reconstruction of the sound-transmitting mechanism of the middle ear.

Tympanoplasty involves re-creation of (1) an air-containing middle ear space, (2) a properly placed, intact and vibratory TM, (3) an intact connection between the oval window and the TM, and, sometimes (4) reconstruction of the EAC.

At present, the material of choice for tympanoplasty is temporalis fascia. This material provides a strong fibrous framework for epithelization, is resistant to infection, will not be rejected by the patient's immune system, and results in a repair of nearly equal thickness to the original TM. Temporalis fascia can be easily manipulated into position and can be precisely shaped. Perichondrium is an excellent second choice when a cartilage graft will be used or if temporalis fascia is unavailable. Alternately, vein grafts have been used with similar success rates to temporalis fascia. The main disadvantage of vein grafts is that a separate surgical field must be prepared.

Tympanoplasty can be performed through the earcanal or through a postauricular approach. The choice of surgical approach for a small central TM perforation depends on the condition of the ossicles and on the location of the perforation. Perforations in the posterior half of the TM in the absence of mucosal disease can be approached through the earcanal (transcanal) provided the middle ear mucosa is normal and the ossicular chain is intact and mobile. Often the middle ear mucosa can be inspected under a high-power microscope through the existing perforation.

One way to determine the condition of the ossicular chain is by placing a paper patch over the perforation. If the hearing is normal when the hole is patched and the patient experiences no discomfort, tinnitus, or fullness, a normal middle ear beyond the known perforation is assumed. With a normal middle ear, repair of the perforation alone can successfully restore hearing to its premorbid state. Typically the patch is left in place at least a week to evaluate the middle ear. Alternately, the remainder of the middle ear can be evaluated by the placement of a thin, angled endoscope through the perforation to visually inspect the ossicular chain, middle ear mucosa and eustachian tube orifice. CT scanning may also be used to evaluate aeration of the mastoid cavity and middle ear space.

Very anterior central perforations and situations in which the integrity of the ossicular chain and middle ear mucosa is in question require the postauricular approach. The postauricular approach provides a better angle of view for visualizing the anterior aspect of the middle ear space and enables the surgeon to evaluate and repair any ossicular pathosis that may be present. Tympanoplasty with accompanying ossiculoplasty should always be performed by the postauricular approach.

Once the approach and type of repair have been determined, preoperative audiograms are obtained and the risks and benefits of surgery are discussed in detail with the patient. The risks of surgery include sensorineural hearing loss, tinnitus that may appear or worsen after surgery, failure of the TM graft, injury to the facial nerve, infection, bleeding, and reaction to the anesthetic.

Whether the TM repair is performed through the earcanal or through the postauricular approach, the principles of tympanoplasty remain the same. These principles include the creation of a framework that bridges the perforation and is stable. This framework acts to allow the migration of healthy epithelium along with an adequate vascular supply that will restore the middle ear transformer in a sterile environment.

The achievement of these principles depends on (1) the freshening of the edges of the perforation to stimulate new blood supply and epithelial growth, (2) a framework that is resistant itself to infection and that will survive until a local blood supply is established, (3) adequate coverage of the perforation without slippage of the graft, and (4) the creation of an aerated middle ear space free of infection with healthy middle ear mucosa. Given the best-case scenario, approximately 90% of perforations will be successfully closed on the first surgical attempt.

For successful tympanoplasty, the surgery must be performed in a sterile environment, usually in an operating room. Injections of epinephrine solution are made within the earcanal skin to help prevent excessive bleeding. The perforation is visualized with a microscope, and the edges of the perforation are freshened or removed. The middle ear mucosa on the underside of the TM is roughened to encourage adhesion of the graft and epithelial growth of the mucosa along the underside of the graft. Incisions in the canal skin are made to allow elevation of the TM and anulus from the bony tympanic ring while preserving a strip of canal skin with an adequate blood supply and a healthy source of epithelial cells. If the middle ear is accessed through the postauricular approach, the incision behind the ear is carried to the edge of the bony EAC. The skin of the posterior EAC is then elevated to the level of the canal incisions. The remaining canal skin and anulus are then elevated to the level of the malleus handle and turned forward to provide adequate visualization of the middle ear space and ossicular chain. Key to the procedure is visualization of the underside of the TM anterior to the perforation to ensure placement of the graft well beyond the margins of the perforation.

The middle ear is packed with a dissolvable gelatin sponge to hold the graft in place while it adheres to the TM remnant. The ET orifice is often packed with the gelatin sponge as well to prevent negative pressure on the graft during the healing and epithelialization process. The gelatin sponge will take 2 to 4 weeks to dissolve, and its presence can contribute to an initial conductive hearing loss during this time.

For an underlay technique, the graft is then cut to appropriate size and placed on top of the gelatin sponge and underneath the remaining TM. The graft is cut long enough so that it extends along the posterior bony canal wall beyond the original canal incision. The reflected TM with the anulus still attached is then unfolded on top of the graft. The posterior canal skin strip (created during the initial incisions) is then placed on top of the new TM graft helping to secure it in place and providing a blood supply and source of squamous epithelium. Care is taken to unravel all the edges of the TM remnants and the canal skin to avoid burying any squamous epithelium. The earcanal is then packed to hold all the elements in place. Choices for packing include dissolvable gelatin sponge, antibiotic ointment, expanding cellulose sponges, or gauze strips. If a postauricular incision has been used, it is closed at this time and the ear is dressed with a mastoid dressing. For the transcanal approach, packing of the earcanal is adequate to control any bleeding, and the donor site is covered with a sterile dressing.

Large central perforations, such as those resulting from longstanding chronic infection, tuberculosis, or slag burns to the TM may be repaired with a similar underlay technique, provided there remains a large anterior remnant of TM under which a graft could be securely anchored. More frequently, these larger perforations will leave little viable TM remnant and will require an overlay graft technique. In skilled hands the overlay and underlay techniques have equal failure and complication rates and the choice of technique is entirely based on the anatomy of the remaining TM and the surgeon's preference. Overlay grafting requires the presence of at least some of the malleus handle to keep the graft from lateralizing in the canal.

Absence of the malleus handle necessitates accompanying ossiculoplasty (reconstruction of the ossicular chain) for an optimal hearing result. The overlay technique requires a post-auricular approach and drilling of the bony anterior canal wall bulge to completely visualize the anterior anulus. Removal of the anterior canal wall skin and its later replacement as a free skin graft allows drilling of the anterior canal wall while maintaining its epithelial covering. All squamous epithelium must be denuded from the TM remnant in order to prevent trapping of epithelium and subsequent intratympanic cholesteatoma from forming.

Temporalis fascia is used as the grafting material and must be cut to fit the edges of the anulus in the anterior canal exactly. The fascia graft is tucked underneath the handle of the malleus and then pulled up on top of the denuded anulus. Gelfoam within the middle ear space holds the graft lateral to the promontory, and the earcanal is packed to hold the graft in its placed position. Overlay graft techniques are also used for anterior perforations with too little anterior remnant to support an underlay graft.

Tympanoplasty *with ossicular reconstruction* is usually undertaken because damage has occurred to the ossicular chain and to the TM. Regardless of the cause, erosions of the ossicular processes can occur without affecting the overall function of the ossicular chain or causing hearing loss. When the mobility or continuity of the ossicular chain are compromised, however, ossicular reconstruction becomes an important option. Adequate exposure of the middle ear is necessary to fully evaluate and reconstruct the middle ear. Therefore tympanoplasty with ossicular reconstruction is usually performed through a postauricular incision.

The choice of which ossicular reconstruction device is used is made on the basis of the repair needed and the surgeon's preference. Often the damage to the ossicles cannot be fully assessed before surgery and the choice of prosthetic cannot be made until the surgeon has explored the middle ear. The incus is the most common ossicle to require replacement.

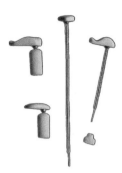

Figure 9–6 Ossicular chain prostheses. *Right top and center,* total ossicular replacement prostheses (TORP, from stapes footplate to TM or malleus). *Right bottom,* incudostapedial joint prosthesis. *Left top and bottom,* partial ossicular replacement prostheses (PORP, from head of stapes to TM or malleus handle).

The lenticular process has a tenuous blood supply that is easily compromised by chronic infection (Fig. 9–6).

PATHOLOGICAL CONDITIONS OF THE EUSTACHIAN TUBE

The most common type of ET dysfunction is obstruction. Because the ET is actively opened, disease affecting the ET tends to prevent the opening of the ET and frequently leads to disease of the middle ear and mastoid.

Patulous Eustachian Tube

In abnormal patency of the ET, the ET is open at rest or, to a lesser extreme, has a lower opening pressure than normal. This can lead to a higher incidence of otitis media because nasal secretions have easier access to the middle ear than with normal ET function. Nose-blowing, sniffing, sneezing, and crying all create pressure at the ET opening, which may be greater than the opening pressures of a patulous ET resulting in the forced entry of nasal secretions into the middle ear space.

Symptoms of a patulous ET consist of hearing respiratory noises in the ear, tinnitus, and paradoxical stuffiness in the affected ear. Autophony (hearing one's own voice echoing in the ear) is the most common complaint with patulous ET. Exercise, loss of weight, and fatigue aggravate the symptoms. They improve with nasal stuffiness, as seen with allergy or upper respiratory infection. TM movements in synchrony with respirations can be seen on physical examination. In some patients, the autophony is so loud that it interferes with normal hearing. (Falk & Magnusm, 1994). A careful history will distinguish dysacusis (distorted hearing) from true autophony.

Weight loss is the most common cause of a patulous ET. As little as 6 pounds of weight loss can cause a loss of tissue mass in the peritubal area potentially leading to patulous ET (Pulec, 1967). Pregnancy has been found to be associated with patulous ET (the cause of this association is unclear at this time). Scarring of nasopharynx, as in radiation treatments, atrophy of nasopharyngeal muscles as seen in multiple sclerosis and

---

PEARL

- Repair of a perforated TM does not ensure improvement of a conductive hearing loss.
- Pathosis within the middle ear does not always cause hearing loss.
- Because of poorer ET function, young children have a lower expected rate of success for tympanoplasty than adults.
- Surgery may be recommended to prevent future pathosis, even in the presence of normal hearing.

cerebral palsy, and dysfunction of tensor veli palatini are all also thought to be contributors to the cause of patulous ETs.

Tympanograms can document mobility of the TM during respiration, indicating that the ET is not closing passively as is seen with normal physiology. Treatment of a patulous ET is offered in severe cases only. Such treatment includes placement of irritating substances into the ET orifice at the nasopharynx to cause scarring within the tube and to decrease its patency (Virtanen & Palva, 1982). Injection of Teflon into the wall of the cartilaginous ET through the nasopharynx has also been tried; however, this can be risky because of the proximity of the carotid artery to the medial wall of the ET. Teflon has been shown to migrate years after its placement and is no longer a standard treatment. Obliteration of the ET orifice within the middle ear can be a permanent solution if the condition is severely disturbing the patient's ability to function (Dyer & McElveen, 1991). ET obliteration requires concomitant placement of a permanent tympanostomy tube to avoid chronic effusion and to avoid barotrauma to the middle ear.

Palatal Myoclonus

Because of the anatomical connections between the ET and the palatal muscles, a condition known as "palatal myoclonus" or chronic spasm of the palate can lead to opening and closing of the ET. This causes a sensation of clicking or a pulsating tinnitus. Treatment of the palatal muscles leads to resolution of the symptoms. This may involve partial paralysis of these muscles with botulinum toxin injections or use of antispasmodic, antiseizure, or muscle-relaxing medications.

Eustachian Tube Obstruction

Anatomical ET obstruction occurs with pathosis in the nasopharynx that obstructs the nasopharyngeal opening of the ET. Tumors of the nasopharynx and other tumors extending into the nasopharynx can obstruct the ET. Hypertrophy of the lymphoid tissue, normally present at the nasopharyngeal orifice of the ET and hypertrophy of the adenoid bed can occur with chronic infections, diseases that cause lymphoid hypertrophy, lymphoma, leukemia, or immunodeficiency syndromes.

The ET can also be obstructed in the nasopharynx by scarring of the orifice as a result of radiation treatments, inadvertent injury during adenoidectomy, or other nasopharyngeal surgeries. Chronic infections such as sinusitis can cause hypertrophy and polyp formation within the mucosa of the nasopharynx creating obstruction as well.

Anomalies of the muscles that would normally open the ET orifice in the nasopharynx can also effectively act as an anatomical obstruction to the ET opening. Such anomalies are seen with craniofacial syndromes, clefting of the palate, musculoskeletal syndromes, and neurological syndromes.

Treatment of ET obstruction usually involves treatment of the associated middle ear disease that invariably accompanies such obstruction. Placement of tympanostomy tubes is the most common otologic treatment. Treatment of the diseases of the nasopharynx causing obstruction of the nasopharyngeal orifice of the ET can lead to resolution of the obstruction and normal ET function. Improvement of ET function after cleft palate repair is an example of this.

SPECIAL CONSIDERATION

- **Patulous ET syndrome is treated only in severe cases.**
- **ET dysfunction can be caused by nasopharyngeal disease. More commonly, it results from recurrent middle ear infection.**
- **Medical treatment of ET dysfunction seeks to normalize the respiratory tract mucosa.**
- **Surgical treatment of ET dysfunction usually includes tympanostomy tubes.**
- **Tympanostomy tubes relieve the symptoms of ET dysfunction but only rarely improve long-term ET function.**

Adenoidectomy is frequently recommended when the adenoids obstruct the nasopharynx.

MUCOSAL DISEASE

Mucosal diseases can affect the ability of the middle ear to clear infection or effusions. These diseases can, in themselves, cause disruption of the normal transformer function of the middle ear, resulting in conductive hearing loss and chronic symptoms for the patient. They can also lead to serious complications and pathosis beyond the middle ear.

Effusions

OME is defined as persistent fluid in the middle ear space after an episode of acute otitis media (AOM). OME can be associated with a single episode of AOM and can been seen in the setting of recurrent or frequent infections, ET obstruction, or mucosal disease in the absence of prior infection. Middle ear effusion is identified by otoscopic examination and can cause a conductive hearing loss in some patients. Up to 90% of children will clear a middle ear effusion within 3 months of an otitis media, with most clearing their effusions within 1 month (Teele et al, 1980).

Evaluation of the circumstances contributing to the presence and persistence of fluid in the middle ear is essential when deciding on the treatment options. ET dysfunction, either from a stable anatomical abnormality or from local mucosal changes caused by a particular disease process, is the most common cause for effusion in the middle ear. The fluid can be serous (thin and transparent), mucoid (thick and transparent), or mucopurulent (thick and opaque that indicates infected or infected secretions). OME is more frequent in the winter months when upper respiratory infections occur more often, especially in confined areas like day-care centers. The presence of virus in the upper respiratory tract causes inflammation in the middle ear, ET and nasal mucosa. This can cause dysfunction of the ET and help prevent clearance of fluid from the middle ear space. Viral infections can present in the middle ear as AOM in the absence of other upper respiratory symptoms. Alternately, OME can occur in association with an upper respiratory viral infection in the absence of any otologic symptoms of infection.

The effusion resulting from an episode of AOM or acute upper respiratory illness is usually treated initially with watchful waiting. Because 90% of children with an acute effusion will clear an untreated effusion within 3 months (Teele et al, 1980), effusions that persist longer than 2 or 3 months should be considered for treatment. Children with symptoms associated with their effusions (unsteadiness, vertigo, discomfort, and hearing loss are the most commonly reported symptoms) are often treated more aggressively, with earlier use of medical or surgical management to help clear the effusion.

Medical management of acute effusions with symptoms includes antimicrobials, antihistamines in the presence of known allergy, steroids, and decongestants. Some clinicians will also offer their patients politzerization or inflation of the ET. Clinical practice guidelines on otitis media with effusion (OME) in children have been published by the U.S. Department of Health and Human Services (Stool et al, 1994). The specific management depends on the patient's medical history (e.g., language delay, allergic history, immune disorders, anatomical anomalies, adenoid hypertrophy, age of the patient) and the type of effusion present.

Of the current medical therapies, only the use of antibiotics has consistently been shown to be of benefit in the clearing middle ear effusion. The use of steroids is controversial, and although theoretically steroids should improve ET function and clearance of fluid from the middle ear space, the clinical trials have not shown consistent benefit. Steroids in the treatment of OME are not recommended in the previous guidelines.

With moderate-to-severe symptoms, children are offered myringotomy with or without tube placement, depending on their prior otologic history and the presence of other confounding factors. Myringotomy is also offered when the effusion persists despite medical management or if symptoms do not improve with medical management. The development of atelectasis or severe retraction of the TM in the setting of OME will also prompt the otologist to recommend myringotomy and tube placement in an attempt to prevent complications that are more serious. Children may have frequent AOM develop in the presence or absence of middle ear effusion. Frequent infections with clearing of any fluid in the intervals between infections define recurrent AOM. Recurrent AOM has also been implicated in language delay and decreased quality of life for children. Recurrent AOM or OME in the presence of adenoid hypertrophy warrants consideration of adenoidectomy (removal of the lymphoid tissue pad from the posterior wall of the nasopharynx) in addition to myringotomy and the placement of tubes.

Effusions of the mucoid or mucopurulent type are thicker and can be more difficult to clear. Mucoid and mucopurulent effusions may be a sign of underlying mucosal or systemic disease. Mucosal disease and anatomical obstructions should be treated when possible before myringotomy or the placement of tubes to help prevent complications.

The Controversy of Prophylactic Antibiotics

Recurrent acute otitis media is middle ear infection occurring not fewer than once every 2 months with normal examinations between the episodes. Antibiotics in reduced dosages over long periods of time have historically been used in children with recurrent OM. Recent concern over emerging antibiotic resistance, especially in the streptococci species, has lead to a re-evaluation of the practice of prescribing antibiotics both to treat acute OM and as prophylaxis (Barnett & Klein, 1995; Heikkinen & Ruuskjanen, 1998). Major factors in the controversy over the treatment of children diagnosed with OM include the 60% rate of spontaneous resolution of untreated, uncomplicated OM, the difficulties of accurately diagnosing OM in a primary care setting, and the difficulty in separating bacterial from viral OM.

Recent studies have shown only a modest effect of antibiotics on acute OM in children and a lack of significant effect of antibiotics for OM with effusion (Williams et al, 1993). Despite this compelling compilation of more than 1600 patients, many physicians continue to overprescribe antibiotics to a large population of patients. Efficacy of prophylactic antibiotic treatment in some children with frequent infections has been controversial (Legler, 1991). More recent studies indicate that tympanostomy tubes are more effective than antibiotic prophylaxis (Bergus & Lofgren, 1998) and that antibiotic prophylaxis is no more effective than placebo (Roark & Berman, 1997). Most patients with OM will resolve their infections without sequelae. Because the overuse of antibiotics in the community has resulted in the increasing development of antibiotic-resistant strains, the use of prophylactic antibiotics should be limited (Poole, 1998). Children who are still acquiring language and who have frequent or severe infections should be referred to an otolaryngologist for workup and treatment. Tympanostomy tubes are strongly recommended in such patients. It is believed that avoidance of exposing children to multiple drugs can help to reduce the rate of antibiotic-resistant bacterial strains in the community.

CONTROVERSIAL POINT

- Chronic OME has not been shown to respond significantly to antibiotics.
- OME can cause language delay in young children and should be aggressively managed.
- OME can exist in the absence of a history of AOM.
- Antibiotic prophylaxis for OM in children should be considered short term and only for the child with mild disease.
- The overuse of antibiotics for OM prophylaxis is believed to significantly contribute to the increasing prevalence of antibiotic-resistant bacteria in OM.
- Because large clinical trials have not shown consistent benefit, steroid use for OME should be based on individual patient considerations only.

Acute Bacterial Otitis Media and Mastoiditis

Bacterial invasion of the middle ear space can occur by way of the ET, through a perforation, or by direct invasion of the

TM. The development of an infection, after such an invasion has occurred, depends on several factors. These include the degree of the immune response of the host to the invasion, the virulence of the invading organism, and the effectiveness of the treatment given. The range of infection extends from mild inflammation with few symptoms to severe suppuration with necrosis of tissues and possible inner ear and intracranial complications that can threaten the patient's hearing and even the patient's life.

The most common bacteria causing acute OM are streptococcus, staphylococcus and moraxella infections. Even more frequent are viral infections of the middle ear space. Bacterial infections are treated with antibiotics. In cases where infection is not responsive to first-line therapy, tympanocentesis (drawing out of fluid from the middle ear with a needle) can help relieve pressure buildup behind the TM and provide a means of identifying the responsible microbial. Frequent infections are often treated more aggressively with newer antibiotics; failure of resolution of pain, erythema, or fever warrants a change in medications or a switch to intravenous therapy to prevent complications. Despite the high incidence of OM, true emergencies arising from complications of OM have become rare.

Factors associated with an increased incidence of OM include unrepaired cleft palate, craniofacial abnormalities, immune deficiency syndromes, ciliary dysfunction, nasotracheal or nasogastric intubation, and nasal obstruction. Cleft palate is a congenital deformity in which the two shelves of the palate do not fuse during development, resulting in improper alignment of the muscles involved in palatal function. Some of the muscles of the palate (tensor and levator veli palatini) insert on the nasal end of the ET, resulting in opening of the ET during elevation of the palate, as in swallowing. When the palatal muscles are misaligned, as in cleft palate, they cannot act effectively on the ET and result in ET dysfunction. Surgical correction of palatal clefts often results in improved ET function. Pathological conditions that may have developed before a surgical correction for cleft palate are not always reversible, and OM or chronic problems related to ET dysfunction may persist. Craniofacial abnormalities are also associated with increased incidence of OM. They often are associated with cleft palate but also contribute separately to OM by altering the anatomical relationships of the middle ear, ET, and nasopharynx.

Edema, acute inflammatory cell invasion, and engorgement of the vascular structures of the middle ear mucosa cause thickening of the TM and local obstruction of the ET orifice in the middle ear. The cilia of the middle ear and ET are often damaged by these changes in the mucosa, and this destruction of cilia further hampers the clearance of secretions and debris from the middle ear space. Intubation of the nasopharynx obstructs the normal clearance of secretions from the nasopharynx and allows backflow of infected secretions, increasing the likelihood of infection of the middle ear space.

logical changes can occur. These changes can involve the TM, middle ear mucosa, or ossicles. Severe complications of acute bacterial infections include bacterial invasion of the inner ear through the round window membrane, facial nerve infection with facial weakness, thrombosis of the sigmoid sinus, extradural abscess, and brain abscess.

Prolonged infection can lead to resorption of bone after osteitic invasion with mastoiditis, ossicular destruction, and exposure of the dura to bacterial invasion and facial paralysis. Evidence of destruction of the mastoid's trabeculated bone on radiographic studies is an indication for surgical intervention. Patients may present with destruction of the mastoid cortex by an infective focus with edema, pain and inflammation of the overlying skin, and subperiosteal abscess formation. Infection that breaks through the mastoid cortex and tracks down into the neck forms Bezold's abscess.

Treatment of these serious complications involves complete eradication of the infecting organisms. Intravenous antibiotics, surgical removal of infected bone and tissue (debridement), wide-field myringotomy, drainage of abscesses, and removal of infected clot are all part of the treatment armamentarium of these life-threatening complications. Bacterial or suppurative labyrinthitis can lead to encephalitis or meningitis and is frequently treated aggressively with emergency labyrinthectomy (surgical exenteration of the labyrinth). This procedure, although it causes unilateral deafness, can be lifesaving. Patients with acute coalescent mastoiditis may also require surgical treatment if intravenous antibiotics fail to provide a rapid eradication of the infection. Severe complications of otitis media occur in less than 3% of children with AOM (Culpepper, 1997).

SPECIAL CONSIDERATION

- **Normal ciliary function is necessary for mucosal and middle ear health.**
- **Craniofacial anomalies are associated with an increased incidence of otitis media.**
- **The most common bacteria causing AOM are streptococcal, staphylococcal and Moraxella infections.**
- **Resistant strains of *streptococcus* in the community limit the effectiveness of many commonly used antibiotics for otitis media.**
- **Despite a vast array of antibiotics, complications of otitis media continue to occur.**
- **Complications from bacterial otitis media can be life threatening and may require emergency surgery.**

Complications of Otitis Media

Most acute infections will resolve without any permanent changes to the middle ear structures or mucosa. If, however, infections become recurrent or chronic, irreversible patho-

Chronic Otitis Media and Cholesteatoma

Infections that persist longer than 6 weeks are, by definition, chronic infections. COM can cause changes to the TM. Often chronic infections result in perforations to the TM, either with or without chronic drainage. The perforation can range from pinpoint to a total loss of the membrane. The severity of the infection is not necessarily related to the amount of loss of the TM. Changes to the membrane, other than perforation, can be evident on otoscopic examination, with thickening, hypervascularity, scarring, retractions, and loss of the normal landmarks.

Chronic infections involve the mastoid cavity and are often characterized by drainage from a perforated TM. Drainage also occurs from deep retraction pockets in the TM. When they organize within the middle ear or mastoid, such infections may develop into what is called a cholesterol granuloma—a locally destructive process. Foul-smelling drainage is a sign of anaerobic infection or *Pseudomonas* infection. Granulation tissue, polypoid mucosal changes, and local edema are all frequently seen in the setting of chronic infection. Granulations forming on dura through dehiscences of the tegmen indicate infection of the epidural space. Aggressive treatment with intravenous antibiotics, mastoid debridement, and close follow-up is needed.

Cholesteatoma formation is commonly associated with COM. Cholesteatoma is a lesion arising from trapped squamous epithelium within the temporal bone. Congenital cholesteatomas are thought to arise in the absence of infection. They originate in epithelial rests trapped within the temporal bone during development. Most cholesteatomas are acquired (secondary), with squamous epithelium implanted or growing into the temporal bone. This commonly occurs through a perforation in the TM, during tympanostomy tube placement, or as a result of squamous changes to the middle ear mucosa from chronic infection. As the top layers of the trapped epithelium shed or desquamate, the accumulated keratin debris collects to form a cyst. This cholesteatoma cyst continues to expand as long as the epithelial cells are viable. Expansion of the cyst leads to pressure on the surrounding bone.

Infection of cholesteatoma either through a TM perforation or in conjunction with an acquired otitis media cannot be adequately treated with antibiotics and topical medications, primarily because no blood is supplied to the center of a cholesteatoma. Substances that are produced in association with the edge of the cyst erode the bone and surrounding tissues, often carrying infection outside the temporal bone. Collagenases and other substances prevent local scarring from impeding the growth of the cyst. Cholesteatoma, left without treatment, will erode through the mastoid cortex, destroy the ossicles, and invade the oval and round windows and the otic capsule, causing sensorineural hearing loss and vertigo.

Cholesteatoma has been shown to erode through the tegmen, invade the dura, and eventually the brain. Fistulas of the semicircular canals, dehiscence (uncovering of the bone) of the facial nerve, and invasion into the facial nerve are commonly found in patients with extensive or long-standing cholesteatomas. These patients rarely have facial nerve symptoms but have intermittent vertigo and sensorineural hearing loss. Further sensorineural hearing loss and injury to the facial nerve can occur during removal of cholesteatoma.

Cholesteatoma originating in the middle ear space can erode through the attic and tympanic ring and present within the external canal or at the level of the TM. Often the drainage and discomfort associated with an infected cholesteatoma are the first clues to its presence. COM and cholesteatoma are frequently seen together. Untreated cholesteatoma can lead to

significant morbidity and mortality. Currently no medical therapy is available for cholesteatoma, and a chronic ear drainage that does not clear up with medical therapy should initiate a search for a hidden cholesteatoma within the mastoid or attic space.

Surgical Treatment of Chronic Otitis Media and Cholesteatoma

Mastoidectomy or surgical exenteration of the mastoid air cells and opening of the antrum is the basic operation offered for complicated otitis media, COM, and cholesteatoma. In the case of AOM with complications, the goal of surgery is to remove areas of infection and provide aeration to the mastoid and middle ear space with a minimum of morbidity for the patient. For COM and cholesteatoma, surgical goals include complete eradication of squamous debris or exteriorization of the epithelium to prevent accumulation or formation of future cholesteatoma cysts, eradication of infection, and, when possible, repair or reconstruction of the middle ear mechanism.

An operating drill is used to open the mastoid cortex at its lateral surface just behind the auricle and to carefully and systematically remove the septations of the mastoid to clean out any areas of trapped infected secretions. Landmarks for this dissection include the bony posterior canal wall, the thin layer of bone over the dura of the temporal lobe, and the sigmoid sinus. Once all these landmarks have been identified and fully defined, the dissection is continued with smaller burrs, through Koerner's septum to expose the antrum.

Within the antrum of the mastoid, the horizontal semicircular canal can usually be found protruding laterally at the level of the vertical facial nerve. As the antrum is opened widely, the short process of the incus can be seen within the fossa incudis. In the case of serious infection or suspected extensive cholesteatoma, the facial recess is often carefully opened to further help aerate the middle ear and to visualize the tympanic recess. This is the area where infection and cholesteatoma can hide, causing problems and recurrence of disease, but is also the area where the facial nerve is at most risk for injury during mastoid surgery. In acute disease and in the first surgery for moderate cholesteatoma or COM, the canal wall is left intact. This operation widely opens the mastoid and antrum, eradicates disease, and preserves the integrity of the external canal and TM. If all the disease has been removed, a canal wall intact procedure will leave the patient with the potential for normal middle ear function.

Tympanoplasty to reconstruct the middle ear mechanism is deferred in the case of acute infection or extensive cholesteatoma. Tympanoplasty can be concurrently attempted in an ear with COM if minimal infection is present and the surgeon believes there has been complete removal of all cholesteatoma. (See the section on tympanoplasty.)

In ears with long-standing chronic infections that have failed previous surgical attempts and in ears with extensive cholesteatoma invading critical structures (facial nerve, oval window, the labyrinth, or involving the dura), the canal wall is taken down to exteriorize the mastoid bowl and any remaining epithelial matrix. Complete removal of the contents of the middle ear and closure of the ET orifice along with a canal wall down mastoidectomy constitutes a radical mastoidectomy. Radical mastoidectomy is reserved for extensive cholesteatoma causing oval or round window niche destruction, fistulas of the cochlea, exposure of the tympanic facial nerve, or extension of cholesteatoma into the ET orifice.

Preservation or reconstruction of a middle ear space and ossicular chain with canal wall down mastoidectomy is called a modified radical tympanomastoidectomy. The ET is left open in a modified radical tympanomastoidectomy. The extent of the surgical procedure is determined by the need to preserve the hearing mechanism while lowering the risk of a recurrence or serious complication of the disease process.

SPECIAL CONSIDERATION

- Cholesteatoma is an invasion of squamous epithelium into the temporal bone structures where it is normally not present.
- The optimal treatment for cholesteatoma and COM is tympanomastoidectomy.
- Attempts are made, where possible, to reconstruct the middle ear.
- Cholesteatoma causing facial nerve, dural, or labyrinthine dehiscence, involving the oval or round windows, or the ET necessitates more radical surgery.
- Cholesteatoma within the facial recess can be treated with a modified radical tympanomastoidectomy or with a facial recess approach, leaving the canal wall intact.
- A radical mastoidectomy does not leave any middle ear space and usually results in a maximal conductive hearing loss.

Tympanosclerosis

Chronic infections or other chronic inflammatory conditions of the TM and middle ear mucosa cause submucosal and subepithelial fibrosis and thickening. Deposits of hyalin and calcium called tympanosclerosis appear on the TM and within the middle ear mucosa as white patches and can lead to a change in compliance of the TM and middle ear transformer. Occasionally new bone formation can occur within the TM in association with this process. Coalescent tympanosclerosis involving a significant portion of the pars tensa or extending to the ossicular chain can be a major cause for conductive hearing loss in affected individuals.

Tympanosclerotic patches of the TM are avascular and will not be able to provide a blood supply to a graft. If tympanoplasty is contemplated for a perforation in the presence of significant tympanosclerosis of the TM remnant, that involved remnant will need to be replaced. The placement of a larger graft and the presence of well-vascularized epithelial strips are required in this situation to avoid postoperative failure of the repair. If most of the TM is involved with tympanosclerosis, a lateral graft technique with complete replacement of the diseased TM is usually required for successful repair.

Tympanosclerosis within the middle ear mucosa must be removed when it involves the ossicular chain or obstructs the oval or round windows. No specific medical management exists for the prevention or treatment of tympanosclerosis of the TM or middle ear mucosa. Timely treatment of AOM with systemic antibiotics may be effective in reducing the amount of TM scarring resulting from recurrent infection and thus in the resultant amount of tympanosclerosis. Ossicular replacement prostheses are used when tympanosclerosis fixes the ossicular chain, necessitating removal of the involved ossicle for hearing restoration.

OSSICULAR DISEASE

Ossicular disease can present in the setting of otitis media, as an isolated event or as part of a systemic disease. The TM is commonly normal and clues to the presence of the disease are based on the patient's history and on audiometric examinations coupled with the physical examination.

Otosclerosis

Otosclerosis (OS) is a disease of the stapes footplate and bony labyrinth. It usually occurs in the second or third decade of life. This disease is often noted only when stapes involvement causes hearing loss. A familial association has been shown in some cases (Larsson, 1960). OS is bilateral in more than 80% of affected individuals with slight female predominance (Cawthorne, 1955). OS can progress more rapidly during pregnancy (Cawthorne, 1955; Gristwood & Venobles, 1983). Disease involving the oval window will eventually cause fixation of the footplate with an associated conductive hearing loss, as a result of the failure of transmission of sound waves from the TM to the oval window. Early in otosclerosis, fibrous connections develop between the oval window niche and the bony footplate, causing a mild conductive hearing loss. As bony ankylosis of the stapes footplate occurs, a conductive hearing loss of up to 40 dB is seen. Fixation of the anterior portion of the footplate is the most common lesion seen at surgery. Because OS can involve the bony labyrinth, sensorineural losses and vestibular disturbances are also seen in some patients with OS.

On microscopic examination of otosclerotic lesions, the initial process involves resorption of bone around vessels replaced by new, immature, collagen-poor bone. This remodeling of bone progresses irregularly, creating foci of OS within the normal bone. The resorption of bone with increased perivascular spaces is the "active" or spongiotic phase of the disease. These increased perivascular spaces form connections with the submucosal vessels, resulting in increased blood flow and an increase in the capillary vessels within the submucosa. It is this increase in capillary vessels that is responsible for Schwartze's sign, a reddish hue on the promontory seen through the TM indicating active disease (Rüedi, 1969). The increase in blood flow over the promontory also causes tinnitus, occasionally pulsatile, in some patients. As the new collagen-deficient bone is laid down, the bone becomes sclerotic.

Within a single portion of the labyrinth, both active and mature regions of OS may exist. In some patients, this process is particularly active, and bone within the cochlea becomes involved, causing sensorineural hearing loss by encroaching on the nerve fibers (Richter, 1980; Sando et al, 1974). Sensorineural hearing loss is also thought to occur through inner ear damage by inflammatory mediators released by otosclerotic foci within the labyrinth. Approximately 7% of temporal bones examined by Schuknecht and Barber (1985) had involvement of the round window niche by otosclerotic lesions. Once a patient notices significant handicap from progressive hearing loss caused by OS, he or she comes to the attention of the audiologist and otologist or otolaryngologist.

The actual diagnosis of ossicular fixation can be confirmed only at surgery by directly visualizing otosclerotic foci within the oval and round window niches and by palpation of a non-mobile stapes. Once the stapes is fixed, the round window reflex is absent. Surgical options for mature disease have ranged from lateral semicircular canal fenestration and stapes mobilization procedures in the first half of this century to the stapedectomy and small fenestra stapedotomy procedures that are commonly practiced today. OS involves the footplate and superstructure of the stapes in varying degrees, depending on the stage of the disease and on the individual. The range of disease that can cause conductive pathological conditions includes isolated foci of OS at the anterior or posterior edge of the oval window, bipolar involvement at both ends of the footplate, narrowing of the oval window niche, and complete obliteration of the round window niche by otosclerotic bone.

Whenever possible, small fenestra stapedotomy provides the best result with the smallest surgical risk. The stapedotomy technique can be performed with the patient under local or general anesthesia, depending on the surgeon and the patient's preference. Incisions are made in the canal wall skin and a tympanomeatal flap of canal wall skin in continuity with the TM is elevated. The fibrous anulus is then elevated from the tympanic ring, and the skin flap along with the anulus and the posterior portion of the TM is reflected anteriorly. This opens the middle ear space just over the incudostapedial joint in the posterior superior quadrant. If an overhang of the bony tympanic ring obscures the view of the oval window, it must be drilled or curetted away.

Successful placement of the fenestra of the footplate and of the stapes prosthesis depends on direct visualization of the incudostapedial joint and the posterior portion of the oval window niche. Once the stapedial tendon is in view, the surgeon will have an adequate view of the posterior footplate in the oval window niche. The ossicular chain is then palpated to determine whether the lateral ossicles are mobile and if, in fact, the stapes itself is the fixed ossicle. Lack of footplate mobility and lack of a round window reflex are the two ways to confirm a fixed footplate.

Once the diagnosis has been established, the operation changes from an exploratory tympanotomy to a stapedotomy. If the OS has completely obliterated the oval window niche and its location (along with the location of the facial nerve running above the oval window) cannot be precisely determined, the surgeon will close without proceeding with the stapedotomy. If the round window niche is completely obliterated by otosclerotic disease, the surgery will also be aborted. Such situations will prevent correction of the hearing loss despite otherwise excellent technique, and the risk/reward ratio for the surgery becomes unacceptable. An aberrant facial nerve that crosses the footplate or courses between the crura of the stapes will also cause the surgeon to terminate the surgery. This situation puts the facial nerve at an unacceptable risk for injury if the stapedotomy is attempted.

If the situation is favorable and the surgeon chooses to proceed with stapedotomy, the next step is to safely remove the stapes superstructure. This is accomplished by lysing the stapedial tendon, separating the incostapedial joint, and fracturing the stapes suprastructure. A laser is often used for these procedures because it is precise, hemostatic, and does not create pressure on the footplate. These elements help to prevent complications during surgery.

The distance from the footplate to the long process of the incus is measured, and a hole is then made with a laser in the posterior portion of the footplate. Care is taken to use the laser just to vaporize the bone over the vestibule and to avoid penetration of the perilymph by the laser light. The stapedotomy created with the laser is then enlarged with a rasp or with picks to 0.8 mm. A stapes prosthesis is then placed into the stapedotomy hole and crimped around the long process of the incus. This recreates the connection between the TM and the vestibule. Proper sizing of the prosthesis is critical to a good result, and each manufacturer's prosthesis is sized differently. Finally, a soft tissue seal is created around the base of the prosthesis (Fig. 9–7).

The goal of medical treatments for OS is to mature the spongiotic lesions and prevent new lesions from beginning. Medications include oral sodium fluoride for rapidly maturing active foci and prevention of new lesions. As with all

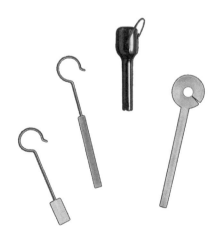

Figure 9–7   Stapes prostheses. Examples of different stapes prostheses.

conductive pathological conditions, the patient may forego surgery and purchase hearing aids.

PEARL

- **OS can be inherited.**
- **Progression of disease is frequently associated with progressive hearing loss.**
- **Small fenestra stapedectomy is currently the surgical treatment of choice.**
- **Progression of disease can be slowed with sodium fluoride.**
- **OS involving the round window or obliterating the oval window niche is nonoperative.**

Ossicular Erosion

Air-bone gaps of 50 dB or more are a sign of ossicular discontinuity or immobility, especially in the presence of a closed middle ear space. Ossicular discontinuity can be the result of trauma or loss of the blood supply to bone caused by infection, cholesteatoma, or tympanosclerosis. Occasionally, a retraction of the TM onto the head of the stapes will bypass an ossicular discontinuity, resulting in near normal hearing despite significant middle ear pathosis.

COM commonly leads to erosion or resorption of the ossicles. Pathologically, the inflammatory reaction of the mucosa to chronic infection can extend to involve the ossicles causing an osteitis (or direct inflammatory reaction within the bone). The long process of the incus that normally articulates with the head of the stapes is at greatest risk for resorption once osteitis occurs because of its relatively poor blood supply. Resorption of the lenticular process initially leaves only a fibrous band to connect the long process of the incus with the stapes, resulting in a conductive loss. Once a significant amount of bone is lost from the long process of the incus, the result is ossicular discontinuity.

In the presence of an intact TM, ossicular discontinuity causes a maximum conductive loss of 50- to 60-dB. Occasionally, ossicular discontinuity exists in the absence of infection. A severe blow to the head can dislocate the ossicles as a result of transmitted force alone or associated with a temporal bone fracture. The incus is most often dislocated during trauma. Fractures of the stapes superstructure or of the malleus neck are associated with more severe head traumas.

Ossicular discontinuity is also seen in congenital malformations of the middle ear. Congenital absence of the ossicles or a portion of the ossicles often leads to discontinuity of the ossicular chain. Because the embryological origins of each ossicle are from more than one branchial arch, abnormalities of the branchial arches (also called branchial arch syndromes) can lead to ossicular abnormalities and conductive hearing loss. Absence of one of the ossicles or part of an ossicle can be seen in isolation with no other noted congenital abnormalities.

Abnormal formation of the ossicles and/or fusion of the ossicular chain is commonly seen in atresia of the earcanal but can be found (rarely) in an otherwise normal individual. Treatment of ossicular discontinuities and malformations is with surgical repair or replacement of the ossicles (ossiculoplasty), often in conjunction with surgery for canal stenosis or atresia. Hearing aids are also offered as treatment to some patients.

SYSTEMIC DISEASE AFFECTING THE MIDDLE EAR

Systemic disease can present for the first time with otologic symptoms. Many systemic diseases can affect the middle ear. The most common ones are presented here.

Osteogenesis Imperfecta

Osteogenesis imperfecta is also known as van der Hoeve's syndrome. This genetically transmitted disorder of collagen formation is inherited as an autosomal dominant disease with variable severity. The most severe form results in multiple fractures occurring during fetal development and is incompatible with life. The spectrum has been divided into four types (Sillence, 1981). Type I is the only form in which hearing loss is frequent, with close to 100% of patients experiencing significant air-bone gaps by middle age (Kosoy & Maddox, 1971).

Although these patients have been described as having stapes fixation consistent with otosclerosis, the disease of osteogenesis imperfecta is usually quite different from OS (Brosnan et al, 1977). The microscopic structure of the bone in osteogenesis imperfecta is immature with osteoid that is disordered and less dense than normal, providing a weak underlying structural support for the bone. The ossicles can exhibit areas of thinning with increased fragility (Nager, 1988). They then become susceptible to pathological fractures and erosion and can be so delicate as to be ineffective in the transmission of sound energy (Armstrong, 1984). When this fragility is noted, the conductive hearing loss is often due to incudostapedial joint separation.

In osteogenesis imperfecta the footplate of the stapes has been described as being thick and chalklike and frequently immobile in the oval window (Brosnan et al, 1977). Occasionally, true otosclerotic foci are found to be fixing the stapes (Armstrong, 1984; Sando et al, 1981). When OS exists in the setting of osteogenesis imperfecta, it has been shown to be more aggressive (Nager, 1988; Sando et al, 1981). Despite the presence or absence of OS, a careful stapedectomy is the treatment for the fixed footplate. In these patients the success rate for closure of the air-bone gap is lower than for patients with stapes fixation but without osteogenesis imperfecta. As with OS, these patients can choose hearing aids for treatment of their conductive hearing loss. Sodium fluoride, although used in early OS, has not been shown to affect the outcome in patients with stapes fixation caused by osteogenesis imperfecta.

Arthritis

The ossicles are susceptible to arthritic conditions because they have joints that contain cartilage. Both the incudomalleal and the incudostapedial joints are diarthrodial joints.

They, like all other diarthrodial joints, are susceptible to the degeneration associated with aging, autoimmune processes, accumulation of deposits, and inflammation. Autoimmune reactions and changes diagnostic for rheumatoid arthritis have been found to involve the cartilage of the ossicular joints (Belal & Stewart, 1974). Treatment of the ensuing pain and conductive hearing loss from joint fixation can include ossiculoplasty and nonsteroidal anti-inflammatory medications. The patient's candidacy for surgery depends on the severity of the disease.

Wegener's Granulomatosis

Wegener's granulomatosis is a systemic disease of the connective tissue that has been shown to be caused by inflammatory reactions around blood vessels. Involved tissue shows necrotizing granulomas on microscopic pathological examination. In the middle ear Wegener's granulomatosis can manifest as otitis media, either of the serous or suppurative type. Suppurative otitis media is often associated with thickening or perforation of the TM and granulations within the middle ear and mastoid. Unilateral serous otitis media can be an early manifestation of this disease. Often the middle ear effusion will not respond to the usual medical therapy or to placement of ventilating tubes, and this may be a clue that a systemic process is responsible for the effusions. Surgery of the mastoid (used in severe cases with recurrent bacterial infections) can help to maintain an aerated middle ear space but is not indicated in most cases. Management is for the systemic disease and involves immune suppressants such as cyclophosphamide and steroids as needed.

Other systemic granulomatous diseases such as sarcoid, polyarteritis nodosa, systemic lupus, tuberculosis, and syphilis can lead to granulomatous lesions of the middle ear. Such lesions can interfere with hearing by obstructing the ET, blocking normal mucociliary flow within the middle ear, physically preventing motion of the ossicular chain or TM, and acting as a nidus for infection with associated effusion.

Tuberculosis

Tuberculosis (TB) is caused by a mycobacterial infection that is transmitted by airborne particles and can be ingested through the unpasteurized milk of cows. In immunocompromised individuals TB infection of the middle ear and mastoid is becoming a more common diagnosis, despite the advent of vaccination programs, aggressive treatment with antituberculous medications, and containment of outbreaks. TB infections of the middle ear can be the result of the ET admitting infected secretions, hematogenous spread, or lymphatic spread. TB otitis media is typically painless. A purulent middle ear effusion develops early in the course of the disease, causing a conductive hearing loss. The TM may appear thickened or red. If the infection progresses, inflammation, fibrosis, and granuloma formations occur as the body's defenses respond to the mycobacteria and its irritative capsule.

TB can present as AOM. More commonly, however, TB is seen as a chronic middle ear infection because the initial phase of middle ear infection is usually silent. A profuse immune response to the TB organism can cause erosion of the ossicular chain and usually leads to multiple perforations of the TM associated with a thin gray discharge. Coalescence of the TM perforations can leave a large central perforation or complete loss of the TM. Polypoid granulations not responsive to usual treatments for otitis media are common. Extension of this infection into the mastoid cavity with the accompanying mucosal response frequently occurs. Facial nerve involvement with paralysis is rarely seen. As the systemic infection progresses, regional lymph nodes become infected and fistulas that drain necrotic material can develop. The clinical hallmark of TB is a caseating necrotic granuloma, typically involving the lung and other upper respiratory sites such as the middle ear. Middle ear TB infection without pulmonary manifestation of the disease is uncommon.

Diagnosis of mycobacterial infection is made on culture or stain of acid-fast bacilli from infected material. Clinically the disease may mimic other granulomatous disorders such as Wegener's disease, and histological examination with acid-fast staining is required to make the diagnosis. Mastoidectomy performed in the absence of systemic treatment will often lead to a chronically draining infected cavity with the disease progressing to adjacent sites. Once the patient has been diagnosed and is taking appropriate antituberculous medication, tympanomastoidectomy may become necessary to remove necrotic sequestered bone, to aid in healing, and to reconstruct the middle ear.

Syphilis

Syphilis is caused by a microorganism called *Treponema pallidum*, a spirochete. The two types of syphilis are congenital syphilis and acquired syphilis. Congenital syphilis has an early form (presenting from birth to 3 years of age) and a late form (presenting in childhood to early adulthood). Acquired syphilis has three stages: primary, secondary, and tertiary syphilis. Syphilitic infection of the ear is termed otosyphilis and can involve the middle ear, mastoid, and the inner ear. Congenital syphilis is transmitted from mother to fetus in utero. The otologic manifestations are not distinguishable from acquired syphilis. The infection reaches the otologic structures by hematogenous spread.

Early otosyphilis is characterized by inflammatory tissue accumulating around the site of infection. As scarring and fibrosis of the tissues occurs, the characteristic "gumma" of syphilis forms with a necrotic center surrounded by a raised fibrotic area. Spirochetes can be demonstrated under darkfield microscopy in scrapings from accessible lesions (including perilymph), and serologic testing is positive for antibodies to the organism. Typically, areas of bony involvement are scattered throughout the temporal bone. Both the inner and middle ear can be involved and infection of the eighth cranial nerve is frequently seen (Martinez & Mooney, 1982). Within the middle ear, fibrosis in the submucosa, involvement of the ossicles with deformities, and fusions of the joints can be found. Infection of the TM causes perforation and scarring and can be accompanied by cholesteatoma. Middle ear involvement in syphilis often results in conductive hearing loss. When the inner ear is involved, patients can present with Meniere's-type symptoms, low-frequency hearing loss, sudden sensorineural hearing loss, and vestibular symptoms.

Because of the inaccessibility of lesions of the middle and inner ear, the diagnosis of otosyphilis is made with serologic tests. Two types of serologic testing for syphilis are currently available. Antibody levels to a lipid response occurring during syphilitic infection can be measured with the Venereal Disease Research Laboratory (VDRL) test and the rapid plasma reagin (RPR) test. These tests are typically positive in early congenital syphilis and in the secondary stage of acquired syphilis but can become nonreactive in the later stages of the disease. These two reagin tests (VDRL and RPR) are not specific for syphilis and false positive results occur in up to 40% (Hughes & Rutherford, 1986). Antibody levels to specific treponemal antigens can be measured by the fluorescent treponemal antibody absorption test and the microhemagglutination assay for treponemal pallidum. These antibody titers to specific treponemal antigens are positive in 100% of cases of secondary syphilis and will persist in later stages of the disease.

For all stages of both congenital and acquired syphilis, the treatment of choice is intramuscular injection of penicillin G. For patients with penicillin sensitivity, other antibiotics such as erythromycin, tetracycline, and cephalosporins can be used. The dose and time course of treatment varies with the stage of disease (Dobin & Perkins, 1983; Tamari & Itkin, 1951). Infants with congenital syphilis and positive titers of antibody in the cerebral spinal fluid (CSF) are treated for a minimum of 10 days. Asymptomatic infants and those with normal CSF and early acquired otosyphilis can be treated with a single dose of penicillin. Treatment for late-stage infections with otic manifestations includes up to 3 weeks of penicillin. Concomitant steroids are also given for associated sensorineural hearing loss because the prognosis for hearing recovery has been shown to improve with steroid treatment (Balkany & Dabs, 1978).

Immotile Cilia Syndromes

Immotile cilia syndromes are genetic diseases that result in a microscopic defect in the cell structures normally responsible for ciliary function. The cilia of mucosal cells beat in an organized way to move secretions in a specific direction. In the upper respiratory tract, ciliated cells help to clear secretions from the middle ear and ET, from the sinuses, and from the nasal cavity and nasopharynx. When these specialized cell structures are not functioning normally, the mucus produced in the upper respiratory tract is stationary. Without the normal clearance mechanisms, water is absorbed from the mucus blanket and the mucus becomes viscous. It then can act as a medium for bacteria to grow and to obstruct a normally open space. Immotile cilia can be seen with Kartagener's syndrome and in diseases such as cystic fibrosis.

In the middle ear immotile cilia syndromes are manifest as chronic mucoid otitis media. Associated middle ear atelectasis is common and can result in cholesteatoma if severe retractions occur. A similar picture can be seen when genetically normal cilia are damaged by chronic infection of the middle ear mucosa.

With immotile cilia, effusions are difficult to clear from the middle ear space even when the ET is patent and opening normally. Treatment involves active removal of the effusion through myringotomy, placement of wide-bore tympanostomy tubes, and the instillation of antibiotic and steroid drops to reduce the viscosity of the effusion and the inflammation of the mucosa. Some patients may require steroids to improve the conductive hearing loss, but effusions with associated hearing loss tend to recur in these patients once the steroids are discontinued. Perforations resulting from previous infections are often left open, with aural hygiene, observations, and water precautions as the basic treatment. Many patients will also require frequent suctioning of their gluelike effusions to minimize their hearing loss.

Immunoglobulin Deficiency

Immunoglobulins are essential components of the immune system that act to protect and defend the body against foreign invading organisms. Specific deficiencies in the production and secretion of immunoglobulins usually are present in the first decade of life and significantly affect the body's ability to fight off infection. All the major classes of immunoglobulins have been found in middle ear effusions. IgA and IgG are found in high concentrations in the middle ear, and these levels are routinely higher than those seen in the circulation.

IgA is normally produced by lymphoid tissues in the upper respiratory tract mucosa. It is secreted locally in the middle ear and is the main immunoglobulin found in middle ear effusions. These molecules are produced with a specific affinity for certain antigens (or portions of infecting microbials). IgA has been shown to interfere with a microbial's ability to adhere to the mucous membranes and can help stop viral invasion of local cells. IgG is the most common immunoglobulin found in the blood. In the middle ear IgG is found in effusions of both patients with COM and AOM. The lymphoid tissues of the middle ear are thought to locally produce IgG.

Immunoglobulins are known to directly affect the severity of an episode of otitis media. The clearance of fluid from the middle ear after an acute infection has been shown to be associated with the levels of immunoglobulins in the middle ear effusion. Most children and adults with recurrent episodes of otitis media have normal concentrations of immunoglobulins and have no apparent defects in their immune systems either locally within the middle ear or systemically. Usually some other reason can be identified to explain the recurrent infections (often ET dysfunction). However, a few patients have an otherwise undiagnosed immunodeficiency syndrome. IgA and IgG deficiencies will predispose an individual to recurrent sinus, pulmonary, and middle ear infections. Occasionally, no other signs or infections are present except recurrent otitis media to suggest an underlying immunodeficiency, and many of these patients are misdiagnosed. Once a deficiency of IgA or IgG has been identified, adjunctive treatment of recurrent otitis media in conjunction with the usual treatment options should include replacement of immunoglobulins during periods of infection. For patients with chronic or recurrent severe infections, treatment with replacement of immunoglobulins can be given at regular intervals.

Infection with Human Immunodeficiency Virus

Today, with the recent epidemic of human immunodeficiency virus (HIV) infection in the United States, middle ear disease is on the increase. HIV infection has been shown to affect the T-cell and B-cell components of the immune system and the complement system and the ability of cells to phagocytose and kill invading microorganisms. They tend therefore to have an increased number of bacterially caused otitis media and may fail to completely clear microbials from effusions in the middle ear. Most middle ear infections in HIV-infected individuals are caused by the common pathogens of otitis media. In addition, HIV-infected individuals are also at risk for infection with unusual, opportunistic, or particularly virulent microbials. For this reason, these patients should be treated aggressively with intravenous antibiotics if they fail an initial course of oral medications. An essential component in the treatment of otitis media with HIV infection is aspiration of the middle ear contents for culture. Because of the risk for recurrent infections in the setting of immunocompromise, the placement of tympanostomy tubes should be considered with caution. A chronic effusion with mild hearing loss can be inadvertently converted into a chronically draining ear with a perforation that is resistant to healing. Perforation of the TM in an immunocompromised individual puts that person at an increased risk for chronic mastoiditis and its associated complications.

PITFALL

- **The failure to search for systemic disease in patients with usual or COM can lead to permanent changes in hearing and more severe otologic disease.**
- **Wegener's disease of the middle ear causes suppurative otitis media with chronic effusions and middle ear granulomas that are difficult to treat locally.**
- **Otosyphilis (both congenital and acquired) can lead to middle ear fibrosis and effusions.**
- **TB otitis media, usually painless with large or multiple TM perforations and thin grayish discharge, fails to improve with conventional treatments.**
- **Patients with immotile cilia syndromes will have recurrence of their symptoms without tubes and frequent aural hygiene measures.**
- **The pathogens commonly causing otitis media in HIV-infected individuals are generally the same as those pathogens commonly causing otitis media in non-HIV-infected individuals.**

TUMORS OF THE MIDDLE EAR

Tumors of the middle ear are rare. When present, they cause hearing loss and middle ear disease through mechanical obstruction of normal structures or through displacement or destruction of those structures. Often obstruction of the ET will lead to chronic effusions.

Leukemia

Leukemic infiltrates are found in the submucosa of the middle ear in patients with chronic leukemic syndromes (Zechner & Altmann, 1969). They act to cause thickening of the TM with chronic, often suppurative effusions and recurrent bleeding into the middle ear and mastoid process. Conductive hearing loss is a common complaint in these patients. The effusions are treated with methods to improve ET function such as Valsalva maneuvers and decongestants. Tympanostomy tubes may be placed to relieve pressure and conductive hearing loss, but the risk of recurrent infections and chronically draining ears is high in these immunocompromised individuals. Radiation and chemotherapy are the mainstays of treatment for leukemia.

Glomus Tumors

Glomus jugulare, tympanicum, or vagale tumors arise from paraganglioma cells of the jugular bulb, the middle ear portions of the vagus nerve (Arnold's nerve), or the glossopharyngeal nerve (Jacobson's nerve) (Ogura et al, 1978). Ten percent of these tumors are familial (Parkin, 1981), and about 10% of glomus tumors have been found to be bilateral (Spector et al, 1975). These glomus tumors are the most common tumors of the middle ear. They present with a history of aural pulsation, pain, fullness, tinnitus, hemorrhage, and/or symptoms of cranial neuropathy. When these tumors arise from the jugular bulb (as about 85% do), they can cause lower cranial nerve palsies and destruction of the skull base. They can extend to the intracranial space and erode into the otic capsule.

Treatment options for glomus tumors include surgical removal, embolization (placement of blocking substances into blood vessels feeding the tumor), and radiation treatment. Occasionally glomus tumors can produce catecholamines and surgical manipulation can be risky in an unstable patient (Schwaber et al, 1984). Radiation treatment is primarily reserved for those patients who are not surgical candidates or who refuse surgery (Konefal et al, 1987). Radiation is also used in patients with recurrent disease that cannot be completely resected. Embolization can be offered as the main treatment or in conjunction with other treatments such as surgery and radiation. Surgery is frequently preceded by angiogram with embolization of major feeding vessels to reduce the blood loss and aid in preserving vital structures of the skull base.

Surgery for glomus tumors is based on the degree of involvement of the skull base and any intracranial involvement (Jackson et al, 1982). This surgery is usually a team effort. The surgical team consists of a neurotologist, head and neck surgeon, and neurosurgeon. Because these tumors arise in the skull base and neck, they frequently involve cranial nerves and the carotid artery. Attempts to preserve these vital structures make surgery laborious and lengthy. Control of the major vessels is achieved in the neck, and the involved structures (usually those of the jugular foramen and the facial nerve) are followed up to the skull base. An extensive mastoidectomy with skeletonization of the carotid artery within the temporal bone is frequently needed. This portion of the surgery involves careful dissection of the facial nerve from the stylomastoid foramen through tumor to the geniculate ganglion. The facial nerve must often be transposed (moved out of its bony canal) to remove the medial aspect of the tumor. Transposition of the facial nerve always results in postoperative paralysis. The lower cranial nerves must all be identified in the neck and or at the brain stem and traced through tumor whenever possible. Injury to these nerves often results in permanent deficits in speech, swallowing, and shoulder motion.

When the tumor extends intracranially, a craniotomy with careful dissection from above the skull base may be necessary but adds to the risk and difficulty of the procedure. Injury or involvement of the carotid artery puts the patient at risk for stroke. Injury to the carotid artery can occur during removal of the tumor from the carotid sheath. Preoperative temporary occlusion of the carotid artery with a balloon catheter on the involved side can help to determine whether the patient can tolerate an attempt at total tumor removal from the surface of the vessel. If necessary, the tumor may be left behind to avoid unacceptable morbidity from surgery. A second surgery, or radiation therapy, is often necessary if the residual tumor grows. Patients with large glomus tumors of the skull base may receive a tracheotomy during surgery to protect the airway in anticipation of swallowing and vocal cord dysfunction after surgery. Because complete tumor removal becomes more difficult as the tumors become more extensive, close follow-up with CT or MRI and physical examinations is maintained in all these patients.

Adenomas of the Middle Ear

Primary adenomas of the middle ear are rare. They are benign tumors that arise from the glands found naturally in the middle ear mucosa and are usually slow growing. They are often discovered during the workup for conductive hearing loss or otitis media with effusion. Treatment of these tumors is surgical. Most adenomas of the middle ear do not respond well to radiation or chemotherapy. Mastoidectomy and tympanoplasty are the most common surgical procedures performed for these tumors. Postoperative CT scans should be obtained to follow any potential recurrences. Although extremely rare, these tumors can be aggressive, destroying bone and recurring when the resection is incomplete. Despite their benign pathology, they can be life threatening when they extend intracranially.

Basal Cell Carcinoma

Basal cell carcinoma is a slow-growing, locally invasive neoplasm of the basal cells of the skin. It is most commonly seen in men older than 60 and usually results from sun exposure. It can arise in the external auditory canal and often extend into the subcutaneous tissues and middle ear before the tumor is discovered. This tumor is a malignancy with a tendency to invade soft tissues and bone if left untreated in its early stages. The tumor advances with invading fingers. Once it has extended past the skin, a resection with wide margins and postoperative radiation treatments may be needed to prevent recurrence.

Other tumors found in the middle ear include rhabdomyosarcoma, melanoma, and benign neuromas. Discussion of these tumors has been left out here because they are rare.

TRAUMA

Trauma can cause TM pathosis, with tears in the membrane related to temporal bone fractures. Temporal bone fractures can also cause hemotympanum. Other types of perforations can be seen with external trauma from foreign bodies being forced through the TM through the external canal. Slag burns (such as seen in welders) and small batteries (usually placed by children in their ears) cause a necrosis of the TM and middle ear mucosa. Pressure trauma from blasts, sound, or a closed blow to the ear all can cause large or total perforations.

Temporal Bone Fractures

Transverse fractures of the temporal bone are often the result of a blow to the occiput. The fracture can run across the labyrinth or through the middle ear. The hearing loss is usually sensorineural, and total; facial paralysis occurs about half of the time; hemotympanum is common. These fractures tend to occur in conjunction with serious head trauma, and the hearing impairment and facial nerve injuries can go unrecognized and untreated for extended periods.

In longitudinal fractures the external canal is often lacerated, the TM may be torn and the ossicles are often injured. Only 25% of these patients will have facial nerve injury. With either of these fractures or with mixed fractures the ossicles may be damaged or dislocated. A CT scan will help determine whether such an injury has occurred. Treatment of ossicular injury or dislocation with or without TM injury is nonurgent middle ear exploration with tympanoplasty and ossiculoplasty as needed (Figs. 9–8 and 9–9). Facial nerve injuries resulting from temporal bone trauma require rapid intervention, especially when acute. Facial paralysis from temporal bone trauma can be *delayed* for up to several weeks. This usually is indicative of a better prognosis for recovery than immediate paralysis. When the facial nerve has been disrupted at a fracture line or contused severely, the patient experiences immediate paralysis. Decompression of the injured segment (removal of the surrounding bony canal) and anastomosis (reattachment of severed ends) or grafting (placement of a connecting nerve between severed ends) can improve the final outcome.

Temporal bone fractures can result in CSF leak either from the EAC or from the nasal cavity through the ET. Acutely, bleeding associated with the head injury can obscure a CSF leak. CSF leaks are of concern because they indicate possible intracranial injury and can lead to meningitis. CSF leaks are usually initially managed conservatively with bedrest, head elevation, and avoidance of straining. Two weeks of such treatment will determine whether the leak will close spontaneously. If conservative measures fail, lumbar drainage of the CSF or surgical repairs of the leak at the skull base are indicated. Once a CSF leak is recognized or suspected, nothing that is not sterile should be placed in the ear. Unsterile cotton, ear drops, wicks, unsterile ear swabs, irrigations, or ear probe tips can all introduce bacteria into the ear and through the leak to the meninges. These should be avoided until the leak has closed.

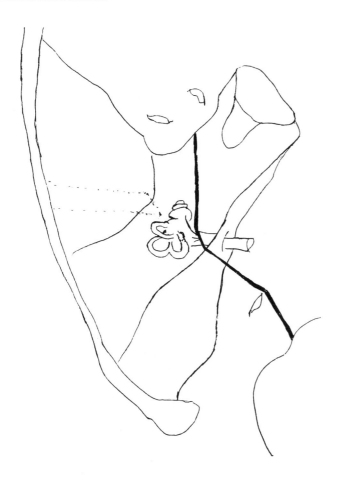

Figure 9–8 Schematic drawing of a longitudinal temporal bone fracture. The fracture line usually extends from the petrous apex, lateral to and around the bony labyrinth and along the EAC. These fractures frequently cross the facial nerve and ossicular chain and can tear the TM.

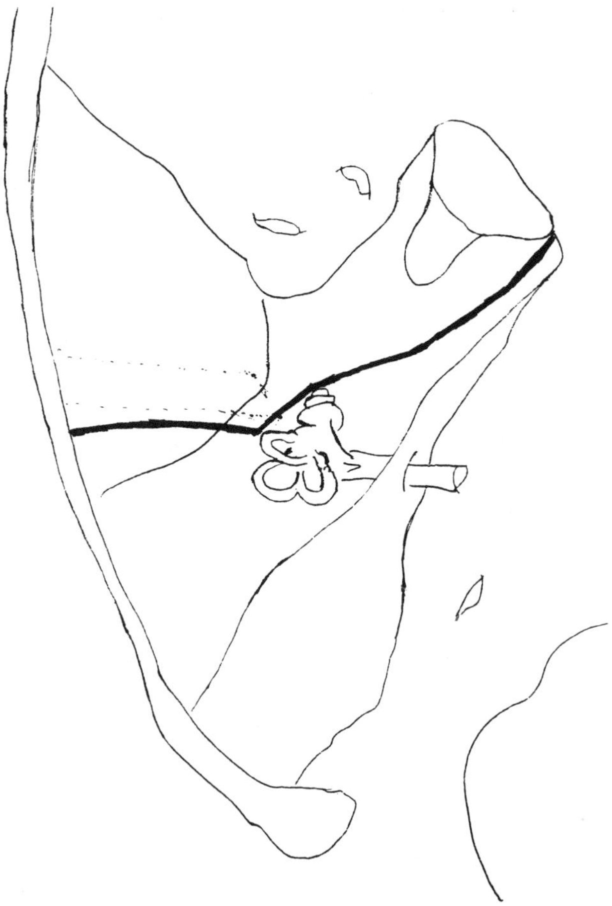

Figure 9–9 Schematic drawing of a transverse temporal bone fracture. The fracture line usually extends from the foramen magnum across the internal auditory canal, medial to the bony labyrinth, and only rarely involves the middle ear.

Perilymph Fistulas

Perilymph fistulas can occur spontaneously and are a more common cause of sudden hearing loss in children than in adults. Patients present with a sudden decrease in hearing, tinnitus, and/or vertigo. Such leaks of perilymph into the middle ear can be sequelae of barotrauma in susceptible individuals. Spontaneous perilymph fistulas can be associated with inner ear malformations.

A search for associated malformations should be undertaken in children with sudden hearing losses attributed to fistulas. Bedrest will frequently lead to resealing of the fistula with resolution of the vertigo. Hearing can be stabilized with fistula closure (spontaneous or surgical) but often does not recover completely. If recovery does not occur after 1 week of bedrest, the patient can opt for exploratory tympanotomy with fat, vein, or fascia placed as a patch over the fistula. Patients with proven fistulas may need further patching if recurrent symptoms or progression of symptoms after patching develop.

Barotrauma to the Middle Ear

Usually barotrauma results in inflammation of the middle ear and mastoid process because of the rapid development of negative pressure within the middle ear/mastoid system. Such pressure causes edema of the mucosa and TM retraction (Farmer, 1985). The negative pressure can draw fluid transudate into the middle ear space from the tissues, creating an effusion. Bleeding into the middle ear can result from a rapid high negative pressure. Often such middle ear barotrauma causes pain, hearing loss, tinnitus, and sometimes vertigo. With barotrauma from diving, the TM can rupture from rapid pressure differentials of as little as 100 mm Hg (Farmer, 1982). Patients with ET dysfunction are at increased risk for barotrauma of the middle ear with only mild-to-moderate stress, such as gradual airplane descent or when diving.

Barotrauma also can occur in susceptible individuals from rapid elevator rides from high floors or when traveling over mountains. Mechanical obstruction of the ET by nasal edema from upper respiratory infection or allergy can contribute to or worsen ET dysfunction and lead to barotrauma during flight. Restoration of normal ET function with drainage of the effusion will usually correct the problem.

Prevention of barotrauma during air travel in individuals with known ET dysfunction can be facilitated with the use of Valsalva maneuvers during airplane descent or the placement of tympanostomy tubes to equalize the pressure on both sides of the TM. Diving should be avoided in individuals with ET dysfunction, chronic ear disease, or a history of stapedectomy.

COMPLICATIONS OF SURGERY

Surgery of the temporal bone can be complicated and risky. Often diseases of the middle ear and mastoid process obscure or eliminate the usual landmarks, putting the patient at risk for intraoperative and postoperative complications. Occasionally, the disease process is the cause of a problem that must be addressed at surgery to ensure the patient's best possible outcome.

Facial Nerve Complications

Extensive cholesteatoma can be a particularly damaging disease. The facial nerve can be uncovered, displaced, or invaded by this disease, which often acts like a malignancy of the temporal bone. This puts the facial nerve at high risk for injury from infection, local compression, and cholesteatoma removal.

Immediate recognition of facial nerve injury, or transection with immediate repair, gives the patient the best chance for recovery of acceptable facial function. If the facial nerve can be anastomosed primarily, this is done immediately. Transposition of the facial nerve out of its bony canal changes its orientation. When the neuronal fibers regrow, they rarely can find their original paths. This leads to synkinesis and incomplete recovery of facial function. In the worst case the nerve is injured such that a portion of the nerve is absent and length is insufficient for a primary anastomosis. In such a case an interposition graft, usually taken from the greater auricular nerve, is anastomosed between the cut edges of the facial nerve. The result is facial motion with obvious asymmetry at rest in the best of circumstances. Delays in repairing a transected facial nerve can lead to scarring and neuroma formation at the transection site or failure to find both ends of the nerve.

Incomplete Removal of Cholesteatoma

If cholesteatoma intimately involves the facial nerve or fenestrates (cause a hole to form into) the cochlea or labyrinth, it becomes necessary to leave cholesteatoma matrix (the layer of living epithelial cells) over the involved structure to avoid a serious complication. Failure to properly exteriorize this remaining matrix will invariably lead to a recurrence of the cholesteatoma with the potential for further damage of the involved structures.

The solution of exteriorizing the matrix of cholesteatoma that is purposely left behind sometimes includes sacrifice of the middle ear structures in a radical mastoidectomy procedure and a permanent, surgically created, conductive hearing loss. Only rarely can a radical mastoid cavity be revised,

with an attempt to recreate an air-containing middle ear space and ossicular reconstruction. Most commonly the ET orifice is obliterated or scarred after surgery, and the only option for rehabilitation of the hearing is hearing aids.

Mastoid cavities with remaining tight corners or small air cells within the mastoid tip can become infected. Trapping of moisture, cerumen, and squamous debris within a deep or creviced mastoid cavity or behind a high facial ridge can create optimal conditions for bacterial growth. Infections that are persistent within a mastoid cavity cause chronic drainage, can invade intracranially, and usually require a surgical revision or obliteration of the mastoid cavity. Persistent infections can also indicate recurrence of cholesteatoma, which also requires surgical revision.

Postoperative Dizziness and Hearing Loss

Surgery of the middle ear often involves manipulation of the ossicular chain. Occasionally, a fistula of the lateral semicircular canal is present. Both manipulations of the ossicular chain and of tissues on or near a lateral canal fistula can result in disturbance of the perilymph of the labyrinth and result in postoperative dizziness that can be disabling.

Manipulation of the stapes during stapedectomy can disturb the perilymph of the vestibule and result in postoperative dizziness. The treatment for such postoperative dizziness is bedrest and head elevation for 2 to 5 days. In the case of stapedectomy when the vestibule has been opened, a noninfectious serous labyrinthitis (inflammatory reaction within the inner ear) can develop and cause delayed postoperative dizziness. In these cases a short course of steroids is added to the postoperative regimen and helps to resolve the dizziness. Dizziness immediately after stapedectomy can result if the prosthesis, placed during the procedure, is too long. This dizziness will persist beyond the first postoperative week and often requires reoperation. Careful measurements before placement of the prosthesis are essential in preventing this complication.

The lack of an adequate seal around the stapes prosthesis will result in a persistent postoperative perilymph fistula, with intermittent or continuous vertigo and, possibly, a decline in hearing. Usually, additional bedrest and head elevation will be enough to allow a soft tissue seal to develop, closing the leak. Infections of the middle ear space shortly after stapedectomy are of particular concern because any opening in the footplate puts the patient at risk for both labyrinthitis and meningitis until an adequate seal at the oval window has occurred. Perioperative antibiotics, careful timing of surgery in children, and the placement of oval window tissue seals can help prevent this very serious complication.

Any time surgery is performed on the structures of the ear, the potential for a permanent sensorineural hearing loss exists. Surgery on the oval and round windows such as stapes surgery or surgery for perilymph fistulas carries the highest risk because this surgery occurs at the middle inner ear interface. Surgery for extensive or aggressive cholesteatoma also carries a high risk of hearing loss if a labyrinthine fistula is present. Once an opening into the perilymphatic space is made or discovered during surgery, care must be taken to avoid suctioning of the perilymph from the vestibule. If the vestibule is kept clean of bone dust and cholesteatoma debris and the pressure of the perilymph fluid is not significantly reduced, there is usually no residual affect on the function of the inner ear. Children with inner ear malformations, who undergo stapes surgery, can often have perilymph gushers from the direct effect of CSF pressure on the perilymph. Opening the vestibule in this situation can lead to rapid drops in perilymph pressure, severe dizziness, and permanent profound hearing loss. Obtaining a preoperative CT scan that adequately evaluates the inner ear structures will help the surgeon predict a potential complication. Surgery should be avoided, if possible, in these children.

Postoperative Scarring

Scarring of the middle ear mucosa and fixation of portions of the TM and ossicles can occur in some individuals. This scarring results from abnormal healing of denuded middle ear mucosa. This can be minimized by removing only diseased middle ear mucosa and by placing material, such as absorbable gelatin film or silicone elastomer, between the promontory and the undersurface of the TM. Scarring around the ossicles can be very difficult to prevent in susceptible individuals. Removal of mucosa from the surface of the ossicles can lead to devascularization of these structures and loss of bone mass. The long processes of the incus and the incudostapedial joint are at particular risk for this process. Over time, such devascularization will create bone loss with ossicular discontinuity and an associated conductive hearing loss. Scarring can also occur in the external auditory canal, causing stenosis. Stenosis can prevent adequate visualization of a mastoid cavity, cause accumulation of debris and cerumen in the external canal, and contribute to a conductive hearing loss. We have found the laser particularly useful in removing scars from the external canal safely, while helping to prevent recurrence of the stenosis. Stenosis of the external canal can be prevented by removing conchal cartilage during a meatoplasty (always performed in conjunction with a canal wall down procedure), by the application of permanent sutures to hold the meatal skin open, and by minimizing trauma to the external canal skin during middle ear surgery.

Drainage After Tympanostomy Tubes

Chronic drainage from a tympanostomy tube occurs because of infection of the middle ear mucosa, foreign body reaction to the material of the implant, systemic mucosal disease, or occult cholesteatoma. Drainage that fails to respond to topical antibiotic/antiinflammatory combinations can be due any of these causes. From 6 to 40% of ears with tympanostomy tubes will drain (Balkany et al, 1980; Gates et al, 1986). If not responsive to topical antibiotics, resolution of this problem requires removal of the tube (often with placement of a second tube of alternative material). Metal tubes are often used in cases of refractory drainage. Fluoroplastic tubes have also been shown to resist infection. Occult cholesteatoma must be ruled out with CT scanning when the suspicion is high. Occasionally the tympanostomy tube will become colonized with unusual bacteria that do not respond to topical therapy.

Culture of the drainage will usually identify any persistent microbial, and removal of the existing tympanostomy tube will be necessary to stop the drainage. Care should be taken when considering placing a tympanostomy tube for effusion or conductive hearing loss in the presence of systemic disease. Unless the systemic disease is well controlled, the middle ear mucosa will continue to discharge and the patient will just be trading one problem for another. (See section on mucosal disease.)

Persistent Perforation After Tympanostomy Tubes

Failure of closure of the perforation resulting from tympanostomy tubes is treated like a perforation from any other cause. With observation and water precautions, the perforation can be managed indefinitely, barring other complications (like the development of cholesteatoma). Once surgery is considered, the size and location of the perforation determine the optimal treatment.

Lateralization of the TM

Hearing loss can also occur if the TM lateralizes and separates from the ossicular chain, or prosthesis, as it heals from tympanoplasty. Lateralization of the TM can occur when a large perforation is repaired. Failure to place the graft under the malleus handle during lateral grafting and lack of an appropriate length of the malleus handle remnant lead to lateralized grafts. Grafting of the anterior TM without recreation of the anterior sulcus will also lead to anterior blunting, with an associated air-bone gap. Lateralization can also occur when a short total replacement prosthesis is used or if the prosthesis tips over. Ossicular reconstruction must be redone with a longer prosthesis.

Reoperation

Postoperative infections can be particularly troublesome, resulting in new or recurrent perforation (failed tympanoplasty). Extrusion of the prosthesis, scarring, or thickening of the TM and the development of ET or attic obstruction also contribute to infection and to a persistent conductive hearing loss after surgery with failure of the tympanoplasty.

If the dura of the middle or posterior fossa is injured during mastoid or middle ear surgery, CSF leakage or brain herniation can occur. Most commonly, these rare complications must be treated with corrective surgery. Herniated nonviable brain tissue must be carefully amputated and any openings in the dura repaired. Neurosurgical consultation and involvement in the treatment of such complications is critical to proper handling.

Bleeding

Dehiscence of the vascular structures of the skull base into the middle ear puts these structures at risk during middle ear and mastoid surgery. The carotid canal forms the medial portion of the bony ET and dehiscences of this bone can expose the carotid artery at the ET entry into the middle ear. The carotid artery can become inadvertently injured during probing or packing of the ET, especially during obliteration of the ET for radical mastoidectomy or surgery for glomus tumors. Injury to the carotid artery puts the patient at risk for stroke, future bleeding, and possible death.

The jugular bulb sits in the hypotympanum and is usually covered by bone. Congenital dehiscence; erosion of the covering bone by infection, cholesteatoma, or tumor; and aggressive drilling in the hypotympanum can injure the jugular bulb. Myringotomy in the inferior quadrant of the TM can create a hole in an unrecognized dehiscent jugular bulb. Jugular injuries can cause severe bleeding, clot formation into the lateral sinus with brain edema, and lower cranial neuropathies.

Bleeding is controlled, for both the jugular bulb and the carotid artery, with packing material such as surgical cellulose or thrombin-soaked gelatin foam. This material assists in clot formation. Often further exposure of the carotid artery is needed to maintain control of the bleeding. In severe cases ligation of the vessels may be necessary to control bleeding.

CONCLUSIONS

This chapter has provided the reader with the most commonly used medical and surgical managements of diseases affecting the middle ear. Some of these diseases are poorly understood and research is ongoing to improve the treatment options and aid in prevention. Overuse of antibiotics remains a source of altered strains of pathogens, which are becoming more difficult to treat medically. Surgical treatments are currently the mainstay for most middle ear diseases. Future management will involve improved surgical techniques and newer medical and therapeutic regimens to increase our success in treating these pathological conditions.

REFERENCES

ARMSTRONG, B.W. (1984). Stapes surgery in patients with osteogenesis imperfecta. *Annals of Otology, Rhinology, and Laryngology, 93*;634–635.

BALKANY, T.J., BARKIN, R.M., SUSUKI, B.H., & WATSON, W.J. (1980). A prospective study of infections following tympanostomy tube insertion. *Archives of Otolaryngology, 106*; 645–647.

BALKANY, T.J., & DABS, P.E. (1978). Reversible sudden deafness in early acquired syphilis. *Archives of Otolaryngology, 104*;66–68.

BARNETT, E.D., & KLEIN, J.O. (1995). The problem of resistant bacteria for the management of acute otitis media. *Pediatric Clinics of North America, 42*(3);509–517.

BEKESY, G. VON (1960). *Experiments in hearing.* New York: McGraw-Hill Book Co.

BELAL, A., & STEWART, T.J. (1974). Pathological changes in the middle ear joints. *Annals of Otology, Rhinology and Laryngology, 83*;159–167.

BELLUCCI, R.J. (1981). Congenital aural malformations: Diagnosis and treatment. *Otolaryngology Clinics of North America, 14*;95–124.

BERGUS, G.R., & LOFGREN, M.M. (1998). Tubes, antibiotic prophylaxis, or watchful waiting: A decision analysis for managing recurrent acute otitis media. *Journal of Family Practice, 46*(4);304–310

BROSNAN, M., BURNS, H., JAHN, A.F., & HAWKE, M. (1977). Surgery and histopathology of the stapes in osteogenesis imperfecta tarda. *Archives of Otolaryngology, 103*; 294–298.

CAWTHORNE, T. (1955). Otosclerosis. *Journal of Laryngolology and Otology, 69*;437–456.

CULPEPPER, L. (1997). Routine antibiotic therapy of acute otitis media: Is it necessary? *Journal of the American Medical Association, 278*;1643–1645.

DAMIANI, J.M., DAMIANI, K.K., & KINNEY, F.E. (1979). Malignant external otitis with multiple cranial nerve involvement. *American Journal of Otology, 2*;115–118.

DOBBIN, J.M., & PERKINS, J.H. (1983). Otosyphilis and hearing loss: Response to penicillin and steroid therapy. *Laryngoscope, 93*;1540–1543.

DYER, R.K., & MCELVEEN, J.T. (1991). The patulous eustachian tube: Management options. *Archives of Otolaryngology–Head and Neck Surgery, 105*;832–835.

FALK, B., & MAGNUSON, B. (1994). Eustachian tube closing failure. *Archives of Otolaryngology, 110*;10–14.

FARMER, J.C. (1982). Otologic and paranasal sinus problems in diving. In: P.B. Bennet, & D.H. Elliott (Eds.), *The physiology and medicine of diving* (3rd ed.) (pp. 507–536). London: Baillière Tindall.

FARMER, J.C. (1985). Eustachian tube function and otologic barotrauma in eustachian tube function: Physiology and role in otitis media. *Annals of Otology, Rhinology, and Laryngology, 94*;45–47.

GATES, G.A., AVERY, C., PRIHODA, T.J., & HOLT, G.R. (1986). Post-tympanostomy otorrhea. *Laryngoscope, 96*;630–634.

GRAHAM, M.D., & KNIGHT, P.R. (1981). Atelectatic tympanic membrane reversal by nitrous oxide supplemented general anesthesia and polyethylene ventilation tube insertion. A preliminary report. *Laryngoscope, 91*;1469–1471.

GRISTWOOD, R.E., & VENABLES, W.N. (1983) Pregnancy and otosclerosis. *Clinics in Otolaryngology, 8*(3);205–210.

HANSON, J.R., ANSON. B.J., & STRICKLAND, E.M. (1962). Branchial sources of the auditory ossicles in man. *Archives of Otolaryngology, 76*;200–215.

HEIKKINEN, T., & RUUSKJANEN, O. (1998). Otitis media. *Current Opinion in Pediatrics, 10*(1);9–12.

HUGHES, G.B., & RUTHERFORD, I. (1986). Predictive value of serologic tests for syphilis in otology. *Annals of Otology, Rhinology and Laryngology, 95*;250–259.

JACKSON, C.G., GLASSCOCK, M.E., & HARRIS, P.F. (1982). Glomus tumors: Diagnosis, classification, and management of large lesions. *Archives of Otolaryngology, 108*(7);401–410.

KONEFAL, J.B., PILEPICH, M.V., SPECTOR, G.J., & PEREZ, C.A. (1987). Radiation therapy in the treatment of chemodectomas. *Laryngoscope, 97*(11);1331–1335.

KOSOY, J., & MADDOX, H.E. (1971). Surgical findings in van der Hoeve's syndrome. *Archives of Otolaryngology, 93*;115–122.

LAMBERT, P.R. (1990). Congenital absence of the oval window. *Laryngoscope, 100*(1);37–40.

LARSSON, A. (1960). Otosclerosis: A genetic and clinical study. *Acta Otolaryngologica Supplement (Stockholm), 154*;1–86.

LEGLER, J.D. (1991). An approach to difficult management problems in otitis media in children. *Journal of the American Board of Family Practice, 4*(5);331–339.

MARTINEZ, S.A., & MOONEY, D.F. (1982). Treponemal infections of the head and neck. *Otolaryngology Clinics of North America, 15*;613–620.

MOREANO, E.H., PAPARELLA, M.M., ZELTERMAN, D., & GOYCOOLEA, M.V. (1994). Prevalence of facial canal dehiscence and of persistent stapedial artery in the human middle ear: A report of 1000 temporal bones. *Laryngoscope, 104*(3, part 1);309–320.

NAGER, G.T. (1988). Osteogenesis imperfecta of the temporal bone and its relation to otosclerosis. *Annals of Otology, Rhinology, and Laryngology, 97*;585–593.

OGURA, J.H., SPECTOR, G.J., & GADO, M. (1978). Glomus jugulare and vagale. *Annals of Otology, Rhinology, and Laryngology, 87*;622–629.

PARKIN, J.L. (1981). Familial multiple glomus tumors and pheochromocytomas. *Annals of Otology, Rhinology, and Laryngology, 90*;60–63.

POOLE, M.D. (1998). Declining antibiotic effectiveness in otitis media—A convergence of data. *Ear, Nose and Throat Journal, 77*;444–447.

PULEC, J.C. (1967). Abnormally patent eustachian tubes: Treatment with injection of polytetrafluoroethylene (Teflon) paste. *Laryngoscope, 77*;1543–1554.

RICHTER, E.(1980). Quantitative study of human Scarpa's ganglion and vestibular sensory epithelia. *Acta Otolaryngologica (Stockholm), 90*;199–208.

RICHTER, E., & SCHUKNECHT, H.F. (1982). Loss of vestibular neurons in clinical otosclerosis. *Archives of Otorhinolaryngology, 234*(1);1–9.

ROARK, R., & BERMAN, S. (1997). Continuous twice daily or once daily amoxicillin prophylaxis compared with placebo for children with recurrent acute otitis media. *Pediatric Infectious Disease Journal, 16*(4);376–381.

RÜEDI, L. (1969). Otosclerotic lesion and cochlear degeneration. *Archives of Otolaryngolology, 89*;364–371.

SANDO, I., HEMENWAY, W.G., MILLER, D.R., & BLACK, F.O. (1974). Vestibular pathology in otosclerotic temporal bones: Histopathological report. *Laryngoscope, 84*(4);593–605.

SADE, J., & BERCO, E. (1976). Atelectasis and secretory otitis media. *Annals of Otology, Rhinology and Laryngology, 85*;66–72.

SADE, J., LUNTZ, M., & PITASHNY, R. (1989). Diagnosis and treatment of secretory otitis media. *Otolaryngology Clinics of North America, 22*(1);1–14.

SANDO, I., MYERS, D., HARADA, T., HINOJOSA, R., & MYERS, E.N. (1981). Osteogenesis imperfecta tarda and otosclerosis. A temporal bone histopathological report. *Annals of Otology, Rhinology, and Laryngology, 90*;199–203.

SCHUKNECHT, H.F., & BARBER, W. (1985). Histologic variants in otosclerosis. *Laryngoscope, 95*;1307–1317.

SCHWABER, M.K., GLASSCOCK, M.E., & NISSEN, A.J. (1984). Diagnosis and management of catecholamine secreting glomus tumors. *Laryngoscope, 94*;1008–1015.

SILLENCE, D. (1981). Osteogenesis imperfecta: An expanding panorama of variants. *Clinics in Orthopedics and Related Research, 159*;11–25.

SINGER, D.E., FREEMAN, E., HOFFERT, W.R., KEYS, R.J., MITCHELL, R.B., & HARDY, A.V. (1952). Otitis externa, bacterial and mycological studies. *Annals of Otology, Rhinology, and Laryngology, 61*;317–330.

SPECTOR, G.J., CIRALSKY, G.J., & MAISEL, R.H. (1975). Multiple glomus tumors in the head and neck. *Laryngoscope, 85*;1066–1075.

STOOL, S.E., BERG, A.O., BERMAN, S., CARNEY, C.J., COOLEY, J.R., CULPEPPER, L., EAVEY, R.D., FEAGANS, L.V., FINITZO, T., FRIEDMAN, E.M., GOERTZ, J.A., GOLDSTEIN, A.J., GRUNDFAST, K.M., LONG, D.G., MACCONI, L.L., MELTON, L., ROBERTS, J.E., SHERROD, J.L., & SISK, J.E. (1994). *Otitis media with effusion in young children. Clinical Practice Guidelines, Number 12.* AHCPR Publication No. 94-0622. Rockville, MD: Agency for Health Care Policy and Research, Public Health Service, U.S. Department of Health and Human Services.

TAMARI, M.J., & ITKIN, P. (1951). Penicillin and syphilis of the ear. *Eye Ear Nose Throat Monthly, 30*;252–261,301–309,358–366.

TEELE, D.W., KLEIN, J.O., & ROSSNER, B. (1980). Epidemiology of otitis media in children. *Annals of Otology, Rhinology, and Laryngology, 89*(Suppl. 68);5–6.

TONNDORF, J., & KHANNA, S.M. (1970). The role of the tympanic membrane in middle ear transmission. *Annals of Otology, Rhinology, and Laryngology, 79*;743–753.

VIRTANEN, H., & PALVA, T. (1982). Surgical treatment of patulous eustachian tube. *Archives of Otolaryngology, 108*;735–739.

WAJNBERG, J. (1987). The true shape of the tympanic membrane. *Journal of Laryngology and Otology, 101*(6);538–541.

WEVER, E.G., & LAWRENCE, M. (1954). *Physiological acoustics.* Princeton, NJ: Princeton University Press.

WILLIAMS, R.L., CHALMERS, T.C., STANGE, K.C., CHALMERS, F.T., & BOWLIN, S.J. (1993). Use of antibiotics in preventing recurrent acute otitis media and in treating otitis media with effusion. A meta-analytic attempt to resolve the brouhaha. *JAMA, 270*(11);1344–1351.

ZECHNER, G., & ALTMANN, F. (1969). The temporal bone in leukemia: Histological studies. *Annals of Otology, Rhinology, and Laryngology, 78*;375–387.

PREFERRED PRACTICE GUIDELINES

Professionals Who Perform the Procedure(s)

▼ Team approach

▼ Audiologists

▼ Otolaryngologists and/or otologists

Expected Outcomes

▼ Relief of the symptoms of middle ear disease.

▼ Improvement of conductive hearing loss.

▼ Prevention of the complications of middle ear disease.

▼ Cure of infections.

Clinical Indications

▼ Fullness, pressure, pain, itching, drainage, hearing loss, dizziness, tinnitus.

▼ Incidental effusion, conductive hearing loss, or TM abnormality.

Clinical Process

▼ Referral to otolaryngologist or otologist and audiology team.

▼ Clinical evaluation.

▼ Audiological evaluation.

▼ Imaging studies, where appropriate.

▼ Blood testing, where appropriate.

▼ Referrals to primary care or other specialists, when appropriate.

▼ Medical management and surgical options discussed with patient.

▼ Treatment plan formulated and modified on the basis of the patient's response.

▼ Follow-up.

Documentation

▼ Medical history.

▼ Audiometric evaluation, reflex testing, tympanogram.

▼ Pneumatic otoscopic examination, microscopic examination, where appropriate.

▼ Complete head and neck examination.

▼ Imaging studies.

▼ Response to treatment documented in the chart.

Chapter 10

Medical and Surgical Treatment of Neural Hearing Loss

J. Gail Neely and Mark S. Wallace

Outline

Introduction
Red Flags in a Busy Office Practice
Diseases Causing Neural Hearing Losses
Medical and Surgical Treatment of Specific Diseases Causing Neural Hearing Loss
  Lesions Detectable by Imaging
  Lesions Not Detectable by Imaging
Conclusions
References
Preferred Practice Guidelines

INTRODUCTION

Neural hearing loss is defined in this chapter as any audiometric evidence of a lesion referable to the eighth nerve or low brain stem. "Lesion" is defined as any anatomical or physiological deviation from normal. Because the human cost is so great; false positive results are tolerated much better than false negative results. Even the slightest hint of a neural lesion must be evaluated; neural lesions are not often purely neural.

To understand how diseases of the ear might cause neural hearing loss and possible lesions of other proximate nerves and of the conductive system of the middle ear, a brief review of the relevant anatomy may help. Looking at the anatomy like a surgeon might in planning an approach to a lesion, the ghosted outline of the labyrinth and the facial nerve are seen anterior to the sigmoid sinus, and the posterior aspect of the jaw joint is seen to be the anterior wall of the external auditory canal. The floor of the middle cranial fossa forms the roof of the jaw joint, middle ear, and mastoid. Surgical approaches may go anterior to the sigmoid sinus, through the mastoid, and around the labyrinth into the posterior fossa, a retrolabyrinthine approach, or may go above the labyrinth into the middle fossa and subsequently into the posterior fossa by means of a middle fossa approach. The posterior fossa may also be reached by going through the labyrinth and, at times, the cochlea, in a translabyrinthine or transcochlear approach, respectively. The posterior fossa may be approached posterior to the sigmoid sinus in a retrosigmoid or suboccipital approach (Fig. 10–1).

Looking at the skull base with the calvarium (top of the skull) and the brain removed, cranial nerves V through XII are seen to course through or about the temporal bones, which form most of the lateral walls of the posterior fossa and much of the middle fossa (Fig. 10–2).

A posterolateral view with the bone removed shows the intimate relationship of the cochlea, vestibular labyrinth, eighth nerve, and facial nerve with each other and the other

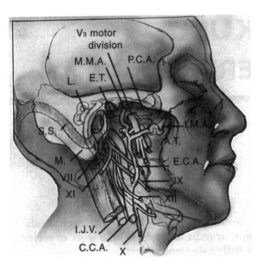

P.C.A. - Petrous Cartoid a.
M.M.A. - Middle Meningeal a.
I.M.A. - Internal Maxillary a.
A.T. - Auriculo-temporal n.
E.C.A. - External Cartoid a.
XI - Accessory n.
IX - Glossopharyngeal
X - Vagus n.
C.C.A. - Common Cartoid a.
I.J.V. - Int. Jugular v.
VII - Facial n.
M. - Mastoid
S.S - Sigmoid sinus
L. - Labyrinth
E.T. - Eustacian tube
XII Hypoglossal n.

Figure 10–1 Artist's illustration of a lateral skull base view with surface landmarks and ghosted deep anatomy. (From Pensak [1997], with permission.)

Audiology: Treatment. Edited by Valente, Hosford-Dunn, and Roeser. Thieme Medical Publishers, Inc., New York © 2000

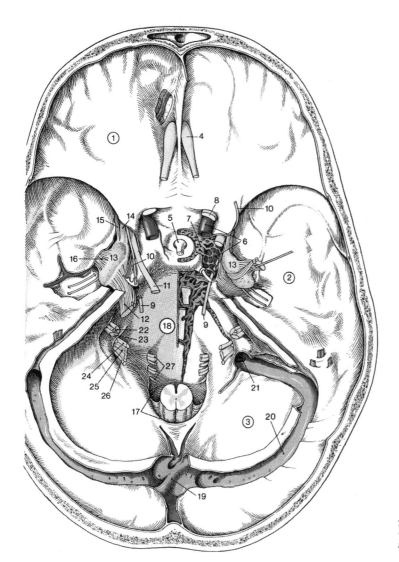

Figure 10–2 Illustration of skull base seen from above. (From Roeser [1996], with permission.)

nerves, cerebellum, pons, and medulla oblongata (Fig. 10–3).

In Figure 10–4, a drawing graphically illustrates how the facial nerve is intimately related to all parts of the ear, the posterior fossa internal auditory canal, the labyrinth, the middle ear by the stapes, and the mastoid. In Figure 10–5, a facial recess approach from the mastoid to the middle ear and from the middle fossa to the middle ear along the facial nerve are illustrated; the facial nerve is a surgical landmark in most surgical approaches to the temporal bone. A closer view of the relationship of the facial nerve to the stapes is seen in Figure 10–6.

These patients may have minimal-to-profound auditory, vestibular, or facial motor complaints. They may, and often do, present with conductive hearing loss with or without middle ear effusion. For example, a patient may demonstrate perfectly normal pure tone thresholds and word recognition but show reflex decay or elevated reflex thresholds at 500 Hz along the afferent limb of the reflex arc, or they might show normal pure tone thresholds, speech and impedance audiometry, but a delay of only wave V on auditory brain stem audiometry (ABR) ipsilateral to subjective tinnitus. These two examples are real patient presentations; each had large

solitary vestibular schwannomas with brain stem compression. A patient may have middle effusion and a mild neural hearing loss and have a large petroclival meningioma. Or a patient might have bilateral moderate-to-severe noise-induced hearing loss for which he or she has regularly been followed and fitted with hearing aids for 20 years; later, a mild progressive difference in the word recognition scores may be discovered in one ear without any change in pure tone thresholds. This patient was found to have a 2-cm solitary vestibular schwannoma on that side.

The primary focus of medical audiology is to determine the site and the degree of each independent lesion affecting the auditory system and to monitor those lesions throughout the course of the disease. Conductive or long-standing sensory hearing losses do not immunize the patient from a host of serious illnesses capable of causing a superimposed neural hearing loss.

Repeated measurements of all the audiometric parameters, important in the initial diagnosis, are always required to accurately assess the clinical course of the disease for diagnostic confirmation, management planning, disease, and therapeutic monitoring. In the management of complex otological

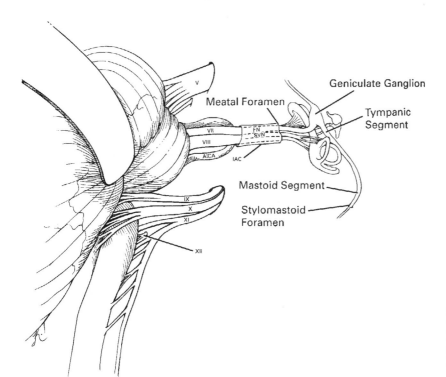

Figure 10–3 Artist's illustration of a posterolateral view of posterior fossa showing cranial nerves V to XII. (From Rubinstein et al [1997], with permission.)

and neurotological cases, it is a serious error to failure to obtain a full audiogram, including speech thresholds, word recognition, and impedance audiometry with the full array of reflex measures in both the contralateral and ipsilateral conditions for both ears and reflex decay assessment throughout the clinical course. Any of these variables may change independently and can have major implications on the progressive or retrogressive pathophysiology of the disease.

Professionally skilled medical audiologists are crucial partners with medical specialists, knowledgeable about ear diseases, for the diagnosis and for monitoring the medical and surgical management of the neurotological patient; every patient with a hearing loss is, or can become, a neurotological patient.

PEARL

The primary objective of an audiological assessment is to determine the site of lesions within the auditory system and the degree to which they are involved. To do this, a full audiogram, including speech and impedance audiometry, is required initially and again every time audiological assessment is clinically necessary.

RED FLAGS IN A BUSY OFFICE PRACTICE

The following are a few "red flags" that may occur in a busy practice that may alert the audiologist to a serious problem. Some of the "red flags" that can occur are seen in Table 10–1. These are some of the more common ones and are presented as helpful hints in a busy practice. However, the way to understand and to evaluate these patients is to have a thorough

---

PITFALL

On repeat testing during the clinical course of the disease, it is a serious error to obtain only pure tone thresholds. Each audiometric variable can change independent of the others; this can have important medical implications.

---

knowledge of the anatomy and the physiology of these integrated systems and be ever vigilant to identify the slightest deviation from normal and to triangulate all the signs and symptoms to one site of lesion capable of explaining them all. Later confirmation requires special tests designed to specifically prove the lesion. Slight deviations from the expected clinical course of simple, uncomplicated, common diseases are often the only clue that a serious problem exists or has arisen.

PEARL

Minimal, subtle, or transient signs and symptoms, with recovery, do not mean the lesion is gone or that is not serious.

DISEASES CAUSING NEURAL HEARING LOSSES

This chapter is organized into the following diseases visible on imaging studies:

Bone diseases of adjacent bone
    Paget's disease

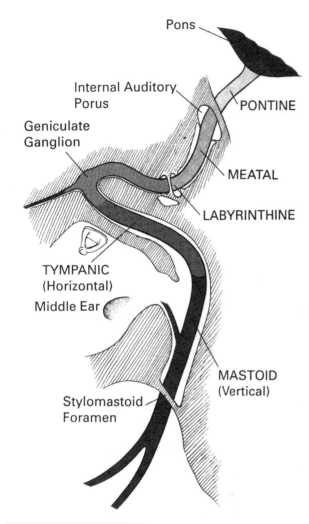

Pons

Internal Auditory
Porus

PONTINE

Geniculate
Ganglion

MEATAL

LABYRINTHINE

TYMPANIC
(Horizontal)

Middle Ear

MASTOID
(Vertical)

Stylomastoid
Foramen

Figure 10–4 Graphic illustration of the intratemporal course of the facial nerve. (From Gulya [1997], with permission.)

Osteopetroses
Monostotic fibrous dysplasia
Growths or neoplasia of the primary neural tissues or adjacent tissues
    Solitary vestibular schwannomas (acoustic neuromas)
    Neurofibromatosis II (NF2)
    Facial nerve schwannomas
    Fifth nerve schwannomas
    Meningiomas
    Cholesteatomas (epidermoids) of the deep petrous bone
      or meninges
    Petrous cholesterol granulomas
    Chondromas and chondrosarcomas
    Chordomas
    Jugulotympanic paragangliomas (glomus tumors)
    Jugular foramen schwannomas
    Brain stem gliomas
    Primary or metastatic malignancies of the temporal bone
Trauma
    Temporal bone fractures
Vascular lesions
    Vascular loop compression

Aneurysms
Stroke
Diseases that do not create a discrete anatomical lesion detectable on imaging but are definable by history and special laboratory tests follow.

Aging/neural degenerative diseases
    Neural presbycusis
    Cranial neuropathies
    Primary cochlear neuron degeneration
    Secondary cochlear neuron degeneration
    Leukodystrophies
    Multiple sclerosis
Collagen/immunological/allergic diseases
    Polyarteritis nodosa
    Rheumatoid arthritis
    Wegner's granulomatosis
    Cogan's syndrome
    Vogt-Koyanagi-Harada syndrome
    Relapsing polychondritis
    Giant cell arteritis
    AIDS
    Paraneoplastic neuropathy
    Lymphomatoid granulomatosis
    Sarcoidosis
    Systemic lupus erythematosus
Inflammatory/infectious diseases
    Intracranial complications of suppurative otitis media
    Meningitis, bacterial
    Mycoplasma and viral infections
    Fungal infections
    Syphilis
    Lyme disease
Developmental/genetic/congenital diseases
    Congenital syndromes with hereditary hearing loss
    Nonsyndromic hereditary hearing losses
    Prenatal and perinatal noxious events
Idiopathic diseases

The imaging studies most often used are computed tomography (CT), magnetic resonance imaging (MRI), magnetic resonance angiography (MRA), conventional angiography, and conventional radiography of the skull or chest. CT is used when looking at bone is the primary concern. MRI is predominantly useful to look at the nerves and brain without bone obscuring the view. MRA is used to look at large arteries and venous sinuses. Conventional angiography is required when a detailed look at the vessels is needed. Standard radiographs are still useful to look at the skull and the chest; a number of diseases, for example, tuberculosis, sarcoidosis, and Wegner's granulomatosis, may affect the lungs and the auditory system.

Special laboratory tests often used are noninvasive and electrophysiological tests of cardiac and vascular function; cultures or serological tests for viral, spirochetal, rickettsial, bacterial, or deep fungal infections; blood tests for function of the immune systems, metabolic systems, hemapoietic system; and toxicological tests. Physiological tests of other systems are sometimes also required, such as the vestibular system, the visual system, and the renal system.

Diagnostic tests are either anatomically based, meaning they are designed to look at distortions of anatomy, or

Facial Recess Approach

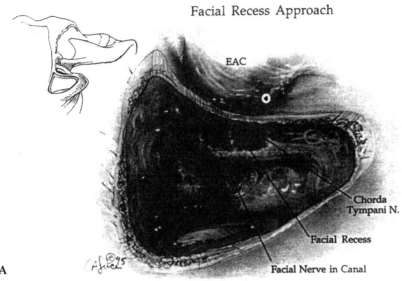

EAC

Chorda Tympani N.

Facial Recess

Facial Nerve in Canal

A

Middle Fossa Approach

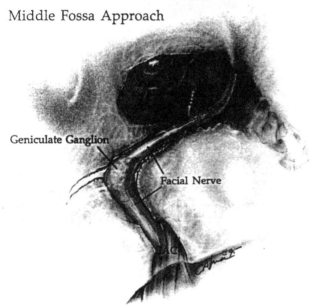

Geniculate Ganglion

Facial Nerve

B

Figure 10–5 **(A)** Diagram of the facial recess approach from the mastoid to the middle ear and **(B)** middle fossa exposure of the facial nerve in the labyrinthine and tympanic segments. (From Huang & Lambert [1997], with permission.)

physiologically based, designed to look at the physiology of a system or region. It takes both kinds of tests, combined, to fully identify the disease and its extent. The history, taken by a physician with depth of knowledge in the systems involved, remains the most important single tool for diagnosis. The audiologist is a crucial partner in this venture because of their expertise in accurately defining the site and degree of specific independent lesions within the auditory system. The first question in diagnosis is, Where is the lesion?

Each symptom or sign is defined as a three-dimensional object in space on its separate time line; the duration of each episode and frequency of occurrence is mentally graphed on the x axis, the intensity is graphed on the y axis, and the quality is graphed on the z axis. Patterns of aggregates of signs and symptoms are then compared with known patterns of specific diseases. When a match is found, a new diagnostic menu is generated to explore the specific diseases that can match that exact scenario. Ultimately, by the use of this technique and by filtering it with an in-depth knowledge of the anatomy and physiology of the systems involved, a diagnostic impression is

formulated, which contains a differential diagnostic list in which each disease must be confirmed or rejected.

The clinical course during treatment is also a vital part of the process of confirmation and surveillance to ensure resolution of the disease and to ensure no new diseases arise without detection.

MEDICAL AND SURGICAL TREATMENT OF SPECIFIC DISEASES CAUSING NEURAL HEARING LOSS

Lesions Detectable by Imaging

Bone Diseases of Adjacent Bone

Paget's Disease

Paget's disease is a autosomal dominant polyostotic (meaning more than one separate bone) bone disease of laminar

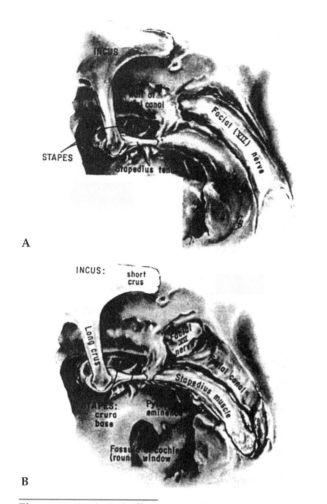

A

B

Figure 10–6   Artist's illustration of the facial nerve in relation to the stapes and stapedial muscle **(B)** and tendon **(A)**. (From Arts [1997], with permission.)

bone of the neurocranium, sacrum, spine, pelvis, femur, and tibia. It deforms the local architecture by progressive osteoclastic osteolytic (meaning bone destruction by special cells adjacent to bone called osteoclasts) bone resorption and replacement with fibrous and vascular tissue, followed by osteoblastic (special cells adjacent to bone that build bone) new bone formation, which creates a mosaic pattern of an excess, but weak, bony mass.

Conductive and sensory hearing loss are far more common than neural hearing loss. The cause of these losses is not clear; obliteration of the round window niche with fibrous tissue or with a markedly enlarged jugular bulb and sigmoid sinus may be implicated. Bony distortions of the skull base can result in basilar impressions, resulting in vertebrobasilar ischemia (under perfusion of tissues), compression of cranial nerves, or cerebral or cerebellar dysfunction (Schuknecht, 1993a).

Treatment is predominantly medical by calcitonin, sodium etidronate, mithramycin, or the combination of calcitonin and sodium etidronate. The objective of treatment is to arrest progression of the disease and symptoms. Surgery can be hazardous and ineffective, except in few select cases (Cheung & Jackler, 1994).

Osteosarcoma, fibrosarcoma, or giant cell tumor transformation can arise from a Paget's lesion (Cheung & Jackler, 1994). A rapid or unusual change in symptoms causing pain, pathological fractures, or bone enlargement should alert the caregiver to this possibility.

Osteopetroses

Osteopetroses are a group of hereditary metabolic bone diseases generally classified, by time of clinical onset and clinical course, into a congenital (early onset), or lethal, form and a tarda (delayed onset), or adult form; the former is transmitted in an autosomal recessive fashion and the later is autosomal dominant, except *Albers-Schönberg disease*, which is autosomal recessive. The tarda form may involve all the skull, type I, such as *Engleman's disease*, or only the skull base, type II (Cheung & Jackler, 1994).

The disease obliterates spaces and foramina (anatomical holes or passages in bone), resulting in compression neuropathies and conductive and neural hearing losses.

Medical treatment is ineffective; surgical intervention can be helpful. Reconstruction of the external earcanal, middle ear space, and ossicular reconstruction can be useful. Facial nerve decompression can be effective to avoid progressive or recurrent paralysis; decompression of the internal auditory canal might be effective in stabilizing neural hearing losses but remains to be proven (Cheung & Jackler, 1994).

Monostotic Fibrous Dysplasia

Fibrous dysplasia is a progressive bone disease of uncertain cause in which marrow and bony septae are replaced by fibro-osseous proliferation in which osteoblastic and osteoclastic activity abound. Fibrous dysplasia may be classified into polyostotic and monostotic (affecting only one bone) forms; the monostotic form is the one that may involve the temporal bone (Schuknecht, 1993a).

These lesions must be differentiated from bone lesions resulting from hyperparathyroidism by blood chemistry tests showing normal serum levels of calcium, phosphorus, and alkaline phosphatase.

Conductive hearing loss, from stenosis of the external auditory canal, with or without an entrapped canal cholesteatoma, and cosmetic deformity from a laterally expanding temporal bone are the predominant symptoms and signs from monostotic fibrous dysplasia. Sensorineural hearing loss is unusual.

No medical treatment exists for this disease; surgery is the only effective intervention, when necessary to open the external auditory canal or to resculpture the lateral temporal bone for cosmesis. Surgical decompression of the internal auditory canal or facial nerve is theoretically useful, but yet to be proven (Cheung & Jackler, 1994).

Because neural compression is unusual, if nerve compression or pain were to begin to occur in an established case, malignant transformation to osteosarcoma, fibrosarcoma, or chondrosarcoma should be considered. By the same token, if a patient with fibrous dysplasia were to begin to complain of pulmonary symptoms, lung metastasis should be ruled out because these unusual malignancies frequently metastasize to the lungs.

TABLE 10–1 "Red flags" indicating a potentially serious problem

"Red Flag"	Explanation
An audiometric retrocochlear finding that seems to have spontaneously resolved	Serious things can get better without disappearing.
A chronically draining ear with fever or pain	Such ears rarely present this way unless a complication or cancer is present.
A nose that runs unilaterally	Unilateral rhinorrhea may indicate a foreign body, severe infection, cancer, or a cerebrospinal leak.
Reduced ability to attend or inconsistent results	Serious developmental, psychiatric, cardiovascular, pulmonary, renal, central nervous system disease, drug or alcohol abuse, or dangerously excessive medication can present this way.
Minimal or no hearing loss with subtle retrocochlear signs	Little correlation exists between tumor size and hearing loss; any retrocochlear sign is too much.
Long duration, circumstantially "explained," hearing loss that has not been medically evaluated	It is not unusual for large benign tumors to exist and slowly and progressively enlarge without changing the pure tone thresholds in moderate to profoundly affected ears; this has been observed to occur in long persistent, nonprogressive mild losses as well.
Asymmetrical pure tone thresholds, unilateral tinnitus, or asymmetrical word recognition scores	Very subtle asymmetries may be the only presentation of serious disease; ABR or imaging is usually necessary to resolve the issue. The size of the lesion does not have to correlate with the audiometric dysfunction. Evidence is increasing that ABR may give false-negative results in some of these lesions.
Facial paralysis or twitching	All facial paralysis is not Bell's palsy; tumors, infections, and trauma may present this way with little other signs or symptoms. Bell's palsy, per se, is treatable for better outcome if seen very early.
A child that complains of dizziness	Children are not often dizzy, especially when they lie down. Brain stem gliomas may initially present with only this symptom. Children may have other treatable, or dangerous, causes of dizziness similar to adults.
Hoarseness persisting for 2 weeks or that frequently recurs	Base of skull or other discrete or systemic lesions capable of causing neural hearing loss may initially have hoarseness; a good example is the glomus jugulare tumor extending along the tenth nerve into the posterior fossa.
Retro-orbital pain behind one eye	Such pain tends to come from deep orbital or petroclival infections or tumors that may or may not be associated with neural hearing loss, but are urgently serious.
Double vision or diplopia	A host of petrous apex, neural, or brain stem lesions may present this way.

(continued)

TABLE 10–1 (continued) "Red flags" indicating a potentially serious problem

"Red Flag"	Explanation
Anyone less than the age of 40 presenting with the slightest eighth nerve finding	Young people may have large bilateral acoustic tumors and many other neurofibromas and meningiomas intracranially and within their spine, characteristic of NF2, and present only with the slightest hearing loss.
Persistent or frequent headaches, especially severe ones and those that awaken the patient	Headaches that awaken a patient are associated with a high incidence of intracranial pathological findings.
An unusually dark hue to the middle ear	A high-lying jugular fossa, dehiscent of bone, or blood behind the eardrum from a base of skull fracture present this way.
Unilateral ear infections or unilateral serous otitis media	Acute, recurrent otitis media or chronic serous otitis media are usually bilateral; when these occur unilaterally, it is imperative to investigate the nasopharynx and petrous apex for the presence of nasopharyngeal cancer, petrous apex tumors, or occult cholesteatomas. These will often not be otherwise apparent.
Unsteady gait, ataxia	Ataxia is not caused by inner ear disease; the brain or spinal cord is implicated. Even when the patient is severely vertiginous, off balance, and deviating to the involved side, this passes and persistent ataxia does not occur.
Rapidly progressive losses over weeks, months, or 2 years	Such losses are dangerous if proven to be neural and often reversible if proven to be sensory.
Vague symptoms of dizziness or an off-balance feeling	Most of the time these symptoms are not associated with serious disease; however, these symptoms associated with a neural hearing loss are often from dangerous disease.
Falling down or passing out (becoming unconscious), with or without dizziness	Inner ear problems do not make people fall down, with the rare exception of the otolithic crisis of Tumarkin, or pass out. These signs are usually from cardiovascular or central nervous system disease.

SPECIAL CONSIDERATION

Some bone diseases can, on rare occasions, undergo malignant transformation. If you are following a case of a defined bone disease and the patient shares with you that an area of bone seems to be expanding or has become painful, immediate investigation, which may require biopsy, is indicated.

CONTROVERSIAL POINT

Hearing conservation surgery may increase the risk of incomplete tumor removal. If incomplete removal does happen, is that important?

Growths or Neoplasia of the Primary Neural Tissues or Adjacent Tissues

Solitary Vestibular Schwannomas ("Acoustic Neuromas")

Schwannomas, also known as neurinomas or neurilemmomas, originate from Schwann cells comprising the neurilemmal, rather than the glial, portion of cranial and peripheral nerves. Common usage, albeit erroneous, has led to the terms *acoustic neuromas* or *acoustic tumors*. Eighth nerve schwannomas arise within the vestibular nerve and expand within the trunk of the eighth nerve and its branches in all directions, destroying some fibers, infiltrating between others, encasing some fibers in the peripheral substance of the tumor mass, and dispersing and displacing other fibers on the surface of the tumor in large or very small aggregates. Because of this pathobiology, excellent function can be maintained even in very large tumors (Gulya, 1994; Neely, 1981). Figures 10–7 and 10–8 demonstrate small and large solitary vestibular schwannomas and the value of gadolinium-enhanced MRI to detect these tumors.

Treatment of these tumors is predominantly by surgical removal. In certain cases, however, such as in small tumors in elderly or medically unstable patients, tumors are followed without treatment for years, until death occurs from other causes or the tumor grows in such a way to make intervention mandatory, such as emerging hydrocephalus. The long-term efficacy and safety of highly focused radiation, gamma knife, to control the growth of these tumors is currently being explored as an alternative intervention; the disadvantages of this modality are the persistence of the tumor mass, the potential for facial and cochleovestibular nerve deterioration, and the uncertainty of control (meaning the tumor is still visibly present, and it is uncertain when or if it will break through the treatment and begin to grow again).

Three surgical approaches are appropriate for tumors of any size, large or small; the approach primarily depends on the surgical objective and the experience of the surgeon. *Middle fossa approaches* and *retrosigmoid, retrolabyrinthine approaches* are usually used for hearing conservation. *Translabyrinthine or the extended transcochlear approaches* are used when hearing conservation is not a feasible objective; the advantage of these approaches is that bone alone is removed to expose the tumor and identify the facial nerve, rather than brain displacement or removal.

Hearing conservation is potentially feasible in small tumors (questionably, the total medial to lateral length of 1.5 cm, including the intracanalicular portion) with good auditory function (arguably, pure tone average of 50 dB HL or

better, and word recognition of 50% or better); the disadvantage of attempting to save hearing is the potential for leaving tumor behind, which might regrow into a significantly large tumor. The cochlear nerve may not be definable, even when preoperative function is excellent (pure tone average 30 dB HL or better and word recognition scores of 80% or better). Albeit, sparing the cochlear nerve anatomically is far easier than sparing its function. The vascular supply to the cochlear nerve and cochlea is very tenuous and runs in the plane between the tumor and any remaining portion of the cochlear nerve; dissection on the nerve itself, which is the way to be sure that all the tumor is removed, usually destroys this vascular supply. Thus sparing hearing usually requires saving a thin layer of nonspecific tissue over the cochlear nerve; this layer may easily contain tumor (Neely, 1984). Intraoperative monitoring is crucial for the delicate management of this nerve and vascular supply.

Vestibular dysfunction is always present in these tumors; however, stimulated responses from the superior division of the vestibular nerve may be quite normal. Resection of these tumors almost always requires resection of the complete vestibular nerve. If little vestibular function remains preoperatively, little if any vertigo or imbalance occurs postoperatively. On the other hand, if reasonably good vestibular function exists preoperatively, the patient may have spontaneous vertigo for several days, positional vertigo for several weeks, and some sense of instability for a few months. Vestibular compensation, however, is usually very rapid and complete in a matter of a few weeks. Vestibular exercises emphasizing movement of the head on the neck and early ambulation are very important for rapid recovery.

The primary objectives of surgical resection are to completely remove the tumor and to spare the anatomy and function of the facial nerve. The facial nerve is displaced about the circumference of the tumor, often markedly lengthened, and always flattened into a thin ribbon. Dissection along the facial nerve-tumor interface can be relatively easy or extremely difficult, even in small tumors, depending on the degree to which the tumor shares vessels with the tumor and the degree to which it is attached to the tumor by fibrous bands; currently, this interface can not be determined preoperatively. The initial postoperative function of the facial nerve predominantly depends on tumor size and the tumor-nerve interface; ultimate facial function can be very good, even if immediately postoperatively the face is paralyzed. Intraoperative monitoring is crucial for the delicate management of this nerve. It is unusual for the facial nerve to be infiltrated by tumor; however, this can happen. If any preoperative facial dysfunction is present and if the tumor is a vestibular schwannoma, the nerve is invaded and cannot be saved; if the nerve is preoperatively normal, the odds are very high that the nerve can be spared (Neely & Neblett, 1983).

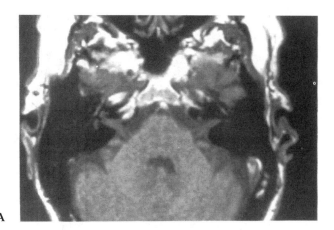
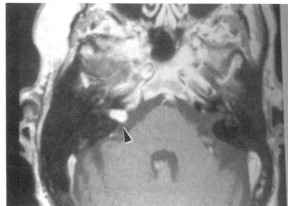

A

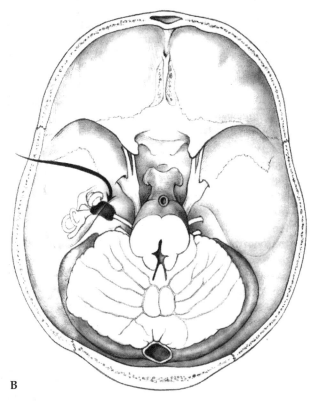

B

Figure 10–7 **(A)** MRI without contrast and with contrast, gadolinium, showing a small right intracanalicular solitary vestibular schwannoma; **(B)** the illustration shows the tumor drawn on the left for easy comparison with the MRI, which by convention, shows the patient's right side on the examiner's left. (From Lustig & Jackler [1997], with permission.)

Neurofibromatosis II

Hereditary bilateral vestibular schwannoma syndrome, or neurofibromatosis type 2 (NF2), once called "central neurofibromatosis," is an uncommon autosomal dominant disorder, transmitted on chromosome 22, presenting with bilateral acoustic tumors. Neurofibromatosis type 1 (NF1), once called "peripheral neurofibromatosis" of von Recklinghausen, is a more common autosomal dominant disorder, also transmitted on chromosome 22, but does not have acoustic tumors. NF2 patients frequently have multiple other brain and spinal cord tumors, such as meningiomas, multiple cranial and spinal nerve schwannomas, ependymomas, astrocytomas, cataracts, and some cutaneous neurofibromas; any or all of these may be occult and without symptoms. Anyone younger than the age of 40 with an "acoustic neuroma" is suspect for NF2 and should have an ophthalmological examination and be considered for full head and spine MRI with gadolinium

enhancement. Family members should also be considered at risk (Miyamoto et al, 1994).

NF2 vestibular schwannomas, compared with solitary vestibular schwannomas, may be much larger before symptoms are manifest, multicentric, more infiltrative of the eighth and of the seventh nerve, more expansive of the internal auditory canal, and more invasive of air cells and marrow spaces (Gulya, 1994). Figure 10–9 illustrates bilateral tumors in a young adult.

Treatment, like for the solitary vestibular schwannomas, is predominantly surgical with the initial approach directed at any life-threatening problems. Because of the tumor characteristics, hearing conservation with total tumor removal may be impossible, even in small tumors. Because all schwannomas have an unpredictable growth rate, some enlarging rapidly, when to operate on these particular cases and whether to attempt total tumor removal is a serious consideration in each case. If some cochlear nerve can be spared, cochlear

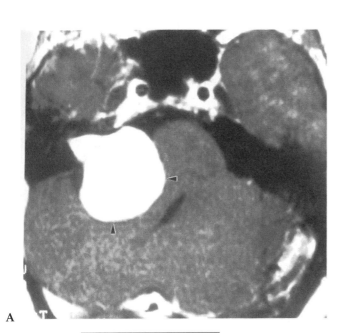

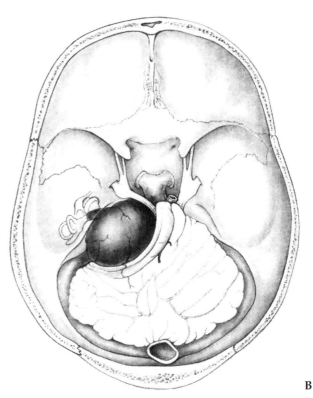

Figure 10–8 **(A)** MRI with contrast, gadolinium, showing a large solitary vestibular schwannoma; **(B)** the illustration shows the tumor drawn on the left for easy comparison with the MRI, which by convention, shows the patient's right side on the examiner's left. (From Lustig & Jackler [1997], with permission.)

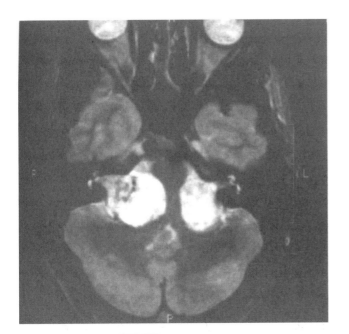

Figure 10–9 MRI with gadolinium, showing bilateral vestibular schwannomas in a young adult with NF2. (From Roland & Marple [1997], with permission.)

implantation can be considered at the risk of tumor recurrence. Brain stem auditory implantation may offer an additional option in selected cases (Miyamoto et al, 1994).

CONTROVERSIAL POINT

Because bilateral neurofibromas of the eighth nerve almost invariably lead to bilateral profound sensorineural hearing loss either from the disease or its treatment and because a few isolated cases of successful tumor removal or stabilization with irradiation with hearing conservation, when and how to intervene in NF2 remains challenging and controversial.

Facial Nerve Schwannomas

Schwannomas of the facial nerve (seventh cranial nerve) are much less common than schwannomas of the eighth nerve and may occur anywhere along the nerve from the intracranial segment to the distal branches in the parotid gland. Progressive facial paresis (partial paralysis) or paralysis is a common symptom; however, they may cause no paralysis or present as sudden-onset "Bell's palsy" and actually recover completely or partially. They can present as middle or external auditory canal masses, looking very much like a cholesteatoma. In the internal auditory canal they may present as an acoustic tumor and in the face they may present as a parotid mass; however, they often occur at the area of the geniculate ganglion and can extend "dumbbell-like" into the middle and posterior fossa through the petrous apex. These can present as a conductive hearing loss from impingement on the medial surface of the ossicular chain, easily misdiagnosed as otosclerosis (Neely & Alford, 1974).

Because any manipulation of the tumor usually results in a complete facial paralysis, usually requiring a nerve graft to restore function, treatment is a delicate balance between the degree of current facial paralysis, the expected outcome from a nerve graft, the fact that many nerve fibers may be destroyed before even mild paresis is seen, and effectiveness of nerve grafts depend on restoration of function within 2 years of denervation. Resection of the tumor with a restorative graft, which may take 1 year for maximal function, may be approached transmastoid, transmastoid-extradural middle fossa, translabyrinthine, transmastoid-parotid, or parotid depending on the location and extent of the tumor. Watchful waiting is very appropriate in some cases (O'Donoghue, 1994). Focused high-intensity irradiation, gamma knife, is being evaluated currently; the long-term effects of this approach have yet to be well established.

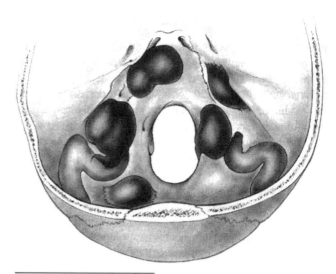

Figure 10–10 Artist's illustration showing common locations of meningiomas that are associated with the temporal bone. (From Lustig & Jackler [1997], with permission.)

CONTROVERSIAL POINT

Because even the slightest manipulations of these tumors can result in total facial paralysis and a poor outcome, even with nerve grafting, and because the longer a partial paralysis exists, the poorer the outcome with grafting, when to intervene in facial nerve schwannomas is controversial.

Fifth Nerve (Trigeminal) Schwannomas

Fifth nerve schwannomas are rare. They are usually solitary; however, they may be associated with other schwannomas, such as in NF2, and, in contrast to seventh and eighth nerve schwannomas, may rarely be malignant. Because of the possibility of malignancy, special immunohistochemical staining of the surgical specimen is necessary (Shaw & Fisch, 1994).

These tumors may be asymptomatic, incidentally discovered, or may present with trigeminal facial pain, paresthesias (unusual sensations, like tingling or burning), and numbness. They often begin in the sensory ganglion but may involve the motor fibers for mastication (chewing) and extend into the middle fossa, posterior fossa, or both; in doing so they may cause ophthalmoplegia (paralysis of the nerves that control eyeball movement) or eighth nerve dysfunction.

Treatment, like for most schwannomas, is surgical resection. A subtemporal, intradural approach or large postauricular (type C) or preauricular (type D) infratemporal fossa approach to the paracavernous, petrous apex, and posterior fossa clival region is usually required, depending on the site and extent of lesion. The type C approach usually requires obliteration of the middle ear and oversewing of the external auditory canal. The objective of the infratemporal fossa approaches is to obtain a more lateral view with less brain retraction (Post & McCormick, 1996; Shaw & Fisch, 1994).

Meningiomas

Meningiomas arise from arachnoid meningothelial cells in a variety of intracranial locations and are usually benign. Four

characteristic locations from which meningiomas arise relative to the temporal bone are (1) internal auditory canal, (2) jugular foramen, (3) geniculate ganglion, and (4) greater and lesser petrosal nerves (Nager, 1993a) (Fig. 10–10). They are usually globular, encapsulated tumors tightly adherent and invasive of dura but not of brain and often highly vascular from the adjacent dural vascular supply. However the papillary type, occurring in younger people, is aggressive and, because of its propensity to invade brain and metastasize, is considered malignant. Malignant meningiomas do occur and often show malignant characteristics histologically; however, brain invasion or metastasis can occur without histologically malignant-looking lesions. Immunohistochemistry (special immunological staining of histological tissue preparations after the tumor has been removed) is important to differentiate tissue types and benign from malignant (Haddad & Al-Mefty, 1996a).

Posterior fossa, or infratentorial, meningiomas may be subdivided into six groups according to location: (1) petroclival, (2) cerebellopontine angle, (3) cerebellar convexity, (4) fourth ventricle, (5) foramen magnum, and (6) jugular foramen (Haddad & Al-Mefty, 1996b). Any of these meningiomas may mimic vestibular schwannomas by direct impingement on or by distortion of the eighth nerve, or they may occur simultaneously with NF2 bilateral eighth nerve schwannomas. Those most often associated with eighth nerve signs are the cerebellopontine angle group, which are differentiated from the petroclival group by their relative position to the fifth nerve. Petroclival meningiomas are anteromedial to the fifth nerve, and cerebellopontine angle meningiomas are posterolateral to it. The cerebellopontine angle group can be divided into two subgroups by their relative position to the seventh and eighth nerves: the medial subgroup (anteromedial to VII and VIII) and the lateral subgroup (posterolateral to VII and VIII) (Glasscock et al, 1994; Haddad & Al-Mefty, 1996b). Those directly involving the eighth nerve are easiest to suspect because they

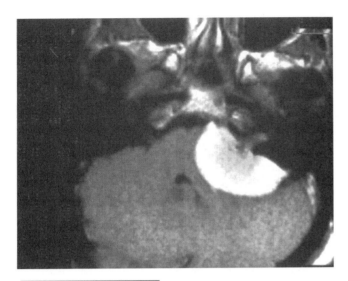

Figure 10–11 MRI with gadolinium, showing a large left cerebellopontine angle meningioma. (From Roland & Marple [1997], with permission.)

produce early signs of a neural lesion. Petroclival meningiomas, however, can become quite large before even very subtle auditory, vestibular, or any other symptoms raise suspicion because space for them to expand before they compromise neural structures is considerable. Figure 10–11 illustrates a large cerebellopontine angle meningioma.

Treatment is surgical resection; the approach depends on the site and extent of the lesion and the residual function of the involved nerves. Approaches may be limited to the suboccipital, retrosigmoid posterior fossa approach or the middle fossa approach, or combinations of both with or without transpetrosal and transtentorial extensions; translabyrinthine or transcochlear approaches with or without more posterior or superior extensions can reduce brain retraction or resection (Glasscock et al, 1994; Haddad & Al-Mefty, 1996b).

Treatment for recurrent or incompletely resected tumors may include radiotherapy. The discovery of hormone receptors in these tumors has stimulated research into a variety of drugs that may prove useful in reducing cell proliferation. Drugs currently under study are bromocriptine, mifepristone, and trapidil (Haddad & Al-Mefty, 1996a).

PITFALL

Meningiomas can get quite large and have slight symptoms. They are easily missed or underestimated.

Cholesteatomas (Epidermoids) of the
Deep Petrous Bone or Meninges

Congenital epidermoids, or congenital cholesteatomas, may be divided into four groups: mesotympanic, perigeniculate, petrous apex (extradural, cranial, or diploic), and cerebello-

pontine angle (intradural, intracranial). By far the most common are those that arise in the mesotympanum of the middle ear, which rarely cause neural hearing loss. Those arising in the perigeniculate (more lateral to the otic capsule) and petrous apex (more medial to the otic capsule) locations erode bone to impinge on the facial nerve, inner ear, and eighth nerve but usually remain extradural even if they expand into the posterior or middle fossae. Those arising in the cerebellopontine angle may become quite large before presenting like vestibular schwannomas. Facial twitching is very common in all three (De La Cruz & Doyle, 1994; Schuknecht, 1993b; Schwaber, 1990).

Because of the proximity to the eustachian tube, like many other mass lesions in the petrous apex or protympanum, mesotympanic, perigeniculate, and petrous apex cholesteatomas may present as a unilateral serous middle ear effusion, with or without sensorineural loss, emphasizing the need to evaluate unilateral effusions or mixed hearing losses very carefully relative to each component of the anatomy and hearing loss.

Treatment is surgical and is designed to remove the mass totally or to marsupialize it (marsupialize means to remove the lateral wall of the cyst and all tissues lateral, or external, to the cyst so that the contents of the cyst are exposed to the outside). The surgical approach is designed to accommodate the remaining function and the exact site and extent of the lesion. A transtympanic, transmastoid approach, with extradural middle fossa or posterior fossa perilabyrinthine extensions, may be used to resect or marsupialize the lesions limited to the osseous and extradural areas, which have function and in which the anatomy makes this appropriate. Otherwise, a translabyrinthine or transcochlear approach may be necessary. For intradural lesions, approaches for vestibular schwannomas are used; marsupialization is not an option; however, incomplete resection occasionally is necessary.

As is appropriate in all mass lesion resections, periodic and perpetual surveillance is required for the possibility of recurrence. Total removal with sparing of function is possible in those cases with favorable anatomy.

SPECIAL CONSIDERATION

Petrous apex lesions can obstruct the eustachian tube and present only as unilateral serous otitis media.

Petrous Cholesterol Granulomas

Petrous apex cholesterol granulomas are slowly expanding bone-erosive lesions in the petrous apex formed by foreign body tissue reaction about cholesterol crystals as a consequence of red cells, the source of the cholesterol, in the presence of a relative vacuum. They are primarily composed of yellow or dark brownish fluid and semisolid small masses of foreign body granulomas containing cholesterol crystals. As these painless, occult lesions expand, they may compress the eighth nerve or nerves adjacent to the apex, such as the fifth or sixth nerves.

Complete resection of these lesions is not usually possible or necessary. Surgical drainage with aeration into the middle ear or mastoid is effective (Thedinger & Jackler, 1994). Infracochlear or infralabyrinthine approaches through an enlarged external auditory canal or mastoidectomy with stenting the opening is usually sufficient. These are reasonably short but extremely complex procedures in which the internal carotid artery, dura, facial nerve, or jugular bulb can be injured; this surgery requires an experienced neurotological surgeon. Reaccumulation of fluid and recurrence of symptoms is possible although not common. Careful and perpetual surveillance is necessary.

Chondromas and Chondrosarcomas

Chondromas are rare benign tumors of hyalin cartilage arising from areas of synchondroses (where embryonic cartilage origin bones join) within the base of skull. They may arise from or extend into the cerebellopontine angle from primary sites as distant as the parasellar region and compress the eighth nerve, mimicking signs and symptoms of solitary vestibular schwannomas. As they expand within the petrous bone, they create a radiographically lytic (bone destructive) lesion with irregular margins. Rarely they may become malignant and metastasize (Nager, 1993b).

Chondrosarcomas, are rare malignant tumors of cartilage arising from areas of endochondral ossification within the base of skull. The degree of malignancy tends to correlate with the histological findings. These tumors are difficult to distinguish from benign chondromas; histological examination of the surgical specimen is crucial in this differentiation (Nager, 1993c).

Treatment is surgical resection using one or more of the extradural or intradural approaches to skull base. Preservation of neural function is expected if the anatomy of the lesion allows. Unresected, these lesions can become quite large.

Treatment of chondrosarcomas with total removal was once considered impractical or impossible; however, with infratemporal fossa or transcochlear approaches, these can sometimes be totally resected. Preservation of neural function is not the primary concern in these tumors. These are relatively radioresistant (not susceptible to irradiation); however, some response is seen with high doses of irradiation (Thedinger & Jackler, 1994).

Chordomas

Chordomas are uncommon, but less rare than chondromas, and derive from aberrant remnants of the notochord; these tend to arise in children and young adults. The embryonic notochord is predominantly midline; however, these tumors may originate or extend to lateral locations. They occur in the vertebrae, sacrococcygeal area (the pelvic bone), and the spheno-occipital region of the skull. In the skull base they may involve the sella (sella turcica, wherein sits the pituitary gland), clivus, or petrous apex and become quite large, compressing cranial nerves. They may involve the seventh and eighth nerve within the petrous bone or with the cerebellopontine angle. They may present like a vestibular schwannoma; however, imaging shows a large destructive lesion in the petrous bone. These lesions are clinically difficult, if not impossible, to differentiate from chondromas, except chordomas are more

common. Rarely they may become malignant and metastasize (Nager, 1993d).

Treatment is surgical resection using one or more of the extradural or intradural approaches to skull base. Preservation of neural function is expected if the anatomy of the lesion allows. Often, these lesions are soft and can be evacuated almost totally with suction; recurrences can occur. Unresected, these lesions can become quite large.

Jugulotympanic Paragangliomas (Glomus Tumors)

Paragangliomas are tumors arising from one or more of the small aggregates of branchiomeric (taking origin from the embryonic branchial arches), extra-adrenal (not within the adrenal glands), paraganglia (small aggregates of these special cells, also called glomus bodies in the ear) along the glossopharyngeal and vagus nerves, from the temporal bones to the aortic arch. The tumors may arise and remain limited to the middle ear over the promontory, hypotympanum external to the jugular bulb, or in the adventitia (fibrous tissue on the external surface of a vessel) of the jugular bulb. They may extend from these sites of origin to involve the other sites, the mastoid, the internal carotid artery, the infralabyrinthine and petrous apex regions, and extend intracranially into the posterior fossa, extradurally or intradurally. The usual presentation of these tumors is pulsatile tinnitus and conductive hearing loss. However, if the tumor mass invades the pars nervosa (the portion of the foramen associated with cranial nerves IX, X, XI and the origin of the cochlear aqueduct) of the jugular foramen, it can compress, invade, and paralyze the ninth, tenth, and eleventh cranial nerves (Fig. 10–12). It can extend along these nerves intradurally into the posterior fossa and compress the seventh and eighth nerves, manifesting much the same as a solitary vestibular schwannoma. These tumors are usually single, isolated tumors; however, they may be multicentric (occur in several places simultaneously), ipsilateral, or bilateral. The most common combination is a tumor in the temporal bone and one ipsilaterally at the bifurcation of the external and internal carotid artery as a carotid body tumor. These tumors may be differentiated in two classes, sporadic (without current evidence of hereditary transmission; these are most common) and hereditary; the hereditary group are much more commonly multicentric. Hereditary tumors may be associated with the multiple endocrine neoplasia type II (MEN II/A), which includes pheochromocytomas, medullary thyroid carcinoma, and parathyroid hyperplasia; patients with a paraganglioma should be evaluated for multicentricity and, if found, should be evaluated for these other lesions (Nager, 1993e).

Treatment for paragangliomas is predominantly surgical; however, in special circumstances, their growth can be arrested with irradiation. The surgical approach is tailored to the site and extent of the lesion; the usual approaches are transtympanic, transmastoid, or infratemporal fossa approaches, with or without rerouting of the facial nerve. Those that extend intracranially may require two operations, one to deal with the extracranial portion, the other to deal with the intracranial portion; however, often the complete mass can be operated on at one operation. Preoperative embolization (instilling small particles by arteriography into the tumor to occlude much of the vascular supply) is very helpful to reduce bleeding in these extremely vascular tumors (Horn &

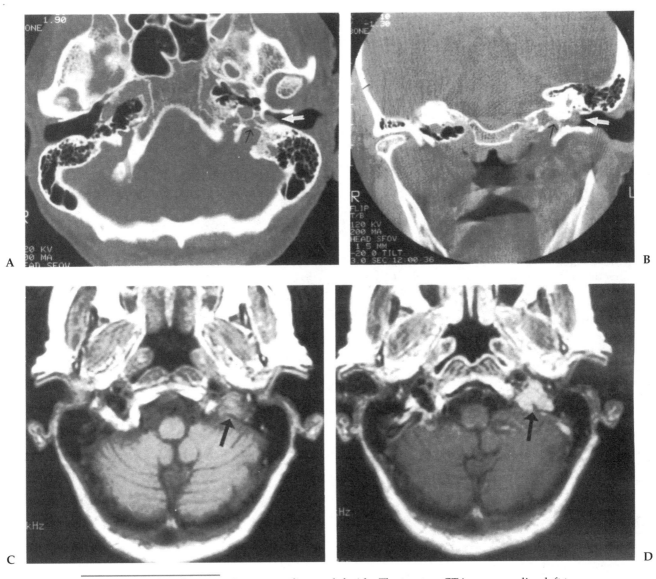

Figure 10–12 Jugulotympanic paragangliomas, left side. The top two CT images, reading left to right, **(A)** axial and **(B)** coronal views, respectively, demonstrate a left middle ear mass (*white arrow*) and erosion of the superolateral bony wall of the jugular foramen (*black arrow*). The bottom two MRI images, reading left to right, **(C)** T1-weighted image without contrast and **(D)** T1-weighted image with contrast, gadolinium, demonstrate that the CT findings are due to highly vascular jugular foramen mass that fills the jugular bulb and extends into the middle ear. (From Cornelius [1997], with permission.)

Hankinson, 1994). Intraoperative hemostasis (control of bleeding) and excellent blood-free visualization can be achieved by bipolar cautery under a saline blanket; with this technique coupled with embolization, blood transfusion is usually not required; however, blood should be available if needed (Neely, 1990). Salvage and restoration of eighth nerve function is often possible; however, if the lower cranial nerves (IX, X, XI) are preoperatively involved by tumor invasion, return of function is not possible. Additional procedures, on a temporary or permanent basis, may be required for voice and deglutition (swallowing) restoration.

> **PEARL**
>
> **Multiple or bilateral glomus tumors or carotid body tumors suggest a probable hereditary origin or the possibility of MEN II/A.**

Jugular Foramen Schwannomas

Schwannomas of the jugular foramen are rare; they may be divided into three general groups, depending on their growth pattern: (1) those that extend immediately into the posterior fossa, with or without paralysis of cranial nerve IX, X, and/or XI, with or without compression and displacement of the eighth nerve with retrocochlear signs and symptoms; (2) those that primarily extend inferiorly into the neck, usually with dysfunction of cranial nerve IX, X, and/or XI; and (3) those extremely rare ones that remain within the jugular fossa (Horn & Hankinson, 1994).

Treatment is surgical resection of the tumor. If preoperatively involved, cranial nerve IX, X, and/or XI cannot be saved; however, return of function of the eighth nerve can occur with resection of the compressing tumor (Neely, 1979).

Brain Stem Gliomas

Intrinsic (originating within the brain, in contrast to extra-axial lesions like vestibular schwannomas or meningiomas) brain tumors, such as brain stem gliomas, can occasionally involve the audiologist in the evaluation for "dizziness," which, in fact may rather be vomiting, with or without ataxia. It is important to be ever vigilant in the search for a diagnosis in children presumed to have inner ear dizziness or vertigo. Intraoperative monitoring and posttreatment surveillance in these cases may also involve the audiologist (Dennis et al, 1985; Jerger et al, 1975; Jerger et al, 1980).

Brain stem gliomas are classified into two types: (1) diffuse intrinsic infiltrating tumors and (2) focal, exophytic (bulging outward) tumors. The diffuse variety tends to be malignant astrocytomas or glioblastoma multiforme. These have a very poor prognosis and are treated with chemotherapy and radiotherapy. The focal, exophytic variety are low-grade astrocytomas or gangliogliomas and tend to be cystic or solid. These have a much better prognosis and are treated surgically by resection and cyst evacuation (Hoffman & Goumnerova, 1996).

PITFALL

Brain stem gliomas can be very subtle and present only as minor dizziness.

Primary or Metastatic Malignancies of the Temporal Bone

Primary malignant neoplasms of the temporal bone are derived from the various tissues in and about the bone. These are (a) squamous cell or basal cell carcinomas from skin, (b) adenoid cystic carcinomas or adenocarcinomas from glandular structures in the skin or mucosa, (c) embryonal rhabdomyosarcomas presumed to be from primitive skeletal muscle, (d) chondrosarcomas from developmental cartilage, and (e) osteogenic sarcoma from bone (Schuknecht, 1993c).

These lesions generally arise lateral to the neural structures of hearing and balance. Treatment is surgical resection with or without irradiation. Involvement of the eighth nerve is a very poor prognostic sign and usually suggests nonresectability.

Metastatic lesions to the temporal bone are by hematogenous (blood-borne) dissemination and thus can occur anywhere vascular nourishment is present, including the eighth nerve. These lesions usually occur late in the course of a known primary lesion. However, metastasis to any of the temporal bone contained structures may be the first sign of

metastasis from a known primary lesion or may the first sign of any disease at all. This fact serves to emphasize the absolute requirement for a precise medical diagnosis in any hearing loss. Primary lesions tending to metastasize to the temporal bone are in order: breast, kidney, lung, stomach, larynx, prostate, and thyroid. Most of these lesions are radiographically lytic; however, lesions from the prostate or breast may be osteoblastic (Schuknecht, 1993c). Treatment of these lesions is usually palliative (for comfort, not cure) by chemotherapy or irradiation.

SPECIAL CONSIDERATION

Lytic bone lesions are malignant until proven otherwise.

Trauma

Temporal Bone Fractures

Temporal bone fractures are generally classified into longitudinal or transverse. Longitudinal fractures occur through the external auditory canal, often tear the tympanic membrane, and fracture longitudinally through the shock-absorbing pneumatized spaces of the middle ear and mastoid lateral to the otic capsule. Transverse fractures, however, fail to take advantage of the shock-absorbing characteristics of the external canal, tympanic membrane, and lateral pneumatized spaces and fracture through the hardest bone in the body, the otic capsule, and petrous bone from foramen to foramen through the vestibule, often right through the facial nerve and transmit trauma directly to the intracranial contents (Figs. 10–13 and 10–14).

Either can create a cerebrospinal fluid (CSF) leak that externalizes through the torn tympanic membrane as CSF otorrhea and/or down the eustachian tube as CSF rhinorrhea. Often CSF leaks are obvious if looked for; however, they may be occult. Meningitis, although not extremely common, can occur immediately or be delayed for months or years (Schuknecht, 1993d).

Immediate treatment is usually confined to caring for any brain, facial nerve, or other associated injuries. Later care may be directed at any persistent CSF leaks, perilymph fistulas with fluctuating or progressive sensory hearing loss with or without constant instability, persistent positional or episodic vertigo, ossicular discontinuity, or entrapment cholesteatomas or external auditory canal stenoses.

It is always wise to inform the patient of and be personally diligent for delayed meningitis, especially during the onset of an acute ear infection months or years later; the earlier meningitis can be identified, the better the chances of survival. Early signs of meningitis are headache, with or without confusion, and a generalized feeling of illness, with or without diaphoresis (profuse sweating). Classic later signs are fever and stiff neck. Rapid deterioration to coma and death may follow.

Vascular Lesions

Vascular Loop Compression

Little doubt exists that vascular compression of cranial nerves by aneurysms, ectatic vessels, and vascular loops does occur, giving rise to symptoms specific to those nerves. The difficulty is to differentiate these causes from other causes giving the same symptoms. In the posterior fossa tic douloureux (trigeminal neuralgia), hemifacial spasm, and glossopharyngeal neuralgia are, perhaps, more generally recognized as originating from this mechanism. There is some consideration that tinnitus, fluctuating hearing loss, episodic or positional vertigo, or constant imbalance may arise from vascular compression of portions of the eighth nerve; however, differentiating this cause from a host of other causes convincingly awaits improved diagnostic techniques.

Treatment is by microvascular decompression of the nerve involved by moving the offending vessel(s) and wedging pieces of soft Teflon felt (Dow Co., Midland, MI) between the nerve and the vessel(s). This requires surgical entry into the posterior fossa (Jannetta, 1996; Schwaber, 1994).

Aneurysms

Seventh and eighth nerve signs and symptoms are rare, even in aneurysms of the posterior fossa circulation; however, headache, dizziness, diplopia (double vision), and transient cerebral ischemic attacks are not rare symptoms of aneurysms, with or without sentinel bleeding (small amount of bleeding

signaling much more severe bleeding to come). These same symptoms can be present in patients being evaluated for hearing loss or dizziness and should be taken seriously and evaluated. An aneurysm rupture can have a mild headache and stiff neck or can be quite dramatic with the sudden onset of severe headache and rapid onset of coma.

Treatment of aneurysms are predominantly surgical by microvascular hemostatic clip application (Peerless et al, 1996; Weir & Macdonald, 1996).

Stroke

Stroke is defined as a "sudden, nonconvulsive, focal neurological deficit" (Adams et al, 1997e). The principle underlying cause is cerebrovascular arteriosclerotic disease, although aneurysms and arteriovenous malformations may participate. Strokes are classified clinically as thrombotic (blood clot originating within the vessel), embolic (clot originating somewhere else and moving to the affected vessel), or hemorrhagic (rupture in the blood vessel). It is important to remember that transient ischemic attacks are warning attacks of generalized arteriosclerosis and indicate not only a higher probability of a full-blown stroke but also of a myocardial infarct. Chronic hypertension increases the probability of both stroke and heart attacks; birth control pills in patients with migraine increase the chances of stroke.

The audiologist may encounter a patient being evaluated for dizziness, tinnitus, transient unilateral blindness, or speech and language problems that may, in fact, be having these symptoms as a result of transient ischemic attacks.

Treatment of transient ischemic attacks is focused on reducing risk factors, such as smoking, hypertension, birth

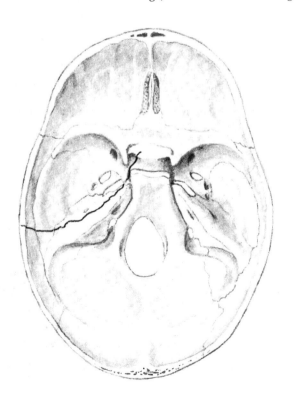

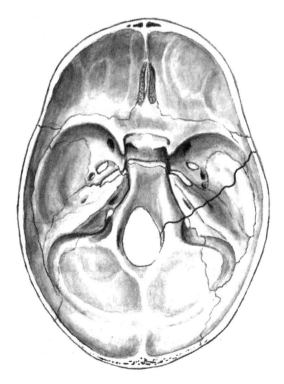

A   B

Figure 10–13   Drawings of **(A)** a longitudinal temporal bone fracture and **(B)** a transverse temporal bone fracture. (From Jahrsdoerfer & Ghorayeb [1996], with permission.)

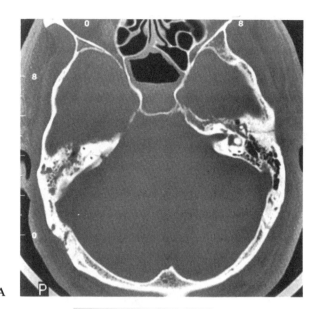
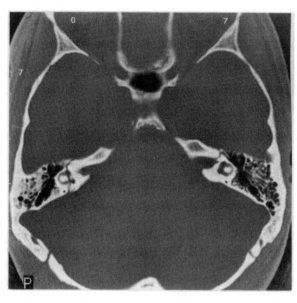

Figure 10–14 **(A)** CT showing a left longitudinal fracture through the superior wall of the external canal, right side of the left image and **(B)** CT showing a right transverse fracture through the horizontal semicircular canal, left side of the right image. (From Huang & Lambert [1997], with permission.)

control pills, and diets high in cholesterol, and the prophylactic (preventive) use of aspirin. Definite ischemia may require thrombolytic agents, anticoagulants, and occasionally surgical remedies for occluded cervical vessels. Treatment of embolic strokes must look closely at the usual origin of the embolic thrombus, the heart. Atrial fibrillation, old infarctions, and valve disease are common cardiogenic causes of occult thrombi capable of embolizing. Hemorrhagic strokes require extensive monitoring and care of the comatose patient, control of the hypertension, and occasionally surgical evacuation of cerebral or cerebellar hematoma or clipping an offending aneurysm or intraluminally occluding an arteriovenous malformation (Adams et al, 1997e).

> ### SPECIAL CONSIDERATION
>
> **Transient ischemic attacks can be a warning not only of an impending stroke but also of a heart attack.**

Lesions Not Detectable by Imaging

Neural lesions may not create a mass or anatomical distortion detectable by imaging techniques. Cellular, or subcellular, dysfunctions of the primary auditory neurones and pathways can also manifest as neural auditory defects. Cellular dysfunctions in other systems may be genetically or physiologically related to the auditory neuronal function. Leads to these disorders come from a careful and professionally done history; confirmation requires specific tests determined by this medical sleuthing. These tests are too numerous to list and such a list would be meaningless. Where appropriate, some indication

will be given about these in this chapter; however, this chapter is focused on treatment.

Aging/Neural Degenerative Diseases

Neural Presbycusis

Schuknecht classified presbycusis into four types: sensory, neural, strial, and cochlear conductive. Neural presbycusis is defined by a progressive loss of word recognition in the presence of stable pure tone thresholds (i.e., phonemic regression) (Schuknecht, 1993e) (Fig. 10–15).

Currently, no medical or surgical treatment exists for this disorder; however, it should be emphasized that this is a clinical diagnosis of exclusion, requiring that no other identifiable lesion exists in the inner ear, nerve, or low brain stem causing the progressive loss. Auditory hallucinations of indistinct music or garbled sound, with or without hyperacusis, may occur from lesions of the pons; more complex and distinct auditory hallucination of music or voices may arise from temporal lobe lesions or seizures; conversely, certain sounds may incite temporal lobe seizures (Adams et al, 1997a).

> ### PEARL
>
> **Four types of presbycusis exist, one of which results in neural hearing loss. However, other causes of neural hearing losses must be excluded, even in the elderly.**

Cranial Neuropathies

Acute cochlear neuritis and acute vestibular neuritis have sudden, spontaneous onset of neural-type lesion and are the

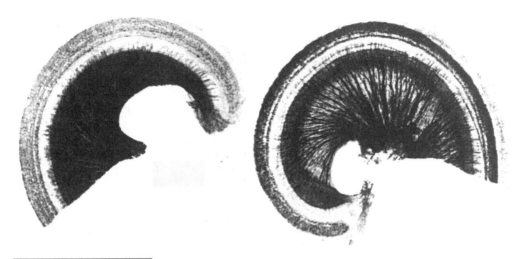

Figure 10–15 Neural presbycusis. Two stained-surface preparation dissections of the osseous spiral lamina and basilar membrane, showing normal population of nerve fibers on the left and reduced cochlear nerve fibers on the right. (From Roland & Marple [1997], with permission.)

result of a direct viral attack on the cochlear nerve or one of the vestibular nerves. Acute cochlear neuritis presents as a sudden idiopathic sensorineural hearing loss. Vestibular neuritis presents as a sudden onset of constant severe vertigo without auditory symptoms, which remains severe for days, gradually reducing to intermittent positional vertigo, and ultimately resolving over weeks to months. Diabetic cranial neuropathies, conversely, are the result of microangiopathies usually affecting the III, IV, or VI cranial nerves; however, the vestibular nerve may be involved and may have the same symptoms of vestibular neuritis (Schuknecht, 1993f).

Multiple cranial neuropathies must be assessed carefully with the exact location of the lesions and associated dysfunctions defined precisely relative to temporal and spatial characteristics. Primary neuropathies must be differentiated by clinical pattern and exclusion of other diseases mentioned in this chapter; in addition, the site of neuropathy must be identified as extra-axial or intra-axial. Secondary lesions on the surface of the brain stem involve adjacent cranial nerves, often unilaterally and sometimes painfully, and involve long sensorimotor tracks much later; whereas lesions occurring within the brain may rapidly involve the long sensorimotor tracks and cranial nerves bilaterally (Adams et al, 1997b).

Steroids or antiviral agents have been used for the presumed viral-induced illnesses; steroids may be contraindicated in the diabetic patient. Good diabetic control is the principle treatment for diabetic neuropathies.

PITFALL

Multiple cranial neuropathies must be evaluated carefully to ensure they are primary rather than a result of other diseases.

Primary Cochlear Neuron Degeneration

Isolated bilateral primary cochlear neuron degeneration in aging subjects is neural presbycusis (Schuknecht, 1993f).

However, many hereditary diseases may be associated with progressive neural hearing loss. These diseases are classified by type of inheritance and clinical presentation; most, but not all, of these diseases are also associated with dysfunction in other organ systems. The other organs or systems involved are vestibular, renal, skin, skull and mandible, retina, optic nerve, multiple cranial nerves, central sensory or motor, cognitive brain, skeletal muscle, gonadal, lens, dental, and musculoskeletal systems. Epilepsy, diabetes mellitus, and diabetes insipidus are specific diseases that may accompany these hereditary syndromes (Adams et al, 1997a).

Prevention and treatment of the cochlear nerve loss is not yet possible with medicine or surgery; however, cochlear prosthesis or brain stem auditory prosthesis implantation may be necessary. It is very important to remember that the other system disorders must be identified and treated, whenever possible, sometimes to save the life of the patient. Another important principle to keep in mind is that one disease does not "immunize" an individual against additional diseases.

Secondary Cochlear Neuron Degeneration

Secondary (retrograde) cochlear neuron degeneration occurs as a function of degeneration and collapse of the inner phalangeal cells and pillar cells, which in turn injure the dendrites and ultimately cause retrograde neural degeneration; this may occur at a considerable time after the loss of the hair cells. Certain diseases that cause terminal injury to the hair cells may spare neurons more than other diseases; sudden deafness, Meniere's disease, ototoxic drugs, and temporal bone fractures spare cochlear nerve fibers more than measles, suppurative labyrinthitis, and syphilis (Schuknecht, 1993f).

Currently, no medical or surgical treatment halts or prevents secondary degeneration. Cochlear prosthesis or brain stem auditory prosthesis implantation may be necessary to assist function.

Leukodystrophies

Leukodystrophies are almost always fatal in early infancy or early childhood; however, unusual cases may survive into the third decade of life. These diseases are congenital or early-onset, postnatal rapidly progressive demyelinating diseases of the white matter of the central nervous system. Auditory brain stem responses may show only wave I (Igarashi et al, 1976; Schuknecht, 1993b).

At present, no treatment, except supportive, for this tragic group of diseases exists.

Multiple Sclerosis

Although MRI can often detect larger lesions suggesting multiple sclerosis, diagnosis is principally made on the basis of clinical presentation and course and CSF analysis. Thus it is included in this section of the chapter.

Multiple sclerosis is one a group of demyelinating diseases that meet the following criteria for inclusion: destruction of myelin sheaths of nerve fibers, relative sparing of other neural cellular components, perivascular inflammatory infiltration, specific distribution of lesions to perivenous white matter, and relative lack of wallerian neural degeneration. The cause may be a delayed, viral-reactivated autoimmune reaction to a previous viral insult years before.

The pathology of these scattered lesions, from a millimeter to several centimeters in size, with a perventricular predilection, is initially myelin destruction with astrocytic reaction and infiltration of mononuclear cells and lymphocytes; later these "plaques" become a matted fibroglial scar. Fluctuating and recurring symptoms arise from surrounding waxing and waning edema and conduction blockade; ultimately, the demyelination areas create more permanent dysfunction. Some sporadic remyelination does occur.

Weakness, fatigue, numbness, tingling, diplopia, evidence of internuclear ophthalmoplegia, dizziness, and ataxia are common presenting symptoms; scanning speech, nystagmus, and intention tremor (Charcot's triad) is a classic, but late, presentation. Sudden or fluctuating neural hearing loss may rarely be the only, but more commonly an associated, symptom.

Diagnosis is made by demonstrating symptomatic lesions separated in time and anatomical locus, MRI evidence of demyelinated periventricular lesions, and CSF abnormalities such as an elevated CSF/serum "immunoglobulin G (IgG) index," oligoclonal IgG electrophoretic bands, and a high concentration of myelin basic protein during an acute attack.

Treatment of acute exacerbations for more rapid resolution of symptoms is by adrenocorticotropic hormone (ACTH), methylprednisolone, prednisone, cyclophosphamide, or beta-interferon. However, long-duration, continued use of these agents has not yet proved to change the ultimate course of the disease or prevent recurrences. Much therapeutic research is ongoing in this potentially debilitating disease (Adams et al, 1997c; Schuknecht, 1993f).

Collagen/Immunological/Allergic Diseases

Polyarteritis nodosa, rheumatoid arthritis, Wegner's granulomatosis, Cogan's syndrome, Vogt-Koyanagi-Harada syndrome, relapsing polychondritis, giant cell arteritis, AIDS, paraneoplastic neuropathy, lymphomatoid granulomatosis, sarcoidosis, systemic lupus erythematosus, and others are immune system disorders that can affect the middle ear, inner ear, eighth nerve, or brain. In some of these diseases and others not listed, the underlying mechanism seems to be a humoral or activated cellular, or hypersensitive, immunological response against specific antigens in specific locations. Tissue antigens, present from gestation and compatible with the body's immune defenses, in some cases become altered by a viral infection or are released by tissue-damaging infection or trauma to be sequestered elsewhere. These newly altered or sequestered antigens are no longer compatible, and the body launches an immunological attack on the antigens, damaging the tissue in which the antigens reside, often by a progressive vasculitis and granulation tissue proliferation. The body's immune system itself can become ineffective, such as in AIDS, which allows an unprotected assault by many organisms and cellular and tissue responses that ordinarily would not occur (Campbell et al, 1983; Schuknecht, 1993g).

Treatment is by titrating (adjusting medication to achieve and maintain an effect using as little or as much of the medication as required at that time interval) dosages and durations of corticosteroids, such as prednisone, immunosuppressive drugs, such as cyclophosphamide, or rapidly emerging antiviral agents given continuously or intermittently during clinical exacerbations. Clinical control is often possible with stabilization or reversal of clinical symptoms and signs; cure is usually not possible. The role of the audiologist is crucial in monitoring therapeutic efficacy in cases in which the auditory system is affected.

SPECIAL CONSIDERATION

It is crucial to determine whether immunological inner ear disease is associated with a systemic collagen disease. The later can be devastating to vital structures for life.

Inflammatory/Infectious Diseases

Intracranial Complications of Suppurative Otitis Media

Acute or chronic middle ear infections can spread intracranially and can be fatal. Extracranial or intracranial complications of suppurative ear disease may be suspected when an acute ear infection lasts more than 1 week, an acute infection recurs within 2 weeks of treatment, or a chronic ear infection gets worse, especially if there is a foul discharge that persists even with treatment. The intracranial complications are extradural granulations or abscess, sigmoid sinus thrombophlebitis (inflammation of the wall of the vessel, with or without partial or complete occlusion), brain abscess, subdural abscess, meningitis, and otitic hydrocephalus (increased intracranial pressure without meningitis or brain abscess). Any can result in a neural hearing loss as a result of active infection, associated intracranial pressure, or early or late sequelae, from the infection.

Treatment is surgical drainage and exenteration of the ear disease, intravenous antibiotics, and surgical drainage of intracranial abscesses. An exception to this rule is some brain abscesses respond to antibiotics alone. Neural dysfunction resulting from pressure or toxicity often recover; whereas dysfunctions resulting from direct infection of the specific conducting tissue usually do not (Neely, 1993a; Neely, 1993b; Neely, 1994; Neely & Doyle, 1994).

PITFALL

Failure to suspect an impending complication can result in serious morbidity or mortality.

Bacterial Meningitis

Bacterial meningitis usually occurs as a result of hematogenous dissemination from the respiratory system. Devastating effects from the bacteria can occur throughout the central nervous system, the cranial nerves, and the inner ears.

Treatment is predominantly life support and specific intravenous antibiotics given in high enough doses and for a long enough duration. Systemic steroids have been shown to reduce sequelae, such as deafness (McIntyre et al, 1997).

CONTROVERSIAL POINT

The use of steroids in bacterial meningitis remains controversial.

Mycoplasma and Viral infections

Mycoplasma organisms, influenza viruses, mumps, measles (rubeola), rubella, herpes zoster virus, herpes simplex virus, cytomegalovirus, and Epstein-Barr virus (mononucleosis) can have systemic influenza symptoms, a skin eruption, hemorrhagic painful blebs on the tympanic membrane or face, swollen salivary glands, or many other symptoms suggesting a systemic illness with generalized or localized manifestations. Any of these can also cause single or multiple cranial nerve deficits or meningoencephalitis, which can be sudden and stable or progressive (Adams et al, 1997b; Schuknecht, 1993h).

Treatment is generally supportive; however, antiviral medications are being developed very rapidly and medications such as acyclovir may have some use in some of the viral infections. Steroids can, at times, reduce inflammation and sequelae. *Mycoplasma*, somewhat between bacteria and viruses, are responsive to the macrolides (erythromycin, azithromycin, clarithromycin) or tetracycline (Fairbanks, 1996).

Fungal Infections

Fungi can cause brain or cranial nerve infection. The patient is often immunocompromised, either from disease, such as AIDS, or from medications to suppress organ rejection, and becomes infected by opportunistic fungi. *Cryptococcus* sp. (cryptococcosis), *Aspergillus* sp. (aspergillosis), and *Phycomycetes* sp. (mucormycosis) are some of the fungal species that can penetrate deeply and infect tissues. Commonly, these originate in the lungs or nose and paranasal sinuses and spread hematogenously or by direct extension to the intracranial cavity. Rapidly progressive central nervous system or cranial nerve destruction by the organisms and by invasive vasculitis can be fatal (Adams et al, 1997d; Schuknecht, 1993h).

Treatment is predominantly by systemic use of rather toxic antifungal medications, such as amphotericin B and, occasionally, by extensive local debridement, as in cases of mucormycosis (Fairbanks, 1996; Johnson, 1993).

Syphilis

A spirochete (a special family of bacteria named for their long flowing hairlike architecture), the *Treponema pallidum*, causes syphilis. This organism reproduces in the early stages only every 30 to 33 hours; in later stages, it may lay dormant for years and rarely reproduce. It is only during reproduction that penicillin can kill this organism; therefore once infected, if any organisms were missed in the initial treatment, the patient may have delayed disease develop.

The two types of transmission stratify syphilis into *acquired syphilis*, acquired after birth, or *congenital syphilis*, transmitted to the fetus by the mother.

In both strata, clinical stages of the disease are characterized by time from exposure and clinical signs. Clinical stages in *acquired syphilis* are: (a) primary (initial local chancre, or ulcerated sore, at entry site [e.g., the labia or penis]), (b) secondary (several weeks later a rash, lymphadenopathy, and systemic fever and illness), (c) latent (recurrence of symptoms years later; early latent is within 2 years and late latent is greater than 2 years later), and (d) tertiary (3 to 10 years after onset, specific target organ destruction: "benign" tertiary syphilis of bone, skin, and viscera; cardiovascular syphilis; and neurosyphilis). Clinical stages in *congenital syphilis* are: (a) early (infantile) (skin rash and blisters and liver and spleen enlargement), (b) late (tardive) (late childhood or adulthood, specific target organ destruction: "saddle nose," "saber shins," interstitial keratitis, Hutchinson's notched teeth, sudden deafness (Schuknecht, 1993h). Any stage after the initial chancre in either stratum can cause hearing loss from infection of the eighth nerve or inner ear.

Treatment is with large doses of penicillin. Hearing loss is treated with long-duration steroids. Steroids are begun at high levels and titrated so that the maximal hearing improvement or stabilization is first achieved, then the dose is slowly decreased over many weeks to months to define the optimum lowest dose to maintain effect and minimize the serious side effects and possible complications from long-duration steroids. If ever the medication can be discontinued, any sudden loss or progressive loss is considered a medical emergency and high, or higher, doses are reinstituted (Darmstadt & Harris, 1989).

Lyme Disease

Lyme disease, named after Lyme, Connecticut, a town in which the first recognized cases were identified, is a systemic disease caused by a spirochete, *Borrelia burgdorferi*, transmitted by a common deer tick vector. Initially, a rash and influenza-type symptoms occur. Weeks or months later, this neurotropic organism may cause dysfunction of cranial nerves and can cause a chronic meningitis (Adams et al, 1997d). Treatment is by tetracycline or doxycycline orally.

Developmental/Genetic/Congenital Diseases

When evaluating an adult or child with hearing loss, it is prudent to look carefully at their overall appearance, especially their face, eyes, skin, hair, ears, face, skeletal structure, and evaluate basic functions of the thyroid, kidneys, heart, and nervous system. If something is wrong with one or more of these areas, it is probable that they have a syndromic type of hereditary hearing loss.

Congenital Syndromes with Hereditary Hearing Loss

In Adams et al (1997a) Table 15–1, pages 296–299, hereditary cochlear and cochleovestibular atrophies are organized into two groups: type I, progressive hearing loss with involvement of kidneys, skin, or bones; type II, hearing loss with retinal disease. Of the 37 diseases listed, 21 are associated with neural hearing loss.

Medical treatment consists of searching for and addressing dangerous, correctable, or controllable associated conditions. Some of these associated conditions are Meniere-type symptoms, proteinuria (proteins in the urine), uremia (excess urea in the bloodstream) or renal failure, potential for hyperthermia. Progressive neural foramina stenosis amenable to decompression, stapedial fixation amenable to stapedotomy, potential for CSF gusher after stapes surgery or trauma, susceptibility for long bone fractures, cataracts, and glaucoma are other associated problems. Additional associated diseases are diabetes mellitus, exudative retinitis, epilepsy, potential for excessive sunburning, sudden death from cardiac dysrhythmia, skin ulceration or infection, dental deterioration, kyphoscoliosis, indifference to pain leading to severe injury, severe inner ear dysplasia with abnormal dehiscences into the intracranial cavity potentially leading to recurrent meningitis, and diabetes insipidus (Adams et al, 1997a; Grundfast & Toriello, 1998; Neely, 1985). Medical treatment may eventually extend to cochlear or brain stem implantation.

Nonsyndromic Hereditary Hearing Losses

All sensorineural hearing losses in adults and children should be considered to derive from a definable disease, some of these dangerous to life. Many of those deemed unexplained, or idiopathic, after thorough investigation, are, indeed, genetic and often hereditary.

Khetarpal and Lalwani (1998) suggest a diagnostic algorithm that includes the following:

- A thorough history and physical examination
- Complete diagnostic audiometry
- A more detailed medical examination of the unexplained cases, including:
  - A pregnancy history
  - Postnatal history
  - Family history
  - Otological examination
  - Eye examination
  - Laboratory tests for:
    - Renal and thyroid function
    - Diabetes
    - Anemia
    - Infection
    - Syphilis
    - Immunological and autoimmune disease
    - Specific viral disease, such as CMV and rubella
    - Electrocardiogram
    - High-resolution CT of the temporal bones

Nonsyndromic hereditary hearing losses are identified and further classified by inheritance pattern, audiometric characteristic, vestibular signs/symptoms, and radiographic findings (Khetarpal & Lalwani, 1998).

The specific identification of the type of hereditary hearing loss may lead to therapeutically important implications, beyond managing the hearing loss with amplification, special education, and cochlear implantation in profound cases. For example, a small proportion of Meniere's disease cases, which can respond to medical or surgical treatment, may present with an autosomal dominant inheritance pattern for sensorineural hearing loss. Mondini dysplasias, which can be seen in some cases of syndromic or nonsyndromic hereditary sensorineural hearing losses, can be severe enough to create a defect in the otic capsule medially through the vestibule into the internal auditory canal and laterally through the stapedial footplate into the middle ear; this can predispose the patient to have a delayed onset of recurrent meningitis with middle ear infections (Neely, 1985). Unusual sensitivity to aminoglycoside antibiotics or diabetes mellitus can result from mitochondrial genetic defects causing sensorineural hearing loss. Otosclerosis, familial conductive hearing loss, and X-linked progressive mixed hearing loss can all be associated with genetic defects capable of causing sensorineural hearing loss, and the conductive loss is potentially treatable with surgery; however, in the X-linked cases, the probability of a CSF gusher through the stapedial surgical defect is increased and can have serious consequences for persistent CSF leak, recurrent meningitis, and damage to the membranous labyrinth, resulting in profound deafness on that side.

Prenatal and Perinatal Noxious Events

Symptomatic, or usually asymptomatic, maternal infection during the first trimester with rubella, cytomegalovirus (CMV), toxoplasmosis, or syphilis can result in a severe or progressively severe-to-profound sensorineural hearing loss. These often have congenital inner ear, eye, cardiac, and nervous system birth defects. Diagnosis is made by the characteristic array of defects, history of rash or infection of the mother in the first trimester, and early serological testing of the neonate (Irving & Ruben, 1998).

No effective medical treatment exists against congenital rubella; however, surgery to correct the cataracts or heart defects can help in some cases. Immunizing against rubella, even in adults, has proven an effective way to prevent congenital rubella.

Congenital CMV is treatable with the antiviral foscarnet (Walsh et al, 1995).

Congenital toxoplasmosis may be treated with pyrimethamine and sulfadiazine, spiramycin combined with pyrimethamine and sulfadiazine, or spiramycin alone for approximately 1 year beginning the first months of life (Roizen et al, 1995; Vergani et al, 1998).

Congenital syphilis is treated with high doses of penicillin as mentioned earlier in this chapter.

Perinatal trauma, infection, or anoxia may cause sensorineural hearing loss. A seriously ill neonate may receive ototoxic aminoglycosides or diuretics for survival; they may become hypoxic, or high levels of unconjugated bilirubin may develop, which stains the basal ganglia in the brain in a condition known as kernicterus. Aggressive pulmonary ventilation, antibiotics, blood exchange transfusions, and careful monitoring of drug levels are all ways of keeping the infant alive and preventing hearing loss. Once the hearing loss occurs, very little more can be done to improve the hearing (Irving & Ruben, 1998).

Idiopathic Diseases

Most of the named diagnoses believed to be idiopathic (having an unknown cause) associated with sensorineural hearing loss affect the inner ear, not the eighth nerve or brain stem. However, in the experience of one of us (JGN) over the past 26 years several instances during each clinic day occur in which an eighth nerve lesion is demonstrated without a clear cause. This is graphically illustrated in the review of articles assessing the false positive and false negative rates of the ABR versus MRI in identifying solitary schwannomas of the vestibular nerve (Gordon & Cohen, 1995; Mangham, 1997; Wilson et al, 1997). The focus is usually on how poorly the ABR does in relationship to the MRI in identifying these tumors; this, by the way, is not this author's experience. An interesting way to look at these data is to see how poorly the MRI identifies a demonstrated eighth nerve lesion as defined by ABR. This observation would seem to be a fruitful area of future research. One might easily hypothesize that genetic

causes would account for a reasonably large proportion of these lesions.

CONTROVERSIAL POINT

Most retrocochlear lesions defined by audiometry remain idiopathic. This is a fruitful area for further research.

CONCLUSIONS

Audiological assessments are crucial in the initial evaluation and subsequent therapeutic monitoring of neural hearing losses. Because the primary purpose is to determine which components are changing and to what degree, a full diagnostic audiogram, including impedance audiometry in the ipsilateral and in the contralateral condition and speech audiometry, is mandatory at each evaluative session; shortcuts are not acceptable.

The specific diagnosis of the cause of the hearing loss has important medical ramifications relative to the cause of the hearing loss, per se, and other potentially associated medical conditions that can result in increased morbidity and, in some cases, mortality.

REFERENCES

ADAMS, R.D., VICTOR, M., & ROPPER, A.H. (1997a). Deafness, dizziness, and disorders of equilibrium. In: R.D. Adams, M. Victor, & A.H. Ropper (Eds.), *Principles of neurology,* (pp. 284–310). St. Louis: McGraw-Hill.

ADAMS, R.D., VICTOR, M., & ROPPER, A.H. (1997b). Diseases of the cranial nerves. In: R.D. Adams, M. Victor, & A.H. Ropper (Eds.), *Principles of neurology,* (pp. 1370–1385). St. Louis: McGraw-Hill.

ADAMS, R.D., VICTOR, M., & ROPPER, A.H. (1997c). Multiple sclerosis and allied demyelinative diseases. In: R.D. Adams, M. Victor, & A.H. Ropper (Eds.), *Principles of neurology* (pp. 902–927). St. Louis: McGraw-Hill.

ADAMS, R.D., VICTOR, M., & ROPPER, A.H. (1997d). Infections of the nervous system (bacterial, fungal, spirochetal, parasitic) and sarcoid. In: R.D. Adams, M. Victor, & A.H. Ropper (Eds.), *Principles of neurology* (pp. 695–741). St. Louis: McGraw-Hill.

ADAMS, R.D., VICTOR, M., & ROPPER, A.H. (1997e). Cerebrovascular disease. In: R.D. Adams, M. Victor, & A.H. Ropper (Eds.), *Principles of neurology* (pp. 777–873). St. Louis: McGraw-Hill.

ARTS, H.A. (1997). Anatomy of the ear. In: P.S. Roland, B.F. Marple, & W.L. Meyerhoff (Eds.), *Hearing loss* (pp. 1–25). New York: Thieme Medical Publishers.

CAMPBELL, S.M., MONTANARO, A., & BARDANA, E.J. (1983). Head and neck manifestations of autoimmune disease. *American Journal of Otolaryngology, 4*;187–216.

CHEUNG, S.W., & JACKLER, R.K. (1994). Diffuse osseeous lesions of the temporal bone. In: R.K. Jackler & D.E. Brackmann (Eds.), *Neurotology* (pp. 1189–1202). St. Louis: Mosby.

CORNELIUS, R.S. (1997). Temporal bone imaging. In: G.B. Hughes & M.L. Pensak (Eds.), *Clinical otology* (pp. 75–87). New York: Thieme Medical Publishers.

DARMSTADT, G.L., & HARRIS, J.P. (1989). Luetic hearing loss: Clinical presentation, diagnosis, and treatment. *American Journal of Otolaryngology, 10*;410–421.

DE LA CRUZ, A., & DOYLE, K.J. (1994). Epidermoids of the cerebellopontine angle. In: R.K. Jackler & D.E. Brackmann (Eds.), *Neurotology* (pp. 823–833). St. Louis: Mosby.

DENNIS, J.M., NEELY, J.G., & SCHWARTZ, D.M. (1985). Somatosensory evoked potential monitoring in the operating room. *The Hearing Journal, 39*(11);15–20.

FAIRBANKS, D.N.F. (1996). *Pocket guide to antimicrobial therapy in otolaryngology–head and neck surgery.* Alexandria, VA: Committee on Medical Devices and Drugs. The American Academy of Otolaryngology–Head and Neck Surgery.

GLASSCOCK, M.E., III, MINOR, L.B., & MCMENOMEY, S.O. (1994). Meningiomas of the cerebellopontine angle. In: R.K. Jackler & D.E. Brackmann (Eds.), *Neurotology* (pp. 795–822). St. Louis: Mosby.

GORDON, M.L., & COHEN, N.L. (1995). Efficacy of auditory brain stem response as a screening test for small acoustic neuromas. *American Journal of Otology, 16*(2);136–139.

GRUNDFAST, K.M., & TORIELLO, H. (1998). Syndromic hereditary hearing impairment. In: A.K. Lalwani & K.M. Grundfast (Eds.), *Pediatric otology and neurotology* (pp. 341–363). Philadelphia: Lippincott-Raven.

GULYA, A.J. (1994). Pathological correlates in neurotology. In: R.K. Jackler & D.E. Brackmann (Eds.), *Neurotology* (pp. 109–129). St. Louis: Mosby.

GULYA, A.J. (1997). Anatomy and embryology of the ear. In: G.B. Hughes & M.L. Pensak (Eds.), *Clinical otology* (pp. 3–34). New York: Thieme Medical Publishers.

HADDAD, G., & AL-MEFTY, O. (1996a). Meningiomas: An overview. In: R.H. Wilkins & S.S. Rengachary (Eds.), *Neurosurgery.* Vol. 1. (pp. 833–841). St. Louis: McGraw-Hill.

HADDAD, G., & AL-MEFTY, O. (1996b). Infratentorial and foramen magnum meningiomas. In: R.H. Wilkins & S.S. Rengachary (Eds.), *Neurosurgery* (Vol. 1) (pp. 951–958). St. Louis: McGraw-Hill.

HOFFMAN, H.J., & GOUMNEROVA, L. (1996). Pediatric brain stem gliomas. In: R.H. Wilkins & S.S. Rengachary (Eds.), *Neurosurgery* (Vol. 1) (pp. 1183–1194). St. Louis: McGraw-Hill.

HORN, K.L., & HANKINSON, H. (1994). Tumors of the jugular foramen. In: R.K. Jackler & D.E. Brackmann (Eds.), *Neurotology* (pp. 1059–1068). St. Louis: Mosby.

HUANG, M.Y., & LAMBERT, P.R. (1997). Temporal bone trauma. In: G.B. Hughes & M.L. Pensak (Eds.), *Clinical otology* (pp. 251–267). New York: Thieme Medical Publishers.

IGARASHI, M., NEELY, J.G., ANTHONY, P.F., & ALFORD, B.R. (1976). Cochlear nerve degeneration coincident with adrenocerebroleukodystrophy. *Archives of Otolaryngology, 102;*722–726.

IRVING, R.M., & RUBEN, R.J. (1998). The acquired hearing losses of childhood. In: A.K. Lalwani & K.M. Grundfast (Eds.), *Pediatric otology and meurotology* (pp. 375–385). Philadelphia: Lippincott-Raven.

JAHRSDOERFER, R.A., & GHORAYEB, B.Y. (1996). Temporal bone trauma. In: H.H. Naumann, J. Helms, C. Herberhold, R.A. Jahrsdoerfer, E.R. Kastenbauer, W.R. Panje, & M.E.J. Tardy, (Eds.), *Head and neck surgery* (Vol. 2) Ear (pp. 131–157). New York: Georg Thieme Verlag.

JANNETTA, P.J. (1996). Posterior fossa neurovascular compression syndromes other than neuralgia. In: R.H. Wilkins & S.S. Rengachary (Eds.), *Neurosurgery* (Vol. III) (pp. 3227–3233). St. Louis: McGraw-Hill.

JERGER, J., NEELY, J.G., & JERGER, S. (1980). Speech, impedance, and auditory brain stem response audiometry in brain stem tumors. Importance of a multiple test strategy. *Archives of Otolaryngology, 106;*218–223.

JERGER, S., NEELY, J.G., & JERGER, J. (1975). Recovery of crossed acoustic reflexes in brain stem auditory disorder. *Archives of Otolaryngology, 101;*329–332.

JOHNSON, J.T. (1993). Infections (paranasal sinuses). In: C. Cummings, J. Fredrickson, L. Harker, C. Krause, & D. Schuller (Eds.), *Otolaryngology–head and neck surgery* (pp. 929–940). St. Louis: C.V. Mosby.

KHETARPAL, U., & LALWANI, A.K. (1998). Nonsyndromic hereditary hearing impairment. In: A.K. Lalwani & K.M. Grundfast (Eds.), *Pediatric otology and neurotology* (pp. 313–340). Philadelphia: Lippincott-Raven.

LUSTIG, L.R., & JACKLER, R.K. (1997). Benign tumors of the temporal bone. In: G.B. Hughes & M.L. Pensak (Eds.), *Clinical otology* (pp. 313–334). New York: Thieme Medical Publishers.

MANGHAM, C.A. (1997). Expert opinion on the diagnosis of acoustic tumors. *Otolaryngology–Head and Neck Surgery, 117*(6);622–627.

MCINTYRE, P.B., BERKEY, C.S., KING, S.M., SCHAAD, U.B., KILPI, T., KANRA, G.Y., & PEREZ, C.M. (1997). Dexamethasone as adjunctive therapy in bacterial meningitis. A meta-analysis of randomized clinical trials since 1988. *Journal of the American Medical Association, 278*(11);925–931.

MIYAMOTO, R.T., ROOS, K.L., & CAMPBELL, R.L. (1994). The neurofibromatoses. In: R.K. Jackler & D.E. Brackmann (Eds.), *Neurotology* (pp. 787–793). St. Louis: Mosby.

NAGER, G.T. (1993a). Meningiomas. In: G.T. Nager (Ed.), *Pathology of the ear and temporal bone* (pp. 620–670). Philadelphia: Williams & Wilkins.

NAGER, G.T. (1993b). Chondromas. In: G.T. Nager (Ed.), *Pathology of the ear and temporal bone* (pp. 793). Philadelphia: Williams & Wilkins.

NAGER, G.T. (1993c). Mesenchymal neoplastic processes. In: G.T. Nager (Ed.), *Pathology of the ear and temporal bone* (pp. 448–482). Philadelphia: Williams & Wilkins.

NAGER, G.T. (1993d). Chordomas. In: G.T. Nager (Ed.), *Pathology of the ear and temporal bone* (pp. 794–814). Philadelphia: Williams & Wilkins.

NAGER, G.T. (1993e). Jugulotympanic paragangliomas. In: G.T. Nager (Ed.), *Pathology of the ear and temporal bone* (pp. 743–778). Philadelphia: Williams & Wilkins.

NEELY, J.G. (1979). Reversible compression neuropathy of the eighth cranial nerve from a large jugular foramen schwannoma. *Archives of Otolaryngology, 105;*555–560.

NEELY, J.G. (1981). Gross and microscopic anatomy of the eighth cranial nerve in relationship to the solitary schwannoma. *Laryngoscope, 91;*l5l2–l53l.

NEELY, J.G. (1984). Is it possible to totally resect an acoustic tumor and conserve hearing? *Otolaryngology–Head and neck surgery, 92;*162–167.

NEELY, J.G. (1985). Classification of spontaneous cerebrospinal fluid middle ear effusion: Review of 49 cases. *Otolaryngology–Head and Neck Surgery, 93*(5);625–634.

NEELY, J.G. (1990). *The role of microcoagulation in the resection of vascular base of skull tumors* (pp. 1475–1479). XIV World Congress of Otorhinolaryngology, Head and Neck Surgery. Madrid, Spain/Berkeley, CA: Kugler & Ghedini Publications.

NEELY, J.G. (1993a). Complications of temporal bone infections. In: C. Cummings, J. Fredrickson, L. Harker, C. Krause, & D. Schuller (Eds.), *Otolaryngology–head and neck surgery* (Vol. 4) (pp. 2840–2864). St. Louis: C.V. Mosby Co.

NEELY, J.G. (1993b). Intratemporal and intracranial complications of otitis media. In: B. Bailey (Ed.), *Head and neck surgery—otolaryngology* (pp. 1607–1622). Philadelphia: J.B. Lippincott Co.

NEELY, J.G. (1994). Surgery of acute infections and complications. In: D. Brackmann, C. Shelton, & M. Arriaga (Eds.), *Otologic surgery* (pp. 201–210). Philadelphia: W.B. Saunders Co.

NEELY, J.G., & ALFORD, B.R. (1974). Facial nerve neuromas. *Archives of Otolaryngology, 100;*298–301.

NEELY, J.G., & DOYLE, K.J. (1994b). Facial nerve and intracranial complications of otitis media. In: R.K. Jackler & D.E. Brackmann (Eds.), *Textbook of neurotology* (pp. 905–918). St. Louis: Mosby-Year Book.

NEELY, J.G., & NEBLETT, C.R. (1983). Differential facial nerve function in tumors of the internal auditory meatus. *Annals of Otology, Rhinology, and Laryngology, 92;*39–41.

O'DONOGHUE, G.M. (1994). Tumors of the facial nerve. In: R.K. Jackler & D.E. Brackmann (Eds.), *Neurotology* (pp. 1321–1331). St. Louis: Mosby.

PEERLESS, S.J., HERNESNIEMI, J.A., & DRAKE, C.G. (1996). Posterior circulation aneurysms. In: R.H. Wilkins & S.S. Rengachary (Eds.), *Neurosurgery* (Vol. II) (pp. 2341–2356). St. Louis: McGraw–Hill.

PENSAK, M.L. (1997). Revision skull base surgery. In: V.N. Carrasco & H.C.I. Pillsbury (Eds.), *Revision otologic surgery* (pp. 143–159). New York: Thieme Medical Publishers.

POST, K.D., & MCCORMICK, P.C. (1996). Trigeminal neurinomas. In: R.H. Wilkins & S.S. Rengachary (Eds.), *Neurosurgery* (Vol. II) (pp. 1545–1552). St. Louis: McGraw-Hill.

ROESER, R.J. (1996). *Roeser's audiology desk reference: A guide to the practice of audiology*. New York: Thieme Medical Publishers.

ROIZEN, N., SWISHER, C.N., STEIN, M.A., HOPKINS, J., BOYER, K.M., HOLFELS, E., METS, M.B., STEIN, L., PATEL, D., MEIER, P., et al. (1995). Neurologic and developmental outcome in treated congenital toxoplasmosis. *Pediatrics, 95*(1);11–20.

ROLAND, P.S., & MARPLE, B.F. (1997). Disorders of inner ear, eighth nerve, and CNS. In: P.S. Roland, B.F. Marple, & W.L. Meyerhoff (Eds.), *Hearing loss* (pp. 195–256). New York: Thieme Medical Publishers.

RUBINSTEIN, J.T., & GANTZ, B.J. (1997). Facial nerve disorders. In G.B. Hughes & M.L. Pensak (Eds.), *Clinical otology* (pp. 367–380). New York: Thieme Medical Publishers.

SCHUKNECHT, H.F. (1993a). Disorders of bone. In: H.F. Schuknecht (Ed.), *Pathology of the ear* (pp. 365–414). Philadelphia: Lea & Febiger.

SCHUKNECHT, H.F. (1993b). Developmental defects. In: H.F. Schuknecht (Ed.), *Pathology of the ear* (pp. 115–189). Philadelphia: Lea & Febiger.

SCHUKNECHT, H.F. (1993c). Neoplastic growth. In: H.F. Schuknecht (Ed.), *Pathology of the ear* (pp. 447–498). Philadelphia: Lea & Febiger.

SCHUKNECHT, H.F. (1993d). Trauma. In: H.F. Schuknecht (Ed.), *Pathology of the ear* (pp. 279–301). Philadelphia: Lea & Febiger.

SCHUKNECHT, H.F. (1993e). Disorders of aging. In: H.F. Schuknecht (Ed.), *Pathology of the ear* (pp. 415–446). Philadelphia: Lea & Febiger.

SCHUKNECHT, H.F. (1993f). Neural disorders. In: H.F. Schuknecht (Ed.), *Pathology of the ear* (pp. 319–344). Philadelphia: Lea & Febiger.

SCHUKNECHT, H.F. (1993g). Disorders of the immune system. In: H.F. Schuknecht (Ed.), *Pathology of the ear* (pp. 345–363). Philadelphia: Lea & Febiger.

SCHUKNECHT, H.F. (1993h). Infections. In: H.F. Schuknecht (Ed.), *Pathology of the ear* (pp. 191–253). Philadelphia: Lea & Febiger.

SCHWABER, M.K. (1990). Acoustic neuroma and tumors of the cerebellopontine angle. In: M.E. Glasscock & G.E. Shambaugh, Jr. (Eds.), *Surgery of the ear* (pp. 535–570). Philadelphia: W. B. Saunders Co.

SCHWABER, M.K. (1994). Vascular compression syndromes. In: R.K. Jackler & D.E. Brackmann (Eds.), *Neurotology* (pp. 881–903). St. Louis: Mosby.

SHAW, C., & FISCH, U. (1994). Benign tumors of the infratemporal and pterygopalatine fossae. In: R.K. Jackler & D.E. Brackmann (Eds.), *Neurotology* (pp. 1069–1100). St. Louis: Mosby.

THEDINGER, B.A., & JACKLER, R.K. (1994). Lesions of the petrous apex. In: R.K. Jackler & D.E. Brackmann (Eds.), *Neurotology* (pp. 1169–1187). St. Louis: Mosby.

VERGANI, P., GHIDINI, A., CERUTI, P., STROBELT, N., SPELTA, A., ZAPPAROLI, B., & RESCALDANI, R. (1998). Congenital toxoplasmosis: Efficacy of maternal treatment with spiramycin alone. *American Journal of Reproductive Immunology, 39*(5); 335–340.

WALSH, J.E., ABINUN, M., PEIRIS, J.S., APPLETON, A.L., & CANT, A.J. (1995). Cytomegalovirus infection in severe combined immunodeficiency: Eradication with foscarnet. *Pediatric Infectious Disease Journal, 14*(10);911–912.

WEIR, B., & MACDONALD, R.L. (1996). Intracranial aneurysms and subarachnoid hemorrhage: An overview. In: R.H. Wilkins & S.S. Rengachary (Eds.), *Neurosurgery* (Vol. II) (pp. 2191–2213). St. Louis: McGraw–Hill.

WILSON, D.F., TALBOT, J.M., & MILLS, L. (1997). A critical appraisal of the role of auditory brain stem response and magnetic resonance imaging in acoustic neuroma diagnosis. *American Journal of Otology, 18*(5);673–681.

PREFERRED PRACTICE GUIDELINES

Professionals Who Perform the Procedure(s)

▼ Skilled and certified audiologist knowledgeable in medical audiology

Expected Outcomes

▼ Good iterative working relationship with a medical specialist for the diagnosis. Medical diagnoses are complete, accurate, and expedient.

Clinical Indications

▼ Any patient complaining of hearing loss should be fully evaluated to define the medical cause of the complaint.

Clinical Process

▼ Crucial to a proper diagnostic evaluation is a complete case history, comprehensive audiogram, including ipsilateral and contralateral stapedial reflexes and speech audiometry, and a skilled otological examination.

Documentation

▼ A formal recording of the tests used, the results obtained, and an interpretation of the data describing the site of lesions and the degree of lesions is required. In addition, written evidence that the patient received a recommendation for a medical specialist evaluation is necessary, and a follow-up progress note to document due diligence was used to ensure the safety of the patient.

Chapter 11

Medical and Surgical Treatment of Cochlear Hearing Loss

J. Gail Neely and Mark S. Wallace

Outline

Cochlear hearing loss may be caused by a wide variety of medical problems. Cochlear hearing loss may be due to metabolic disorders, immunologic disorders, ototoxic medication, trauma, infection, neoplasm, presbycusis, developmental abnormalities, and unknown causes (i.e., idiopathic). Medical and surgical management is based on identification of the underlying cause of the hearing loss. In the identification process, the first issue is to determine the site of the lesion (an anatomical or physiological variation from normal), the second issue is to determine the degree of the lesion, and the third issue is to determine the cause of the lesion. Without a precise understanding of the magnitude and site of the lesion, diagnostic and treatment algorithms cannot move forward. The audiologist is crucial in the determination of the specific sites and the degrees of auditory lesions within a given individual. With this information, the otolaryngologist may begin to determine the cause(s) and institute treatment. This chapter will discuss the management of lesions (i.e., pathological conditions, disorders) arising within the cochlea. The reader may refer to the Chapters 2 and 5 in *Diagnosis* for introductory information on these two topics to supplement the information in this chapter.

METABOLIC DISORDERS

Diabetes, renal (i.e., kidney) disease, hypothyroidism (i.e., underactive thyroid gland), disorders of bone formation, hyperphosphatemia/hypophosphatemia (too much or too little phosphate in the blood), and vitamin D deficiency may be associated with sensorineural hearing loss. Although some investigators suggest Meniere's disease is due to an autoimmune phenomenon, others believe that Meniere's disease is due to a defect in regulation of ions and water in the inner ear fluid spaces. It is generally agreed that endolymphatic hydrops (excessive accumulation of endolymph) within the cochlea and/or vestibule is the histopathological correlate of clinical Meniere's disease (Fig. 11–1).

Audiology: Treatment. Edited by Valente, Hosford-Dunn, and Roeser. Thieme Medical Publishers, Inc., New York © 2000

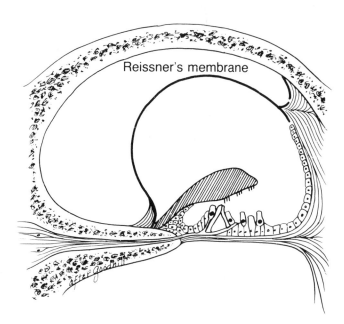

Figure 11–1 Illustration of histopathology of Meniere's disease demonstrating distention of the endolymphatic space with bulging of Reissner's membrane. (From Schwaber [1997], with permission.)

Meniere's Disease

Meniere's disease, in its classical form, describes an aggregate of signs and symptoms in which the patient has recurrent episodes of vertigo lasting minutes to hours, with associated fluctuating roaring tinnitus, aural fullness, and sensory hearing loss. These episodes may be accompanied by nausea and vomiting. Meniere's disease typically is unilateral and presents with a rising audiometric configuration. Early in the disease, the patient's hearing is usually preserved between attacks. The course of this illness is highly variable. Some patients may have a few mild episodes, whereas others may endure numerous debilitating episodes and gradually lose hearing over time. In some cases the illness is said to "burn out" over time with fewer, less intense, occurrences as the patient's hearing decreases. Twenty percent of the patients will have a family history of Meniere's disease. Forty percent of patients have bilateral disease develop. Meniere's disease may occur at any age; however, its onset is most common in the third to sixth decade of life (Roland & Marple, 1997).

Medical Treatment

Meniere's disease is not curable; however, 75 to 85% of patients respond to medical treatment. The goals of treatment are to alleviate symptoms during the acute attack and to reduce the frequency of recurrence. Labyrinthine suppressants such as antihistamines (meclizine), benzodiazepines (Valium), anticholinergics (scopolamine), and antiemetics (perchlorperazine maleate [Compazine] and promethazine [Phenergan]) are used to control acute symptoms of vertigo, nausea, and vomiting. Low-salt diet and avoidance of caffeine and alcohol may be useful in reducing recurrences.

In addition, triamterene with hydrochlorothiazide (Dyazide), a diuretic used to treat mild hypertension, has been found to reduce recurrences in some patients (Roland & Marple, 1997).

Surgical Treatment

For those patients who fail conservative medical therapy, surgical options may be considered. It should be remembered that 20 to 40% of patients with Meniere's disease will have bilateral involvement. Therefore any surgical procedure that would potentially compromise hearing must be carefully considered. Surgical options for Meniere's syndrome have been divided into two categories: *enhancement* or *ablative*. Although still somewhat controversial, enhancement surgery is usually directed toward reducing the pressure within the endolymphatic sac by means of different surgical techniques. *Endolymphatic sac surgery* has a lower risk of hearing loss and an increased chance of stabilizing hearing, and control of symptoms of vertigo are between 68 and 92% (Pensak & Friedman, 1998). Because of its lower risk of hearing loss, this surgery may be cautiously considered in patients with vertigo originating in a better hearing ear or those with bilateral disease. Two procedures on the endolymphatic space are endolymphatic sac decompression and endolymphatic sac shunt. Endolymphatic sac decompression involves complete mastoidectomy and removal of the bony confines of the endolymphatic sac. The shunt operation involves mastoidectomy, exposure of the endolymphatic sac, and placement of a wedge of silicone elastomer sheeting into the sac, in theory shunting the excess endolymphatic fluid out of the sac (Fig. 11–2).

Ablation of the vestibular system may be accomplished through several techniques, including chemical ablation, vestibular neurectomy, or labyrinthectomy. It is generally believed that ablative techniques are better at controlling symptoms of vertigo but have higher risks of hearing loss and postoperative disequilibrium. *Chemical ablation* may be accomplished with high-dose intramuscular streptomycin or transtympanic administration of gentamicin or streptomycin (Fig. 11–3). Gentamicin and streptomycin are antibiotics that have known vestibulotoxic properties. However, these aminoglycosides do possess some cochleotoxic properties that are responsible for the higher risk of hearing loss than endolymphatic sac surgery or vestibular neurectomy. Serial audiograms and caloric testing may be useful in evaluating the effects of aminoglycoside therapy. Less frequent gentamicin injection schedules allowing for better hearing monitoring have been shown to yield a lower rate of severe hearing loss (Kaasinen et al, 1998; Youssef & Poe, 1998). Titrated intramuscular streptomycin may be considered for patients with active bilateral disease; whereas transtympanic aminoglycoside therapy may be considered for patients with unilateral disease.

Vestibular neurectomy, or division of the vestibular nerve, has been accomplished by various craniotomy approaches, middle cranial fossa (Fig. 11–4), retrolabyrinthine, and retrosigmoid (Fig. 11–5). Vestibular nerve section is believed to control symptoms of vertigo in 95% of patients with Meniere's disease with a relatively low risk of profound hearing loss. After surgery, patients require admission to the intensive care unit followed by a hospital stay of a few days. In addition, a high incidence of postoperative disequilibrium may require

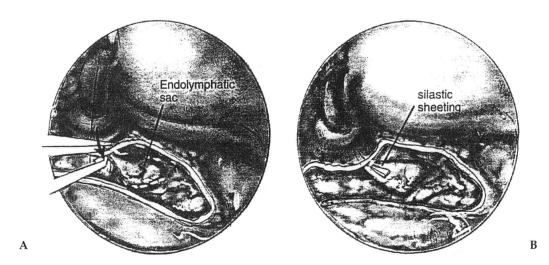

Figure 11–2 Artist's drawing of transmastoid endolymphatic sac (ES) decompression and shunt operations, right ear. **(A)** ES decompression by removing posterior fossa bone to expose the sac. **(B)** ES shunt procedure by opening the lumen of the exposed sac and placing a small wedge-shaped silicone elastomer sheet in the lumen to maintain an open, shunted sac. (From Wackym & Monsell [1997], revision with permission.)

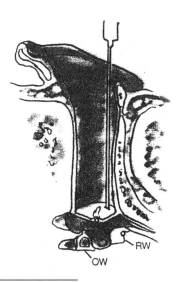

Figure 11–3 Illustration of intratympanic gentamicin injection through the tympanic membrane. The middle ear is filled, and the gentamicin enters the perilymphatic space by diffusion through the round window (*RW*). OW, Oval window. (From Wackym & Monsell [1997], with permission.)

intensive rehabilitation. The reader is referred to Chapter 21 in this volume. Furthermore, vestibular nerve section, by any approach, is associated with risks related to craniotomy, such as cerebrospinal fluid leak, meningitis, stroke, other cranial nerve injury, and even death. Vestibular neurectomy may be considered an option for patients who have failed endolymphatic sac surgery and who have useful hearing.

Ablation of neural input from the inner ear may be accomplished by *labyrinthectomy*, the surgical removal of the vestibular labyrinth (Fig. 11–6). This may be considered an option for patients with profound hearing loss and unilateral

disease (Langman & Lindeman, 1998). Labyrinthectomy offers good control of vertigo without the risks of craniotomy; however, it does eliminate hearing in that ear (Kartush & Larouere, 1998; Liston et al, 1991; Roland & Marple, 1997).

PEARL

The initial treatment for Meniere's disease is aimed at medical control of symptoms. Generally, invasive techniques with lower surgical risk and risk of hearing loss may be considered for those patients who initially have medical therapy fail. Invasive techniques associated with a higher risk of hearing loss or associated complications may be considered in patients who have a permanent severe loss or those in whom more conservative therapy has failed.

Each patient should be evaluated individually, with therapy directed to the highest benefit/risk ratio for that patient.

Diabetes Mellitus

Diabetes is a disorder of carbohydrate metabolism resulting in difficulties controlling blood glucose. An association exists between sensorineural hearing loss and diabetes. In addition, an association exists between the interaction of diabetes and hypertension (a common problem in the diabetic patient) in the pathogenesis of sensorineural hearing loss (Duck et al, 1997). The mechanism by which diabetes may participate in producing hearing loss is unclear. Possible explanations include (1) microangiopathic (small vessel disease) changes to the inner ear blood supply, (2) primary diabetic neuropathy

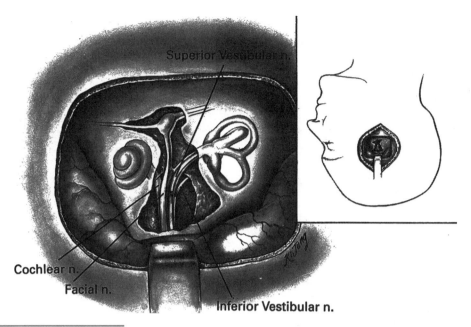

Figure 11–4 Artist's drawing of middle fossa vestibular nerve section, right ear. (From Schwaber [1997], with permission.)

(Friedman et al, 1975), (3) neuropathy caused by involvement of the vasa nervorum (vessels supplying the sensory organ or nerve, per se), and (4) alterations in the inner ear glucose metabolism. Some reports correlate diabetic hearing loss with general vascular disease and the severity of diabetes. No correlation exists between hearing loss and the duration of diabetes, insulin dosage, and family history of diabetes. No treatment reverses or prevents diabetic cochlear hearing loss except, perhaps, good diabetic control (Meyerhoff & Liston, 1991; Monsell et al, 1997).

Renal Disease

As with diabetes, the exact mechanism of sensorineural hearing loss commonly seen in patients with renal disease is unclear. Metabolic abnormalities, such as accumulation of uremic toxins, electrolyte imbalance, osmotic shifts during dialysis, or endocrine abnormalities, are believed to contribute to the inner ear hearing loss. Fluctuation in low-frequency hearing is occasionally observed after dialysis; however, hearing loss is not proportional to elevated blood urea nitrogen or serum creatinine levels. Other possible explanations for hearing loss seen in patients with renal failure may be associated with the use of ototoxic diuretics/antibiotics (Gendeh et al, 1998), anemia (Shaheen et al, 1997), presence of infection, coexisting diabetes, hypertension, small vessel disease, and hemodynamic changes associated with dialysis and kidney transplantation. No treatment reverses or prevents cochlear hearing loss associated with renal disease except, perhaps, good control of the renal disease (Meyerhoff & Liston, 1991; Monsell et al, 1997).

Hypothyroidism

The mechanism causing sensorineural hearing loss associated with low levels of thyroid hormone (hypothyroidism) is also poorly understood. *Endemic cretinism* is a congenital form of hypothyroidism caused by a lack of iodine. Affected children have goiter, mental retardation, and mixed hearing loss. Thyroid hormone supplementation may improve the mental retardation, but not the hearing loss.

Athyroid cretinism results from abnormal lack of development of the thyroid gland. During development, the fetal metabolism is supported by maternal thyroid hormone crossing the placenta. However, shortly after birth the infant becomes hypothyroid. *Adult* forms of *hypothyroidism* may occur after infections, radiation, surgery, or drug treatment. Occasionally, the sensorineural hearing loss associated with hypothyroidism is improved with thyroid hormone supplementation (Meyerhoff & Liston, 1991; Monsell et al, 1997).

PITFALL

In patients with early hearing loss, failure to identify and treat hypothyroidism may result in deafness.

Cochlear Otosclerosis

Otosclerosis is usually associated with a conductive hearing loss that presents with progressive hearing loss. Lesions of this disease of otic capsule bone usually cause fixation of the stapes footplate. However, these lesions may spread extensively within the otic capsule and cause sensory hearing loss and conductive hearing loss. If the cochlear hearing loss occurs without the conductive component, it is known as *cochlear otosclerosis*; otherwise, it may be described as oval window and labyrinthine otosclerosis. Rarely does otosclerosis cause a sensorineural loss without a conductive hearing loss. Oral sodium fluoride may be given in attempt to stabilize

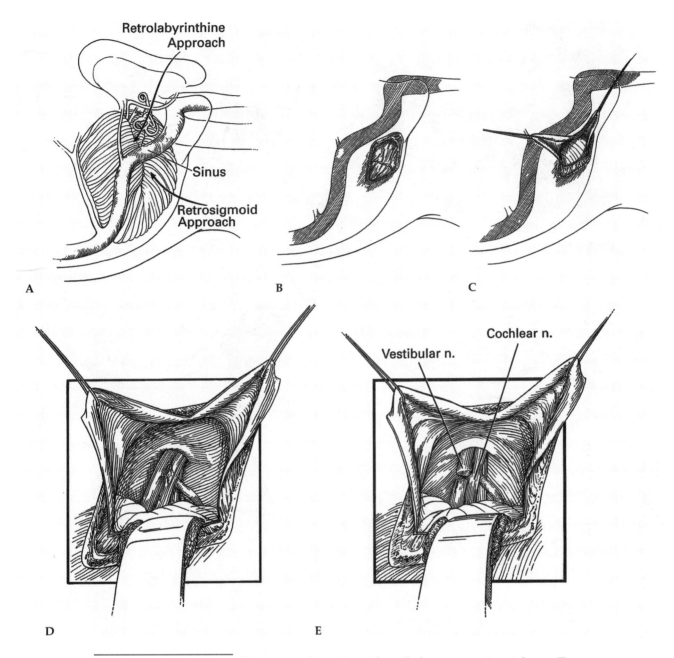

Figure 11–5 (A–E) Artist's illustrations of retrosigmoid vestibular nerve section, right ear. (From Schwaber [1997], with permission.)

hearing. Serial audiograms are used to monitor hearing during sodium fluoride therapy (House, 1997, 1998).

Other Metabolic Disorders

Other metabolic disorders, such as vitamin D deficiency, hypophosphatemia/hyperphosphatemia, and abnormalities in bilirubin metabolism, are known to be associated with sensorineural hearing loss. Some patients with adrenocortical insufficiency have symptoms of Meniere's disease thought to

be due to a defect in regulation of sodium (Meyerhoff & Liston, 1991).

IMMUNOLOGIC DISORDERS

Autoimmune Inner Ear Disease

Clinically, autoimmune inner ear disease (AIED) presents as bilateral, asymmetric progressive sensorineural hearing loss over a period of days to months. Although AIED may occur at any age, it is more frequently seen in the middle-aged

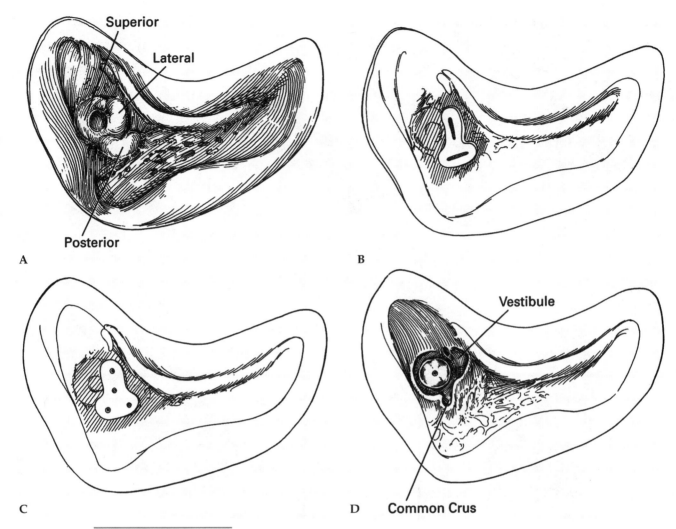

Figure 11–6 Artist's illustrations of transmastoid labyrinthectomy, right ear. **(A)** The labyrinth is exposed. **(B)** The lateral and posterior canals are opened. **(C)** Most of curve of the canals are removed. **(D)** The superior canal is opened and the medial wall of all the canals are followed to open and exenterate the vestibular contents. (From Schwaber [1997], with permission.)

female. It may occur in association with other systemic autoimmune diseases such as Wegener's granulomatosis, Cogan's syndrome, polyarteritis nodosa, rheumatoid arthritis, ulcerative colitis, Crohn's disease, systemic lupus erythematosus, ankylosing spondylitis, multiple sclerosis, relapsing polychondritis, and postvaccination serum sickness. The hearing loss may be fluctuant but is progressive and not sudden (less than 72 hours). In addition, half of the patients may have vestibular symptoms, making the initial diagnosis difficult to separate from Meniere's disease. In fact, many patients with classic Meniere's disease have been shown to have serologic testing suggestive of AIED (Bassiouni & Paparella, 1991; Harris, 1998; Meyerhoff & Liston, 1991; Rauch, 1998; Roland & Maple, 1997).

AIED is thought to occur when the patient has antibodies, autoantibodies, or a cell-mediated immune response develop against their own cochlear and/or vestibular antigens, which then causes an inflammatory response damaging the inner ear (Harris et al, 1997). An immune-mediated cause has been considered to be the cause of idiopathic, progressive, bilateral,

sensorineural hearing loss because of its high incidence of responsiveness to steroid treatment. Audiometric evaluation should demonstrate cochlear hearing loss of at least 30 dB at any frequency, with evidence of progression in at least one ear on serial audiograms performed in less than or equal to 3 months apart. Progression should be at least 15 dB hearing loss at one frequency, 10 dB hearing loss at two or more frequencies, or significant change in the word recognition score.

Excluding retrocochlear causes of the hearing loss with auditory brain stem response (ABR) testing and/or magnetic resonance imaging (MRI) is important to avoid missing the diagnosis of multiple sclerosis or acoustic neuroma before initiation of treatment of AIED. Blood tests that may be useful include complete blood count, erythrocyte sedimentation rate, antinuclear antibody titer, rheumatoid factor, syphilis serology, thyroid function testing, C-reactive protein, C3 and C4 compliment levels, Raji cell assay for circulating immune complexes, and immunoglobulin levels. Although somewhat controversial in its clinical usefulness, the lymphocyte transformation test may be helpful in determining the patient's own lymphocyte response to inner ear antigens. Western blot assays for the patient's own antibodies against 68-kD inner ear protein antigen is becoming one of the standards to confirm this disease.

Initial therapy for patients whose hearing loss is suspected to be autoimmune mediated consists of a therapeutic trial of high-dose anti-inflammatory steroid (prednisone 40 to 60 mg daily) for 3 to 4 weeks. Audiograms are performed at patient presentation and again in 3 weeks. If the patient's discrimination scores or thresholds have significantly improved (greater than or equal to 15 dB at one frequency or 10 dB at two or more consecutive frequencies), the patient is believed to be a steroid responder and is treated for an additional 1 to 2 months with a slightly reduced dose. The objective is to determine the maximum hearing improvement possible before beginning to reduce the medication significantly. Subsequently, the steroid dose is gradually decreased. The patient's hearing is monitored with serial audiograms. The objective in this titration phase is to keep the improved hearing and reduce the medication to reduce complications. Potential complications associated with long-term use of anti-inflammatory steroids include gastritis, bleeding gastric ulcer formation, weight gain, hypertension, diabetes, liver dysfunction, and psychiatric problems. Careful monitoring is mandatory. Occasionally, hearing improvement is not demonstrated, but hearing stabilization is seen; therefore the same technique is used is these cases. Hearing stabilization is, of course, difficult to substantiate unless the progression is very rapid. The ultimate goal is to arrest the disease and stop prednisone treatment. If the hearing loss begins to recur during dose reduction, the dose must be increased and the following additional medications should be considered.

Plasmapheresis or cytotoxic agents may be considered in patients with relapse during or after steroid taper or patients who show little or no response to anti-inflammatory steroids. Methotrexate (Sismanis et al, 1997), an antineoplastic chemotherapy agent with immunosupressive effects, has been used successfully alone or in combination with prednisone to reduce hearing loss or preserve hearing in AIED in adults and children. Potential complications of methotrexate therapy include bone marrow suppression, nausea, vomiting, diarrhea, oral ulceration, acute pneumonitis, and hepatic fibrosis. Serial blood counts, liver/kidney function testing, and urinalysis may be useful in avoiding toxicity.

Cyclophosphamide, also an antineoplastic chemotherapy agent with immunosupressive effects, has been used to treat AIED. Because of its significant risk of causing urinary tract malignancies and infertility, it is rarely used to treat children or young adults. Other potential complications include bone marrow suppression, opportunistic infection, hair loss, and hemorrhagic cystitis.

Plasmapheresis may be considered in cases that do not respond to other forms of therapy. Plasmapheresis removes autoantibodies and circulating immune complexes from the patient. Patients should be treated with immunosuppressive drugs while undergoing plasmapheresis. Appropriate consultation with the otolaryngologist, hematology/oncologist, and rheumatologist should be ongoing during the treatment of AIED with cytotoxic agents and plasmapheresis (Bassiouni & Paparella, 1991; Harris, 1998; Luetje & Berliner, 1997; Meyerhoff & Liston, 1991; Rauch, 1998; Roland & Marple, 1997).

Cogan's Syndrome

Cogan's syndrome is a disorder generally affecting young adults characterized by a sudden onset of interstitial keratitis and vestibuloauditory symptoms. Interstitial keratitis presents with eye pain, blurred vision, and lacrimation. Associated vestibuloauditory symptoms include vertigo, tinnitus, and sensorineural hearing loss occurring concomitantly. These symptoms usually occur with a sudden onset with waxing and waning and progressive hearing loss.

The cause of this disease is believed to be of cell-mediated autoimmune origin, with the autoimmune response being directed at the eye and ear. Cogan's syndrome may be associated with polyarteritis nodosa, which is discussed later.

Treatment is directed at suppressing the immune response with steroids, methotrexate, cyclophosphamide, and rarely plasmapheresis (Harris, 1998). Cochlear implantation in patients with Cogan's syndrome and sensorineural hearing loss is being studied (Cinamon et al, 1997; Minet et al, 1997).

PITFALL

Failure to identify and treat Cogan's syndrome can result in blindness and deafness.

Polyarteritis Nodosa

Polyarteritis nodosa is a systemic necrotizing vasculitis of small and medium-sized arteries thought to be of immune complex deposition in origin. It most commonly affects middle-aged individuals, with a male/female ratio of approximately 2:1. Vessels of the kidneys, heart, liver, gastrointestinal tract, peripheral nerves, mesentery, testes, and skeletal muscles are commonly involved. Symptoms include fever, weight loss, fatigue, abdominal pain, skin lesions, and joint pain. In addition, symptoms of renal failure, myocardial infarction, heart failure, and cardiac dysrhythmia may develop. Hearing loss, although not always present, may be mixed, conductive, or sensorineural, depending on vessel involvement.

Diagnosis by arteriography may demonstrate segmental narrowing of small and medium-sized vessels in the gastrointestinal tract. Biopsy of involved tissue may demonstrate necrosis, polymorphic infiltrate, thrombosis, and small vessel aneurysm formation. Treatment options consist of corticosteroids, cytotoxic agents, and/or plasmapheresis (Burns & Meyerhoff, 1991).

Vogt-Koyanagi-Harada Syndrome

Vogt-Koyanagi-Harada syndrome is believed to be an autoimmune-mediated response against melanocytes contained in the eye, skin meninges, and the inner ear. Symptoms include sensorineural hearing loss, vertigo, depigmentation of the hair and skin with uveitis and nonbacterial meningitis (Harris, 1998). Treatment options are similar to that of polyarteritis nodosa.

Wegener's Granulomatosis

Classic Wegener's granulomatosis consists of necrotizing granulomas with systemic vasculitis affecting the upper and lower respiratory tracts and kidneys. Common problems associated with this illness are sinusitis, epistaxis (nosebleeds), otalgia, and hearing loss (Dekker, 1993; Fenton & O'Sullivan, 1994). Eighty-seven percent of patients with Wegener's granulomatosis have pulmonary disease. Left untreated the illness is rapidly fatal, with renal involvement being the most frequent cause of death. Hearing loss is the presenting feature in 6 to 15% of the cases.

Early diagnosis and treatment are important in improving the long-term prognosis. Unfortunately, no single laboratory test is diagnostic for Wegener's granulomatosis. Complete blood count, erythrocyte sedimentation rate, urinalysis antinuclear antibodies, rheumatoid factor, creatinine level, sinus CT scan, and chest x-ray films are useful during the initial diagnostic process. Cytoplasmic staining anticytoplasmic antibodies have been found to be elevated in patients with active disease, and changing levels may correlate with activity of disease. Intranasal or lung biopsy specimens may show the pathological features of granulomatous changes, small and medium vessel vasculitis, and necrosis.

Treatment is often directed by a rheumatologist. Combinations of anti-inflammatory steroids, cyclophosphamide, methotrexate, and trimethoprim-sulfamethoxazole have been used to induce remission. Surgery, other than diagnosis by biopsy, is only useful in controlling occurrences of complications: sinusitis, otitis media, dacrocystorhinits, proptosis, subglottic stenosis, and renal failure (Amedee & Jabor, 1998).

Sarcoidosis

Sarcoidosis is an inflammatory disease of unknown cause affecting multiple organ systems, particularly the lower respiratory tract. Noncaseating granulomas and Langhans giant cells may be identified in any organ system. Respiratory failure, lymphadenopathy, splenomegaly, hepatic dysfunction, and cutaneous lesions may be seen in patients affected by this disease. Perivascular lymphocytic infiltrate, demyelinization, and axonal degeneration of cranial nerves VII and VIII have been identified in temporal bone sections of a patient with sarcoidosis. Patients with Heerfordt's disease, a variant of sarcoidosis, have uveitis, parotid enlargement, and bilateral facial paralysis (Lee & Goodrich, 1987). Central nervous system involvement is seen in nearly 10% of patients with sarcoidosis. Treatment consists of corticosteroids (Burns & Meyerhoff, 1991).

Poststapedectomy Granuloma

A noninfectious process that may occur 2 to 6 weeks after stapedectomy is foreign body granuloma formation at the site of the stapes implant. Typically patients experience sensory and conductive hearing loss with significant reduction in word recognition scores. Patients may experience vertigo and tinnitus. A gray or erythematous mass in the posterior-superior quadrant of the middle ear space noted on otoscopy combined with the appropriate history is helpful in making the early diagnosis (Burns & Meyerhoff, 1991; Glasscock et al, 1993).

PEARL

Early and complete surgical excision may stabilize or reverse permanent sensorineural hearing loss in cases with poststapedectomy granuloma.

OTOTOXICITY

Numerous medications are known to cause hearing loss. However, most clinical ototoxic hearing loss is caused by the aminoglycoside antibiotics, loop diuretics, and antineoplastic agents. Hearing loss, tinnitus, and balance instability are symptoms of ototoxicity. Hearing loss from ototoxic antibiotics is sensorineural and initially seen in the high frequencies. Hearing loss with loop diuretics usually produces a flat or gradually sloping hearing loss (Irving & Ruben, 1998; Roland & Marple, 1997; Stringer et al, 1991). Although most ototoxic drugs have both cochleotoxic and vestibulotoxic properties, some are predominantly cochleotoxic whereas others are predominantly vestibulotoxic (Table 11–1) (Irving & Ruben, 1998).

Aminoglycoside Antibiotics

Aminoglycosides are a group of antibiotics that are used to treat many gram-negative bacterial, staphylococcal, and mycobacterial infections (Manji, 1987). The choice of an antibiotic depends on the kind of pathogen (bacteria, virus, fungus etc.), the sensitivity of the particular pathogen, and the side effects and potential complications of each antibiotic. Some aminoglycosides are more vestibulotoxic than cochleotoxic, whereas the reverse is true about others. The hearing loss associated with the aminoglycosides is usually bilateral, symmetrical, permanent, and initially in the high frequencies. Hearing loss may be seen in the first few days of treatment or several months after the completion of therapy (Stringer et al, 1991). The outer hair cells of the basal turn are most vulnerable to injury, corresponding to the high-frequency hearing loss seen with aminoglycoside treatment. The magnitude of hearing loss is related to dose, rate of infusion,

TABLE 11–1 Drugs that cause cochleotoxicity and vestibulotoxicity

Cochleotoxicity
Dihydrostreptomycin
Neomycin
Kanamycin
Vancomycin
Erythromycin
Quinine
Cisplatin
Vestibulotoxicity
Streptomycin
Gentamicin

From Irving and Ruben (1998).

serum peak and trough levels (i.e., serum high and low levels measured at various times after dosing), and duration of treatment. However, toxic affects can be idiosyncratic, meaning they may occur in a given individual even when no clear reasons exist why such toxicity should be seen. In addition, these events may prove to be genetic, meaning that the individual is genetically predisposed to the toxic effects of a specific compound.

These antibiotics are excreted in the urine and can also be nephrotoxic (i.e., toxic to the kidney). In addition, any renal impairment may allow increased circulating levels of drug and increase the risk of ototoxicity. Streptomycin, neomycin, cactinomycin, kanamycin, gentamicin, tobramycin, amikacin, netilmycin, and sisomycin are examples of aminoglycoside antibiotics.

In the past, streptomycin was primarily used to treat tuberculosis (Manji, 1987). It is rarely used today because of its potent vestibulotoxic side effects. However, because of its relatively selective vestibulotoxicity, streptomycin has been used to chemically ablate the peripheral vestibular system in carefully selected patients with intractable Meniere's disease (Roland & Marple, 1997).

Gentamicin, used for many gram-negative bacterial infections, also is more likely to be vestibulotoxic than ototoxic (Manji, 1987; Roland & Marple, 1997). Gentamicin may also be used to create vestibular ablation when infused into the middle ear space through a myringotomy in carefully selected patients with intractable Meniere's disease (Roland & Marple, 1997).

Treatment for Aminoglycoside Ototoxicity

If ototoxicity is identified, the medication must be discontinued, unless no alternative treatment exists for a serious disease. Unfortunately, little can be done to reverse or arrest ototoxicity from aminoglycoside antibiotics once it has begun. It is possible for hearing loss to progress after the discontinuation of the medication; however, ototoxicity often spontaneously stops at some level.

Prevention of Aminoglycoside Ototoxicity

Ideally, monitoring audiometry (i.e., complete audiologic evaluation including tympanogram, acoustic reflexes, reflex thresholds, and high-frequency audiometry) would be completed before potentially ototoxic drugs were administered and repeated periodically during treatment. In addition, complaints of dizziness or tinnitus should be reported to the physician. The physician uses this information to evaluate antibiotic selection and dosing.

Factors that increase the risk of aminoglycoside ototoxicity are advanced age, renal failure, pre-existing hearing loss, concurrent noise exposure, hypertension, previous aminoglycoside therapy, fever, simultaneous use of other ototoxic agents, and aminoglycoside treatment for longer than 10 days. Concomitant use of furosemide, ethacrynic acid, and mannitol have been shown to potentiate aminoglycoside ototoxicity. Ototoxic effects of the aminoglycosides initially affect the vestibular system and the basal turn of the cochlea. Ultra-high-frequency audiometry may identify high-frequency hearing loss while still at a reversible stage. In addition,

electronystagmography has been advocated to determine early vestibulotoxicity with gentamicin and streptomycin; bedside vestibular tests, such as the head thrust or tandem Rhomberg, have proven to be most sensitive. Unfortunately, patients undergoing aminoglycoside therapy are seriously ill and many are not able to cooperate with bedside audiometry or vestibular testing. In the future, monitoring toxicity by measurement of otoacoustic emissions (not requiring patient cooperation) may be useful. Although no reliable method exists to avoid aminoglycoside ototoxicity, measurement of serum peak and trough levels currently remains important to avoid potentially ototoxic levels (Fausti et al, 1998; Roland & Marple, 1997; Stringer et al, 1991).

> ### PEARL
>
> **The best way to "treat" ototoxicity is to identify it early and take steps to prevent its progression (i.e., change medicine, dose, dose-frequency).**

Interestingly, the concomitant use of iron-chelating agents with aminoglycoside administration has been shown to prevent ototoxicity in laboratory animals (Sha & Schacht, 1997). Clinical trials will be needed to see whether this will be of benefit to humans.

Nonaminoglycoside medications that have potentially ototoxic or vestibulotoxic side effects are erythromicin, vancomycin, loop diuretics, antineoplastic agents, anti-inflamatory agents, and antimalarial agents. These will be discussed in the following.

Erythromycin

Erythromycin is a macrolide antibiotic used to treat many common upper and lower respiratory tract infections and Legionnaire's disease. Symptoms of erythromycin ototoxicity include hearing loss, tinnitus, and, rarely, vertigo. Coexisting advanced age, hepatic or renal failure, Legionnaire's disease, and doses greater than 4 g/d predispose patients to ototoxicity. Symptoms of ototoxicity are potentially reversible with discontinuation of therapy (Roland & Marple, 1997; Stringer et al, 1991).

Vancomycin

Vancomycin, in the intravenous form, is used to treat serious infections caused by *Staphylococcus aureus*. Vancomycin may be cochleotoxic and vestibulotoxic. Its side effects may be transient or permanent. Its ototoxic effects have been associated with pre-existing hearing loss, high doses, and renal dysfunction. As with most of the ototoxic medications, monitoring audiometry may be useful in identifying early ototoxicity (Arky, 1995).

Other Antibiotics

Other antibiotics with known ototoxic effects are minocycline, chloramphenicol, polymyxin B, pharmacetin, and colistin (Stringer et al, 1991).

Loop Diuretics

Loop diuretics, used to treat fluid overload, congestive heart failure, pulmonary edema, and hypertension, may produce transient or permanent hearing loss. The risk of hearing loss is increased with rapid dosing, renal impairment, or concomitant use of other ototoxic medications. Furosemide, ethacrynic acid, and bumetanide are examples of loop diuretics. Cautious dosing in patients with renal impairment and treatment with other ototoxic medications may reduce the risk of ototoxicity (Roland & Marple, 1997; Stringer et al, 1991).

Antineoplastic Agents

Cisplatin, bleomycin, 5-fluorouracil, and nitrogen mustard are antineoplastic agents known to cause ototoxicity. These chemotherapeutic agents are used to treat leukemia; lymphoma; and cancers of lung, head and neck, breast, ovary, testicle, gastrointestinal tract, and connective tissue (Fischer, 1987). Cisplatin, the most studied, causes hearing loss, tinnitus, and instability. The higher frequencies are affected early and progress to low-frequency hearing loss as toxicity continues. Tinnitus and early hearing loss may be reversible. Vestibular toxicity does occur. The risk of ototoxicity increases with rapid dosing, cumulative doses more than 400 mg, renal impairment, volume depletion, intracranial radiation, and concomitant use of other ototoxic medications. High-frequency audiometry may be useful as an early detection of ototoxicity (Stringer et al, 1991). The only treatment for antineoplastic ototoxicity is to discontinue the medication, if possible.

Anti-Inflammatory Agents

Aspirin, an anti-inflammatory salicylate, is used to treat everyday aches and pains and rheumatoid arthritis. Tinnitus and sensory hearing loss occur with higher doses and high blood levels. The hearing loss is rarely more than 40 dB and is typically flat. These effects are reversible with decreasing or discontinuing therapy. The effects are so predictable that physicians have used tinnitus and hearing loss to determine effective dosages. Other nonsteroidal anti-inflammatory agents may also cause sensory hearing loss; however, the hearing loss and tinnitus from these agents may not be reversible (Roland & Marple, 1997; Stringer et al, 1991).

Antimalarials

Quinine and chloroquinine have been used to protect against malaria. They are capable of producing tinnitus and sensorineural hearing loss that is dose related. Their toxicity is usually reversible with termination of therapy (Roland & Marple, 1997).

TRAUMA

Head injury (temporal bone fracture and concussion), noise trauma, and barotrauma may cause cochlear hearing loss. The sensorineural hearing loss may be transient or permanent. Hearing loss is the most common sequella of head injury. Twenty to 40% of patients with head injury have hearing loss. Ten to 24% of patients with head injury have high-

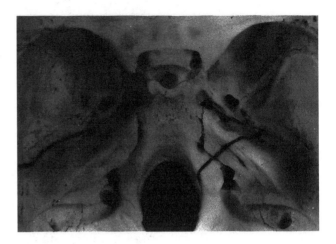

Figure 11–7 Photograph of skull base, viewed from above, with a longitudinal fracture *(left)* and a transverse temporal bone fracture *(right)* drawn onto the bone. (From Huang & Lambert [1997], with permission.)

frequency sensorineural hearing loss. Nearly 15% of patients with brain concussion, without skull fracture, have hearing loss (Friedman & Luxford, 1998).

Temporal Bone Fractures

Transverse and longitudinal temporal bone fractures causing neural (retrocochlear) hearing loss are discussed elsewhere in this textbook. Sensorineural hearing loss (cochlear or retrocochlear) occurs more commonly with transverse temporal bone fractures (Figs. 11–7 and 11–8). Cochlear hearing loss occurring with temporal bone fractures may be due to a direct fracture through the otic capsule, as in transverse fractures, a perilymphatic fistula from disruption of the stapes in the oval window, or by labyrinthine concussion.

Head injury causing labyrinthine concussion may occur with or without associated skull fracture. Labyrinthine concussion describes a nonfracture injury to the labyrinthine capsule that results in vertigo, disequilibrium, with or without hearing loss, aural fullness, and tinnitus. Vestibular abnormalities identified by electronystagmography and platform posturography and sensorineural hearing loss can be helpful with diagnosis. Recovery depends on associated injury but is usually complete in weeks.

Treatment of hearing loss from head trauma is usually directed at restoration of middle ear function if the ossicles are fixed or separated and the repair of perilymphatic fistulas, is suspected and ultimately found at surgery. Vestibular rehabilitation may be useful in hastening recovery. The reader may refer to the Chapter 21 in this volume. Differentiating between labyrinthine concussion, posttraumatic endolymphatic hydrops, and perilymph fistula may be difficult. Surgical exploration for *perilymph fistula* (PLF) should be considered in patients with head trauma who continue to have fluctuating hearing loss and vertigo (Roland & Marple, 1997). After head trauma, some patients have typical attacks of what appears to be Meniere's syndrome (posttraumatic endolymphatic hydrops): vertigo, aural fullness, hearing loss that may last hours (DiBiase & Arriaga, 1997). The treatment

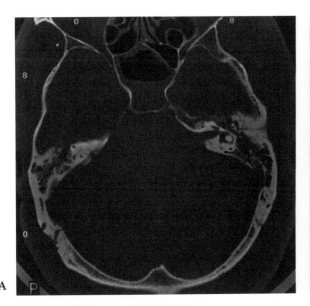 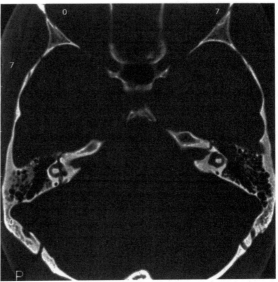

A   B

Figure 11–8 **(A)** Axial computed tomography (CT) showing a left longitudinal temporal bone fracture. The fracture extends along the external auditory canal toward the incus and head of malleus in the epitympanum. **(B)** Axial CT showing a right transverse temporal bone fracture through the labyrinth. (From Huang & Lambert [1997], with permission.)

of posttraumatic endolymphatic hydrops is the same as the treatment for Meniere's disease.

Perilymph Fistula

PLF is an abnormal communication between the labyrinth and the middle ear spaces that can allow passage of perilymph into the middle ear spaces, air into the labyrinth, or a mixture of perilymph and endolymph if a tear is present in the membranous labyrinth. The most common site for PLF is the oval window followed by the round window; however, cholesteatomas or fractures may produce fistulas directly into the cochlea or, more commonly, into the horizontal semicircular canal. PLFs may also be congenital. They can also occur bilaterally. The congenital form is associated with craniofacial malformation, birth trauma, and inner ear malformations such as large vestibular aqueduct syndrome and common cavity deformity as in Mondini dysplasia. Acquired PLFs are associated with head trauma, noise trauma, barotrauma (swimming/diving, nonpressurized airline travel, scuba diving, skydiving, forceful nose blowing, and sneezing), recent ear surgery, cholesteatoma, or tumors of the middle ear, and vigorous physical activity.

Symptoms

Symptoms include fluctuating or progressive sensorineural hearing loss and fluctuating or progressive vertigo or disequilibrium. Symptoms seem to be improved in the morning or after periods of rest and worsen in the evening or after prolonged periods of activity. Symptoms tend to be persistent and insidious without the well-defined symptom-free intervals seen with Meniere's disease. However, the patient may be symptom free for periods of time punctuated by recurrence after strenuous physical activity, minor trauma, straining, or nose blowing (Black & Pesznecker, 1998; Bluestone, 1998; Brookhouser, 1996).

Evaluation

The history and physical examination may raise the index of suspicion. Audiometry, vestibular testing, ABR, electrocochleography, and CT scan of temporal bones can help confirm or dispel suspicion. Unfortunately, no preoperative test or findings on physical examination are diagnostic of PLF. The "gold standard" for *diagnosis* is visualization, during exploratory tympanotomy, of clear fluid leaking from a definite opening in the inner ear. However, even during surgery, the differentiation between accumulation of perilymph, transudate, cerebrospinal fluid, irrigation, or anesthetic solutions in the middle ear space is difficult. Western blot assays for beta$_2$-transferrin (a marker believed to be unique to perilymph and cerebrospinal fluid) have been advocated to help with this problem; however, no widely available rapid analysis technique has been developed (Brookhouser, 1996; Roland & Marple, 1997).

Treatment

Initial management of PLF is directed at reducing intracranial pressure with bedrest and head elevation; avoidance of straining, lifting, and bending with the head down; stool softeners; vestibular suppressants; and sedation. In patients whose hearing loss continues to progress despite conservative management, a trial of carbogen therapy is considered by some authors before surgical exploration (Black & Pesznecker, 1998). Closure of the PLF is indicated for prevention of bacterial meningitis and control of progressive hearing and vestibular loss.

Surgical exploration may be performed with the patient under local anesthesia, with sedation, or under general anesthesia. A tympanomeatal flap is elevated, exposing the middle ear space. The oval and round windows are observed for direct leakage of fluid. Care is taken to keep the operative field dry of transudate, blood, irrigation, and local anesthetics. If no obvious fluid can be seen directly escaping the inner ear during active or passive Valsalva maneuvers, the middle ear space is observed for persistent reaccumulation of fluid. Fluid may be sent for analysis at a later time. If a fistula is found, the mucosa about the fistula is removed manually or with a laser, and the fistula is repaired with previously harvested loose areolar tissue, muscle with or without various combinations of cryoprecipitated fibrinogen, bovine collagen, and bovine thrombin. The argon laser may be used to "weld" the graft tissue in place (Black & Pesznecker, 1998; Roland & Marple, 1997).

In the immediate postoperative period the patient is confined to strict bedrest with head elevation, avoidance of the Valsalva maneuver, stool softeners, and, where appropriate, vestibular suppressants, and sedation. Over a period of time, depending on the symptoms and surgical findings, the patient may gradually return to normal activity with some restrictions, including avoidance of activities known to increase intracranial pressure.

Noise Trauma

Sound, ranging from high-intensity, short-duration, to lower intensity, long-duration exposure may result in cochlear (sensory) hearing loss that is either transient or permanent. Tinnitus and threshold shifts after noise exposure are indications of cochlear injury that may contribute to permanent threshold shifts (Roland & Marple, 1997).

Sudden, extremely intense sounds can tear the membranous labyrinth; this is termed noise trauma. More commonly, less intense sound over longer durations resulting in hearing loss is known as noise-induced hearing loss.

Permanent cochlear hearing loss from intense sound may be ameliorated with amplification. However, prevention is the principal focus in this disorder.

PEARL

Noise trauma is distinctly different than noise-induced hearing loss.

The reader may refer to Chapter 22 in this volume for use of hearing protection to reduce effects of noise exposure. Genetic predisposition for noise-induced hearing loss seems to be very important. Thus individuals who seem to have a more rapid or greater hearing loss for the amount of noise exposure should be especially told of this predisposition and warned of the consequences for themselves specifically.

Barotrauma

Barotrauma occurs when the ear is subjected to (1) sudden changes in pressure or (2) more gradual changes in pressure that cannot be equalized by the eustachian tube. Activities such as scuba diving, skydiving, airline travel, severe sneezing, lifting, straining at the stool, and vigorous sexual activity may be associated with cochlear hearing loss. Barotrauma causing cochlear hearing loss is much less common than the conductive hearing loss from sudden middle ear effusion. The sensorineural hearing loss that occurs may be partial or complete.

Causes may included perilymphatic fistulas, rupture of the membranous labyrinth, and/or intralabyrinthine hemorrhage. Initial treatment is directed at avoidance of activities associated with sudden changes in external or internal increases of pressure across the middle or inner ear, such as the Valsalva maneuver, coughing, sneezing, and airline travel. Patients with symptoms that persist after conservative treatment may require surgical exploration (Hough & McGee, 1991).

INFECTIONS

Cytomegalovirus

Infection with cytomegalovirus (CMV), a herpes-type virus, is the most common *congenital infection* occurring in 1 to 2% of live newborns in the United States. It is the most common cause of early acquired sensorineural hearing loss in infants and children. Most infections in adults and children with intact immune systems are asymptomatic. Ninety to 95% of CMV neonatal infections are asymptomatic. However, 1 to 5% have CMV inclusion disease and may have multi-organ disease, causing dysfunction of the brain, liver, spleen, eye, and inner ear. One in 1000 congenitally infected asymptomatic patients have sensorineural hearing loss beyond the first year of life. Five to 15% of these patients eventually have mild-to-moderate bilateral hearing loss. Hearing loss is poorer at the high frequencies. Fowler and others found that asymptomatic congenital CMV infection is likely a leading cause of sensorineural hearing loss in young children. Furthermore, among CMV-infected children with an earlier hearing loss, further deterioration in hearing occurred in 50% (Fowler et al, 1997).

CMV infections *acquired after birth* in nonimmunocompromised patients rarely progress to sensorineural hearing loss. CMV infections in the immunocompromised patient may lead to more serious complications associated with multi-organ system involvement. CMV may be passed transplacentally during an acute infection or during reactivation of a latent infection in mothers who previously demonstrated immunity. A 20-fold increase is found in parental infection in families with a child actively excreting virus and a 10-fold increase in parental infection in day-care workers.

Diagnosis of CMV in the newborn may be made by (1) isolation of virus in urine, saliva, or umbilical cord blood; or (2) detection of CMV DNA by polymerase chain reaction. Detection of neonatal immunoglobulins to CMV may be helpful if performed in the first weeks of life. Active infection is treated with acyclovir, gancyclovir, or foscarnet sodium (Brookhouser, 1996; Davis, 1998; Irving & Ruben, 1998).

Toxoplasmosis

Toxoplasma gondii is an obligate intracellular protozoan parasite that can infect humans or other warm-blooded species. It is commonly acquired after ingestion of material contaminated with feces from infected cats, which are a reservoir for the oocyst-containing parasites. Nonimmunocompromised adults and children may experience a flulike illness. The fetus of a first-time infected mother may have congenital toxoplasmosis develop. Ninety to 95% of subclinically infected infants may eventually have symptoms of infection develop up to 16 years of age, predominantly retinal and choroid problems. Hearing loss occurs in 25% of these patients if not treated. In these untreated cases the progressive hearing loss is due to the continued inflammatory response within the cochlea caused by the presence of the organism. Five to 10% of congenitally infected neonates are born with severe complications of toxoplasmosis with involvement of the central nervous system and eye.

Diagnosis is made on clinical suspicion, serologic testing of the mother and infant, and occasionally CT scan of the neonate brain.

Spiramicin is used to treat mothers until definitive diagnosis. If infection is confirmed, a regimen of pyrimethamine-sulfonamide is initiated. Pyrimethamine-sulfonamide is alternated with spiramicin and continued for 1 year in the infected neonate. Patients with acquired immunodeficiency syndrome (AIDS) with toxoplasmosis are treated with pyrimethamine, trisulfapyrimadines, prednisone, and clindamycin. Risk of infection may be reduced by immunizing kittens with antitoxoplasma vaccine and heating food to at least 70 degrees for 10 minutes (Brookhouser, 1996; Irving & Ruben, 1998).

Congenital Rubella

Rubella virus infection during pregnancy may lead to a wide variety of congenital problems, ranging from delayed sensorineural hearing loss to congenital heart defects, ocular defects, hepatosplenomegaly, thrombocytopenia, microcephaly, mental or motor retardation, long bone radiolucencies, interstitial pneumonitis, encephalitis, and low birth weight. The severity of complications is associated with duration of infection during pregnancy. First trimester infections are associated with worse outcomes than third trimester infections.

The classic triad of the congenitally infected infant is congenital hearing loss, cataracts, and cardiac defects. The sensorineural hearing loss is usually flat in configuration and severe or profound. Fifty percent of infants born with symptomatic congenital rubella have hearing loss. Infants born with infection later in the pregnancy may be asymptomatic at birth. Ten to 20% of these asymptomatic children have hearing loss that may be progressive.

Clinical suspicion should be elevated in the patient with congenital hearing loss with a mother that had a history of skin rash during pregnancy. Diagnosis of congenital rubella may be made by (1) isolation of rubella virus or detecting rubella RNA from urine or throat cultures, (2) detection of neonatal IgM antibodies in the first weeks of life, (3) detection of increasing antirubella antibody titer in the first few months of life, and (4) ophthalmologic examination may reveal pigment abnormalities diagnostic of rubella embryopathy.

Unfortunately, no treatment for preventing the sequellae of congenital rubella infection exists after infection occurs. However, prevention of rubella infection with the introduction of the rubella vaccine has significantly reduced the incidence of congenital rubella in this country (Brookhouser, 1996; Davis, 1998; Irving & Ruben, 1998).

Mumps (Epidemic Parotitis)

The mumps virus causes a flulike illness with sore throat, chills, fever, malaise, and parotid gland swelling in children and young adults. Deafness that occurs with mumps usually occurs at the end of the first week of parotitis. It is unilateral in 80% of the cases and is usually profound and permanent. Tinnitus and fullness in the affected ear are common.

Mumps may be diagnosed by viral isolation from throat cultures or cerebrospinal fluid (CSF) or detection of a rise in mumps antibody titers between acute and convalescent titers. At present, no treatment exists for mumps infection; however, mumps vaccine given at an early age prevents infection in later life (Brookhouser, 1996; Davis, 1998).

Measles

Measles is a highly communicable viral disease causing fever, sore throat, cough, and rash in the pediatric to young adult age group. It is caused by the rubeola virus. Deafness occurs in 0.1% of patients with measles. The bilateral and usually abrupt onset of hearing loss occurs at the time of the rash. Usually a greater degree of hearing loss is seen in the higher frequencies. No specific treatment for measles or its associated hearing loss exists. Measles and deafness caused by measles is now rare because of the widespread use of the rubeola vaccine (Davis, 1998).

Varicella-Zoster Virus

The varicella-zoster virus is a *herpesvirus* that is identical to the virus that causes chickenpox (varicella) and shingles (zoster). Infections by this virus (herpes-zoster oticus or Ramsay Hunt syndrome) cause painful vesicular eruptions of the earcanal and external ear, facial paralysis, and occasionally sensorineural hearing loss and vertigo. Sensorineural hearing loss occurs in 6% of these patients.

The diagnosis is based on a high level of clinical suspicion. Herpes-zoster oticus can be confirmed by the isolation of virus from vesicles, detection of virus DNA in vesicle fluid or CSF, and demonstration of multinucleated giant cells in vesicle scrapings. Treatment consists of local care of the vesicles, acyclovir, and anti-inflammatory steroids (Davis, 1998; Kinney et al, 1997; Rubinstein & Gantz, 1997; Schaitkin et al, 1998; Wackym & Cyr, 1998).

Human Immunodeficiency Virus

AIDS is caused by the human immunodeficiency virus (HIV). Sensorineural hearing loss is seen in 49% of HIV-infected patients. Worsening cochlear and vestibular dysfunction is correlated with longer durations of infection. The cause of sensorineural hearing loss in HIV-infected patients is due to (1) use of potentially ototoxic medication (Marra et al, 1997); (2) opportunistic infection; (3) neoplastic processes affecting the temporal bone, internal auditory canal, and central nervous system; (4) idiopathic causes; (5) central nervous system infections or demyelination. Potentially ototoxic medications used to treat HIV complications are aminoglycosides, amphotericin B, azydothymidine, pentamidine, and azythromycin. HIV-infected patients are predisposed to syphilis and cryptococcal meningitis, which can cause sensorineural hearing loss.

Otosyphilis should be considered in any HIV-infected patient complaining of hearing loss or vertigo. Patients may complain of sudden, progressive, or fluctuating hearing loss with or without tinnitus, aural fullness, or disequilibrium. Diagnosis may be made with FTA-ABS fluorescent treponemal antibody absorption test (FTA-ABS) and Venereal Disease Research Laboratory test (VDRL).

Treatment of otosyphilis in the HIV-infected patient should consist of high-dose penicillin given over several weeks. Corticosteroids, normally used in treating non-HIV otosyphilis, should be used with caution in the HIV population because they may worsen the pre-existing immunocompromised condition. In addition, previously treated HIV-syphilis patients may have reactivation of latent syphilis; therefore recurrent otosyphilis should be suspected in any treated patient with cochleovestibular complaints.

Sensorineural hearing loss caused by *cryptococcal meningitis* may have headache, nausea/vomiting, disorientation, and cranial nerve abnormalities. Hearing loss is the most common cranial nerve abnormality and may be the initial presenting symptom. Cryptococcal meningitis causes a predominantly retrocochlear hearing loss. Diagnosis can be made by serum cryptococcal antigen and evaluation of CSF by lumbar puncture. Cryptococcal meningitis is treated with amphotericin B and 5-fluorocytosine followed by life-long suppression with fluconazole.

Central auditory dysfunction unrelated to cryptococcal meningitis is a common cause of sensorineural hearing loss in the patient with HIV and is related to demyelination of the central auditory tract. Evaluation of sensorineural hearing loss in the HIV-infected patient should include a thorough history, head and neck examination, pure tone audiometry with evaluation of stapedial reflex, and word recognition scores. In addition, electronystagmography may be useful in the evaluation of patients with disequilibrium. VDRL test, FTA test, serum cryptococcal antigen, antinuclear antibodies, erythrocyte sedimentation rate, and rheumatoid factor may be useful. MRI or CT scan should precede lumbar puncture in patients with neurological signs or symptoms.

Treatment of HIV-infected patients with hearing loss should concentrate on the underlying cause of hearing loss. Caution should be exercised with the use of anti-inflammatory steroids because of their inherent risk of worsening immunosuppression (Monsell et al, 1997).

Other Viruses and *Mycoplasma*

Adenovirus, influenza virus, and *Mycoplasma* (a nonviral cause of pneumonia) have been associated with sensorineural hearing loss. In addition, sudden sensorineural hearing loss occurs in the presence of an upper respiratory tract infection in 25% of patients. Epidemiologic clusters of upper respiratory tract infections associated with sensorineural hearing loss have been observed (Roland & Marple, 1997).

Meningitis

Meningitis is caused by inflammation of the brain or spinal cord and may be caused by bacteria, viri, or more rarely disseminated fungal infections, disseminated malignancies, and chemicals or toxins. Symptoms of meningitis are fever, headache, stiff neck, and vomiting. This may progress to disorientation, coma, or death. One third of all noncongenital hearing loss is due to complications of bacterial meningitis.

Persistent sensorineural loss occurs in 10% from bacteria or their toxin invading the inner ears from the CSF. Deafness may occur at any point during the course of meningitis; however, it commonly occurs early. Bacteria most commonly associated with sensorineural hearing loss after meningitis are *Streptococcus pneumoniae, Neisseria meningitides,* and *Haemophilus influenzae.*

Diagnosis is made by history, physical examination, and CSF evaluation and culture from lumbar puncture.

Treatment is aimed at appropriate antibiotic therapy and corticosteroids. Corticosteroids reduce the inflammatory process in the labyrinth, therefore lessening the chances or intensity of hearing loss (Davis, 1998).

Labyrinthitis

Labyrinthitis is due to an inflammatory process within the labyrinth. It may be secondary to direct invasion by bacteria, viri, spirochetes, protozoa, or fungi or their toxic effects. The types of labyrinthitis are stratified into perilabyrinthitis and endolabyrinthitis. Perilabyrinthitis is caused by substances entering the perilymph and defined by what enters the fluid. In *serous* labyrinthitis, toxins enter; in *suppurative* labyrinthitis, bacteria enter; and in *chronic* labyrinthitis, soft tissue enters, like the matrix of a cholesteatoma. Endolabyrinthitis is from hematogenous dissemination of viri to the membranous labyrinth. End-stage obliteration of the labyrinth with fibrous tissue is called fibrous labyrinthitis, and obliteration with new bone is known as labyrinthine ossificans. *Serous labyrinthitis* is one of the most common complications of otitis media. It is caused by bacterial toxins entering the labyrinth from an adjacent acute otitis media. These toxins may enter the inner ear from the CSF in cases of meningitis.

Clinically, the patient experiences vertigo, tinnitus, and sensorineural hearing loss associated with otitis media or meningitis. The accompanying irritative nystagmus beats toward the affected ear until it rapidly becomes paralytic to the labyrinth and reverses direction. The cochleovestibular symptoms can be reversible. Treatment for serous labyrinthitis includes supportive care, appropriate antibiotic coverage, and myringotomy in patients with bacterial otitis media. It can rapidly progress to bacterial labyrinthitis and meningitis.

PEARL

Sudden onset of severe vertigo, tinnitus, nausea and vomiting with sudden hearing loss in the setting of an acute or chronic otitis media indicates that labyrinthitis has developed. Within a very short time, this can progress to meningitis.

Suppurative labyrinthitis occurs with direct bacterial invasion of the labyrinth. Signs and symptoms are exactly the same as serous labyrinthitis; however, recovery does not occur and meningitis can rapidly result. Therefore patients with these signs and symptoms and an ear infection should be considered a medical emergency. The ultimate recovery profile will determine whether it is suppurative or serous.

Treatment for suppurative labyrinthitis consists of hospitalization, hydration, vestibular suppressants, and appropriate antibiotic therapy. Antibiotic selection depends on the results of culture obtained from the patient and the specific antibiotic sensitivities of the cultured organism. When acute otitis media is the source of infection, myringotomy for drainage and bacterial identification is necessary. Mastoidectomy may be required to resolve a subacute or chronic infection.

Chronic labyrinthitis is a complication of chronic middle ear disease, characteristically with cholesteatoma, resulting in fistula through the otic capsule, usually over the horizontal semicircular canal. Other causes of fistula are granulation tissue, cholesterol granuloma, and tumors of the middle ear. A patient with a history of chronic ear disease presenting with fluctuating mild vertigo or hearing loss that is worsened by the Valsalva maneuver, or pressure on the ear should be suspected of having a labyrinthine fistula. A positive fistula test is found by creating positive or negative pressure in the external auditory canal that causes vertigo with nystagmus. Patients with this problem are predisposed to suppurative labyrinthitis. Mastoidectomy is usually required to resolve this problem (Bassiouni & Paparella, 1991; Bluestone & Klein, 1996; Roland & Marple, 1997; Slattery & House, 1998; Wackym & Cyr, 1998).

PITFALL

Failure to make the diagnosis of labyrinthine fistula may result in permanent loss of cochleovestibular function.

Labyrinthine fibrosis and ossification are a common sequellae to suppurative labyrinthitis. This process begins within months of a suppurative labyrinthitis and is caused by fibrous replacement of the inner ear structures. This fibrous process is followed by bony replacement of the labyrinth. Clinically, deafness is complete, the incapacitating vertigo has disappeared, and the patient may continue to have mild disequilibrium.

Although little can be done to stop ossification, it is important to recognize its early development in potential cochlear implant patients. Insertion of the complete electrode array is difficult once labyrinthine ossification begins. In addition, performance of patients implanted after the ossification process is poorer than those implanted before ossification. Temporal bone CT and/or MRI confirms labyrinthine fibrosis and/or ossification (Bassiouni & Paparella, 1991; Bluestone & Klein, 1996; Roland & Marple, 1997).

Fungal Infections

Fungal infections of the labyrinth are rare. Species associated with fungal labyrinthitis are *Candida, Mucor, Cryptococcus,* and *Blastomyces.* Infections of this nature usually occur in patients with immunocompromise (i.e., AIDS and transplant patients), diabetes, leukemia, or terminal illness. The source of infection may be middle ear, meninges, or blood borne. When possible, treatment is directed at correcting the underlying cause and administration of intravenous amphotericin B (Bassiouni & Paparella, 1991).

Syphilis

Otitic syphilis is caused by the spirochete *Treponema pallidum.* Often the presenting symptoms are similar to those of Meniere's disease: fluctuating progressive sensorineural hearing loss, aural fullness, tinnitus, and vertigo. However, otitic syphilis has a higher incidence of bilateral disease. Syphilis as a cause of sensorineural hearing loss occurs during the late congenital and tertiary acquired stage of syphilis.

Symptoms are due to a resorptive osteitis of the labyrinth that can destroy the inner ear, cause hydrops, or cause fistulization of the bony labyrinthine wall. A positive Hennebert's sign (vertigo and nystagmus with pressure applied to the earcanal) and Tullio's phenomenon (vertigo seen with high-intensity sound) can be associated with otosyphilis.

Diagnosis is suspected if there is a positive FTA-ABS or VDRL test result in a patient with these symptoms. Neurosyphilis must be excluded or confirmed by evaluating the CSF for organisms and/or positive CSF, FTA-ABS, and VDRL test findings.

Treatment consists of high-dose, long-term penicillin and anti-inflammatory corticosteroids (Arts, 1998; Brookhouser, 1996; Monsell et al, 1997; Roland & Marple, 1997).

PEARL

In patients with fluctuating hearing loss with or without vertigo, it is important to consider syphilis a treatable disease.

MALIGNANCY

Malignancies invading the temporal bone may be classified into those originating in the temporal bone (primary) or metastasizing to the temporal bone from other sites (secondary or metastasis). They are uncommon and rarely cause a sensorineural hearing loss until the labyrinth is involved. Squamous cell carcinoma is the most common malignancy involving the temporal bone in adults (85%). The remaining 15% of adult temporal bone malignancies are due to basal cell carcinomas, glandular tumors, regionally invasive cancers, and metastases. In the pediatric population rhabdomyosarcoma is by far the most common temporal bone malignancy followed by leukemia, fibrosarcoma, Ewing's sarcoma, and aggressive papillary adenoma.

Metastatic tumors to the temporal bone may originate from carcinomas of the breast, kidney, thyroid, lung, bone, and gastrointestinal tract. Also metastasis from melanoma, leukemia, and lymphomas occur occasionally.

Pain is the most common and noteworthy symptom of temporal bone malignancy followed by hearing loss, pruritus, bleeding, headache, tinnitus, and vertigo. Typical signs of temporal bone malignancy are earcanal ulcerated mass, aural drainage, periauricular swelling, facial paralysis, and cervical adenopathy. Diagnosis is usually made by biopsy with additional information from CT and MRI scanning.

Treatment for most temporal bone malignancies usually consists of local measures (i.e., wound care and control of infection) and options of surgical resection, radiation therapy, and chemotherapy. It should be remembered that many anti-neoplastic agents are capable of causing ototoxicity. These are discussed elsewhere in this chapter.

Hematopoietic malignancies such as lymphoma and leukemia may involve the temporal bone and have a granular friable mass in the earcanal or middle ear space, thickened tympanic membrane, otitis media, hearing loss, mastoiditis, and facial nerve paralysis. Acute lymphocytic leukemia produces more otologic symptoms than the other leukemias. Involvement of the temporal bone occurs in 20% of patients with leukemia. The temporal bone is affected by leukemic infiltrates, hemorrhage, and infection. Leukemic infiltrate of the labyrinth is rare.

Treatment is directed at controlling the leukemia and any secondary infection. Chemotherapy, culture, antibiotics, myringotomy and tube placement, and mastoidectomy may become necessary. Aural complications usually improve with treatment of the underlying leukemia (Cass, 1996; Doyle, 1998; Pensak & Friedman, 1997).

PRESBYCUSIS

Presbycusis describes the loss of hearing associated with the aging process. Schuknecht has defined four histopathologic types: sensory, neural, strial, and cochlear conductive (Schuknecht, 1993). *Sensory presbycusis* is due to flattening and atrophy of the basal turn of the organ of Corti because of loss of hair cells and supporting cells. It produces a progressive bilateral, sharply sloping high-frequency sensorineural hearing loss that begins in middle age.

Neural presbycusis is initially due to atrophy of the spiral ganglion and nerves of the osseous spiral lamina in the basal turn of the cochlea. Neural presbycusis produces a moderate sloping high-frequency hearing loss that is bilateral and gradual in progression. The organ of Corti is usually intact compared with sensory presbycusis. Speech discrimination scores are disproportionately worse than pure tone thresholds, making amplification more difficult.

Strial presbycusis is due to atrophy of the stria vascularis producing a flat sensorineural hearing loss with preservation of word recognition scores. Word discrimination scores are usually preserved until pure tone averages exceed 50 dB HL.

Cochlear conductive presbycusis is believed to be due to excessive stiffness of the basilar membrane; however, histopathological findings are absent. It produces an elevation of pure tone thresholds and decrease in word recognition scores. Audiometric evaluation demonstrates a bilateral linear gradually sloping sensorineural hearing loss.

At present, little can be done to prevent or slow the progression of presbycusis. However, moderately severe hearing loss, or worse, is usually not because of aging alone. After the occurrence of significant hearing loss, amplification or cochlear implantation may be the only treatment options available (Goodwin et al, 1998; Monsell et al, 1997). The reader may refer to Chapters 5, 6, 12, 13, 16, and 17 in this volume.

SUDDEN IDIOPATHIC SENSORINEURAL HEARING LOSS

Sudden sensorineural hearing loss is defined by a sensorineural hearing loss of 30 dB HL or greater over at least three audiometric frequencies occurring within 3 days or less. With the exception of presbycusis, most of the previously discussed causes of sensorineural hearing loss (infections, neoplasms, trauma, ototoxicity, immunologic, metabolic, and developmental) may have what initially appears to be idiopathic sudden sensorineural hearing loss. It is the duty of the practitioner to attempt to identify the source of any hearing loss by thorough history, physical examination, appropriate audiometric evaluation, laboratory examination, and diagnostic imaging. A careful patient history will identify a cause in 10 to 15% of these sudden cases. The "diagnosis" of sudden idiopathic hearing loss can only be made when other identifiable causes of hearing loss are ruled out.

Sudden sensorineural hearing loss occurs in approximately one patient per 5000 population per year. It is likely that more cases actually occur than present clinically because of possible spontaneous resolution before obtaining medical advice. No predilection for either ear or sex exists. No apparent occupational predisposition exists. The degree of hearing loss is variable and usually unilateral. Ten percent are bilateral. Seventy percent of patients with sudden deafness present with tinnitus, and 40% have some form of vertigo or disequilibrium. Two-thirds of patients improve without treatment within 2 weeks. Fifteen percent of patients with hearing loss progress. A poorer prognosis for recovery is associated with severity and duration of hearing loss, presence of vertigo, advanced age, and reduced word recognition scores. In addition, the shape of the audiogram appears to have some relationship to prognosis. Rising and trough configurations have a better prognosis for recovery than sloping or flat configurations.

When identifiable, treatment of sudden sensorineural hearing loss is based on the cause. Treatments of sudden idiopathic sensorineural hearing loss are numerous, based on suspected cause. Viral infection, labyrinthine hypoxia, and autoimmune disease have been suggested as potential factors. In the past treatment regimens have aimed at (1) improving blood flow or oxygenation to the inner ear, (2) fighting possible viral infection, (3) reducing inflamation or autoimmune response, (4) preventing further injury (rest), and (5) reducing the potential causes of hydrops. The current, generally accepted approach includes an initial trial of bedrest, anti-inflammatory corticosteroids, low-salt diet, and a diuretic. Others would consider the addition of oral antiviral medication and the vasodialating properties of Carbogen, an inhaled mixture of oxygen and carbon dioxide. When medical therapy fails and there is suspicion of PLF, surgical exploration may be warranted (Arts, 1998).

HEREDITARY/DEVELOPMENTAL

One in 1000 children are born with a significant sensorineural hearing loss. Congenital hearing loss may be due to genetic and nongenetic causes. Twenty-five percent of congenital hearing losses are due to a nongenetic identifiable complication such as intrauterine injury from infection, hypoxia, exposure to ototoxic medication, radiation, and metabolic disorders. Fifty percent of congenital hearing impairment is hereditary.

Genetic hearing loss is transmitted by autosomal recessive, autosomal dominant, and X-linked inheritance. Seventy-five to 90% of genetic hearing losses are transmitted in the autosomal recessive pattern. Genetic (hereditary) hearing loss should be suspected in patients with a "U-shaped" ("cookie-bite") audiogram or patients with immediate relatives with premature hearing loss.

Genetic hearing loss may be divided into syndromic and nonsyndromic categories. Syndromic hearing loss implies hearing loss associated with other clinically detectable abnormalities, whereas nonsyndromic hearing loss implies hearing loss alone. Approximately 30% of congenital genetic hearing losses are associated with syndromes. More than 200 syndromes have been identified that are associated with neurosensory hearing loss. Congenital hearing impairment should be considered the first sign of a syndrome.

Some patients with syndromic hearing loss have more apparent associated dysmorphic features of the head and neck and cutaneous or musculoskeletal systems. Other associated malformations may be more difficult to detect (i.e., cardiac or renal abnormalities). *Waardenburg's syndrome*, an autosomal dominant inherited disorder, may present with sensorineural hearing loss and abnormalities of pigmentation such as white forelock, premature graying of hair, or two eyes of different color (heterochromia iridis). In addition, craniofacial abnormalities such as high broad nasal root, confluent eyebrows, and lateral displacement of the medial canthi of the eyes (dystopia canthorum) may be evident.

A patient with *Pendred's syndrome* may have a congenital hearing loss with an enlarged thyroid gland (goiter). On further investigation the patient may actually have hypothyroidism.

Patients with *branchio-oto-renal syndrome* may have hearing loss, malformed pinna, preauricular pits, and/or branchial cleft cysts or fistulas. Identification of this disorder is important because many patients also have renal anomalies.

Goldenhar syndrome patients have varying degrees of *hemifacial asymmetry* or mandibular hypoplasia, with mixed hearing loss. On further examination, these patients may possess abnormalities of the ocular, renal, skeletal, and central nervous system.

However *symmetric* malar hypoplasia with underdeveloped zygomatic arches (small cheekbones), mandibular hypoplasia (small mandible), downward sloping eyelids, microtia (small ears), aural meatal atresia (narrow earcanals) with mixed or sensorineural hearing loss describe *Treacher Collins syndrome* (mandibulofacial dysostosis).

A patient with sensorineural hearing loss and a family history of renal failure or hematuria (blood in the urine) might have *Alport's syndrome*. This includes hereditary progressive glomerulonephritis and sensorineural hearing loss. Interestingly, this syndrome affects women more commonly and men more severely. Fifty to 75% of affected males have end-stage renal failure develop by 20 to 40 years of age and require extensive treatment for the renal disease.

Young congenitally hearing-impaired children who are slow to sit, stand, or walk may be experiencing an additional vestibular disorder and difficulty with vision. The suspicion of *Usher's syndrome* should be entertained. This syndrome may accompany a constellation of symptoms ranging from poor night vision to blindness, mild sensorineural hearing loss to deafness, and normal balance to complete loss of vestibular function. More than 50% of cases of combined blindness and deafness are due to Usher's syndrome

(sensorineural hearing loss and retinitis pigmentosa). Diagnosis may be assisted by a complete ophthalmologic examination and electroretinography.

An obese patient who has progressive sensorineural hearing loss may have undiagnosed *Alstrom's syndrome*, an autosomal recessive disorder that may eventually have diabetes, retinal degeneration, and eventual blindness develop and require medical management of the diabetes.

A child being evaluated for congenital bilateral profound deafness with a history of syncopal attacks (complete loss of consciousness) and sudden lapses of consciousness or family history of a sibling with sudden unexplained death in childhood may have the autosomal recessively inherited disorder of *Jervell and Lange-Nielson*. This disorder includes hereditary sensorineural hearing loss and abnormalities in electrical conduction of the heart that may result in a lethal dysrhythmia. Electrocardiograms of these patients will have an abnormally prolonged QT interval. Syncopal attacks begin at ages of 3 to 5 years; before the development of appropriate cardiac medication, most affected individuals died by age 15 (Arts, 1998; Bauer & Jenkins, 1998; Brookhouser, 1996; Grundfast, 1996; Grundfast & Toriello, 1998; Khetarpal & Lalwani, 1998; Reilly et al, 1998; Schoem & Grundfast, 1998).

PEARL

It is important to recognize syndromic hearing loss to identify coexisting potentially treatable medical conditions and provide information for possible genetic counseling and identification of family members with undiagnosed genetically related medical problems.

Although little can be done to treat congenital hearing loss, early identification of patients with syndromic hereditary hearing loss often leads to early diagnosis and treatment of associated medical problems and, in many cases, avoidance of complications. An undiagnosed hereditary hearing loss should lead to a more detailed patient and family history. Questions to ask patients and families of suspected congenital sensorineural hearing loss are as follows:

1. Is there a family history of earlier than normal hearing loss (less than 30 years of age) (possible hereditary hearing impairment)?
2. Is there anyone in the family with eyes spaced widely apart, different colored eyes, premature graying of hair, unusual areas of depigmentation of skin (possible Waardenburg's syndrome)?
3. Is there a family history of night blindness or retinal disorders (possible Alstrom's syndrome or Usher's syndrome)?
4. Is there anyone on either side of the family with goiter (possible Pendred's syndrome)?
5. Is there any family history of sudden unexplained death in child or adolescent relatives? Is there any history of syncope or sudden loss of consciousness in this child? Is there anyone in the family with severe hearing impairment and an abnormal heart rhythm (possible Jervell and Lange-Nielson syndrome)?

6. Is there any history of delayed or difficulty sitting, standing, or walking in this patient (possible Usher's syndrome)?

7. Is there any family history of hematuria or renal failure (possible Alport's syndrome) (Brookhouser, 1996; Grundfast & Toriello, 1998)?

Any patient with a significant history of hereditary hearing loss should be evaluated by a pediatrician, otolaryngologist, audiologist, and so forth, with appropriate consultations to the clinical geneticist, urologist, cardiologist, ophthalmologist, and endocrinologist for further evaluation and treatment.

Management of the patient with congenital hearing loss includes early amplification, preschool aural rehabilitation, and special educational programs. In patients with syndromic hearing loss, it is important to initiate appropriate treatment and prevention strategies for associated medical problems.

Surgery for correcting associated craniofacial defects and conductive hearing loss may be necessary. In congenitally deaf patients in whom adequate aural rehabilitation fails, early cochlear implantation may be a reasonable option. The only absolute contraindication to cochlear implantation is aplasia of the auditory nerve, which is easily identified on CT scan (Grundfast & Lalwani, 1992; Reilly et al, 1998).

CONCLUSIONS

Cochlear hearing loss may be due to a multitude of factors. It is the responsibility of the practitioner to identify the cause of hearing loss and to evaluate the other potential associated medical ramifications to treat the patient as a whole. Complete audiological assessments are crucial in the initial evaluation and subsequent therapeutic monitoring of sensorineural hearing losses.

REFERENCES

AMEDEE, R.G., & JABOR, M.A. (1998). Wegener's granulomatosis. In: G.A. Gates (Ed.), *Current therapy in otolaryngology–head and neck surgery* (pp. 378–381). St. Louis: Mosby.

ARKY, R. (1995). *Physician's desk reference* (pp. 1371). Montvale: Medical Economics Data Production Company.

ARTS, H.A. (1998). Differential diagnosis of sensorineural hearing loss. In: C.W. Cummings, J.M. Fredrickson, L.A. Harker, C.J. Krause, M.A. Richardson, & D.E. Schuller (Eds.), *Otolaryngology–head and neck surgery* (Vol. 4) (pp. 2908–293). St. Louis: Mosby.

BASSIOUNI, M., & PAPARELLA, M.M. (1991). Labyrinthitis. In: M.M. Paparella, D.A. Shumrick, J.L. Gluckman, & W.L. Meyerhoff (Eds.), *Otolaryngology* (Vol. 2) (pp. 1601–1618). Philadelphia: W. B. Saunders.

BAUER, C.A., & JENKINS, H.A. (1998). Otologic symptoms and syndromes. In: C.W. Cummings, J.M. Fredrickson, L.A. Harker, C.J. Krause, M.A. Richardson, & D.E. Schuller (Eds.), *Otolaryngology–head and neck Surgery* (Vol. 4) (pp. 2547–2558). St. Louis: Mosby.

BLACK, F.O., & PESZNECKER, S.F. (1998). Perilymphatic fistula. In: G.A. Gates (Ed.), *Current therapy in otolaryngology–head and neck surgery* (pp. 71–78). St. Louis: Mosby.

BLUESTONE, C. (1998). Perilymphatic fistula in children. In: G.A. Gates (Ed.), *Current therapy in otolaryngology–head and neck surgery* (pp. 67–71). St. Louis: Mosby.

BLUESTONE, C.D., & KLEIN, J.O. (1996). Intratemporal complications and sequelae of otitis media. In: C.D. Bluestone, S.E. Stool, & M.A. Kenna (Eds.), *Pediatric otolaryngology* (Vol. 1) (pp. 583–635). Philadelphia: W.B. Saunders.

BROOKHOUSER, P.E. (1996). Diseases of the inner ear and sensorineural hearing loss. In: C.C. Bluestone, S.E. Stool, & M.A. Kenna (Eds.), *Pediatric otolaryngology* (Vol. 1) (pp. 649–670). Philadelphia: W.B. Saunders.

BURNS, D.K., & MEYERHOFF, W.L. (1991). Granulomatous disorders and related conditions of the ear and temporal bone. In: M.M. Paparella, D.A. Shumrick, J.L. Gluckman, & W.L. Meyerhoff (Eds.), *Otolaryngology* (Vol. 2) (pp. 1529–1559). Philadelphia: W.B. Saunders.

CASS, S.P. (1996). Tumors of the ear and temporal bone. In: C.D. Bluestone, S.E. Stool, & M.A. Kenna (Eds.), *Pediatric otolaryngology* (Vol. 1) (pp. 707–718). Philadelphia: W.B. Saunders.

CINAMON, U., KRONENBERG, J., HILDESHEIMER, M., & TAITELBAUM, R. (1997). Cochlear implantation in patients suffering from Cogan's syndrome. *Journal of Laryngology and Otology, 111*(10);928–930.

DAVIS, L.E. (1998). Infections of the labyrinth. In: C.W. Cummings, J.M. Fredrickson, L.A. Harker, C.J. Krause, M.A. Richardson, & D.E. Schuller (Eds.), *Otolaryngology–head and neck surgery* (Vol. 4) (pp. 3139–3152). St. Louis: Mosby.

DEKKER, P. (1993). Wegener's granulomatosis. *Journal of Otolaryngology, 22*(5);346–347.

DiBIASE, P., & ARRIAGA, M. (1997). Post-traumatic hydrops. *Otolaryngology Clinics of North America, 30*(6);1117–1122.

DOYLE, K.J. (1998). Tumors of the temporal bone. In: A.K. Lalwani, & K.M. Grundfast (Eds.), *Pediatric otology and neurotology* (pp. 505–513). Philadelphia: Lippincott-Raven.

DUCK, S., PRAZMA, J., BENNETT, P., & PILLSBURY, H. (1997). Interaction between hypertension and diabetes mellitus in the pathogenesis of sensorineural hearing loss. *Laryngoscope, 107*(12);1596–1605.

FAUSTI, S., HENRY, J., HAYDEN, D., PHILLIPS, D., & FREY, R. (1998). Intrasubject reliability of high-frequency (9-14 kHz) thresholds: Tested separately vs. following conventional-frequency testing. *Journal of the American Academy of Audiology, 9*(2);147–152.

FENTON, J., & O'SULLIVAN, T. (1994). The otologic manifestations of Wegener's granulomatosis. *Journal of Laryngology and Otology, 108*(2);144–146.

FISCHER, D.S. (1987). Cancer chemotherapy. In: K.J. Lee (Ed.), *Essential otolaryngology: Head and neck surgery* (pp. 839–853). New York: Medical Examination Publishing Company.

FOWLER, K., McCOLLISTER, F., DAHLE, A., BOPPANA, S., BRITT, W., & PASS, R. (1997). Progressive and fluctuating sensorineural hearing loss in children with asymptomatic congenital cytomegalovirus infection. *Journal of Pediatrics, 130*(4);624–630.

FRIEDMAN, R.A., & LUXFORD, W.M. (1998). Injuries of the auricle, middle ear, and temporal bone. In: A.K. Lalwani, & K.M. Grundfast (Eds.), *Pediatric otology and neurotology* (pp. 443–453). Philadelphia: Lippincott-Raven.

FRIEDMAN, S., SCHULMAN, R., & WEISS, S. (1975). Hearing and diabetic neuropathy. *Archives of Internal Medicine, 135*(4);573–576.

GENDEH, B., GIBB, A., AZIZ, N., KONG, N., & ZAHIR, Z. (1998). Vancomycin administration in continuous ambulatory peritoneal dialysis: The risk of ototoxicity. *Archives of Otolaryngology–Head and Neck Surgery, 118*(4);551–558.

GLASSCOCK, M.E., SHAMBAUGH, G.E., & JOHNSON, G.D. (1993). Operations for otospongiosis (otosclerosis). In: M.E. Glasscock, G.E. Shambaugh, & G.D. Johnson (Eds.), *Surgery of the ear* (pp. 389–418). Philadelphia: W.B. Saunders.

GOODWIN, W.J., BALKANY, T., & CASIANO, R.R. (1998). Special considerations in managing geriatric patients. In: C.W. Cummings, J.M. Fredrickson, L.A. Harker, C.J. Krause, M.A. Richardson, & D.E. Schuller (Eds.), *Otolaryngology–head and neck surgery* (Vol. 1) (pp. 314–326). St. Louis: Mosby.

GRUNDFAST, K.M. (1996). Hearing loss. In: C.D. Bluestone, S.E. Stool, & M.A. Kenna (Eds.), *Pediatric otolaryngology* (Vol. 1) (pp. 249–283). Philadelphia: W.B. Saunders.

GRUNDFAST, K.M., & LALWANI, A.K. (1992). Practical approaches to diagnosis and management of hereditary hearing impairment (HHI). *Ear, Nose, and Throat Journal, 71*(10);479–493.

GRUNDFAST, K.M., & TORIELLO, H. (1998). Syndromic hereditary hearing impairment. In: A.K. Lalwani, & K.M. Grundfast (Eds.), *Pediatric otology and neurotology* (pp. 341–363). Philadelphia: Lippincott-Raven.

HARRIS, J., HEYDT, J., KEITHLEY, E., & CHEN, M. (1997). Immunopathology of the inner ear: An update. *Annals of the New York Academy of Science, 830*;166–178.

HARRIS, J.P. (1998). Autoimmune inner ear disease. In: A.K. Lalwani, & K.M. Grundfast (Eds.), *Pediatric otology and neurotology* (pp. 405–419). Philadelphia: Lippincott-Raven.

HOUGH, J.V., & MCGEE, M. (1991). Otologic trauma. In: M.M. Paparella, D.A. Shumrick, J.L. Gluckman, & W.L. Meyerhoff (Eds.), *Otolaryngology* (Vol. 2) (pp. 1137–1160). Philadelphia: W.B. Saunders.

HOUSE, J.W. (1997). Otosclerosis. In: G.B. Hughes, & M.L. Pensak (Eds.), *Clinical otology* (pp. 241–249). New York: Thieme Medical Publishers, Inc.

HOUSE, J.W. (1998). Otosclerosis. In: C.W. Cummings, J.M. Fredrickson, L.A. Harker, C.J. Krause, M.A. Richardson, & D.E. Schuller (Eds.), *Otolaryngology–head and neck surgery* (Vol. 4) (pp. 3126–3135). St. Louis: Mosby.

HUANG, M.Y., & LAMBERT, P.R. (1997). Temporal bone trauma. In: G.B. Hughes, & M.L. Pensak (Eds.), *Clinical otology* (pp. 251–267). New York: Thieme Medical Publishers, Inc.

IRVING, R.M., & RUBEN, R.J. (1998). The acquired hearing losses of childhood. In: A.K. Lalwani, & K.M. Grundfast (Eds.), *Pediatric otology and neurotology* (pp. 375–385). Philadelphia: Lippincott-Raven.

KAASINEN, S., PYYKKO, I., & AALTO, H. (1998). Intratympanic gentamicin in Meniere's disease. *Acta Otolaryngologica (Stockholm), 118*(3);294–298.

KARTUSH, J.M., & LAROUERE, M.J. (1998). Meniere's disease: Surgical therapy. In: G.A. Gates (Ed.), *Current therapy in otolaryngology–head and neck surgery* (pp. 81–86). St. Louis: Mosby.

KHETARPAL, U., & LALWANI, A.K. (1998). Nonsyndromic hereditary hearing impairment. In: A.K. Lalwani, & K.M. Grundfast (Eds.), *Pediatric otology and neurotology* (pp. 313–340). Philadelphia: Lippincott-Raven.

KINNEY, W.C., KINNEY, S.E., & VIDIMOS, A.T. (1997). Disorders of the auricle. In: G.B. Hughes, & M.L. Pensak (Eds.), *Clinical otology* (pp. 177–189). New York: Thieme Medical Publishers, Inc.

LANGMAN, A.W., & LINDEMAN, R.C. (1998). Surgical labyrinthectomy in the older patient. *Archives of Otolaryngology–Head and Neck Surgery, 118*(6);739–742.

LEE, K.J., & GOODRICH, I. (1987). Related neurology. In: K.J. Lee (Ed.), *Essential otolaryngology–head and neck surgery* (pp. 803–814). New York: Medical Examination Publishing.

LISTON, S.L., NISSEN, R.L., PAPARELLA, M.M., & DA COSTA, S.S. (1991). Surgical treatment of vertigo. In: M.M. Paparella, D.A. Shumrick, J.L. Gluckman, & W.L. Meyerhoff (Eds.), *Otolaryngology* (Vol. 2) (pp. 1715–1732). Philadelphia: W.B. Saunders.

LUETJE, C., & BERLINER, K. (1997). Plasmapheresis in autoimmune inner ear disease: Long-term follow-up. *American Journal of Otology, 18*(5);572–576.

MANJI, R. (1987). Antimicrobials. In: K.J. Lee (Ed.), *Essential otolaryngology–head and neck surgery* (pp. 855–869). New York: Medical Examination Publishing.

MARRA, C., WECHKIN, H., LONGSTRETH, W., REES, T., SYAPIN, C., & GATES, G. (1997). Hearing loss and antiretroviral therapy in patients infected with HIV-1. *Archives of Neurology, 54*(4);407–410.

MEYERHOFF, W.L., & LISTON, S.L. (1991). Metabolic hearing loss. In: M.M. Paparella, D.A. Shumrick, J.L. Gluckman, & W.L. Meyerhoff (Eds.), *Otolaryngology* (Vol. 2) (pp. 1671–1687). Philadelphia: W.B. Saunders.

MINET, M., DEGGOUJ, N., & GERSDORFF, M. (1997). Cochlear implantation in patients with Cogan's syndrome: A review of four cases. *European Archives of Otorhinolaryngology, 254*(9–10);459–462.

MONSELL, E.M., TEIXIDO, M.T., WILSON, M.D., & HUGHES, G.B. (1997). Nonhereditary hearing loss. In: G.B. Hughes, & M.L. Pensak (Eds.), *Clinical otology* (pp. 289–312.) New York: Thieme Medical Publishers, Inc.

PENSAK, M.L., & FRIEDMAN, R.A. (1997). Malignant tumors of the temporal bone. In: G.B. Hughes, & M.L. Pensak (Eds.), *Clinical otology* (pp. 335–343). New York: Thieme Medical Publishers, Inc.

PENSAK, M., & FRIEDMAN, R. (1998). The role of endolymphatic mastoid shunt surgery in the managed care era. *American Journal of Otology, 19*(3);337–340.

RAUCH, S.D. (1998). Sensorineural hearing loss: Medical therapy. In: G.A. Gates (Ed.), *Current therapy in otolaryngology–head and neck surgery* (pp. 51–55). St. Louis: Mosby.

REILLY, P.G., LALWANI, A.K., & JACKLER, R.K. (1998). Congenital anomalies of the ear. In: A.K. Lalwani, & K.M. Grundfast (Eds.), *Pediatric otology and neurotology* (pp. 205–210). Philadelphia: Lippincott-Raven.

ROLAND, P.S., & MARPLE, B.F. (1997). Disorders of inner ear, eighth nerve, and CNS. In: P.S. Roland, B.F. Marple, & W.L.

Meyerhoff (Eds.), *Hearing loss* (pp. 195–256). New York: Thieme Medical Publishers, Inc.

RUBINSTEIN, J.T., & GANTZ, B.J. (1997). Facial nerve disorders. In: G.B. Hughes, & M.L. Pensak (Eds.), *Clinical otology* (pp. 367–380). New York: Thieme Medical Publishers, Inc.

SCHAITKIN, B.M., SHAPIRO, A., & MAY, M. (1998). Disorders of the facial nerve. In: A.K. Lalwani, & K.M. Grundfast (Eds.), *Pediatric otology and neurotology* (pp. 457–475). Philadelphia: Lippincott-Raven.

SCHOEM, S.R., & GRUNDFAST, K.M. (1998). Oculoauditory syndromes. In: A.K. Lalwani, & K.M. Grundfast (Eds.), *Pediatric otology and neurotology* (pp. 365–374). Philadelphia: Lippincott-Raven.

SCHUKNECHT, H.F. (1993). Disorders of aging. In: H.F. Schuknecht (Ed.), *Pathology of the ear* (pp. 415–446). Philadelphia: Lea and Febiger.

SCHWABER, M.K. (1997). Vestibular disorders. In: G.B. Hughes, & M.L. Pensak (Eds.), *Clinical otology* (pp. 345–365). New York: Thieme Medical Publishers, Inc.

SHA, S., & SCHACHT, J. (1997). Prevention of aminoglycoside-induced hearing loss. *Keio Journal of Medicine, 46*(3);115–119.

SHAHEEN, F., MANSURI, N., AL-SHAIKH, A., SHEIK, I., HURAIB, S., AL-KHADER, A., & ZAZGORNIK, J. (1997). Reversible uremic deafness: Is it correlated with the degree of anemia? *Annals of Otology, Rhinology, and Laryngology, 106*(5); 391–393.

SISMANIS, A., WISE, C., & JOHNSON, G. (1997). Methotrexate management of immune-mediated cochleovestibular disorders. *Archives of Otolaryngology–Head and Neck Surgery, 116*(2); 146–152.

SLATTERY, W.H., & HOUSE, J.W. (1998). Complications of otitis media. In: A.K. Lalwani, & K.M. Grundfast (Eds.), *Pediatric otology and neurotology* (pp. 251–264). Philadelphia: Lippincott-Raven.

STRINGER, S.P., MEYERHOFF, W.L., & WRIGHT, C.G. (1991). Ototoxicity. In: M.M. Paparella, D.A. Shumrick, J.L. Gluckman, & W.L. Meyerhoff (Eds.), *Otolaryngology* (Vol. 2) (pp. 1653– 1669). Philadelphia: W.B. Saunders.

WACKYM, P.A., & CYR, D.G. (1998). Vertigo, dizziness, and disequilibrium. In: A.K. Lalwani, & K.M. Grundfast (Eds.), *Pediatric otology and neurotology* (pp. 423–439). Philadelphia: Lippincott-Raven.

WACKYM, P.A., & MONSELL, E.M. (1997). Revision vestibular surgery. In: V.N. Carrasco, & H.C. Pillsbury (Eds.), *Revision otologic surgery* (pp. 108–133). New York: Thieme Medical Publishers, Inc.

YOUSSEF, T., & POE, D. (1998). Intratympanic injection for the treatment of Meniere's disease. *American Journal of Otology, 19*(4);435–442

PREFERRED PRACTICE GUIDELINES

Professionals Who Perform the Procedure(s)

▼ Skilled and certified audiologist knowledgeable in medical audiology.

Expected Outcomes

▼ Good iterative working relationship with a medical specialist for the diagnosis. Medical diagnoses are complete, accurate, and expedient.

Clinical Indications

▼ Any patient complaining of hearing loss should be fully evaluated to define the medical cause of the complaint.

Clinical Process

▼ Crucial to a proper diagnostic evaluation is a complete case history, comprehensive audiogram, including ipsilateral and contralateral stapedial reflexes and speech audiometry, and a skilled otologic examination.

Documentation

▼ A formal recording of the tests used, the results obtained, and an interpretation of the data describing the site of lesions and the degree of lesions is required. In addition, written evidence that the patient received a recommendation for a medical specialist evaluation is necessary, and a follow-up progress note to document due diligence was used to ensure the safety of the patient.

Chapter 12

Selection and Fitting of Conventional Hearing Aids

Catherine V. Palmer, George A. Lindley, IV, and Elaine A. Mormer

The authors of this chapter teach students how to select and evaluate assistive technology including hearing aids. To meet that goal, students must be provided with a framework within which to think about fitting amplification because fitting hearing aids is a quickly changing art and science. This chapter has been approached in the same manner (see Palmer [1998] for a complete description of a hearing aid curriculum). The basic framework consists of what audiologists need to measure, up-front decisions that have to be made regarding the hearing aids, ordering/selecting the hearing aids, fine-tuning/verification of the selection, orientation/follow-up, and measuring the benefit provided by the hearing aids. It is essential to interrelate the various components. For instance, measurements related to the patient must be used to order the hearing aids and to verify performance. Audiologists will always need to measure something about the auditory system or decide to use average data. Hearing aids will have to be obtained and preset. Some sort of verification is necessary to ensure that the audiologist has done what was planned. Finally, an evaluation will be necessary to establish that the hearing aids have made an impact on the individual in some positive way. The following information describes a reasonable way to approach selecting, fitting, and evaluating conventional hearing aid technology.

For the purposes of this text, conventional hearing aids are defined by what they are not. Conventional hearing aids are not programmable by means of a computer interface or handheld programmer. Conventional hearing aids contain the high-level circuitry found in analog programmable or digital hearing aids if chosen carefully. On the other hand, programmable and digital hearing aids tend to contain high-level circuitry as the standard. The difference between programmable hearing aids and conventional hearing aids is that one must choose desired hearing aid responses before receiving the conventional hearing aid. Whereas programmable hearing aids offer room for error because one can manipulate various parameters (compression ratio, gain, crossover frequency, etc.),

Audiology: Treatment. Edited by Valente, Hosford-Dunn, and Roeser. Thieme Medical Publishers, Inc., New York © 2000

conventional hearing aids can be thought of as less flexible and in need of more precise ordering specifications. Although conventional hearing aids could contain more than one memory (each memory's response specified on ordering), they typically contain only one memory. Conventional hearing aids were considered deserving of a separate chapter because they differ from programmable hearing aids in how the audiologist interacts with the hearing aid specifications and the manufacturer.

If one is unsure how to manipulate various programmable parameters, the approach outlined may serve as a good starting point whether ordering conventional technology or programming digitally programmable technology. This may be especially true when fitting young children with programmable technology. Because children may not be able to provide enough feedback regarding the response of the hearing aids, one would like to start with the best possible fit, which may come from following the guidelines regardless of the technology being fit.

THE GOALS OF THE HEARING AID FITTING

The goals of hearing aid fittings do not change whether one is fitting conventional, programmable, or digital technology. Most audiologists can agree on the following set of goals for a hearing aid fitting: sounds are audible, comfortable but not uncomfortable, the hearing aids provide good sound quality and a safe listening environment, and amplification meets the patient's communication needs and the patient's expectations. Most also would add that hearing aids should improve speech recognition in quiet and noise, but this most likely is included in the patient's communication needs and expectations. The goals do not change depending on the technology choosen. How the goals are met may change slightly.

The goals of each fitting (some will apply to all fittings and some will be specific to the individual) should be defined before hearing aid selection in that they should dictate much of the selection and measurement procedures. The goals should dictate how the hearing aids ultimately will be assessed. In other words, if sound quality is essential, selection is impacted (one might want circuitry that demonstrates low distortion including compression output limiting) and the individual's perception of sound quality should be incorporated into the verification procedure. If audibility is important, circuitry that can make a wide range of input signals audible (e.g., wide dynamic range compression) might be selected, and the individual's ability to hear soft, average, and loud sounds might be assessed during the hearing aid fitting. A mechanism should be available for measuring each of the goals of the hearing aid fitting whether the goal is physical (fit of the earmold) or subjective (improving the quality of an individual's life).

EVALUATION AND MEASUREMENT OF THE AUDITORY SYSTEM, ENVIRONMENT, AND INDIVIDUAL

At a minimum, one must document an individual's ear-specific thresholds as a function of frequency to start the fitting process. But there is more about the auditory system, the listening environment, and the individual that may assist in the selection and fitting of hearing aids.

EVALUATION OF THE AUDITORY SYSTEM

At present, some clinicians and researchers are advocating measurement of an individual's loudness growth to assist in the selection of a hearing aid's response. Loudness growth may be interpolated by measuring an individual's threshold and uncomfortable loudness level. This assumes a fairly linear growth of loudness between the two end points. These data are not mandatory but can be used in selection programs such as National Acoustics Laboratory (NAL-R) (Byrne & Dillon, 1986) and Desired Sensation Level (DSL [i/o]) (Cornelisse et al, 1994). The Visual Input Output Locator Algorithm (VIOLA) of the Independent Hearing Aid Fitting Forum (IHAFF) (Valente & VanVliet, 1997) program mandates loudness growth functions at two or more frequencies (500 and 3000 Hz, minimally). This entails having an individual judge the loudness of warble tones from threshold to uncomfortably loud (Cox, 1995). Individual loudness growth curves do not assume that individual loudness growth functions are linear from the threshold of detection to the threshold of discomfort and perhaps, more importantly, that comfortable loudness is half way between the threshold of detection and the threshold of discomfort (see also Kamm et al, 1977; Mueller & Bentler, 1994; Pascoe, 1989; Ricketts & Bentler, 1996; Valente et al, 1997).

The amount of auditory data that one collects will depend on one's interest in individual-specific measures and which hearing aid fitting program is being used. For instance, if a clinic is using FIG6 (Gitles & Niquette, 1995, named after Figure 6 in Killion & Fikret-Pasa, 1993) exclusively, it does not make sense to collect individual loudness growth data because it cannot be used in the FIG6 program. On the other hand, using FIG6 exclusively implies that this group of clinicians does not believe that the need for individual loudness growth data is supported in the literature, for their particular clinical population, and/or for the technology that they are fitting. This chapter focuses on fitting conventional hearing instruments, and it already has been noted that this implies less flexibility. One may be comfortable using a hearing aid fitting program with average data as a starting point because programmable instruments can be fine-tuned through a variety of verification procedures. One may become less comfortable with this protocol when using conventional instruments that cannot be manipulated to such a large extent.

Investigators also are examining clinical measures that might define an individual's ability to make use of returned audibility, especially at frequencies with hearing loss greater than 60 dB HL (e.g., Turner et al, 1997). This type of evaluation might assist the clinician in knowing which frequencies should be pursued with amplification. For instance, if a clinician knows that making sound audible at 4000 Hz will not assist a particular patient, the time in the hearing aid fitting will focus on audibility at the lower frequencies. In addition, an individual who cannot benefit from audibility at most of the high frequencies might become a reasonable candidate for a transposition hearing aid (a hearing aid that transposes the inaudible high frequencies to low-frequency sound). Although these types of tests are not widely clinically available and some controversy exists over whether adaptation should be considered (the individual might need a lengthy period of exposure to the newly audible signal before being able to make use of it), they may become an important part of making up-front decisions in the selection of hearing instruments.

EVALUATION OF INDIVIDUAL COMMUNICATION NEEDS AND THE LISTENING ENVIRONMENT

Palmer and Mormer (1997) provide a systematic approach to hearing instrument orientation and adjustment. As part of that program, several forms for gathering patient information are presented. Specifically, the *Hearing Demand, Ability, and Need Profile* (Fig. 12–1) is used as a systematic interviewing tool that should define the patient's current communication abilities and demands, as well as the patient's communication needs. Communication needs are identified as a function of situation (alerting, one-to-one communication, etc.), hearing aid use, and listening environment. This worksheet allows data to be collected and analyzed easily. The results of the worksheet should lead directly to hearing solutions. These might include hearing aid features and/or assistive technology. For instance, difficulty in one-to-one communication because of background noise might lead one to consider directional microphone technology for the hearing aids, whereas difficulty in large group situations caused by distance might lead to coupling an assistive device to a hearing aid that is equipped with direct audio input (DAI) or telecoil technology (see Chapter 19 in this volume). This type of measurement is used extensively in making up-front decisions regarding the hearing aid. The form is revisited after the hearing aids have been fit and worn for several months to evaluate whether all the individual's communication needs have been met or whether further technology and/or communication strategies need to be pursued.

The *Patient Expectation Worksheet* (Fig. 12–2) is used to document the patient's expectations of the forthcoming intervention (hearing aids, assistive technology, communication strategies, etc.). This form is adapted from the *Client Oriented Scale of Improvement (COSI)* developed by Dillon et al (1997). The patient generates five specific expectations. The clinician may have to assist the patient in creating specific expectations as opposed to general goals. For instance, "hearing better in noise" is too general. The patient should be questioned until a specific situation can be identified (e.g., "understanding what my five-year-old daughter says at the dinner table"). The patient then indicates how he or she is performing currently and how he or she expects to perform after intervention. The clinician uses a check mark to indicate what would be considered a reasonable expectation given the patient's audition and the technology being pursued. This creates a forum for assisting the patient in forming realistic expectations if the clinician's check mark and the patient's expectation are not in agreement. It also can provide a meaningful discussion of some of the up-front decisions regarding the hearing aids that

the patient has made. For instance, if the patient insists on pursuing monaural amplification when binaural amplification is indicated, the clinician can demonstrate that the level of success expected in noisy situations is lower as a result of this decision. This helps all parties understand that the up-front decisions made regarding the hearing aid will directly affect the outcome of the hearing aid fitting.

The *Patient Expectation Worksheet* is used as a tool to further assist in up-front decision making on the basis of the patient's communication goals. The expectations are used as an outcome measure in that the patient will indicate how he or she is performing after the intervention (short period of hearing aid use, etc.). If the patient is not meeting or exceeding the realistic expectations that were recorded on the sheet, the clinician and patient work to understand what further remediation needs to be implemented. Again, this can be a valuable counseling tool. If the patient indicates that dinner conversation is still a problem and the clinician's interview reveals that the television is on during dinner, an obvious recommendation would be to eliminate the television. If the individual is doing everything according to plan and dinner conversation is still difficult, a directional microphone (if not already included) or an assistive device might be considered. Once all the individual's communication goals are met, the individual may generate new goals that he or she had not thought of until communication began to improve.

Because a lack of speech recognition tasks that will be sensitive enough to document change before and after hearing aid fitting exists and it is questionable whether one speech recognition task could measure all the possible benefits of wearing appropriate amplification, the clinician may want to use a measurement of hearing handicap or hearing aid benefit as an outcome measure. The authors routinely use the *Abbreviated Profile of Hearing Aid Benefit* (APHAB) (Cox & Alexander, 1995) to further assess communication needs that may be addressed by the variety of up-front decisions made in the hearing aid selection process. Perhaps more importantly, the before and after APHAB scores are compared to provide a benefit score that can be used to document the hearing aid fitting outcome. Alternately, the absolute post-APHAB scores can be compared with results from normally hearing young (Paul & Cox, 1995) or aging (Cox, 1997) individuals.

EVALUATION OF INDIVIDUAL PHYSICAL MEASUREMENTS

Real-ear measures play a role in both diagnostic measures made before ordering the hearing aids and in verification measures. See Chapter 3 in this volume for a detailed description of real-ear measures. The amplification goal must be established at the time of measurement to realistically expect success in the verification process. For example, if one intends to verify the fitting with insertion gain measurements [real-ear-aided response (REAR) minus the individual's real-ear-unaided response (REUR)], one would want to measure the REUR to be included in the selection of the hearing aid and select a fitting protocol allowing for its incorporation. In addition, the fitting protocol should include insertion gain targets for use in verification. The hearing aid fitting goal should be

HEARING DEMAND, ABILITY, AND NEED PROFILE

[adapted from Healey, J. (1992) and Palmer, C.(1992)]

Name:

Age	Description of Communication Milestone/Activity	Communication Problem is Present…. With Hearing Aid:							The Problem is Due to…				Current Compensation
		on HOME	off	on WORK	off	on TRAVEL	off	Hearing	Noise	Distance	Visibility	(describe)
	ALERTING											
	telephone bell											
	doorbell											
	door knock											
	alarm clock											
	smoke alarm											
	siren											
	turn signal											
	personal pager											
	PERSONAL COMMUNICATION											
	telephone											
	tv/stereo/radio											
	one-to-one(planned)											
	one-to-one(unplanned)											
	group											
	large room											
	OTHER ACTIVITIES											
	clubs/games:											
	lessons:											
	sports:											

Further information (e.g, status of hearing aids, telecoil, DAI,communication environment):

Recommendations (Assistive Technology, Communication Strategies, Environmental Manipulation):

Figure 12–1 Hearing Demand, Ability, and Need Profile. (Used with permission from High Performance Hearing Solutions, Supplement to the Hearing Review, 1, 1997.)

Patient Expectation Worksheet

I am successful in this situation…

Goal (list in order of priority)	Hardly Ever	Occasionally	Half the Time	Most of the Time	Almost Always
1.					
2.					
3.					
4.					
5.					

C = how the client functions currently (pre-treatment or with current technology/strategies)

E = how the client expects to function post intervention (HA, ALD, strategies, etc.)

√ = level of success that the audiologist realistically targets

A = how the client/family actually perceives level of success post fitting

Figure 12–2 The Patient Expectation Worksheet. (Used with permission from *High Performance Hearing Solutions, Supplement to the Hearing Review*, 1, 1997.)

consistent across procedures and must be understood early on for the correct measurements, selection procedure, and verification measures to be used.

Compromises are made each time average data are used regarding a patient's responses or regarding individual ear characteristics (see also Libby, 1985; Valente et al, 1995; Valente et al, 1997). These compromises may be worth making for the sake of time management, but it is important to understand that a choice is being made. With conventional fittings, time may be better used up-front to obtain accurate measures because the conventional hearing aid may not be flexible enough to correct for deviations in response from targets as a result of individual ear differences from average. The real-ear measurements that may add to the accuracy of the hearing aid fitting are described later in this chapter, and case examples are provided to illustrate what may be gained from inclusion of individual-specific data in the hearing aid ordering process.

Armed with the evaluation data (auditory system, communication environment, and individual's needs) the clinician is ready to make the up-front decisions required before selecting and ordering a hearing aid.

UP-FRONT DECISIONS

Up-front decisions are not specific to conventional hearing aids. These are decisions that must be made in the selection process of any hearing aid. The difference may be in when the decision can be made. For instance, with the Siemens MUSIC programmable hearing aid you can create a linear or wide dynamic range compression (WDRC) response depending on how you manipulate the compression ratio parameter. With the Phonak programmable line, peak clipping, output compression limiting, and WDRC are programmable parameters, so the decision of how to output limit the hearing aid does not have to be made before selection of the hearing aid. With conventional technology, these decisions will have to be made up-front or the decision of what potentiometers to order to allow these choices must be made up-front. The up-front decisions are made through a combination of information gleaned from the *Hearing Demand, Ability, and Need Profile* (Fig. 12–1), *Patient Expectation Worksheet* (Fig. 12–2), *APHAB*, audiometric data, clinical experience, and empirical data. The patient will be involved in making some of these decisions. The realistic expectations that were documented on the *Patient Expectation Worksheet* may have to be modified on the basis of some of the up-front decisions that are dictated by the patient. This provides a meaningful format for discussion of an individual's preferences.

The list of up-front decisions is constantly changing in view of new technology and new research. Items are deleted and items are added. Table 12–1 provides a current list of up-front decisions and a line to record the decision made (or action taken). Although the experienced clinician may not fill out this list every time hearing aids are dispensed, the wise

TABLE 12–1 Decisions to be made before ordering a hearing aid

Decision	Action
BTE vs ITE vs ITC vs CIC	
CROS, BICROS, transcranial	
Air vs bone conduction	
Frequency transposition	
Cochlear implant	
Implantable	
Spare	
Monaural vs binaural	
Binaural summation	
Microphone type/location	
Earmold material/type/color	
Earmold length/vent	
Sound channel	
Bandwidth	
Volume control	
Receiver type	
Compression options	
Output limiting	
Multichannel	
Ability to fine-tune	
Controls for fine-tuning	
Remote control	
Multimemory	
Analog vs digital	
Previous experience	
Coupling ALDs	

clinician will review this list periodically to make sure that concious decisions backed by patient and/or empirical data are made for every item.

FITTING PROTOCOLS FOR SELECTING CONVENTIONAL HEARING AIDS

Regardless of the type of circuitry fit, the audiologist must derive appropriate fitting targets that can be used to determine the electroacoustic characteristics of the hearing aid before ordering the hearing aid and to verify that the fitting goal has been met. With conventional hearing aids, it becomes important to identify how the hearing aids should function before fitting as less flexibility for adjustment will be available on the day of the fitting. Fortunately, the audiologist has a large number of fitting strategies to choose from. Unfortunately, little research is available comparing the relative aided performance of individuals fit using these strategies. Therefore the audiologist must

choose the appropriate fitting strategy on the basis of past experience, amount of time available, and available resources.

Fitting protocols differ in theoretical approach, amount of data necessary for implementation, and amount of data provided in the end (see Chapters 4, 5, 6, 13, and 25 in this volume for detailed information). One must know what measurements would be needed to use each fitting technique, the differences in what each fitting technique recommends, how each fitting technique meets the requirements of our original goals for a patient, and what verification/validation techniques each fitting protocol demands to stay in line with the goals of the fitting technique. For example, Table 12–2 (from Lindley & Palmer, 1997) provides a comparison of the three fitting protocols and illustrates what information must be entered into each fitting protocol (e.g., threshold in dB HL, loudness discomfort levels [LDLs], etc.), as well as what information is produced by each fitting protocol (e.g., real-ear targets, coupler targets).

Some choices depend on the type of circuitry to be fit. For example, when fitting a WDRC hearing aid, it is beneficial to use a fitting strategy that provides targets for more than one

TABLE 12–2 A comparison of three hearing aid fitting methods

Method*	DSL	VIOLA/IHAFF	FIG6
Required audiometric data	Thresholds (minimum) also can enter LDLs, RECD, REDD, REUR	Loudness contour data at two frequencies (minimum)	Thresholds across frequencies
Data can be collected via dB HL or dB SPL?	Headphones, insert earphones, sound field Both	Headphones or insert earphones Both	Headphones or insert earphones dB HL
Average dynamic range and/or loudness growth data used?	Depends on what measures are entered. LDLs are predicted if not entered	No, individual data are used or tester may enter average data	Yes Yes
Target information provided	REAR, REAG, 2-cc coupler targets at several input levels; aided sound field target	2-cc coupler target at several input levels	REIG and 2-cc targets at several input levels
Specific compression parameters provided?	Yes	Yes, but dispenser also may enter hearing aid information to see how closely it matches targets	Yes
Can be used with AGC and linear hearing aids?	Yes	Yes, but will likely not come close to meeting target	Yes, but will likely come close to meeting target
Recommends specific efficacy measures (other than matching a target)	No	Yes	No
For additional information	(519) 661-3901	Hearing Aid Research Laboratory, University of Memphis www.ausp.memphis.edu/harl	1-888-FIG6-HLP

*The Hearing Aid Selection (HAS) program contains all three of the above-mentioned programs and includes the ability to implement individual-specific measures. The HAS is available from Support Syndicate for Audiology, 108 South 12th Street, Pittsburgh, PA 15203 (E-mail: mrauterkus@sportsurf.net).

input level (i.e., DSL[i/o], IHAFF, FIG6) (Cornelisse et al, 1994; Cox, 1995; Gitles & Niquette, 1995; Lindley & Palmer, 1997). With WDRC, the goal is to restore audibility of speech sounds and to restore a normal sense of loudness perception. These fittings are three-dimensional. Gain varies as a function of frequency and input level. As such, it becomes necessary to determine how the hearing aid should operate at soft, average, and loud input levels. Conversely, many fitting strategies are designed specifically for fitting linear hearing aids (i.e., NAL-R, POGO) or provide an option for fitting linear hearing aids (DSL[i/o]) because only one target is provided on the basis of a conversational level input (Byrne & Dillon, 1986; Lyregaard, 1988). With linear processing, the goal is to make conversational speech sounds audible without having loud sounds amplified to an uncomfortable level. These fittings are two-dimensional. Gain varies as a function of frequency.

The focus of this section will be on methods that can be used with many fitting strategies in customizing the hearing aid order. When determining appropriate hearing aid characteristics, it is important to have a good estimate of how the hearing aids will function in a given individual's ear. A 2-cc coupler response is required when selecting and ordering conventional hearing aids. This is the only way to communicate the desired response of the hearing aids to the manufacturer. Because the fitter will have limited flexibility to change the response of the hearing aids, the process of identifying the 2-cc coupler target takes on special importance when fitting conventional technology. By determining a priori what 2-cc coupler response will lead to the desired response in the individual's ear, the need for major potentiometer adjustment on the day of the fitting will be avoided.

DERIVING A CUSTOM 2-CC COUPLER RESPONSE

There are several points in the prefitting process where either average-based data (Bentler & Pavlovic, 1989) or individual-based data can be used in deriving appropriate targets. Average-based data work well when an individual is close to average; however, if an individual differs significantly from average, as individuals often do, the fitting targets derived may not be accurate. This may not be a problem with programmable hearing aids because a great deal of adjustment flexibility is available to the audiologist. A conventional hearing aid, however, may not accommodate significant changes that may be necessary on the day of the fitting if the hearing aid is not functioning in the real ear as predicted (Feigin et al, 1989; Hawkins et al, 1990; Lewis & Stelmachowicz, 1993).

Does inclusion of individual-specific data guarantee better fit hearing aids or a more satisfied hearing aid user? When individual data allow us to use the full dynamic range of the individual (not limiting needlessly low) or allows us to be confident in the acoustic parameters of a hearing aid fit to an individual who can provide limited subjective data (e.g., child, patient with Alzheimer disease, etc.), we probably have a better fit. Palmer et al (1991) examined whether it was preferable, on the basis of recognition and sound quality judgments, for hearing aids to mimic an individual's external ear (REUR and eardrum impedance). Continuous discourse and multispeaker babble were recorded at the eardrums of 10 subjects with various earcanal and eardrum characteristics and various hearing sensitivity. These recordings were manipulated for each subject to produce four hearing aid configurations. The hearing aid responses included an average earcanal response, an average earcanal response and compensation for individual eardrum impedance, individual earcanal data and no compensation for individual eardrum impedance, individual earcanal data and compensation for individual eardrum impedance. Subjects rated 16 presentations of each condition in terms of absolute sound quality (0 to 100%) and recognition (0 to 100%). Results indicated that it was preferable on the basis of recognition judgments for a given hearing aid to mimic the external ears of three subjects. For four of the subjects mimicking the external ear was not preferable, but it also was not detrimental. For two of the subjects, poorer recognition ratings resulted from mimicking the individuals' external ears. A lack of difference between the individual external ear response and the average (Knowles Electronic Manikin for Auditory Research [KEMAR]) response resulted in a lack of difference in ratings across listening conditions, although the presence of a difference between the individual external ear response and the average (KEMAR) response did not guarantee a difference in ratings across listening conditions. Results indicated that sound quality and recognition preferences differed for each subject and appeared to be related to certain subject variables, including external ear characteristics and amount of dB difference in particular frequency regions between conditions.

So it is not clear that these individual measures will provide more satisfied patients. It is clear that a lack of individual measures incorporated in target generation can produce the need for greater manipulation of the selected hearing aid during the fitting process. Therefore the clinician fitting conventional technology may want to consider inclusion of individual measurements in generating 2-cc coupler targets to minimize the need for hearing aid adjustments to match real-ear verification targets at the time of fitting.

Table 12–3 lists measures that can be applied at various stages of the hearing aid fitting process. Depending on the fitting strategy, some or all of these measures are used when deriving appropriate hearing aid fitting targets, although the audiologist may not realize this because average-based values are often automatically applied. Individual-specific measures can be applied instead either by direct entry into the actual fitting protocol software applications (e.g., DSL[i/o], HAS) or through the use of some simple calculations. These measures are not time consuming and can be obtained in most clinical settings using available hardware. The potential benefits of and methods for incorporating these measures into the various fitting strategies will be discussed. Case examples will be provided to show how these measures can be applied in clinical situations.

AUDIOMETRIC DATA

All fitting strategies require entry of various audiometric measures (i.e., thresholds, LDLs, loudness contour data, etc.) to derive appropriate fitting targets. Traditionally, these measures have been obtained with insert or TDH series earphones in dB HL. When thresholds are plotted on an audiogram, they are plotted in dB HL. Hearing aid data, however, are presented in dB SPL referenced to a 2-cc coupler. Somehow, the audiometric information obtained in dB HL not only must be transformed to dB SPL but it must be dB SPL re a 2-cc coupler. This allows identification of appropriate 2-cc coupler and real-ear verification targets.

Typically, transformations based on average data are used. Using this method, the real-ear dB SPL value near the eardrum is predicted from the measured dB HL value on the basis of mean values obtained from large numbers of individuals. Valente et al (1991), however, have shown that at a given dB HL value, the actual real-ear dB SPL value recorded in the ear can vary considerably among individuals, sometimes by as much as 30 dB. This variance is related to individual differences in earcanal size and shape and differences in tympanic membrane compliance.

If an individual differs significantly from average, problems on the day of the fitting may be encountered. For example, if LDLs are obtained in dB HL, an average-based transformation will be used to change those values into dB SPL. These predicted dB SPL values may be substantially larger or smaller than the actual dB SPL value in the individual's ears. As such, the prescribed saturation sound pressure level (SSPL) with a 90 dB SPL input (SSPL90) for the hearing aid may be too high or too low, both of which could have a negative impact on the success of the fitting. The clinician may meet the coupler target for SSPL90 exactly, yet have a patient who cannot tolerate a 90 dB SPL input. Conversely, the SSPL90 may be set too low, and a 90 dB SPL input may not be perceived as too loud. In this case, the individual's full dynamic range is not taken advantage of because the hearing aid could likely allow sounds to come through louder without reaching the individual's LDL.

TABLE 12–3 Transformations that may be applied during selection of an appropriate 2-cc coupler response. These transformations can be based on average-based data or individual-specific data.

Measure	Definition	Application	Clinical Example
Audiometric information in real-ear dB SPL	Intensity value measured using a probe microphone near the eardrum at threshold, LDL, etc.	Audiometric data in real-ear db SPL can be entered directly into some fitting protocol's software. Avoids use of transformation from data obtained in dB HL to real-ear dB SPL.	Can be used in conjunction with RECD to obtain individual specific 2-cc coupler targets using IHAFF software.
Real-ear-to-dial difference (REDD)	Difference between the intensity in dB HL on the audiometer dial and the intensity level in dB SPL measured near the eardrum.	Can be applied to audiometric data obtained in dB HL (i.e., thresholds, LDLs) to transform to real-ear dB SPL. Otherwise, an average-based transformation is used.	Can be entered directly into DSL[i/o] to transform audiometric data in dB HL to real-ear dB SPL.
Real-ear-unaided-response (REUR)	Outer earcanal resonance as measured using probe microphone.	Can be used in deriving individual specific insertion gain or coupler gain targets. Typically an "average" REUR is used. Also used by DSL[i/o] when deriving appropriate targets from thresholds obtained in the sound field.	Applying the difference between an individual's REUR and the average REUR to FIG6 2-cc coupler targets.
Real-ear-coupler-difference (RECD)	Difference between the output of a hearing aid or insert earphone measured in the earcanal versus a 2-cc coupler.	Can be applied to insertion gain targets or real-ear output targets in deriving appropriate 2-cc coupler targets.	Applying the difference between an individual's RECD and the average RECD to FIG6 2-cc coupler targets.
Coupler response for flat insertion gain (CORFIG)	REUR-RECD-microphone location (i.e., BTE, CIC)	Correction factor that is added to REIG targets to obtain appropriate 2-cc coupler target.	Adding CORFIG value to NAL-R REIG target to derive 2-cc coupler target.
Measures of dynamic range	Loudness discomfort levels Loudness contour	Used in determining SSPL90 of a linear hearing aid or appropriate compression ratios with a WDRC hearing aid.	Using individual specific dynamic range data vs average-based data.

The audiologist can use two methods to remove the need for average-based data at this level. With both methods, a probe microphone system is necessary. By placing a probe microphone near the eardrum during audiometric testing, individual specific real-ear dB SPL values can be obtained (Humes et al, 1996). With this method, the audiologist can continue to plot threshold values in dB HL on the audiogram. For the purposes of hearing aid fitting, however, the audiologist can record the threshold values in real-ear dB SPL by noting the level measured by the probe microphone in the real-ear. Remember that the reference microphone of the real-ear system should be disabled during measurement. This same setup can be used when obtaining LDLs or loudness contour data.

Another option would be to determine the real-ear-to-dial difference (REDD). As the name implies, this measure is the difference between the audiometer dial in dB HL and the real-ear value in dB SPL obtained using a probe microphone. With

a probe microphone near the earcanal, the REDD is determined by subtracting the audiometer dial reading in dB HL from the intensity value recorded in the earcanal. By presenting a series of tones across frequency at a given intensity level, the audiologist can quickly determine frequency-specific REDD values. Once obtained, the REDD can be applied to all audiometric data (e.g., LDLs) obtained in dB HL when converting to dB SPL. Again, this removes the need for average-based transformations. Remember, these two methods have provided real-ear dB SPL data. Hearing aids are ordered using data obtained in 2-cc couplers; therefore the final target data must still be referenced to a 2-cc coupler through further real-ear measures or by using average-based conversions.

The two procedures should provide identical data. For the first, every response is measured in dB SPL. In the second, individual-specific correction values are obtained and then applied to all dB HL results. These measures can be performed with a separate audiometer and real-ear system. Depending on the clinic layout, placement of the systems may be awkward. Systems such as the Madsen Auricle combine the systems and automatically record both the HL and SPL data.

CLINICAL EXAMPLE OF REAL-EAR-TO-DIAL DIFFERENCE

DSL[i/o] allows for entry of audiometric data in dB HL or in real-ear dB SPL. When entered in dB HL, average, age-appropriate transformation data are used to change the audiometric data obtained in dB HL to dB SPL. Other programs may use adult average data at all times. This is why entry of an individual's birth date is required with DSL[i/o]. In addition, the audiologist can enter the REDD, and these values will be applied instead of the average values. DSL[i/o] uses audiometric values such as thresholds and upper limits of comfort in determining an individual's dynamic range. Verification and coupler targets are then generated with the goal of keeping soft, average, and loud speech within the individual's dynamic range.

Table 12–4 shows the 2-cc coupler data of a hearing aid derived with DSL[i/o] software. In the top half of Table 12–4, the transformation from dB HL to dB SPL was made on the basis of average data. In the bottom half of Table 12–4, individual specific REDD values were entered and applied in transforming audiometric data from dB HL to dB SPL. The REDD values entered are −2 standard deviations (SD) from the mean REDD values obtained in the Valente et al (1994) study for ER-3A earphones. When the dB HL to dB SPL transform is predicted, the data recommend a more powerful hearing aid and greater compression than would have been recommended when the individual-specific REDD are considered.

TABLE 12–4 Hearing aid recommendation data when an average-based versus an individual-specific REDD is used

	500 Hz	1000 Hz	2000 Hz	3000 Hz	4000 Hz
Average based					
SSPL90	101	103	106	110	108
Full-on gain	20	26	32	38	37
Use gain	10	16	22	28	27
Compression ratio	1.5	1.8	2.0	2.7	3.0
Individual specific					
SSPL90	98	100	100	101	97
Full-on gain	10	21	25	27	22
Use gain	−1	11	15	17	12
Compression ratio	1.1	1.6	1.6	1.9	1.8

In this case, had the dB HL to dB SPL been predicted, output targets would have been considerably higher than needed, and the patient likely would have complained that the hearing aid was too loud. Of course, a young child may not be able to voice these complaints. Looking at the hearing aid recommendation data, substantial differences exist in desired SSPL90, full-on gain, use gain, frequency response, and compression ratio. Thus manipulation of a volume control would not necessarily rectify the differences between these two recommendations for the same individual. A conventional hearing aid may not be flexible enough to make these modifications, making incorporation of these real-ear pecularities in the derivation of the coupler target an efficient use of time and energy.

REAL-EAR-TO-COUPLER-DIFFERENCES/ REAL-EAR-UNAIDED RESPONSE/ COUPLER-RESPONSE FOR FLAT INSERTION GAIN (CORFIG)

The preceding section described obtaining individual-specific measures that can be used to gather data in dB SPL at the eardrum or in converting data in dB HL to dB SPL at the earcanal through the use of individual specific REDD values. Hearing aid targets and electroacoustic data, however, are provided in dB SPL referenced to a 2-cc coupler, not to an individual's eardrum. Therefore even with these individual measures applied, a conversion must still take place to create data referenced to a coupler for hearing aid ordering purposes. The output of a hearing aid is typically greater in an individual's ear than in a coupler in the mid to high frequencies. However, substantial variation exists in the general population. Individual real-ear-to-coupler-differences (RECDs) are affected by factors such as earcanal volume and middle ear immittance characteristics that have an impact on eardrum impedance (Feigin et al, 1989; Fikret-Pasa & Revit, 1992; Hawkins et al, 1990; Palmer et al, 1991). For example, the output of a given hearing aid will be greater in the earcanal of a child versus an adult because of the smaller earcanal volume in children. As such, it becomes necessary to determine what 2-cc coupler response will lead to the desired output in the individual's earcanal. Unless entered directly, average-based data rather than individual-specific data are used in predicting an appropriate 2-cc coupler response. As with the dB HL to dB SPL transformation, the transformation from dB SPL in the earcanal to dB SPL in the coupler is derived from mean data obtained on a large number of individuals. This may lead to problems when an individual deviates significantly from average (Fikret-Pasa & Revit, 1992; Palmer et al, 1991). One way to avoid this potential problem is through the use of two measures, the *RECD* and/or the *REUR*. The need to use one or both of these measures will depend on what type of targets will be used during the verification stage.

When output measures (i.e., REAR) will be used for real-ear verification, the audiologist needs to know what 2-cc coupler response a hearing aid should exhibit to achieve the desired real-ear output. The RECD is a measure that serves to quantify the difference in the hearing aid response obtained in a 2-cc coupler versus the response obtained in a real-ear as measured using a probe microphone. Some real-ear systems can automatically calculate the RECD. For those that do not, it is a relatively simple measure to obtain. The 2-cc coupler response of an insert earphone (or hearing aid) is determined in the test box. Using probe microphone measures, the audiologist determines the frequency response of the same insert earphone in an individual's ear. The RECD is then determined by subtracting the response obtained in the coupler from the response obtained in the real-ear. A stock hearing aid also could be used by determining the frequency response in the test box versus the individual's ear when coupled with a stock earmold or the individual's earmold. See Table 12–5 for three examples for obtaining RECD.

Clinical Example of Application of RECD

Using the DSL[i/o] software, it becomes relatively easy to incorporate individual-specific RECD values. DSL[i/o] gives the audiologist the option of using predicted or custom RECD

values. Table 12–6 shows the hearing aid recommendations for a WDRC hearing aid for an example patient when RECD is predicted and when the individual-based RECD was entered. As can be seen in this table, prescribed gain is higher, most notably at 4000 Hz, when the patient's actual RECD is entered.

Clinical Example of Application of RECD in Conjunction with Audiometric Data Obtained in Real-Ear dB SPL

When entering data into the Contour Test portion of the IHAFF software (see Chapters 5 and 6 in this volume for specific information regarding the IHAFF protocol), the audiologist is given the option of entering loudness contour data in dB HL or in real-ear dB SPL. When entered in dB HL, average-based values are used to transform the data into dB SPL as

TABLE 12–5 Suggested protocol for obtaining RECD through the use of insert earphones, the individual's earmold, or a stock hearing aid

---

A. Insert earphones

Step 1. Place probe microphone in ear to measure output from audiometer through the insert earphone. (Disable the reference microphone and loudspeaker on the real-ear system.)

Step 2. Input discrete frequencies at 70 dB HL and document the probe microphone SPL.

Step 3. Subtract previously measured (with probe microphone) SPLs with insert earphones attached to the HA-1 coupler (with foam tip) or tube attached to the HA-2 coupler in the test box from the individual's levels (Step 2).

Step 4. Apply the correction factor obtained in Step 3 to all individual SPL measurements used in ordering or verifying the hearing aid response. For example, apply the RECD to LDLs measured in dB SPL (or transformed from dB HL to dB SPL through the REDD) to determine the desired maximum output of a hearing aid in a 2-cc coupler.

Suggested protocol for obtaining RECD with the individual.

B. Individual's earmold

Step 1. Place probe microphone in ear to measure output from the audiometer through the insert earphone line/tube connected to the ear mold sound channel. (Disable the reference microphone and loudspeaker on the real-ear system.)

Step 2. Input discrete frequencies at a constant level 70 dB HL and document the probe microphone SPL for each.

Step 3. Measure the output of the audiometer in the 2-cc coupler. The output of the audiometer is routed through the insert earphone line/tube to the earmold sound channel. The earmold is coupled to an HA-1 coupler. The probe microphone is placed in the coupler to measure output in dB SPL.

Step 4. Subtract results from Step 3 from the results from Step 2.

Step 5. Apply the correction factor obtained in Step 4 to all individual SPL measurements used in ordering or verifying the hearing aid response. For example, apply the RECD to LDLs measured in dB SPL (or transformed from dB HL to dB SPL through the REDD) to determine the desired maximum output of a hearing aid in a 2-cc coupler.

C. Stock hearing aid (Hawkins & Mueller, 1992)

Step 1. Equalize sound field and calibrate probe tube.

Step 2. Place probe tube in earcanal 25 to 30 mm past the tragal notch.

Step 3. Place hearing aid on the patient and set the volume control wheel (VCW) to a mid position. Obtain a REAR with a 60- to 70-dB SPL signal (level is important only in that the hearing aid should not be in saturation).

Step 4. Remove the hearing aid without changing the VCW.

Step 5. Measure the output of the hearing aid and earmold in a 2-cc coupler (HA-1) with the same input intensity as used in the REAR measurement.

Step 6. Subtract the 2-cc coupler output from the REAR, producing the RECD.

TABLE 12–6 Hearing aid recommendation data when an average-based versus an individual-specific RECD is used

	250 Hz	500 Hz	1000 Hz	2000 Hz	3000 Hz	4000 Hz
Average based						
SSPL90	91	98	97	100	102	95
Full-on gain	11	9	15	21	28	23
Use gain	1	−1	5	11	18	13
Compression ratio	1.2	1.1	1.3	1.3	1.7	1.6
Individual specific						
SSPL90	95	97	101	105	112	111
Full-on gain	15	19	20	26	38	40
Use gain	5	9	10	16	28	30
Compression ratio	1.2	1.1	1.3	1.3	1.7	1.6

measured in an HA-1 coupler. The audiologist can customize the procedure by obtaining loudness contour data in real-ear dB SPL or by applying an individual-specific REDD to data obtained in dB HL. The individual's RECD then can be applied to the data to convert from real-ear dB SPL to dB SPL referenced to an HA-1 coupler (see Table 12–7). Thus individual-specific data can be used in the VIOLA portion of the IHAFF protocol.

REAL-EAR-INSERTION-GAIN

When real-ear-insertion-gain (REIG = REAR − REUR) targets are used, the RECD can be used in conjunction with the REUR to determine an appropriate 2-cc coupler response. The REUR is a probe microphone measure that represents the resonance characteristics of the outer ear without a hearing aid inserted. This natural resonance is lost when a hearing aid is inserted and needs to be accounted for when deriving appropriate gain targets. For example, if a NAL-R REIG target prescribes 20 dB of gain at 3000 Hz, and the individual's REUR is 10 dB at 3000 Hz, the hearing aid itself would need to provide 30 dB of gain at 3000 Hz (NAL prescription [20 dB] + gain lost with insertion of hearing aid [10 dB]).

The importance of incorporating individual-specific REUR measures into the fitting process is demonstrated in Figure 12–3. Here, the REUR obtained from the left ear of a patient is shown along with an average REUR obtained using KEMAR. For this patient, if average-based data (KEMAR) had been used, prescribed coupler gain would have been approximately 10 dB less than required by the patient to meet the REIG target. When deriving an appropriate 2-cc coupler response that allows the dispenser to arrive close to meeting the REIG target, there is a need to account for both the REUR and the RECD.

To account for an individual's REUR and RECD, the CORFIG is determined and applied to the prescribed REIG target to derive an appropriate 2-cc target (Killion & Revit, 1993). The CORFIG is determined by subtracting the individual's RECD and an appropriate microphone correction factor from the individual's REUR. This is done at all frequencies for which the audiologist wants a target gain value.

In essence, it is unfair to the manufacturer of the conventional hearing aid if one plans to verify the hearing aid's response with REIG if the individual's REUR was not accounted for in the original coupler targets. The hearing aid could match the requested coupler targets (the only data the manufacturer has) and yet be far off from the REIG targets if average REUR is used to create the coupler targets, wheres individual REUR is used when obtaining REIG for verification.

TABLE 12–7 Applying RECD when using VIOLA fitting software

Step 1. Obtain loudness contour data in real-ear dB SPL or apply individual-specific REDD to data obtained in dB HL to transform to real-ear dB SPL.

Step 2. Obtain the individual's RECD (see Table 12–5).

Step 3. In the Contour/Stimulus menu, change the "THR units entered in:" setting from "data entered in dB HL" to "data entered in dB SPL."

Step 4. Enter the individual's threshold data in dB SPL.

Step 5. Replace the default audiometer correction values with the individual's RECD as a function of frequency in the Contour/Stimulus menu.

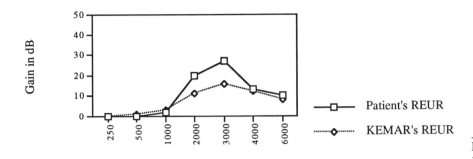

Figure 12–3 Average REUR versus an individual REUR.

Clinical Example of Application of CORFIG

An example patient (Fig. 12–4) was fit binaurally with behind-the-ear (BTE) hearing aids using FIG6. By entering this individual's thresholds into the FIG6 software, insertion gain targets (Table in center of Fig. 12–4) and coupler targets (graphs to the left of Fig. 12–4) for a BTE instrument were derived for both ears. The hearing aids were adjusted to the coupler targets before the verification portion of the hearing aid fitting (Fig. 12–5). Verification consisted of real-ear measurement and subjective ratings of loudness. Using probe microphone measures, REIG was determined at several input levels. As can be seen in Figure 12–6, REIG fell short of the target in the higher frequencies, most notably at 4000 Hz (this was true for the soft and loud REIG targets as well). Thus even though the hearing aids were adjusted to the prescribed coupler targets, when real-ear measures were performed, the real-ear targets were not met. Therefore this individual likely has a REUR and/or RECD that differs from normal.

In this case the hearing aids used were not flexible enough to allow for the manipulations to the frequency response necessary to meet the target. In addition, loudness judgments of continuous discourse by the patient revealed that speech was not being perceived as loud enough. In Table 12–8, the patient's CORFIG was determined by subtracting his RECD and the BTE microphone response from his REUR. The difference between the individual's CORFIG and the average CORFIG is shown in Figure 12–7. Note the large difference in the high frequencies that lead to insufficient prescribed gain when the average-based CORFIG was used. At this point, the individual's CORFIG values could be added to the insertion gain targets to derive the appropriate coupler gain response (see Table 12–9). The resultant values represent the desired coupler gain target for a 65 dB input with the individual-specific CORFIG values incorporated. Substantial differences exist between the original coupler target and the individual-specific coupler target, most notably in the high frequencies (see Fig. 12–8). By ordering a hearing aid that will come close to meeting the new coupler targets, it is likely that the REIG targets will be met as well. And, indeed, that was the case for this patient. Loudness judgments also revealed appropriate loudness perception for comfortable and loud continuous discourse.

The preceding example can be applied to any insertion or coupler gain targets provided by insertion-gain–based fitting strategies (i.e., NAL-R, POGO, etc.). All that is needed are insertion gain targets, the individual's REUR and RECD, and appropriate microphone correction values (see Appendix).

DYNAMIC RANGE MEASURES

The preceding sections have shown how individual-specific measures can be used in transforming values obtained in dB HL to real-ear dB SPL and 2-cc coupler data. Another aspect of hearing aid fitting in which either average-based data or individual-based data can be used concerns dynamic range measures. For many fitting strategies, measures of dynamic range are used in deriving fitting targets. For WDRC hearing aids, depending on the fitting strategy used, loudness contour data or LDLs are used in determining appropriate compression ratio(s). VIOLA, for example, requires that loudness contour data be obtained from threshold to LDL (Cox, 1995; Palmer & Lindley, 1998). DSL[i/o], however, determines an appropriate compression ratio using threshold and LDLs. With linear hearing aids, LDLs are typically used in deriving an appropriate SSPL90.

When dynamic range information is not obtained, this information is often predicted on the basis of threshold data. Some fitting protocols (e.g., FIG6) do not allow the dispenser to enter dynamic range information and rely solely on average-based data. This can lead to problems on the day of the fitting if an individual's dynamic range differs substantially from average. The audiologist needs to consider the adjustment capability of the hearing aids to be ordered when deciding on an appropriate fitting strategy and whether individual-specific dynamic range measures are a necessity. When adjustment flexibility is limited, individual-specific dynamic range measures easily can be justified, assuming the individual can perform the task. As alluded to throughout this chapter, dynamic range measures, just as threshold data, can be customized through the use of individual-specific transformations as described previously.

LIMITATIONS OF INDIVIDUAL-BASED TRANSFORMATIONS WHEN DERIVING 2-CC TARGETS

Most of the transformations described previously do not take into account venting characteristics (i.e., diameter, length) nor do

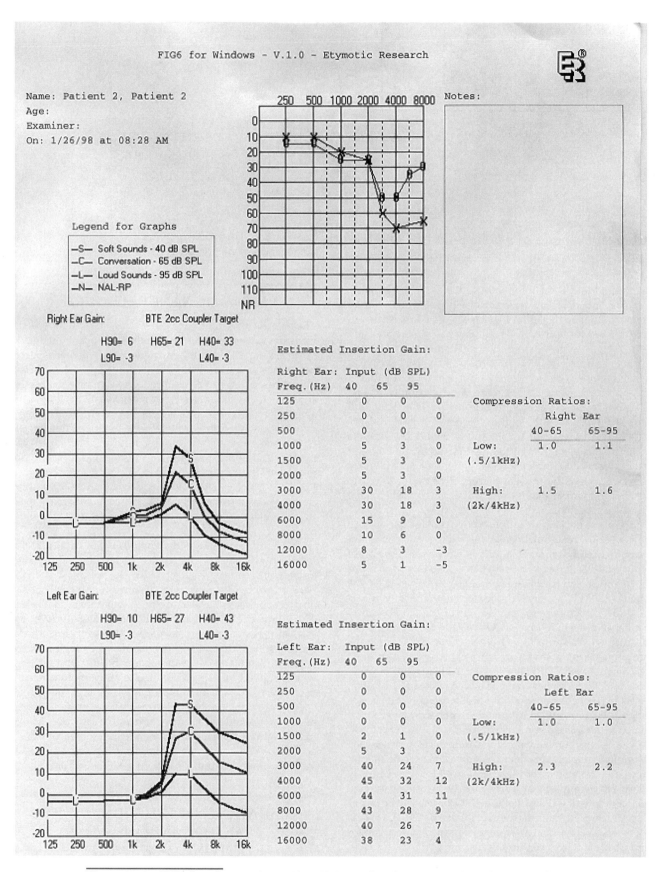

Figure 12–4 FIG6 data for a patient with a REUR and real-ear-to-coupler difference different from average.

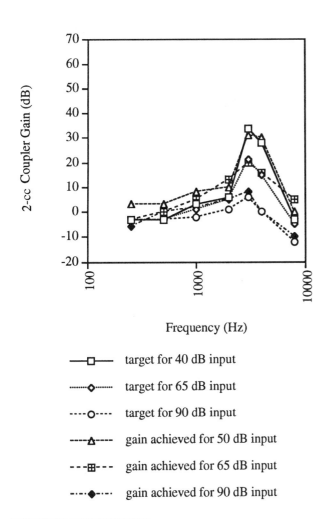

Frequency (Hz)

——□—— target for 40 dB input

·········◇········· target for 65 dB input

----○---- target for 90 dB input

----△---- gain achieved for 50 dB input

- - -⊞- - - gain achieved for 65 dB input

----◆---- gain achieved for 90 dB input

Figure 12–5 Gain achieved in a patient's hearing aid versus the target coupler gain at three input levels.

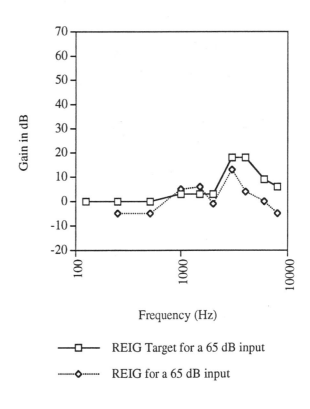

Frequency (Hz)

——□—— REIG Target for a 65 dB input

·········◇········· REIG for a 65 dB input

Figure 12–6 REIG obtained from the patient versus the target REIG.

they account for various canal lengths. Thus when individual-specific REURs and RECDs are obtained and the 2-cc targets are met, real-ear targets may not be exactly matched without further adjustment to the hearing aid. When RECD is measured with the individual's earmold, the vent response will be included. By using individual-specific transformations, the audiologist can reduce, but not eliminate, differences between performance in the coupler and performance in the real-ear. When possible, it is always beneficial to verify using real-ear measures.

However, in cases where this is not possible, the individual-specific 2-cc targets represent the best starting point. In addition, at least one software package, HAS (de Jonge, 1996), and DSL [i/o], allows for entry of various earmold characteristics and provides the predicted effect on the real-ear response. Audiologists also can consult published data that provide correction factors for various earmold characteristics. See Chapter 2 in this volume, which provides detailed information regarding earmold acoustics.

SOFTWARE APPLICATIONS

How easily the preceding measures can be applied in deriving 2-cc coupler targets will depend on how a particular

fitting strategy is incorporated into clinic routine. Typically, 2-cc coupler targets are derived using software applications, real-ear systems, or through manual calculation using a worksheet. The use of software applications facilitates the incorporation of the measures described above.

Many software applications are available for use in deriving fitting strategies and some are more limited in their ability to accommodate individual data than others. Some software packages are specific to a particular strategy (i.e., VIOLA portion of the IHAFF; FIG6; DSL[i/o]), whereas in others, the audiologist can choose from a number of possible fitting strategies (i.e., HAS which includes NAL-R, FIG6, VIOLA, and DSL[i/o]) (de Jonge, 1996). Some software packages allow for direct entry of thresholds in dB SPL, RECD, REDD, REUR, and/or LDL's (DSL[i/o], HAS). Some software packages only allow for entry of thresholds in dB HL (i.e., FIG6), whereas in HAS, the user can enter REDD and RECD and these are automatically applied to FIG6 fitting targets. It is beyond the scope of this chapter to review every possible software package available. See Table 12–2 for ordering information regarding the software packages described in this chapter. Table 12–10 provides a list of considerations when selecting a fitting protocol.

Armed with 2-cc coupler data, hearing aid circuitry, and other options (e.g., compression output limiting, telecoil) identified in the patient evaluation, the clinician is ready to order a conventional hearing aid. Once the clinician has chosen one or more manufacturers, it is time to examine the specification sheets to see whether one of the hearing aids in the product line will meet the patient's needs. The next

TABLE 12–8   Calculating individual CORFIG

Frequency (Hz)	Patient's REUR −	Patient's RECD −	BTE Microphone Response =	Resulting Individual CORFIG
250	0.0	0.0	0.8	−0.8
500	2.0	−5.0	1.6	5.4
1000	0.0	−0.0	1.6	−1.5
2000	14.0	−1.8	2.8	13.0
3000	18.0	−2.9	2.8	18.1
4000	20.0	−7.2	3.2	24.0
8000	10.0	−5.0	3.9	11.1

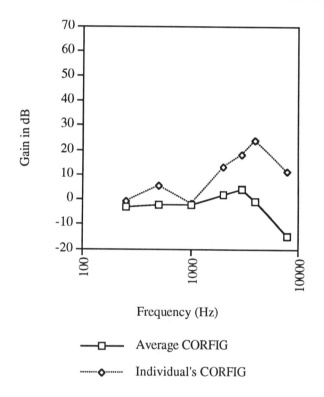

Average CORFIG

Individual's CORFIG

Figure 12–7   Average CORFIG versus the individual's CORFIG.

section introduces the use of manufacturers' specification sheets, which is essential when ordering conventional hearing aids.

PEARL

Maintain relations with two or three manufacturers whose products cover most of your patients' needs. Each time you try a new manufacturer you will be required to expend considerable time learning to understand their product line, specification sheets, and company policies.

UNDERSTANDING MANUFACTURERS' SPECIFICATION SHEETS

Components of the Specification Information

Because conventional hearing aids are often chosen from a review of the manufacturer's specification information, it is important to correctly interpret the data that are presented. The information itself is usually compiled in a binder referred to as the specification book or in a software format that can be accessed by computer disk, compact disc, or the World Wide Web (WWW). The data provided serve as the means by which the audiologist understands the physical and electroacoustic capabilities of each instrument. The data usually begin with general information on features of the instrument such as the number of channels, type of signal processing, range of hearing loss covered, and types of available potentiometers. An ANSI (1987) technical summary is included. This summary can be somewhat misleading because its data may reflect the combined available responses of a group of hearing aid matrices. It is, however, a good starting point from which one can further evaluate the suitability of the instrument in meeting the fitting goal. The specification data then show gain curves and input/output curves as measured in a 2-cc coupler, using given source signals, potentiometer settings, and volume control settings when appropriate. Thus these data show a sampling of the responses available from the instrument. With any adjustment to one or more of the variable controls (e.g., volume control, compression ratio potentiometer, tone control) the actual response will be different from that shown in the data. An example of hearing aid specification data is shown in Figure 12–9.

Labeling of Specification Data

Labeling of the specification data is critical to the accurate interpretation of the hearing aid characteristics. When reviewing the gain and input/output curves presented by the manufacturer, the reader should first look for labels identifying the values represented on the vertical and horizontal axis, the frequency and intensity of the source signal, the volume control setting (usually full-on), and the position of any potentiometer settings. In this manner, target fitting data may be more easily compared with that displayed by the manufacturer.

TABLE 12–9   Determining desired 2-cc coupler gain target using individual CORFIG

Frequency	Real-Ear-Insertion Gain target	+	Individual's CORFIG	=	Desired 2-cc gain target
250	0.0		−0.8		−0.8
500	0.0		5.4		5.4
1000	3.0		−1.5		−1.5
2000	3.0		13.0		16.0
3000	18.0		18.1		36.1
4000	18.0		24.0		42.0
8000	6.0		11.1		17.0

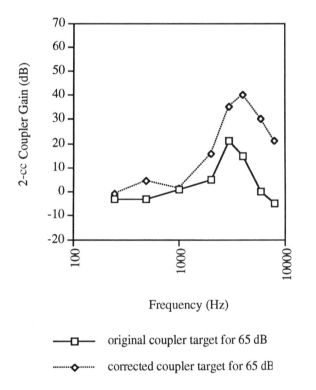

—□— original coupler target for 65 dB

·······◇······· corrected coupler target for 65 dB

Figure 12–8 Coupler target based on average data versus the coupler target based on individual data.

The Matrix Approach

With the increased popularity of custom in-the-ear (ITE) hearing aids in the 1980s, it became possible for manufacturers to provide a variety of hearing aid responses available in a few different shell styles. Thus audiologists could become more involved in the fitting process by actually choosing parameters of the hearing aid, such as the gain, output, and the slope of the response. These response parameters were organized into groups called matrices. One matrix would be specified by the audiologist or manufacturer as the response most likely to meet the fitting target. The matrices available for a given hearing instrument are usually represented by a series of three numbers corresponding to the gain, output, and slope, respectively (Table

12–11). When ordering a particular hearing aid for a patient, the audiologist can specify the matrix to be used, or the manufacturer will make the choice for the audiologist. Some manufacturers include matrix selection in the computer software that is supplied with their hearing aids. Thus the audiologist is able to enter patient data and a desired fitting formula, and a recommendation for the most appropriate instrument and matrix is automatically generated.

PRIORITIZING POTENTIOMETERS

Potentiometers on conventional hearing aids are controls that can be manipulated by a screwdriver to change the response of the hearing aid. BTE hearing aids usually are delivered with a preselected number of screw-set potentiometers. In some BTE instruments, the fitter may request alternate potentiometers. In ITE and smaller custom-type shells, size limitations often dictate the number of possible potentiometer options. For this reason, it is necessary to prioritize the capabilities that are desired for the instrument. The potentiometer capabilities are important to consider because they will dictate the electroacoustic flexibility in the hearing aid/earmold system. Other electroacoustic flexibility will come from options in the shell or earmold plumbing system (see Chapter 2 in this text). For example, the use of a variable venting (VV) system will allow the audiologist to manipulate the low-end frequency response without requiring placement of a low-cut potentiometer. Aside from the volume control, screw-set potentiometers often provide the only electroacoustic flexibility in the conventional hearing aid circuitry. In addition, they serve as the vehicle through which fine-tuning of the fitting can be achieved.

Thus caution and attention to detail are advised when choosing which potentiometers to order and the positions at which they should be set. Each manufacturer uses terminology that is not necessarily consistent with other manufacturers when referring to available potentiometers. For example, one company may refer to a potentiometer that increases or decreases the SSPL90 as the maximum power output (MPO) control, whereas another calls it the P control, and another designates it as AOP. At present, no standard format exists for referring to such controls. The fitter needs to understand what parameter of the response will be affected by a given adjustment. In addition, different manufacturers choose different

TABLE 12–10 What to consider when selecting a fitting protocol

1. Are there data to support the efficacy or validity of the protocol?

2. Is the protocol device independent?

3. Is the protocol software driven (ease, time saver)?

4. Does the protocol allow you to enter data in the format in which you collect data (HL, SPL, insert earphones, TDH-50 earphones, sound field, etc.)?

5. Does the protocol have a mechanism for applying individual data (RECD, REDD, etc.)?

6. Does the protocol's goal match your goal?

7. Does the protocol provide coupler targets that allow you to order/preset a hearing aid?

8. Does the protocol provide verification data in the format in which you like to verify (REIG, output, subjective loudness targets, etc.)?

9. Does the protocol handle the technology you are fitting (e.g., multiple targets for WDRC instruments, etc.) and the style (e.g., BTE, ITE, ITC, CIC) you are fitting?

10. Does the fitting protocol provide a mechanism for dealing with a conductive component? One may have to contact the fitting protocol designer to find out the mechanism.

11. Does the protocol provide options for fitting conductive losses and does the protocol account for binaural summation?

approaches to achieve the intended response adjustments from a potentiometer. For example, a potentiometer labeled H may suggest a high-frequency emphasis that is incorporated in the response when set to maximum. However, a variety of ways exist that such an emphasis could be achieved. One way would be to decrease the low-frequency gain. Others could be to increase the gain for high-frequency input or to broaden the response to include higher frequencies. To effectively use the potentiometers one needs to understand how the adjustment in the response is achieved. This information should be explained in the specification sheets provided by the manufacturer. Coupler or real-ear verification is the only way to know exactly what has changed in the hearing aid response after a potentiometer is manipulated.

The setting of the potentiometer adjustments becomes a factor at the point when the audiologist is ready to compare the 2-cc coupler targets to the response of a hearing aid that has been ordered and received in the office. Some manufacturers include a potentiometer adjustment guide in their computer software, showing the fitter the recommended settings for the given hearing loss and hearing aid. This assumes that the manufacturer is using the same fitting protocol (e.g., FIG6, DSL[i/o], VIOLA) to produce targets. That will not always be the case. Most likely, the audiologist will need to consult the manufacturer product information for guidance as to the operation of the potentiometers. Once again, each manufacturer may use their own convention for such descriptions. For example, a potentiometer labeled TK is often designated as the threshold knee point control. The labeling on such a potentiometer is often shown as − for minumum and + for maximum. Without reading the product literature carefully, one could have difficulty understanding whether the minimum TK position actually refers to the lowest available threshold knee value or the minimum available amount of compression (actually the maximum threshold knee value). Certainly, one can alleviate some of

this confusion by implementing adjustments in the potentiometers and observing changes in the response, as measured in the hearing aid test box. When available, the manufacturer's computer software often will illustrate the electroacoustic changes that take place with potentiometer control adjustments. These graphic simulations do not eliminate the need for objective verification of the actual hearing aid response but do illustrate the general direction of the change.

MAKING USE OF DATA FROM THE FITTING FORMULA IN SELECTING CONVENTIONAL INSTRUMENTS AND OPTIONS

As noted previously, the outcome of a hearing aid fitting formula is a prescribed hearing aid response as would be measured in a 2-cc coupler. Once derived by means of the formula, the clinician must identify an appropriate commercially available hearing aid that will closely approximate this prescribed response. For a BTE, the hearing aid is either ordered from the manufacturer by telephone or chosen from a stock of previously purchased instruments. For a custom product, a detailed order form that is unique to each manufacturer is completed. The process of selecting and ordering an appropriate instrument with which the targets will be met will be examined in this section.

The data presented in Figure 12–10 (Mr. Patient) will be used in this description. On the basis of his individual listening needs, cosmetic preferences, and financial resources, we have decided to fit binaural conventional ITC hearing aids. Although the fitting is binaural, the data from the right ear will be presented for the purposes of this example. Fitting targets will be derived using the DSL[i/o] procedure. This will be used to determine the suitability of a given hearing aid and to fill out an order form for the instrument. To complete

SOUND F/X CUSTOM / MINI CANAL • CANAL • HALF SHELL • FULL SHELL

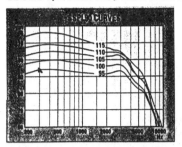

Input sound pressure level: 90 dB   Volume Control: full on
G_L Parameter: +   G_H Parameter: +   F Parameter: −
TK Parameter: −   P Parameter: +

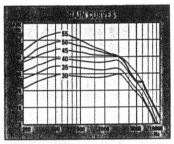

Input sound pressure level: 50 dB   Volume Control: full on
G_L Parameter: +   G_H Parameter: +   F Parameter: −
TK Parameter: −   P Parameter: +

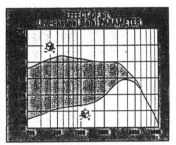

Input sound pressure level: 50 dB   Volume Control: full on
G_H Parameter: +   F Parameter: +
TK Parameter: −   P Parameter: +

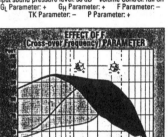

Input sound pressure level: 50 dB   Volume Control: full on
G_L Parameter: +/−   G_H Parameter: +/−
TK Parameter: −   P Parameter: +

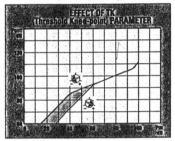

Input sound pressure level: 50 dB   Volume Control: full on
G_L Parameter: +   G_H Parameter: +
F Parameter: −   P Parameter: +

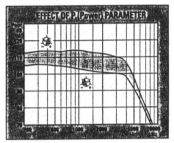

Input sound pressure level: 100 dB   Volume Control: full on
G_L Parameter: +   G_H Parameter: +
F Parameter: −   TK Parameter: −

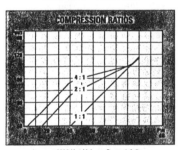

Input at 2000 Hz   Volume Control: full on
G_L Parameter: +   G_H Parameter: −/+   F Parameter: −
TK Parameter: −   P Parameter: +

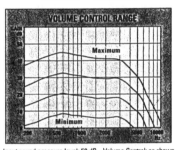

Input sound pressure level: 50 dB   Volume Control: as shown
G_L Parameter: +   G_H Parameter: +   F Parameter: −
TK Parameter: −   P Parameter: +

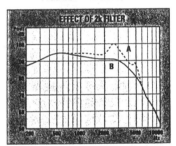

Input sound pressure level: 50 dB   Volume Control: full on
"A" unfiltered, not recommended   "B" filtered, standard

SOUND FX ANSI TECHNICAL DATA	
Frequency Range	100-8000 Hz
Reference Test Gain	- 5-46 dB
HF - Average Gain (50 dB in)	5-46 dB
HF - Average SSPL90	92-109 dB
Zinc Air Premium Battery Life 13	175-380 h
312	85-180 h
10A	75-90 h
Current Drain	0.6-1.3 mA
Output with Inductive Input at 1 kHz	82-102 dB
Peak	83-104 dB
Equivalent Input Noise at RTP Typical 24 dB	<28 dB
Total Harmonic Distortion	
500 Hz	typical 1% <6%
800 Hz	typical 1% <6%
1600 Hz	typical 1% <6%
Attack Time	<220 ms
Release Time	500 ms
Compression Ratio	1:1 to 4:1

CUSTOM PRODUCTS

SOUND F/X

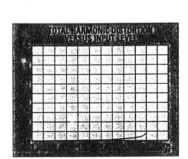

Input at 1600 Hz   Volume Control: full on
G_L Parameter: +   G_H Parameter: +   F Parameter: −
TK Parameter: −   P Parameter: +

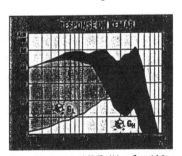

Input sound pressure level: 50 dB   Volume Control: full on
This insertion gain is similar to the functional gain for an
average adult with a closed earmold.

Figure 12–9   Unitron specification sheet for the Sound FX.

TABLE 12–11 Matrix options on the Unitron Specification Sheet

Sound FX Custom Matrix Selections	
Sound FX	Sound FX H
Mini canal 95/30-5/F/X	95/30-5/F/XH
100/35-10/F/X	100/35-10/F/XH
105/40-15/F/X	105/40-15/F/XH
Canal 95/30-5/F/X	95/30-5/F/XH
Half shell 100/35-10/F/X	100/35-10/F/XH
105/40-15/F/X	105/40-15/F/XH
110/45-20/F/X	110/45-20/F/XH
Concha 95/35-5/F/X	95/35-5/F/XH
100/40-10/F/X	100/40-10/F/XH
105/45-15/F/X	105/45-15/F/XH
110/50-20/F/X	110/50-20/F/XH
115/50-25/F/X	115/50-25/F/XH
115/55-25/F/X	

this process one must (1) understand the data obtained from the formula, (2) understand the descriptions and data on circuits and options shown in the manufacturers' product literature, and (3) order an instrument with options that will allow us execution of fitting strategy by characteristics and/or controls on the hearing aid and meet any additional needs identified through our assessment (*Hearing Demand, Ability, Needs Profile, Patient Expectation Worksheet, APHAB*).

Figure 12–9 illustrates the manufacturer's specifications on the hearing aid model and circuit chosen for Mr. Patient's right ear. This particular hearing aid was chosen for a number of reasons. Having two separate channels with some controls will allow the audiologist to address the different gain as a function of input in the low-frequency and high-frequency regions of this patient's audiogram. The parameters within these channels can be controlled independently, allowing for good flexibility in the instrument. In addition, the wide variety of responses displayed on the specification sheet are very well labeled, avoiding the confusion of guessing where the potentiometers are set or at what level the volume control is adjusted.

Figure 12–10 shows a printout of the DSL[i/o] targets derived for Mr. Patient's right ear. The data that are most useful for comparing with manufacturer specifications are the SSPL90, the Full-On Gain (reserve 10 dB), and the compression ratio. Begin by comparing the SSPL90, shown from 250 Hz to 6000 Hz on the printout, to that displayed in the manufacturer's specification sheet. The corresponding curve appears in the upper left-hand corner of Figure 12–9. Because the Hearing Aid Recommendation DSL[i/o] targets are generated assuming a full-on volume control, it would be tempting to make a direct comparison between the values in the DSL[i/o] printout and those displayed in the specification sheet. This would be misleading, however, because the positions of the adjustable parameters, such as the low-channel gain (GL), TK, crossover frequency (F), and high-channel gain (GH) must be considered (gain is changed through manipulation of the compression ratio). The SSPL90 curve assists in assessing the suitability of this instrument for the target, and

it will also help select the matrix number, as the lines labeled with matrix maximum output designators across the SSPL90 curves are examined.

It may appear that low-frequency gain is too high when selecting the manufacturer's gain curve. However, the curve labeled "Effect of GL Parameter" (Fig. 12–9) shows that an adjustment made to reduce the low channel gain could result in a reasonable approximation of the target.

PITFALL

When comparing manufacturer's frequency-response curves to desired coupler targets be sure to consider the volume control setting and the input level of the source signal.

DSL[i/o] shows compression ratios for each test frequency (1.4 to 4.2). It would be unusual to find a conventional hearing aid capable of this many different compression ratios. Thus this information can be averaged across frequencies or frequency bands and the results compared with the hearing aid under consideration. In Mr. Patient's case, all the CR values, except that found at 6000 Hz (4.2) fall within the capability of the hearing aid chosen. This is illustrated by the manufacturer in the graph labeled "Compression Ratios" in Figure 12–9, showing that the CR can vary from 1:1 (linear) to 4:1 for a 2000 Hz input. Manufacturers typically display an input/output curve (where compression ratios can be viewed/calculated) only for 2000 Hz. With a multiple-channel instrument, it is important to know the CR for the low-frequency and high-frequency channel and perhaps, more importantly, whether they can be manipulated independently. The CR range for the low-frequency channel is not provided in the specifications for this hearing aid and would have to be obtained by contacting the manufacturer.

CONTROVERSIAL POINT

Audiologists and manufacturers may tout the benefits of targeting the compression ratio in the hearing aid. This parameter is intimately tied into the gain and output characteristics of a nonlinear hearing aid. Some would argue that by first targeting the appropriate gain and output values, the compression ratio will necessarily fall at the appropriate value.

The adjustment of the compression ratios in this hearing aid is accessed by means of the GL parameter. This is a good illustration of how the gain in a channel is directly related to the compression ratio. The DSL[i/o] printout for Mr. Patient specifies a 40 dB compression threshold. Compression threshold is selected from a list of possibilities by the clinician using the DSL[i/o]. The graph labeled "Effect of TK" in Figure 12–9 illustrates that such a threshold knee should be possible. Once again, considering the function of each potentiometer, it would appear that the F (crossover) and GL parameters will assist in reaching the targets.

```
                        University of Western Ontario
                                  Canada

                            Patient Information

    Patient ID : Patient 1              Street :
          Name :  ,                       City :
    Birth Date : 11-dec-1928        State/Prov. :
  Professional :                       Country :
  Today's Date : 15-Jul-1998, 17:05:40   Phone :
```

ASSESSMENT DATA (dB HL)

RIGHT EAR		.25	.50	.75	1.0	1.5	2.0	3.0	4.0	6.0
	Threshold	20	35	37	40	50	55	65	70	80
	Upper Limit									
	Exponent									
	RECD									
	REUR									
	REDD									

HEARING AID RECOMMENDATION

RIGHT EAR
Selection Method : DSL [i/o]

```
HEARING AID                    OTHER                          OTHER
    Style : ITC                Transducer : ER3               Speech : Cox/Moore
    Make :                     HL to SPL : Predicted          Compr. Thresh : 40
    Model :                    HA Style : ITC                 Loudness : Predicted
  Serial # :                   Circuit : WDRC (fixed CR)
                               RE to 2cc : Predicted          Max. Out : Predicted
```

		.25	.50	.75	1.0	1.5	2.0	3.0	4.0	6.0
	SSPL-90	92	102	102	102	104	108	110	108	106
	Full-On Gain (Reserve 10 dB)	15	22	23	24	29	35	38	37	40
	User Gain (Input 65 dB)	5	12	13	14	19	25	28	27	30
	Comp. Ratio	1.4	1.6	1.6	1.7	2.0	2.2	2.7	3.0	4.2

VERIFICATION DATA

RIGHT EAR
Hi-Level (Coupler Output)

		.25	.50	.75	1.0	1.5	2.0	3.0	4.0	6.0
	Target 90 dB	88	93	93	93	97	101	103	100	101
	Measured 90 dB									

Mid-Level (Coupler Gain)

		.25	.50	.75	1.0	1.5	2.0	3.0	4.0	6.0
	Target 80 dB	1	7	7	8	11	17	19	17	18
	Measured									
	Target 65 dB	5	12	13	14	19	25	28	27	30
	Measured									
	Target 50 dB	9	18	19	20	26	33	38	37	41
	Measured									

Low-Level

		.25	.50	.75	1.0	1.5	2.0	3.0	4.0	6.0
	Aided SF 0°	8	13	12	15	18	21	25	25	25
	Measured									

Figure 12–10   The DSL[i/o] coupler target recommendations for the example patient's right ear.

SPECIAL CONSIDERATION

Never shy away from calling a manufacturer for further clarification or information on product features. Often, product features or custom modifications are possible that are not described in the specification materials.

The manufacturer's software for the example hearing aid does allow for the fitter to enter a choice of hearing aid fitting formulas including the DSL[i/o]. The resulting computerized recommendation for Mr. Patient's hearing loss includes the F and GL potentiometers, with a 110/45-20/FX matrix. As noted previously, the numbers in the matrix (Table 12–11) refer to peak output and gain of the hearing aid response. In the case of Mr. Patient the DSL[i/o] SSPL90 (Fig. 12–10) recommendation shows a peak output of 110 dB at 3000 Hz in the right ear. Thus the matrix option that begins with the number 110 is chosen. The second number in the matrix refers to the peak gain of the response. In an instrument such as the one that has been chosen, this value may vary greatly, depending on the adjustments that are made by means of the potentiometers. Thus this manufacturer designates the gain value by showing the range of peak gain that is possible (Fig. 12–9). The peak value shown in the DSL[i/o] Full-On Gain recommendation (Fig. 12–10) is 40 dB at 6000 Hz. Realistically, the hearing aid that has been chosen only responds out to about 5000 Hz, so the peak value below 5000 Hz would be more appropriate (38 dB at 3000 Hz). The canal matrix showing the range of 45- to 20-dB of gain would be appropriate for this fitting. In this particular hearing aid the slope is not designated in the matrix because it is so variable with the potentiometer adjustments. The company refers to the slope as F/X when listing the matrix options. So the matrix selected would be 110/45-20/F/X (Table 12–11).

CONTROVERSIAL POINT

Some audiologists choose to let the manufacturer select the matrix for the fittings that are ordered. They argue that, given the 2-cc coupler target, the manufacturer can best understand the ability of the product to meet the target. Others feel strongly that the fitter should select the matrix and should not leave this role to the manufacturer.

As illustrated in the preceding example, the intent of the hearing aid fitting formula used in this example is not to select a particular hearing aid but rather a particular electroacoustic response. One is limited to hearing aids that are commercially available. The chosen fitting formula serves as a guide by which to select a hearing aid that will later be fine-tuned to produce the desired response. Even when choosing conventional hearing aids, the manufacturer's fitting software can further serve as a guide to choosing a particular model, potentiometer, and potentiometer settings. Once the clinician is comfortable that the hearing aid described in the specifications contains all the needed features and can provide the required electroacoustic response, the hearing aid must be ordered.

SPECIAL CONSIDERATION

Some fitting strategies assume that no volume control is included because the hearing aid is adjusting gain as a function of input so targets are in use-gain. Add 10 dB (reserve gain) to obtain targets that can be compared with manufacturers' full-on gain specifications.

FACING THE ORDER FORM

When a custom hearing aid is ordered, the final link from the audiologist to the hearing aid manufacturer is the order form itself. Martin (1998) lamented that the process of ordering hearing aids could be improved by using specialized checklists in addition to the standard order forms. The authors recommend that order forms be previewed while the patient is still in the office. This will reduce the need to telephone patients later, wondering whether items such as removal notches or windscreens should be included.

PEARL

Preview the order form before the patient leaves the office so you will not forget to ask questions relevant to requesting special options or features on the instruments.

As noted earlier, each manufacturer uses a different format for the layout and design of the order form. It is critical that product literature, including specification sheets and general product information, be reviewed before attempting to use a given manufacturer's order form. Before filling in any information, the entire order form should be examined. Determine first the circuit type, potentiometers, and other options. Then determine the nomenclature by which these features are referred to by that company. For example, the Starkey Sequel order form lists the Starcoil with Switch as a control option available on this hearing aid. One would have to refer to the circuit option guide, a booklet distributed along with the specification book, to know that the Starcoil is Starkey's name for a telecoil. For another example, look at the Unitron Sound FX order form shown in Figure 12–11. This form is filled out for the hearing aids to be ordered for Mr. Patient.

A section of the form allows for entry of a desired Matrix. If 2-cc target data are being supplied (from DSL[i/o], VIOLA, FIG6, or some other fitting protocol), the manufacturer is being left with the decision of which is the most appropriate matrix. In this example the values were taken directly from the DSL[i/o] printout. The authors currently send the desired 2-cc targets (the printout from the fitting protocol can be used) because manufacturers may be able to create 2-cc responses closer to the actual targets than what are displayed in the specification book. The audiologist may want to discuss this option with a given manufacturer; the authors have had success with both Phonak and Argosy using this method.

PEARL

When sending a target(s) to a manufacturer, make sure you inform the manufacturer what type of target it is (e.g., 2-cc versus real-ear, use versus full-on gain). In addition, do not worry about filling out the patient's audiogram, speech testing results, specifications of previous hearing aids, and so on on the order form. Provide the manufacturer with the 2-cc coupler targets. If you are confident in your target selection, you do not need to supply all the other supporting data.

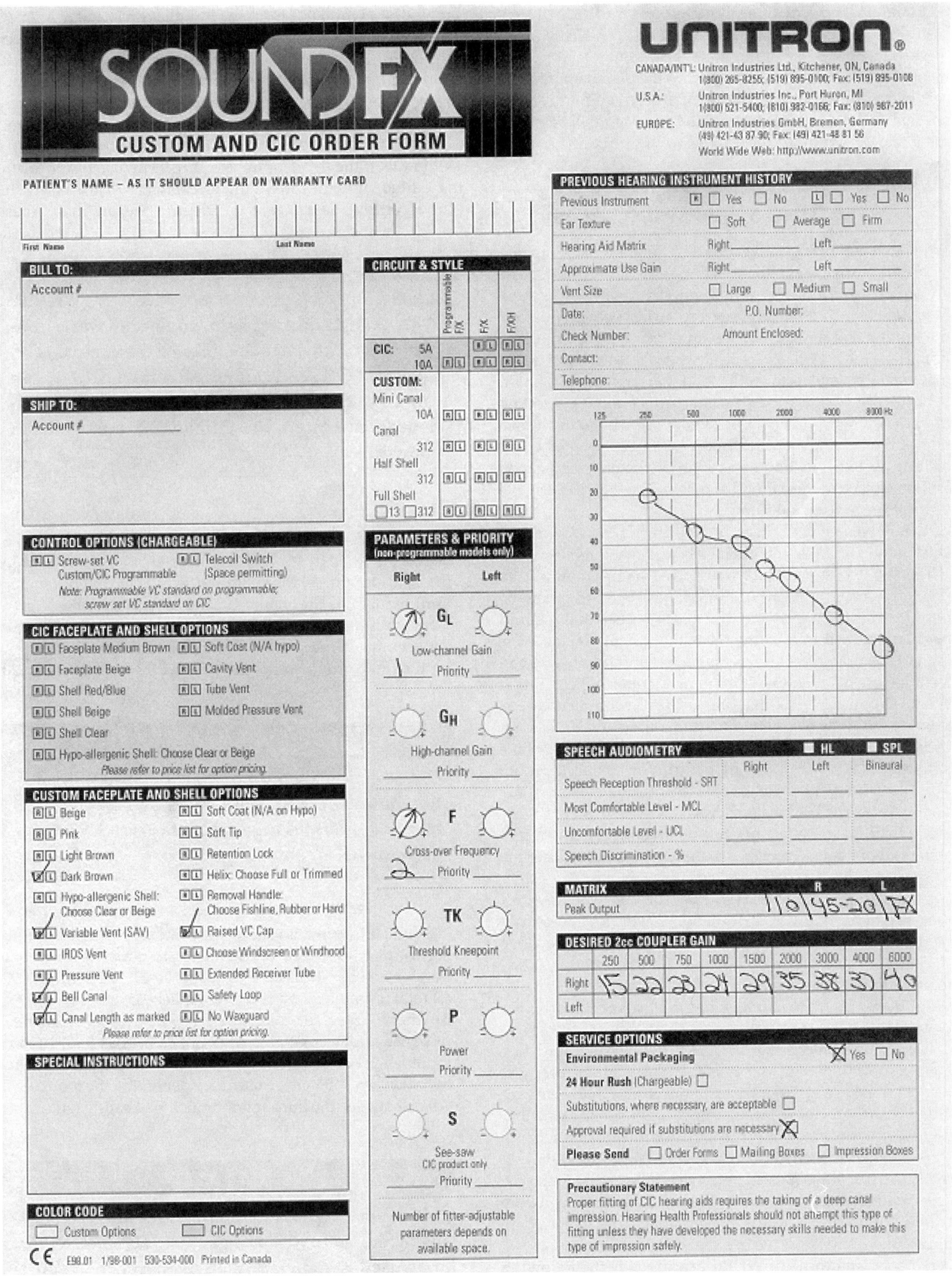

Figure 12–11 Sound FX custom product order form.

In the end the goal of the fitting process is to order instruments that meet the electroacoustic, cosmetic, and fiscal needs of the patient and to communicate these requirements in the most effective and efficient manner to the manufacturer. The earmold impressions (in the case of an ITC) and order form are sent to the manufacturer and the next step will be evaluating and presetting the hearing aids when they arrive.

PRESETTING THE HEARING AIDS

Whether one is fitting conventional or programmable hearing aids, time working with the patient is saved if the hearing aids are preset before arrival of the patient. If the presetting is accurate, time in the verification session can be spent on minimal fine-tuning and maximal counseling. Presetting is especially important for a pediatric patient where real-ear verification may not be possible (e.g., if the child will not tolerate the test) and patient opinion may not be forthcoming. Presetting implies having a set of coupler targets that will guide the setting of the hearing aids and will serve to verify whether the hearing aids are functioning as desired. The final verification will take place in the ear and will be dictated by the original goals of the hearing aid fitting.

Before presetting the hearing aids, the hearing aids should be set with all of the potentiometers and the volume control wheel (VCW) (if included) to provide maximum output. In this condition, a standard ANSI (1987) test box run should be performed (see Chapter 1 in this volume). These data should be compared with the coupler data that came with the hearing aid (assuming the hearing aid was set full-on when collecting these data) and with the manufacturer's specification sheet. The ANSI (1987) hearing aid test recommendations provide the allowance between the manufacturer's measurements and the resulting hearing aid measurements. Make sure that the hearing aids are performing to specification. This is a quick way to ensure that the hearing aids are functioning properly. The concern always exists that either a hearing aid left the manufacturer functioning improperly or that some sort of damage occurred in transit. In addition, listen to the hearing aids through a personal listening mold or listening stethoscope. The ANSI (1987) test run does not provide a measure of all types of distortion and will not necessarily identify hearing aids with some intermittent problems. Move the hearing aid around and listen. If all looks good, proceed to presetting the hearing aids. As stated previously, this initial set of measures may help identify problems with particular manufacturers.

Depending on the manufacturer, the hearing aids may have arrived with data for presetting. The manufacturer will have based these settings either on the targets that were provided with the order or by entering the audiometric data into a fitting protocol to which the particular manufacturer prescribes. Either way, these settings are probably a good starting place. Review the requested potentiometers by examining the specification sheet or by using the manufacturer's software to see how changes in the potentiometer are expected to impact the response of the hearing aids.

At a minimum, with WDRC hearing aids the following should be measured in the coupler: (a) frequency response (gain or output depending on how the chosen fitting protocol provides target data) for three input levels (whatever levels were used to generate the targets), (b) SSPL90 curve (to check the limiting), (c) total harmonic distortion for a quiet (45 dB) and loud (90 dB) input, (d) circuit noise (equivalent input noise level), and (e) telecoil response. The audiologist may want to obtain input/output curves for a low (500 Hz) and high (3000 Hz) frequency to document compression threshold and ratio. If the three input level targets match, this measure is redundant. If the three input level targets do not match, the input/output data may help identify the problem. These

---

PEARL

With WDRC hearing aids, do not be overly concerned with the actual values of the compression threshold (CT) and compression ratio (CR). If you can adjust the hearing aid to meet your level-dependent targets, the CT and CR must be close enough.

---

measures are meant to be compared directly to the coupler targets provided by the fitting protocol that was used to order the hearing aid. Manipulate the available potentiometers until the targets are matched as closely as possible. Agreement within 3 dB is excellent. More than 7 dB difference between the hearing aid's response and the original targets is cause for concern and perhaps for return of the hearing aid.

PEARL

Use a hearing aid test box that allows for the selection of a variety of input levels and types of signals and provides input/output curves for a range of frequencies (not just 2000 Hz).

A linear hearing aid should be evaluated with the following coupler measures: (a) frequency response (gain or output) for a moderate input level (65- to 70-dB SPL), (b) SSPL90, (c) total harmonic distortion for a quiet (45 dB) and loud (90 dB) input, (d) circuit noise, and (e) telecoil response. A linear response implies that gain does not change as a function of input level, but a high-frequency and low-frequency input/output curve still may be useful in identifying the input level, which engages the output limiting of the hearing aid.

PITFALL

Make sure you verify the hearing aid responses using the same type of signal and signal level that was used to generate the targets for the coupler and real-ear.

In the following sections the example hearing aid (Unitron Sound FX) has been adjusted using the GL and F potentiometers that were ordered and the volume control to match the coupler targets generated by DSL[i/o]. Figure 12–9 provides all the coupler data needed to preset the hearing aids. Measure the output of the hearing aid with a 90-, 80-, 65-, and 50-dB SPL input signal. Make sure that the type of signal used in the coupler measures is the same as was used in creating the targets. In DSL[i/o] the user selects these parameters and the user will see the selections on screen. Figure 12–12 illustrates the coupler measurements made with the example hearing aid. The measured values can be entered into DSL[i/o] for graphical comparison to the prescribed values (see Fig. 12–13; the coupler values are automatically transformed to real-ear values). In this case the actual values obtained are in good agreement with the prescribed values. This provides an ideal documentation of the coupler response. Some of the coupler measurement systems will calculate the target for the fitting protocol that is being used or will allow entry of particular targets.

If the level-dependent gain or output targets are being met and the hearing aids are being limited at the appropriate output, the combination of compression threshold and ratio must be appropriate. If, on the other hand, the gain or output targets are not met, the compression threshold and ratio that can be deduced from an input/output curve may be instructive in what needs to be manipulated.

ASSESSING THE FUNCTION OF THE TELECOIL OR OTHER COUPLING TO ASSISTIVE TECHNOLOGY

In the beginning of this section, assessing the telecoil response was included in the list of items to check using the coupler. If a telecoil has been ordered, its frequency response should be documented. Although the clinician does not have any method of changing the telecoil response in the conventional hearing aid, a weak response should motivate the clinician to return the hearing aid until a reasonable telecoil response is obtained. The telecoil should produce the same response as the microphone response with some additional low-frequency emphasis. A weak telecoil response would provide significantly less gain than the microphone response. Including a telecoil option is not useful if the telecoil is not functioning. Although the ANSI (1987) test recommends a single telecoil measurement with a 1000 Hz signal, this is not adequate for evaluation of the response.

One way to evaluate the response of the telecoil is to set it up for testing with an assistive listening device using a neckloop. Place the hearing aid (set to telecoil) in the middle of a neckloop (positioned as if it were on an ear and neck) connected to the receiver of an assistive listening device and connect the hearing aid to the 2-cc coupler. The test box microphone is inserted into the 2-cc coupler. This equipment can be sitting outside the test box on a padded surface. Inside the test box, connect the microphone of the assistive listening device to the transmitter. This is the unit that will pick up the signal generated inside the test box. The FM signal will be transmitted to the receiver coupled to the hearing aid, and the test box microphone will pick up and record the response. Make sure the

hearing aid, assistive listening device transmitter, and receiver are all turned on and have good batteries. An 80 dB SPL signal is reasonable because it mimics the input level at the microphone of an assistive device. This will not necessarily mimic a telephone signal, but the measurement will document the frequency response of the telecoil. Returning inadequate telecoils will assist in educating manufacturers about the importance of this component of the hearing aid. A direct audio input or built-in FM receiver could be tested in the same manner.

FINE-TUNING/VERIFICATION OF THE SELECTION

The conventional hearing aids that were ordered have arrived and have been preset to approximate the coupler targets supplied through the fitting protocol of choice. The patient is scheduled for the hearing aid fitting and arrives expecting to go home with new hearing aids. It is time to verify the hearing aids' responses in the patient's ears and verify any other features that were part of the original goal of the fitting. The goal of the hearing aid fitting and the data collected for ordering the hearing aids will dictate how the hearing aid verification should be conducted. If one has chosen to fit linear technology, assessing loudness ratings across input levels to verify the fitting not only does not make sense but also is unfair to the manufacturer from whom the hearing aids were ordered. On the other hand, if the original goal was to restore normal loudness perception, some sort of evaluation to determine whether this has been achieved would seem to be essential.

REAL-EAR MEASUREMENTS

Real-ear verification should follow the procedures used to create the targets. If the measurement system includes the selected fitting algorithm, targets will appear on the same screen where the individual real-ear data are presented. This is ideal in that the clinician is not looking back and forth between papers to see if the data look the same. Some measurement systems will allow the audiologist to enter the actual targets even though the system does not calculate these. Either method provides good documentation in terms of matching the real-ear target. Regardless of the coupler data, the real-ear is where the hearing aids work. A pediatric patient who tolerated RECD also may tolerate real-ear measurements (depending on how quickly they can be done).

PEARL

For easier verification and good record-keeping, purchase a coupler and real-ear system that produce targets using the fitting algorithm you prefer, or at a minimum, allow you to enter absolute targets for several input levels. Check to see the manufacturer's track record of updating their target selections as new fitting protocols are introduced and/or modified.

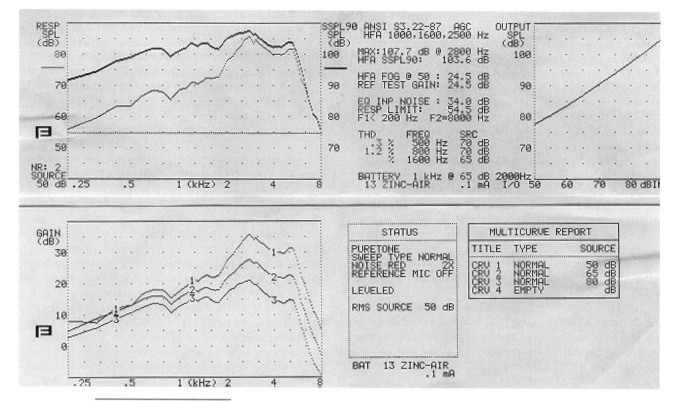

Figure 12–12   Coupler data used to preset the hearing aid according to a fitting protocol.

If the patient will not tolerate any type of real-ear measurements, RECD and coupler target matching take on even more importance. Even if the audiologist cannot perform an entire real-ear test battery (REAR, REUR or a family of REAR curves), try to obtain one REAR sweep to identify if the hearing aid is producing a smooth frequency response. This may save time troubleshooting feedback problems.

FIG6 provides insertion gain targets, which means that REUR and REAR should be collected for the patient using the signal type and level (40-, 65-, and 95-dB SPL) used in the FIG6 program. If the audiologist manipulated the FIG6 coupler target using RECD and individual REUR, he or she should expect a good match between the measured and targeted insertion gain. If these measures were not included, the REIG may not match the target. The clinician must then use whatever features were included on the hearing aids to make adjustments. Generally, the error will require an adjustment in gain in the low and/or high frequencies as opposed to a large change in limiting, compression ratio, or compression threshold.

DSL[i/o] provides REAR targets in the form of a Verification SPL-O-Gram. If the measurement system does not provide DSL[i/o] targets and they cannot be entered in absolute value, the clinician can enter the values from the REAR measurements into the original DSL[i/o] fitting patient file, and these curves will be presented along with the targets. These will be the curves labeled "M" along with the input level. A family of REAR curves should be generated with a soft (50 dB SPL), moderate (65 dB SPL), and loud (90 dB SPL) signal. The SPL-O-Gram provides the auditory dynamic range of the patient (threshold to UCL) with targets displayed in the audible area. The clinician may be less concerned with matching the exact target and more concerned with presenting soft, moderate,

and loud signals within the audible range and with frequency responses producing the general shape of the targets. The SPL-O-Gram is a strong tool for verification and for counseling because of its relationship with audibility. Just because one matches a REIG target does not mean that the signal is audible to the patient. For example, if an individual has an 80 dB HL threshold at 4000 Hz and normal-hearing out to 2000 Hz, NAL-R would try to restore one third of the loss, which would produce a 50- to 60-dB HL aided threshold. Obtaining enough gain to achieve this and thereby matching the insertion gain target would not lead to audibility of a soft conversational level speech signal in that frequency region. With the DSL[i/o] verification data, a statement regarding audibility can be made. For severe hearing losses, one may find that soft sounds cannot be made audible across the frequency range. In this case the SPL-O-Gram is a good counseling tool to instill realistic expectations for the individual.

The VIOLA does not provide any real-ear verification strategy. As previously mentioned, REAR sweep will identify the smoothness of the real-ear response and may save time in troubleshooting later. If LDLs were measured in SPL during the assessment, a REAR with a 90 dB SPL input also can be used to verify that the limiting of the hearing aid is appropriate.

LOUDNESS GROWTH

If the goal of the fitting was to restore a normal loudness growth (soft sounds are perceived as soft, moderate sounds are perceived as comfortable, and loud sounds are perceived

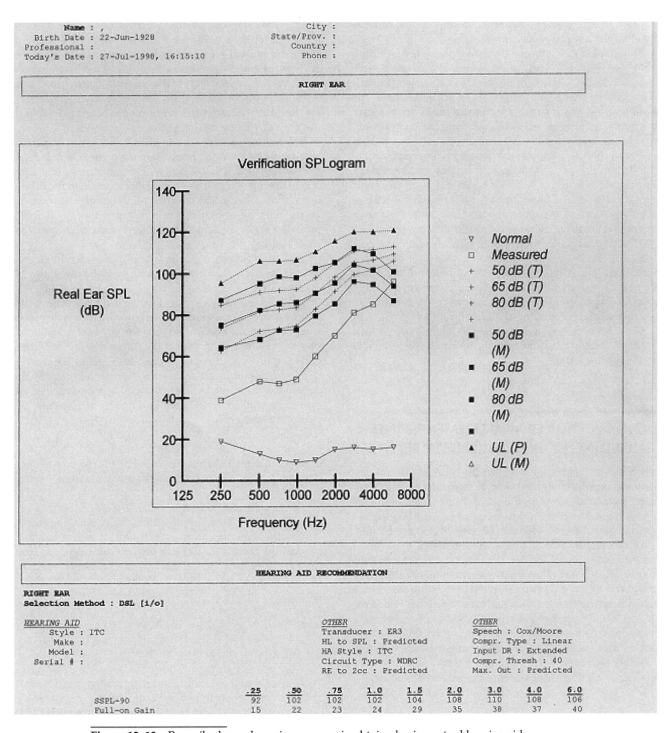

Name : ,
Birth Date : 22-Jun-1929
Professional :
Today's Date : 27-Jul-1998, 16:15:10

City :
State/Prov. :
Country :
Phone :

RIGHT EAR

Verification SPLogram

Real Ear SPL
(dB)

Frequency (Hz)

▽ *Normal*
□ *Measured*
+ *50 dB (T)*
+ *65 dB (T)*
+ *80 dB (T)*
+
■ *50 dB (M)*
■ *65 dB (M)*
■ *80 dB (M)*
■
▲ *UL (P)*
△ *UL (M)*

HEARING AID RECOMMENDATION

RIGHT EAR
Selection Method : DSL [i/o]

HEARING AID
Style : ITC
Make :
Model :
Serial # :

OTHER
Transducer : ER3
HL to SPL : Predicted
HA Style : ITC
Circuit Type : WDRC
RE to 2cc : Predicted

OTHER
Speech : Cox/Moore
Compr. Type : Linear
Input DR : Extended
Compr. Thresh : 40
Max. Out : Predicted

	.25	.50	.75	1.0	1.5	2.0	3.0	4.0	6.0
SSPL-90	92	102	102	102	104	108	110	108	106
Full-on Gain	15	22	23	24	29	35	38	37	40

Figure 12–13   Prescribed coupler gain versus gain obtained using actual hearing aid.

as loud, but not uncomfortable), the patient should participate in a procedure designed to verify these responses. Figure 12–14 provides the data that the authors use for these purposes. If the goal is to return a normal growth of loudness, one would want to compare the perception of the hearing aid user to the average perceptions of individuals with normal-hearing. The graphs in Figure 12–14 represent the mean loudness ratings for warble tones presented monaurally and continuous discourse (speech) presented monaurally and binaurally.

These data are in dB SPL and were obtained in the sound field. In the monaural condition the nontest ear must be occluded and/or masked. The patient's ratings are marked on each graph. The clinician may want to verify with all of the warble tones or may just assess speech. At a minimum, it is useful to verify the monaural and binaural conditions of speech. In a case where the REIG or family of REAR curves was not exactly on target and further manipulation was not possible, loudness perception verification may lead the clinician to accept the compromise in response or provide data that the compromise is unacceptable.

The graphic display can be very helpful when deciding what needs to be changed regarding the hearing aid's response. The separation of frequencies allows the clinician to identify if a change is needed in a low or high channel. The input levels at which targets are met will enable the clinician to identify if compression threshold and/or compression ratio needs to be adjusted. Remember that a change in gain without a change in limiting is a change in compression ratio. The data in Figure 12–14 were collected using 10 normally hearing adults listening in the test booth that is used for hearing aid verification. The authors advise that each test site collect these data in their own booths and with their own equipment because differences in results may occur.

This type of patient participation verification can be a powerful counseling tool for the first time user of WDRC technology. The clinician can be comfortable indicating that the goal of the fitting has been met (i.e., the patient perceives a range of input levels at appropriate levels). The patient may not immediately thank the clinician for returning the soft sound of his or her refrigerator that has not been heard for a decade, but these data may help encourage the individual to try the hearing aids.

FINAL COUPLER MEASUREMENTS AND RECORDING OF POTENTIOMETER SETTINGS

When the clinician is satisfied that the hearing aids are performing appropriately and any changes in response have been made (and verified), the set of coupler measurements reported previously should be repeated and the hearing aid settings should be recorded for purposes of documentation.

Some combination of the above-mentioned verification procedures are completed before instructing the patient about the hearing aids and allowing the patient to simply sit and listen and try the controls (e.g., VCW). If the hearing aids do not produce appropriate verification data, time is wasted if the patient has already been instructed and has provided feedback about the hearing aids. The clinician should make sure that the individual will be leaving with the hearing aids before investing time into instruction because this would have to be repeated if the hearing aids were returned and reordered.

ORIENTATION

Now that the hearing aids' responses have been modified if necessary and verified in some meaningful way (meeting fitting strategy generated targets, matching data from normal listeners, etc.), it is time to introduce the patient to the hearing aids. Palmer and Mormer (1997) provide a detailed process for hearing aid orientation. The details will not be repeated here, but the essential items will be outlined. See also Chapter 14 in this volume for an in-depth discussion of the hearing aid orientation. The patient must be comfortable with the hearing aids before leaving the session (removal, insertion,

volume control wheel, telecoil switch, on/off switch, battery). Being comfortable could mean knowing not to use the telecoil switch for normal listening until the 2-week follow-up if this is a new user and one more setting will be too much to handle in the first weeks. During the orientation time, play some continuous discourse (in quiet and noise at varying levels) for the patient in order to experience the hearing aid and to use the VCW if one was provided.

The authors do not seek to elicit a great deal of patient opinion at this time. The hearing aid's response rarely is modified at this time. This, of course, is a matter of opinion; the opinion being who is the expert at this moment in the fitting: the individual who has matched all the targets or the individual listening to all of this new sound? Palmer et al (1998) provide a review of data that may shed light on this question. New hearing aid users may not have heard a variety of sounds at different input levels in particular frequency regions for more than a decade, and previous users may be used to different signal processing (e.g., going from linear to WDRC). Trying to modify the hearing aid's response to the patient's wishes may result in a hearing aid that provides no gain for quiet sounds and no gain for any high frequencies (the authors have witnessed this). Patient-specific modifications (other than discomfort) are better left to the 2-week follow-up appointment, unless they are so important to the patient that he or she will not try the hearing aids. In these cases, the clinician may want to attempt to fine-tune the patient's hearing aid. This entails providing less gain initially (especially in the high frequencies) and then slowly adding the gain as the patient adjusts to the hearing aid. Oticon is an example of a manufacturer who builds this type of adaptation into their recommendations for initial and final hearing aid settings.

The *Hearing Aid Wearing Schedule* (Fig. 12–15) is reviewed with the patient. This type of schedule may not be appropriate for the experienced user. The patient is instructed to increase the hearing aid wearing time and increase up to more difficult listening experiences. Listening experience H and I (Fig. 12–15) are taken from the *Patient Expectation Worksheet* (Fig. 12–2) and will be different for every patient. This type of schedule provides the patient with needed instructions for using the new technology. The *Hearing Aid Commentary* (Fig. 12–16) is used to list the situations that the individual has identified as important (from the *Hearing Demand, Ability, and Need Profile* and the *Patient Expectation Worksheet*). With a conventional hearing aid, only one configuration may be available for the patient to judge. Some patients may want to compare their ability with one hearing aid versus two or with their hearing aids set to microphone versus coupled to an assistive device by means of the telecoil. The patient is meant to record thoughts regarding each listening category (filled in by the audiologist and patient during orientation) as a function of configuration (if appropriate). This form is used to stimulate discussion and lead to recommendations during the 2-week follow-up appointment.

Before leaving with the new hearing aids, the patient is scheduled for a 2-week follow-up visit. The patient is instructed to contact the clinic before this time if questions or concerns arise. Whenever possible, the patient should be contacted 1 to 2 days after fitting by telephone to inquire about success or difficulty.

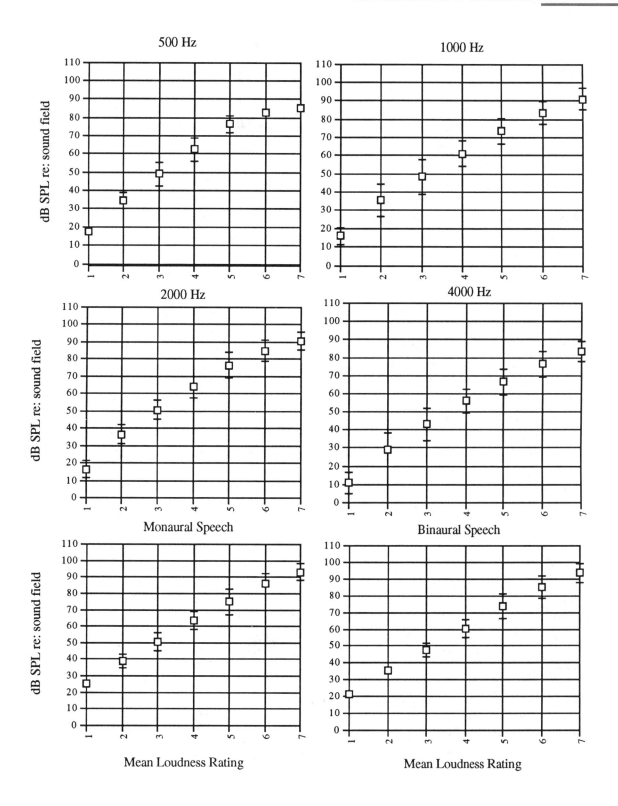

Figure 12–14 Loudness growth functions (500, 1000, 2000, 4000 Hz warble tones and monaural and binaural continuous discourse) from normal-hearing subjects for purposes of verification.

Hearing Aid Wearing Schedule

Days of Use	Maximum In	Minimum Out	Maximum In	Listening Category
Day 1	1 hour	1 hour	1 hour	
Day 2	2 hours	1 hour	2 hours	
Day 3	3 hours	1 hour	3 hours	
Day 4	4 hours	1 hour	4 hours	
Day 5	5 hours	1 hour	5 hours	
Day 6	6 hours	1 hour	6 hours	
Day 7	7 hours	1 hour	7 hours	
Day 8	8 hours	1 hour	8 hours	
Day 9	9 hours	1 hour	9 hours	

A. Inside your home, listening to quiet household sounds (e.g., water from faucet, toilet flushing, doorbell ringing, fan...).

B. Radio, television, quiet conversation with low background noise.

C. Quiet indoor work activities at home or office.

D. Quiet outdoor activities (e.g., gardening, walking, visiting in backyard).

E. Group conversation, dinner table discussion, entertaining visitors, driving car.

F. Theater, worship, classroom, other group listening.

G. Noisy work activities, back seat of car.

H. Other: _____.

I. Other: _____.

Figure 12–15   Hearing Aid Wearing Schedule.

CONTROVERSIAL POINT

The VIOLA and FIG6 will routinely require almost no gain in the low frequencies when hearing is close to normal in this range. The audiologist must consider whether this is appropriate given the amount of (or lack of) venting that will be provided with the particular ear mold or style of hearing aid and the balance between the amount of high-frequency and low-frequency gain.

FOLLOW-UP/EVALUATION OF BENEFIT

The checklist provided in Figure 12–17 guides the clinician through the follow-up appointment. Use of this type of form provides excellent documenation of what has been discussed and recommended with a patient. Action plans are made for any areas that are not satisfactory and these action plans will dictate when the patient needs to be seen next. If any hearing aid (or earmold) modifications are made as a result of the follow-up appointment, updated coupler data should be completed and maintained in the patient's records along with the final hearing aid settings.

Verification is different from evaluating the benefit of the hearing aids (validation). Just because all the targets are achieved does not necessarily result in a successful or satisfied patient. At present, the authors depend on post-test measures of the *Patient Expectation Worksheet* and *APHAB* to provide outcome measures. The *Patient Expectation Worksheet* (Fig. 12–2) has strong face validity for the patient who is filling out his or her perceived level of success. An audiologist can feel confident in the methods of hearing aid fitting when he or she can say that the patient's clearly defined expectations have been met.

The APHAB also is readministered to determine a benefit score. The software that provides the VIOLA has a computerized scoring verison of the APHAB, which makes it easy to score and plot results. The subsection results can be used to document the outcome of the hearing aid fitting. Perhaps more importantly, reactions to individual questions on the APHAB can guide the audiologist to further solutions that may be necessary for the hearing aid user.

Hearing Aid Commentary

Listening Category	Configuration 1	Configuration 2	Configuration 3	Configuration 4	Configuration 5

Figure 12–16 Hearing Aid Commentary.

Palmer and Mueller (1999) introduced the *Profile of Aided Loudness (PAL)* to be used as a validation tool for a hearing aid fitting, when the goal was to return normal loudness perception. The loudness restoration verification procedure (Fig. 12–14) may document that the hearing aid user perceives warble tones and continuous discourse in a sound booth similarly to individuals with normal-hearing. This does not necessarily translate into a restoration of loudness in the individual's listening environment. It also does not address the individual's reaction to loudness restoration. The PAL provides a list of sounds that have been judged as "very soft," "soft," "comfortable but slightly soft," "comfortable," "comfortable but slightly loud," "loud but OK," or "uncomfortably loud" by a large group of normally hearing individuals. The items included in the profile revealed good test/retest reliability and consistency in loudness rating across subjects (differing by gender and age). The audiologist has the hearing aid wearer rate the perceived loudness of each of the listed sounds and the satisfaction with the loudness of the sound. For instance, the refrigerator could be perceived as soft, but the individual could be unhappy with that perception. The results of the loudness rating are plotted against the perceptions of the normally hearing individuals. This allows the audiologist to judge whether the perception is in the appropriate range and indicates appropriate modifications (e.g., if everything is being perceived as too loud). The satisfaction results are used for counseling purposes. For instance, if the loudness perception for an item is in agreement with the normative data yet the individual is not satisfied, the normative data are useful in counseling the patient that most normal-hearing individuals perceive the sound the same way.

Choose validation procedures that relate directly to the original goals of the hearing aid fitting. For example, if the goals were related to individual expectations, a final evaluation of whether the expectations were met makes sense. However, if the goal is related to hearing in background noise, the background noise subscale of the APHAB may provide the most appropriate data. Finally, if the goal was to equalize loudness perception (i.e., all input signals should be perceived as comfortable), do not compare the hearing aid user to normally hearing individuals.

CONCLUSIONS

The individual with hearing loss enters into a process with the audiologist. The audiologist must present the hearing aid fitting as a process. The outcome does not focus on whether the individual will be a hearing aid wearer or not. The outcome focuses on what will be the right combination of technology and other interventions for the individual, and these solutions will be found through the hearing aid fitting process. The process continues as the individual's needs change, as the communication environment changes, and as technology changes.

Checklist for 1 to 2 Week Follow-Up Visit

ITEM	OUTCOME	ACTION PLAN	✓
Hearing Aid Commentary			
Hours Worn Per Day			
Able to Insert Aid			
Able to Remove Aid			
Cleaning & Maintenance			
Situations of Best Success			
Situations of Least Success			
Assistive Devices			
Aural Rehab Follow-Up			
Review Telephone Use			
Memory/Features Options			
Warranty Expiration			
Insurance Information			
Consent Form Signed			

✓ = Check off item if outcome is positive or when action plan is successfully completed.

_____   _____
Patient Signature   Date

_____   _____
Dispenser Signature   Date

Figure 12–17   Checklist for one to two week follow-up visit.

ACKNOWLEDGMENTS

Thanks to the people at Unitron, in particular Ted Venema and Carol Zaccatto, for their assistance with the figures related to their product. Thanks to Gus Mueller and Tom Powers of Siemens for their support (intellectual and financial) for a project that supplied the data in Figure 12–14. Thanks to Melissa Nascone and Tara Dudley for their work in producing the hearing aid fitting protocol as a manual and as Figure 12–18. Thanks to all of our students and the professionals in the Pittsburgh area who push us to systematically think about hearing aid evaluation, selection, fitting, and verification.

Appendix

Correction factors for microphone location used in FIG6. Data were obtained in a diffuse field and are courtesy of Killion (1988). Some additional sources for average-based values include Bentler and Pavlovic (1989), Hawkins and Mueller (1992), and Killion and Revit (1993).

TABLE 12A–1   Correction factors for microphone location

Frequency (Hz)	BTE	Avg ITE	Full ITC	Small ITC
250	0.4	0.5	0.5	0.5
500	1.0	1.3	1.5	1.2
1000	1.6	1.6	2.0	2.0
2000	2.8	2.7	3.4	3.8
3000*	2.9	3.7	4.9	6.3
4000	3.2	5.4	7.7	9.5

*Values actually obtained at 2918 Hz.

REFERENCES

AMERICAN NATIONAL STANDARDS INSTITUTE. (1987). *Specification of hearing aid characteristics* (ANSI S3.22-1987). New York: ANSI.

BENTLER, R.A. (1991). Programmable hearing aid review. *American Journal of Audiology, 2;*25–28.

BENTLER, R.A., & PAVLOVIC, C.V. (1989). Transfer functions and correction factors used in hearing aid evaluation and research. *Ear and Hearing, 10*(1);58–63.

BYRNE, D., & DILLON, H. (1986). The National Acoustics Laboratories' (NAL) new procedure for selecting the gain and frequency response of a hearing aid. *Ear and Hearing, 7;*257–265.

CORNELISSE, L.E., SEEWALD, R.C., & JAMIESON, D.G. (1994). Wide-dynamic-range-compression hearing aids: The DSL[i/o] approach. *Hearing Journal, 47*(10);23–29.

COX, R.M. (1995). Using loudness data for hearing aid selection: The IHAFF approach. *Hearing Journal, 48*(2);10,39–44.

COX, R.M. (1997). Adminstration and application of the APHAB. *Hearing Journal, 50*(4);32–48.

COX, R.M., & ALEXANDER, B. (1995). The abbreviated profile of hearing aid benefit. *Ear and Hearing, 16;*176–183.

DE JONGE, R. (1996). Microcomputer applications for hearing aid selection and fitting. *Trends in Amplification, 1*(3); 86–114.

DILLON, H., JAMES, A., & GINIS, J. (1997). Client oriented scale of improvement (COSI) and its relationship to several other measures of benefit and satisfaction provided by hearing aids. *Journal of the American Academy of Audiology, 8;*27–43.

FEIGIN, J.A., KOPUN, J.G., STELMACHOWICZ, P.G., & GORGA, M.P. (1989). Probe-tube microphone measures of earcanal sound pressure level in infants and children. *Ear and Hearing, 10*(4);254–258.

FIKRET-PASA, S., & REVIT, L.J. (1992). Individualized correction factors in the pre-selection of hearing aids. *Journal of Speech and Hearing Research, 35*(2);384–400.

GITLES, T., & NIQUETTE, P. (1995). FIG6 in ten. *Hearing Review, 2*(10);28–30.

HAWKINS, D.B., COOPER, W.A., & THOMPSON, D.J. (1990). Comparisons among SPLs in real-ears, 2-cc and 6 cm^3 couplers. *Journal of the American Academy of Audiology, 1;*154–161.

HAWKINS, D.B., & MUELLER, H.G. (1992). Test protocols for probe-microphone measurements. In: H.G. Mueller, D.B. Hawkins, & J.L. Northern (Eds.), *Probe microphone measurements* (pp. 269–278). San Diego: Singular Publishing Group.

HEALY, J. (1992). *Americans with Disabilities Act: An evolutionary force in your case management. The ABCs of the ADA Conference on the Americans with Disabilities, American Speech-Language-Hearing Association,* Washington, D.C. (May, 1992).

HUMES, L.E., PAVLOVIC, C., BRAY, V., & BARR, M. (1996). Real-ear measurement of hearing threshold and loudness. *Trends in Amplification, 1*(4);121–135.

KAMM, C., DIRKS, D., & MICKEY, M. (1977). Effect of sensorineural hearing loss on loudness discomfort level and most comfortable listening judgments. *Journal of Speech and Hearing Research, 21;*668–681.

KILLION, M.C. (1988). Personal communication re: FIG6 average correction values.

KILLION, M.C., & FIKRET-PASA, S. (1993). The 3 types of sensorineural hearing loss: Loudness and intelligibility considerations. *Hearing Journal, 46*(11);31–34.

KILLION, M.C., & REVIT, L.J. (1993). CORFIG and GIFROC: Real-ear to coupler and back. In: G.A. Studebaker, & I. Hochberg (Eds.), *Acoustical factors affecting hearing aid performance* (pp. 65–85). Boston: Allyn & Bacon.

LEWIS, D., & STELMACHOWICZ, P. (1993). Real-ear to 6 cm^3 coupler differences in young children. *Journal of Speech and Hearing Research, 36;*204–209.

LIBBY, E. (1985). The LDL to SSPL90 conversion dilemma. *Hearing Instruments, 36*(8);15–16.

LINDLEY, G.A., & PALMER, C.V. (1997). Fitting wide dynamic range compression hearing aids: DSL[i/o], the IHAFF protocol, and FIG6. *American Journal of Audiology, 6*(3);19–28.

LYREGAARD, P.E. (1988). POGO and the theory behind. In: J. Jensen (Ed.), *Hearing aid fitting: Theoretical and practical views* (pp. 81–94). Proceedings of the 13th Danavox Symposium, Copenhagen.

MARTIN, R. (1998). Introducing a new tool for ordering hearing aids. *Hearing Journal, 51*(2);66–68.

MUELLER, H.G., & BENTLER, R. (1994). Measurements of TD: How loud is allowed? *Hearing Journal, 47*(1);10, 42–44.

PALMER, C. (1992). Assistive devices in the audiology practice. *American Journal of Audiology, 2*(37);37–57.

PALMER, C. (1998). Curriculum for graduate courses in amplification. *Trends in Amplification, 3*(1);6–44.

PALMER, C., & LINDLEY, G. (1998). Reliability of the contour test in a population of adults with hearing loss. *Journal of the American Academy of Audiology, 9;*209–215.

PALMER, C., & MORMER, E. (1997). A systematic program for hearing aid orientation and adjustment. *Hearing Review Supplement, 1;*45–52.

PALMER, C., & MUELLER, H.G. (1999). Profile of aided loudness: A validation prodedure. *The Hearing Journal, 52*(6);34–41.

PALMER, C., NELSON, C., & LINDLEY, G. (1998). The functionally and physiologically plastic adult auditory system. *Journal of the Acoustical Society of America, 103*(4); 1705–1721.

PALMER, C., WILBER, L., KILLION, M., & CANTER, J. (1991). Influence of external ear characteristics on intelligibility and quality judgments. *American Speech-Language-Hearing Association Convention.* Atlanta, GA. (November, 1991). (Abstract) *ASHA, 33*(10),187,1991.

PASCOE, D. (1989). Clinical measurements of the auditory dynamic range and their relation to formulas for hearing aid gain. In: J.H. Jensen (Ed.), *Hearing aid fitting: Theoretical and practical views* (pp. 129–152). Proceedings of the 13th Danavox Symposium, Copenhagen.

PAUL, R., & COX, R. (1995). Measuring hearing aid benefit with the APHAB: Is this as good as it gets? *American Journal of Audiology, 4*(3);10–13.

RICKETTS, T., & BENTLER, R. (1996). The effect of test signal type and bandwidth on the categorical scaling of loudness. *Journal of the Acoustical Society of America, 99;*2281–2287.

TURNER, C., KWON, B., TANAKA, C., & KNAPP, J. (1997). Further studies in high-frequency amplification. *Second Biennial Hearing Aid Research and Development Conference sponsored by the National Institute on Deafness and Other Communication Disorders and the Department of Veterans Affairs.* Bethesda, MD. (September, 1997).

VALENTE, M., FABRY, D., & POTTS, L. (1995). Recognition of speech in noise with hearing aids using dual microphones. *Journal of the American Academy of Audiology, 6*;440–449.

VALENTE, M., POTTS, L., & VALENTE, M. (1997). Differences and intersubject variability of loudness discomfort levels measured in sound pressure level and hearing level for TDH-50P and ER-3A earphones. *Journal of the American Academy of Audiology, 8*;59–67.

VALENTE, M., VALENTE, M., & GOEBEL, J. (1991). Reliability and intersubject variability of the real-ear unaided response. *Ear and Hearing, 12*(3); 216–220.

VALENTE, M., & VANVLIET, D. (1997). The Independent Hearing Aid Fitting Forum (IHAFF) Protocol. *Trends in Amplification, 2*(1);6–35.

PREFERRED PRACTICE GUIDELINES

Listed below is, in the opinion of the authors, the preferred practice guideline for the selection and fitting of conventional hearing aids:

Professionals who perform the procedure(s)

▼ Audiologists

Expected Outcomes

▼ The hearing aids are physically comfortable in the user's ears.

▼ The hearing aid fitting with wide dynamic range circuitry provides appropriate amplification so that soft input levels are judged as soft, moderate input levels are judged as comfortable, and loud input levels are judged as loud. The hearing aid fitting with linear circuitry provides amplification so that moderate input levels are comfortable and loud input levels are not uncomfortable.

▼ The hearing aids are limited in such a way that the hearing aid user does not judge a 90 dB SPL signal as uncomfortably loud and/or report excessive distortion with a loud input.

▼ The hearing aid user or a caregiver is able to insert, use, remove, and care for the hearing aids.

▼ The individual's communication needs are surveyed and solutions for identified problems related to hearing are offered.

▼ Use of the hearing aids improves the individual's quality of life.

▼ The audiologist is perceived as a hearing health provider who can be contacted in the future to discuss and provide further hearing-related solutions (e.g., alerting devices, personal listening devices, group listening devices).

▼ The patient or caregiver is knowledgable regarding their rights under the law to access employment, public accomodations, transportation, education, and public activities.

Clinical Indications

▼ Hearing aid fitting is conducted for individuals of all ages who have been identified through an audiologic assessment as having a nonmedically treatable hearing loss. In addition, individuals not wishing to pursue medical treatment for a medically treatable hearing loss may pursue amplification.

Clinical Process

▼ See Figure 12–18 for a schematic of the clinical process.

▼ Basic audiological evaluation

▼ Individual and environmental evaluation

▼ Up-front decisions related to hearing aid features

▼ Earmold impression (for earmold of BTE or shell)

▼ Dynamic range assessment and assessment of acoustic properties of the ear (RECD, REDD, REUR depending on the fitting rationale and population)

▼ Selection and use of a fitting formula on the basis of patient data and fitting goals

▼ Identify commercially available hearing aids through use of specifications and order the hearing aids on the basis of target data generated by the fitting formula

▼ Hearing aid adjustment and test box validation according to selection data

▼ Patient verification (includes patient perception of a variety of input levels and real-ear measures) dependent on the fitting protocol used

▼ Electroacoustic measures to document final response after patient verification

▼ Systematic hearing aid orientation and suggested wearing schedule

▼ Follow-up including review of hearing aid commentary, checklist of hearing aid functions, postexpectation results, posthearing aid benefit inventory results

▼ Modifications based on follow-up

▼ Ongoing communication with the hearing aid user (and/or family) through office newsletters, reminder appointments for hearing aid checks, battery program, etc.

Documentation

▼ Documentation includes all survey/inventory results (history, *Hearing Demand, Ability, and Needs Profile, Patient Expectation Worksheet, Hearing Aid Benefit Inventory*).

▼ Documentation includes all assessment results whether audiometric (e.g., thresholds, dynamic range, LDLs) or real-ear (e.g., RECD, REDD, REUR).

▼ Documentation includes all information related to the ordering and receiving of the earmold and hearing aid (e.g., coupler targets, order form, invoice, hearing aid coupler data from the manufacturer).

▼ Documentation includes all presetting and verification data whether generated from the coupler, the individual's real ear, behavioral evaluation, and/or the individual's auditory perceptions (e.g., loudness rating, sound quality judgments).

▼ Documentation includes a record of compliance with state and federal guidelines/laws/regulations for hearing aids.

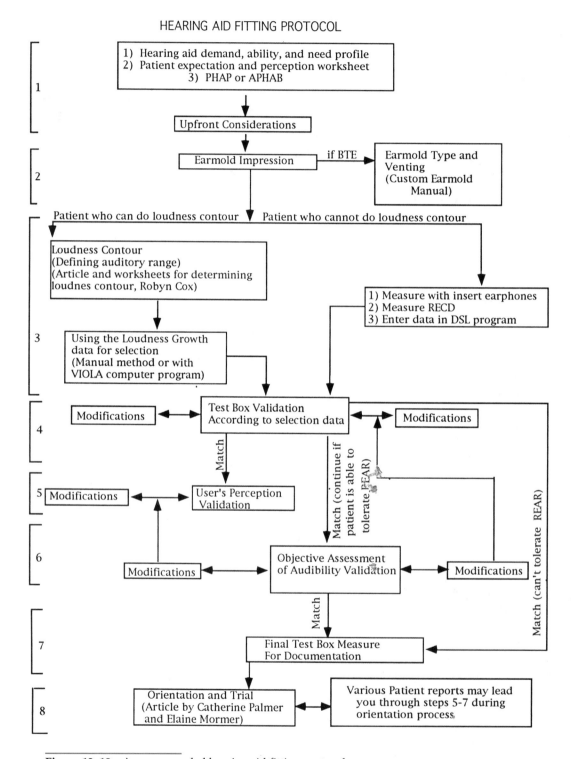

Figure 12–18   A recommended hearing aid fitting protocol.

Chapter 13

Selection and Fitting of Programmable and Digital Hearing Aids

Robert W. Sweetow

The increased flexibility granted to the hearing health professional and the user of programmable and digital instruments provides a broader, and sometimes different, array of fitting strategies. Some of these methods are based on existing procedures used for conventional analog devices (see Chapters 4, 5, and 12). Other fitting and selection procedures can be approached in a more novel manner. Each listener with impaired hearing presents his or her own unique set of acoustic needs. Clinical determination regarding which adjustable parameters are applicable to a specific patient must be assessed on an individual basis. Because it would be extremely difficult to offer all the potentially useful features in one system, the array of individual demands underscores the need for the availability of several programmable and digital systems from which the appropriate selection can be made.

It is not the intent of this chapter to find a "winner" among commercially available hearing aid systems. Indeed, during the time it took to complete this chapter, several newer programmable and digital systems have been introduced. It is with certainty that additional systems will be available before this textbook is published. In fact, any attempt to select a "winner" among programmable or digital hearing aids is unnecessary because one of the great advantages of these devices is their diversity. Therefore philosophies, strategies, and techniques discussed in this chapter will focus on the features and fitting strategies of programmable and digital systems that make them unique, rather than on specific makes and models of the hearing instruments. Before proposing strategies for selection and fitting of digital and programmable hearing aids, a brief explanation of why such systems are needed will help lay the foundation for much of the strategic rationale.

THE NEED FOR PROGRAMMABLE AND DIGITAL HEARING AIDS

In the same manner that computers have become an integral part of our society, programmable and digital hearing aids are now poised to dominate the future of wearable amplification. At the time this chapter was prepared, more than 60 programmable and 8 digital hearing aid models were available (Strom, 1998). However, through 1997 digital and programmable hearing aids accounted for less than 20% of the overall sales of wearable amplification. This is a somewhat surprising statistic considering that only 53% of conventional hearing aid users report overall satisfaction with amplification, whereas as many as 90% are satisfied with certain advanced technologies that will be discussed shortly (Kochkin, 1996). These data underscore the reality that either technology or fitting strategies need to improve. The most commonly reported complaints from hearing aid users continue to be that hearing instruments do not yield adequate recognition of speech in noisy environments, work only in limited situations, introduce feedback, or have poor sound quality. When one analyzes the complexity of the elements comprising hearing impairment, it is not surprising that conventional hearing aids have not been able to satisfy the needs of the user. Table 13–1 lists some of the characteristics of hearing loss.

The progression from conventional analog instruments to digitally programmable hybrid devices and then to the newest digital hearing aids has been dictated by the needs of listeners with impaired hearing as much as by the availability of new technology. *Conventional hearing aids* can be defined as analog instruments that amplify, filter, and limit output with a fixed set of parameters manipulated by means of on-instrument potentiometers, switches, or rotary controls. Many of these

433

TABLE 13–1   Characteristics of hearing loss

- Reduced sensitivity
- Altered loudness perception
- Increased susceptibility to noise interference
- Impaired frequency discrimination
- Altered intensity resolution
- Reduced temporal integration
- Altered pitch perception
- Impaired localization

devices have rather active filters and some increase their flexibility by means of a switch or potentiometer that allows for a certain amount of decrease/increase in either the high-frequency or low-frequency gain. This, in essence, allows the hearing aids to function as dual-response devices. However, it is important to recognize that it does not allow the degree of flexibility in establishing the parameters of the responses or "programs" that true programmable, multiple program devices have. For patients who experience fluctuations in their hearing or, more commonly, need to hear in a wide variety of acoustic environments, single response (memory) conventional instruments have limitations (Libby & Sweetow, 1987). Thus manufacturers began introducing a family of Automatic Signal Processing (ASP) devices that automatically alter their electroacoustic characteristics, depending on the spectrum and amplitude of the incoming signal. The benefit of such instruments is based on the assumption that most, although not all, background noises are comprised of predominantly low-frequency energy. In other words, ASP hearing aids automatically reduce low-frequency gain when the low-frequency input reaches a certain level. An example of an automatic low-frequency reduction response is shown in Figure 13–1. Note that the solid curve represents the frequency response when the input is relatively low, but as the input increases and exceeds a predetermined level, the low-frequency gain decreases (as depicted by the dotted line frequency response). This type of signal processing is sometimes referred to as "automatic noise reduction," but because *both* the signal and

the noise are reduced by the same amount, the input signal-to-noise ratio (SNR) is preserved at the output. In many instances the "perceptual" SNR is enhanced, however, because the low frequencies of the noise may be annoying, whereas the low frequencies of the speech signal carry minimal weight in terms of intelligibility (French & Steinberg, 1947). Reports in the literature are conflicting regarding the value of ASP aids, but the abundance of studies suggests that they do not usually result in significant improvement in speech recognition compared with conventional linear hearing, unless (a) the conventionals provide an inappropriate frequency response or excessive maximum output for the subject's needs; or (b) the background noise is limited to the low frequencies (Tyler & Kuk, 1989; Van Tasell et al, 1988). Unfortunately, in the real world, noise is not conveniently limited only to the low frequencies. So, although ASP circuitry might reduce annoying background sounds, it may do little in enhancing intelligibility.

In addition, many conventional devices have single-band compression circuitry designed to minimize discomfort and reduce distortion. This means that once a predetermined input (or output level) is reached, gain will be reduced across all amplified frequencies. Conventional hearing instruments thus can be relatively successful in compensating for reduced sensitivity, somewhat less successful in addressing altered loudness perception, and even less successful in solving the problem of noise interference. Virtually no attempts are made with conventional hearing aids to restore normal function for the remaining abnormalities cited in Table 13–1.

As evidenced by the lack of satisfaction among wearers, listeners with impaired hearing require more flexibility, finer tuning, and greater processing power than can be provided by conventional analog instruments. Furthermore, considering the popularity of digital recording technology, as exemplified by compact discs, it is no surprise that a serious effort was made to produce digital hearing aids. Unfortunately, engineers found that the battery consumption required to power digital hearing aids exceeded that provided by the 1.3 to 1.5 volt batteries used in conventional instruments by anywhere from 10 to 100%. As a result, the size of digital aids would have had to be cumbersome and unlikely to be accepted by our cosmetically conscious society. One company did introduce a "body-borne" style digital hearing aid, but it never reached the necessary acceptance level and lasted for about a year in the marketplace.

In the late 1980s, technology produced a compromise, however, with the introduction of *digitally programmable hearing aids*. With these instruments, signals remain processed by analog components as in the case with conventional amplification. This type of amplification is considered hybrid (combination analog and digital) because digital technology is used to *program* the hearing aids. In addition to enhancing precision and quality control, hybrid hearing aids allow for an increase in the electroacoustic flexibility of the aids, both for the audiologist and user.

The advantages of digitally programmable instruments include ease of adjustment, multiple programs, advanced compression parameter control, multiple band (multichannel) compression, and long-term flexibility. Each of these features will be discussed in detail with regard to programming strategy later in the chapter.

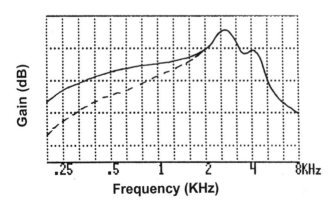

Figure 13–1 Frequency responses from a hearing aid having automatic signal processing. Solid curve is for a 60 dB SPL input; dashed curve is for a 75 dB SPL input.

Digitally programmable instruments provide benefits that further address loss of sensitivity and altered loudness perception. They are still somewhat limited, however, because even though they are programmed by a computer (the digital portion), they still operate in an analog fashion. This means that signals entering the hearing aid microphone are amplified and filtered by a variety of electronic components. Because hearing is such a complex sense, the extent of filtering and amplifying required to partially correct a hearing impairment adds to the limitations of the hearing instrument by producing distortion and noise. Thus additional and alternate processing strategies and power are needed to resolve the remaining factors listed in Table 13–1.

In 1997, the first ear-level *digital hearing instruments* became commercially available. As of 1998, there were at least eight models on the market. By 2000, it is expected that there will be more than 20 models.

SPECIAL CONSIDERATION

In addition to the potential for superiority that exists from advanced technology, the movement toward modern digital technology is important because it may help alter the common public perception of hearing aids as being overpriced, antiquated, and less than useful in many acoustic environments.

CHARACTERISTICS OF PROGRAMMABLE HEARING AIDS

As mentioned earlier, programmable hearing aids incorporate many characteristics and features not found in conventional devices. Some of the most useful include the following.

Programmability and Ease of Adjustment

If the listener's hearing, communicative environments, or auditory needs change, these hearing aids can be reprogrammed. Programming is accomplished either by a dedicated programmer (used only for that particular manufacturer's hearing products) or by a personal computer. Software and cabling for coupling to the hearing aids are supplied by the manufacturer. Many programmable hearing aids now use a "universal" software (NOAH) and hardware interface (HI-PRO) that will be discussed in detail later in this chapter.

Multiple Programs

Some programmable hearing aids offer multiple programs so that at the touch of a button on the hearing aids or a remote control, the electroacoustic characteristics can be instantaneously changed to (hopefully) allow for improved performance in a particular acoustic environment. Among current models, the number of programs available in a specific instrument ranges from two to eight. Frequency responses of a multiple program aid offering four responses are depicted in Figure 13–2. It can be noted in this figure, for example, that programs A through C differ mainly in their low-frequency

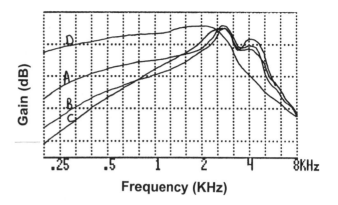

Figure 13–2 Frequency responses from a hearing aid with four programs. Curves *A* to *C* are for progressively noisier acoustical environments and curve *D* is designed for telephone use.

gain, with presumably response A best for quiet environments, programs B and C for environments with high background noise levels, and program D for telephone listening (when a t-coil is not a viable alternative).

The usefulness of multiple programs is not limited to providing choices to the user in a variety of acoustic environments. Some audiologists also use it as a means of gradually introducing variations in the amplified sound to the new user. For example, some patients with high-frequency loss initially find that a sharply rising high-frequency response sounds too tinny. The listener might prefer a program that incorporates a flatter and broader frequency response that more closely resembles what the patient has been accustomed to hearing (as in program A). As the wearer becomes more acclimated to amplification, he or she may then switch to a different program (such as program B or C) that has been programmed to filter out the low frequencies and provide a high-frequency emphasis that is believed to be more appropriate for his or her hearing loss. Additional programs may be programmed to provide similar frequency responses but different compression characteristics.

Advanced Control of Compression Characteristics

It is essential to prevent the amplified signal from reaching the loudness discomfort level of the wearer. One method of limiting the output is with peak clipping (linear amplification). Linear amplification provides for constant gain, regardless of input level, until the output (gain plus input level) reaches a certain, predetermined ceiling level. At this level, further increases in input no longer produce any increase in output. Unfortunately, once the aid reached this saturation point, the energy must be redistributed into other frequency regions, thus producing distortion. An alternative output-limiting approach that is useful in minimizing distortion is compression (sometimes referred to as automatic gain control or AGC). In compression circuits, gain is automatically reduced once a predetermined level (on the basis of either the input or the output level) is reached, so that hearing aids never enter into saturation. Compression is described in detail in Chapters 1, 4, 5, 6, and 12. Although this is an improvement over peak clipping in terms of minimizing amplitude distortion such as harmonic and intermodulation, an inevitable degree of temporal distortion is introduced during the activation and release of the compression function that may be disadvantageous for listeners with severe and profound hearing loss (Boothroyd et al, 1988).

Two-stage (input/output) compressors, wide dynamic range compression (WDRC), curvilinear compression, and the ability to program compression threshold and kneepoint are found in various programmable systems. In addition, many incorporate variable or adjustable attack or release times. Digitally programmable hearing aids can be adjusted to specify the parameters of these advanced compression and automatic signal processing functions. If the desired electroacoustic parameters have been appropriately defined by the proper clinical test battery and if the programming is completed properly, the need for frequent volume control manipulations is greatly minimized (or even eliminated).

A potential shortcoming of traditional compression circuits is that they are single band. Thus as stated earlier, the activating input triggers a gain reduction across the entire frequency range, often reducing the gain of the high frequencies to the extent that the important consonant sounds are no longer in the audible range of the listener (Barfod, 1976; Moore, 1990; Villchur, 1973).

Multiband (Multichannel) Compression

Attempts have been successful at increasing high-frequency amplification for soft inputs (Killion, 1990) but are still limited by the single channel design. To resolve this shortcoming some manufacturers introduced hearing aids that contain multiple compression circuits acting independently for two or more frequency bands.

Two major benefits to multiband compression exist. First, because the pattern of recruitment for any given individual cannot be predicted on the basis of a pure tone audiogram, it is beneficial to have adjustable characteristics for various parameters such as *compression kneepoint* (activation level), *compression ratio* (the extent to which the gain is reduced), and *release time* (how quickly the hearing aids return to linear amplification once the activating signal ceases). In this way, frequency regions with recruitment (i.e., usually the high frequencies) can use compression circuitry, whereas other frequency regions showing less recruitment (i.e., usually the low frequencies) can be amplified in a linear manner or use less aggressive methods of compression.

The second, and perhaps main, advantage of multiband compression is that an invasive noise that may be restricted to certain frequencies (i.e., the low frequencies) produces a decrease in gain only for those frequencies, without affecting the remaining regions (i.e., the high frequencies). Thus the weaker high-frequency consonants could still remain audible. Figure 13–3 depicts frequency responses for single, dual, and three band instruments. Notice that the gain decreases across the entire frequency range for the single band instrument even though the input signal is a narrow band signal centered around 500 Hz. With the two band instrument, only the lower half of the frequency response is affected, and with the three channel instrument only the frequencies located in the lowest band are affected.

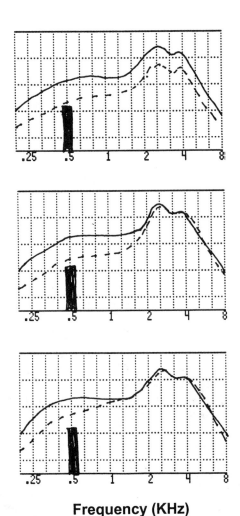

Frequency (KHz)

Figure 13–3 Frequency responses from hearing aids containing single band (*top*), dual band (*middle*), and three band (*bottom*) compression. In each case a narrow band noise centered around 500 Hz activated the compression function. Solid line is the original frequency gain response. Dashed lines represent the change in the response following stimulation with the 500 Hz signal.

In addition to the obvious advantage of preselecting a different amount of gain for various frequency regions, hearing aids having multiple channels of compression also can adaptively adjust the amount of gain in specific frequency regions as a function of the input signal. For example, low-frequency gain can decrease simultaneously with an increase in high-frequency gain. This is the concept embodied by WRDC in which very low input signals (i.e., 40- to 50-dB SPL) may be amplified linearly, but high input sounds receive little or no electronic processing. With this design, the hearing aid operates in a nonlinear fashion throughout the entire dynamic range of the listener. This electroacoustic feature often helps audibility, although not necessarily word recognition in noise because the spectral distribution of environmental noises are broadband. Moore (1990), however, notes that the acoustically impaired ear has about 10 critical bands that process information (the normal ear has 35). He theorizes that unless the hearing aid has more than 10 bands, it will do little to reduce the masking effects of background noise. He asserts that adaptive filtering may be as effective in noise reduction as multiband AGC. Despite Moore's theoretical construct, there continue to be a large number of multiband hearing aid users who report enhanced listening comfort in noise. Such improvement is often not achieved with single band instruments.

Despite patient reports of the superiority of these multiband compression systems, improvement is not always demonstrated in the laboratory, office, or clinic. Barfod (1976) and Lippman et al (1981) contend that multiband compression is not superior to linear amplification, providing proper frequency shaping has been achieved with linear signal processing. However, Villchur (1978) disagrees and believes the research studies supporting these conclusions are flawed. He contends that realistic evaluation of multiband compression must take into account the following factors: (a) Speech test materials do not reflect the true dynamic range of speech in "real life." The speech test materials have more restricted dynamic range than does "real-life" speech, thus there are limited intersyllabic and word-to-word amplitude changes; (b) when compared with linear hearing aid systems, the linear reference must use frequency shaping that is realistic and remains within the sound comfort level of the patient; and (c) multiband compression should be restricted only to those patients who demonstrate reduced dynamic range. These issues may account for the lack of "objectively measured" superiority in light of the reported "subjective" superiority. A study by Sousa and Turner (1998) suggested that the greatest benefit of having more than one band of compression is the ability to achieve audibility of soft sounds without overamplifying loud sounds. This audibility may not be as attainable with either linear or single channel compression. The benefit of the use of multiband compression, coupled with the low compression kneepoints needed to achieve audibility without producing overamplification of intense inputs was shown by Valente et al (1997) in their comparison of two different dual band instruments versus single channel linear hearing aids. In this study, superiority was demonstrated for both objective and subjective data.

Many multiband instruments allow the dispenser to alter the bandwidth and location of the crossover frequency according to the specific needs of the individual wearer. In other words the dispenser may decide to divide the bands in a dual band system at a crossover frequency of 1000 Hz if, for example, the patient had a flat audiometric configuration with a hearing loss of 20 dB at 1000 Hz and below but then decreased to a flat configuration with a hearing loss of 60 dB at 1500 Hz and above. Then kneepoint and ratio could be set for the near-normal-hearing loss at 1000 Hz and below and separately for the 60 dB hearing loss at 1500 Hz and above. Unfortunately, the audiometric configuration does not always provide such a clean and easy decision. In these more difficult (and often typical) cases crossover frequency, kneepoint, and ratio are determined by the results of the clinical test battery and patient preferences. Adjustment of the crossover frequency can help not only in frequency shaping for various input levels but also for enhanced loudness restoration.

Long-Term Flexibility

Conventional analog hearing aids have an average life expectancy of 3 to 5 years. It remains to be seen whether the life expectancy of programmable aids will be the same or longer because many of the components (i.e., microphones and receivers) are used in both. It is likely, however, that if a patient's hearing fluctuates significantly, even a well-functioning nonprogrammable aid will have to be replaced to maintain pace with changes in the patient's hearing level. Consider, for example, patients with Meniere's syndrome, hormonal fluctuation, or progressive loss caused by ototoxicity. Often the extent of necessary electroacoustic changes exceeds that obtainable even with conventional analog aids having active filtering potentiometers. Programmable and digital aids can more readily meet the changing amplification needs of these patients.

Not only can the dispenser produce great changes by reprogramming the instrument but the use of hearing aids having multiple programs can also assist the patient *and* the dispenser by allowing for programming of *anticipated* changes without necessitating frequent return visits for reprogramming procedures.

An additional advantage of programmable aids for fluctuating hearing can be shown for patients reporting sudden hearing loss. For these patients dramatic changes in sensitivity and audiometric configuration often occur within the first few months after onset. It is not clinically practical to change to other hearing aids while waiting for the hearing level to stabilize.

A tier system can be constructed to illustrate a (debatable) hierarchy of programmable and digital features. Although the precise structure of a pyramid, such as the one depicted in Figure 13–4, is arguable, it is likely that at the base would be found devices that, although programmed on either a dedicated or personal computer, function primarily as an electronic screwdriver with flexibility only for frequency shaping and output limiting. Progressing up the pyramid are hearing aids containing adjustable kneepoints or compression ratios. Still further up are hearing aids containing multiple programs or multiple channels. In addition, hearing aids containing multiple or directional microphones, albeit not a parameter necessarily requiring programmability, would contribute to an elevated placement on the pyramid.

CHARACTERISTICS OF DIGITAL HEARING AIDS

Digitization means that incoming analog signals received by the microphone are sent through a preamplifier to an analog to digital (A/D) converter where the signals are converted to a series of binary digits (0's and 1's). These numbers are then manipulated by the digital signal processing (DSP) unit according to a set of instructions (algorithms) that are either preset or programmed by the fitter. A new set of binary digits is formed, which then is reconverted from digital to analog (D/A) as it exits the receiver and enters the earcanal.

In addition to all the features already cited for digitally programmable hearing aids, digital hearing aids have characteristics that cannot be attained with conventional or digitally programmable analog systems. Among the more prominent are the following.

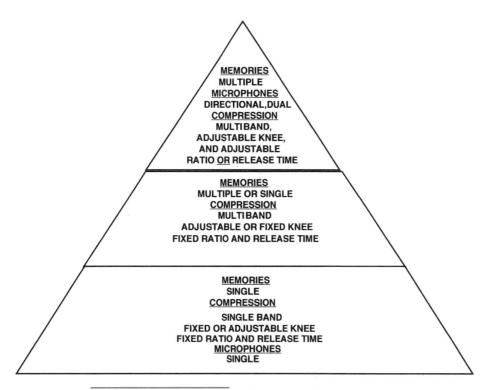

Figure 13–4   An example of a "hierarchy of programmable hearing aids."

Fine-Tuning of Frequency Response

Frequency shaping among relatively independent bands is superb in digital hearing aids because no limitations are based on filter skirts or cascading. Limitations remain, however, because of the use of analog microphones and receivers. Even so, the ability to match targets for highly unusual audiometric configurations is enhanced by the presence of multiple frequency-shaping bands. At the time of this writing digital devices are available that have as many as seven relatively independent frequency bands (but only two compression bands), and one is due out soon that promises 16 bands of compression. An example of the ability for a hearing aid like this to match a target for even highly unusual audiometric configurations is shown in Figure 13–5.

Active Feedback Control

Digital processing allows for determination of the maximum allowable gain before producing feedback. Also, digital technology can minimize feedback by introducing digitally induced phase reversal of the oscillating signal.

Multiple Microphones and Beamforming

Hearing aids having multiple microphones can amplify signals originating from in front of the listener while partially suppressing amplification of sounds originating from the sides and behind the wearer. This concept of amplifying primarily from a selected "beam" of space represents perhaps

the greatest potential for true signal to noise enhancement. Although the use of directional or multiple microphones do not require digital processing, the ability to maintain phase relationships and stable acoustic and electrical delays make digitization a logical associate to this exciting technology.

Noise Reduction Strategies

Noise reduction strategies can go beyond simple gain reduction determined as a function of the intensity level of the input signal. Some digital systems expand the use of spectral and amplitude detection to include temporal analysis in their speech/noise detection algorithms.

PEARL

In reality, analog hearing aids can do all the things a digital system can do, however, it would require excessive size, power consumption, or both. Moreover, increasing the processing functions of an analog system will decrease the SNR of the instrument. This decrease can be largely avoided with digital technology. Therefore digital is clearly the technology of the future where advanced processing is concerned.

Recall earlier that a hierarchy of programmable instruments was discussed. Differentiation among digital hearing aids can similarly be done on the basis of characteristics.

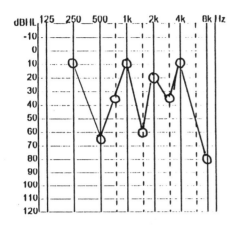

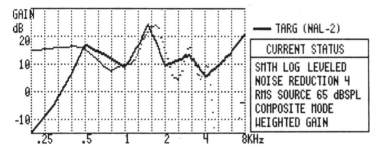

Figure 13–5 Target match (*bottom*) obtained from a digital hearing aid with seven bands of frequency shaping for the hypothetical audiogram (*top*) shown.

However, because all the digital systems currently available contain multiple bands, adjustable compression ratios, highly flexible frequency shaping, and in some cases, adjustable kneepoints, the differentiation among digital systems is based on differences in either (1) the algorithm, and/or (2) the hardware features.

Algorithms for currently available digital hearing aids include variations in release times for various bands, speech versus noise differentiation based on the modulation pattern of the incoming signal in a number of bands, and/or a host of others yet to be introduced. For example, two of the 1998 vintage digital hearing aids divide the incoming signal into either three or four frequency bands, analyze the amplitude, spectral, *and* temporal modulation pattern in each of the bands; use a statistical analysis to interpret whether the input in each of the bands is dominated by speech (a slower modulation pattern than noise) or noise; and then increase or reduce the gain in each band accordingly.

Furthermore, the digital hearing device can either incorporate a closed platform or an open platform. *Closed algorithm platforms* have an inherent processing rule set that cannot be changed by the dispenser or wearer; performance parameters can be adjusted but are limited to the engineered performance of the digital chip. *Open algorithm platforms* allow a variety of algorithms to be loaded into a single instrument. This would seem like a great advantage; however, it should be recognized that open platforms cannot accommodate improvements requiring hardware changes (such as dual microphones and better receivers). Also, as more powerful processing schemes are developed, digital signal processor chips may need to be upgraded (just like a 286 computer cannot adequately handle Windows 95). No clear consensus exists as to what is the superior algorithm for a given

individual. It is possible that numerous algorithms are needed to fulfill the requirements of a very heterogeneous hearing-impaired population. In defense of open platforms, however, it is reasonable to assume that giving the user the ability to choose among several algorithms may prove to be informative not only to the user but to the fitter as well.

SPECIAL CONSIDERATION

The benefit of a digital hearing instrument is a function of the algorithm.

Among the hardware considerations are the presence of directional or multiple microphones, the sensitivity of the telecoil, and the presence or absence of a remote control versus an "on-instrument" control versus a fully automatic function. As stated earlier, although the presence of these hardware features is not restricted to digital products, the combination of flexible programming and advanced algorithms may certainly be synergistic with microphone technology.

CANDIDACY FOR PROGRAMMABLE AND DIGITAL HEARING AIDS

Because of the flexible nature of programmable and digital hearing aids, an appropriate system will probably provide a suitable fit for nearly every mild to severely hearing-impaired patient. However, this statement does not imply that all hearing aid candidates require a digitally programmable system.

Because there may be considerable expense in terms of monetary cost to the patient, as well as time spent by the dispenser, one must determine whether a given patient needs a programmable or digital instrument.

CONTROVERSIAL POINT

Unless the hearing health professional can present supporting clinical data that the most suitable instrument for the patient is a programmable or digital device, there may be little justification for its selection. If goals can be reached with conventional analog aids, it may be the simplest and most economical path.

SELECTION OF A SPECIFIC DEVICE

The fact that many digital and programmable hearing aids are available affords the dispenser with a wide choice of features from which to choose. The first step in selecting a particular device is to establish which programmable features are applicable for a specific patient. These features must be assessed on an individual basis and cannot be assumed entirely on the basis of hearing impairment "classification" only. Each hearing deficit will likely require its own fitting algorithm. Hecox (1988) points out that no single signal processing approach will work for most patients. Thus *versatility* is the key word. Effectively using the versatility inherent in programmable and digital hearing aids depends on the dispenser's knowledge of the interaction between the hearing aid's available features and the accurate measurement of the perceptual and psychoacoustic needs of the patient. Significant improvement is needed in the clinical evaluation of perceptual and psychoacoustic deficits, as well as the strengths of listeners with impaired hearing, to improve algorithms.

The needs assessment of an individual with impaired hearing must encompass both *subjective* (obtained by the case history and questionnaires or surveys) and *objective* (obtained by the clinical testing) data collection. The following questions are some of the more important to consider.

How often is the patient exposed to noisy environments and how do these environmental noises affect the patient's performance?

The patient who rarely is subjected to environmental noise may not require an amplification system with multiple programs, multiple microphones, or algorithms designed to identify and reduce noise. For this patient, it may be more important to concentrate on other features, such as additional flexibility in frequency shaping provided by multiple bands, or increased sensitivity of the telecoil and so forth. Patients not adversely affected by noise may prefer the sound quality of wide-band systems appropriate for their type and magnitude of hearing loss. It may not be necessary to markedly reduce low-frequency amplification if a patient with a relatively flat audiometric configuration seldom converses in a communicative environment in which noise is present. Furthermore, certain advanced algorithms for minimizing noise may have a deleterious effect on other listening environments. (For example, algorithms based on temporal modulation patterns may misinterpret music for background noise and reduce the gain.)

How loud or disturbing are the changing environmental conditions? How large are the rooms in which listening takes place? How far away are the speakers? Are the rooms highly reverberant?

The dispenser should obtain a description of the most difficult listening environments. Tape recordings may augment the patient's verbal description. Answers to these questions can be primary indicators of the need for certain features such as full dynamic range compression, directional or multiple microphones, or adjustable and/or adaptive release times. It should be recognized, for example, that highly reverberant environments minimize the benefits from multiple and directional microphones and that longer release times may provide more subtle effects while maintaining sounds at a comfortable level.

Are multiple programs really better?

As mentioned earlier, conflicting data exist regarding whether automatically adjusting hearing aids provide substantial improvement in speech perception and word recognition. Some of the pitfalls inherent in automatically adaptable responses can be avoided by allowing the user to select among programs according to their own preferences. Kochkin's 1996 data suggested that users often assign hearing aids having multiple programs superior ratings. Keidser (1996) showed that multiple programs are useful primarily for users that present flat audiometric configurations. She indicated that normal-hearing in the low frequencies tended to negate the benefit from multiple programs. It is possible that part of this preference is related to psychologic factors, such as ability to produce an audible change, as much as true improvements in the ability to recognize speech in noisy environments.

Does the patient have difficulty understanding conversation over the telephone? How important is telephone use for the patient? Does, or will, the patient use assistive listening devices requiring telecoils?

The telecoil sensitivity listed by manufacturers of digital and programmable systems covers a rather broad performance range. Some systems have no telecoil at all. If the patient relies on the microphone input only, an in-the-ear hearing aid might be more susceptible to feedback, particularly when conversing over the telephone. If so, it may be necessary to use a multiple-program system that has one program dedicated to telephone use by modifying the frequency response to roll-off the frequencies above 2500 Hz. Also, the Americans with Disabilities Act (Carey, 1992) has made the availability of assistive listening devices more accessible, and telecoil use should be given high priority.

Has the patient had previous experience with hearing aids? Was the patient satisfied with the particular aid previously tried? If not, why not? Was the previous hearing aid a linear device?

If the patient was a satisfied user of linear hearing aids, the introduction of amplification containing compression may be initially unacceptable. This is a common occurrence because the patient was accustomed to receiving consistently greater acoustic gain. Some of the current compression systems may provide for greater gain for low inputs but progressively less gain as the input increases. Counseling may resolve the issue or it may be helpful to use multiple programs with similar frequency responses but different compression (versus linear) characteristics. The compression ratio or kneepoint may need to be altered gradually or introduced to a less dramatic extent. The dispenser must also accept the fact that some users never accept compression. This may be particularly true for listeners with severe or profound losses.

Does the patient have an unusual audiometric configuration?

Certain programmable hearing aids have as many as 13 bands for frequency shaping (not to be confused with independent compression bands). A greater number of bands will allow for finer tuning of the frequency response.

Does the patient have external earcanals that might increase the likelihood of feedback?

Patients who have excessive hair in their earcanals or canals highly susceptible to cerumen accumulation are among those more likely to experience feedback problems. It is intuitively obvious that to prevent feedback, one should strive to achieve a more complete acoustic seal of the external auditory meatus. Unfortunately, improving the acoustic seal may magnify the occlusion effect, increase the tactile sensation intrameatal pressure, and create greater insertion loss. Venting the earmold or in-the-ear shell may reduce these unwanted effects but at the same time increase the possibility of acoustic feedback. If one cannot reduce feedback through acoustic modification, another tactic often used is electro-acoustic modification. Many conventional hearing aids have "feedback reduction" potentiometers. Typically, these operate by one of two tactics. Either they shift the peak away from the feedback producing frequency or they reduce the high-frequency gain. In either case, feedback may be minimized at the expense of rendering certain high-frequency speech sounds inaudible.

PITFALL

Even though there are great advantages to hearing aids with low kneepoints designed to increase gain for low-intensity input signals, the likelihood of feedback may be enhanced with these devices.

Some multiband hearing aids allow for a reduction of a fairly narrow band of frequencies from which feedback is arising so that intelligibility is not sacrificed. Hearing instruments that incorporate active feedback control (as opposed to mere reduction of the high-frequency gain) using in-situ calculations of maximum gain before oscillation or by actual phase reversal of the feedback signal can be appropriate. At present, this type of feedback control is only available in digital hearing aids.

Would the patient prefer (and function better with) hearing instruments that are completely automatic versus devices with volume or program controls? And, if a volume control or program selector is needed, should it be a remote control or on the instrument itself?

For some individuals who either object to or display difficulty manipulating controls at ear level, a remote control may be helpful, providing, of course, that the controls on the remote unit are large and easy to operate. Most remote controls allow the user to make instantaneous changes in volume or program. The remotes differ, however, in terms of their size, shape, and signal transmission characteristics (i.e., frequency modulation (FM) versus ultrasonography). A drawback to those remote controls that use ultrasonographic transmission is that they require a "line-of-sight" and operate most effectively when the remote control is positioned 18 to 24 inches away from the hearing aids. The orientation of the remote to the sensor within the hearing aids might be critical. My clinical experience suggests that more transmission problems may be present when certain spatial conditions exist (i.e., enclosed space in an automobile) for ultrasonic transmission than for FM transmission. Also, interference from security systems that operate at similar carrier frequencies can be present. In addition, certain induction remote controls are interfered with by computers, so an individual who works in this type of environment may be better served by an FM remote or no remote at all.

Certain remote-controlled systems have no volume control on the aids themselves. This means that if the user accidentally misplaces the remote control, it may be impossible to vary the volume control settings. Some manufacturers produce systems that allow for limited manual adjustment of the volume in lieu of the remote control.

For those programmable and digital aids that do not use remote controls, there are also certain considerations. Some systems have no volume control, per se, but instead have separate push buttons or toggle switches that allow the aid to access its various programs. For some users, this physical arrangement is easier to control than a rotary volume wheel. However, for others, it may be confusing because the user cannot determine visually or tactually which program is currently in operation. Some remote controls that offer liquid crystal displays (LCDs) are advantageous because they allow the patient to make rapid visual determinations of which program the aid is operating in and at what particular gain setting. For others, this determination is not important. A momentary pause or audible signal may be present whenever the program is changed that can be displeasing to some users but extremely useful for others who are not certain whether the program has actually changed.

CONTROVERSIAL POINT

At the time of this writing, the movement seems to be away from user controls. Although this is convenient and desirable for many new users, it may be presumptuous for hearing healthcare professionals to assume that we have greater knowledge of the user's preferences than the user.

If the patient is on a limited budget, is he or she better off with two conventional devices than one digital or programmable device?

No clear answer to this question exists, but the same binaural advantages that apply to conventional analog systems also are relevant for digital or programmable hearing aids. For example, binaural amplification is important in minimizing the effects of the head shadow. Placing the aided ear in a position allowing an advantageous azimuth can alter sound pressure level (SPL) by as much as 17 dB between 2500 to 5000 Hz. With proper positioning in an acoustic environment the binaural loudness summation advantage is 2- to 3-dB. In noise, binaural hearing permits the listener to take advantage of interaural phase differences (i.e., masking level differences). Silman et al (1984) and Silverman and Silman (1990) raise the possibility that auditory deprivation of the unaided ear may occur for monaural fittings. Thus withholding a recommendation of binaural amplification may actually present legal ramifications.

Can digital and programmable devices overcome poor selection of style?

Comfort and cosmetic factors are matters of personal taste that must be taken into account regardless of the technology one uses. The same acoustic advantages and limitations of different styles apply regardless of the technology. If a patient's comfort is compromised by a deep fitting within the canal, it will be so whether the aid is digital or analog. If, however, the constraining factor in fitting a small aid such as a completely-in-the-canal (CIC) aid is feedback, devices with finer tuning ability (such as those with multiple frequency-shaping bands) may be helpful because gain can be reduced in a narrow band in which feedback is occurring. This frequency can be determined with probe microphone measures. Furthermore, it is important to note that the greater control obtainable through digital and programmable hearing aids can help minimize adverse effects that might result from a less than optimal fitting. This was demonstrated in a study by Sweetow and Valla (1998) measuring unwanted occlusion perception from CIC devices. They demonstrated that subjective impressions of the occlusion effect can be altered by making subtle changes in the low frequency response or compression parameters. Such subtle changes might not be attainable without the flexibility present in programmable and digital hearing aids.

Are multibands needed?

It is interesting to note that despite the obvious benefits that multiband compression implies (namely selective control for loudness restoration and minimization of gain reduction for frequencies not present in the offending noise spectra), few laboratory experiments have clearly demonstrated the superiority of multibands using objective data (i.e., word recognition scores, or SNR required to achieve a certain percentage of recognition) (Schuchman et al, 1996). However, it is important to note that numerous field studies using subjective data have reported advantages of multiband technology (Horwitz et al 1991; Valente et al, 1998). One can observe either the loudness growth pattern at different frequencies (see next section) or the audiometric configuration to predict how many bands might be appropriate. For example, Figure 13–6 depicts an audiogram of a patient presenting three distinct regions of sensitivity (250 to 750 Hz; 1000 to 2000 Hz;

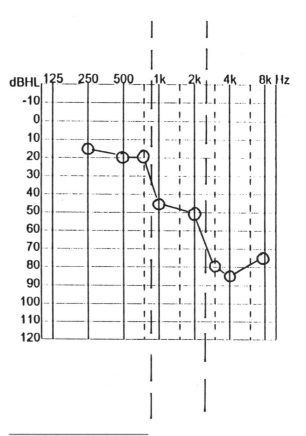

Figure 13–6 Audiogram of a patient for whom three bands of compression would be appropriate. The two vertical dashed lines represent suggested crossover frequencies.

and 3000 to 8000 Hz). For this patient, dual band devices with a crossover frequency of 1500 Hz might produce too little gain at 1000 Hz (if the gain for the low-frequency band was set according to the thresholds at 250 to 750 Hz) and too much gain at 2000 Hz (if the gain for the high-frequency band was set according to the thresholds at 3000 to 8000 Hz). Thus the use of three band instruments might be appropriate, using crossover frequencies at 800 Hz and again at 2500 Hz. This would allow for more appropriate gain settings for all frequencies.

How can the dispenser and patient decide whether the recommended system should be digital or digitally programmable?

This answer should be arrived at by both the patient and the dispenser after extensive discussion and education of the patient. The decision should be based largely on the acoustic needs of the patient. A patient who lives alone and who wants to wear amplification for the sole purpose of watching television does not *require* digital hearing aids. The phrase "you don't need to drive a Rolls-Royce if all you are going to use it for is to drive to the supermarket" is suitable. Presenting options to patients, but framing them realistically in view of their needs, will enhance the credibility of the dispenser. Furthermore, digital, in and of itself, may not be a sufficient cause to add to the expense for a patient. If the processing algorithm is not superior to that which can be provided by an analog system, there may be little justification for using that product.

Once having determined the necessary features for the patient, attention now can be directed toward selection of the specific programmable or digital system for the patient. This decision should incorporate all the following factors—most of which can be ascertained by a careful history or use of a scale such as the Client Oriented Scale of Improvement (COSI) (Dillon et al, 1997).

1. *Which device contains all the necessary features?* No hearing aid has all the possible features. For example, only one of the digital systems currently available has a rotary (on-device) volume control. If it has been deemed that the prospective user should have a volume control, the remaining digital instruments should be ruled out. Here is another example of this decision making process: If both listening to music and noise reduction is a high priority, only one of the two digital systems that uses advanced noise detection algorithms on the basis of temporal input allows the user to turn off the algorithm. This may be important because, as mentioned earlier, use of this algorithm can "trick" the hearing aids into reducing gain by misinterpreting wanted music as unwanted noise. Certainly the need for multiple or directional microphones should be considered. Only two of the currently available digital systems contain this feature, and of those, only one allows for placement of a dual-microphone in an ITE-style hearing aid. Also, if one wants the option of having the hearing aids function in either a directional or omnidirectional mode, the number of devices available becomes even further limited. Or, if the patient needs multiple programs, certain models will be ruled out. In addition, the number of desired bands may help determine the selected device because not all instruments offer the required number.

2. *Does the preferred style contain all the necessary features?* A patient who attends lectures and who plans on using assistive listening devices may not be well served by an ITC or CIC that does not have a telecoil capability or direct auditory input (DAI). Similarly, these small devices cannot accommodate multiple or directional microphones. In fact, at the time of this writing, only one programmable aid and one digital aid offer directional or multiple microphones in full shell ITE aids. This can be an important consideration. For example, Killion et al (1998) found that patients with sloping hearing losses obtained more improvement from the use of dual microphones than subjects with flat audiometric configurations. Thus one must prioritize the desire for a style versus the desire for features. In addition, not all of the products are available in all of the styles. At the time of this writing, only two of the digital products are available in CICs (although this number is certain to increase quite soon).

3. *Are there other devices that have the same features and quality that may be more affordable?* At least one of the currently available digital hearing aids uses algorithms and features that are no different than those found in digitally programmable units at a lesser price. Furthermore, some features available may be superfluous. Multiple programs add to the cost of hearing aids; if the patient is not going to use more than one program, why not order less expensive, single program devices that have similar sound processing?

4. *Does the audiometric configuration dictate the need for certain devices?* As mentioned earlier, certain reverse slope or unusual audiometric configurations may require the need for devices offering extreme flexibility in frequency shaping.

Some of the more advanced devices on the market may not offer this flexibility, particularly if they are confined to single or dual bands. Therefore choosing hearing aids that incorporate at least three bands of compression or seven or more bands of frequency shaping may take priority. Only a small number of products incorporate this feature, so this too will help limit the selection process.

Another point to consider is that the internal noise levels of programmable and digital hearing aids may vary over a significant range. So, if a patient has frequency regions of normal or near-normal thresholds, hearing aids that have internal noise levels that are higher than the individual's threshold (in SPL) at any frequency should be used with caution.

5. *How comfortable is the dispenser with the product, the programming of the product, and the manufacturer?* The rapid increase in the number of available digital and programmable hearing aids makes it difficult for even the most ambitious dispenser to stay focused on all the important aspects of programming. Dispensers may be best served by becoming proficient at programming a limited number of digital and programmable products rather than trying to have a vague familiarity with all. Certainly, a mastery of the NOAH platform (discussed later in this chapter) for one manufacturer tends to furnish a foundation for other models, but no substitute exists for experience. So a dispenser may be wise in selecting and grasping the important programming parameters and idiosyncrasies of just enough hearing aids so that all the important features described previously are covered. Just as important, the dispenser needs to ensure that he or she has a good working relationship with the manufacturers.

PROGRAMMING STRATEGIES

The programming of hybrid hearing aids originally required use of a dedicated programmer. Because of the potentially overwhelming expense required for a dispenser using an ever increasing number of programmable devices, an attempt was made to create a "universal" programming platform that would allow a personal computer user to program hearing aids made by a number of manufacturers. In 1993, a group called HIMSA (Hearing Instrument Manufacturers' Software Association) developed software (NOAH) to be interfaced with a small piece of hardware (HI-PRO) that is shown in Figure 13–7. Today, more than a dozen manufacturers produce hearing aids (programmable and digital) using the NOAH platform. This common software platform operates with a central database for patient records, audiological data, and dedicated fitting and measurement modules. Dispensers obtain software modules from the selected manufacturers and then load these programs into their personal computer under the NOAH "Setup" menu. Although differences exist among each manufacturer's software, knowledge of NOAH, along with the ability to follow on-screen instructions, allows dispensers to program most of the devices available. Because of early discrepancies in the complexity of programming, many manufacturers now offer various "levels" of programming complexity from the "first fit" proprietary algorithms,

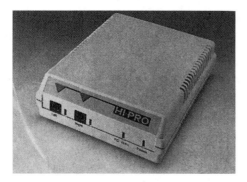

Figure 13–7   HI-PRO hardware interface.

requiring little more than input of the audiogram, to more complex levels, allowing options for adjustments of a variety of parameters such as number of programs, kneepoint, ratio, and crossover frequencies for multiband devices. Several manufacturers have chosen to also provide a dedicated programmer (usually handheld and portable) either instead of NOAH or in addition to it for the dispenser's convenience (i.e., ReSound, Widex, Siemens).

The principles of prescribing gain and output described in Chapters 4, 5, 6, and 12 also apply to digital and programmable hearing aids. The major difference is that with digital and programmable devices, greater flexibility and more options are available to the dispenser. Recognizing that a key advantage of many systems described in this chapter is flexibility, one must keep in mind that algorithms and prescriptive fitting formulas calculated by even the most sophisticated computer or software program should be viewed only as starting points in the final-tuning of the hearing aid response. Fine-tuning following the initial programming may be even more important than the initial fitting. It is essential that this be emphasized to the patient, so that realistic expectations regarding the initial fitting can be established and maintained.

The ensuing section will begin with a discussion of initial programming strategies, continue with suggestions for setting multiple programs, and will conclude with a discussion of fine-tuning strategies based on patient observations. Each section will consider frequency response issues and output (and/or compression) parameters.

Initial Programming

Three methods can be used during the initial programming of hearing aids: behavioral measures (functional gain and loudness discomfort levels), prescriptive formula approaches, and manufacturers' algorithms.

Behavioral Measures

Functional Gain

Use of behavioral thresholds and *functional gain* (the difference between aided and unaided threshold) for setting frequency response has several limitations. First, because these measures are made at threshold, the hearing aids may not be operating with the compression characteristics that would typically be functioning during most suprathreshold listening situations. In other words, gain could be overestimated

(because for many hearing aids having low input compression kneepoints, such as WDRC systems), gain is highest for softer input levels). It also should be noted that the level of compression operating in the hearing aid may be affected by the user's threshold. For example, if a the hearing aid has curvilinear compression with a kneepoint of 45 dB SPL, and the individual's aided threshold is 60 dB HL, the input to the hearing aid at threshold would activate the compression circuit and the gain will be reduced relative to its maximum potential. On the other hand, for the same hearing aid, if the user has an aided threshold of 20 dB, the input to the hearing aid will be below the kneepoint, and the aid would function in its linear mode with its maximum gain potential. In the first example, a 45 dB kneepoint would *not* be advisable for an individual with such a severe loss. Second, if thresholds are particularly good (better than 20 dB HL), the ambient noise level, even in a sound-treated booth, may be high enough to produce masking, thus elevating the true aided threshold. Therefore the use of functional gain measures should be considered as adjunctive, at best, to the other two approaches. However, if functional gain is all that is available, a basic rule of thumb would be that the goal is to bring the aided thresholds as close to 20 dB HL as possible. Better thresholds will probably be wasted in the real world because of ambient noise levels.

When using functional gain measures, be sure to compare "apples to apples." In other words, because the measures are made in the sound field, pure tones cannot be used (because of standing waves). The choice of narrow-band noises versus warbled pure tones may be dictated on the basis of the bandwidth of the narrow-band noises available. For example, a one-third narrow-band noise may activate more than one frequency band in a multiband hearing aid. Thus it may be desirable to use warbled pure tones presented from a 0 degree azimuth from at least 1 m away for both unaided and aided sound field measures. Also, be certain to eliminate the nontest ear from the measurements by properly using masking or attenuating earmuffs.

Because digital and programmable devices allow for precise frequency tuning, threshold measures should be made at interoctave, as well as octave, frequencies to ensure smoothness. Even with these additional measures, it must be recognized that possible peaks and valleys in the response may exist between the tested frequencies. As such, it is essential that frequency-response curves be measured in a hard-walled coupler to detect such irregularities, keeping in mind that even this procedure may fail to detect unwanted resonances produced by the coupling system (earmold or shell) and the real earcanal.

Loudness Discomfort Measures

If the aided output exceeds an individual's loudness discomfort level (LDL), it is likely that the hearing aids will be rejected. Aided LDLs should be measured for speech and for at least two frequencies (500 and 3000 Hz). More frequencies should be added when only behavioral methods are available. Detailed discussions of measuring loudness discomfort can be found elsewhere in Chapters 4, 5, 6, and 12 and will not be described here, but a reasonable approach is that prescribed by Hawkins et al (1987). Perhaps the most important aspect to using LDLs is that one must be consistent in the measurement approach for both unaided and aided measures.

The same caveats expressed for sound field behavioral thresholds apply to LDLs, specifically that aided output may exceed LDLs at frequencies not conveniently located at octave or interoctave locations. So here, too, OSPL 90 (output SPL with a 90 dB input) curves need to be measured in a hard-walled coupler to detect irregularities, again keeping in mind that this may fail to predict unwanted resonances produced by the coupling system and the real earcanal.

Prescriptive Formulas

Setting Frequency Response

Real-ear measures and prescriptive formulas (along with their associated ear-to-coupler conversions) provide a method with which one can ascertain whether the three basic goals required for any successful hearing aid fitting are fulfilled. These goals are as follows:

1. Allowing "soft" (i.e., 50 dB SPL) sounds to be audible
2. Allowing average input signals (i.e., 65 dB SPL) to be judged as comfortable
3. Not allowing "loud" sounds (i.e., 85 dB SPL) to be judged as uncomfortable

Probe microphone measures are described earlier in Chapter 3. It was stated previously that the flexibility of digital and programmable hearing aids allows the hearing health professional to achieve remarkably close target gain matches. There are important issues regarding target gains and prescriptive formulas for digital and programmable hearing aids, however, that must be considered.

1. *Optimum frequency response changes as a function of signal input level. Ideally, recommended target gains should restore audibility and comfort for soft, moderate and loud acoustic signals.* A number of prescriptive fitting formulas are described in Chapters 6, 7, and 13. As mentioned, the first popular formulas were POGO (Prescription of Gain and Output), Libby, 1/3 gain, (National Acoustics Laboratory) NAL, and NAL-R. (Berger et al, 1980; Byrne & Dillon, 1986; Libby, 1986; McCandless and Lyregaard,1983). Mueller (1998) states that NAL-R continues to be the most frequently used formula in use today, despite the fact that this first generation of prescriptive fitting formulas was based on threshold data and for a single input intensity level for 1970 style BTE peaked frequency response with narrow bandwidth hearing aids with linear gain and volume controls (Newman & Levitt, 1990). Thus direct measures of comfort, as suggested by Skinner (1979) and Cox (1983), are essentially ignored. Moreover, many of the principles that these prescriptive formulas were based on may not be applicable for modern, nonlinear multiband hearing aids (Ludvigsen, 1998). Furthermore, it is critical to note that none of these formulas have been validated in terms of their effectiveness for long-term patient satisfaction or benefit.

Given that most digital and programmable hearing aids use compression (and many no longer contain volume controls), a single input level is not sufficient to define their function. Therefore use of these formulas is probably not appropriate and certainly not adequate. At present, several fitting approaches can be used to help determine whether audibility has been achieved without exceeding comfort levels (Cornelisse et al, 1995; Cox, 1985; Hawkins et al, 1989; Killion, 1995; Killion & Fikret-Pasa, 1993; Loven, 1991; Skinner et al, 1982). Refer to Chapters 4, 5, 6, and 12 for details. All the newer formulas described in these chapters consider either prescribed real-ear insertion gain (REIG), real-ear aided response (REAR), or coupler gain for multiple input levels. Some of these prescriptions can be calculated directly from coupler measures, others require probe microphone measures, or a combination of these approaches can be used if the dispenser uses real-ear-to-coupler differences (RECD). In addition, some of the newer formulas assume the patient has average loudness growth (for example FIG6), whereas others (IHAFF's VIOLA) are based on results from the CONTOUR test and accordingly consider the loudness growth pattern of the specific patient rather than predictions from average group results. Considering the variance in individual loudness growth patterns, as well as differences among individual's earcanal resonances, average group results can produce significant discrepancies for a given individual.

2. *No one prescriptive formula is correct for all individuals.* The targets prescribed by the various formulae differ considerably. For example, the higher target gain prescribed by POGO or Berger may be preferred for providing audibility for a patient with a severe or profound loss (who is receiving linear amplification), but the NAL-R formula may be more appropriate for ensuring both audibility and comfort for those with a mild or moderate loss. Similarly, the optimum formula for a mildly sloping loss may not be the same as the optimum formula for a sharply sloping loss. The full on 2-cc coupler gain prescribed by some of these formulas is depicted in Figure 13–8. Please note that the older linear formulas prescribe gain for a single input level, whereas the nonlinear formula (DSL[i/o]) prescribes gain for multiple input levels. In this figure, however, only a single prescribed response prescribed for an average conversational input intensity is given.

3. *Most current real-ear devices only provide prescribed targets on the basis of the "linear" formulas.* Although the trend is changing, most real-ear devices still do not provide automatic calculations using FIG6, DSL[i/o], or VIOLA. As a result, for simplicity sake (and to conserve time) many dispensers continue to use a single intensity level (60- to 70-dB SPL) as a starting point and then observe the changes in gain resulting from lower and higher input intensities. For example, if a target match is made for a 65 dB SPL input using NAL-R and a compression ratio of 2:1 is desired, the gain for a 45 dB SPL input should be approximately 10 dB greater than for the 65 dB SPL input, and the gain for an 85 dB SPL input should be approximately 10 dB less than the gain for the 65 dB SPL input. If possible (on the basis of the ambient noise level in the room in which the probe microphone equipment is situated), it would be reasonable to measure either insertion gain or REAR using 45-, 65-, and 85-dB SPL input levels. The use of a 45 dB SPL input would allow the hearing aid to produce its maximum gain for all but a few of the hearing aids (specifically those digital systems that allow for a kneepoint lower than 45 dB SPL). Also, this intensity level is equivalent to a soft conversational input that should be audible to the hearing aid user. The 65 dB SPL input approximates average conversational speech levels and

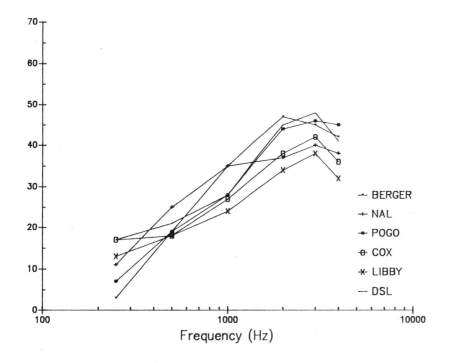

Figure 13–8 Full-on 2-cc coupler gain prescribed by several prescriptive formulas for a gradually sloping hearing loss.

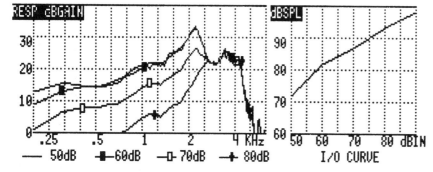

Figure 13–9 Frequency response curves and I/O function illustrating 2:1 compression ratio.

should be perceived as comfortable to the wearer. The 85 dB SPL input signal should place the hearing aids into saturation and should not be judged as uncomfortable by the wearer. An illustration of these relationships is shown in Figure 13–9. If the maximum gain produced by the hearing aid cannot be obtained using real-ear measures because the lowest measurable input level still places the aid into compression, the fitter can simply move the kneepoint to a level above the input level or can adjust the compression ratio to linear (i.e., 1:1). After the soft input measure is completed, the desired compression parameters can be reset for further measures. It is important to recognize that although observation of the relationships of these curves verify that the compression is working, it does not verify that the 45 dB SPL input signal is audible, the 65 dB SPL input signal is comfortable, or the 85 dB SPL input is loud but not uncomfortable. FIG6, DSL[i/o], and VIOLA make these assumptions on the basis of average group data, but, as stated earlier, none of these has been validated. Thus subjective statements must be elicited from the individual patient to substantiate these conclusions.

4. *One must guard against creating a false sense of security encouraged by prescriptive formulas.* Despite the use of the term "expert fitting systems" by one manufacturer of digitally programmable aids, there is no assurance the dispenser is an "expert" or that the manufacturer's algorithm represents an "expert" prescription. It is imperative that one does not get so enamored with sophisticated technology that the critical role of realistic patient counseling (Downs, 1991) in conjunction with all hearing aid fittings is overlooked.

5. *Matching a target gain recommended by a prescriptive formula (or computer-specified algorithm) is only the* initial *step in the fitting process.* Fine-tuning beyond the specified target is essential if the user's acoustic needs are to be met. Stelmachowicz et al (1998) showed most experienced users of a two-band WDRC system found that both FIG6 and DSL[i/o] *overestimated* the preferred high-frequency gain. This may be because DSL[i/o] and FIG6 are based on the average group data collected by Pascoe (1985) in which he established the LDL as uncomfortable (as opposed to the more common practice of establishing LDL as "loud, but OK"). As a result, the dynamic range of these formulas is probably wider than it would be for most hearing-impaired listeners, and the calculated compression ratio is thus lower (more linear), resulting in greater prescribed gain because the dynamic range is wider than most patients would prefer. It also is interesting to note, however, that the preferred settings often did not produce adequate audibility index results. Thus it must be recognized that personal preferences (i.e., comfort versus audibility)

should override formula data, at least for the initial fitting, if one is to have any chance at allowing the new user to feel that the hearing aids are providing a satisfactory fit.

No doubt exists that the interfacing of probe microphone real-ear measures with programmable hearing aid response greatly enhances the fitting procedure (Sweetow & Mueller, 1991). However, if the dispenser does not have a real-ear system, reasonably simple conversions can be made (Hawkins et al, 1990) so that functional gain and 2-cc coupler targets are based on the average real-ear characteristics. Although less ideal than using the individual's real ear, additional modifications can be made on the basis of certain assumptions regarding differences in earcanal resonance and RECDs (especially important when comparing an adult's ear to a child's ear). Then, functional gain can be plotted against a normal conversational speech spectrum. This concept is covered in great detail in Chapters 3, 4, 5, 6, and 12.

Having expressed all the above warnings regarding real-ear measures, attention is now directed to the fact that even early versions of digital and programmable aids can achieve most target gain requirements with remarkable accuracy. Mueller and Jons (1989) studied deviations from NAL-R targets for more than 500 nonprogrammable ITE hearing aids after a REIG target match was achieved at 2000 Hz. They found that target gain at 4000 Hz was rarely achieved. It was usually missed at 3000 Hz as well. They reported that the amount of deviations from target gain occurring within the 90th percentile was 8 dB at 1500 Hz, 9 dB at 3000 Hz, and 13 dB at 4000 Hz. The deviations from target gain that fell within the 70th percentile was 4 dB at 1500 Hz, 6 dB at 3000 Hz, and 9 dB at 4000 Hz. Sweetow and Mueller (1991) examined target gain matches using a single-band programmable BTE hearing aid. They found that REIG deviated from target gain by no more that 6 dB at any frequency for high-frequency and gradually sloping losses and by no more than 8 dB at any frequency for the more difficult-to-match reverse slope notch and cookie bite audiometric configurations. One must be cautious in making direct comparisons between these two sets of findings. In addition to the limited sample size of the Sweetow and Mueller (1991) data, versatility in available acoustic coupling modifications is inherently greater when using BTE aids. Theoretically, however, the individually programmed target gain match should be no worse than the "best case" achievable by fitting a nonprogrammable instrument.

Digitally programmable and digital hearing aids featuring multibands for frequency response or for compression can achieve even closer target matches. As mentioned previously, one currently available digital hearing aid contains seven bands for frequency shaping. A distinction should be made between hearing aids having multibands for frequency shaping versus multibands of compression. Although the bands function in both capacities for some systems, others such as the one described here has only two bands for compression with seven bands for frequency shaping. This device is capable of matching even the most unusual audiometric configurations as was shown previously in Figure 13–5. Certain limitations still apply, however. For example, when fitting a patient with a precipitous hearing loss, even digital aids, despite their theoretical ability to provide a infinitely sharp slope, are still restricted by the use of analog receivers. Thus if a patient has more than a 30 dB difference between thresholds octave frequency, it may not be possible (or even

desirable) to produce such a sharp slope in the frequency response. Indeed, providing gain to frequencies for which the remaining auditory fibers are nonfunctional (Sweetow, 1994) may increase the likelihood of acoustic feedback without enhancing speech recognition. Thus it may be best to simply ignore attempts to achieve targets for thresholds exceeding 100 dB HL.

PEARL

When presetting the frequency response of digital and programmable hearing aids (i.e., before the patient arrives), it is important to observe the coupler response to ascertain that are no irregularities be perceived by the listener as unpleasant. As with real-ear measures, coupler measures should be performed at multiple input levels.

Finally it is important to remember that all of the prescriptive formulas (new and old) are predicated on the use of monaural data for sensorineural losses. Therefore it is wise to reduce overall gain by 3- to 5-dB when fitting binaurally and to add 20 to 25% of the air-bone gap up to a maximum of 8 dB for conductive loss (Valente et al, 1996).

Setting Compression and Output Characteristics
Compression kneepoint (also called compression threshold), compression ratio, crossover frequency, attack and release times, and maximum output levels are parameters that work in connection with the frequency response to determine whether the three basic goals (audibility for soft speech, comfort for conversational speech, and no discomfort for loud speech) are achieved. Prescriptive approaches generally do not define a suggested compression kneepoint. The available kneepoints vary over a wide range, depending on the system. Programmable aids offer kneepoints as low as 45 dB SPL. Some digital hearing aids operate according to algorithms that can produce a compression kneepoint as low as 20 dB SPL. This low threshold seems to minimize pumping and "breathing" effects often heard in conventional AGC aids by keeping the aid in compression most of the time. It also allows for full dynamic range compression. With single channel AGC systems, the user's own voice can trigger compression when kneepoints of 60- to 70-dB SPL are used, thus producing an unwanted overall decrease in gain. Considering the "give-and-take" nature of most conversational situations, the compression kneepoint may have to be set at a higher (or lower) level in to avoid annoying "pumping and fluttering." Kuk (1998) shows that the effect of increasing the compression kneepoint in dynamic range hearing aids is to reduce the gain for low-level inputs (below the kneepoint) while maintaining constant gain above the kneepoint. For other compression systems, however, increasing the kneepoint will allow the hearing aid to remain in a linear mode for a wider range of input intensities.

Although it is reasonably safe to assume that a sensorineural impaired individual will have some degree of loudness recruitment, no way short of clinical assessment can determine at which frequencies and to what degree recruitment is occurring. Establishment of *compression ratio* can be based either on average loudness growth data and predicted by certain available prescriptive formulas (i.e., FIG6 [Killion, 1995], DSL[i/o] [Cornelisse et al, 1995]) or by formulas designed to incorporate individual loudness growth data (i.e., VIOLA [Cox, 1995]). Obviously, collection of loudness data on individuals is more time consuming. However, the reality is that patients having identical audiograms may present significantly different loudness growth patterns. Many programmable systems allow the dispenser to either adjust the compression ratio or to adjust the compression kneepoint. A few will allow for adjustment of both. This is particularly helpful when trying to match a target for at least three input levels. Otherwise only two of the targets might be achieved. Although the Loudness Growth by Octave Band (LGOB) test (Pluvinage & Benson, 1988) was specifically designed for one manufacturer's programmable system, it can be used to estimate compression parameters for nearly all of the programmable systems. The use of multibands provides the fitter the ability to be precise in specifying which frequencies should have certain compression kneepoints and compression ratios. Having the ability to provide linear amplification for one band, a 3:1 ratio for another band, and perhaps a 2:1 ratio for a third band can be essential for the patient who recruits at a different rate for different frequencies.

No current prescriptive formulas dictate the setting of *crossover frequency(s)*. These will often be established on the basis of either the manufacturer's suggestions (to be discussed shortly) or on the basis of individual loudness growth test results. In addition, as described earlier and illustrated in Figure 13–6, examination of the audiogram may help direct the dispenser toward selection of crossover frequencies. In this example, it would be logical to have a crossover frequency between 750 and 1000 Hz and then another crossover frequency above 2000 Hz.

Considerations relating to *attack and release* times can have a significant effect on the acceptance of an amplification system. None of the currently used prescriptive formulas make suggestions for these parameters. Certain manufacturers' software, however, do present suggestions. Some additional guidelines will be offered later in this chapter in the "fine-tuning" section.

The importance of setting the *maximum output* parameter is to ensure that the hearing aids do not saturate at audible levels and that the maximum output is below the LDL. A variety of approaches (Cox, 1983; Hawkins et al, 1989) are available to help select OSPL90 (formerly called SSPL90) and real-ear output. VIOLA determines the maximum gain levels on the basis of individual loudness growth measures (the CONTOUR test; Cox, 1995). DSL[i/o] uses either average data or the dispenser entry of the individual's LDL to predict the maximum allowable levels. Once a determination is made as to what the output level is that should not be exceeded, it is necessary to verify the output level in the patient's earcanal. This can be done by establishing a real-ear saturation response (RESR) with a 90 dB SPL input using both complex noise inputs and a swept pure tone input (Revit, 1991).

Manufacturer's Algorithms

Each hearing aid programmed with the NOAH platform has prescribed settings on the basis of manufacturer's algorithms.

Some of these settings are based on known formulas such as FIG6, DSL[i/o], or NAL-R. Others are based on a proprietary algorithm.

Although each manufacturer's software has variations, NOAH-based programming generally entails following a logical sequence. A typical sequence of steps might include the following:

- First screen: enter patient (client) data
- Second screen: enter audiogram (some manufacturer's algorithms use airbone gap data in their gain and output calculations, some do not); enter maximal comfort level (MCL) and uncomfortable listening level (UCL) data (here again, some manufacturer's algorithms use MCL and UCL data in their gain and output calculations, some do not)
- Third screen: select the manufacturer
- Fourth screen: select the specific instrument from the manufacturer's line
- Fifth screen: select acoustic variables (i.e., vent size, bore, and hook); choose viewing options (binaural or monaural; desired coupler readings or KEMAR); choose number of programs; select the fitting formula (NAL-R, POGO, DSL[i/o], etc., or the manufacturer's proprietary algorithm); set the parameters (including frequency response at a variety of input levels, compression kneepoint, compression ratio, crossover frequency(s), etc.); or request "initial, quick, or automatic" fit
- Sixth screen: activate the second program (for multiple-program devices); set as desired or request manufacturer's algorithm for the desired "comfort" programs (see the next section); program the instrument(s)
- Seventh screen: program the remote control
- Eighth screen: check binaural balance; save and exit

A partial list of the variety of other options include muting the hearing aids, autorelating the multiple programs to the first (basic program), telecoil programming, setting the switch tone level and frequency, locking the volume control, determining the maximum gain before feedback, reading the current settings in the hearing aid, and a host of others. It is obviously impossible to detail all the programming options available from all the programmable and digital hearing aids on the market. Some of the manufacturers provide manuals that should be carefully read before fitting any of these hearing aids. Others provide "help" screens in the software. These are typically quite useful for both initial fitting purposes and for fine-tuning.

Figure 13–10 shows a sample step-by-step menu screen from NOAH. Figure 13–11 illustrates two targets (MCL and UCL), crossover frequencies (the two heavy vertical lines at 750 and 2100 Hz), and anticipated real-ear responses that would occur on the basis of the selected parameters.

PITFALL

It is hazardous to assume that that the response characteristics prescribed by the manufacturer's algorithms or depicted on the programming screen will actually match those found in the real-ear.

① Title bar

② Menu bar

③ Tool bar

④ Status bar

⑤ Customer's name / Function *

⑥ Display monaural/binaural

⑦ Selected side left/right

⑧ Selected PiCS model or Classic Family

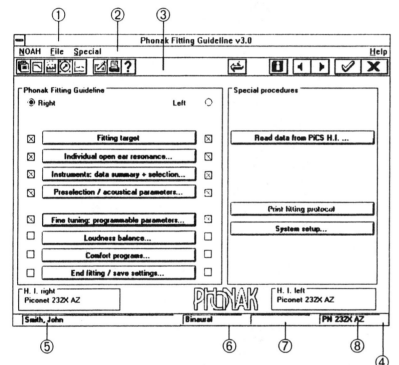

Figure 13–10   A menu screen from NOAH. This screen depicts the step-by-step procedural menu from the Phonak PFG software.

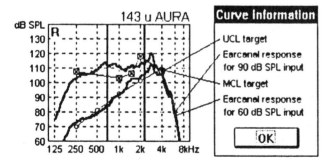

Figure 13–11   A programming screen from NOAH parameters (from the Danavox Danafit software). This screen depicts targets on the basis of MCL and UCL, crossover frequencies (the two heavy vertical lines at 750 and 2100 Hz), and anticipated real-ear responses that would occur based on the selected parameters.

In addition to NOAH, dedicated programmers are used for certain systems. Most of these systems also require input of the audiogram and a selection of a variety of features

before calculation of the manufacturer's algorithm. An example of a screen showing prescribed coupler gain as a function of two input levels (50- and 80-dB) for one of the dedicated programmers is depicted (Fig. 13–12). These prescribed data were calculated by the ReSound P3 handheld programmer based solely on the inputted audiometric thresholds. The ReSound proprietary algorithm thus suggests that in the low-frequency band (below 2000 Hz) the user requires an overall gain of 8 dB for a 50 dB input and a gain of 2 dB for an 80 dB input. This translates into a compression ratio (CR) of 1.3:1. That is, for a 30 dB range in input (50- to 80-dB), output is only changing by 24 dB. In the high-frequency band (above 2000 Hz) the user requires an overall gain of 12 dB for an 80 dB input and a gain of 26 dB for a 50 dB input. This translates into a compression ratio (CR) of 1.9:1. That is, for a 30 dB range in input (50- to 80-dB), output is changing by 16 dB.

A handy feature of some, though not all, programming systems is real-time adjustments. These immediate changes are particularly helpful when comparing two programs (i.e., paired comparisons) or when reducing feedback. Systems having a delay rely too much on the memory of the user in

PITFALL

It is interesting to note that many of the manufacturer's algorithms fail to match the high-frequency targets called for by some of the prescriptive formulas. This is likely not an accident. Probably, manufacturers recognize that too much high-frequency gain may result in feedback or immediate rejection by a new user. Thus they wisely underprescribe gain with the understanding that more gain can be added later as the user becomes more accustomed to amplification.

	Gain	
	Low frequency	High frequency
80 dB in	2	12
50 dB in	8	26
Compression ratio	1.3	1.9
Crossover frequency	2.0	

Figure 13–12 A screen (adapted from the ReSound P3 dedicated programmer) showing selection of gain for a low (50 dB) and high (80 dB) input levels, along with compression ratios and crossover frequency for a two channel instrument.

making subjective comparisons. Real-time adjustments also help speed the fitting and verification process.

One manufacturer's software prescribes variations in the prescribed parameters on the basis of whether the user is a new hearing aid user or an experienced user. For example, one parameter that might be adjusted would be to initially provide the new user with less high-frequency gain. This may produce greater acceptance. It is then recommended that the gain be increased to reach the prescribed target as the user becomes more accustomed to amplification. This concept considers acclimatization issues and has been found to be very useful for this author.

A final issue that is often incorrectly overlooked is the cabling system connecting the hearing aids to the programming hardware. Most cables terminate in either a battery pill or a pin connector. When the connection is appropriate, all the cables work effectively. However, dispensers are well aware that a considerable range of coupling effectiveness exists that can become a significant issue because it is quite embarrassing and time inefficient when the connections become undone during a critical time in the fitting process.

Multiple Program Strategies

One of the useful features available in some digital and programmable hearing aids is the capacity to use multiple programs. As stated earlier, no single hearing aid has proven to be optimal for all listening environments. Therefore many programmable devices offer the patient choices of acoustic response to best interface with the environment in which listening is taking place. This concept is not entirely new. For years, some conventional analog hearing aids have offered user-manipulated tone control switches.

The optimal number of multiple programs to meet listening needs is unknown. No research data support the concept that the more memory choices the better. It is possible that too many choices might confuse the user and create difficulty in rapidly selecting the "right" program choice. Even so, the psychological advantage of offering the patient some "control" over the listening environment is significant. The number of available memory choices for listeners vary from two to as many as eight. Systems with multiple programs can be used effectively for aural rehabilitation and hearing aid orientation purposes. Consider the report cited by Sweetow and Mueller (1991). An individual had normal-hearing through 1500 Hz and was seen in conjunction with the fitting of binaural hearing aids. His primary hearing difficulty occurred during group meetings in which he was frequently involved. At the time of the fitting, target gain was calculated and the instrument was programmed accordingly. The patient, however, objected to this response saying that it sounded "tinny" and did not think the use of the hearing aids made a significant difference in his hearing ability. By manipulating the low-cut and slope adjustment features, the patient was given remote control over three additional responses even though logic suggested that these additional responses would be a poor choices, particularly in noise. However, as the patient became accustomed to programmable hearing aid use, he gradually increased his use of the audiologist's suggested response by progressing through the additional responses. The flexibility of providing four different settings led to amplification acceptance that may not have occurred had the patient been offered only the single prescribed frequency response.

Procedures for setting multiple program hearing aids are based on subjective information gathered during the interview of the patient. In addition, fitting strategies should consider the patient's audiometric configuration and the coupling (i.e., earmold, tubing or shell) configuration used. The dispenser also may want to reserve one program for telephone use. The astute dispenser will obtain the relevant information from the patient to ascertain just how many listening environments require a separate program of their own. If the device has no volume control, the number of programs might be increased so that, for example, a listener might have two programs set for relatively quiet environments, one yielding more gain than the other, and then two more programs set for listening in noise, again with one program yielding more gain than the other (Fabry, 1996). Thus, in effect, the program selection acts as a pseudo volume control.

The following are examples of some *general* guidelines I have used for setting multiple programs. These proposals are relative to the basic program, which for this example is considered to be listening in quiet based on the NAL-R prescription. It should be emphasized that these are merely suggested guidelines. It is important to recognize that differences in programs should be demonstrated to the patient while the background environments the program is designed for is simulated. Otherwise, the program may sound too similar to the basic program or may sound detrimental for the quiet environment.

Comfortable listening in noise: set to −9 to −12 dB regarding the basic program in the low frequencies and increase the high-frequency gain in 2- to 3-dB step intervals (be sure to check that feedback is not occurring and/or that the patient is finding the amplified sound too harsh or tinny). If the hearing aid has two channels, raise the crossover frequency one step at a time. If the basic program called for more gain in the high-frequency band than the low-frequency band (as is common), raising the crossover frequency will have the effect of sharpening the slope of the frequency response. Lower the maximum output in all bands by 5 dB. Ask the patient to confirm loudness by establishing that he or she chooses a rating of "comfortable, but slightly loud" in background noise. I use a variety of signals generated from the 3M/Sonar Sound Pro II CD, including female conversation in noise, restaurant noise, and traffic noise. Patients are positioned at a 0 degree azimuth from the loudspeaker, and the primary signal (usually speech) and background noise are at a calibrated SPL of 75 dB (to simulate the increased noise levels typically found in noisy environments). Other CDs and cassette tapes are also commercially available or can be recorded by the dispenser. Also, the release time may be adjusted depending on the patient's reports of the type of environmental noise he or she is typically exposed to. For example, an individual who is exposed to a fairly constant level of background noise may prefer a longer release time. An individual exposed to frequent transient background signals may prefer shorter release times. When possible, I will use variable release times, if available. Variable or adaptive release time means that the hearing aids automatically adjust their release times, depending on the duration of the input signal that activated the compression. That is, short-duration inputs (i.e., a spoon or fork clanking) produce a short release time and a longer release time is provided for inputs having longer durations (i.e., machinery noise). This concept, explained by Smriga (1986), will be discussed later in this chapter. Specific manufacturers may have software offering "help" screens, may recommend suggestions for multiple programs in the manual, or may have proprietary algorithms. An example of one manufacturer's corrections for "listening in noise" (relative to the basic "listening in quiet") is shown in Table 13–2.

Car or wind noise: reduce the low frequencies in 2- to 3-dB step intervals and simulate the environment.

Music: flatten the frequency response or add low frequencies in 2- to 3-dB step intervals, increase the dynamic range (i.e., 60 dB versus 30 dB for speech) by slowly raising the kneepoint or gradually lowering the compression ratio making the processing more linear (i.e., closer to 1:1). Make all adjustments in small steps and allow the patient to listen to the type of music he or she prefers.

Telephone: reduce the high-frequency gain above 3000 Hz.

Reverberant environments: reduce the low frequencies and shorten the release time. Remove the patient from the unrealistic acoustic environment of a test room and allow him or her to listen to your adjustments in a larger, more echoic atmosphere.

Sensitivity to paper rustling or dishes rattling: use treble increase for lower input levels (TILL) processing (i.e., increase the gain for low-input high frequencies and decrease the gain for high-input low frequencies). Shorten release times.

TABLE 13–2 One manufacturer's corrections for "listening-in-noise" program (relative to the basic "listening-in-quiet" program)

Frequency	Correction
250	−9 dB
500	−5 dB
1000	−3 dB
1500	+1 dB
2000	+3 dB
3000	+5 dB
4000	+7 dB

Keidser (1996) concluded that "high-frequency compression is preferred for ease of understanding multiple talkers, whose voices differ in overall level, in quiet environments. The annoyance of low-frequency background noise can be reduced by low-frequency compression, whereas a frequency response steeper than the NAL response makes it easier to understand speech in low-frequency background noise... a frequency response flatter than the NAL response can be used to make a high-frequency background noise less annoying."

Some multiple programs are specified by processing terms rather than by situational terms. For example, one can do the following:

- Use Bass Increase for Low-input Levels (BILL) to minimize spread of masking and wind noise
- Use Treble Increase for Low-input Levels (TILL) to normalize loudness perception for mild-to-moderate losses who have normal loudness perception at high intensities. This may be particularly helpful for patients who are sensitive to loud high frequencies such as paper rustling or dishes rattling
- Use variable release time for fluctuating noise environments

Some patients may also benefit from having either a visual or audible prompt to allow them to be aware of what program the hearing aids are in. Remote controls with LCDs or with two-position or three-position switches can be valuable. In the absence of a remote control, some multiple-program instruments have audible switch tones (of different frequencies and perhaps different intensities) that are activated when moving from one program to another.

Before leaving the section on initial programming, it should be mentioned that no prescriptive procedures are specific to the telecoil response. In fact, only a few digital and programmable systems allow for independent programming of the telecoil. Given the importance of the t-coil and assistive listening devices (ALDs), this is surprising and hopefully will change with future advances in technology. When this option is available, it is reasonable to try to set the frequency response of the t-coil to approximate the frequency response of the hearing aid.

When patients decide to obtain hearing aids with multiple programs, they often have expectations of clearly perceptible changes between the programs. They may be disappointed when differences are subtle. It is crucial that the patient be counseled that some differences in programs will only be noticeable in certain acoustic environments. For example, in a quiet environment, memories programmed for reduction of noise may not sound different from the basic program. Recordings of various sounds should be used to demonstrate multiple programs. One software program (SoundPro) contains a variety of calibrated CD-quality sounds (restaurant noise, music, traffic, loud speech, loud noises, soft-spoken woman's voice, etc.) and can be quite useful. It is also helpful to use real-ear measures to visually display differences to the patient. Figure 13–13 depicts 2-cc coupler readings of four memories programmed to differ only in output, not in gain. These programs will sound different in high-intensity environments but will sound identical for moderate input intensities.

Fine-Tuning Strategies

Some hearing aid fitting procedures and processing strategies are designed to improve speech recognition (TILL), reduce background noise (BILL), enhance audibility (POGO), restore normal loudness contours (DSL[i/o]), or heighten comfort (FIG6). However, none have been proven to succeed in all areas (i.e., improve speech recognition, enhance audibility, restore normal loudness contours, *and* heighten comfort). Therefore emphasis must be placed on the individual's prioritized weighting of the importance of these attributes. These priorities should be established during the subjective and objective needs assessment. It is essential to prioritize issues, recognizing that certain compromises (noise reduction vs. speech recognition; recognition vs. tinny sound quality; gain vs. loudness comfort; feedback vs. high-frequency gain, etc.) may be inevitable. Often, the patient will not be in a position to prioritize until he or she has had a chance to wear the hearing aids for a while. This is why initial programming through prescriptive formulas and/or manufacturer's algorithms are good starting points. However, the real challenge to the audiologist arrives when it is time to fine-tune the amplification systems to the preferences of the patient.

Some patients are quite articulate about their likes and dislikes, whereas others require prompting from the dispenser to determine fine-tuning needs. Phrasing questions effectively helps elicit comments that can aid the dispenser in fine-tuning. Often, soliciting comments from spouses and significant others can be of great assistance. It is not adequate for the patient to say "it doesn't sound right." Instead the audiologist must help the patient operationally define the problems. Asking questions such as, "Is speech difficult for you to understand from all talkers, or just from females?" or "Are the background sounds that are bothering you only those that are loud, or are the soft ones also bothersome?" may be useful. Stypulkowski (1994) proposed a method to troubleshoot dual channel instruments that he termed "the quadrant

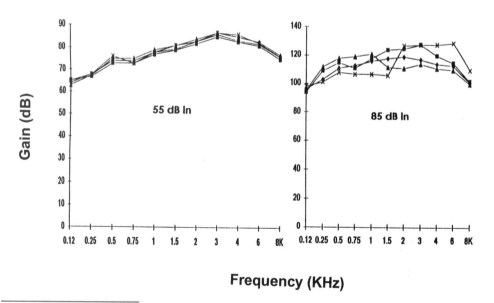

Figure 13–13 Frequency responses for a four-program hearing aid. Note that gain is similar for all four programs for a low-intensity input, but quite different for a high-intensity input.

Loud Sounds	Loud Sounds
Noise Auto traffic Machinery Loud speech LOW-BAND OUTPUT	Dishes Paper rustling Keys or coins rattling Loud speech HIGH-BAND OUTPUT
Soft Sounds	Soft Sounds

Speech
   Quality
   Naturalness
   Balance
 	
LOW-BAND GAIN
	Speech
	   Clarity
	   Consonants
	   Intelligibility
	
	HIGH-BAND GAIN

Figure 13–14 Example of a "quadrant" approach to fine-tuning a two channel programmable hearing aid.

approach." Figure 13–14 is an adaptation of this procedure. As shown, there are four boxes; soft low-band and soft high-band sounds are represented in the lower left and lower right boxes, respectively. In addition, speech quality, naturalness, and balance are also found in the lower left quadrant, whereas speech clarity, consonants, and intelligibility are found in the lower right quadrant. Loud low-band and loud high-band sounds are represented in the upper left and upper right boxes, respectively. The lower left and right quadrants represent low-frequency and high-band gain, respectively; whereas the upper left and right quadrants represent low-band and high-band output, respectively. If the patient's complaints concern aspects listed in the lower right quadrant, for example "consonants don't sound clear," then an appropriate adjustment would be to increase the high-band gain. If, on the other hand, the patient complains that "shuffling of the newspaper sends me through the roof," then the adjustment

should be to reduce the high-band output. Stypulkowski (1994) states that most modifications related to quality or intelligibility of soft speech are related to gain, whereas most adjustments needed for complaints of quality of comfort of loud sounds are related to output.

> **PEARL**
>
> Now that three-band and four band hearing aids are becoming popular, the inventive dispenser can fine-tune even more sensitively by dividing the patient's complaints into soft, moderate, and loud sounds falling into low, middle, and high frequencies. In other words, the four-box approach can be expanded to a nine-box approach (see Fig. 13–15).

Compression Kneepoint

In addition, keep in mind that compression kneepoint and release time can affect gain at low input levels. Kuk (1998) presents an excellent discussion of the interaction of these factors. Even complaints that do not fall neatly into one of the aforementioned boxes can be dealt with by extending the same line of reasoning. For example, if the patient complains that he or she has difficulty hearing speakers from far distances, a TILL philosophy can be adopted because speech originating from a nearby speaker receives less gain. Or, another way to phrase this modification would be to raise the high-frequency gain for soft inputs (i.e., increase the compression ratio) in a wide dynamic range (one that has kneepoints at 40- to 45-dB SPL) system. If the opposite complaint occurs (i.e., the user hears people talking from another table in a restaurant), then soft inputs are receiving too much gain, so compression ratio should be decreased to reduce the difference in gain between close and distant speakers. For older hearing aids with higher kneepoints (i.e., 70 dB and above) and ratios (i.e., 4:1 and higher), raising the kneepoint and

Troubleshooting

	Low	Mid	High
Loud	car door slamming groups street	party	dishes rattling
Avg.	echo reverberation	TV radio telephone	reverberation
Soft	refrigerator	wind noise fan leaves	distant speakers birds feedback

Figure 13–15 Example of a nine-box approach to fine-tuning a three channel programmable hearing aid.

lowering the compression ratio will also provide greater gain for soft input signals.

Release Time

In addition to adjustments in gain, output, kneepoints, and compression ratios, the importance of release time should be weighed. Temporal cues are often overlooked because of the preoccupation with amplifying spectral cues. Crucial formant transition information can be lost or altered during attack and release phases. The patient's ability to detect these rapid frequency changes is crucial. Minifie (1973) reports that some vowels (dipthongs) are perceived by formant transitions and by location of the first two spectral peaks. Consonants are very transient and have rapid spectral fluctuations occurring in the range of 10 to 30 ms. Listeners differentiate voiced from voiceless (i.e., /b/ versus /p/) initial consonants on the basis of voice onset time after the sound burst (voiced = 5 ms, voiceless = 40 to 60 ms). Perception of speech involves the ability to detect brief, silent intervals of ongoing acoustic stimuli. Listeners with sensorineural hearing loss weigh the spectral and temporal cues differently than normal listeners. For normal listeners, spectral cues determine identification of consonants. For listeners with impaired hearing, spectral cues have less influence, whereas time and tilt cues assume greater importance. This is because frequency selectivity is generally more impaired than temporal resolution for the listener with impaired hearing. For severe-to-profound losses, temporal cues may supply the major information. Drechsler and Plomp (1980) suggest elevated temporal resolution in hearing-impaired listeners does not adversely affect speech intelligibility. However, if the hearing aid further degrades temporal cues, perceptual problems could occur. This is precisely what could occur if the release time is too fast (i.e., less than 150 ms for ongoing, though fluctuant background noise) or too slow (i.e., 500 ms or more for transient background). If the release times are not appropriate for the temporal characteristics of the offending background signals, reverberant, ambient, and background noise could fill or smear the important silent intervals.

Several years ago, the concept of adaptive compression was introduced to minimize periods of inaudibility that occur as a result of listening in an acoustic environment characterized by loud transient sounds (Smriga, 1986). In this design, release time varies as a function of the duration of incoming noise. For example, a short burst of noise (such as a spoon dropping on a hard surface) produces a shorter release time than an ongoing noise, such as constant background chatter or machine noise. If the release time is too short, the SNR is decreased. If the release time is too long after transient noises, the hearing aids remain in compression during a period of time in which the listener wants to listen to speech. Such compression activity may render speech components inaudible while the gain recovers to its desired level. Although at the time of this writing only a minority of the programmable systems feature variable release time, several incorporate different release times for the low-frequency versus high-frequency inputs. At least one system allows the dispenser to select among three release times for different frequency bands. At least one of the digital hearing aids contains a form of variable release. For example, one system uses a slow-acting, adaptive release time that becomes fast for signals of short duration and up to 30 seconds for signals whose intensity is fairly stable over time. Release times of this magnitude are not available in any of the hybrid systems.

Another advantage of multiband instruments is that attack times may be longer for lower frequency inputs. High-frequency sounds fluctuate within a time frame of 40 ms, and vowels may last for 500 ms. It is best to activate low-frequency filtering for long-duration sounds and not for fluctuating sounds of less than 40 or 50 ms. If different time constraints are not used for low-frequency versus high-frequency inputs, normal conversational speech could activate an unnecessary adaptive filtered response.

Feedback Reduction

Minimizing feedback in conventional analog systems is often limited to earmold or shell modifications such as reducing vent size or reducing high-frequency gain. Both of these strategies have obvious drawbacks. As mentioned earlier, some programmable and digital devices use multibands in which case reduction in gain is limited to only a narrow band of frequencies around the frequency of the feedback. Others use digital technology and minimize feedback by sensing the oscillation frequency and then producing a similar tone of opposite phase. In addition, some of the digital systems provide for in-situ measurement of the maximum gain allowable without producing feedback. When performing this test, ask the patient to wear a hat (if that is common for him or her), sit near a wall, and chew.

Finally, for the dispenser who finds the preceding discussion to be too complicated to remember, many of the manufacturer's software programs now offer suggestions and apply the appropriate solutions simply by identifying the complaint on the menu.

SPECIAL CONSIDERATION

Earmold modifications are not rendered unnecessary because of the increased flexibility of digital and programmable hearing aids.

Validation Techniques

As described earlier, technological advances such as dynamic range compression, multiband compression, multiple programs, multiple and/or directional microphones, and digital algorithms designed to reduce gain as a function of the temporal characteristics of the input signal hold great promise for enhancing listening comfort or speech recognition in a variety of listening environments. However, many of the traditional electroacoustic and real-ear analysis measures discussed in Chapters 1 and 3 are now no longer adequate to assess the functionality of these new features. As a result, manufacturers of hearing aid analyzers have provided dispensers with new techniques to determine the function of these features. Revit details real-ear measures strategies using newer acoustic signals in Chapter 3. In this section, techniques available to measure these functions will be briefly described.

Dynamic Range Compression

Hearing aids with full dynamic range compression are often characterized as systems having low compression kneepoint (40- to 45-dB SPL), low compression ratio (3:1 or lower), and fast time constants (5 ms or less attack; 50 to 100 ms release). Because most programmable and digital hearing aids use a low compression kneepoint, validation procedures must take into account the fact that most speech signals will activate compression. Thus full gain can only be assessed by using very low-level inputs. For example, the ANSI 3.22 (1987) standard calls for measuring compression aids with a 50 dB SPL input. If the hearing aid has a compression threshold of 45 dB SPL, this aid will already be in compression. Moreover, an increasing number of digital hearing aids will have lower kneepoints. Knowledge of the compression ratio will not even allow for prediction of precise gain levels because the compression may be curvilinear (i.e., compression ratio increases as input level increases) rather than fixed (i.e., compression ratio is constant). Fortunately, some electroacoustic equipment now allow for a rapid succession of frequency responses for different input levels. For example, use of the ANSI 3.42 (1992) standard yields a series of four frequency responses for input levels from 50- to 80-dB SPL (or if desired 40- to 70-, or 60- to 90-dB SPL). Also, it is relevant to note that hearing aids without volume controls may not be able to be tested at reference test gain. For quality assurance, ANSI (1987) standards dictate measuring the hearing aid at its most linear conditions, but this does not reflect the true function of the hearing aids.

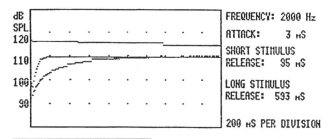

Figure 13–16 Dual time constant display for a hearing aid with variable release compression. The upper curve shows the attack time, the middle curve shows the release time for a short-duration signal; the lower curve shows the release time for a long-duration signal.

can be done, for example, on the Fonix 6500 with a Star option and will result in a dual time constant display of either the attack and release times or of the attack and release times for a short versus a long duration signal (Figure 13–16).

Multiple Programs, Multiple and/or Directional Microphones

As stated earlier, it is helpful to combine visual validation of changes in programs along with live demonstrations of changes occurring in differing acoustic environments. Providing patients with printouts of the responses of different programs from real-ear responses or from coupler measures may help the patient understand subtle differences in addition to supplying them handy instructions relating to the purpose of each of the programs.

Similarly, real-ear measures of hearing aids containing directional or multiple microphones can be performed by having the composite signal emanating first from a speaker at 0 degree azimuth and then from a speaker at 180 degree azimuth so that patients can see, in addition to hear, the suppression of sound originating from behind.

> ## SPECIAL CONSIDERATION
>
> **Remember that the compression ratio measured in a coupler may not be the actual (effective) compression ratio in a real-ear because of venting and release time.**

The fast release times associated with some dynamic range compression instruments allow for use of the default delay time settings (500 ms) for obtaining an input/output function. However, because of the ability to, for example, increase the attack time in certain instruments, it is important to modify the delay time so that it is longer than the attack time. This may require setting it to as high as 3 s.

Similar reasoning can be applied to measuring distortion in high-technology hearing aids. Because of the enhanced frequency-shaping capabilities of these devices, it may be necessary to use the regulations associated with the special purpose average (SPA) frequencies. This would apply, for example, to a hearing aid having no gain through 2000 Hz, but then 30- or 40-dB of gain at 3000 Hz.

Multiband Compression

Compression parameters such as I/O and attack/release times are typically measured using a 2000 Hz tone. If hearing aids have multiple channels, these characteristics should be measured using tones located within each of the channels.

In addition, if multiple (or single program) hearing aids have variable or adaptive release function, time constants should be measured using signals of varying duration. This

Digital Algorithms Designed to Reduced Gain as a Function of the Temporal Characteristics of the Input Signal

Because of the unique nature of two of the digital hearing aids available at the time of this writing (and certainly, more in the near future), gain (or frequency response) may be erroneously measured even in real time because the hearing aid will interpret the composite noise (or pure tone) input signal as noise and will consequently reduce its gain. To avoid this confusion, when using a composite noise, it is necessary to introduce the signal for a short duration (5 to 10 ms) and allow 20 to 30 s before introducing subsequent signals (so that the long release time has a chance to recover). The manufacturers of these products have recently worked with designers of electroacoustic analyzers to introduce methods to measure the basic properties of the instruments by turning off the noise reduction algorithm. However, for the reasons discussed previously, it seems ludicrous to measure the hearing aid when it is not in its usual functioning mode. Recently, Frye Electronics introduced a "Digital Speech-in-Noise" test that uses short bursts of real-time composite noise that are randomly interrupted. These interruptions simulate the temporal fluctuations of speech and thus do not produce a reduction in gain. In addition, the dispenser has the option of adding a continuous pure tone signal (which would be interpreted by the digital instrument as noise) to be mixed with the interrupted composite noise. When the hearing aid detects the pure tone signal, it will enable its noise reduction function and thus reduce gain. The frequency of the pure tone can be varied to induce the noise reduction action in individual channels. This test is not only helpful for the dispenser to be able to verify the noise reduction function, but it is impressive to the patient and therefore a great accessory to counseling.

The classic Carhart approach of measuring monosyllabic word recognition scores in quiet (Carhart, 1946) is no longer considered sensitive enough to discriminate among hearing aids or processing schemes perhaps because it does not take into effect the dynamic range characteristics of speech or fill in between syllables with noise as occurs in real life (Villchur, 1978). Use of sentence materials such as the Speech Perception in Noise (SPIN) test (Bilger et al, 1984) or continuous discourse immersed in noise is closer to reality. As with all other aspects of audiology, use of a battery of tests is preferred. Hence, a combination of real-ear and hard-walled electroacoustic measures, coupled with recognition of continuous discourse in noise, along with subjective survey materials, is prudent.

CONCLUSIONS

Because of the relatively high cost of digital and programmable hearing aids, many patients expect "miracles." Some potential users have been misled, either by other satisfied users, or by overly optimistic advertisements, suggesting that these "high-tech" aids are capable of eliminating background noise. Features unique to programmable systems, such as multiple programs, multiband compression, and adjustable release time can, in fact, improve the patient's perception in noisy listening environments. However, realistic expectations must be conveyed to the listener. These aids *do not* eliminate background noise. It should be indicated to the prospective user that elimination of background noise is neither realistic nor necessarily advisable. A world void of background is analogous to a world limited to black and white. Even listeners with normal-hearing have more difficulty in noise than they do in quiet. They are simply better able at extracting the primary acoustic message and placing it "in front." This, not the elimination of background noise, should be the goal.

Furthermore, given the limitations described in this chapter of prescriptive formulas, it is the opinion of this author that too much time is spent attempting to match hypothetical targets during initial programming sessions and that more time needs to be devoted to *listening* to the needs of the patient. Fine-tuning can only be accomplished successfully when the dispenser truly "hears" what the patient has to say.

REFERENCES

AMERICAN NATIONAL STANDARDS INSTITUTE. (1987). Specifications of hearing aid characteristics (ANSI 3.22-1987). New York: ANSI.

AMERICAN NATIONAL STANDARDS INSTITUTE. (1992). Specifications of hearing aid characteristics (ANSI 3.2-1992). New York: ANSI.

BARFOD, J. (1976). Multi-band compression hearing aids. *Report 11, The Acoustics Laboratory.* Copenhagen: Technical University of Denmark.

BERGER, K., HAGBERG, E., & RANE, R. (1980). A reexamination of the one-half gain rule. *Ear and Hearing, 1;*223–225.

BILGER, R.C., NUETZEL, J.M., RABINOWITZ, W.M., & RZECKOWSKI, C. (1984). Standardization of a speech perception test in noise. *Journal of Speech and Hearing Research, 27;*32–48.

BOOTHROYD, A., SPRINGER, N., SMITH, L., & SCHULMAN, J. (1988). Amplitude compression and profound hearing loss. *Journal of Speech and Hearing Research, 31;*362–376.

BYRNE, D., & DILLON, H. (1986). The National Acoustic Laboratories' (NAL) new procedure for selecting the gain and frequency response of a hearing aid. *Ear and Hearing, 7;*257–265.

CAREY, A.L. (1992). Americans with disabilities act. *ASHA, 34;*5.

CARHART, R. (1946). Tests for the selection of hearing aids. *Laryngoscope, 56;*780–794.

CORNELISSE, L.E., SEEWALD, R.C., & JAMIESON, D.G. (1995). The input/output formula: A theoretical approach to the fitting of personal amplification devices. *Journal of the Acoustical Society of America, 97*(3);1854–1864.

COX, R. (1983). Using ULCL measures to find frequency-gain and SSPL-90. *Hearing Instruments, 34*(7);17–21.

COX, R.M. (1985). A structured approach to hearing aid selection. *Ear and Hearing, 6;*226–239.

COX, R.M. (1995). Using loudness data for hearing aid selection: The IHAFF approach. *Hearing Journal, 47*(2);10,39–42.

DILLON, H., KORITSCHONER, E., BATTAGLIA, J., LOVEGROVE, R., GINIS, J., MAVRIAS, G., CARNIE, L., RAY, P., FORSYTHE, L., TOWERS, E., GOULISA, H., & MACASKILL, F. (1991). Rehabilitation effectiveness I: Assessing the needs of clients entering a national hearing rehabilitation program. *Australian Journal of Audiology, 13*(2);55–65.

DOWNS, D. (1991). Viewpoint: Clinical audiologists have lost sight of their clients. *Hearing Journal, 44*(2);18–23.

DRESCHLER, W., & PLOMP, R. (1980). Relationship between psychophysical data and speech perception for hearing-impaired subjects. *Journal of the Acoustical Society of America, 68;*1608–1615.

FABRY, D. (1996). Clinical applications of multimemory hearing aids. *Hearing Journal, 49*(8);10,53–56.

FRENCH, N.R., & STEINBERG, J.C. (1947). Factors governing the intelligibility of speech sounds. *Journal of the Acoustical Society of America, 19;*90–119.

HAWKINS, D., COOPER, W., & THOMPSON, D. (1990). Comparisons among SPLs in real-ears, 2 cm^3 and 6 cm^3 couplers. *Journal of the American Academy of Audiology, 1;*154–161.

HAWKINS, D., MORRISON, T., HALLIGAN, P., & COOPER, W. (1989). The use of probe tube microphone measurements in hearing aid selection for children. *Ear and Hearing, 10;*281–287.

HAWKINS, D., WALDEN, B., MONTGOMERY, A., & PROSEK, R. (1987). Description and validation of an LDL procedure designed to select SSPL 90. *Ear and Hearing, 8;*162–169.

HECOX, K. (1988). Evaluation of hearing aid performance. *Seminars in Hearing, 9*(3);239–251.

HORWITZ, A., TURNER, C.W., & FABRY, D. (1991). Effects of different frequency response strategies upon recognition and preference for audible speech stimuli. *Journal of Speech and Hearing Research, 34;*1185–1196.

KEIDSER, G. (1996). Selecting different amplification for different listening conditions. *Journal of the American Academy of Audiology, 7;*92–104.

KILLION, M.C. (1990). A high fidelity hearing aid. *Hearing Instruments, 41,*8:38–39.

KILLION, M.C. (1995). Talking hair cells: What they have to say about hearing aids. In: C.I. Berlin (Ed.), *Hair cells and hearing aids* (pp. 3–19). San Diego: Singular Publishing Group.

KILLION, M.C., & FIKRET-PASA, S. (1993). The 3 types of sensorineural hearing loss: Loudness and intelligibility considerations. *Hearing Journal, 46*(11);31–36.

KILLION, M.C., SCHULEIN, R., CHRISTENSEN, L., FABRY, D., REVIT, L., NIQUETTE, P., & CHUNG, K. (1998). Real world performance of an ITE directional microphone. *Hearing Journal, 51*(4);24–38.

KOCHKIN, S. (1996). Customer satisfaction and subjective benefit with high performance hearing aids. *Hearing Review, 3*(12);16,18,22–24,26.

KUK, F.K. (1998). Using the I/O curve to help solve subjective complaints with WDRC hearing instruments. *Hearing Review, 5*(1);8–16,59.

LIBBY, E. (1986). The 1/3 - 2/3 insertion gain hearing aid selection guide. *Hearing Instruments, 37*(3);27–28.

LIBBY, E., & SWEETOW, R. (1987). Fitting the environment: some evolutionary approaches. *Hearing Instruments, 38*(8);8–12.

LIPPMAN, R., BRAIDA, L., & DURLACH, N. (1981). Study of multichannel amplitude compression and linear amplification for persons with sensorineural hearing loss. *Journal of the Acoustical Society of America, 69*, 524–531.

LOVEN, F. (1991). A real ear speech spectrum based approach to ITE preselection/fitting. *Hearing Instruments, 42*;3,6–13.

LUDVIGSEN, K. (1998). *Comparison of fitting rules of nonlinear hearing aids and a digital processing system.* American Academy of Audiology, Los Angeles, CA. (April, 1998).

MCCANDLESS, G., & LYREGAARD, P. (1983). Prescription of gain/output (POGO) for hearing aids. *Hearing Instruments, 34*;(1)16–21.

MINIFIE, F.D. (1973). Speech acoustics. In: F.D. Minifie, T.J. Hixon, & F. Williams (Eds.), *Normal aspects of speech, hearing and language* (pp. 254–282). Englewood Cliffs, NJ: Prentice-Hall.

MOORE, B. (1990). How much do we gain by gain control in hearing aids? *Acta Otolaryngologica, Supplement, 469*;250–256.

MOORE, B. (1996). Perceptual consequences of cochlear hearing loss and their implication for the design of hearing aids. *Ear and Hearing, 7*;411–418.

MUELLER, H.G. (1998). Probe microphone measurements: Yesterday, today, and tomorrow. *Hearing Journal, 51*(4);17–22.

MUELLER, H.G., & JONS, C. (1989). Some clinical guidelines for the fitting of custom hearing aids. *ASHA, 10*;57.

NEWMAN, C., LEVITT, H. (1990). Selection procedures for digital hearing aids. *Seminars in Hearing, 11*(1);79–89.

PASCOE, D. (1985). Hearing aid evaluation. In: J. Katz (Ed.), *Handbook of clinical audiology* (3rd ed.) (pp. 936–948). Baltimore, MD: Williams & Wilkins.

PLUVINAGE, V., & BENSON, D. (1988). New dimensions in diagnostics and hearing aid fittings. *Hearing Instruments, 39*(8);28–30.

REVIT, L. (1991). New tests for signal processing in multiband hearing instruments. *Hearing Journal, 44*(5);20–23.

SCHUCHMAN, G., FRANQUI, M., & BECK, L.B. (1996). Comparison of performance with a conventional and a two-band hearing aid. *Journal of the American Academy of Audiology, 7*;15–22.

SILMAN, S., GELFAND, S., & SILVERMAN, C. (1984). Effects of monaural versus binaural hearing aids. *Journal of the Acoustical Society of America, 76*;1357–1362.

SILVERMAN, C., & SILMAN, S. (1990). Apparent auditory deprivation from monaural amplification and recovery with binaural amplification: two case studies. *Journal of the American Academy of Audiology, 1*(4);175–180.

SKINNER, M. (1979). Speech intelligibility in noise induced hearing loss: Effects of high-frequency compensation. *Journal of the Acoustical Society of America, 67*;306–317.

SKINNER, M., PASCOE, D., MILLER, J., & POPELKA, G. (1982). Measurements to determine the optimal placement of speech energy within the listeners' auditory area. In: G. Studebaker, & F. Bess (Eds.), *The Vanderbilt report* (pp. 161–169). Upper Darby, PA: Monographs in Contemporary Audiology.

SMRIGA, D. (1986). Modern compression technology: developments and applications, Part 2. *Hearing Journal, 39*(7);13–16.

SOUSA, P.E., & TURNER, C.W. (1998). Multichannel compression, temporal cues, and audibility. *Journal of Speech and Hearing Research, 41*;315–326.

STELMACHOWICZ, P., DALZELL, S., PETERSON, D., KOPUN, J., LEWIS, D., HOOVER, B. (1998). A comparison of threshold-based fitting strategies for nonlinear hearing aids. *Ear and Hearing, 19*(2);131–138.

STROM, K. (1998). A review of the 1997 hearing instrument market. *Hearing Review, 55*(3);8–16,72.

STYPULKOWSKI, P.H. (1994). *Fitting strategies for 3M programmable hearing instruments: The quadrant approach.* Minneapolis, MN: 3M Hearing Health publication.

SWEETOW, R.W. (1994). Pitfalls in assessing high-frequency thresholds. *Hearing Journal, 47*(4);10,45–48.

SWEETOW, R.W., & MUELLER, H.G. (1991). The interfacing of programmable hearing aids and probe microphone measures. *Audecibel, 40*(3);11–13.

SWEETOW, R.W., & SHELTON, C.W. (1996). Analysis of time/cost and satisfaction factors for programmable versus conventional hearing aids. *Hearing Journal, 49*(4);51–57.

SWEETOW, R.W., & VALLA, A. (1998). Effects of electroacoustic parameters on Ampclusion in CIC Hearing Aids. *Hearing Review, 4*,(9);8–22.

TYLER, R., & KUK, F. (1989). Some effects of "noise suppression" hearing aids on consonant recognition in speech-babble and low-frequency noise. *Ear and Hearing, 10*;243–249.

VALENTE, M., FABRY, D., POTTS, L., & SANDLIN, R. (1998). Comparing the performance of the Widex Senso with analog hearing aids. *Journal of the American Academy of Audiology, 9*;342–360.

VALENTE, M., POTTS, L., & VALENTE, M. (1996). Clinical procedures to improve user satisfaction with hearing aids. In: H. Tobin (Ed.), *Practical hearing aid selection and fitting* (pp. 75–93). Baltimore: Department of Rehabilitation Research and Development in the Office of the Department of Veteran Affairs.

VALENTE, M., SAMMETH, C.A., POTTS, L., WYNNE, M.K., WAGNER-ESCOBAR, M., CAUGHLIN, M. (1997). Benefit and satisfaction between the Oticon MultiFocus and Resound BT2E. *Journal of the American Academy of Audiology, 8*;280–293.

VAN TASELL, D., LARSEN, S., & FABRY, D. (1988). Effects of an adaptive filter hearing aid on speech reception in noise by hearing-impaired subjects. *Ear and Hearing, 9*;15–21.

VILLCHUR, E. (1973). Signal processing to improve speech intelligibility in perceptive deafness. *Journal of the Acoustical Society of America, 53*;1646–1657.

VILLCHUR, E. (1978). A critical survey of research on amplitude compression. *Scandinavian Audiology Supplement, 6*;305–314.

PREFERRED PRACTICE GUIDELINES

Professionals Who Perform The Procedure(s)

▼ Dispensing audiologists
▼ Adequately trained and licensed traditional hearing aid specialists

Expected Outcomes

▼ Aided performance in quiet should be significantly better than unaided performance in quiet
▼ Aided performance in noise should be significantly better than unaided performance in the same listening environment
▼ Aided performance in noise is *not* going to be as satisfactory as aided performance in quiet
▼ Soft speech should be audible; average speech, comfortable; and loud speech, loud, but not uncomfortable
▼ The earmold should be comfortable
▼ The user's own voice should be "acceptable"
▼ No feedback
▼ All the previous expectations should be achieved to have a successful fitting

Clinical Indications

▼ When the acoustic, occupational, and societal demands and wishes of a patient are such that conventional amplification may not be sufficient

Clinical Process

▼ Selection of appropriate device based on:

1. Necessary features
2. Style
3. Cost
4. Dispenser comfort with the product

▼ Setting frequency response

1. Prescriptive formulas
2. Real-ear measures with multiple input levels
3. Coupler measures with multiple input levels
4. Manufacturer's algorithms

▼ Setting compression and output characteristics

1. Prescriptive formulas
2. Real-ear measures with multiple input levels
3. Coupler measures with multiple input levels
4. Manufacturer's algorithms

▼ Setting multiple programs

1. Prescriptive programs (for noise, music, telephone, etc.)
2. Real-ear measures with multiple input levels
3. Coupler measures with multiple input levels
4. Manufacturer's algorithms

▼ Use of real-ear and coupler measures to assess performance of devices having digital speech/noise recognition algorithms
▼ Minimizing occlusion perception
▼ Counseling regarding realistic expectations, benefits, and limitations

Documentation

▼ Documentation including records of past fittings
▼ Questionnaires and surveys indicating current needs
▼ Electroacoustic and real-ear analyses
▼ Parameter settings
▼ Documentation of compliance with federal and state guidelines
▼ Information regarding ordering and receiving of hearing aids, earmolds, etc.

Chapter 14

Counseling and Orientation Toward Amplification

David Citron, III

Outline

Counseling is perhaps the most overlooked aspect of the process of fitting amplification and at the same time is probably the most important professional service an audiologist can provide for patients and their families (Garstecki & Erler, 1997). Most audiologists perceive counseling as orientation in the care and use of amplification (Wilkinson, 1995). Certainly, this is a critical part of the audiological rehabilitation process. However, it is clear that such a narrow focus on "product solutions" is only one small portion of a set of necessary components of audiological rehabilitation. O'Neill (1988) raised the issue of why so many hearing instrument patients fail to accept and use amplification. Smedley and Schow (1990) investigated this problem by surveying adult hearing aid candidates and found that poor use patterns were secondary to certain aspects of the patient's hearing impairment, the nature of the hearing aid technology, and unrealistic expectations from the use of amplification. Reports from unsuccessful users included "worthless in noisy settings, a damn nuisance, making them nervous, and feeling uncomfortable." It is evident that a large patient population requires counseling support during the amplification process, and it is critical that audiologists deliver these helping skills directly to

their patients or provide an appropriate referral to a mental health professional.

This chapter will provide an extensive overview of the counseling and orientation processes, along with the importance of differentiating these services from each other. An additional goal of this chapter is to furnish the necessary tools for training audiologists in the use of basic helping skills. Audiologists will then be able to deliver hearing instrument fittings in which (1) psychological barriers to the use of amplification are identified, (2) appropriate strategies in managing those barriers are implemented, (3) a balanced picture of the advantages and limitations of amplification are presented to the patient, and (4) management and resolution of psychological barriers occur before hearing instrument fitting. Patients must realize the importance of accepting their hearing impairment and the aspects of adapting to hearing aid use before the actual fitting process.

PEARL

Appropriate management of psychological barriers to the use of amplification will reduce hearing instrument returns and in-the-drawer (ITD) hearing aid nonuse.

COUNSELING VERSUS ORIENTATION

A common mistake made by audiologists is to define counseling as providing information as a part of the hearing aid orientation process. It is easy to see how this misconception occurs, because most dictionaries provide the same ambiguity in their definitions of counseling and orientation. For instance, *The American Heritage Dictionary of the English Language* (1992) and *Webster's New Twentieth Century Dictionary–Unabridged* (1996) define *counseling* as "advice or guidance, especially as solicited from a knowledgeable person." *Orientation* is defined as "an adjustment or adaptation to a new environment, situation, custom, or set of ideas; introductory instruction concerning a new situation." *Merriam-Webster's Collegiate Dictionary* (1993) defines *counseling* as "professional guidance of the individual by utilizing psychological methods, esp. in collecting case history data, using various techniques of the personal interview, and testing

Audiology: Treatment. Edited by Valente, Hosford-Dunn, and Roeser. Thieme Medical Publishers, Inc., New York © 2000

interests and aptitudes," whereas *orientation* is defined as "to set right by adjusting to facts or principles; to acquaint with existing situation or environment." If we apply these principles to audiology and amplification, it appears that we often ignore the "psychological aspects" of the counseling process, particularly *affect* or "emotional"-based phenomena.

Affect

One measure of separation between counseling and orientation is the identification of patient affect. Most audiologists receive little or no training in managing patient affect. Affect can best be described as "feeling" states. Certainly, any of these can be present in our patients, and the keys in audiological counseling are the recognition and management of affective behaviors. When these emotional reactions are unchecked, they can be increased to the point where they cause severe lifestyle and personality changes.

Rezen and Hausman (1985) state that anyone who undergoes a physical or emotional change goes through the same stages of *denial, projection, anger, depression,* and *acceptance.* These categories are similar to those described by Kubler-Ross (1969) for patients coping with death and dying. All patients will not always move from one stage into the other but will experience at least one of the following until they come to grips with their hearing impairment. Defining and understanding these emotional stages are critical in effective counseling.

Denial is an expected initial reaction if someone is faced with a threat to their physical or emotional health. Acceptance of hearing impairment is certainly unpleasant, and denial creates a mechanism for the patient's emotions to "stall for time" to build up the necessary emotional energy to come to grips with their problem. The slow, progressive nature of hearing impairment can make denial an easy alternative because the change in hearing sensitivity is often so gradual that it is frequently not discernible to the patient. Denial can often be carried to extreme lengths by patients to avoid dealing with their hearing impairment. For instance, a spouse can bring to the attention of the patient that he or she did not understand most of the communication that occurred at the social function that they just attended. "Baloney," replies the patient. "The conversations were so boring that I did not care to listen to any of it. I can hear when I want to hear." It is clear that this will almost always cause emotional distress within the family, and it will not change until the patient realizes a problem exists and wishes to deal with it in an effective fashion. Often, patients are stuck in this stage for some time and practice the philosophy of Lucy Van Pelt from "Peanuts" who said, "No problem is so big or so complicated that it cannot be run away from." Denial is not a river in Egypt.

Projection is the next effective avoidance measure and involves shifting the blame for the hearing impairment to another person. A common example of projection is the patient who responds, "I hear fine, people mumble. If everyone would stop their mumbling, I would hear just fine. Especially, my wife." They may also blame the acoustics of the room for not being able to hear the TV unless it is turned to loud levels. This is a similar patient defense mechanism, but many elderly patients are convinced that the youth of the 1990s all mumble and do not produce speech in a clear fashion. Just as in the case of denial, erroneous lack of awareness of the slow, progressive

nature of hearing impairment can lead to projection. The underlying psychological behavior is that nothing is better than a good scapegoat to avoid solving a problem.

Anger typically follows projection and usually involves a general sense of anger at things in general or may be anger directed at a specific individual, most often the significant other in the patient's everyday life. No question exists that anger can cause a breakdown in the most solid family relationships. However, significant others must take care in managing patients who exhibit anger in that they can reinforce the lack of positive behavior in dealing with their hearing impairment. For instance, the husband who tells his wife, "You did not hear anything at the Waxmans' last night and made me feel like a real idiot," can often serve to reinforce the patient's anger and defensiveness. Angry patients may also say: "If you are frustrated to be with me, why don't you go out by yourself?"

Depression develops once the anger is spent and is often accompanied by a sense of isolation and further withdrawal. A sense of lethargy grows, and some patients will be acutely aware that the birds no longer chirp, television seems distorted, and traffic noises once heard from the living room have faded. Patients may internalize their embarrassment of their lack of receptive communication and subsequently impose a long-term isolation. Depressed patients will state, "I know I cannot hear well, but I don't mind having to ask my family to repeat things" or "I just don't think that I can face my friends the Gilmans again because I feel so ashamed of my hearing loss." In some patients, this sense of isolation can last for many years before they seek help for their hearing impairment.

Acceptance occurs when depression fades, and the patient finally realizes that the problem lies not with themselves but with their hearing. This is the only stage in which patients can take action to seek treatment for their hearing impairment. They come to the realization that they do not wish to be deprived of positive life experiences and understand that they cannot communicate effectively in certain situations. It is well documented in the mental health literature that elderly patients manifest denial, projection, anger, and depression as a result of other psychological problems within their lives (Novalis et al, 1993). This can be illustrated with the following case.

Case Vignette

An 80-year-old woman arrived at our facility for amplification consultation accompanied by her daughter. She had recently undergone audiological evaluation at a hospital in Boston, and test results demonstrated a bilateral mild-to-moderately severe sensorineural hearing loss. Although the patient's daughter was completing the necessary forms, the patient sat in the waiting room with her arms folded tightly across her chest, with a sad waxen facial expression. She maintained both postures in the examination room. When asked by the audiologist to "tell me about your hearing loss," she replied, "I'm here because of her," and pointed to her daughter. When asked to elaborate, the patient stated that "I know that I cannot hear well, but I have no problems having to ask people to repeat." Further case history information revealed recent vision deterioration that necessitated an end to driving, as well as a recent move into the daughter's residence. She clearly had no motivation to pursue amplification, and when it was discussed with her that she had to be self-motivated to seek help, the patient asked, "Aren't you going to try to talk me into it?" At the end of the session, the patient did ask if she could speak with two of our patients who were successful users of amplification. After receiving permission from two patients who were similar in age and lifestyle, their names and phone numbers were forwarded to the patient's daughter. Four months passed, and the two patients were never contacted; the patient did return subsequently for amplification consultation, and thanked the audiologist for not "pressuring" her to pursue amplification when she was not motivated.

Clearly, this patient had depression that was a result of a myriad of other issues in her life and not just hearing impairment. If hearing aid use was "pushed," nonuse or a return for credit was likely. In this case she needed time to deal with the recent changes in her life and ultimately was able to accept her hearing impairment. Despite the fact that this patient decided to move in a positive direction to accept her hearing impairment and pursue amplification, the orientation session and follow-up visits illustrated some interesting behaviors.

During the amplification consultation session, the patient was questioned as to whether she was "ready" to pursue hearing aid use. Some degree of apprehension was displayed, and the patient stated that she was not certain that she would be able to physically operate the hearing aids. Practice with replica instruments was helpful to reassure the patient that she could change the battery and insert/remove the instruments with little or no difficulty. As well, she appeared to understand that an adjustment and orientation period was normal for all new users of amplification.

Throughout the course of the fitting session, the patient displayed a constant attitude of apprehension about the entire concept of hearing aid use. When informed that it would take a few weeks to adjust to hearing her voice differently and the audibility of new sounds, she displayed the same physical posture of her arms folded tightly across her chest and stated, "This is all so complicated and overwhelming." In addition to constant reassurance to the patient that these were normal feelings of new users, she was placed on a wearing schedule that would permit a more gradual acclimatization to hearing aid use. Her daughter, who accompanied her to the fitting session, was motivated to provide positive support for her mother during the initial weeks of hearing aid use. Despite all the positive encouragement, the patient requested that she not wear the instruments home and begin a gradual introduction of amplification at home. A follow-up visit was scheduled for 2 weeks.

At the time of the follow-up visit, the patient and her daughter arrived approximately 15 minutes late. After waiting about 10 minutes and remarking to her daughter that "I have not used these that much and do not know if I will keep them," they could not wait any longer and decided to leave the office.

The patient did return for further follow-up 3 weeks later. She reported that she has begun to adapt to hearing new sounds again and has experienced significant improvement in communication. Despite those positive interactions, she stated that it was still "an effort" to use the hearing aids consistently and that in many ways she was "happier without them."

If we examine this patient's history, it is apparent that she is depressed from all the other "issues" in her life and that any change from her depressed state is too large of an emotional jump for her to make. Certainly, her behavior during the fitting session could have been a predictor, but how much user apprehension is acceptable? How much "encouragement" can

we provide before it is clear that we are pushing the patient into something that they do not want and may not use?

Often, patients will have other problems in their lives such as recent loss of spouse, serious illness, or changes in lifestyle that are not related to hearing impairment. Many patients will be able to manage these issues successfully and accept their hearing loss, whereas others will be "stuck." During the course of the interview, patients will make it apparent how they cope with age-related changes in their health and lifestyle. Many will often state, "They call it the golden years . . . it certainly has not been golden for me, but I'm ready to seek help." At the same time, we have seen patients in rehabilitation facilities where relearning to walk, feed themselves, and fasten their clothes are far higher priorities than obtaining amplification. Most of these patients will seek help for their hearing loss when they are less burdened with more pressing medical and personal problems.

Theory of the Psychology of Hearing Impairment

What are the sources of denial, projection, anger, and depression that we observe in many of our patients? A better understanding of the processes that transform individuals into these psychological states can provide valuable assistance for audiologists in learning to manage their patients and assist them in receiving help for their hearing impairment.

One of the more popular theories of the bases of psychological disorders is described by Beck (1979) and is known as *cognitive therapy*. He states that humans manage to approach external forces around them much like a scientist in that they make observations, set up hypotheses, check their validity, and eventually form generalizations that will subsequently serve as a guide for making quick judgments of situations. Throughout the course of their development, humans use the basics of the experimental method without recognizing it. The person acquires an array of techniques and generalizations that enable judgment as to whether he or she is reacting realistically to situations; to resolve conflicts; and to deal with rejection, disappointment, and danger. By virtue of personal experience and emulation of others, the individual learns to make use of the tools of common sense: forming and testing hunches, making discriminations, and reasoning. The individual also uses these tools to fine-tune observations and reasoning over time.

A good example of this process is driving an automobile. We learn that when the traffic signal turns yellow, we slow down and get ready to stop. Of course, a red signal means stop. We also discover how to react quickly to various driving conditions such as cars pulling out quickly in front of us, tailgaters, and operating the vehicle in snow and ice. This "learning and reasoning" may have occurred initially in a small town in Ohio. A further need to test hypotheses and reason may need to occur on moving to Boston. Drivers in Boston believe that a yellow light means "speed up" and will always attempt to speed through the intersection before it turns to red. Often, many drivers will accelerate when the light turns red before their vehicle enters the intersection. This is a part of the standard driving "culture," so that there is virtually no enforcement of this phenomenon by the local police. Unaware of the "culture," new residents will often slow down and stop at a yellow light, only to hear the screeching of brakes and honking horns from the cars behind them who fully intended to run the light. Wise reasoning will cause a change in the new resident's driving habits; they will soon learn that survival dictates that they accelerate when the signal turns to yellow.

Beck (1979) theorizes that psychological disorders occur from ordinary problems such as flawed learning, making incorrect inferences on the basis of insufficient or false information, with an inability to distinguish between imagination and reality. Our inner workings can suppress or twist around the signals from the outside so we may be completely out of phase with what is going on around us. Emotional disturbances can be related to the types of misconceptions an individual has experienced throughout cognitive development. In other words the deviant meanings create the cognitive distortions that form the essence of emotional disorders. This approach to the neuroses is known as *cognitive therapy* because reality testing, insight, learning, and introspection are all basically cognitive processes.

Beck (1979) describes the case of the compulsive hand washer as a good example of cognitive distortions. He spends exorbitant amounts of time scrubbing his hands and other exposed parts of his body. His explanation is that he is concerned that he may have come into contact with a germ that could produce a deadly disease if his exposed skin is not thoroughly scrubbed. The patient may even report that this fear is bizarre, yet he persists even though it has a severe impact on his career, social interactions, and recreation—even sleeping and eating.

On further exploration of the patient's thinking, the following is revealed: We learn that whenever he touches an object that might contain bacteria, he thinks that he may develop a serious disease. Simultaneously, he has a *visual image* of himself dying from the disease in a hospital bed. The combined thought and visual fantasy produce anxiety. To counteract and reduce his fear, he runs to the closest bathroom and starts to wash himself.

In treating these cases, Beck (1979) organizes a procedure in which he induces the patient to touch a dirty object in his presence. It is agreed before the session that there will be no chance for him to scrub his hands. Stripped of the opportunity for eliminating the germ-laden dirt, the patient begins to see himself in the hospital bed dying of the horrible disease. The visual fantasy occurs without warning and is so graphic that the patient actually believes he has the disease. As a result, he starts to cough, feels febrile and weak, and reports peculiar feelings all over his body. By interrupting his visual fantasy, Beck (1979) demonstrates to the patient that he is not sick—he continues to have his full strength, possesses no fever, and achieves breathing without coughing. The sequence of interrupting his visual image and prodding him to make a realistic assessment of his health relieves his fear of having contracted a serious disease and lowers his compulsion to wash his hands. This illustrates what a critical role the processes of visual fantasy and the related physical sensations based on self-suggestion play in certain psychological disorders.

The cognitive therapy theory reported by Beck (1979) has interesting application to the emotional aspects of hearing impairment. As hearing sensitivity deteriorates, the patient will apply the concept of "hypothesis testing." Some awareness may be present that the television is more difficult to perceive; raising the level of the television solves the problem.

Communication in restaurants has started to become more demanding; it must be the poor acoustics in the restaurant. Spouse's and grandchildren's voices appear faint and tough to discriminate; *they* must be mumbling. The resulting erroneous misinterpretation is that nothing is wrong with them, and it must be an external problem, whether it be the acoustics of the room, their spouse not speaking properly, or that the actors do not project their voices properly on the television. Thus the patient's thinking is unrealistic because it is derived from misconceptions that they experience numerous times in their daily environment.

Anger and depression occur as a further response to the fallacious thinking described by Beck (1979). Mistaken thoughts that constitute projection ("it is them—*they* mumble") lead to anger when the hearing-impaired individual is a recipient of "noxious verbal assault," which is an attack on their self-esteem. A significant other such as a spouse is the most common source of the verbal abuse. Typically, they will continually criticize the hearing-impaired person for his or her inability to communicate. The behavior of the offender indirectly exposes the individual to self-devaluation. Anger may be the first reaction: "If you are so embarrassed to go to the Clarks' with me, I can just stay home."

According to Beck (1979), depression develops when the person becomes sensitized by particular varieties of life situations, such as chronic rejection by peers or spouse. It could also be a chain of experiences that the patient views as diminishing in some fashion. Included in these experiences may be those that relate to their hearing impairment: frustration because they cannot always communicate in a consistent fashion; sadness caused by changed relationships with spouse, family, and friends; isolation from activities that they used to enjoy but are now difficult because of the hearing impairment. Patients may regard themselves as inadequate, unworthy, and deficient, and they are susceptible to attributing unpleasant events to their own deficiencies. They often become self-critical and blame themselves for their difficulties. Sadness, hopelessness, apathy, and subsequent loss of motivation can trigger depression.

Treatment of these emotional disorders through cognitive therapy can be integrated into the counseling process. Beck's (1979) protocol involves offering the patient productive procedures for conquering blurred perceptions, blind spots, and self-deceptions. It is called cognitive therapy because the main psychological *problem* and the psychological *treatment* are both concerned with the patient's thinking (or cognitions).

Many methods exist that can assist patients in making more realistic self-evaluations and linking them to their world. Beck (1979) describes an "intellectual" approach that identifies misconceptions, tests their validity, and substitutes more appropriate concepts. The need for change often occurs when the patient recognizes that the rules he or she has relied on to guide thinking and behavior ("people mumble") have served to deceive and defeat. "The "experiential" approach exposes the patient to experiences that are in themselves strong enough to change misinterpretations. Specific application of cognitive therapy techniques for hearing-impaired patients will be described in later sections on interviewing and consultation.

COUNSELING

Carl Rogers (1951), one of the pioneers in modern psychotherapy, stresses the importance of the counseling "relationship." Patients must possess a sense of "safety and freedom" to express their feelings and concerns and feel confident in the skills of their audiologist. The external environment is a critical component in providing comfort to the patient during the hearing aid counseling and selection process.

Comfort and emotional safety begin at the front desk of your facility. Are patients greeted in a timely and friendly fashion? Does the front office staff provide assistance in completing forms? Observe the telephone manners of your staff. How many times are patients placed on hold before they are appropriate served? How quickly can patients receive an appointment? Is there flexibility in scheduling appointments (early mornings, evenings, weekends) to accommodate patient needs? How frequently do patients have to wait past their scheduled appointment times?

Office layout and structure are equally important in creating a "counseling-friendly" environment. Chairs need to be comfortable and have arms so patients can move about in an easy fashion, and soft lighting (incandescent) is preferred for waiting areas. Examination and waiting areas must possess adequate space to accommodate wheelchairs and patients and their families. Magazines and audiology brochures should be current, well-organized, and within easy reach. Examination rooms must be neat and respect patient privacy. Sessions should only be interrupted in case of emergency. These issues may appear to be trivial, but successful counseling and hearing aid orientation can be limited if the professional environment does not create a sense of emotional safety and comfort.

Basics of Helping Skills

Most audiologists possess little or no training in basic helping skills. Our knowledge base of understanding hearing loss, amplification, and follow-up aural rehabilitation is exceptional, but do we know how to be good listeners and integrate our patients' emotions and attitudes in the audiological rehabilitation process? The intent is not for audiologists to become psychologists; the goal is to improve patient care and minimize in-the-drawer (ITD) hearing instruments and those returned for credit. In addition, training and understanding of basic helping skills will help audiologists to determine when patients need to seek further help from mental health professionals.

Helping Skills Model

Carkhuff (1993) has developed an excellent model for training basic helping skills. It is based on his theory that people are constantly undergoing *intra*personal processing, and it is the basic process for human growth and development. *Intra*personal processing involves exploring, understanding, and acting. This is a personal process in which the helpee (patient) relates to personally relevant experiences and transforms them into human actions for human purposes. In a strict sense, *intra*personal processing is quite similar to Beck's (1979) underlying theory behind cognitive therapy. This model will be reviewed in somewhat simplistic fashion; the

PHASES OF INTERPERSONAL PROCESSING

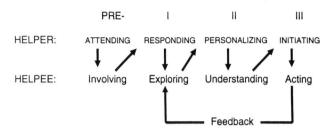

Figure 14–1 Phases of interpersonal processing. (From Carkhuff [1993], with permission.)

goal is to provide specific strategies that audiologists can use to improve their counseling skills.

*Inter*personal processing or helping skills facilitate the *intra*personal processing of others. The phases of interpersonal processing that compose Carkhuff's (1993) model are seen in Figure 14–1. Attending skills involve the helpees in the helping process. Responding skills expedite understanding by the helpees. Personalizing skills facilitate understanding by helpees. Initiating skills encourage acting by the helpees. Feedback that occurs from the helpee's actions recycles the stages of *intra*personal and *inter*personal processing.

Attending (Prehelping)

Attending involves communicating undivided attentiveness to the patient. It also serves to direct the audiologist's listening and observing skills to the patient's verbal and behavioral description of their experiences. As well, it functions to express a strong concern in the experiences of the patients and encourages them to become engaged in the helping process.

Physical attending is another important ingredient of prehelping. It is critical to posture ourselves to give complete and undivided attentiveness to the patient. This involves making eye contact, squaring by fully facing the patient, and leaning forward at least 20 degrees so that our forearms can rest on our thighs. Consistency in attentive behaviors communicates interest in the patient and his or her problems.

Yogi Berra, a member of baseball's Hall of Fame and premier philosopher, once said, "You can observe a lot by watching" (Berra, 1998). Observing consists of viewing the appearance and behavior of the patient. This can begin right in the waiting room by observing the patient's body movements, posture, grooming, and facial expressions. For instance, poor grooming, a slouched appearance, slow body movements, a furrowed brow, and downcast eye movements all suggest low energy level and minimal readiness for helping, whereas fast body movements and fidgeting can indicate anxiety.

Our ability to listen and respond to the verbal expressions of the patient are most critical in the helping process. Certainly, listening is hard work and necessitates deep concentration. Carkhuff (1993) describes numerous ways to sharpen our listening skills, which include having a purpose for listening, suspending our judgments or preexisting attitudes, focusing on the patient and the content, and recalling the patient's verbal and nonverbal expressions while listening for common themes. For instance, we can observe and process the patient's verbal and nonverbal expressions while listening for common themes in the same fashion that we listen for common themes in the patient's experiences with amplification. We often reprogram hearing instruments after we listen to and process patient's verbal descriptions of their amplification experiences. In the same fashion, we learn about patient's emotional attitudes and readiness to seek help from listening and processing their verbal and nonverbal expressions. Some excellent case studies are presented by Carkhuff (1993) to provide practice in developing helping skills.

Stage I: Responding

Responding consists of responding to the content, feelings, and meaning of the patient's expressions. *Responding to content* helps to clarify the basics of the patient's experiences, whereas *responding to feelings* identifies the affect that is a part of the experience. Clarification of the reason for the feeling occurs by responding to meaning.

Naturally, the first step is to respond to the content of the patient's expressions. This is accomplished by using Carkhuff's (1993) "5 Ws":

Who and *what* was involved? *What* did they do? *Why* and *how* did they do it? *When* and *where* did they do it?

This will help the audiologist to organize the patient's thoughts. A good response does not "parrot" back the statement but rephrases the expression in a fresh fashion. An appropriate response format is:

"You are saying that _____."
or
"In other words _____."

Responding to feeling is perhaps the most critical of helping skills because it mirrors the patient's emotional experience of themselves in relation to their everyday world. Most of us are uncomfortable in relating to patients in the affective domain. A simple way to think during patient interchanges is, If I were the patient, how would I feel? Carkhuff (1993) organizes these different emotions into seven different categories: (1) happy, (2) sad, (3) angry, (4) scared, (5) confused, (6) strong, and (7) weak. Table 14–1 provides a breakdown and classification of these feelings. This can provide valuable assistance in expanding our feeling vocabulary. Having a laminated copy of a "feelings table" within easy reach in an examination room can greatly assist the audiologist in the development of good helping skills. It is best to first choose the general feeling category (happy, sad, angry, scared, confused, strong, or weak) and the severity of the feeling (high, medium, or low). We then select the statement that reflects the content and intensity of the feeling. This can then be presented to the patient in the following format:

"You feel (*very sad*)."
With further practice, general feelings can be transferred into more specific feelings:
"When I feel (*depressed*),
I feel (*lost*)."

Because human feelings represent the most basic quality of human experience, it becomes critical for the audiologist to understand and identify the affective forces that patients bring into the hearing rehabilitation process. Learning to respond to emotional issues can help to facilitate appropriate counseling.

Proper responses to the affect and content of the patient's statements are not adequate. According to Carkhuff (1993),

TABLE 14–1 Categories of feelings grouped according to intensity and affect state

Levels of Intensity	Categories of Feelings						
High	**Happy**	**Sad**	**Angry**	**Scared**	**Confused**	**Strong**	**Weak**
	Excited	Hopeless	Furious	Fearful	Bewildered	Potent	Overwhelmed
	Elated	Depressed	Seething	Afraid	Trapped	Super	Impotent
	Overjoyed	Devastated	Enraged	Threatened	Troubled	Powerful	Vulnerable
	___	___	___	___	___	___	___
	___	___	___	___	___	___	___
	___	___	___	___	___	___	___
Medium	Cheerful	Upset	Agitated	Edgy	Disorganized	Energetic	Incapable
	Up	Distressed	Frustrated	Insecure	Mixed-Up	Confident	Helpless
	Good	Sorry	Irritated	Uneasy	Awkward	Capable	Insecure
	___	___	___	___	___	___	___
	___	___	___	___	___	___	___
	___	___	___	___	___	___	___
Low	Glad	Down	Uptight	Timid	Bothered	Sure	Shaky
	Content	Low	Dismayed	Unsure	Uncomfortable	Secure	Unsure
	Satisfied	Bad	Annoyed	Nervous	Undecided	Solid	Bored
	___	___	___	___	___	___	___
	___	___	___	___	___	___	___
	___	___	___	___	___	___	___

Reprinted with permission from Carkhuff, R. (1993). *The art of helping IV*. Amherst, MA: HRD Press.

feelings must be integrated with content to provide patients with emotional meaning to their expressions. It is based on the principle of cause and effect in that every feeling is precipitated by some particular reason or causes.

PEARL

One of the most important objectives in counseling is to recognize the patient's reason for each true feeling.

It is easy to practice responding to feeling and content by using examples in our own lives, then extending them into typical patient expressions:

Feeling	Content
"I feel happy	because I was promoted."
"I feel sad	because my son moved away."
"I feel upset	about my sister's divorce."

Stage II: Personalizing Meaning

Stage II of Carkhuff's (1993) model involved personalizing the meaning of the patient's experiences and expressions. It is probably the most demanding helping skill to master and use during counseling. It tends to happen over a long time and may exceed the format of the typical hearing aid consultation session. However, it can provide the necessary information to assess the emotional stage of the patient and whether the patient is close to setting goals to resolve hearing problems. Personalization consists of introducing the patient's experiences into the responses by use of the format "You feel (*feeling*) because *you* (*meaning, problem or goal*)." We can apply this to the patient with impaired hearing by using the following examples:

Personalizing meaning:
"You feel frustrated because you wish people would stop mumbling."

Personalizing problems:
"You feel sad because you cannot understand your grandchildren."

Personalizing goals:
"You feel upset because you cannot hear at Rotary and you want to stay active." Ultimately, personalizing goals can shift into decision making and action to begin to take positive steps toward problem solving.

Stage III: Initiating to Facilitate Acting

During the final stage of Carkhuff's (1993) helping process, the audiologist assists the patient in a program for action (amplification). It is important for the audiologist to define and focus the patient's personalized goals in developing an action plan. Implementing the program will resolve the patient's problem and achieve his or her goals. Feedback is necessary throughout this stage. Often, a patient will cling to emotional barriers such as depression while initiating solving the hearing problem. This occurred in the case vignette that was described earlier. Feedback involves recycling into those emotions that can serve to block acting. For instance, in the case vignette, even though the patient was willing to pursue amplification, her depression still served to make the

process difficult; every step along the way felt "overwhelming." The plan was subsequently modified to "ease" her into the amplification experience. The acting stage requires hard work and high motivation on the part of the patient. Many will succeed with support and encouragement; others will border the emotional line so that any negative experience during the process (i.e., poor shell fit) will result in termination of the amplification process.

Initial Interview

Certainly, the importance of a thorough patient case history cannot be overstated. It is a starting point to use the basic helping skills that have been described previously; it is the natural place in the counseling process to identify a patient's attitude toward his or her hearing impairment and the use of amplification.

After the medical portion of the case history, the audiologist can begin to inquire about the patient's perception of their hearing impairment and those of significant others. It is critical to include items that will probe for affect-based attitudes. Pertinent questions include:

- *"Tell me about your hearing loss."*
- *"When is it most noticeable?"*
- *"How does your spouse/family feel about it?"*
- *"How does it affect watching television?"*
- *"How does it affect going to church/synagogue?"*
- *"How does it affect the movies/theater?"*
- *"How does it affect social gatherings with family and friends?"*
- *"Have there been any recent changes in your lifestyle over the past few years?"*
- *"What changes in your vision or general health have occurred over the past few years?"*
- *"Have you, any family members, or friends ever used hearing aids?"*
- *"What size and type of instrument(s) were worn and for how long?"*
- *"Tell me about your/their experiences with amplification."*
- *"How do you feel about wearing amplification?"*

This list is not designed to be all-inclusive but will furnish the necessary information concerning the patient's emotional attitude toward their hearing impairment and the use of amplification. For instance, the practitioner can identify whether the individual is in denial, projection, anger, depression, or acceptance; appropriate helping strategies can subsequently be used to address the emotional barriers to amplification. It can also serve to recognize preconceived beliefs the patient may possess about the advantages and limitations of hearing aid use.

Validation of affect can begin to take place during the initial interview. Use appropriate statements such as "I understand how frustrating it is to feel like people are mumbling all the time" or "I know how confined you feel since you have moved in with your daughter." These validation techniques improve the counseling "relationship" and provide an inner sense to the patient that "the audiologist understands what I'm feeling." Management of these affect-based behaviors are best accomplished when the test results are reviewed or during a hearing aid consultation session. Inappropriate intervention early in the counseling process with a statement such as, "People do not mumble; you have a hearing loss" can only serve to create a confrontational counseling relationship.

Postassessment Interview/Consultation

After the completion of the audiological evaluation, it is customary to review the test results with the patient and any significant others. The importance of having the patient understand the audiogram and the effects of hearing loss on communication cannot be overstated. Explanation of the audiometric data needs to be detailed but understandable.

Several different strategies are effective in describing the patient's audiogram and its effects on communication. Harford and Curran (1997) use shading critical areas of the audiogram that affect communication, along with an overlay that contains vowels and critical consonants, which can be laid over the audiogram. This is illustrated in Figures 14–2 and 14–3. Figure 14–2 shows an audiogram with a typical high-frequency sensorineural hearing impairment, with shading in the area of the hearing loss. Figure 14–3 illustrates the critical consonants and vowels that can subsequently be placed over the patient's audiogram. The "Count the Dot" articulation function (Mueller & Killion, 1990) can also be used to show how much critical speech information is missing as a function of the patient's hearing loss. It is necessary for patients who exhibit word recognition scores that are poorer than 70% to understand the limitations of poor word recognition and its impact on hearing aid performance.

Our center uses a modified version of the method described by Harford and Curran (1997). The audiogram and its configuration is reviewed with the patient and significant other. A modified item from the California Consonant Test (Owens & Schubert, 1977) is selected:

cheek, chief, cheese, cheap, cheat.

It is explained to the patient that the softer consonants in our language (/k/ /t/ /z/ /p/ and /f/) supply the critical information in speech, whereas the vowels are much louder and do not carry much information. It is easy for the patient to "see" that by changing one consonant, the meaning of the entire word changes, and the frequency range of the patient's hearing impairment is such that he or she cannot "hear" those softer consonants, especially if the speaker is a woman or child. We also use an anatomical chart to explain how the hair cells are damaged much like a worn carpet and do not "grow back" once they are altered. Often, patients will have the erroneous notion that they have "nerve deafness" and that their "nerve" is just fine. As well, they are often told by their physician that amplification will not help "nerve deafness." The use of the chart and audiogram can act as tools to facilitate patient education and help to indicate to the patient that most successful hearing aid fittings are on individuals who physicians refer to as having "nerve deafness." Certainly, patients can then turn around and educate their family and friends about the erroneous concept of "nerve deafness."

PEARL

The use of visual aids to explain the effect of high-frequency hearing loss on communication will assist in resolving the patient's erroneous assumption that "people are mumbling." Using the term "sensorineural hearing loss" is too technical for most patients. Our practice uses the preferred term "inner ear or hair cell damage."

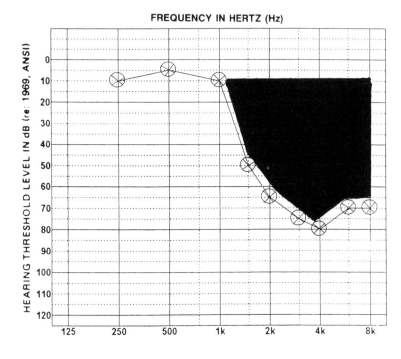

FREQUENCY IN HERTZ (Hz)

Figure 14–2 A typical high-frequency hearing loss with the area of loss shaded. (From Harford & Curran [1997], with permission.)

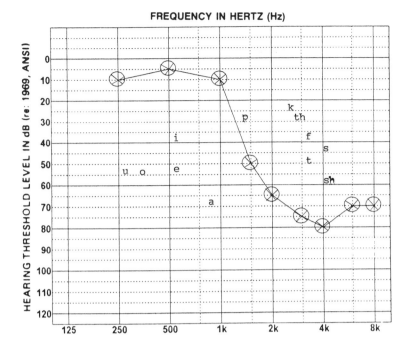

Figure 14–3 A typical high-frequency hearing loss. Critical high-frequency consonants and vowels can be laid over the audiogram in the form of a transparency. (From Harford & Curran [1997], with permission.)

This is also the point in the counseling process in which the principles of Beck's (1979) "erroneous assumptions" can be implemented. It is critical to communicate simply and clearly to the patient that their hearing impairment is very slow in its progression so that they are often unaware that it is changing, and it is very common for others around them to be more conscious of the deterioration in their hearing sensitivity. In addition, it is the softer "information-loaded" consonants that they cannot perceive, so that the false impression they receive is that "people are mumbling." It is also important to share with the patient that their communication problems are often situational, and it is perfectly normal for them to experience an array of environments where they will communicate effectively. In the words of Dr. Mark Ross, "The biggest problem with hearing loss is that you don't know what you don't hear."

An appropriate follow-up to the effects of gradual hearing loss on the perception of softer consonant sounds is to provide a transition into hearing aid consultation. Patients can be questioned about their feelings and attitudes concerning hearing aid use and provided with preliminary basic information about the improvements in hearing aid technology. They can be informed that newer technologies can now boost the softer sounds that they cannot perceive so that they can understand speech in a much clearer fashion without overamplification of the louder, annoying sounds such as dish noises and paper rattling. As a result, they will not have to lower the volume or remove the instruments every time there is a louder sound in their listening environment. Many patients will feel overwhelmed by this process and will require time to digest the information, accept their hearing impairment, and feel comfortable enough to move forward into using amplification. In our practice those patients are given brochures that describe general facts about hearing loss and hearing aids, as well as new technologies and how they differ from conventional instruments. Most are scheduled for a full hearing aid consultation within a week's time, which will review the various hearing aid technologies, sizes, and

fee structure. Those individuals who are still in denial, projection, anger, or depression and are not ready to pursue amplification are also given information and encouraged to return for consultation once they are ready to receive help. Our experience with this population shows that most will return within a time frame that varies from 1 week up to 5 years; others return with instruments purchased elsewhere that are sitting in the drawer. Another group of individuals will continue to search for a reason to avoid dealing with the problem. An audiologist with good helping skills may be able to isolate the patient's emotional barrier that prevents him or her from moving forward; a well-trained mental health professional may be necessary to facilitate positive change in the patient's emotional behavior.

CONSULTATION

A brief review of the patient's audiogram is often necessary when patients return for hearing aid consultation, as well as questions concerning how they feel about wearing amplification. It is critical that the typical patient apprehensions be validated while at the same time creating an emotionally positive atmosphere for evaluating amplification. Dawson (1985) describes the use of the feel-felt-found technique for helping patients to feel more comfortable with pursuing help for their hearing impairment. You can validate the feeling by stating that you understand how they feel and that many other patients have felt the same way about that issue. Finally, you can explain that you have studied the problem and have found a solution. That solution can certainly vary, depending on the specific concern, but will help to avoid confrontation and relate to the patient that you are attentive to their interests.

Personality Typing

Van Vliet (1997) describes an assortment of patient personality types known as high-risk users, which audiologists will frequently encounter during the process of audiological assessment and hearing instrument selection.

IMNB: *I'm not vein, but. . . .* These are individuals who will take one look at a behind-the-ear (BTE) instrument and feel faint. Vanity may not be the only issue for these patients. They may present with feelings that others will perceive them as infirm or disabled if the hearing instruments are "visible." Certainly, completely-in-the-canal (CIC) instruments can provide an alternative for these patients, but in many circumstances they may not be candidates for a CIC fitting because of dexterity issues, earcanal anatomical problems, audiometric constraints, or limitations resulting from above-average cerumen production.

SIHASP: *So, I have a slight hearing problem . . . thank goodness it is not enough for me to use amplification. . . .* The patients are not unlike those in denial or projection. Many patients are not ready to accept their hearing impairment and will often understate their handicap to avoid dealing with it.

DIHTWT: *Do I have to wear two. . . .* It is quite common for patients to feel "twice as deaf" wearing two instruments. In many circumstances, patients have just accepted their hearing impairment so it is a large emotional jump just to use one hearing instrument. Patients will frequently state, "Am I that bad?" Often, they will report that their best friends and relatives only wear one instrument and perform quite well, or they may mention that others remove one instrument in noise because everything is too loud. Financial issues may be a source of concern for patients, but more often it is the psychological "load" of two instruments. It is quite similar to the cane versus walker concept, in which individuals may feel much more handicapped and infirm with a walker than using "just a cane."

ICNST: *I could never spend that. . . .* Many patients are on minimal fixed incomes that may limit their ability to afford amplification. Many programs and foundations exist that can provide assistance to those in need. On a local level, service organizations such as Lions, Rotary International, Kiwanis, Knights of Columbus, or Quota have provided various levels of support. Hear Now, Starkey Foundation, Sertoma, and Miracle-Ear Children's Foundation are among those organizations that furnish financial aid for amplification on a national level. Specific information concerning these national organizations is found in the Appendix.

However, patients will often use financial limitations as an excuse to postpone or avoid dealing with their hearing impairment. Dychtwald and Flower (1989) report that members of the 50+ population: purchase 80% of all luxury travel, gamble more than any age group, spend more per capita in the supermarket than any other age group, own 77% of all financial assets in the United States, and, account for a whopping 40% of total consumer demand! Many individuals would much rather take that trip to Europe than to invest both financially and psychologically in their hearing impairment.

SATYA: *Same as 20 years ago. . . .* Audiologists will encounter patients who enter their offices wearing a 20-year-old linear behind-the-ear instrument with the original earmold and tubing attached. The user will request that the same instrument style, circuit, and original earmold be fitted while they wait. Discussions about new technologies and the importance of comprehensive audiological assessment are fruitless; these patients will reply "My hearing hasn't changed in 20 years . . . if it ain't broke, don't fix it." A formal

waiver may be an option for these patients; certainly detailed documentation in their record is a necessity.

IETLY: *If everyone talked like you. . . .* Most patient communication takes place in quiet rooms at distances that seldom exceed 4 feet; they are often unaware that hearing loss is not "black and white" and that their ability to communicate will depend on the listening environment. Projection will often serve as a convenient roadblock. They will often state, "You speak so clearly, but my husband and children mumble."

IUTIAE: *I understand that I'm an engineer. . . .* Some users have extreme confidence in knowing and understanding the technology to the point where they will attempt to control the entire hearing rehabilitation process. These patients will request a screwdriver so they can operate the instrument's trimmers; others will desire a copy of the programmable software so they can perform their own programming alterations. Many of these users will have unrealistic expectations of even the highest technologies and feel that by adjusting the acoustic characteristics, they can solve all of their problems. A fact-based approach is useful for "engineers"; descriptions of hair cell physiology and of studies that show that sensorineural-impaired patients require a more favorable speech-to-noise ratio (SNR) for accurate communication can be very helpful in managing this group of users.

WDYDBC: *What did you do before computers. . . .* Many patients can be phobic about computers; demonstrating programmable technologies in front of them can cause them to feel "overwhelmed" and that amplification is "much too complicated." Sometimes a simple explanation that before computers we had to keep sending the hearing aids back to the factory for changes may be helpful. For some individuals, the process needs to be made as simple as possible.

Traynor and Buckles (1997) report that identifying the user's personality style through a formal personality evaluation may provide helpful information into their hearing rehabilitative needs. They analyzed the Myers-Briggs Type Indicator (MBTI) (Myers et al, 1993), which is used on a large scale in many industries to furnish information concerning employees and believed that it could be applied to gain knowledge about the patient's personality type, learning style, and coping mechanisms for incorporation into the individual's hearing rehabilitation program.

The MBTI was developed on the basis of the theories of Jung (1974). He suggests that people are different in fundamental ways in that they possess different motivations, purposes, urges, aims, values, needs, impulses, and drives. None of these instincts are ranked as better or more important than another, but their value is in how they influence functional personal choices. Individual preferences for a specific function is indicative of how that person interacts with their instincts. The end result is that an individual can be "typed" according to his or her choices.

The MBTI is composed of 126 questions about individual preferences, diverse situations, and individual reactions to different word pairs. The scores are plotted with a point system that is adjusted according to gender and are presented as a tendency toward one end or the other of four opposite continuums.

Figure 14–4 shows the preference continuums for the MBTI. They are composed of opposite scales of extroversion (E)/introversion (I); sensing (S)/intuition (N); thinking

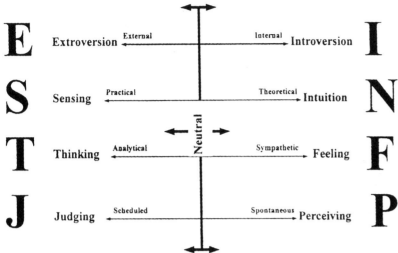

MBTI Preference Continuums

E   Extroversion $\xrightarrow[External]{}$ $\xleftarrow[Internal]{}$ Introversion   I

S   Sensing $\xrightarrow[Practical]{}$ $\xleftarrow[Theoretical]{}$ Intuition   N

T   Thinking $\xleftarrow[Analytical]{}$ Neutral $\xrightarrow[Sympathetic]{}$ Feeling   F

J   Judging $\xleftarrow[Scheduled]{}$ $\xrightarrow[Spontaneous]{}$ Perceiving   P

Figure 14–4   MBTI preference continuums. (From Traynor & Buckles [1997], with permission.)

(T)/feeling (F); and judging (J)/perceiving. Basically, the MBTI scores on these four continuums compose the 16 different personality types. The scores start at zero from the neutral position and become higher as one moves toward each end of the four different continuums. For instance, if the individual scores toward the "I" side of the first continuum and the "S" side of the second, the "F" side of the third and the "P" side of the fourth, the individual's personality type will be scored as ISFP.

Traynor and Buckles (1997) discuss the MBTI personality types in detail and their possible role in the aural rehabilitation process. In a recent study of 30 patients, they found that 80% of those identified by the MBTI as possessing extroverted personalities were satisfied with their first choice of amplification. These patients were often excited about the amplification process and very good communicators with the audiologist about the hearing aid selection process. Introverts, on the other hand, were more interested in receiving a highly detailed explanation of hearing aid technology as opposed to accepting the audiologist's rationale for hearing aid use. They need to be convinced of the benefit of the amplification before they use it. If introverts are comfortable enough in the counseling environment, they may be good candidates for in-office demonstration of the different hearing aid technologies.

Knowing and understanding these personality types is certainly important to serve our patients in a more thorough fashion; the time necessary to administer, score, and interpret a 126-item test can be excessive for most practice settings. Traynor and Buckles state that a retrospective study is necessary with at least 1600 patients to correlate audiological complaint to personality. Future research in personality assessment may assist in providing an amended or abridged version of the MBTI for use by audiologists.

Dawson (1985) describes four different personality styles as they relate to decision making and buying behavior. These individuals may be perfectly motivated to pursue amplification. Learning to understand and interact with individuals who manifest varying personality styles can produce a more successful counseling/orientation session. What follows is a description of these personality types and their application to the processes of counseling and orientation toward amplification.

The Pragmatic

Dawson (1985) describes the pragmatic individual as a fact-driven, bottom-line person. They will always try to get to the point of a topic and are very conscious of time management. As a result, pragmatic individuals will often surround themselves with time-efficiency gadgets like electronic personal organizers. Pragmatics will write their daily reports or read the *Wall Street Journal* while they are waiting in the audiologist's office; that behavior will continue while they wait for their ear impressions to harden. In their offices, they will almost always have their secretaries place their phone calls. As active individuals, pragmatics have difficulty sitting and watching anything; they are doers rather than listeners or watchers. You will not often see them sitting in the bleachers during a baseball game; they will either be on the tennis court or listening to the game on the radio while they write a memo. In a hearing aid consultation session, they will not desire folksy detailed explanations of every hearing aid technology; a quick synopsis of advantages and limitations will be more than sufficient. They will often state their preferences at the beginning of a consultation; many will even try to control the session. Pragmatics are strictly business and will often base any decision, including amplification, on facts. They will desire fee quotations, warranty information, loss damage protection, and service visit policies to be spelled out in very precise terms. The use of "approximately" will not sit well with a pragmatic. Programmable technology may appeal to the pragmatic in that no volume controls need to be adjusted, and many will like the "gadget" concept of multiple memories and remote controls.

The Extrovert

Dawson's (1985) second category are the extroverts who are quite motivated, emotional, very friendly, and easily impressed. Unlike the pragmatic, they enjoy an animated, folksy, humorous approach to life, and they love to share in the emotions of a crowd in a sporting event. They will get very excited over big issues, but will not always think things through in a complete fashion. Their offices are often cluttered with unfinished projects, but extroverts are willing to take risks and have a good sense of the ins and outs of business. Extroverts make quick decisions and are also quite emotional; they will see something they like and take to it almost immediately. They are not afraid to say no, but they will almost always do it in a friendly manner. Much like the pragmatic individual, the extrovert does not like detailed explanations but may need tempering of his or her often emotional responses.

The Amiable

The amiable is the third type of personality described by Dawson (1985). Amiables tend to be creatures of habit and frequently create obstacles around themselves. Many will have unpublished phone numbers and have "No Soliciting" signs on their homes and offices. They often make lifetime bonds to people and attachments to their homes, automobiles, and surroundings. The ambiance of an environment and middle-of-the road personality are often appealing to them. Amiables will have a difficult time buying a new automobile because of their bond to their old car and their fear and discomfort of being pressured by the salesman to trade it in. They tend to be very nice, warm, friendly, and observant people who will always remember the names of your children and identify the mood of a crowd. During a hearing aid consultation session, amiables will often want to have their 10-year-old hearing aid repaired because they do not wish to part with an old friend, or when it finally dies, they will want exactly the same instrument to replace it.

The Analytical

Analyticals comprise the final personality style described by Dawson (1985). The analytical individual is best recognized by their profession; they typically are accountants, engineers, mathematicians, or actuaries. They thrive on detail and are possessed by gadgetry, desiring to be the first on their block to acquire a combination TV remote, garage door opener, and digital cellular phone. Unlike a pragmatic person who seeks results, the analytical searches for causes of a problem. They will pursue every morsel of critical information that even remotely relates to an issue before attacking it. Analyticals are quite methodical and curious, wishing to digest every aspect of a question before they venture forth with a solution. They will devour detailed instrumentation manuals with gusto and will often phone the toll-free help lines with further requests. Because they are obsessed with facts and detail, they are punctual and like to have fees and contracts quoted to the penny. They tend to be withdrawn and prefer gadgets and details to relationships, but once they make a decision it will typically hold up in the most challenging of situations.

Most audiology practitioners have unique stories to share about analytical patients. Even the detailed digital hearing instrument brochures that are geared with an engineering slant are insufficient for some of these patients; they will check out the manufacturer's Web site, annual report, and wish to communicate with the company's director of research and development. Analyticals will also request schematics of the instrument's directional microphones and may ask for a copy of the programming software so they can make their own modifications. Remote controls and multiple memory instruments/microphone arrays can be their best friends. Before the development of programmable technology, analyticals would tend to carry a screwdriver with them to change their trimmer settings. It can be a frustrating experience to work with these patients; using anatomy and hair cell physiology along with constant orientation of the fact that the fitting process is not as "black and white" as they might think can be helpful in managing analyticals.

• • •

These personality styles are not necessarily neat and clean categories. No patients will have all of the attributes of one style of personality without possessing some of the characteristics of the others. Analyzing our own personality and how it fits into Dawson's (1985) scheme can be quite valuable.

Figure 14–5 illustrates how the four personality styles can be graphed according to degree of assertiveness and organizational level. It is divided into quadrants with the analyticals in the upper left-hand corner; the pragmatics in the upper right-hand corner; the amiables in the bottom left corner; and the extroverts in the bottom right corner.

The vertical line on the graph represents the organizational and emotional levels of the various personalities. Dawson (1985) suggests that the pragmatics and analyticals are very organized people who have an excellent sense of time management and completing projects, with very neat work spaces. Decisions are usually made in advance with a fair amount of insight and virtually no emotion.

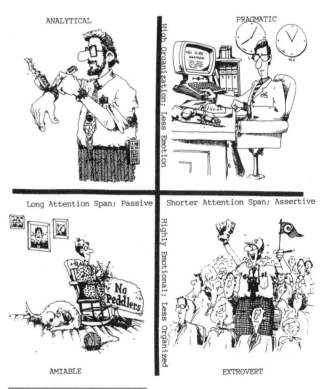

Figure 14–5 Personality styles. (From Dawson [1995], with permission.)

The opposite side of the organizational scale are the amiables and extroverts. They tend to make decisions and plan activities in a more spontaneous fashion, usually on the basis of emotion. Their working and home environments are unstructured, cluttered, and disorganized.

On the horizontal line are the levels of assertiveness and attention span of the four personality styles. High levels of assertiveness are on the right side of the graph. Extroverts and pragmatics possess strong degrees of assertiveness; they will volunteer in group activities because they want to lead. Both are aggressive types and will desire to take charge of situations. Amiables and analyticals, on the other hand, will rather do many other things than be the leader of an activity.

Analyticals and amiables on the left possess longer attention spans. Most analyticals will sit through an hour-long hearing aid consultation loaded with information about digital technology and leave feeling like they have just started the session. Amiables have very long-lasting relationships with everything around them, taking a long time to reach a decision on most issues, but will not analyze things as thoroughly as an analytical.

On the right-hand side of the graph are the extroverts and the pragmatics. They will encounter extreme difficulty sitting through a play or a board meeting and will always feel distracted by other matters that they must accomplish immediately. Pragmatics and extroverts became very unsettled when they have to sit and watch things for extended periods; they are ready to move on to the next life issue. These individuals will look at a proposal and reach a decision quickly, without requiring much time to mull things over.

Dawson (1985) states that conflicts arise when individuals of diverse personalities attempt to negotiate or communicate with each other. The maximum conflict occurs when personality styles in opposite quadrants on the graph interact. If you are a pragmatic or extrovert personality who practices fast decision making and you are in the middle of a hearing aid consultation with an analytical or amiable personality, their slow, methodical decision process will drive you crazy. On the other hand, amiables and analyticals may feel pressured by the fast decisions of pragmatics and extroverts and may abandon or withdraw from seeking further help for their hearing impairment. If you are interacting with a pragmatic, spend less time with small take and anecdotes.

It is apparent that slow decision makers feel threatened by rapid decision makers, and fast decision makers are irritated by methodical decision makers. Patient interaction sessions can flow more smoothly if you can discover the personality style of the patient. A self-assessment is quite valuable; once you have analyzed your own personality style, sources of conflict may be easier to perceive.

Matching Hearing Technology to Patient Needs

Bevan (1997) stresses that the hearing aid fitting system should take into account the needs of the real patient. Most patients will certainly state, "I want to hear better," but the specific lifestyle and communication needs of the patient will determine which specific technology is appropriate. Ask the patient to provide information regarding specific situations in which hearing instruments must solve their communication problems. These may include church, TV, club meetings,

sporting activities, movies, family gatherings, and so forth. In this counseling method the audiologist is an advocate and empowers the patient to make an informed choice.

One of the most successful retailers of discount designer apparel is Sy Syms whose radio and television advertisements feature the tag line "An educated consumer is our best customer." This is stressed to the patient and significant others, and they are briefed in the advancements in hearing aid technology, describing the changes from linear instruments into nonlinear instruments that do not require the use of a volume control and are programmed with a computer, including the innovation of dual microphone technology. It is important that the explanation avoid the use of technical terms and be brief; the sole purpose is to make the patient and significant others aware of the problems of the past and how hearing aid technology has improved. Many patients will enter the consultation session reporting a negative experience with amplification; being sensitive to those experiences and explaining the differences among technologies will help to improve the patient's confidence in pursuing amplification. *It should be emphasized that multiple strategies are available and that the specific amplification solution will depend on the nature of each persons' lifestyle and needs.*

PEARL

Determination of patient goals for amplification should take place before reviewing specific technology solutions.

Setting Realistic Expectations and Goals of Hearing Aid Use

Selection of hearing instrument technology will be made on the basis of the patient's communication needs and lifestyle. A needs assessment can be conducted using the Client Oriented Scale of Improvement (COSI) (Dillion et al, 1997), Abbreviated Profile of Hearing Aid Benefit (APHAB) (Cox & Alexander, 1995), or other self-assessment measure. Use of the COSI (Dillion et al, 1997) provides important information in helping to set patient-specific goals for amplification. A copy of COSI is seen in Figure 14–6. Up to five specific user needs are listed in order of significance at the time of the initial hearing aid consultation. It is critical that the listening needs are stated in a specific condition (e.g., "To communicate better with my spouse in a restaurant" as opposed to "To hear better in noise"). These individual requirements can also assist in selecting a particular type of hearing aid technology for each patient. For instance, if the most critical patient need is to communicate effectively while working in a large exhibit hall, a binaural digital system incorporating optional dual-microphones with multiple memories may be the optimum choice.

At the time of the patient's initial 3- to 4-week postfitting checkup, the COSI is completed. It is possible to measure how well the instruments performed relative to the patient's user requirements. The results can be used to pinpoint problem areas that may require further orientation or in-depth counseling if the patient has unrealistic expectations of hearing aid performance. At the time of the postfitting checkup, the

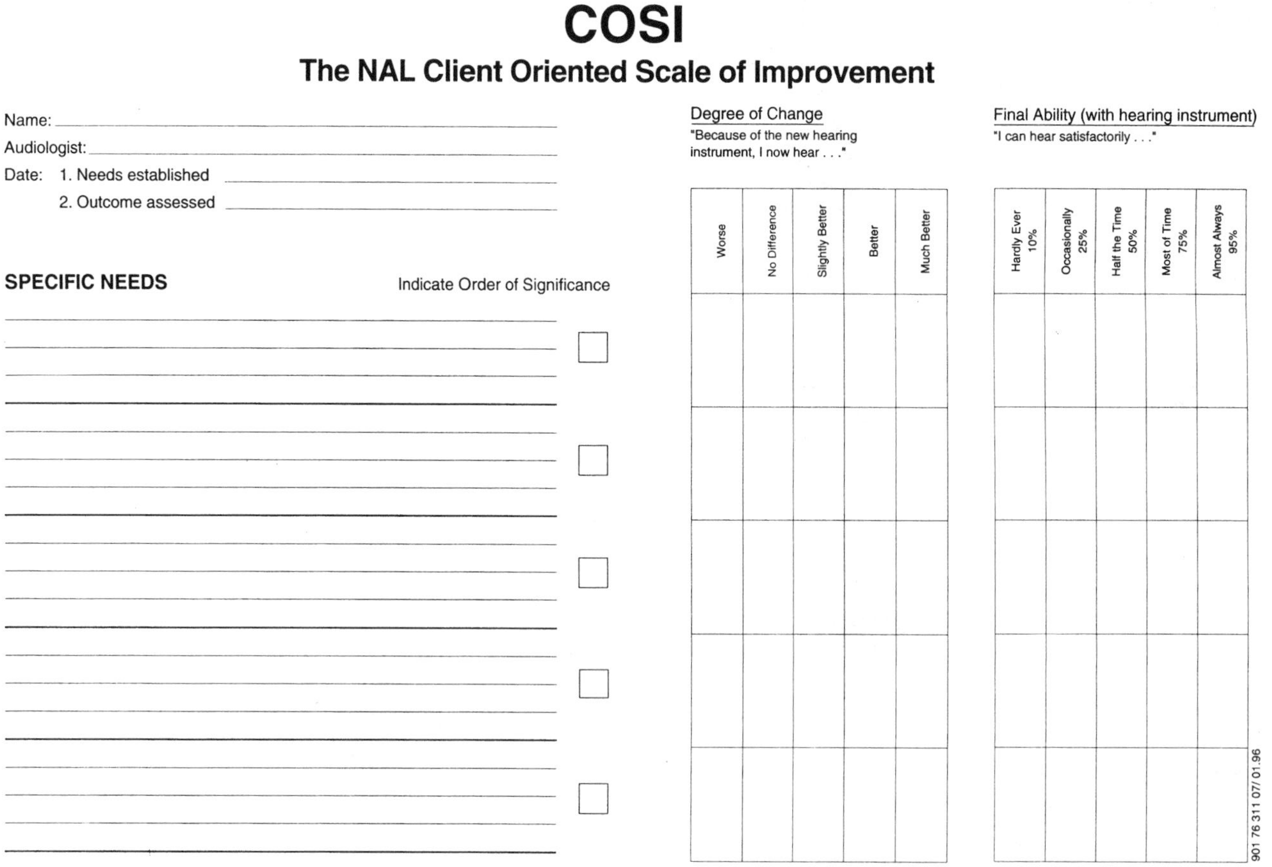

COSI
The NAL Client Oriented Scale of Improvement

Name: _____

Audiologist: _____

Date: 1. Needs established   _____

          2. Outcome assessed   _____

SPECIFIC NEEDS   Indicate Order of Significance

Degree of Change
"Because of the new hearing instrument, I now hear . . ."

Worse	No Difference	Slightly Better	Better	Much Better

Final Ability (with hearing instrument)
"I can hear satisfactorily . . ."

Hardly Ever 10%	Occasionally 25%	Half the Time 50%	Most of Time 75%	Almost Always 95%

901 76 311 07/ 01.96

Figure 14–6   The NAL Client Oriented Scale of Improvement (COSI). (From Dillion et al [1997], with permission.)

patient should reflect on his or her performance with amplification, followed by discussion of a specific degree of change for each particular user need. Final ability with the hearing instruments can also be quantified by having the patient summarize how often he or she can communicate successfully in each of the specific situations.

Conventional instruments may provide significant benefit if the patient's needs are for listening primarily in quiet environments. Many individuals find digitally programmable technology appealing in that it automatically adjusts itself to keep sounds within the comfort range, and many systems do not require a volume control so that the user does not have to worry about making volume adjustments. However, patients need to understand that several follow-up visits are often necessary to "fine-tune" the instruments on the basis of their communication needs, audiometric data, and individual interaction with the technology.

It is important to include the discussion of hearing aid limitations as a part of setting realistic goals for hearing instrument performance. Figure 14–7 describes expected benefits from amplification for both new and experienced users used by Valente and his colleagues at the Washington University School of Medicine's Adult Audiology Division. Copies can be given to users to help ensure realistic expectations from hearing aid use. Often patients will perceive that the hearing aids will "eliminate noise," based in part on some of the early consumer advertising on radio and television. Perhaps the

most significant statement in reviewing expected benefits is that the instruments will perform better in noise than without amplification but not as well as in a quiet environment. A frank discussion of the concept of SNR should contain some basic facts that sensorineural-impaired individuals require a more favorable SNR than normal listeners for effective communication, even with advanced technology instruments (Killion, 1997a). Patients with poorer word recognition will require education on how to use their vision appropriately and manipulate their listening environment to supplement their communication skills.

PEARL

Making the patient aware that hearing instruments are only one component of hearing rehabilitation will help to prevent unrealistic expectations of hearing aid performance.

Many patients fully comprehend the importance of binaural amplification, particularly in helping to optimize communication in the presence of noise. Others will react negatively ("You mean I have to wear two?"). The benefits of binaural amplification are stressed, particularly if their primary goal is improved communication in groups. We also

EXPECTED BENEFITS FROM AMPLIFICATION

- **INEXPERIENCED USERS**
  - **IN QUIET**, AIDED PERFORMANCE WILL BE SIGNIFICANTLY BETTER THAN UNAIDED PERFORMANCE
  - **IN NOISE**, AIDED PERFORMANCE WILL BE SIGNIFICANTLY BETTER THAN UNAIDED PERFORMANCE
  - HOWEVER, AIDED PERFORMANCE **IN NOISE** WILL NOT BE AS GOOD AS AIDED PERFORMANCE **IN QUIET**!
  - **SOFT SOUNDS** WILL BE SOFT, BUT AUDIBLE; **LOUD SOUNDS** WILL BE LOUD, BUT NOT UNCOMFORTABLE!

- **EXPERIENCED USERS**
  - **IN QUIET**, AIDED PERFORMANCE WILL BE SIGNIFICANTLY BETTER THAN AIDED PERFORMANCE WITH THE PREVIOUS HEARING AID
  - **IN NOISE**, AIDED PERFORMANCE WILL BE SIGNIFICANTLY BETTER THAN AIDED PERFORMANCE WITH THE PREVIOUS HEARING AID
  - HOWEVER, AIDED PERFORMANCE **IN NOISE** WILL NOT BE AS GOOD AS AIDED PERFORMANCE **IN QUIET**!
  - **SOFT SOUNDS** WILL BE SOFT, BUT AUDIBLE; **LOUD SOUNDS** WILL BE LOUD, BUT NOT UNCOMFORTABLE!

Figure 14–7 Expected benefits from amplification. (From Washington University School of Medicine, Adult Audiology Division; with permission.)

attempt to create a risk-free environment for patient evaluation in that they are free to return the second instrument if they do not find significant improvement from binaural use. Although some patients will fully understand the benefits of binaural amplification and the fact that they have a risk-free environment for evaluation, numerous patients will feel "twice as deaf" and are not yet ready to consider binaural amplification. Many of these patients have just reluctantly accepted their hearing impairment and feel that monaural amplification is a major emotional step. A large proportion of these individuals will ultimately upgrade from monaural to binaural amplification at a later date, which can vary from 1 month to many years.

In some practices where the patient desires a monaural fitting but a binaural fitting is recommended by the audiologist, patients are required to sign a legal release that states that "binaural amplification results in better long-term performance than one instrument." Typically, the primary basis behind a patient's preference for monaural amplification is the "psychological load" of two instruments. In our practice, we believe that presentation of such a form can serve to place a psychological barrier between the audiologist and the patient. After discussion of the benefits of binaural amplification, detailed notes are entered into the patient record that describe that binaural amplification was discussed and the reason(s) why monaural amplification was chosen.

Conventional Analog Instruments

This type of circuit performs reasonably well in quiet environments where most communication is on a one-to-one basis or the user has a prime goal of making the television or radio easier to understand without having to raise the volume to high levels. The addition of tone trimmers or compression may provide some additional flexibility and make it possible to communicate in small groups with minor amounts of background noise. Conventional instruments are most economical for those patients with financial limitations

but do not provide adequate boost for softer sounds, particularly in large groups where they can distort the output and make speech more difficult to perceive. If the patient has a goal of improved communication in environments that exceed performance in quiet situations, this circuit should be ruled out. Further discussion concerning the selection and fitting of conventional hearing instruments can be found in Chapter 12 in this volume.

Advanced Analog Instruments

Instruments with K-Amp technology (Killion, 1993) and wide dynamic range compression (WDRC) can improve the clarity of speech in many listening environments. These instruments provide maximum gain of softer sounds while at the same time minimizing distortion of higher sound inputs. For a small additional cost, these technologies offer a better alternative than conventional instruments for those patients who desire improved communication in a variety of settings. As well, for listeners with abnormal tolerance problems for loud sounds, these instruments are preferred because they deliver maximum boost for soft sounds and can be set to provide virtually no amplification for loud sounds.

Digitally Programmable Instruments

Digitally programmable technology offers added dimension with the ability to program each instrument according to the listener's individual dynamic range and audiometric profile. The flexibility of the output-limiting characteristics can assist in maximizing speech understanding in noisy listening environments. Acoustical characteristics of programmable instruments can be modified in a more precise fashion to match the hearing profile of the user compared with a conventional instrument that is built with a single acoustical matrix. digitally programmable instruments are also available with a variety of circuit options including WDRC and multiple channels for programming. Modifications can be performed instantly in the practitioner's office if changes are observed in the user's hearing sensitivity without the expense or delay of returning them to the manufacturer for remake or change in matrix. For patients who require improved performance in a variety of listening environments, multiple memories can offer even greater flexibility to solve complex communication problems. Many prospective users find single-memory programmable systems appealing because they are more economical and do not require the use of a volume control.

Digital Signal Processing

Because of the higher sampling rates and processing speeds that are inherent in digital signal processing, these instruments are reported to provide cleaner and clearer sound quality with the intent of maximizing speech recognition, particularly in the presence of noise. Many of these systems feature multiple channels and frequency bands that can serve to provide even greater precision in matching the amplification characteristics to the user's audiometric profile and dynamic range, particularly in those patients who have irregular audiometric configurations that require multiple channels for signal processing. However, recent research has not supported the advantage of improved speech recognition in noise for some of these digital systems. Bentler and Duve (1997), using moderate cocktail party levels of 83 dB SPL, reported that a speaking tube held out to the side of the ear provided a SNR for 50% correct on the Speech Perception in Noise (SIN) test, which was about equal to that of two different all-digital instruments and two high-tech analog hearing aids, one of them a K-Amp instrument. Advantages of all-digital instruments may lie in their ability to maximize audibility and dynamic range rather than to produce large improvements in enhancing SNR (Killion, 1997a). Adding dual-microphones, multiple microphone arrays, and beam-forming microphone technology in coordination with digital programming can provide significant improvement in SNR (Valente, 1998).

Additional information regarding the various hearing instrument technologies are found in Chapters 4, 5, 6, 12, and 13 in this volume.

All these technologies are available in our practice for patient demonstration using behind-the-ear demo units coupled to stock earmolds. The Sound Pro II program, originally developed by 3M, has multiple sound libraries where the patient can listen to soft male or female speech, a child's voice, different environmental sounds, loud noises, and speech in noise to compare conventional versus programmable technologies. Omnidirectional and dual microphone technologies can be contrasted by playing traffic noise behind the user while the Central Institute of the Deaf (CID) sentences are delivered facing the patient. Other demonstrations can involve taking the user to the cafeteria of the facility or outside on a busy street. Although not perfect, these minidemonstrations can provide positive listening experiences under various conditions for patients before fitting, particularly for analytical personality types who require a lot of specific detail before making a decision. These demonstrations can be structured to match the individual's unique communication needs. An additional advantage of the demonstration is that it can

assist patients to realize that they can indeed understand softer voices; this can correct their erroneous assumptions that "people mumble."

Size Preferences

Sam Lybarger, in his timeless "definition of a hearing aid" states, "It is an ultraminiature electroacoustical device which is always too large." Certainly, it is well known that patients are preoccupied as to how they will appear to others while wearing their hearing instruments. This stigma is known as "The Hearing Aid Effect." Johnson and Danhauer (1997) summarize these attitudes as (1) an excuse or form of denial for rejecting amplification, (2) negative experiences from dissatisfied hearing aid users, (3) used as an excuse by patients who have financial limitations to purchase amplification, (4) marketing forces that stress the cosmetics and size of the hearing aids, and/or (5) patients who feel possible adverse reactions to the visual appearance of hearing instruments.

No question exists that counseling patients who are cosmetically sensitive presents a major challenge to practitioners. Certainly, these individuals bring their fear and apprehension into the hearing selection process. Often, many cosmetically sensitive patients are just over the brink of denial and depression. For many, it is a large emotional step just to sit in the audiologist's office. As a result, they may be driven by the fear of stigma so that they have yet to accept their hearing impairment. Others who work in the business world may feel additional apprehension or shame that they will appear weak or infirm if their clients or friends "see" the instruments.

Counseling strategies should focus on validating the cosmetically sensitive patient's emotional attitudes. Beck's (1979) theory of "erroneous thinking" may be the source of the apprehension; the patient fears that he or she will be viewed as disabled and rejected by peers if the instruments are noticeable. In some cases patients can be reassured that most individuals they encounter would view them as a "total person" and would ultimately feel that the patient's hearing impairment may be more conspicuous than the physical visibility of the instruments. Many of these patients can accept this idea and will pursue amplification; others will continue to rank size as their major priority.

In our practice, we treat instrument size as a patient-choice option. All sizes are demonstrated, regardless of the degree of hearing impairment, along with a discussion of the fact that not all sizes are appropriate for all hearing losses. We will gently recommend against the choice of a smaller instrument if it is outside of the patient's fitting range. We keep individual replicas of custom instruments and earmolds for all our professional staff so patients can have a real perception of how they appear in an individual's ear. Patients are also encouraged to interact with the replicas so that they can realize the dexterity necessary to change the battery and operate smaller in-the-canal (ITC) and CIC instruments. They are also informed of the effects of cerumen on the performance of smaller instruments. A stock of earmolds that blend with the user's skin tone are also demonstrated, along with smaller sized BTE hearing aids, which are less conspicuous. The effect of these minidemonstrations can help patients to realize that they may not be able to physically operate smaller instruments and that new smaller-sized BTEs may be more appealing, especially when they can obtain a loaner instrument if repairs are necessary.

Some prospective users will readily understand that not all instrument sizes are appropriate for their hearing impairment; others will continue to be "emotionally stuck." A confrontation that "it must be this size or no instrument" will tend to cause some patients to "shop" for someone who will dispense what they desire, often with limited benefit. The end result is that we will frequently see these patients at a later date when they arrive in our offices complaining that they were "ripped off."

The use of the 30-day "satisfaction guarantee" (60 days in our practice) can serve as a security blanket to provide a low-risk evaluation of hearing aid performance for cosmetically sensitive patients. For some individuals, the experience of inadequate performance may be necessary to provide the evidence that performance is more important than instrument size. Others may be happily satisfied but find themselves at the upper end of the fitting range of programmable CICs, with no capacity to increase the instruments' gain or output. Many of these patients place a low priority on further programming; they tend to live in the present but fully understand that they may need to replace the instruments if any changes are present in their hearing sensitivity. These experiences may be one of the factors that contribute to a higher return rate for CIC instruments; it may be of interest to investigate the percentage of the returns that were ultimately fitted with larger hearing aids. As well, circumstances exist in which experienced ITC or CIC users will reject standard ITE fittings because of insertion difficulties or physical discomfort.

The "Hearing Aid Effect" continues to be an important concern in counseling prospective users. It is certainly critical that we prioritize performance, satisfaction, and the importance of the outcome of "better hearing" as opposed to the "hearing aid." Recent improvements in CIC technology have helped to bridge some of the gaps between cosmetic preference and instrument effectiveness.

ORIENTATION

The primary goal of hearing aid orientation is to furnish the hearing aid user with the necessary information concerning the operation and use of the instruments so that optimum benefit is derived. Extensive amounts of information are presented to the patient, including adapting to hearing aid use, operation of the components, batteries, trouble-shooting techniques, warranty, loss/damage protection, telephone use, limitations, cleaning, wax guard system, and insertion and removal instructions.

In a survey conducted by Eggen and Stanford (1988), they found that the median time to accomplish hearing aid orientation is 30 minutes. Critical variables such as manual dexterity, memory, vision, and aging can certainly have an impact on the success or orientation and subsequent satisfaction in hearing aid use.

Tirone and Stanford (1992) examined the specific amount and type of information that a new user is exposed to during hearing aid orientation. Eighteen new users of ITE amplification were videotaped throughout a hearing aid orientation session. Tapes were reviewed, and "bits of information" presented to the user were counted. "Bits of information" were defined as any new information presented with respect to the patient's amplification device and any demonstration of an adjustable technique. These "bits of information" could be a single word or phrase. The topic areas discussed included batteries, wax guard, physical adjustment, dri-aid kit, warranty/product information, hearing aid adjustment, hearing aid description, trouble-shooting, precautions, cleaning, trial period, accessing facility/fees, and assistive listening devices. Results revealed that the mean number of "information bits" was 93.0, with a range of 61 to 136. In some cases five information bits were presented to the patient in less than 1 minute.

It is apparent from this study that many new users are literally overloaded with much new information that must be integrated and retained to ensure successful hearing aid use. Many elderly patients do not possess sufficient memory to retain all the necessary critical facts concerning hearing aid use. Time management is crucial; information concerning warranty, accessing facilities, fees, and trouble-shooting can be provided in written form. Tirone and Stanford (1992) recommend the use of a programmed videotape on maintenance, cleaning, and physical manipulation of the instruments in addition to one-to-one interaction. Paraprofessionals can also be used to provide extra assistance for patients who require additional training of basic skills.

Ranking the importance of all the necessary information that must be covered during an orientation session is indeed a challenge for the audiologist. Virtually all patients need to practice insertion/removal and operation of the instruments unless a caregiver is present on a consistent basis to provide that function. As well, it is paramount that patients understand the limitations of amplification and the process of relearning to adapt to new sounds. This does not limit the importance of all the other information; it will be based on the unique needs and characteristics of the specific user.

The Orientation Session

PEARL

Just as airline pilots are required to use a "checklist" for items to be confirmed before takeoff, audiologists need a checklist to specify what information is to be covered during a hearing aid orientation/fitting session.

Uniformity of patient care is not only important for audiologists but also for all healthcare practitioners. Many managed care organizations require practice guidelines before issuing contracts to their providers. A comprehensive list of items to be covered during hearing aid orientation and fitting helps to ensure a consistent quality and uniformity of patient care. This is exceptionally important in practice settings where multiple audiologists are providing hearing aid dispensing services. Just as the pilot has a list of safety and airplane function items that need to be confirmed before takeoff, the audiologist needs a similar item inventory so all critical aspects are addressed during a fitting session.

Figure 14–8 is a sample dispensing checkoff sheet. Although it is quite specific, no weighting is given to any of the items. It permits some space for individual interpretation while at the same time defining specific areas to be addressed during the fitting process. Each item on the list will not be reviewed in this chapter, but those factors that involve interaction between the use environment and the patient will be discussed.

Performance Validation

Chapters in this text provide detailed discussion of performance validation with tools such as real-ear measures (Chapter 3), functional gain (Chapter 4), loudness scales (Chapters 6 and 13), and so forth. Certainly, validating optimum acoustical performance is an absolute necessity during a fitting session. Any of these methods are critical tools to demonstrate to the patient how much specific benefit is achieved with amplification.

Expectations and Suggestion for Adapting to Hearing Aid Use

The Occlusion Effect

The effect of hearing aid or earmold placement on the user's voice quality is a well-known process, and its management is discussed in detail in Chapter 2. Certainly, the "hollow, barrel-over-the-head" feeling created by the occlusion effect needs to be minimized, but new users must understand that all hearing aid microphones will pick up and amplify their own voice and that it is a *normal process*, regardless of the instrument's size or type of signal processing. As well, a realistic time frame of patient adaptation to their own voice should be discussed. For some patients, it may take up to 8 weeks before they are completely comfortable with the manner in which they perceive their own voice while using amplification.

Audibility of New Sounds

Another amplification interaction effect is the almost instant audibility of new sounds that the patient may not have perceived for quite some time. This effect is particularly common in WDRC technologies or K-Amp instruments, which have low threshold kneepoints (40- to 50-dB SPL) that provide greater amplification for low-input signals. Patients will typically report that "the hearing aids are making noise," when what the listeners are actually perceiving is a soft sound in the environment that may include the computer fan/hard drive, room ventilator, or footsteps in the hallway. In most circumstances these are sounds that are not audible to the hearing aid user when the instruments are removed but are perceptible to individuals with normal hearing sensitivity.

Gatehouse and Killion (1993) suggest that listeners with impaired hearing require a significant period of time to learn to make optimum use of the new set of speech cues to receive maximum performance from their amplification. They theorize that as a high-frequency sensorineural hearing loss slowly progresses, the neural representation in the cortex of the low-input, high-frequency sounds will no longer receive stimulation. As a result, the brain will begin to "fill in" those gaps with surrounding frequencies and intensities to those areas that are unstimulated. In view of the fact that most sensorineural hearing losses are slowly progressive, the process may take years to run its course.

When the patient is fitted with appropriate amplification, the sounds that were previously inaudible to the user are now perceived and presented to the cortex. If those auditory areas were "filled in" by surrounding frequencies and intensities, it may take a significant amount of time for the "rewiring/ unmapping" of the brain to take place. Gatehouse and Killion (1993) suggest that the time frame for the relearning process can take weeks or even months and may be correlated to how much of the high-frequency information was absent—and for how long.

This pattern is also present in the visual system. Opthalmologists and optometrists (Calnan, 1997; Gustafson, 1998) report that patients who manifest moderate-to-severe vision deficits that are uncorrected will often require gradual refraction changes for optimum vision improvement. They report that a single change in refraction from severe vision deficit to normal will often produce headaches and rejection of the eyeglass/contact lens fitting because the change in visual acuity is too large for the brain to handle in an effective fashion. In addition, it is a well-known fact that bifocals require a period of acclimatization for the visual system to process the changes in visual image that occur when the user "looks down." As well, Calnan (1997) and Gustafson (1998) state that much variability exists among patients with similar visual acuity in how long a period of time is necessary for their visual systems to adapt fully to bifocal use.

PEARL

The nature of the brain rewiring/adaptation process for amplification, with parallels in the visual system, need to be stressed to the patient during all stages of hearing aid counseling/orientation.

The phenomenon of relearning has been confirmed by Cox and Alexander (1992), who showed increases in both measured and perceived benefits from amplification over a 3-month period. Gatehouse (1992) measured speech identification scores in noise for both narrow band and wider band hearing instruments and found that no changes in speech identification abilities occurred over a 16-week period for the narrow band instruments, but performance increased gradually using a wider band condition.

Whether one supports the idea that the brain is rewiring itself or adapting to new stimuli, this new audibility of both speech and nonspeech signals has critical application to the hearing aid orientation process. An individual interaction between the user and the hearing instruments will be unique. It is also important to demonstrate to the patient the difference between "audibility" and "annoyance." Audibility can be defined as the identification of new sounds that have been absent for some time, although annoyance refers to

SOUTH SHORE HEARING CENTER

Hearing Aid Fitting Checklist

Patient: _____ Fitting Date: _____

Audiologist: _____ PC needed: _____

Right Aid: _____ Serial #: _____

Trim Pot Settings: Low Cut _____ Knee _____ High Cut _____ MPO _____ Gain _____

Left Aid: _____ Serial #: _____

Trim Pot Settings: Low Cut _____ Knee _____ High Cut _____ MPO _____ Gain _____

♦ Fitting Verification: Real-Ear Measurement   Functional Gain   Other: _____

♦ Fit modifications:

♦ Reasonable expectations: Noise   Own voice   Speechreading
     Communication strategies   Monaural/Binaural   ALDs

♦ Identification and use of controls
♦ Feedback: Causes and prevention
♦ Cerumen: Cleaning, maintenance and prevention of breakdown, feedback

♦ Battery: Size _____
               Toxicity
               LOBAT / when to change; tracking battery life
               How to change
               Where to purchase: costs

♦ Care of aid: Cleaning
               Turning it off when not in use
               Tips for avoiding loss
               Avoiding water, hairspray, humidity problems, dri-aid kit

♦ Insertion and removal

♦ Telephone use: T-coil   amplified phone   acoustic coupling

♦ Warranty: # of years _____   Hearing Aid Insurance: # of years _____
                              Esco   Manufacturer
   Difference between insurance and warranty explained; replacement fee

♦ Service by appointment

♦ Return policy explained

♦ Follow-up visit issues:

_____
_____
_____
_____

Figure 14–8   Hearing aid fitting checklist.

overamplification of louder sounds such as crackling paper, dishes rattling, traffic noises, etc.

Case Vignette

A 75-year-old man was fit with binaural K-Amp canal instruments after having worn Class A linear canal aids for the past 5 years. The user has a moderate bilateral sensorineural hearing loss with a narrow dynamic range. At 3-week follow-up, he stated that "I'm hearing lots of new sounds and have improved communication over my previous instruments, but in a restaurant I am hearing the person three tables away much better than I can understand my wife who is sitting 3 feet across from me. It is driving me crazy."

Both functional gain in the sound field and real-ear measurements yielded responses consistent with FIG6 targets (Gitles & Niquette, 1995). (FIG6 is also discussed in detail in Chapters 4, 5, and 13.) No discomfort for loud sounds was reported. It was discussed with the patient that until he was fitted with these new instruments, he had minimal audibility for distances in excess of 6 feet because if he tried to raise the volume on his older linear instruments, louder sounds would cause distortion and discomfort. Having opened his "window of sound" with the newer K-Amps, his brain was undergoing a process of trying to "sort out" these newer sounds and was still deciding how to focus its energies. It was stressed to the patient that it may take another month or more for the brain to learn to focus on his wife and "tune out" the patrons located 15 to 20 feet away. We raised the knee control slightly to ease him into the "nonlinear experience," without causing loudness tolerance problems. Further follow-up 8 weeks after fitting revealed a marked reduction in his sense of "distraction" in group listening environments. We were then able to lower the threshold kneepoint and provide him with greater audibility of softer sounds once his brain was more attuned and ready for the change.

It is clearly evident that this large "jump" in audibility, which is experienced by new users of amplification, particularly K-Amp and WDRC instruments, requires significant time of the brain to learn to use and categorize new sounds. Some listeners may need to be introduced gradually to this style of amplification. Where users start will vary significantly, but the audiologist can begin by raising the compression kneepoint by 5- to 10-dB to minimize the effect of too many soft sounds in the initial stage of amplification. Some programmable hearing aid systems are equipped with software called "adaptation managers," where listeners can be introduced to new amplification in small steps, similar to small changes in refraction for eyeglass or contact lens users in the visual system.

Wearing Schedules/User Diaries

Although many users will perform quite well by using their hearing instruments on a full-time basis each day, others may require a more gradual, steady period of acclimatization. Selected hearing aid manufacturers have developed wearing schedules and user diaries to assist selected patients to "ease in" to the process of adjusting to the use of amplification. Palmer and Mormer (1997) use a specific wearing schedule as a part of their hearing aid orientation process. It is a 9-day

schedule that consists of 1 hour of use the first day, followed by a 1 hour "rest period" that is followed by another hour of use. For the second and third days, use time increases in 1-hour intervals, with the same 1 hour "time out." Listening activities during the first 3 days are limited to activities inside the home such as listening to household sounds such as the fan, water running, doorbell ringing, or toilet flushing. Television and radio use and quiet conversation with low background noise are also integrated in the first 3 days of use.

Days 4 and 5 increase the time to 4 to 5 hours of use, followed by the hour of rest, with another 4 to 5 hours of use. Listening activities are increased to include quiet indoor work activities at home or in the work environment. Days 6 and 7 provide the same 1-hour increment in use time and 1 hour time out, with an increase in listening activities to include quiet outdoor activities. By the end of the ninth day, the user is engaged in full-time use with the same 1-hour break period.

It is often difficult to predict which patients will adapt readily to new amplification. Even those who fully understand the process of relearning to hear and integrate new sounds may require gradual increments in use time to accomplish both success and satisfaction with hearing aid use. Others will require a more regimented approach of using the hearing aids consistently each day while fully understanding that the brain will never "rewire" itself if the patient only uses the instruments 1 hour per day. Part-time use can be a facade for denial in that many patients will state, "You mean that I have to use them all the time?. . . My hearing is not that bad!" Many new users will wish to remove the hearing aids in the office right after a thorough and successful fitting/orientation session, not wanting to wear them home. Audiologists will constantly be challenged to identify the difference between psychological acceptance of the hearing impairment in the form of use of amplification and the process of the auditory system physically adjusting to hearing aid use. In our center patients are encouraged to use their instruments full-time, with a brief rest period each day, while stressing that if they do not use the hearing aids consistently, the brain will never accept the change. A wearing schedule similar to that reported by Palmer and Mormer (1997) is subsequently used in situations in which patients require a more gradual introduction to amplification and will not use the schedule as a tool to avoid hearing aid use.

A user diary can be a helpful tool for a new hearing aid patient to provide a structured summary of their experiences with amplification. This can greatly assist the audiologist in providing necessary reprogramming and quantifying benefits from hearing aid use and realistic expectations. Oticon and GN ReSound are among the companies who have structured user diaries.

Hearing Instrument Use in Various Listening Environments

A brief discussion of hearing aid use in different listening environments is a meaningful part of a hearing aid orientation session. Specific situations can be taken from the list of individual patient goals. Instant reassurance to the patient that television communication should be easier without blasting the spouse out of the living room can boost the user's self-confidence. The deleterious effects of poor acoustics and distance should be described to assist the patient in coping with communicating in churches, auditoriums, and theaters. The role of infrared and frequency-modulated systems can be briefly mentioned. More detailed information on assistive listening devices can be found in this volume in Chapter 19. Communication in noise should also be reviewed, with discussion of why individuals with inner ear damage require a more favorable SNR than normal listeners and the importance of binaural amplification in group listening environments. Discussion of performance limitations in everyday environments can help users to form realistic expectations of hearing aid performance. This can go a long way to dispel the myth that newer digital technologies "eliminate noise."

Feedback

Demonstration of the causes and prevention of feedback is critical during hearing aid orientation. Feedback should not interfere with satisfactory hearing instrument performance; this places an additional burden on hearing instrument manufacturers and earmold laboratories to furnish a good-fitting shell and on practitioners to provide good ear impressions. Multiple remakes are not uncommon, particularly in advanced technology instruments. Telephone use must be accomplished without having to remove the instrument because of instrument feedback. Newer programmable technologies are available with "feedback managers" that can assist in reducing feedback without deleterious effects on hearing instrument performance. Conventional instruments have feedback trimmers (high-frequency cut) that can be quite helpful for hearing losses that require large amounts of high-frequency gain. Specific strategies in managing feedback are provided in Chapter 2.

Battery Issues

At present, zinc-air button cells are the preferred choice for most hearing instruments. Certain programmable systems use silver oxide batteries for remote controls. Zinc-air cells tend to dry out in about 60 days once the tab is removed, so that silver oxide cells will provide significantly longer life for long-term, low-drain applications such as remote controls. Some power instruments demonstrate more consistent operation with silver oxide cells or "high-performance" zinc-air batteries. It is important that patients understand the shelf life of a zinc-air cell once the tab is removed; some users will try multiple batteries in an instrument as a means of trouble-shooting and reduce the shelf life on an entire package of batteries to 60 days.

Calculation of the relative battery life of a hearing instrument is rather simple. ANSI (1987) hearing instrument specifications will include a battery drain figure that can then be used to insert into a chart, which is available from most battery manufacturers. This chart is shown in Figure 14–9 and displays battery life in hours or days as a function of cell size and current drain. Specification sheets will typically publish cell drain with the instrument run at full-on gain. Many of the newer hearing instrument test chambers include the ability to calculate specific battery drain.

During a hearing aid orientation session, users can be trained to track the battery life of their instruments. In our practice we instruct patients to place the battery tab onto a calendar when a new cell is inserted so that they can count

the number of days before it loses its power. They are also provided with a miniature plastic case to store a spare cell for quick access. The shelf life of unopened cells often exceeds 2 years; unopened packages do not require refrigeration. Storage should be in a cool, dry location like a desk or dresser, and cells should not be carried loose with other metal objects, which may cause the battery to discharge.

Some circuits provide an internal warning system an audible tone or hum occurs when battery voltage begins to deteriorate. It is our recommendation that all instruments use some sort of battery warning feature. Either Way OK (EWOK) (Killion, 1997b) is another innovative system by which the user can insert the cell into the instrument in either direction; the EWOK circuit will automatically invert the polarity.

Unless it is certain that a caregiver will provide battery insertion/removal, all patients should receive ample practice in changing the battery in their instruments during initial orientation or as a part of preliminary consultation. Many wax loops come with magnets attached to the opposite end; these can provide assistance in battery insertion/removal for patients with more limited dexterity. EWOK can be implemented for those users who consistently damage the instrument from improper battery insertion. Rexton, Inc. also provides a full ITE size instrument that uses a 675 size battery, which only needs to be changed once a year.

Directions concerning battery toxicity are provided to all new users. Virtually all hearing instrument instruction booklets contain the necessary required information. Tamper-resistant battery doors should be used in pediatric fittings, and battery toxicity is a required topic in our "dispensing check-off sheet." Some practices use a signed waiver, which describes the hazards of accidental battery ingestion.

Care of Instruments

Certainly, it is essential that all users be educated concerning the effects of water, humidity, perspiration, and heat on hearing instrument performance. In our practice, nearly all users of BTE instruments are provided with dri-aid kits (seen in Figure 14–10), as well as individuals who are exposed to high humidity or moisture on a consistent basis. More extensive control of moisture and humidity has recently occurred with the introduction of "Dry & Store," an electronic dessicant/sanitizing agent that can be seen in Figure 14–11. The instrument operates with a fan, which causes the air inside the chamber to circulate and increase in temperature. The heat and moving air cause the water molecules to move out of the instruments and into the charged desiccant. A germicidal ultraviolet lamp, which is activated electronically for the last 30 seconds of each hour, also functions to help disinfect the instruments. The total drying/sanitizing cycle takes approximately 6 hours.

Earhooks on BTE instruments should be changed on a regular basis; dirt and moisture can clog the dampers in the earhook, resulting in a deleterious effect on the instrument's frequency response. "Super Seals" (shown in Figure 14–12) are disposable latex sheaths that are mounted onto the case of a BTE instrument to reduce perspiration. Earmold air blowers can be seen in Figure 14–13 and are another important accessory to remove obstructions in earmold tubing for BTE users; earmold tubing that is pretreated with desiccant to

Hearing Aid Battery Life Chart

Life/hrs. $= \dfrac{mAh}{mA}$ (16 hours of use per day)

Battery Drain Current (mA) per ANSI (S3.22 1976)	PRO LINE PREMIUM ZINC AIR*								MERCURY					
	312A 130mAh		13A 255mAh		675A 600mAh		10A 70mAh		R312 60mAh		R13 60mAh		HR675 270mAh	
	Hours	Days	Hours	Days	Hours	Days	Hours	Days	Hours	Days	Hours	Days	Hours	Days
.1mA	1300	81	2550	159	6000	375	700	44	600	37	1000	63	2700	169
.2mA	650	41	1275	80	3000	188	350	22	300	19	500	31	1350	84
.3mA	433	27	850	53	2000	125	233	15	200	13	333	21	900	56
.4mA	325	20	638	40	1500	94	175	11	150	9	250	16	675	42
.5mA	260	16	510	32	1200	75	140	9	120	8	200	13	540	34
.6mA	217	14	425	27	1000	63	117	7	100	6	167	10	450	28
.7mA	186	12	364	23	857	54	100	6	86	5	143	9	386	25
.8mA	163	10	319	20	750	47	88	5	75	5	125	8	338	21
.9mA	144	9	283	18	667	42	78	5	67	4	111	7	300	18
1.0mA	130	8	255	16	600	38	70	4	60	4	100	6	270	16
1.1mA	118	7	232	15	545	34	64	4	55	3	91	6	245	16
1.2mA	108	7	213	13	500	31	58	4	50	3	83	5	225	15
1.3mA	100	6	196	12	462	29	54	3	46	3	77	5	208	13
1.4mA	93	6	182	11	429	27	50	3	43	3	71	5	188	12
1.5mA	87	5	170	11	400	25	47	3	40	3	67	4	180	11
1.6mA	81	5	159	10	375	23	44	3	37	2	63	4	169	11
1.7mA	76	5	150	9	353	22	41	2	35	2	59	4	159	10
1.8mA	72	5	141	9	333	21	39	2	33	2	56	4	150	9

*IMPORTANT NOTE: Maximum battery life with any zinc-air battery will not typically exceed 60 days regardless of what is indicated by the chart. The battery will dry out and no longer be effective.

Figure 14–9 Hearing aid battery life chart. (From Rayovac Corporation, with permission.)

reduce moisture that can build up in the tubing is also available from laboratories. Windscreens are also helpful to help prevent dirt and cerumen particles from entering the microphone, particularly on custom products.

Cerumen Control

Controlling cerumen buildup in the receiver of custom hearing instruments is one of the most common problems faced by dispensing audiologists. On the basis of the high cost of

replacing hearing instrument receivers as a result of cerumen contamination, manufacturers have designed an array of wax guard options. These include "spring dampers," "wax baskets," "wax plungers," "element dampers," which are mounted inside the receiver tubing to prevent the cerumen from clogging the receiver. Further detail concerning these and other wax-prevention systems are described in Chapter 2.

Certainly, patients need to be instructed in detail concerning the effects of cerumen and proper cleaning techniques.

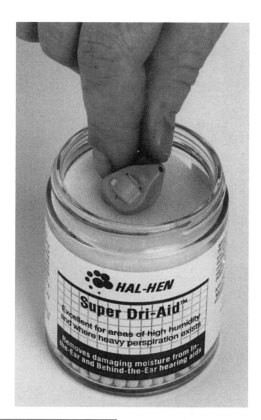

Figure 14–10 Dri-aid kit. (From Hal-Hen Co., Inc., with permission.)

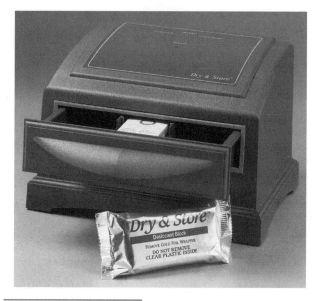

Figure 14–11 Dry & Store electronic hearing instrument desiccant/germicide system. (From Ear Technology Corporation, with permission.)

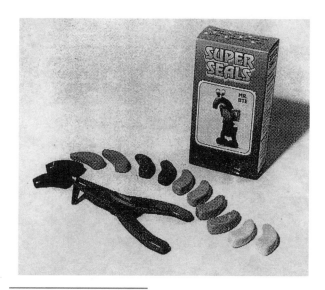

Figure 14–12 Super Seals disposable latex hearing aid covers. (From Hal-Hen Co., Inc., with permission.)

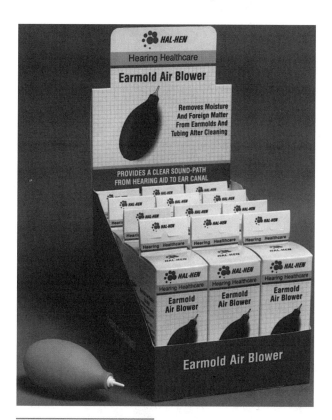

Figure 14–13 Earmold air blower. (From Hal-Hen Co., Inc., with permission.)

Experience in our practice has shown that no one single strategy is effective in controlling cerumen buildup in receiver tubes. Snap-on cerumen filters and extending receiver tubes can cause discomfort in the earcanals of some users; wax springs and baskets can easily become obstructed and can require biweekly replacement in some patients. Others use the wax cleaning tools in a haphazard fashion, often causing collapsed receiver tubes. The use of Ad-hear wax guards

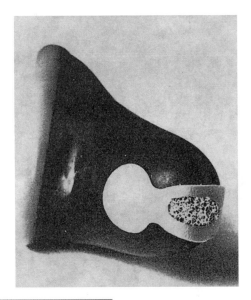

Figure 14–14 Ad-hear wax guard on a CIC hearing instrument. (From Hearing Components, Inc., with permission.)

(Oliveira & Rose, 1994) are shown in Figures 14–14 and 14–15 and can be beneficial for many patients. They provide a barrier to help prevent cerumen and dirt from entering the hearing aid receiver and is something that users can change by themselves; others have difficulty changing the guard or report tactile sensitivity in the earcanal. A swivel wax barrier can be seen in Figure 14–16. The filter/barrier can easily be rotated for simple cleaning of the guard and the hearing instrument receiver tube. Oticon has developed a "wax buster" cerumen cleaning system that is shown in Figure 14–17. The system incorporates a spring-loaded plunger, where the user pushes the tip of the instrument down on a

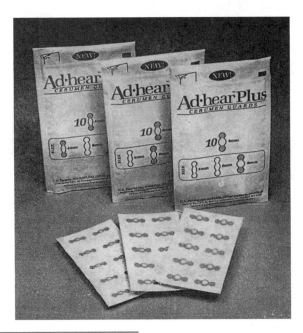

Figure 14–15 Ad-hear wax guards. (From Hearing Components, Inc., with permission.)

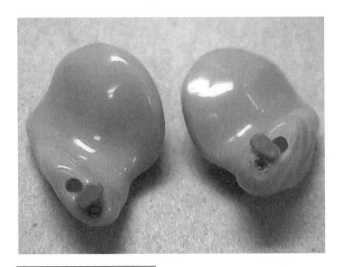

Figure 14–16 Oto-Med wax barrier system. (From Widex Hearing Aid Co., Inc., with permission.)

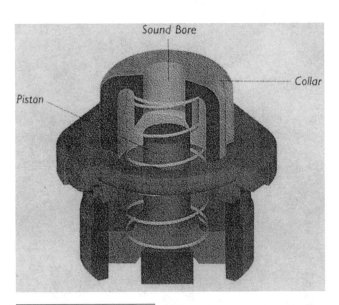

Figure 14–17 Wax buster system. (From Oticon, Inc., with permission.)

paper towel and the piston pushes cerumen debris out of the sound bore. Figure 14–18 shows a snap-on wax guard system developed by GN Danavox. The small cap, which is visible at the tip of the instrument acts, as a wax barrier and can be changed by the user at weekly or monthly intervals. Some manufacturers insert small removable coils into the instrument's receiver tube to help prevent cerumen from spreading into the receiver. Our experiences with these coils have indicated that they clog easily; one new hearing aid user had the instrument coil become completely obstructed with cerumen within 48 hours after his initial fitting. Patients have also pushed the coil with their wax tool or cleaning brush down into the instrument's receiver. In our facility a variety of the above-mentioned techniques are used; we often use the first year of use to assist us in selecting the most effective wax control option for a particular patient.

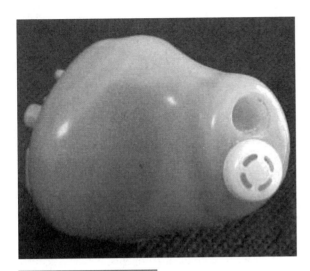

Figure 14–18 Snap-on wax guard system. (From GN Danavox, Inc., with permission.)

Many users use a facial tissue to wipe the earmold or shell of an instrument after removal or before insertion. Although this can be an effective method of removing pieces of cerumen or dirt from the instrument, many facial tissues (i.e., "Puffs") contain perfumes or other additives that can result in dermatitis of the external ear if the instrument is placed into the ear immediately after it is wiped (Cole, 1996). The symptoms can be the same as if the external ear had an allergic reaction to the plastic composition of the shell. Antibacterial wipes are available from supply houses that can be used to clean shells on instruments for patients with draining ears or for infection control. Those wipes can introduce moisture into the hearing aid; the Dry & Store can be helpful for those patients who require routine germicidal treatment. Some users will also use their instruments during sleep; lack of ventilation can often cause severe otitis externa and excessive cerumen problems. It is also a common source of lost/damaged instruments. Alerting devices are a much better alternative for patients who express concerns for monitoring their listening environment during sleep.

Instrument Insertion/Removal

All patients must receive sufficient time to practice instrument insertion and removal. Caregivers and significant others are quite helpful in providing support for patients with limited motor skills and dementia, but under most circumstances, the patient is the responsible individual.

Instrument removal is a preferred place to begin. Most patients perform this task with little or no difficulty; most will use the technique of pushing up from the bottom of the external ear, between the lobe and the antitragus. This typically causes the instrument to slide out of the ear gently, with minimal discomfort. For individuals with firm ear texture or dexterity problems, earmolds and custom shells can be equipped with optional handles and notches to facilitate removal.

For many users, instrument insertion is an extremely demanding task; some patients who live alone use personal listening devices strictly because they are unable to insert and operate any type of traditional hearing aid. Proper hearing aid insertion is a challenge for patients from all walks of life,

including a former U.S. president, whose picture has appeared in numerous magazines and newspapers with his hearing instruments inserted upside down.

Some users with limited vision will require severe color coding or a notch to differentiate the left and right instruments, particularly half-shell, ITC, and CIC instruments. Despite some limited practice during initial hearing aid consultation to screen for dexterity issues, many patients will struggle with insertion. Although some individuals will recognize poor insertion from instrument feedback or "tactile awareness," others will literally have no idea that they are inserted incorrectly, leading to sore spots on the external ear, poor acoustic performance, and/or loss. No one size of instrument is immune; ITE hearing aids will protrude because the helix is not inserted; canal instruments will not be fully seated or will be inserted sideways; BTE earmold tubing will be twisted or the helix will protrude.

We always have the patient use the mirror as a "validator" following their best attempt at insertion. This will reinforce correct insertion technique and will also serve to provide visual feedback to the user to show where they have made a mistake; most will be able to see if the instrument is protruding. The use of a "portable plastic ear" is also helpful for patients to visualize the insertion process. Individuals who experience insertion problems during initial fitting are contacted within 48 hours after orientation and can be scheduled for follow-up before their routine 2-week postfitting visit.

Telephone Use

Proper use of the telephone with hearing instruments is another significant part of the hearing aid orientation process. Unless it is an open fitting incorporating a large vent with large amounts of high-frequency gain, it should not be necessary for users to remove the hearing instrument to use the telephone successfully. Choices of various telephone accessories are described in Chapter 19 on ALDs in this volume.

Choosing between acoustic and inductive coupling for telephone use presents a challenge to the audiology practitioner. Lowe and Goldstein (1982) evaluated speech recognition using the SPIN test for both acoustic and inductive coupling and found no significant differences between the two methods of telephone use, with some users performing better with acoustic coupling, whereas other individuals demonstrated improved speech recognition with inductive coupling. Both coupling methods have advantages and limitation that can affect practical use. Users should be educated concerning compatibility problems with inductive coupling and the use of instruments with certain cellular phones.

Many users require a fair amount of time to activate the telecoil in a BTE instrument and hold the receiver in the correct position for effective communication; some report that the phone stops ringing before they can make the necessary adjustments. Others report that sitting near a computer monitor causes a significant "hum" when the telecoil is active. Many telephones, including certain cellular phones, are not compatible for use with inductive coupling. Recent introduction of the preamp telecoil, however, has provided ease of telephone use for some ITE hearing aid users. Also, certain programmable instruments feature the ability to program a separate frequency response for telecoil use.

Acoustic coupling is also successful for large numbers of users. Acoustic coupling can be limited from feedback that occurs when the handset is positioned on the ear; angling the phone or positioning the receiver a bit higher so it is directly on the hearing aid microphone can be effective in reducing feedback. Patients are also instructed in lowering the volume control on conventional instruments that may accomplish easy telephone use without annoying feedback. Circular pads are also available that mount onto the telephone receiver and create a larger cavity volume, subsequently reducing feedback. Their limitation is that they can interfere with the ability to hang the telephone up properly and cannot be used easily with pay phones.

PITFALL

Feedback should not limit appropriate telephone use; users should be able to use either acoustic or inductive coupling without having to remove their hearing instruments.

Proper determination of the patient's telephone use patterns will identify whether acoustic or inductive coupling is more beneficial; many patients will use both systems. Some users will use acoustic coupling for quick telephone use, while using inductive coupling for noisy environments or assistive device application. Detailed instruction during fitting is important; most patients do not position the phone correctly for effective use. Even with extensive practice during initial orientation, many users will require reinstruction during follow-up. Some states have subsidized programs for patients to acquire amplified handsets or special phones at no charge or for a reduced cost. Erber (1985) provides a comprehensive overview of telephone communication and hearing aid use.

Service Policy

During initial orientation, all users receive written information containing instrument warranty, loss/damage protection, and follow-up visits. The differences between warranty and accidental loss/damage are reviewed in detail; many users think that their loss/damage plan will cover routine repairs. They are also instructed as to the length of time given to cover follow-up services and instrument reprogramming. Many patients who spend the winter months in locations such as Florida, Arizona, or California are given materials so they can ship the instruments to us for repairs if needed. In addition, patients are provided with the names of practitioners in their area, with instructions that they may be charged

for shipping or office visits if the instrument needs servicing or reprogramming, even if the warranty is in effect.

Follow-up visits are extremely important in hearing aid orientation. Typically, they are scheduled for 2 to 3 weeks after initial fitting. Their general purposes are to evaluate patient satisfaction and make certain that the goals of the user are met. The scope of this visit is quite varied and can include any of the following: reprogramming the instrument; remanaging user apprehension, denial, and projection; shell remake or modification; environmental manipulation strategies; discussing realistic expectations; real-ear measurements; functional gain measurements; practice with insertion/removal; cleaning instructions; orientation on telephone use; assistive listening devices; outcome measures; discussion of performance in restaurants and church; and so forth. Certainly, if the prestated realistic goals of the user are met and they plan to use and keep the instruments, they will achieve satisfaction. Long-term success may entail more than just keeping the instruments past the 60-day satisfaction guarantee period. It is best defined by Palmer and Mormer (1997), who describe successful use as when the patient's prestated communication needs are met, combined with the use of hearing instruments, assistive listening devices, counseling, communication strategies, and environment manipulation.

CONCLUSIONS

No doubt exists that counseling and orientation toward amplification are complex processes. Greater knowledge and management of the psychological aspects of hearing impairment and our patients will not only reduce the number of instruments that sit in the drawer but will also improve the proportional number of successful hearing aid users. The audiologist is not intended to become a mental health professional, but we are optimistic that the information contained within this chapter will provide dispensing audiologists with some of the tools that are essential to improve their helping skills and fitting proficiencies.

ACKNOWLEDGMENTS

I thank Robert Beckhardt, M.D., and Herbert Goldberg, Ph.D., for their valuable input in the area of the psychology of hearing impairment.

Appendix
Sources of Financial Assistance for Amplification

1. Hear Now
   9745 E. Hampden Avenue, Suite 300
   Denver, CO 80231-4923
   (303) 695-7797 (Voice/TTY)
   (303) 695-7789 (Fax)
   1-800-748-HEAR
   E-mail: jostelter@aol.com

2. Sertoma International
   1912 E. Meyer Boulevard
   Kansas City, MO 64132
   (816) 333-8300 (Voice)
   (816) 333-4320 (Fax)
   E-mail: infosertoma@sertoma.org
   Web site: http://www.sertoma.org

3. Miracle Ear Children's Foundation
   P.O. Box 59261
   Minneapolis, MN 55459-0261
   1-800-234-5422
   Web site: http://www.miracle-ear.com

4. Starkey Foundation
   c/o Starkey Laboratories, Inc.
   6700 Washington Avenue South
   Eden Prairie, MN 55344
   (612) 941-6401
   1-800-328-8602
   (612) 828-9262 (Fax)

REFERENCES

AMERICAN HERITAGE DICTIONARY OF THE ENGLISH LANGUAGE. (1992). (pp. 427, 1276). New York: Houghton Mifflin.

AMERICAN NATIONAL STANDARDS INSTITUTE. (1987). *Specifications of hearing aid characteristics (ANSI S3.22-1987).* New York: ANSI.

BECK, A.T. (1979). *Cognitive therapy and the emotional disorders.* New York: Meridian Books.

BENTLER, R.A., & DUVE, M. (1997). *Progression of hearing aid benefit over the 20th century.* Poster presented at the annual meeting of the American Academy of Audiology, Fort Lauderdale, FL.

BERRA, Y. (1998). *The Yogi book.* New York: Workman Publishing.

BEVAN, M.A. (1997). Matching hearing technology to hearing needs. *Hearing Reviews Supplement, 1;*32–36.

CARKHUFF, R.R. (1993). *The art of helping VII.* Amherst, MA: Human Resource Development Press.

COX, R.M., & ALEXANDER, G.C. (1992). Maturation of hearing aid benefit: Objective and subjective measurements. *Ear and Hearing, 13(3);*131–141.

COX, R.M., & ALEXANDER, G.C. (1995) The abbreviated profile of hearing aid benefit. *Ear and Hearing 16(2);*176–183.

DAWSON, R. (1985). *You can get anything you want.* New York: Fireside Books.

DILLION, H., JAMES, A., & GINIS, S. (1997). Client oriented scale of improvement (COSI) and its relationship to several other measures of benefit and satisfaction provided by hearing aids. *Journal of the American Academy of Audiology, 827–843.*

DYCHTWALD, K., & FLOWER, J. (1989). *Age wave.* Los Angeles, CA: Jeremy P. Tarcher.

EGGEN, S., & STANFORD, L.S. (1988). *A survey of hearing aid orientation procedures in Michigan audiologists.* Independent study, Mt. Pleasant, MI: Central Michigan University.

ERBER, N.P. (1985). *Telephone communication and hearing impairment.* San Diego, CA: College Hill Press.

GARSTECKI, D.C., & ERLER, S.F. (1997). Counseling older adult hearing instrument candidates. *Hearing Review Supplement, 1;*14–18.

GATEHOUSE, S. (1992). The time course and magnitude of peripheral acclimitization to frequency responses: Evidence from monaural fitting of hearing aids. *Journal of the Acoustical Society of America, 92;*1256–1268.

GATEHOUSE, S., & KILLION, M.C. (1993). HABRAT: Hearing aid brain rewiring accommodation time. *Hearing Instruments, 44(10);*29–32.

GITLES, T.C., & NIQUETTE, P.T. (1995). FIG6 in ten. *Hearing Journal, 2(10);*28,30.

HARFORD, E.R., & CURRAN, J.R. (1997). Managing patients with precipitous high-frequency losses. *Hearing Review Supplement, 1;*8–13.

JOHNSON, C.E., & DANHAUER, J.L. (1997). The "hearing aid effect" revisited: Can we achieve hearing solutions for cosmetically sensitive patients? *Hearing Reviews Supplement, 1;*37–44.

JUNG, C. (1974). *Psychological types.* Princeton, NJ: Princeton University Press.

KILLION, M.C. (1993). The K-Amp hearing aid: An attempt to present high fidelity for persons with impaired hearing. *American Journal of Audiology, 2(2);*52–74.

KILLION, M.C. (1997a). The SIN report: Circuits haven't solved the hearing-in-noise problem. *Hearing Journal, 50(10);*28–32.

KILLION, M.C. (1997b). The EWOK circuit. U.S. Patent #5,623,550 issued April 27, 1997.

KUBLER-ROSS, E. (1969). *On death and dying.* New York: Macmillan Publishing.

LOWE, R.G., & GOLDSTEIN, D.P. (1982). Acoustic versus inductive coupling of hearing aids to telephones. *Ear and Hearing, 3(4);*227–234.

MERRIAM WEBSTER'S COLLEGIATE DICTIONARY. (1993) (pp. 264, 820). Springfield, MA: Merriam-Webster.

MUELLER, H.G., & KILLION, M.C. (1990). An easy method for calculating the articulation index. *Hearing Journal, 43(9);*14–17.

MYERS, I. KIRBY, L.K., & BRIGGS, K.D. (1993). *Introduction to type* (5th ed.). Palo Alto, CA: Consulting Psychologists Press.

NOVALIS, P.N., ROJCEWICZ, S.J., JR., & PEELE, R. (1993). *Clinical manual of supportive psychotherapy.* Washington, DC: American Psychiatric Press.

OLIVEIRA, R.J., & ROSE, D.E. (1994). "Keep your wax guard up." *American Journal of Audiology, 3(1);*7–10.

O'NEILL, J. (1988). Are we marketing the right product? *Hearing Journal, 4(11);*21–22.

OWENS, E., & SCHUBERT, E.D. (1977). Development of the California consonant test. *Journal of Speech and Hearing Research, 20;*463–474.

PALMER, C., & MORMER, E. (1997). A systematic program for hearing instrument orientation and adjustment. *Hearing Review Supplement, 1;*45–52.

REZEN, S.V., & HAUSMAN, C. (1985). *Coping with hearing loss.* New York: Dembner Books.

ROGERS, C.R. (1951). *Client centered therapy: Its current practice, implications and theory.* Boston, MA: Houghton Mifflin.

SMEDLEY, T., & SCHOW, R. (1990). Frustrations with hearing aid use: Candid observations from the elderly. *Hearing Journal, 43;*21–27.

TIRONE, M., & STANDORD, L.S. (1992). *Analysis of the hearing aid orientation process.* Paper presented at the annual meeting of the American Speech-Language-Hearing Association, San Antonio, TX.

TRAYNOR, R.M., & BUCKLES, K.M. (1997). Personality typing: Audiology's new crystal ball. *Hearing Review Supplement, 128;*31.

VALENTE, M. (1998). The bright promise of microphone technology. *Hearing Journal, 51(7);*10–16.

VAN VLIET, D. (1997). *Personality types.* Paper presented at the annual meeting of the Academy of Dispensing Audiologists, Orlando, FL.

WEBSTER'S NEW TWENTIETH CENTURY DICTIONARY—UNABRIDGED. (1966). (pp. 415; 1261). Cleveland, OH: World Publishing.

WILKINSON, D. (1995). Counseling: Every patient is different. *Hearing Journal, 48(7);*63–66.

PREFERRED PRACTICE GUIDELINES

Professionals Who Perform the Procedure(s)

▼ Audiologists

Expected Outcomes

▼ The emotional status of the patient concerning hearing instrument use is identified.

▼ The hearing aid candidate feels safety and freedom to express his or her feelings concerning hearing aid use.

▼ Emotional barriers to successful hearing rehabilitation are managed appropriately.

▼ Appropriate amplification systems are selected and fitted on the basis of the lifestyle, communication requirements, and personality style of the patient.

▼ Patients have an understanding of adaptation/brain rewiring process that occurs with initial hearing aid use.

▼ The hearing aid user has the ability to operate, clean, and maintain his or her hearing instruments.

▼ The hearing aid user has the ability to communicate successfully on the telephone while using the hearing aid without having to remove the instrument.

▼ Patients demonstrate full understanding of the advantages and limitations of hearing instrument use.

▼ Patients comprehend that the hearing instrument is only one part of the total hearing rehabilitation process.

Clinical Indications

▼ Hearing aid fitting is undertaken for all aged individuals as a result of audiological evaluation and successful management of affective barriers to hearing aid use.

Clinical Process

▼ Comprehensive audiological assessment, including case history.

▼ Probing to discover the patient's emotional state regarding hearing impairment and hearing aid use.

▼ Use of cognitive therapy strategies to alleviate the patient's inappropriate thinking regarding his or her hearing impairment.

▼ Referral to mental health professionals when a patient manifests severe denial or depression.

▼ Selection of hearing instrument technology and size on the basis of the patient's emotional attitudes, personality style, audiometric data, lifestyle, and communication goals.

▼ Continuous monitoring and management of the patient's emotional status and personality style throughout the hearing rehabilitation process.

▼ Orientation concerning the occlusion effect, audibility, and other interaction effects experienced by new hearing aid users.

▼ Orientation on the care, operation, and use of the hearing instruments.

▼ Counseling throughout the course of hearing rehabilitation to set realistic goals and understand that hearing aids are only one component of hearing rehabilitation.

Documentation

▼ Documentation contains relevant case history information, audiometric data, dispensing checkoff sheet, specification recommendations, and log of follow-up visits.

▼ Documentation includes confirmation of compliance with all appropriate federal/state laws, regulations, and guidelines for hearing instruments.

▼ Documentation includes all pertinent information concerning the ordering and repair of the hearing aids or earmolds.

▼ Documentation includes all real-ear, functional gain, and other behavioral measures.

Chapter 15

Implantable Hearing Aids

Douglas A. Miller and John M. Fredrickson

It is estimated that at present more than 28 million persons in the United States have a hearing loss severe enough to cause problems in communication (American Speech-Language-Hearing Association, 1996). The severity of these losses range from mild, where problems may only be encountered in situations in which significant background noise is present, to profound, where problems may arise even in the quietest listening situation. Figure 15–1 illustrates the categories of hearing loss, their respective thresholds, and the maximum output level a device should be capable of producing, without distortion, to adequately address each category. Generally, when the loss is sensorineural in nature, air conduction hearing aids are capable of providing significant benefit for persons with mild to moderate hearing loss and to some degree for persons with more severe hearing losses. If the loss is conductive, it can often be corrected by surgical means, or the patient can derive adequate benefit with air conduction hearing aids. Aural rehabilitation and assistive listening devices, which are used effectively in treating less severe hearing losses, as well as tactile aids and *cochlear implants* are the treatments currently available for persons with profound hearing losses. A small subset of the profoundly hearing impaired are those patients with auditory nerve discontinuity for whom *electrode arrays implanted into the brain stem* are currently under investigation.

However, a growing population of patients with moderately severe to severe sensorineural hearing loss (estimated to be some 3 to 4 million in the United States) are often dissatisfied with air conduction hearing aids but have sufficient residual hearing to preclude the use of cochlear implants. This population has been recognized by several research groups, who are working to develop *implantable middle ear hearing devices*.

Another group also has a history of unsatisfactory treatment with air conduction hearing aids. These are patients

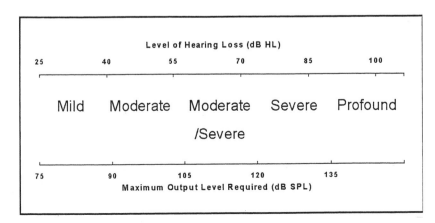

Figure 15–1 Levels of hearing loss and the output level in dB SPL that a device should be capable of generating to provide adequate amplification to effectively treat each category.

489

with recurrent otitis externa or chronic suppurative otitis media, which precludes the placement of an object in the external auditory canal, and persons with an atresia of the outer ear, who have conductive or mixed hearing loss. Implantable bone conduction hearing aids, generally termed *bone anchored hearing aids*, have been developed as a treatment option for this population.

Early work in the field of implantable hearing devices was conducted by Alvar Wilska in 1935, when he placed iron particles on the tympanic membrane and vibrated them with an electromagnetic field, suggesting that mechanical, rather than acoustic, stimulation of the ear was a viable alternative. Even earlier, electrical stimulation of the ear was suggested by Alessandro Volta, who, around 1800, placed an electrode at each ear and reported hearing a sound like rushing water when he applied a current from a battery to the electrodes.

For the moderately severe to severely hearing-impaired, air conduction hearing aids are currently the most commonly used treatment. However, due to feedback, distortion and occlusion effects, these patients are frequently dissatisfied with these aids, often to the point of discontinuing their use. Although this segment of the hearing-impaired population is relatively small, perhaps 15%, this means approximately 3 to 4 million persons in the United States fall within this category. This is the group of patients for whom middle ear implants are attempting to provide improved benefit.

The cochlear implant was developed to treat patients with profound hearing loss. Due to the arduous fitting and training period, which is not always successful, and the fact that residual hearing is destroyed by the electrode insertion, the cochlear implant is not generally deemed appropriate for less severe hearing losses.

Another type of implantable device under development is the auditory brain stem implant. This device is being developed to treat persons who no longer have an intact auditory nerve (e.g., in cases in which a portion of the nerve has been obliterated during the removal of an acoustic neuroma). Like the cochlear implant, this device provides electrical stimulation of the auditory system; however, whereas the point of electrical stimulation with the cochlear implant is the cochlea, the brain stem implant's electrodes deliver an electrical signal directly to the cochlear nucleus complex.

The selection criteria for implantable hearing devices depend on the type of device and the particular characteristics of the hearing loss it was designed to address. At this time, implantable hearing devices are generally considered only when air conduction hearing aids are not able to provide satisfactory performance. The four categories of implantable hearing aids and the types of hearing losses they have been designed to treat are outlined in Table 15–1.

Although it is currently not considered appropriate to recommend an implantable hearing device if the patient can be satisfactorily fitted with an air conduction hearing aid, other considerations may influence the decision not to recommend an implantable device. These include the requirement for surgery, the cost of an implantable device and the related expense, or an assessment predicting no improvement over an air conduction aid. Also, nothing would be gained by fitting an implant if the problem is determined to be central in nature.

CONTROVERSIAL POINT

Much controversy exists as to whether, with the progression of technology in the design and fitting of air conduction hearing aids, implantable devices, particularly middle ear implants, will be appropriate to recommend, given the cost and need for surgery. Some argue that many of the potential benefits of these devices can be implemented in air conduction hearing aids through the use of new technological breakthroughs. On the other hand, additional benefits may be derived from middle ear implants, such as improved sound quality and lack of occlusion effect, that even the most advanced air conduction hearing aid cannot offer. Furthermore, if a fully implantable device is achieved, it also offers more than just a cosmetic advantage, including shielding of the electronics from moisture and weather extremes.

At present, only bone anchored hearing aids and cochlear implants have market approval in the United States. Middle ear implants and auditory brain stem implants are under investigation in several clinical trials. This chapter describes implantable hearing aids in each of these categories, with particular attention to the bone anchored and middle ear implantable devices.

TABLE 15–1 Types of implantable hearing devices and conditions for which they may be indicated

Type of Device	Designed to Treat
Bone anchored implant	Conductive hearing loss caused by outer ear atresia, either congenital or acquired; chronic otitis externa or media
Middle ear implant	Moderately severe to severe sensorineural and mixed hearing loss
Cochlear implant	Profound hearing loss
Brain stem implant	Eighth cranial nerve discontinuity or dysfunction

DESCRIPTION OF IMPLANTABLE HEARING DEVICES

Bone Anchored Hearing Aids

Bone conduction hearing aids provide stimulation of the cochlear fluids by causing the mastoid bone to vibrate at auditory frequencies. Conventional external bone conduction hearing aids are typically attached to the mastoid by means of a headband, which is cosmetically unattractive, can be difficult to attach satisfactorily, and is uncomfortable to wear. Functionally, bone conduction hearing aids must conduct their vibrational energy through soft tissue to reach the mastoid. Because of this, bone conduction hearing aids typically provide limited output and a narrow frequency response as a result of the dampening effect of the soft tissue. As a result, bone anchored hearing aids have been developed as an alternative treatment approach.

The evolution of bone anchored hearing aids can be traced to the 1970s, when dissatisfaction with external bone conduction hearing aids led to a search for a device that offered improved performance. The bone anchored hearing aids is a by-product of Brånemark's work involving load-bearing titanium implants (Portmann et al, 1997) and the dissatisfaction of patients wearing bone conduction hearing aids. Bone anchored hearing aids were first developed in the mid-1970s in Sweden as a *percutaneous approach* (Tjellström & Håkansson, 1995) and later in the mid-1980s in the United States as a *transcutaneous approach* (Hough et al, 1995). The percutaneous technique involves direct contact with the mastoid bone through the skin. The drawback with this approach is that good hygiene is required to prevent inflam-

mation where the implant protrudes through the skin. This technique does, however, provide for greater efficiency in transmitting the vibrational energy to the mastoid. The transcutaneous technique does not require the implant to protrude through the skin, but instead uses a modulated electromagnetic field to cause a magnet anchored to the mastoid beneath the skin to vibrate at auditory frequencies. The difficulty with this technique is that it results in lower efficiency (i.e., reduced output) and poorer frequency response than the percutaneous method.

Bone anchored hearing aids are primarily indicated when a malformation or atresia of the outer ear exists, which can be either a congenital condition or one caused by external trauma. This device may also be recommended when an unresolvable chronic otitis is present, because the earmold or shell of an air conduction hearing aid often causes additional inflammation and prevents drainage.

Specific indications for bone anchored hearing aids based on the manufacturer's recommendations are as follows:

- Conductive or mixed (transcutaneous approach) or mixed, but primarily conductive (percutaneous approach) hearing loss that cannot be adequately fit with air conduction hearing aids due to chronic or recurrent otitis media, otitis externa, or severe malformation or atresia of the outer ear
- Air conduction pure tone average (PTA) greater than 40 dB HL
- Bone conduction PTA (500, 1000, 2000 Hz) no greater than 25 dB HL for the transcutaneous approach and 45 dB HL for the percutaneous approach
- Air conduction speech reception threshold greater than 40 dB HL
- Air conduction speech discrimination score of at least 80%

Types

The two types of bone anchored hearing aids are differentiated by the fact that one houses the transducer used to vibrate the mastoid bone in an external unit with a physical link through the skin to the anchor screw (the percutaneous approach). The other type anchors a magnet to the mastoid bone and causes it, and therefore the mastoid, to vibrate when subjected to an external electromagnetic field (the transcutaneous approach).

The percutaneous design (Fig. 15–2) was developed by Nobel Biocare. Their device, the *BAHA (Bone Anchored Hearing Aid)*, consists of a titanium screw anchored in the mastoid. Attached to this screw is a percutaneous abutment that has a bayonet connector for attaching the transducer and processor. Stimulation is by direct mechanical vibration of the mastoid, and consequently the cochlea, through the percutaneous abutment (Håkansson et al, 1990).

The transcutaneous design (Fig. 15–3) was developed by Hough and Xomed-Treace. This device, the *Audiant*, consists of a titanium encased samarium cobalt magnet anchored to the mastoid bone, which is stimulated electromagnetically by an external energizing coil contained in the processor. However, due to the coil-to-magnet distances dictated by the skin thickness, its performance was inadequate and this device has since been withdrawn from the market (Dormer et al, 1986).

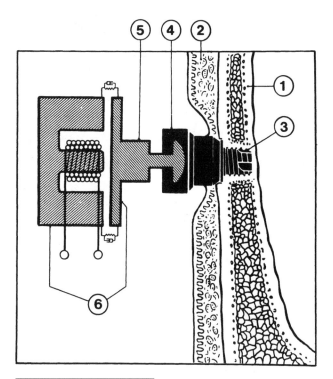

Figure 15–2 Percutaneous bone anchored hearing aid. *(1)* Mastoid bone, *(2)* soft tissue, *(3)* titanium fixture, *(4)* titanium abutment, *(5)* bayonet coupling, *(6)* percutaneous transducer. (From Tjellström & Hakånsson [1995], with permission.)

Middle Ear Implants

Early investigations into directly stimulating the ossicles dates to Wilska in 1935. His experiments with iron particles placed on the tympanic membrane, which he stimulated with an electromagnetic coil, demonstrated that pure tones could be perceived by the subject in this manner (Wilska, 1935). In the late 1950s Rutschmann also successfully stimulated the ossicles by gluing 10 mg magnets onto the umbo and causing them to vibrate via the application of a modulated magnetic field with an electromagnetic coil (Rutschmann, 1959). The Department of Electrical Engineering at the University of Pittsburgh published a paper in 1967 describing the design of an implantable hearing aid. In this paper was a discussion concerning the adaptation of cardiac pacemaker technology for use in an implantable hearing aid. As a consequence of this effort, a patent was granted for an implantable hearing aid. It seems, however, that no device based on this patent was ever fabricated and tested (Goode, 1970). Although initially suggested earlier, devices that were actually placed into the middle ear did not appear until the 1970s (Fredrickson

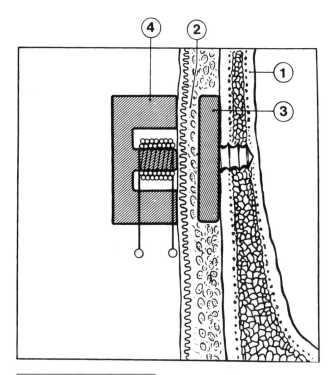

Figure 15–3 Transcutaneous bone anchored hearing aid (Audiant). *(1)* Mastoid bone, *(2)* soft tissue, *(3)* titanium anchored magnet, *(4)* transducer coil. (From Tjellström & Hakånsson [1995], with permission.)

et al, 1973; Goode et al, 1995; Nunley et al, 1976). These early experiments paved the way to develop devices that are now making their way into clinical trials.

Three general types of transducers are used in middle ear implants. Each has its advantages and disadvantages relating to power, efficiency, frequency response, and reliability. The types of transducers are *piezoelectric, electromagnetic,* and *electromechanical.*

Piezoelectric devices make use of the properties of piezoelectric materials, specifically, the property that when a voltage is applied, a deformation of the material results. This deformation provides the mechanical energy to stimulate the ossicular chain or inner ear (Fig. 15–4). Piezoelectric devices are found in two configurations, the *monomorph* and *bimorph.* The monomorph uses the expansion and contraction directly to provide the displacement, whereas a bimorph uses two pieces of piezoelectric materials bonded together with opposite polarities, causing bending of the structure.

The electromagnetic transduction devices consist of a magnet, generally rare earth (either *samarium cobalt* or *neodymium iron boron*), and an energizing coil. The magnet is attached to the ossicular chain, tympanic membrane, or the inner ear (round window or fenestra). A fluctuating magnetic field is generated when the coil is energized by a signal corresponding to an acoustic input. This magnetic field causes the magnet to vibrate (Fig. 15–5). The vibrating magnet then, in turn, causes movement of either the ossicular chain or the cochlear fluids directly. Since the force generated is inversely proportional to the square of the distance between the coil and magnet (e.g., doubling the distance between the magnet and coil results in an output of

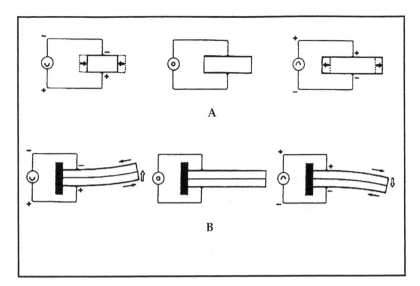

Figure 15–4 How piezoelectric transducers work. Piezoelectric material will contract or expand as a voltage is applied (**A**), depending on the polarity. When two pieces of piezoelectric material are bonded together with opposite polarities (**B**), as a voltage is applied, one shrinks and the other expands. This action causes the bimorph to bend.

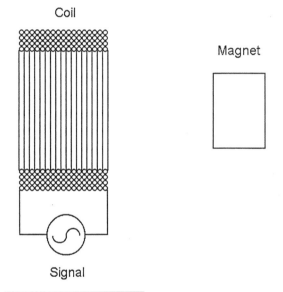

Figure 15–5 Electromagnetic stimulation. The varying magnetic field generated as a signal is introduced into the coil and causes an interaction with the static magnetic field of the magnet. This interaction results in movement of the magnet.

one fourth the force), it is evident that these two components must be maintained in close proximity to one another to realize an efficient system.

Electromechanical transduction is a variation of the electromagnetic type. Because it is often difficult to control the spatial relationship of the magnet and coil with the magnet attached to one portion of the anatomy and the coil attached to another, it is possible that a wide variation in performance will be observed. This is manifested in varying frequency responses and fluctuation of output levels if the relationship between the coil and magnet changes. With the electromechanical device, the energizing coil and magnet are housed within an assembly with an optimized spatial and geometric relationship to avoid this problem. The mechanical energy produced by this type of device is transmitted by a direct connection of the electromechanical transducer to the ossicular chain (Fig. 15–6).

Indications for middle ear implants are widely varied among the many different devices under investigation, and patient selection criteria greatly depend on the type of transducer and the method by which it is implemented. However, unlike bone anchored hearing aids, middle ear implants are targeting the sensorineural hearing-impaired population, as well as some patients with conductive, or mixed hearing losses. Depending on the characteristics of the implant, the device may be recommended for hearing losses ranging from mild to severe, and candidacy may include sensorineural, conductive, or mixed hearing loss categories.

As one example, the piezoelectric device developed by Yanagihara and his colleagues in Japan was implanted in patients with mixed hearing losses of varying degrees caused by chronic otitis media, but who did not have an untreated infection of the middle ear at the time of implantation. Average bone conduction hearing threshold in the frequencies 500, 1000, and 2000 Hz did not exceed 40 dB HL, and the patients had a moderate to severe hearing loss in the

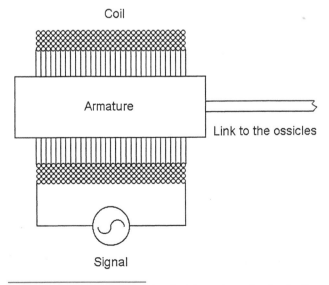

Figure 15–6 An electromechanical transducer is physically linked to the ossicles to transmit the stimulus to the middle ear.

contralateral ear. Prior intraoperative vibratory testing was conducted to assess whether the device would provide benefit superior to that provided by reconstructive middle ear surgery (Yanagihara et al, 1988).

In contrast, selection criteria for the electromagnetic device developed at Case Western Reserve University include patients with symmetrical moderate to severe sensorineural hearing loss who have a normal middle ear and mastoid and have word recognition scores of 60% or better. Magnetic resonance imaging (MRI) is obtained if there is a question of the etiology of a retrocochlear sensorineural hearing loss (Maniglia et al, 1997).

Furthermore, the electromechanical device under investigation by Fredrickson and his colleagues at Washington University in St. Louis is recommended for patients with bilateral, moderate-to-severe nonfluctuating sensorineural hearing loss. The patient should have normal middle ear function with air-bone gaps of less than or equal to 10 dB.

Cochlear Implants

Cochlear implants have become the treatment of choice for profoundly deaf adults and children who obtain little or no benefit from conventional amplification. Sounds are translated into small electric currents that stimulate the auditory nerves in the cochlea and generate hearing sensations. Most notable have been the 3M/House, the Cochlear Corporation Nucleus, and the Advanced Bionics Clarion. As an example, the Nucleus cochlear implant is the result of more than 20 years of research and development, first at the University of Melbourne, Australia, and later by Cochlear Proprietary Limited (Sydney, Australia) in collaboration with the University of Melbourne. Today, Cochlear Corporation's Mini-22 implant system is approved by the United States Food and Drug Administration (FDA) for use in adults and children and, as of 1991, had been implanted in more than 3000 patients worldwide (Patrick & Clark, 1991). For a more

in-depth discussion on cochlear implants, refer to Chapters 16 and 17 in this volume.

Brain Stem Implants

Evolution of auditory brain stem implants stemmed from work with cochlear implants. The auditory brain stem implant was developed to treat patients whose cochlea is disconnected from the brain stem, such as often results from the removal of an acoustic neuroma. Research into the development of this type of device was conducted at the House Ear Institute in the late 1970s, culminating in the implantation of three patients. Early devices were single channel, but more recently, multichannel devices using cochlear implant processors have come under investigation in clinical trials.

According to Otto et al (1998), auditory brain stem implants are indicated for hearing impairment caused by loss of auditory nerve function. This is generally due to the diagnosis and required removal of tumors associated with neurofibromatosis Type 2 (NF2). Indeed, in current clinical trials, this is the only condition for which the brain stem implant is approved. Cochlear implants are not indicated in these patients, since complete tumor removal generally requires the transection of the auditory nerve.

The auditory brain stem implant consists of an electrode array that is placed into the lateral recess in such a way as to provide electrical stimulation of the *cochlear nucleus complex*. Early electrode designs incorporated a single electrode/ground pair. However, more recently, multiple electrode arrays utilizing up to nine electrodes have been developed and implanted. The electrode array is connected by a cable to a subcutaneous receiver unit (Fig. 15–7). The receiver obtains power and signal from an externally worn device based on a cochlear implant processor, which contains the microphone, processor, battery, and transmitter (Shannon et al, 1993).

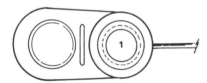

Receiver/stimulator with ground electrode

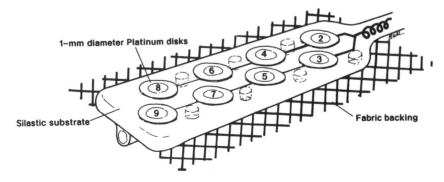

Figure 15–7   The auditory brain stem implant is similar to a cochlear implant except that the electrode array *(bottom)* is placed in the lateral recess where it provides electrical stimulation of the cochlear nucleus complex. The receiver is placed behind the ear just beneath the skin. (From Otto et al [1998], with permission.)

CHARACTERISTICS OF IMPLANTABLE HEARING DEVICES

Advantages

A number of potential advantages of implants exist over air conduction hearing aids, but these vary depending on the type of implant. Because nothing is worn in the earcanal with bone anchored hearing aids, the discomfort of wearing an earmold or hearing aid shell is avoided. The occlusion effect, the impression that bone-conducted sound is louder when the earcanal is tightly closed, is nonexistent with bone anchored hearing aids. In addition, as previously mentioned, problems with otitis of the middle and outer ear are decreased.

The advantages of middle ear implants compared with air conduction hearing aids include better *impedance matching* with the middle ear, resulting in more efficient energy transmission, and the virtual elimination of feedback, which markedly reduces distortion and results in better fidelity. As with bone anchored hearing aids, nothing is placed in the earcanal with most types of middle ear implants.

To expand on the advantages of middle ear devices, the impedance mismatch between the air in the external auditory canal and the cochlear perilymph results in reflection of a significant portion of the amplified sound. To illustrate, 99.9% of incident sound energy at an air-to-water interface is reflected (Fig. 15–8). The ossicular chain acts to improve the impedance mismatch between the air in the earcanal and the fluid in the cochlea, which improves energy transmission; however, there is still a high level of reflected acoustic energy. In a normal-hearing person, there is no issue of feedback and the normal ear has a sensitivity appropriate for the energy that is transmitted through the middle ear to the cochlea. In an impaired ear, however, the amplified acoustic energy reflected from the tympanic membrane can leak past the earmold and be picked up by the microphone of the hearing aid, resulting in feedback. In the worst case this feedback causes an audible squeal that is very unpleasant and reduces intelligibility. It should be noted that even at levels at which the feedback is not audible, distortion can still be introduced, which decreases the fidelity of the signal.

With a middle ear implant, there is direct mechanical stimulation of the ossicular chain, and the device can be designed so as to provide a close impedance match with the middle ear. Therefore the energy is transmitted much more efficiently and with less distortion. Virtually no feedback is present with a middle ear implant, although, since the tympanic membrane acts as a speaker diaphragm, some sound energy is generated in the external earcanal. This signal is, however, sufficiently below the ambient sound level that it causes no discernable feedback. Of course, in the instances in which the ossicular chain is disarticulated, as with the Yanagihara piezoelectric device, no mechanical energy is transmitted to the tympanic membrane, and therefore no sound energy is transmitted to the external earcanal from the middle ear.

Although some middle ear implant designs include components in the earcanal, ideally, the goal is to have nothing placed there. This not only relieves the discomfort associated with wearing an earmold or hearing aid shell, but occlusion effects are also eliminated, because acoustic energy produced by bone conduction transmission is not contained by a closed canal. Finally, elimination of an earmold or hearing aid shell significantly benefits patients suffering from recurrent otitis externa. Otitis media is a contraindication for middle ear implants, and therefore these devices should not be recommended for a patient with chronic or recurrent infections of the middle ear.

In the case of cochlear and auditory brain stem implant candidates, the hearing loss often cannot be satisfactorily treated by air conduction hearing aids. Although high-gain air conduction hearing aids can be fitted with limited success for some patients who are cochlear implant candidates, generally cochlear implants are recommended for patients with no functional hearing. Any type of hearing aid that acts on the outer, middle, or inner ear is not an option for auditory brain stem implant candidates because the acoustic signal cannot reach the cortex as a result of the discontinuity of the auditory nerve. For candidates for these devices, central electrical stimulation is the only avenue of treatment for the affected ear, although a CROS (contralateral routing of signals) or BICROS hearing aid may be fitted. It has been found, however, that few acoustic neuroma patients are satisfied with a CROS hearing aid, although when a hearing loss is present in the other ear, a BICROS can be useful (Pulec, 1994). A more detailed description of the CROS and BICROS technologies is discussed in Chapters 1, 2, and 5 in this volume.

Disadvantages

Some potential disadvantages of implantable hearing devices exist. The first, and most obvious, is that surgery is required for placement of the device. As with any surgical intervention, the possibility of infection or other wound complications and risks associated with anesthesia are present. A disadvantage specific to bone anchored hearing aids involves stimulation of the contralateral ear by bone conduction crossover, reducing the patient's ability to determine the direction from which a sound is emanating. In addition, the patient may experience fatigue because the skull is subjected to constant vibration.

In addition to the initial surgery for implantation, middle ear implants may require further surgery should a device failure occur, in order to correct or remove it. This is a more

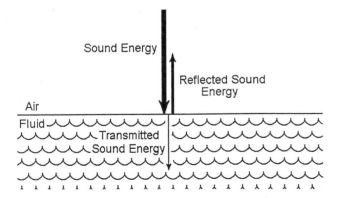

Figure 15–8 Due to the difference in the impedances of air and fluids, most of the sound energy is reflected, rather than transmitted through the air/fluid interface.

relevant issue for middle ear devices than bone anchored implants because they are generally more complex with the inherent possibility for failure.

SPECIAL CONSIDERATION

Battery life in semi-implantable (transcutaneous) devices will generally be shorter than a typical air conduction hearing aid, because the efficiency of transmission of energy through the skin in these devices is typically in the range of 50 to 70%.

The cochlear and auditory brain stem implants have their own unique disadvantages. Unlike bone anchored and middle ear implants, electrical stimulation of the cochlea or cochlear nucleus complex does not provide normal auditory sensation. Also, electrical stimulation of the auditory system is not yet well understood. For these reasons, proper fitting of cochlear and brain stem implants is typically an arduous task. However, improvements in coding strategies have greatly improved the quality of hearing perception. As in the bone-anchored and middle ear implants, the disadvantage of surgical intervention and its associated risks exists; in fact, the risks are greater due to the closer proximity of the surgery to the cranial nerves. There is also the possibility of nonauditory, usually vestibular nerve, stimulation with these devices also exists (Otto et al, 1998).

With all of these devices, at this point in development the necessity for an external component still exists, and consequently, they are still prone to many of the same maintenance and cosmetic issues associated with air conduction hearing aids. However, the eventual goal with most, if not all, of these devices, is the development into fully implantable devices, which will result in a cosmetically appealing option. Finally, implantable devices are expensive, both due to the cost of the device itself and because of the cost of surgery. At present, third-party reimbursement is limited for this category of treatment, although it should improve as the use of implantable devices becomes more widespread.

STATUS OF IMPLANTABLE HEARING DEVICES

Hardware

Microphones

The bone anchored hearing aids fitted to date share microphone technology with air conduction hearing aids, therefore the microphones are typically the electret type used in air conduction hearing aids. In the middle ear devices currently under investigation, generally an air conduction hearing aid is modified to transmit the signal to the implant, therefore the microphones are the same used in the hearing aid. Cochlear implants and brain stem implants share very similar technology, indeed, the brain stem implant under investigation at the House Ear Institute uses modified cochlear implant components to deliver the signal to the electrode array. The microphones used in cochlear implants are also the electret type used in air conduction hearing aids. Further information on electret microphones can be found elsewhere in this volume in Chapter 1.

Signal Processing

Only linear amplification and input compression have been used as signal processing approaches in bone anchored hearing aids to date. As with microphones, signal processing is usually that of a commercially available air conduction hearing aid since an air conduction hearing aid generally is modified to transmit the signal to middle ear implants. This processing may be as simple as linear amplification, or it may be as complex as state-of-the-art multichannel compression and frequency shaping implemented in a fully digital processor. Signal processing in cochlear implants and auditory brain stem implants is of a substantially different nature than that of air conduction hearing aids. It involves determining which electrodes to activate and at what level to produce an auditory sensation. Further information on the signal processing approaches used in electrical stimulation of the auditory system may be found in Chapters 1, 4, 5, 6, and 13 in this volume.

SPECIAL CONSIDERATION

It is important to keep in mind that advances in air conduction hearing aids and fitting techniques can also often be used to improve performance of those implantable devices that act on the conductive pathway of the ear.

Output Transduction

The output medium of implantable devices is one of two types, either vibrational (mechanically transduced) energy as in bone anchored and middle ear devices or electrical energy as in cochlear and brain stem implants. For electrical stimulation, an electrode array is placed either in the cochlea or the brain stem. However, the method for delivering vibrational energy is widely varied, with respect to both the type of transducer and its location.

The first type of transducer used to convert electrical energy to mechanical energy is the piezoelectric transducer. Use of this type is limited to middle ear implants, because its simple design is attractive, but it is not considered to have adequate low frequency power for bone anchored implants. Although a number of piezoelectric materials are available, *lead titanate zirconate* is the material generally chosen as it is one of the most efficient (Dumon et al, 1995; Yanagihara et al, 1983). The development of new piezoelectric materials in the future could improve the performance of devices that use this type of transducer.

Electromagnetic transducers are used for both bone anchored and middle ear implants. Output transduction in electromagnetic types of bone anchored and middle ear implants is a custom-designed electromagnetic coil/magnet configuration. Implementation is varied but of the same general concept. In middle ear implants an electromagnetic coil, placed either externally or implanted near or in the middle ear, is used to stimulate a magnet placed on the ossicular chain or round window membrane. Coils are generally "aircore," that is, wire is not wound around a ferrous metal core. Use of a ferrous core coil increases power output; however, the tendency of the magnet to be attracted to the core causes a bias of the magnet toward the coil when it is not active. One of the concerns with regard to this issue is that the magnet could become dislodged. For this same reason, only a "push" force is generated by the coil. The magnets used in these devices are samarium cobalt or neodymium iron boron. Magnet weight must be kept low, 50 mg or less (Goode, 1989), so as not to cause a "mass-effect," thereby altering the frequency response characteristics of the ossicular chain.

SPECIAL CONSIDERATION

Neodymium iron boron magnets produce a more powerful magnetic field than samarium cobalt and therefore provide a greater output. However, if body fluids come in contact with the neodymium iron boron magnet, the magnetic strength can be significantly reduced because of the chemical interactions.

Electromagnetic transduction is also used in the transcutaneous bone anchored hearing aid (Audiant). The magnet is attached directly to the mastoid bone, and an electromagnetic coil is placed on the overlying skin. Force output realized with the magnet depends on its distance and orientation with respect to the coil. Therefore, coil current requirements increase with magnet distance and misalignment in order to produce the same amount of force.

Similar in concept to the electromagnetic transducer is the electromechanical transducer. Electromechanical transducers are also found in both bone anchored and middle ear implants. Implemented in middle ear implants, this design concept places a small electromechanical transducer into the middle ear and, via a mechanical link with the ossicles, stimulates the ossicular chain. Both custom designed and commercially available transducers have been used. The advantage of this type of device is that it can be designed as a closed magnetic circuit, which is more efficient and can have a more specifically designed frequency response. The disadvantage of this technique is that it is generally a more complex device and more susceptible to fatigue factors. Due to this consideration, the design process is targeted to create a device that functions reliably for the many years an implant will be required to function.

The electromechanical method of transduction is used in the percutaneous bone anchored hearing aid. The transducer is contained in the processor housing and is attached, through the skin, to a titanium abutment anchored to the mastoid bone.

Materials and Issues of Biocompatibility

The materials chosen in the design and construction of any implantable hearing device require careful consideration. Electrical conductors must have good conductivity, be accepted by the body, and be capable of withstanding the hostile corrosive environment. Gold is nearly as good a conductor as copper and is highly resistant to corrosion. In addition, it has been used for many decades in medical devices and instruments due to its superb biocompatibility. A stronger, but less conductive, material often used for electrical conductors is an alloy of 90% platinum and 10% iridium. Pure platinum is also sometimes used. Platinum and iridium are both highly resistant to corrosion and therefore perform exceptionally well in the body. This alloy has also proven to be well accepted by the body. Electrical conductors require, at least in some applications, an electrical insulator. If the conductor may be subjected to bending, the insulator must also be flexible. Polytetrafluoroethylene, more commonly known as *Teflon*, is generally used for this purpose. If the insulator can be rigid or if it is necessary that it be bonded to another metal, such as in an enclosure feedthrough, then a ceramic is the common choice. *Aluminum oxide* is such a ceramic and has a long history of being used in ossicular replacements. Both Teflon and aluminum oxide ceramics are unreactive and well tolerated in the body (Jahnke & Plester, 1981; Stensaas & Stensaas, 1978).

Because in most of these implants it is also necessary to place components into the body that are not biocompatible, these components must be encased in a material that is biocompatible. *Titanium* and *ceramics* are both used in this role. Both are well tolerated, perform well, and have a long history of successful implantation. However, titanium enclosures, which are sealed by welding after the contents are in place, are easier to manufacture. Titanium is also used for structural components, such as mounting platforms and anchors for implanted devices.

Finally, it is sometimes desirable to encapsulate some of the components of an implant in a flexible shell to maintain positional relationships and to provide a soft surface for overlying tissue. *Silicone elastomers* fill this role well. In the 1980s and 1990s, silicone acquired a poor reputation due to problems with breast implants. However, these problems were related to the liquid and gel forms of the material. The cured, solid form of silicone used to manufacture elastomers does not share this trait and has been shown, in exhaustive studies, to be inert and well tolerated by the body (Ng & Linthicum, 1992).

Algorithms and Software

In their current state of development, bone anchored and middle ear implants use an external component that essentially processes sound like any air conduction hearing aid. Indeed, a modified version of a commercial hearing aid is often used. The software and fitting techniques used for programming bone anchored and middle ear implants is usually derived from that currently available in commercial air conduction hearing aids. Because bone anchored hearing aids and middle ear implants can use many of the same techniques as air conduction hearing aids, commercial hearing aid software generally can provide a good starting point. This fitting software is then modified to meet the specific needs and capabilities of the device or is used as provided for fitting the signal processor chosen for use with the device.

The signal processing algorithms used in bone anchored and middle ear implants vary from simple linear amplification to the latest developments in frequency shaping and multichannel compression. Analog, hybrid, and fully digital processing are all being used with these devices, although it is expected that any well developed device would incorporate the best available signal processing technology, with the algorithms optimized for that particular device.

Fitting algorithms for bone anchored and middle ear implants are also essentially based on current knowledge of fitting conventional air conduction hearing aids. These fitting techniques are then adjusted to take into account the differing characteristics of the implanted device.

In contrast, the manner in which sound is processed for electrical stimulation of the auditory system is substantially different from air conduction processing. Simplistically, frequency is coded into electrical impulses that are mapped to the electrode array so as to elicit the sensation of hearing at that frequency. Auditory brain stem implants have drawn from the software developed for cochlear implants. This software is then adapted to the individual peculiarities of that type of device.

The signal processing and fitting algorithms, commonly referred to as coding strategies, that are used in auditory brain stem implants are taken from those laboriously developed for cochlear implants. These are more thoroughly discussed in Chapters 16 and 17 in this volume. As in cochlear implants, electrodes that elicit nonauditory sensation are not used in the auditory brain stem implant's coding scheme and the remaining electrodes are spectrally mapped for coding. Although nonauditory sensations are sometimes experienced with cochlear implants, they are more often experienced with auditory brain stem implants (Otto et al, 1998; Shannon et al, 1993).

Time Requirements

The time required to properly fit an implantable hearing aid varies depending on the type but, in general, requires a preliminary assessment of about 4 weeks to determine if the device would be of benefit and to verify the patient's ability to undergo the requisite surgery. Again, wound healing time varies depending on the type of implant, but in general, 4 to 6 weeks are required for proper healing and fluid to clear from the middle ear (in cases where the middle ear is opened). Processor fitting for bone anchored and middle ear stimulators can be expected to require a similar amount of time as that of air conduction hearing aids. Typically, several months or more are required for fitting devices that deliver electrical stimulation to the auditory system.

Risks

Risks vary with the type of implant and the method in which it is implemented. There is the common risk associated with any surgery of infection or wound complication. Depending on the device there may be risk of disarticulation of the ossicular chain, if indeed that is not done intentionally as in the Yanagihara device. Some procedures require working close to the facial nerve and pose a potential risk of facial nerve injury. In addition, excessive manipulation of the ossicular chain can cause trauma to the inner ear.

It has been suggested that at least some of these devices could eventually be implanted as an outpatient procedure with the patient under local anesthesia. In most cases, however, the surgery will currently be performed with the patient under general anesthesia with the associated risks.

It should be pointed out, however, that if unsatisfactory results occur, bone anchored implants and some middle ear implants can be explanted and the ear returned to its preimplant state, and an air conduction hearing aid may again be fitted.

Placement Procedure

In most cases the implantable hearing devices utilize a surgical approach, including a postauricular incision and some drilling of the mastoid bone. In the case of bone anchored hearing aids, the surgery can be performed relatively quickly, because the procedure is well developed, and only a small and uncomplicated surgical exposure is required for drilling the anchor hole. In the case of middle ear implants, surgery is more involved, requiring the surgeon to identify and preserve important anatomical structures as the middle ear is exposed. Otologists have, however, been entering the middle ear for many decades through the mastoid approach, and it is well described. Cochlear implant surgery additionally requires entering the inner ear, but many of the potential surgical risks involved in cochlear implant surgery have been reduced by many years of experience. Auditory brain stem implants are even more involved, as they require access to the lateral recess. However, these devices are generally placed during the time of tumor removal when this exposure is already developed. Surgery time will obviously vary with the type of device,

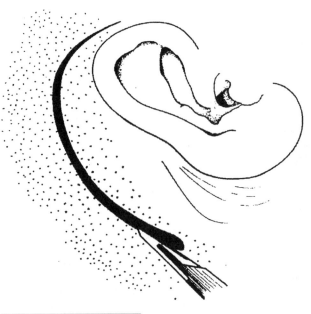

Figure 15–9 A postauricular incision is typically required for most implants.

but 1 to 2 hours is considered to be typical once the procedure is well practiced (Fig. 15–9).

INVESTIGATIONAL RESULTS

Pre-Clinical Investigations

Several groups have been conducting pre-clinical research in the field of middle ear implants. Much data have been collected using a variety of approaches and techniques. The results obtained by these researchers have shown much promise and are now beginning to be carried over into human clinical trials. Some of the more prominent pre-clinical work in this area include the following.

Dumon Group

Dumon and his colleagues at the University of Bordeaux, Bordeaux, France, have used piezoelectric devices implanted in the middle ear. The device is placed in contact with the round window membrane in order to stimulate the cochlear fluids. Twelve guinea pigs were implanted in this study and were evaluated over a 7-month period by auditory evoked potentials. Their results demonstrated responses similar to acoustic stimulation and were stable and reproducible over the entire period.

In an additional study this group also developed a method for placing a piezoelectric device in contact with the ossicular chain without removal of any of the components of the ossicular chain. This was done in human temporal bones, however, it was found that there was not always sufficient space in the middle ear for this approach (Dumon et al, 1995).

Fredrickson/Otologics

Fredrickson and his colleagues at Washington University in St. Louis, Missouri, have developed an electromechanical device (Fig. 15–10) that was implanted in 12 monkeys with up to 2 years of in vivo evaluation. Auditory brain stem responses and distortion product otoacoustic emissions were used to evaluate the performance of the device. Results demonstrated that the electrophysiological responses elicited by mechanical stimulation were similar to those produced by acoustic stimulation and that high intensity signals can be delivered to the middle ear effectively. Histological evaluation of the implanted ear indicated no deleterious effects (Fredrickson et al, 1995, 1996; Park et al, 1995).

Figure 15–11 depicts the Fredrickson device, called the MET, developed for human clinical trials. The external portion of the device utilizes a multichannel digital signal processor that transmits power and signal to the internal portion via a transcutaneous link. Noninvasive testing with an earlier design was accomplished by placing a long drive rod, attached to the transducer, in contact with the umbo. Two subjects with severe sensorineural hearing loss were evaluated in this study. These subjects demonstrated improvements in word recognition scores from 35 and 37% with insert receivers to 54 and 48%, respectively, with the transducer.

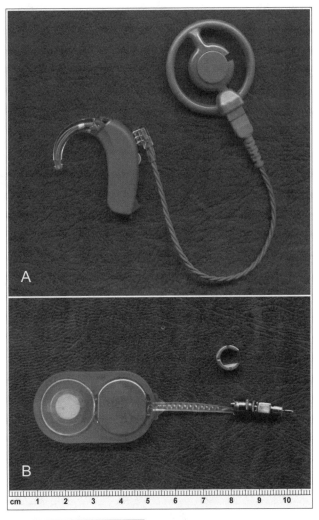

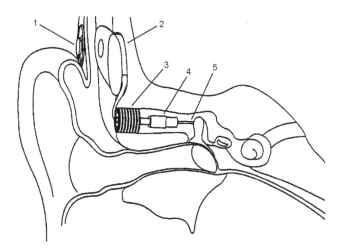

Figure 15–10 Fredrickson Middle Ear Transducer (MET). *(1)* Transmitting coil, *(2)* receiving coil and electronics, *(3)* anchoring and positioning mechanism, *(4)* transducer, *(5)* probe tip coupling the transducer to the incus.

Figure 15–11 MET device. **(A)** External components: microphone, battery, processor, and transmitting coil; **(B)** implanted components: receiver, mounting ring, and transducer.

This group has completed pre-clinical studies and in collaboration with Otologics, LLC of Boulder, CO, has obtained FDA approval, and has begun multi-site human clinical trials with this device in the United States. Concurrent clinical trials will also be conducted in Europe and Japan.

Hough Group

Hough and his colleagues at the Hough Ear Institute in Oklahoma City, Oklahoma, placed magnets on the ossicular chain of guinea pigs and stimulated them with an external electromagnetic coil. Performance was evaluated by auditory nerve action potentials. Positive results with the animal investigations led to testing on patients undergoing surgery for otosclerosis and chronic tympanic membrane perforation. During surgery, magnets were temporarily placed on the ossicular chain and stimulated with an electromagnetic coil placed in the external auditory canal. Hearing thresholds and word recognition were evaluated, after which the magnet was removed and the surgery proceeded normally. These intraoperative results led to approval for a limited clinical trial. In the clinical trials patients were implanted with neodymium iron boron magnets and had good early results. However, degradation of the magnets caused them to cease functioning after approximately 3 months. Replacement with samarium cobalt magnets of similar strength recovered electromagnetic function. However, since the samarium cobalt magnets were larger in order to provide the same magnetic strength as the neodymium iron boron magnets, mass damping of the ossicular chain was experienced. Because this caused decreased function of the normal acoustic pathway, it was deemed unacceptable and the magnets were removed (Baker et al, 1995).

Maniglia/Wilson Greatbatch

Maniglia and his colleagues at Case Western Reserve University in Cleveland, Ohio, have developed an electromagnetic device that was implanted in seven cats and was evaluated for approximately 9 months of in vivo operation. This device consists of a titanium encapsulated magnet attached to the ossicular chain, which is stimulated by a small electromagnetic coil placed in close proximity in the attic of the middle ear (Fig. 15–12). Auditory brain stem responses were obtained to evaluate performance of this device. Results showed comparable thresholds to acoustic stimuli, and histological evaluation demonstrated no adverse effects to the middle ear (Maniglia et al, 1995, 1997).

The results of this work have led to FDA approval for clinical trials with this device. However, only one patient has been implanted due ro inadequate power output (Personal communication, Maniglia, 1998). This group is continuing their experiments.

Spindel Group

Spindel and his colleagues at University of Virginia in Charlottesville, Virginia, are another group investigating stimulation of the cochlear fluids via the round window. Their investigations involve a magnet placed on the round window

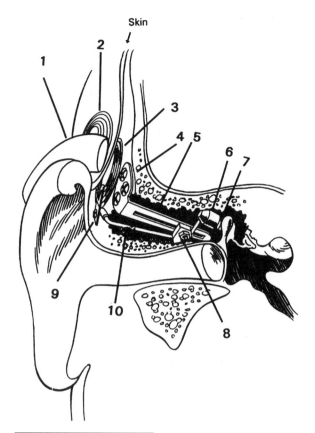

Figure 15–12 Maniglia electromagnetic ossicular stimulator. *(1)* External unit, *(2)* transmitting antenna, *(3)* receiving antenna, *(4)* horizontal support, *(5)* vertical support, *(6)* titanium encased electronics and electromagnetic coil, *(7)* titanium encased magnet attached to the incus, *(8)* locking system, *(9)* feedthrough, *(10)* malleable titanium tubing. (From Maniglia et al [1997], with permission.)

membrane of the guinea pig. Thirteen guinea pigs were implanted and stimulated by an external electromagnetic coil. Auditory brain stem responses in these animals demonstrated magnetic stimuli results comparable to those obtained acoustically (Spindel et al, 1995).

Welling and Barnes/St. Croix Medical

Welling and Barnes at Ohio State University in Columbus, Ohio, evaluated a piezoelectric device similar to the one used by Yanagihara. They intraoperatively stimulated the ossicular chain, the round window, and a fenestrated superior semicircular canal in four cats. Cochlear microphonic results demonstrated good correlation between mechanical and acoustic stimulation (Welling & Barnes, 1995).

Additional investigations into middle ear devices are discussed in the following section on human clinical trials. As previously mentioned in some of the preceeding discussions of preclinical investigations, middle ear devices are just beginning to enter human clinical trials. The status of investigations into middle ear devices is summarized in Table 15–2.

TABLE 15–2 Status of the more prominent middle ear devices under investigation

Primary Investigator	Supporting Company	Investigation Site	Type of Device	Current Status
Dumon		Bordeaux, France	Piezoelectric	Conducting animal and cadaver experiments
Frederickson	Otologics	United States, Germany, and Japan	Electromechanical	Conducting human clinical trials
Hough		Oklahoma City, Oklahoma	Electromagnetic	Limited human clinical trials, returned to device development
Maniglia	Wilson Greatbach	Cleveland, Ohio	Electromagnetic	Began human clinical trials, insufficient output caused return to device development
Perkins	ReSound	Redwood City, California	Electromagnetic	Conducted limited human trials, discontinued because of insufficient benefit
Spindel		Charlottesville, Virginia	Electromagnetic	Conducting animal experiments
Ball	Symphonix	San Jose, California	Electromechanical	Conducting human clinical trials
Kartush & Tos	Smith Nephew Richards	Denmark and United States	Electromagnetic	Conducted human clinical trials, discontinued because of insufficient benefit
Welling & Barnes	St. Croix Medical	Columbus, Ohio	Piezoelectric	Conducting animal experiments
Yanagihara	Rion	Japan	Piezoelectric	Continuing long-term human clinical trials

Clinical Investigations

At present several implantable hearing devices are under investigation in clinical trials around the world. Each category of implant (bone anchored, middle ear, cochlear and auditory brain stem) is represented in clinical trials. This has been an area of active investigation and, as mentioned, in the previous section on preclinical investigations, several groups are nearing human clinical trials.

Two bone anchored hearing aids have been investigated in human clinical trials. One of each type, percutaneous and transcutaneous, has been evaluated in a large patient population worldwide, and both have received market approval by the regulatory bodies of several countries.

Nobel Biocare BAHA

This device has been implanted in more than 3000 patients with more than 10 years follow-up; the first patients were implanted with the BAHA in 1977 (Fig. 15–13). This device has been widely investigated, resulting in a well-developed system and surgical procedure. Results have shown that it performs well when used in accordance with manufacturer's suggested guidelines. It provides improved hearing

thresholds and speech recognition scores relative to unaided hearing in patients unable to wear an earmold and is considered more comfortable to wear than conventional external bone conduction devices. It can be seen in Table 15–3 that the BAHA provides significant improvement in both thresholds and word discrimination over the unaided condition, and most patients reported the BAHA to be more comfortable to wear than the conventional bone conduction hearing aid (Håkansson et al, 1990, 1994; Tjellström & Håkansson, 1995).

Xomed Audiant

The Audiant was introduced in 1985 by Hough and developed in conjunction with Xomed-Treace. Results have shown the Audiant (Fig. 15–14) to be an adequate treatment if selection criteria are rigorously adhered to. It does not perform as well at lower frequencies (below 1000 Hz) as a conventional bone conduction hearing aid but does display somewhat better performance at higher frequencies. Table 15–4 shows two typical cases, indicating that the Audiant provides improved pure tone and speech thresholds but no significant difference in performance over a conventional bone conduction hearing aid. Patients did indicate that some improvement in comfort occurred with the Audiant compared with a conventional

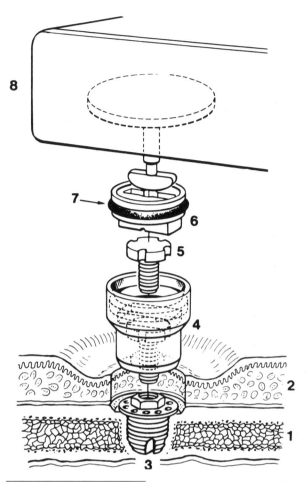

Figure 15–13 Nobel Biocare BAHA. *(1)* Mastoid bone, *(2)* skin and subcutaneous tissue, *(3)* titanium bone implant, *(4)* titanium abutment, *(5)* connection screw, *(6)* plastic insert, *(7)* silicone O-ring, *(8)* sound processor. (From Håkansson et al [1990], with permission.)

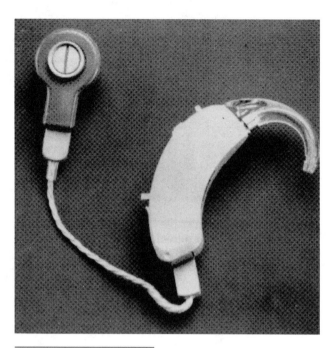

Figure 15–14 The Xomed Treace Audiant bone anchored bone conduction device. (From Pulu [1994], with permission.)

bone conduction hearing aid. However, the Audiant's limited power has relegated it to a rather small population and subsequently Xomed Treace has removed this device from the market (Pulec, 1994; Roush & Rauch, 1990; Tange et al, 1994).

Human clinical trials are being conducted with four middle ear devices, with others just beginning or approved to begin. The four described here have been conducting clinical trials sufficiently long enough to have accumulated data on

their performance. Each of these devices has a unique approach to stimulating the middle ear.

Yanagihara/Rion

Yanagihara and his colleagues at Ehime University and Teikyo University in Japan, in collaboration with Rion Company, have performed clinical trials with a partially implanted piezoelectric device, the PIHA (Fig. 15–15). Results in more than 80 patients with over 10 years of follow-up have been presented in numerous papers and lectures and have demonstrated patient satisfaction with this device. To illustrate, in Table 15–5 it can be seen that speech discrimination scores were generally improved with the implant compared with an air conduction hearing aid

TABLE 15–3 Mean performance of the Nobel Biocare BAHA compared with unaided and a conventional bone conduction device for a large group of subjects

Device	Pure Tone Average*	Word Discrimination[†]
Unaided	58.5 dB HL (SD = 12.7)	8.4% (SD = 16.1)
Bone conduction HA	31.2 (10.7)	43.9 (22.1)
BAHA	29.1 (9.4)	50.2 (21.9)

* Average sound field warble tone thresholds (average of 500, 1000, 2000, 3000 Hz), $n = 122$.
[†] Average word discrimination scores in noise presented at 63 dB SPL (S/N = 6 dB), $n = 110$.
  Adapted from Håkansson et al (1994), with permission.

TABLE 15–4 Performance of the Xomed-Treace Audiant compared with unaided and a conventional bone conduction device for two subjects

Device	Subject 1		Subject 2	
	PTA	SRT	PTA	SAT*
Unaided	52.5 dB HL	60 dB HL	72.5 dB HL	60 dB HL
Bone conduction HA	16.3	15	28.8	15
Audiant	15.0	15	31.3	15

*Speech reception thresholds (SRT) were not obtainable because of the patient's poor command of English; therefore speech awareness thresholds (SAT) were obtained instead.
Adapted from Roush and Rauch (1990), with permission.

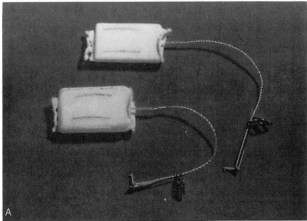

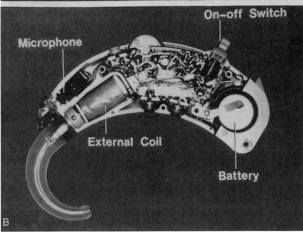

Figure 15–15 Yanagihara implantable hearing aid. **(A)** Implanted receiver and piezoelectric transducer; **(B)** external components housed in a BTE shell. (From Yanagihara et al [1995], with permission.)

using the same signal processing circuitry and microphone as the implant (Kodera et al, 1994). Although limited output capabilities have restricted implantation to patients with mild-to-moderate hearing losses, there has been a general approval of the device, and most continue to use it regularly.

The primary shortcomings of this device are the necessary removal of the incus for implantation (Fig. 15–16), its lack of

sufficient power for patients with greater degrees of hearing loss, and reported frequency responses no better than that of an air conduction hearing aid (Gyo et al, 1990; Suzuki et al, 1987, 1994; Yanagihara et al, 1984, 1995).

Kartush-Tos/Smith Nephew Richards

A variation of the electromagnetically stimulated magnet attached to the ossicular chain is to encapsulate the magnet in a total ossicular replacement prosthesis (TORP) as shown in Figure 15–17 or a partial ossicular replacement prosthesis (PORP). To activate the magnet, an electromagnetic coil is placed in a custom earmold in the earcanal (Fig. 15–18). This device has been used in patients with a mixed hearing loss where surgical replacement of all or part of the ossicular chain was performed. Although the device alleviates feedback, it still requires the placement of an object in the external canal. Performance of this device has not provided sufficient benefit, and Smith Nephew Richards has discontinued their support of the device (Kartush & Tos, 1995; Kartush et al, 1991; McGee et al, 1991).

Ball/Symphonix

The Vibrant Soundbridge, developed by Ball of Symphonix Devices in San Jose, California, consists of an electromagnetic "shaker" that has been termed a Floating Mass Transducer (FMT). This device is attached to the incus by crimping a titanium strap around the long process (Fig. 15–19). Vibration of the device is transmitted to the ossicles, thereby delivering stimuli to the middle and, subsequently, inner ear. Approximately 100 patients have been implanted in the United States and Europe with results pending (Gan et al, 1997).

Perkins/ReSound Corporation

Although not technically an implant, a unique device should also be mentioned that provides mechanical stimulation of the middle ear. This is a system developed by Perkins in collaboration with ReSound Corporation, in which a magnet attached to a thin silicone diaphragm was placed on the tympanic membrane of human volunteers (Fig. 15–20). It was held in place by the surface tension of a drop of mineral oil applied to the tympanic membrane. A coil placed in the earcanal was used to drive the magnet. Results were promising, but maximum functional gain was considered to be inadequate

TABLE 15–5   **Speech discrimination scores of six subjects (% correct). Test materials were tape-recorded nonsense monosyllable lists presented at 70 dB SPL.**

Subject	1	2	3	4	5	6
MEI	90	86	82	80	70	56
Hearing aid	82	86	88	58	56	36
MEI (w/noise)	82	86	68	72	66	48
Hearing aid (w/noise)	76	82	66	56	56	36

MEI, Middle ear implant.
Adapted from Kodera et al (1994), with permission.

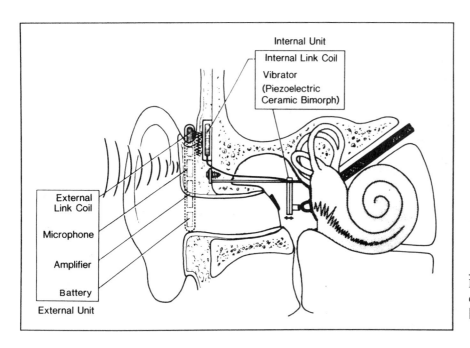

Figure 15–16   Yanagihara piezo-electric device. (From Yanagihara et al [1987], with permission.)

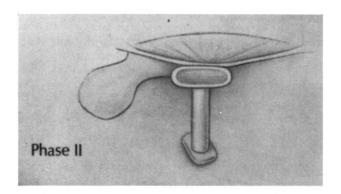

Figure 15–17   An example of the TORP electromagnetic device. The magnet is housed within the TORP near the tympanic membrane. (From Kartush & Tos [1995], with permission.)

for any but mild hearing losses. To eliminate the need for an object in the earcanal, experiments with a coil worn around the neck were also conducted; however, this too had functional gain of only approximately 25 dB, with poorer performance above 2000 Hz (Perkins, 1996).

Many varied clinical trials investigating cochlear implants are in progress around the world. The reader is referred to Chapters 16 and 17 in this volume for further information on cochlear implant clinical trials.

At present, only one auditory brain stem implant is under investigation. This is a difficult and exhausting area to research, with a narrow patient population, and although a need for work in this area exists, support has not been readily available. However, the group investigating this device, the House Ear Institute and Cochlear Corporation, has a long history of working with cochlear implants, which have several similarities.

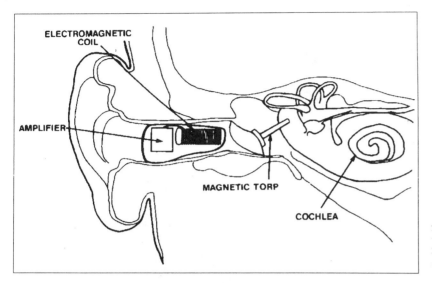

Figure 15–18. Smith Nephew Richards magnetically stimulated ossicular prosthesis. (From Tos et al [1994], with permission.)

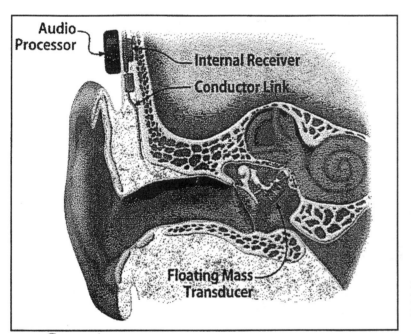

Figure 15–19 Symphonix Vibrant Sound-Bridge middle ear implant. (Source: Symphonix Literature.)

House Ear Institute/Cochlear Corp

Twenty-six patients were fitted with the auditory brain stem implant (Fig. 15–21) from 1992 through 1996. Performance on sound-only sentence recognition tests as high as 58% correct was reported, and some patients were even able to converse on the telephone. Most of the patients scored above chance in identifying environmental sounds, and all patients demonstrated that the auditory cues they received from the implant improved sentence recognition over lipreading alone. Figure 15–22 illustrates the degree to which the auditory brain stem implant can aid a patient's ability to communicate.

Concern about electrode migration led to MRI studies to verify electrode stability. Only one case of electrode migration was found, however, in that case auditory performance was unaltered and it was assumed the movement was due to brain stem and electrodes moving together as they shifted

into the empty space previously occupied by the tumor. The electrode arrays have been shown to be stable for 10 years (Otto et al, 1998; Shannon et al, 1993).

CONCLUSIONS

Although at this time, implants may not be deemed appropriate for patients with mild to moderate hearing losses who can be satisfactorily fitted with air conduction hearing aids, they do have the potential to provide a significant benefit for the moderate to severely hearing-impaired population who are dissatisfied with air conduction hearing aids.

The fitting technique and signal processing approaches for bone anchored and middle ear implants are similar to that of air conduction hearing aids, because the stimulus achieves

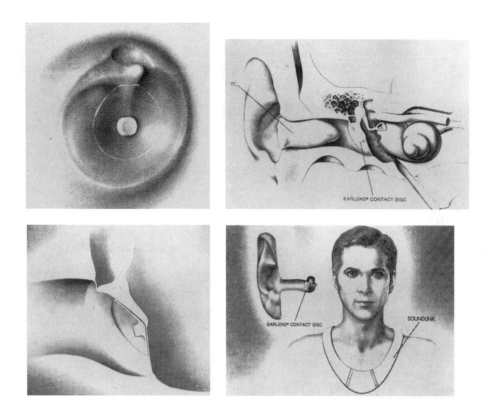

Figure 15–20 The EarLens system developed by Perkins and ReSound. A magnet, contained within a conical silicone disk, is placed on the external surface of the tympanic membrane. An energizing coil is then worn, either in the earcanal or around the neck. (From Perkins [1996], with permission.)

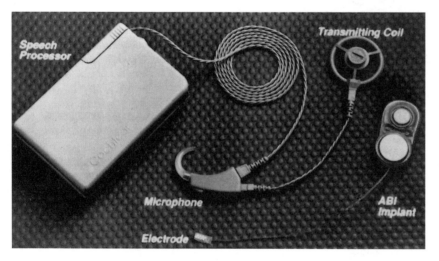

Figure 15–21 The House Ear Institute/Cochlear Corporation auditory brain stem implant. This device is based on a Nucleus cochlear implant manufactured by Cochlear Corporation. The cochlear electrode array of the Nucleus device is replaced with an array designed to be placed on the cochlear nucleus complex of the brain stem. (From Otto et al [1998], with permission.)

the same end result, that is, vibration of the cochlear fluids. Further developments in these areas will most certainly be made as the benefits and capabilities of these devices are better understood.

At this time, the effectiveness of bone anchored hearing aids is fairly well known. Although they are useful for a small segment of the population who have a relatively intact inner ear, they do not provide great benefit for patients with sensorineural hearing loss of any great degree.

The effectiveness of middle ear implants is just now being truly evaluated. Other than the piezoelectric device of Yanagihara, there have not yet been any major long-term clinical studies of a middle ear implant. In the case of Yanagihara's work, the patients expressed an appreciation for the quality of sound and most continue to use their device, but the degree of hearing loss that can currently be treated is relatively mild. In addition, the removal of a portion of the ossicular chain makes the procedure undesirable for patients with a normal middle ear.

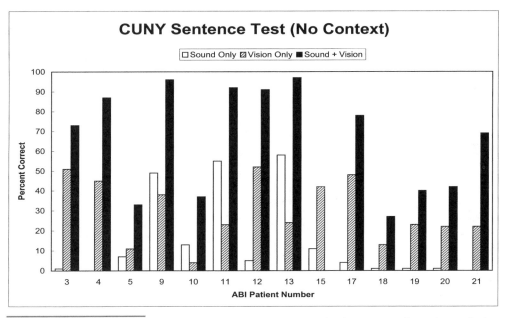

Figure 15–22 Percent correct recognition of sentences (sound only, vision only, and sound plus vision modes) on CUNY Sentence Test without context for patients using an auditory brain stem implant. (From Otto et al [1998], with permission.)

The cost of bone anchored hearing aids and middle ear implants are currently expected to be approximately equivalent to that of a state-of-the-art air conduction hearing aid, although there is an additional cost for the surgical procedure. However, device and audiological costs are expected to be similar. Auditory brain stem implants are expected to be similar to that of cochlear implants, although it should be easier to obtain reimbursement for surgical costs, because the surgery is required to remove the tumor.

Third party reimbursement through insurance and the government Medicare and Medicaid programs continues to be a major issue for implantable hearing devices. The ground was initially broken for third party reimbursement by cochlear implants; however, the percentage of the costs reimbursed still tends to be an issue for cochlear implants and this obstacle still needs to be overcome. It is anticipated that, although new types of implantable hearing devices will have to gain approval individually, they will find it easier to receive third party reimbursement due to precedents set by cochlear implants.

Future

Implantable hearing instruments are still in their infancy, although the cochlear implant already is relatively well established. Great potential exists in this area, and good reason exists to expect these devices to be an important addition to the audiologist's arsenal of tools for treating hearing loss. The fidelity, comfort, cosmesis, and convenience that will eventually come with a well developed, fully implantable device will greatly enhance the quality of life of the hearing impaired person. It could be debated that when implantable hearing devices reach a fully mature state, they could become an alternative to conventional hearing aids, providing the hearing impaired person with significantly improved performance.

Clearly, future signal processing developments in air conduction hearing aids can also be adapted for use in implantable devices. Higher processing speeds and lower power consumption of new DSP (digital signal processing) circuits will provide greater flexibility in frequency shaping and permit a wider frequency response. They will allow more complex compression algorithms to be implemented, providing an improved match to the patient's dynamic range. These more powerful processors will also allow improvements in signal-to-noise ratio by methods such as processing multiple microphone inputs, a technique already in use in air conduction hearing aids.

Development of the battery and microphone technology that would permit a fully implantable hearing device is well underway. Cardiac pacemaker companies have already produced prototype implantable rechargeable batteries. These batteries produce no by-products during charging and remain functional for more than 1000 charging cycles, making them suitable for use in the body. The prototypes now available would require daily recharging, most likely done while the person is sleeping. Although this is considered to be adequate for a practical device, higher capacity batteries can be expected to evolve that will increase the time between recharging.

Microphones that are constructed of biocompatible materials (or encased in them) are also being investigated. Techniques for placing these microphones in order to avoid a loss of sensitivity due to fibrosis or migration are also under consideration. The challenge in developing an implantable microphone may lie in enclosing a conventional, most likely electret, microphone in a biocompatible case in such a way as to not reduce its sensitivity. Alternately, a microphone constructed completely of biocompatible materials could be used. Research is currently underway that could result in just such a microphone. These researchers are using modern microchip technology is used to construct a microphone from silicon, a ceramic material that has been used successfully in the body for many years.

With further development of these technologies, a fully implantable device will be realized. With it would come the higher fidelity that these devices can deliver, the comfort of having no object placed in the external auditory canal and the elimination of any external component, thus allowing the patient to conceal the impairment. The convenience of minimal maintenance (only battery recharging) and less opportunity for damage to the device are also present. Finally, a significant benefit would be the ability of the hearing-impaired person to use the hearing device in environmental conditions that most of today's air conduction hearing aids cannot cope with, such as swimming, going out in the rain, or taking a shower.

REFERENCES

AMERICAN SPEECH-LANGUAGE HEARING ASSOCIATION. (1996). Communication Facts: Prevalence of hearing loss in the United States.

BAKER, R.S., WOOD, M.W., & HOUGH, J.V.D. (1995). The implantable hearing device for sensorineural hearing impairment: The Hough Ear Institute experience. *Otolaryngology Clinics of North America, 28*(1);147–153.

DORMER, K.J., RICHARD, G., McGEE, M., HOUGH, J.V., & SHEW, R.L. (1986). An implantable hearing device: Osseointegration of a titanium-magnet temporal bone stimulator. *American Journal of Otology, 7*(6);399–408.

DUMON, T., ZENNARO, O., ARAN, J.M., & BEBEAR J.P. (1995). Piezoelectric middle ear implant preserving the ossicular chain. *Otolaryngology Clinics of North America, 28*(1);173–187.

FREDRICKSON, J.M., COTICCHIA, J.M., & KHOSLA, S. (1995). Ongoing investigations into an implantable electromagnetic hearing aid for moderate to severe sensorineural hearing loss. *Otolaryngology Clinics of North America, 28* (1);107–120.

FREDRICKSON, J.M., COTICCHIA, J.M., & KHOSLA, S. (1996). Current status in the development of implantable middle ear hearing aids. *Advances in Otolaryngology, 10*:189–203.

FREDRICKSON, J.M., TOMLINSON, D.R., DAVIS, E.R., & ODKUIST, L.M. (1973). Evaluation of an electromagnetic implantable hearing aid. *Canadian Journal of Otolaryngology, 2*;53–62.

GAN, R.Z., WOOD, M.W., BALL, G.R., DIETZ, T.G., & DORMER, K.J. (1997). Implantable hearing device performance measured by laser Doppler interferometry. *Ear Nose Throat Journal, 76*(5);297–299,302,305–309.

GOODE, R.L. (1970). An implantable hearing aid. State of the art. *Transactions of the American Academy of Ophthalmology and Otolaryngology, 74*(1);128–139.

GOODE, R.L. (1989). Current status of electromagnetic implantable hearing aids. *Otolaryngology Clinics of North America, 22*(1);201–209.

GOODE, R.L., ROSENBAUM, M.L., & MANIGLIA, A.J. (1995). The history and development of the implantable hearing aid. *Otolaryngology Clinics of North America, 28*(1);1–16.

GYO, K., YANAGIHARA, N., SAIKI, T., & HINOHIRA, Y. (1990). Present status and outlook of the implantable hearing aid. *American Journal of Otology, 11*(4);250–253.

HÅKANSSON, B., LIDEN, G., TJELLSTROM, A., RINGDAHL, A., JACOBSSON, M., CARLSSON, P., & ERLANDSON, B.E. (1990). Ten years of experience with the Swedish bone-anchored hearing system. *Annals of Otology, Rhinology, and Laryngology (Supplement), 151*;1–16.

HÅKANSSON, B.E., CARLSSON, P.U., TJELLSTROM, A., & LIDEN, G. (1994). The bone-anchored hearing aid: Principal design and audiometric results. *Ear Nose Throat Journal, 73*(9); 670–675.

HOUGH, J.V.D., HOUGH, D.A., & McGEE, M. (1995). Long-term results for the Xomed Audiant bone conductor. *Otolaryngology Clinics of North America, 28*(1);43–52.

JAHNKE, K., & PLESTER, D. (1981). Aluminium oxide ceramic implants in middle ear surgery. *Clinics in Otolaryngology, 6*(3);193–195.

KARTUSH, J.M., McGEE, T.M., GRAHAM, M.D., KULICK, K.C., LAROUERE, M.J., & HEIDE, J. (1991). Electromagnetic semi-implantable hearing device: An update. *Archives of Otolaryngology– Head and Neck Surgery, 104*(1);150.

KARTUSH, J.M., & TOS, M. (1995). Electromagnetic ossicular augmentation device. *Otolaryngology Clinics of North America, 28*(1);155–172.

KODERA, K., SUZUKI, J., NAGAI, K., & YABE, T. (1994). Sound evaluation of partially implantable piezoelectric middle ear implant: Comparative study of frequency responses. *Ear Nose Throat Journal, 73*(2);108–111.

MANIGLIA, A.J., KO, W.H., GARVERICK, S.L., ABBASS, H., KANE, M., ROSENBAUM, M., & MURRAY, G. (1997). Semi-implantable middle ear electromagnetic hearing device for sensorineural hearing loss. *Ear Nose Throat Journal, 76*(5);333–338,340–341.

MANIGLIA, A.J., KO, W.H., ROSENBAUM, M., FALK, T., ZHU, W.L., FRENZ, N.W., WERNING, J., MASIN, J., STEIN, A., & SABRI, A. (1995). Contactless semi-implantable electromagnetic middle ear device for the treatment of sensorineural hearing loss. Short-term and long-term animal experiments. *Otolaryngology Clinics of North America, 28*(1);121–140.

McGEE, T.M., KARTUSH, J.M., HEIDE, J.C., BOJRAB, D.I., & CLEMIS, J.D. (1991). Electromagnetic semi-implantable hearing device: Phase I. Clinical trials. *Laryngoscope, 101* (4 Pt. 1);355–360.

NG, M., & LINTHICUM, F.H. JR. (1992). Long-term effects of Silastic sheeting in the middle ear. *Laryngoscope, 102*(10); 1097–1102.

NUNLEY, J.A., AGNEW, J., & SMITH, G.L. (1976). A new design for an implantable hearing aid. *ISA Transactions, 15*(3);242–245.

OTTO, S.R., SHANNON, R.V., BRACKMANN, D.E., HITSELBERGER, W.E., STALLER, S., & MENAPACE, C. (1998). The multichannel auditory brain stem implant: Performance in twenty patients. *Otolaryngology–Head and Neck Surgery, 118*;291–303.

PARK, J.Y., COTICCHIA, J.M., & CLARK, W.W. (1995). Use of distortion product otoacoustic emissions to assess middle ear transducers in rhesus monkeys. *American Journal of Otology, 16*(5);576–90.

PATRICK, J.F., & CLARK, G.M. (1991). The Nucleus 22-channel cochlear implant system. *Ear and Hearing 12*(4 Suppl); 3S–9S.

PERKINS, R. (1996). Earlens tympanic contact transducer: A new method of sound transduction to the human ear. *Archives of Otolaryngology–Head and Neck Surgery, 114*(6);720–728.

PORTMANN, D., BOUDARD, P., & HERMAN, D. (1997). Anatomical results with titanium implants in the mastoid region. *Ear Nose Throat Journal, 76*(4);231–234,236.

PULEC, J.L. (1994). Restoration of binaural hearing with the audiant implant following acoustic neuroma surgery. *Ear Nose Throat Journal, 73*(2);118–23.

ROUSH, J., & RAUCH, S.D. (1990). Clinical application of an implantable bone conduction hearing device. *Laryngoscope, 100* (3);281–285.

RUTSCHMANN. (1959). Magnetic audition: Auditory stimulation by means of alternating magnetic fields acting on a permanent magnet fixed to the eardrum. *IRE Transactions Med Electron, 6*;22–23.

SHANNON, R.V., FAYAD, J., MOORE, J., LO, W.W., OTTO, S., NELSON, R.A., & O'LEARY, M. (1993). Auditory brain stem implant: II. Postsurgical issues and performance. *Otolaryngology–Head and Neck Surgery, 108*(6);634–642.

SPINDEL, J.H., LAMBERT, P.R., & RUTH, R.A. (1995). The round window electromagnetic implantable hearing aid approach. *Otolaryngology Clinics of North America, 28*(1); 189–205.

STENSAAS, S.S., & STENSAAS, L.J. (1978). Histopathological evaluation of materials implanted in the cerebral cortex. *Acta Neuropathologica, 41*(2);145–155.

SUZUKI, J., KODERA, K., NAGAI, K., & YABE, T. (1994). Long-term clinical results of the partially implantable piezoelectric middle ear implant. *Ear Nose Throat Journal, 73*(2); 104–107.

SUZUKI, J., YANAGIHARA, N., & KADERA, K. (1987). The partially implantable middle ear implant, case reports. *Annals of Otology, Rhinology, and Laryngology, 37*;178–184.

TANGE, R.A., ZUIDEMA, T., V.D. BERG, R., & DRESCHLER, W.A. (1994). Experiences with the new Audiant XA-II implant and the behind-the-ear (BTE) device. *Journal of Otology, Rhinology and Laryngology, Related Spec, 56*(2);78–82.

TJELLSTRÖM, A., & HÅKANSSON, B. (1995). The bone-anchored hearing aid. Design principles, indications, and long-term clinical results. *Otolaryngology Clinics of North America, 28*(1);53–72.

TOS, M., SALOMON, G., & BONDING, P. (1994). Implantation of electromagnetic ossicular replacement device. *Ear Nose Throat Journal, 73*(2);92–6, 98–100, 102–3.

WELLING, D.B., & BARNES, D.E. (1995). Acoustic stimulation of the semicircular canals. *Otolaryngology Clinics of North America, 28*(1);207–219.

WILSKA, A. (1935). Ein methode zur bestimmung der horsch wellanamplituden des trommelfells bei verscheiden frequenzen. *Skandinavisches Archives of Physiology, 72*;161–165.

YANAGIHARA, N., ARITOMO, H., YAMANAKA, E., & GYO, K. (1987). Implantable hearing aid. Report of the first human applications. *Archives of Otolaryngology–Head and Neck Surgery, 113*(8);869–872.

YANAGIHARA, N., GYO, K., & HINOHIRA, Y. (1995). Partially implantable hearing aid using piezoelectric ceramic ossicular vibrator. Results of the implant operation and assessment of the hearing afforded by the device. *Otolaryngology Clinics of North America, 28*(1);85–97.

YANAGIHARA, N., GYO, K., SATO, H., YAMANAKA, E., & SAIKI, T. (1988). Implantable hearing aid in fourteen patients with mixed deafness. *Acta Oto-Laryngologica (Supplement), 458*; 90–94.

YANAGIHARA, N., GYO, K., & SUZUKI, K. (1983). Perception of sound through direct oscillation of the stapes using a piezoelectric ceramic bimorph. *Annals Otology, Rhinology, and Laryngology, 92*(3 Pt. 1);223–227.

YANAGIHARA, N., SUZUKI, J., GYO, K., SYONO, H., & IKEDA, H. (1984). Development of an implantable hearing aid using a piezoelectric vibrator of bimorph design: State of the art. *Otolaryngology–Head and Neck Surgery, 92*(6);706–712.

ADDITIONAL SUGGESTED READING

ABEL, S.M., & TSE, S.M. (1987). Pre-implant evaluation of speech and hearing. *Journal of Otolaryngology, 16*(5); 284–289.

BONDING, P., JONSSON, M.H., SALOMON, G., & AHLGREN, P. (1992). The bone-anchored hearing aid. Osseointegration and audiological effect. *Acta Oto-Laryngologica (Supplement), 492*;42–45.

BRACKMANN, D.E. (1981). Recent advances in neuro-otology. *Archives of Otolaryngology–Head and Neck Surgery 4*(1);22–28.

CHMIEL, R., CLARK, J., JERGER, J., JENKINS, H., & FREEMAN, R. (1995). Speech perception and production in children wearing a cochlear implant in one ear and a hearing aid in the opposite ear. *Annals of Otology, Rhinology, and Laryngology (Supplement), 166*;314–316.

CHMIEL, R., & JERGER, J. (1995). Quantifying improvement with amplification. *Ear and Hearing, 16*(2);166–175.

CHUTE, P.M. (1997). Timing and trials of hearing aids and assistive devices. *Archives of Otolaryngology–Head and Neck Surgery, 117*(3 Pt. 1);208–213.

CLARK, G.M., BLAMEY, P.J., BROWN, A.M., GUSBY, P.A., DOWELL, R.C., FRANZ, B.K., PYMAN, B.C., SHEPHERD, R.K., TONG, Y.C., & WEBB, R.L., et al. (1987). The University of Melbourne—Nucleus multi-electrode cochlear implant. *Advances in Otology, Rhinology, and Laryngology, 38*;V–IX,1–181.

COUNTER, S.A., BORG, E. BREDBERG, G., LINDE, G., & VAINIO, M. (1994). Electromagnetic stimulation of the auditory system of deaf patients. *Acta Oto-Laryngologica, 114*(5); 501–509.

DORMER, K.J., BRYCE, G.E., & HOUGH, J.V. (1995). Selection of biomaterials for middle and inner ear implants. *Otolaryngology Clinics of North America, 28*(1);17–27.

DORMER, K.J., RICHARD, G.L., HOUGH, J.V., & NORDQUIST, R.E. (1981). The use of rare-earth magnet couplers in cochlear implants. *Laryngoscope, 91*(11);1812–1820.

ESSELMAN, G., COTICCHIA, J.M., WIPPOLD, F.J., FREDRICKSON, J.M., & VANNIER, M.W. (1994). Computer-stimulated test fitting of an implantable hearing aid using implantable hearing aid using three-dimensional CT scans of the temporal bone: Preliminary study. *American Journal of Otology, 15*(6);702–709.

ESTREM, S.A., & THELIN, J.W. (1988). Skin tolerance and adaptation following implantation of the Xomed Audiant bone conductor. *American Journal of Otology, 9*(5);393–395.

GEERS, A.E. (1997). Comparing implants with hearing aids in profoundly deaf children. *Archives of Otolaryngology–Head and Neck Surgery, 117*(3 Pt. 1);150–154.

GOODE, R. (1991). Implantable hearing devices. *Medical Clinics of North America, 75*(6);1261–1266.

GOODE, R.L. (1995). Current status and future of implantable electromagnetic hearing aids. *Otolaryngology Clinics of North America, 28*(1);141–146.

GYO, K., GOODE, R.L., & MILLER, C. (1987). Stapes vibration produced by the output transducer of an implantable hearing aid. Experimental study. *Archives of Otolaryngology– Head and Neck Surgery, 113*(10);1078–1081.

GYO, K., SATO, H., YUMOTO, E., MURAKAMI, S., & YANAGIHARA, N. (1997). Masking the protrusion of the receiver-stimulator of electronic implants in otology. *Ear Nose Throat Journal, 76*(5);316–318,320.

GYO, K., YANAGIHARA, N., & ARAKI, H. (1984). Sound pickup utilizing an implantable piezoelectric ceramic bimorph element: Application to the cochlear implant. *American Journal of Otology, 5*(4);273–276.

HÅKANSSON, B., TJELLSTRÖM, A., & ROSENHALL, U. (1985). Acceleration levels at hearing threshold with direct bone conduction versus conventional bone conduction. *Acta Oto-Laryngologica, 100*(3–4);240–252.

LEJEUNE, R., VINCENT, C., LOUIS, E., LEJEUNE, J.P., VANEECLOO, F.M., ROUCHOUX, M.M., & FRANCKE, J.P. (1997). Anatomic basis for auditory brain stem implant. *Surgical Radiologic Anatomy, 19*(4);213–216.

LEVITT, H., BAKKE, M., KATES, J., NEUMAN, A., SCHWANDER, T., & WEISS, M. (1993). Signal processing for hearing impairment. *Scandinavian Audiology (Supplement), 38*;7–19.

MANIGLIA, A.J., KO, W.H., ZHANG, R.X., DOLGIN, S.R., ROSENBAUM, M.L., & MONTAGUE, F.W. JR. (1988). Electromagnetic implantable middle ear hearing device of the ossicular-stimulating type: Principles, designs, and experiments. *Annals of Otology, Rhinology, and Laryngology (Supplement), 136*;3–16.

MYLANUS, E.A., & CREMERS, C.W. (1994). A one-stage surgical procedure for placement of percutaneous implants for the bone-anchored hearing aid. *Journal of Laryngology and Otology, 108*(12);1031–1035.

MYLANUS, E.A., CREMERS, C.W., SNIK, A.F., & VAN DEN BERGE, N.W. (1994). Clinical results of percutaneous implants in the temporal bone. *Archives of Otolaryngology–Head and Neck Surgery, 120*(1);81–85.

MYLANUS, E.A., SNIK, A.F., & CREMERS, C.W. (1995). Patients' opinions of bone-anchored vs. conventional hearing aids. *Archives of Otolaryngology–Head and Neck Surgery, 121*(4); 421–425.

NIEHAUS, H.H., HELMS, J., & MULLER, J. (1995). Are implantable hearing devices really necessary? *Ear Nose Throat Journal, 74*(4);271–274,276.

NUNLEY, J.A., AGNEW, J., & SMITH, G.L. (1976). A new design for an implantable hearing aid. *Biomedical Scientific Instruments, 12*;69–72.

PARK, J.Y., CLARK, W.W., COTICCHIA, L.M., ESSELMAN, G.H., & FREDRICKSON, J.M. (1995). Distortion product otoacoustic emissions in rhesus (Macaca mulatta) monkey ears: Normative findings. *Hearing Research, 86*(1–2);147–162.

PONTON, C.W., DON, M., EGGERMONT, J.J., WARING, M.D., KWONG, B., & MASUDA, A. (1996). Auditory system plasticity in children after long periods of complete deafness. *Neuro Report, 8*(1);61–65.

PORTILLO, F., NELSON, R.A., BRACKMANN, D.E., HITSELBERGER, W.E., SHANNON, R.V., WARING, M.D., & MOORE, J.K. (1993). Auditory brain stem implant: electrical stimulation of the human cochlear nucleus. *Advances in Otology, Rhinology, and Laryngology, 48*;248–252.

PULEC, J.L. (1994). The totally implantable hearing aid. *Ear Nose Throat Journal, 73*(2);69.

ROBINSON, K., GATEHOUSE, S., & BROWNING, G.G. (1996). Measuring patient benefit from otorhinolaryngological surgery and therapy. *Annals of Otology, Rhinology, and Laryngology, 105*(6);415–422.

SAIKI, T., & GYO, K. (1990). Audiological evaluation of the middle ear implant—speech discrimination under noise circumstances. *Nippon Jibiinkoka Gakkai Kaiho [J Oto-Rhino-Laryng Soc Japan], 93*(4);566–571.

SAIKI, T., GYO, K., & YANAGIHARA, N. (1990). Audiological evaluation of the middle ear implant—temporal auditory acuity. *Nippon Jibiinkoka Gakkai Kaiho [J Oto-Rhino-Laryng Soc Japan], 93*(3);413–419.

SEIDMAN, D.A., CHUTE, P.M., & PARISIER, S. (1994). Temporal bone imaging for cochlear implantation. *Laryngoscope, 104*(5 Pt. 1);562–565.

STEPHAN, K., & WELZL-MULLER, K. (1992). Stapedius reflex in patients with an inner ear prosthesis. *International Journal of Artificial Organs, 15*(7);436–9.

SUZUKI, J., KODERA, K., & YANAGIHARA, N. (1985). Middle ear implant for humans. *Acta Oto-Laryngologica, 99*(3–4); 313–317.

SUZUKI, J., KODERA, K., & YANAGIHARA, N. (1983). Evaluation of middle-ear implant: A six-month observation in cats. *Acta Oto-Laryngologica, 95*(5–6);646–650.

SUZUKI, J., SUZUKI, M., KODERA, K., & KAGA, K. (1988). Transplants and implants for major ear anomalies. *Acta Oto-Rhino-Laryngologica Belgica, 42*(6);784–788.

THOMAS, J. (1996). Speech and voice rehabilitation in selected patients fitted with a bone anchored hearing aid (BAHA). *Journal of Laryngology and Otology (Supplement), 21*;47–51.

TJELLSTRÖM, A., & GRANSTROM, G. (1995). One-stage procedure to establish osseointegration: A zero to five years follow-up report. *Journal of Laryngology and Otology, 109*(7); 593–598.

TJELLSTRÖM, A., LINDSTROM, J., HALLEN, O., ALBREKTSSON, T., & BRANEMARK, P.I. (1983). Direct bone anchorage of external hearing aids. *Journal of Biomedical Engineering, 5*(1);59–63.

VERNON, J. BRUMMETT, B., DOYLE, P., & DENNISTON, R. (1970). Cochlear potential evaluation of an implantable hearing aid. *Surgical Forum, 21*;491–493.

WADE, P.S., HALIK, J.J., & CHASIN, M. (1992). Bone conduction implants: Transcutaneous vs. percutaneous [published erratum appears in *Archives of Otolaryngology–Head and Neck Surgery* 1992 Apr; 106(4);412–3]. *Archives of Otolaryngology–Head and Neck Surgery, 106*(1);68–74.

WEBER, B.A., & ROUSH, J. (1991). Implantable bone-conduction hearing device: practical considerations. *Journal of the American Academy of Audiology, 2*(2);123–127.

YANAGIHARA, N., YAMANAKA, E., & GYO, K. (1987). Implantable hearing aid using an ossicular vibrator composed of a piezoelectric ceramic bimorph: Application to four patients. *American Journal of Otology, 8*(3);213–219.

ZHAO, F., STEPHENS, S.D., SIM, S.W., & MEREDITH, R. (1997). The use of qualitative questionnaires in patients having and being considered for cochlear implants. *Clinics in Otolaryngology, 22*(3);254–259.

Chapter 16

Cochlear Implants in Children

Patricia M. Chute and Mary Ellen Nevins

The medical, audiological, and educational management of children with profound hearing loss has been dramatically altered by the introduction of cochlear implants (Nevins & Chute, 1996; Staller et al, 1991; Waltzman et al, 1986). Children who are congenitally profoundly deaf are now provided with technological options that can, in most cases, afford them better access to speech and language through audition. The process of receiving a cochlear implant involves the combined efforts of audiologists, speech-language pathologists, educators, and otologists for the implantation of the device. This medical/surgical/educational treatment, however, requires monitoring throughout the lifetime of the child. Healthcare institutions that were once responsible solely for the diagnosis of hearing impairment are currently involved in the comprehensive (re)habilitation of children with hearing loss in an unprecedented manner. As implant technology has matured, the demands of time and money on healthcare systems has become greater. In light of the recent healthcare revolution, the long-term responsibility of organizations supporting the health and well-being of its clients is unknown. Likewise, the impact of cochlear implant technology on the education of children with profound hearing loss is still evolving. In the educational sector, early studies point to successful integration of implant recipients into the mainstream at younger ages (Francis et al, 1997; Nevins & Chute, 1996). It is likely, however, that a generation of children with implants must pass through the educational system before the final outcomes of implantation can be measured. Despite the lack of generational studies, overall performance of children and adults with cochlear implants has been impressive enough to support three manufacturers in the United States.

At present, cochlear implantation is an option available to profoundly deaf children whose hearing levels are 90 dB HL or greater. This group is still estimated at 1% of the deaf and hard-of-hearing population in the United States or approximately 1 million individuals (Schow & Nerbonne, 1995). New trends in population evolution and healthcare delivery may begin to change these numbers substantially. First, individuals emigrating to the United States have been reaching out to family members in their native country to assist them in accessing healthcare service unavailable in their homeland. Furthermore, cultural mores of marriage and family and responsibility to care for those with special needs may create extended families with the desire for medical intervention. As more states embrace the concept of universal newborn hearing screening, the number of younger children who are identified as having a hearing loss will increase. Thus an additional responsibility exists for providing a range of services for deaf and hard-of-hearing children that includes not only cochlear implants but also hearing aids and other sensory devices.

In the final analysis the number of children who receive cochlear implants will be most affected by (a) changes in hearing aid technology, (b) the comparison of hearing aid

Audiology: Treatment. Edited by Valente, Hosford-Dunn, and Roeser. Thieme Medical Publishers, Inc., New York © 2000

benefit to performance with cochlear implants, (c) financial and technical support of medical and government agencies, and (d) the impact of the Deaf Community. Any of these issues can have a direct effect on the number of children seeking and receiving cochlear implants. Each of these issues will be addressed as factors to be considered when choosing cochlear implantation for a child.

RECENT ADVANCES IN HEARING AID TECHNOLOGY

Hearing aid technology has changed substantially over the last decade (see Chapters 1, 6, and 13 in this volume) as devices have become smaller and have provided better performance in difficult listening situations. Advanced signal processing and programmability have provided hearing aid wearers with instruments that offer choices depending on the listening environment; multiple memory hearing aids that offer better hearing in a diversity of auditory conditions are currently available. Cosmetically, hearing aids have become smaller and more efficient. For a small segment of the hearing aid population, hearing aids can be implanted when warranted (see Chapters 13, 14, 16, and 25).

Hearing aids and frequency modulated (FM) systems still support most individuals who have hearing loss. They are the preferred treatment alternative for children whose hearing impairment is mild to moderate. It should be noted that some children with severe-to-profound hearing loss are also capable of performance that enables them to develop good speech, language, and listening skills (Boothroyd, 1993). Generally speaking, however, the effectiveness of these sensory aids becomes compromised as the degree of impairment increases.

Although FM systems can provide children with more direct signal input (see Chapter 20), their physical size often makes them less acceptable as children become older. Recently, FM systems have become miniaturized and located in more traditional behind-the-ear (BTE) model hearing instruments. This enables children to have access to improved signal-to-noise ratios (SNR) without the need for cumbersome equipment. Despite good performance in some children with these devices, there remains a group of children who are unable to obtain substantial benefit from these traditional types of amplification.

COMPARING HEARING AID BENEFIT TO IMPLANT PERFORMANCE

Predicted benefit from conventional amplification systems often was the criterion by which decisions regarding school placement and mode of communication was made (Moores, 1987; Quigley & Kretschmer, 1982). Children unable to develop acceptable speech skills were placed in educational systems that offered manual communication and therefore did not require the use of hearing aids. Those children demonstrating the ability to process some speech through their hearing aids were placed in oral schools recognized for their ability to use residual hearing for speech production. Researchers working with profoundly deaf children explored the wide spectrum of ability found in children in these oral schools.

In 1985, Boothroyd classified performance in a group of profoundly deaf students at an oral school for the deaf. He found that children who were profoundly deaf with some measurable hearing were often capable of developing adequate speech and listening skills. Children with the greater hearing losses (more than 110 dB HL) did the poorest of the group. Geers and Moog (1987) developed categories of speech perception in an effort to predict whether a deaf child would be capable of developing spoken language. They determined that children who were capable of better speech perception ability were more likely to develop understandable speech. In an attempt to provide a direct comparison between hearing aid benefit and cochlear implant performance, Osberger et al (1993) identified three distinct groups of hearing aid users within the profound hearing loss group. Subjects were categorized on the basis of pure tone average and were systematically compared with a group of children who received cochlear implants. These three groups consisted of children whose pure tone averages were (1) between 90- and 100-dB hearing threshold level (HTL) (2) between 101- and 110-dB HTL, and (3) greater than 110 dB HTL. Overall, children with cochlear implants performed better than the children within the two poorer hearing groups. Children with cochlear implants performed as well as and, in some cases, better than the children whose hearing losses were between 90- and 100-dB HTL. Results such as these coupled with steady improvement in processing strategies have driven the movement of audiological requirements upward on the audiogram from the corner audiogram to flat losses of 90 dB HL. This, in effect, creates a larger pool of audiological candidates and has resulted in an overall increase in children receiving cochlear implants. A list of audiological candidacy guidelines follows:

1. The child must be between the ages of 18 months and 17 years.
2. The child must present with a profound bilateral sensorineural hearing loss.
3. The child must demonstrate little or no benefit from appropriate binaural hearing aids.
4. The child must participate in a 3- to 6-month hearing aid trial if there has been no previous aided experience.

FINANCIAL AND TECHNICAL SUPPORT FOR IMPLANTS

With growing numbers of parents seeking implantation for their children, the financial support from third-party private and public insurers has become a critical consideration. Because implants are approved for use in children, most healthcare insurers support this technology. Although the amount of state and federal support in this country for this technology varies, patient access to implants is more widespread than a decade ago. Because a discrepancy often exists in gross charge billed by the implant facility and the actual payment issued from the insurance provider, in some circumstances costs are borne by the consumer. However, support for cochlear implantation varies from state to state and country to country. For example, in England and Canada (Summerfield & Marshall, 1995) the government supports the total cost of implantation through the national health ministries.

With regard to access, the number of cochlear implant centers in the United States has grown to approximately 200 (personal communication, Cochlear Corporation, 1998) from the initial eight centers involved in the grassroots technology movement of the late 1970s and the early 1980s. To become a cochlear implant center, it is recommended (but not required) that personnel attend a training workshop sponsored by the manufacturer. Implant companies support local centers by providing technological assistance and reimbursement services. Because technical and financial support is now available on a more extensive basis, the number of children receiving implants each year is increasing dramatically. This has created a great deal of opposition from within the Deaf Community because the number of children with the potential to become cultural and linguistic members of the Deaf Community has decreased commensurately.

OPPOSITION FROM THE DEAF COMMUNITY

Deaf Community leaders have long opposed the implantation of children. A position paper issued by the National Association of the Deaf (NAD) deplored the cochlear implant process in young children. Harlan Lane (1992) likened implantation to questionable practices in the past such as reproductive regulation on deaf adults and medical experimentation on deaf children. Because of federal legislation preceding this technological advance, enrollment figures of children in schools for the deaf in the United States over the past 20 years have dropped more than 50% (Craig & Craig, 1975; Gallaudet University, 1994). Concerned by this enrollment trend at state centers of deaf culture (i.e., state schools for the deaf), the Deaf Community views the implant as a further threat to its existence and actively urges parents to reject it for their children.

The cochlear implant must be viewed within the context of any new and emerging technology. There will be advocates who embrace it with confidence, whereas opponents will question it and resist change. Parents must be aware of the risks and benefits of implantation and understand it within its medical, educational, social, and political contexts (Nevins & Chute, 1996). Implantation for a young deaf child should be decided on with full knowledge of all the implications of that choice. Professionals and parents who are considering this technology have a responsibility to educate themselves so that decisions regarding implantation for an individual child are made on the basis of factual information and not emotion.

It is the purpose of this chapter to bring the reader through the various aspects of implantation: implant design, candidacy, surgical issues, device activation, care and maintenance, habilitation, parental and school roles, performance, educational achievements, implants in special populations, and future considerations. It is intended to provide a knowledge base on many of the issues that face parents, teachers, and allied health professionals who work in the field of deafness and (re)habilitation of children.

COCHLEAR IMPLANT DESIGN

Basic Implant Function

A cochlear implant incorporates a number of internal and external components. The internal portion is composed of electrodes, a receiver stimulator, an antenna, and a magnet. Externally, there is a microphone, an external transmitter, cords, and a body worn or BTE speech processor. Implants function in a manner similar to a hearing aid; however, the final transmission of the signal in the cochlea is markedly different. Incoming sounds are detected by a microphone that is placed in a headset worn by the patient. Signals received from the microphone are transmitted through a cord to the speech processor where they are analyzed using an algorithm specific to that device. The processed signal is then forwarded through the cord to the external transmitter that is placed in apposition over the internal receiver. The transmitter and receiver are held in place through external and internal magnets. The signal is sent by means of FM transmission through the skin to the internal receiver. The information is frequency analyzed and delivered to the electrodes in a manner that is specific to the speech processing strategy of the particular device. Because the normal auditory system consists of a great number of functioning hair cells distributed throughout the cochlea, multiple sites of stimulation would be more representative of the incoming signals than a single site. Therefore, any attempt at artificially stimulating the neural elements remaining in deafened cochleas is best accomplished at numerous locations.

History and Development

Early implant work by Dr. William House concentrated on the use of a single electrode and developed into the first commercially available system known as the *3M/House Implant*. Early versions of this device used a transcutaneous (across the skin) system that was coupled through an elaborate arrangement of a headband or eyeglasses with a cuplike extension in which the transmitter was held. In the early 1980s, Dr. Jack Hough developed a rare earth magnet that could be surgically implanted without creating interference with the internal receiver. This magnet forever changed the face of implantation because transmission across the skin could be more precise and occur without slippage. Adults who used the *3M/House* device reported improved speechreading ability, environmental sound discrimination, and improved quality of life (Bilger et al, 1977). Investigation of this device was expanded to include the pediatric population.

The first implant used in children in the United States was the *3M/House* system. Although this system received approval in adults by the Food and Drug Administration (FDA), it was never approved for use in children. This occurred because of a combination of factors including 3M's disinterest in remaining in the cochlear implant market and the more impressive results that were being obtained using the Nucleus 22 multichannel system. Results using multichannel stimulation in adults demonstrated some speech understanding without the aid of visual cues. For this reason, Cochlear Corporation, the manufacturer of the Nucleus 22 channel device began clinical trials in the pediatric population. This device was eventually approved by the FDA in 1989 for use in the pediatric population. Worldwide, this device represents the largest number of users for both adults and children (personal communication, Cochlear Corporation, 1998).

Cochlear implants available today for the pediatric population represent the advances that were made in technology over the past two decades. Each system differs from the other on a number of features, and decisions regarding the choice of a device should be made by well-informed parents. Features that need to be considered when choosing a cochlear implant include the following: FDA status, electrode configuration and material, presence of telemetry, magnetic resonance imaging (MRI) compatibility, number of electrode sites, reliability, programmability, warranty, cost of maintenance, cosmetics, speech-processing strategy, and flexibility. Additional factors that parents may consider pertain to the level of company support of the product and its projection of future product development.

Currently Available Devices

At present, four systems are manufactured by three companies that are available for children in the United States. These include the Nucleus 22 and 24 System manufactured by Cochlear Corporation, the Clarion System manufactured by Advanced Bionics Corporation, and the Med El Combi 40+ System manufactured by Med El Corporation. The Nucleus 22 and 24 and the Clarion have received premarket approval status from the FDA for use with children. Premarket approval status allows the device to be implanted by any center in the

United States. This is preceded by an investigational status that restricts implantation to those centers participating in data collection studies. At present, the Med El Combi 40+ is engaged in investigative trials in the pediatric population. Knowledge of FDA status of a device is important when choosing an implant because some insurance carriers will not support the implantation of a product that has not been approved.

Cochlear Corporation Devices

The steady progression of technological advances made within the field of implantation can be observed by comparing and contrasting devices available in the past 15 years. Figure 16–1 shows an array of implant devices manufactured by Cochlear Corporation; the earliest available device, the Nucleus 22, appears on the left. The most recent implant device released from Cochlear is the 24 ESPrit, an ear level implant pictured at the bottom right. It is important to note that the release of new products does not always result in obsolescence of the previous model. It is therefore necessary to understand the workings of each individual device.

The Nucleus 22 channel device has gone through hardware and software changes since it was first introduced commercially in 1983. Internally, the device consists of a silicone-encased receiver stimulator and 22 band electrodes made of platinum (Patrick & Clark, 1991). This pioneer system does not support any type of telemetry (i.e., a remote method of electronically monitoring the integrity of the internal receiver). Telemetry is an especially important feature to have in a device for young children who are unable to report that a device is not functioning. The Nucleus 22 can be ordered in an MRI-compatible format, which requires that the magnet be removed from the packaging. The reliability of the internal receiver of the original Nucleus 22 device was poorer in children than in the adult population with a cumulative survival rate of approximately 92%. The cumulative survival rate of an implant is the percentage of implants still functioning after each year of implant use. Subsequent changes in the design of

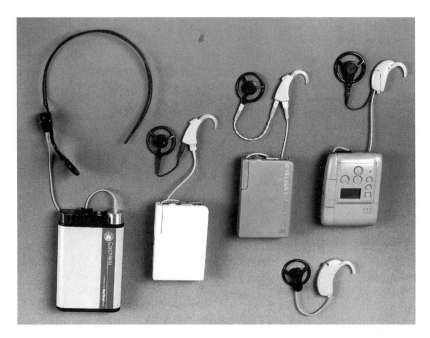

Figure 16–1   Cochlear implant devices available from Cochlear Corporation. From the far left: Nucleus 22, with WSP; Nucleus 22 with MSP; Nucleus 22 with SPECTRA; Nucleus 24 SPrint; and the Nucleus 24 ESPrit at bottom right. (Courtesy of Cochlear Corporation.)

the antenna have assisted in increasing the survival rate to close to 98% (Cochlear Corporation, 1996).

Externally, the original speech processor was a large unit requiring three AA batteries and was known as the WSP (wearable speech processor). The speech processing strategy used a feature extractor that identified the fundamental frequency, first formant, and second formant of the speech signal (Dowell et al, 1990). In 1989 the overall size of the unit was substantially decreased and became known as the MSP (mini speech processor). It required only one AA battery and also introduced a new speech processing strategy known as MPEAK (Multi Peak). This strategy delivered supplementary high-frequency information to the cochlea. In addition to the fundamental frequency, first formant, and second formant, three high-frequency bands were added to improve speech discrimination (Patrick & Clark, 1991; Skinner et al, 1991). In 1994, a second speech processing strategy was added to the programs, although the size of the processor remained unchanged. This strategy was known as SPEAK (Spectral Peak) and was introduced in the speech processor known as the Spectra (McKay & McDermott, 1991). This latest advance abandons the feature extraction scheme and analyzes the whole speech waveform and identifies the 6 to 10 maximal peaks. The pulses are delivered at an adaptive rate up to 300 pulses/s. All patients implanted with the original Nucleus 22 channel device were able to take advantage of these upgrades in technology without undergoing additional surgical intervention.

Each of the cochlear implant systems mentioned previously can provide only one program at a time to the user despite the fact that a variety of coding strategies are available. Although the WSP is no longer available, Cochlear Corporation continues to provide equipment to its customers and all WSP users were offered a free upgrade to an MSP. The MSP is still supported by the manufacturer despite the fact that several more generations of speech processors have been introduced. The cost of maintenance of the MSP and Spectra is minimal and includes the price of replacing the rechargeable batteries once a year and the cords if they should become damaged. The internal receiver is warranteed for 10 years and the external components for 3 years.

In 1997 Cochlear Corporation introduced its next generation of software and hardware in the device called the Nucleus 24. Although this device presently uses the SPEAK processing strategy, additional strategies will be incorporated and available in the near future. The Nucleus 24 internal receiver is constructed of material similar to that of the Nucleus 22, and the device is slightly larger but thinner in profile. It is MRI compatible in that it has a removable magnet that can be reinserted if necessary. It incorporates a traditional telemetry system to monitor electrode integrity and a neural telemetry system that will record neural potentials from within the cochlea. Neural telemetry will provide the programming audiologist with additional information on the stimulability of the individual electrodes and may result in better programming for young children. The cumulative survival rate for this device is noted to be at 99%.

The speech processor for the Nucleus 24 is available in two forms: a body processor known as the *SPrint* and ear-level processor known as the *ESPrit* (see Fig. 16–2). The body processor can store four different programs at one time and provides an audible alarm for parents to warn them that the battery requires replacing. (This alarm can be changed to a personal alarm as the child gets older.) The unit can be used

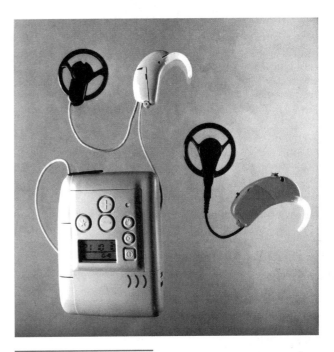

Figure 16–2 The latest generation implant devices from Cochlear Corporation: The Nucleus 24 SPrint (*left*) and ESPrit (*right*). (Courtesy of Cochlear Corporation.)

with one or two rechargeable AA batteries that require recharging daily and replacement yearly. Although the initial strategy used with this device is the SPEAK coding strategy, new speech processing strategies are currently under investigation in the adult population. These are not yet available for children. The newer strategies will introduce a high-speed continuous interleaved sampling strategy (CIS) and an advanced combined encoder (ACE) strategy. (For additional information concerning these strategies, the reader is directed to Chapter 18 in this volume).

The BTE model, *ESPrit*, can store two separate speech-processing programs but can only use the SPEAK strategy at present. Data comparing performance with the body processor and the BTE model demonstrate equivalent results (Staller et al, 1998) when using the SPEAK strategy. Power is supplied to the BTE by two 675 batteries that can last up to 2 weeks. Maintenance of both the *SPrint* and the *ESPrit* is relatively low and consists of battery replacement and cords if damaged. The warranty is for 10 years on the internal equipment, 3 years for the *SPrint*, and 2 years for the *ESPrit*.

Advanced Bionic Corporation Device

The Clarion Multi-Strategy implant system of Advanced Bionics Corporation has been available for the pediatric population since 1995. The internal receiver is encased in ceramic and consists of 16 ball electrodes situated in pairs in a pre-coiled array (Kessler & Schindler, 1994). Although it is not MRI compatible in its traditional manufactured form, it can be ordered without the magnet for special individuals. It incorporates a bidirectional telemetry system that monitors electrode impedance to determine device function (Zilberman & Santogrossi, 1995). The device is capable of delivering both pulsatile and analog signals depending on patient choice and performance. Recent changes to the internal receiver were made in an attempt to fit more subjects with the compressed analog strategy. The compressed analog strategy, now referred to as SAS (simultaneous analog strategy) is another type of speech-processing strategy that has been demonstrated to be beneficial in a subset of cochlear implant users. The CIS strategy that the system presently uses runs at 813 pulses/s across eight channels. Upcoming software changes will incorporate a series of hybrid strategies that will combine certain aspects of CIS along with SAS.

Reliability of the initial series of internal receivers was contaminated by a poorly manufactured batch of ceramic casings that were subject to breakage from minor head trauma. Revisions in the manufacturing process has since corrected this problem, bringing the cumulative survival rate to approximately 98% (personal communication, Advanced Bionics Corporation, 1998).

The external components of the Clarion are designed somewhat differently from the Nucleus device. The headset includes a microphone and external transmitter in a single unit. It is connected by a cord to the speech processor, which is a body-worn device (see Fig. 16–3). The speech processor, originally known as the *1.2*, has recently undergone cosmetic and function changes with the newer version *S-Series*. The *S-Series* processor can store up to three separate programs and contains an audible or personal alarm to signal the need for battery replacement. Also, an audible alarm can be activated to alert parents if the headset should become dislodged from the child's head. The *S-Series* is powered by a special lithium battery that lasts approximately 12 to 14 hours and is provided by the manufacturer. With the exception of the alarm systems and battery power, the *S-Series* speech processor is similar to the *1.2*.

Warranties for the Clarion device are similar to the Nucleus devices. The cost of maintenance of the unit is slightly greater

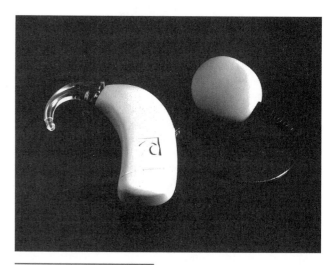

Figure 16–4 Prototype of the Clarion Ear Level Processor. (Courtesy of Advanced Bionics Corporation.)

because of the higher price of the lithium batteries for the *S-Series* and the rechargeable battery packs for the *1.2* series. Development of an ear level processor is underway, and a prototype of the device is shown in Figure 16–4 (personal communication, Advanced Bionics Corporation, 1998).

Med El Corporation Device

The most recent device to become available for children in the United States is the Med El Combi 40+. The internal receiver is made up of 24 electrode contacts arranged as 12 pairs in a straight array (Zierhofer et al, 1995). Like the Clarion, the receiver stimulator and antenna are encased in ceramic. The device uses a telemetry system to measure both impedance and voltage spread across electrodes to monitor device function. It is capable of delivering a high-speed *CIS* signal at 1500 pulses/s and a strategy known as *N of M*. This latter strategy selectively chooses which electrodes will be included in the map on the basis of certain programmed parameters. Reliability problems with the Med El Combi 40+, which arose in Europe because of a poorly manufactured batch of internal receivers, has since been corrected.

The external components consist of a body-worn processor (see Fig. 16–5) or an ear-level unit (currently in field trials in Europe; see Fig. 16–6), an external transmitter, and a microphone. These are physically similar to the Nucleus device in that there are two separate pieces. A cord connects the headset to the speech processor that is capable of storing three programs, has an audible and personal alarm to signal battery change, and is powered by two rechargeable AA batteries. Warranties for the internal and external components are similar to the other two devices. The cost of maintenance is low and consists of battery and cord replacement.

Although differences exist among the four devices, all have provided upgrades through changes in software. Historically, speech-processing strategies have changed substantially over time among and within devices. As more information becomes available, researchers and software engineers will continue to fine-tune these strategies in an attempt to provide better speech understanding without the

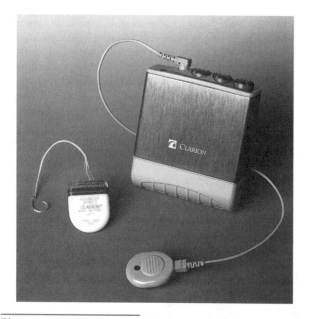

Figure 16–3 The Clarion S-Series Implant System shown with the internal device. (Courtesy of Advanced Bionics Corporation.)

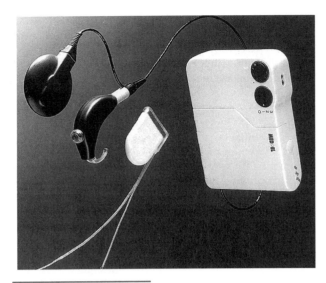

Figure 16–5 The Med El Combi 40+ Implant System. (Courtesy of Med El Corporation.)

need for additional surgery. As newer strategies become available, trials must be performed in adult implant users before they can be distributed for use with children. Choosing the device that best suits the needs of an individual child is a decision that parents must make as they progress through the implant process.

PROCESS OF IMPLANTATION

Candidacy Selection

The process of implantation can be viewed as a series of stages through which the child and parents must pass. These stages include candidacy, surgery, device activation, and habilitation. The first of these stages, candidacy, is critical to the success of implantation in children. The proper selection of children for implantation should be performed by a multidisciplinary team of professionals with knowledge of deaf-

ness and childhood development for speech, language, and audition (Fraser, 1991). Team members should include an audiologist, speech-language pathologist, surgeon, and, when possible, an educator of the deaf. Many teams also include a psychologist and a social worker. Although the fundamental criteria for implantation is based on audiological performance, centers experienced with cochlear implants in children have identified other factors that can contribute to successful use of the implant (Dowell et al, 1995; Hieber et al, 1997; Moog et al, 1994; Niparko et al, 1997). These factors may include medical/radiological integrity, speech and language capabilities, educational environment, and parental/ child expectations.

Audiological criteria for implantation is driven by performance with traditional forms of amplification such as hearing aids, FM systems, vibrotactile aids, and frequency transposition aids. Children must have had access to an adequate trial (at least 3 to 6 months) with these conventional forms of amplification, as well as adequate training with the aids, before an implant can be considered. Good preimplant listening experiences suggesting a history of consistent hearing aid use coupled with extensive opportunities for developing auditory skills contribute to the positive decision regarding implant candidacy. In other words, children being considered for implantation must be using amplification on a daily basis and be enrolled in programs that value audition.

PEARL

Audiologic criteria are the first to be evaluated when considering a particular child for an implant. Once hearing testing confirms that the child is audiologically a candidate, evaluation in other areas begins.

The role of vibrotactile aids during this candidacy period should be considered. In a survey of 14 major implant centers across the country it was reported that more than 75%

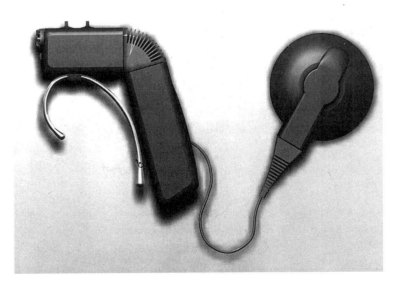

Figure 16–6 Ear level processor for the Med El Combi 40+ in trials in Europe. (Courtesy of Med El Corporation.)

used this type of device during the preimplant training period; however, the percentage of children using vibrotactile aids *within* each center ranged from 1 to 6%. Approximately 40% of the centers used transpositional technology. However, only 3.5% of the children at any given center had access to these devices. The most popular device used during the preimplant period was an FM system for children and hearing aids for adults (Chute, 1997).

Regardless of the device used in the preimplantation period, the measurement of hearing aid benefit from traditional amplification is the key factor considered when choosing an implant candidate. Linguistically appropriate test materials (see Table 16–1 for a listing of tests) that assess auditory speech perception have been standardized on a population of deaf and hard-of-hearing children and assist in measuring hearing aid benefit and skill growth over time. Designed for children at a variety of language levels, tests were developed for youngsters using conventional hearing aids, tactile aids, and cochlear implants. Test procedures fall into two basic categories known as closed-set and open-set measures of speech perception. Although the selection criteria for each implant vary somewhat with respect to the particular tests used to assess benefit, the FDA now allows children with minimal open set speech recognition to obtain a cochlear implant. Guidelines for the Nucleus 24 clinical trials permitted a score of less than or equal to 20% on either the Multisyllabic Lexical Neighborhood Test (MLNT) or the Lexical Neighborhood Test (LNT).

Children with some residual hearing have also successfully received implants in the past, and although a range of performance has been seen in this group, the overall results have been impressive. Skinner (1994) reviewed 24 children who had some residual hearing and found that despite variations in performance, most of the children were able to obtain a level of performance that surpassed their previous performance with hearing aids. Similar findings were reported by Brackett and Zara (1997) and Zwolan et al (1997).

Special Considerations for Very Young Children

The dilemma facing implant teams today is in trying to assess children who are less than 2 years old for implantation.

Although the FDA has recently approved implantation for children 18 months of age for the Nucleus 22 and 24 device, once any device is approved, surgeons may go "off label," and use the device in other populations. When a device is used "off-label," it means that it is being used in a population for which approval has not been granted. For example, in cases of children who were deafened from meningitis and present with ossifying cochleas before the age of 18 months, the device can be implanted once medical necessity is demonstrated. In Europe, the youngest child on record to receive a cochlear implant was 7 months old; deafness was the result of meningitis. This child was implanted after sequential radiological studies indicated that the cochleas were ossifying as a result of the meningitis (Bertram et al, 1996).

Audiological assessment of very young children is performed in two ways: measurement of functional gain afforded by the hearing aids and the use of questionnaires designed to assess daily listening and speaking experiences. Speech perception measures are generally not obtainable because of the paucity of language these youngsters demonstrate. In an attempt to evaluate some of the functional aspects of communication in these children, Robbins et al (1991) developed two qualitative instruments. The Meaningful Auditory Integration Scale (MAIS) and the Meaningful Use of Speech Scale (MUSS) are questionnaires that use parental report across a wide range of subjects with respect to an individual child's hearing aid use and attempts at communication. Responses to this questionnaire assist the implant team in making decisions about implantation for a particular child.

In addition to the measures previously discussed, some implant centers use electrophysiological techniques to support the decision to implant and choose an ear for implantation. Kileny (1991) uses the electrical auditory brain stem response (EABR) to obtain input-output functions across a variety of pulsatile stimuli. Depending on the threshold and slope of these functions, decisions regarding ear of implantation are made at the time of the surgery. Studies comparing the postimplant electrical threshold level and the EABR have been performed by a number of investigators and have demonstrated differences with some indicating good correlation (Abbas & Brown, 1991) and others indicating weaker correlations (Shallop et al, 1991).

TABLE 16–1 Linguistically appropriate tests of speech perception

Test Name	Approximate Age At Administration
Early Speech Perception Test	
Low Verbal Version	2–4 y
Standard Version	6 y and older
Glendonald Auditory Screening Procedure	4 y and older
Monosyllable-Trochee-Spondee Test	4 y and older
Multisyllabic Lexical Neighborhood Test (MLNT)	4 y and older
Lexical Neighborhood Test (LNT)	4 y and older
Audiovisual Feature Test	5 y and older
Northwestern University Children's Perception of Speech	6 y and older
Word Intelligibility by Picture Identification	6 y and older
Phonetically Balanced Kindergarten Test	6 y and older

In many experienced centers audiological criteria for implantation serve as the gatekeeper for the child to gain entry to the implant process. Professionals at these centers have identified a number of additional elements that are evaluated in candidacy selection. Other factors that need to be considered for determining candidacy include chronological age, duration of deafness, medical/radiological findings, multiple handicapping conditions, speech and language abilities, family structure and support, expectations of the family (parents and child), educational environment, and availability of support services. With the intent of providing an organized listing of all factors considered for candidacy, a tool known as the ChIP (Children's Implant Profile) was developed to aid in the decision-making process (Hellman et al, 1991; Nevins & Chute, 1996). The ChIP is based on a retrospective review of a large number of cases from the Implant Center formerly located at Manhattan Eye, Ear and Throat Hospital and is used as a counseling aid for both parents and professionals.

Decisions regarding candidacy should be made on the basis of input from each of the team members in their respective areas of expertise so that an individual profile on the ChIP is generated. This profile identifies the areas that must be remediated before a child can be considered for cochlear implant surgery. In most cases it assists in the decision of *when* to implant as opposed to *whether* to implant (Osberger et al, 1991). Once a center recommends a child for candidacy, the final decision to implant any given child remains with the parents. Teams providing information and support to parents at the candidacy stage establish a solid foundation for the ongoing relationship required between families of implant recipients and implant centers during the postimplantation period.

Surgical Preparation for Implantation

The surgical stage of the implant process represents one of the most stressful for parents. Therefore hospital procedures and the logistics of the hospital stay should be carefully reviewed with the family by the implant personnel. In addition, children themselves should be counseled regarding the procedure using conceptually and linguistically appropriate materials. Clarke School for the Deaf has developed a storybook that outlines the process using pictures. Some of the manufacturers provide coloring books for this purpose as well. A number of teams use stuffed animals and/or dolls to role-play the events with the child. Every attempt should be made to include the child during this stage. Clearly, older children must be informed about the surgical aspects of the implant and the postoperative appearances of the wound.

Practical consideration concerning postoperative management should be reviewed immediately before and after surgery. Parents should be reminded that the child will have a large bandage on the head after the surgery; therefore pajamas and clothing for the trip home should be the type that button down the front. Postoperatively, information about bathing, physical activities, and return appointments also need to be addressed. It is recommended that this information be provided to the parents in both spoken and written form. Finally, parents are assigned an activation appointment approximately 1 month after surgery.

Cochlear Implant Activation

The initial "mapping" or "tune up" of the cochlear implant system uses standard pediatric testing techniques incorporating traditional reinforcement paradigms. The procedure requires the child to respond to an electrical signal that is delivered to each electrode individually. The mapping or programming procedure requires that the child's speech processor be connected to an interface box that communicates with a computer. The headset (which includes the microphone and the transmitter coil) is placed on the child's head over the area of the internal receiver. Because profoundly deaf children often have a better perception of low-frequency sound, it is customary to begin with a low-frequency electrode. The initial task is to determine the threshold level for a particular electrode. Electrical pulses are delivered to a designated electrode at a particular current level determined by the audiologist who adjusts the levels by means of a control knob or keyboard. The units used to measure these levels vary from one device to the other and do not equate with decibel levels.

Once the child acknowledges hearing a sound or is behaviorally observed to have heard one, an assessment of threshold is made. For very young children, standard observational procedures are used; play audiometry is used with older children. The lowest level that a child consistently identifies sound sensation is designated at the *threshold or T-level*. These levels are obtained for each of the active electrodes.

In addition to the T-levels for each electrode, an assessment of *comfort level* (known as a *C-level or M-level*) is also determined. Because many children do not have a well-developed concept of sound, assessing comfort may be too abstract a task, making C-levels difficult to obtain. In an attempt to obtain an objective measure of the C-level in children research has been conducted using the electrically elicited stapedial reflex (also known as the electroacoustic reflex threshold, EART). Hodges et al (1991) and Spivak and Chute (1994) used standard tympanometric recordings to measure middle ear muscle reflexes when stimulating the implanted ear. These measurements were successfully used to provide clinicians with a more objective assessment of C-levels. Agreement between C-levels and EARTs for the Nucleus 22 channel system was quite high. It should be noted that use of the EART with Clarion device may result in an underestimation of M-levels (Chute et al, 1997). It is still possible, however, to create a map with these levels and ensure that the signal delivered to the electrode is not uncomfortable.

PITFALL

Once a child receives a speech processor programmed to his or her individual specifications, it may never be used by another implant recipient.

When threshold and comfort levels have been obtained for each of the electrodes, a program is developed using the manufacturer's software. This program is referred to as a *map* and is somewhat similar to the frequency specifications of a conventional hearing aid (Myres & Kessler, 1992). However, it is much more specific to an individual patient because it contains the threshold and comfort levels and the frequency boundaries for each of the programmed electrodes. Under no circumstances should one child be given another child's map because it might cause an uncomfortable sensation.

All recent implant systems support speech processors that can store more than one program. Multiple storage capacity enables the user to try different maps in different listening situations. These programs are accessed by means of control knobs or buttons depending on the device. For example, one map may enhance higher frequencies, whereas another may delete some low-frequency information that may be perceived as noise. Multiple map storage capacity has allowed children to optimize some of the map features in a shorter period of time. This may contribute to better performance at earlier intervals. Multiple map storage capacity enables the mapping procedure to become a more interactive one calling for the involvement of parents and teachers. Informed decisions regarding ideal map choices can be made with input from the local educational professional or therapist who is following the child on a daily basis. Minor changes in current levels can be built into the stored programs so that children do not have to return to the implant center as frequently.

Responses at Activation

The range of performance that can occur after children have experienced their first stimulation with a cochlear implant can vary substantially. Some children are able to detect a wide range of speech signals in structured situations upon activation of the device. Another group of children are able to discriminate patterns of speech immediately in structured situations. The third group of children will wear the speech processor but will show no awareness to sound and the final group resists wearing the device even when it is turned off.

Setting early therapeutic goals for children directly after the tuning will be child driven and depend on the child's age, responsiveness, and cognitive/linguistic ability. Children who are capable of immediately detecting signals in structured situations can be taught using a variety of speech input and begin training for pattern recognition. On the opposite end of the spectrum are the children who refuse to wear the device. These youngsters require the implementation of a wearing program in an attempt to get the device activated and begin sound introduction. Parental commitment to the management program suggested by the implant center is crucial; networking parents with others who have had similar experiences may be helpful.

Map Changes

Despite the availability of multiple map storage capacity, the need for children to return for readjustment of their implant is a required part of the postimplant process. Periodically, as a child's auditory perceptual performance changes, his map may also need adjustment. This requires the child to return to the implant facility so that new T- and C-levels can be obtained and new programs can be written to the microchip of the speech processor. Generally, most implant centers request that children return for frequent follow-up visits for the first 6 months of implant use. As the child's responses with the implant stabilize, the need for additional mapping sessions decreases.

The linguistic constraints of very young children and their lack of auditory experience often prevent them from indicating when a remapping is necessary. In these instances observations by the parents and teachers are invaluable in signaling when a mapping change is warranted. Certain signs indicate a need for remapping that teachers and parents should recognize. In an effort to hear better, children may suddenly begin to increase the sensitivity or volume from its designated setting. Changes in speech production, a decrease in vocalizations, or loss of speech features that the child was previously able to produce may all be indicators that remapping is necessary. Finally, if the child suddenly develops physical symptoms (e.g., an eye or facial twitch or sensation in the neck or tongue), an appointment with the implant center should be made immediately. Physical manifestations or unusual sensations may require the deletion of electrodes that are causing problems.

Parents, school personnel, and implant center facilities must work together to determine the need for remapping of any individual child. Without good communication, children may go for long periods with maps that are not appropriate and, in some cases, useless.

Care and Maintenance

In addition to monitoring the effectiveness of a child's individual map, it is important that parents and teachers become aware of methods to properly maintain the external components of the cochlear implant system. If the device is carefully maintained on a daily and weekly basis, many simple problems that can arise will be avoided. Many of the procedures used to maintain and care for cochlear implant equipment are similar to those used with conventional hearing aids. Although the burden of maintaining the unit generally rests on the child's parents and/or the child, teachers should also be aware of some of the issues of daily maintenance, especially for the very young child with an implant.

As with any electronic equipment, the foremost avoidable problems are related to physical abuse and moisture. Although most children wear their speech-processing unit in some type of pouch or carrier, wearing the processor on the chest may make it more subject to abuse. It is preferable to situate the processor on the child's back in a protective pouch, especially for the very young, active child. This pouch is usually connected by means of a harness and is worn under the clothing. This safeguards the unit in two ways. First, it removes the processor from the child's reach preventing unwanted adjustment to the dial settings. Second, it protects the unit from exposure to damaging elements (e.g., water and food). Device manufacturers have begun to build some safety precautions directly into their software. For example, the Nucleus 24 SPrint body processor has a feature that allows the clinician to lock out the controls, effectively making the controls childproof. Similarly, the Clarion software provides the clinician with a method of setting the volume control so that it does not go beyond a certain level (Fryauf-Bertschy, 1992; Tye-Murray et al, 1994).

If the speech processor has been subject to physical abuse while at school, either intentionally or accidentally, the functioning of the device should be checked and the parents informed of the situation. Intentional abuse to the speech processor should be reported immediately to both the parents and the implant facility to determine the cause of the problem and resolve it. If a child is removing the unit in the classroom and deliberately throwing it, it may be map-related or behavior-related. Map-related problems should be addressed by the implant center, whereas behavioral problems may require implementing behavior modification techniques at home and in school.

If, despite all best intentions, the speech processor and/or headset has gotten wet while the child is at school, the teacher can provide some immediate care for the unit. First, the teacher should make certain that moisture has truly created a problem with the functioning of the unit. Determining processor function is easy if the child is able to articulate the breakdown. If the child is unable to tell the teacher that the processor sounds acceptable and the child's level of auditory perception is still at the rudimentary stage, the unit should be turned off and the parents should be informed. If a dri-aid kit is available at school, the teacher should remove the battery and place the entire speech processor and headset into the dri-aid kit. No other attempts should be made by the teacher to dry out the unit. Parents have been trained in procedures to be used when this occurs (Nevins & Chute, 1996; Tye-Murray, 1996).

Although excessive moisture in the headset or speech processor will create certain problems to the units, extreme dryness with a subsequent buildup of electrostatic discharge (ESD) can also create problems. In classrooms or homes that are hot and dry, some simple precautions can be taken to help guard against problems caused by ESD. Carpeting can be sprayed with a solution of 50% fabric softener and 50% water. Humidifiers can also used to increase moisture.

On the playground, buildup of ESD when using plastic equipment, specifically slides, has generated concern. Children with cochlear implants should either remove their devices when using this equipment or should be counseled against playing on them. There have been some instances of map contamination or map loss after playing on plastic apparatus. Because it is not a consistent finding, it is difficult to determine the exact combination of factors that may contribute to the problem. If a child has been in the playground and suddenly exhibits changes in his functional ability with the implant, the teacher should notify the parent. The parent should be instructed to contact the implant facility to have the processor checked. Often all that is required is rewriting of the map to the speech processor.

Children using computers can be protected by the use of antistatic mats under the chair and the keyboard and an antistatic shield over the screen. Van de Graaf generators that are often on display at science museums must be avoided because these generate a large amount of ESD (Cochlear Corporation, 1996). An amusement park ride known as the "Drop Zone" must also be avoided because it uses a magnetic break system to stop the ride.

Troubleshooting the Device

Parents and teachers (and child, if age appropriate) should have some exposure to methods that are used to troubleshoot the implant. The amount and type of exposure may depend on the implant facility servicing the child. At the very least, literature on how to perform these procedures should be made accessible; booklets provided by the manufacturers are available on request. In addition, it is preferable that "hands-on" practice of troubleshooting techniques be provided.

Inevitably, the cochlear implant, like many other mechanical devices, will not function properly at some point or cease to function completely. Teachers and therapists must realize that they should not panic if this happens. Knowledge of how the system works should allow for troubleshooting the unit quickly and efficiently. It is important to remember that there can be more than one piece of equipment malfunctioning at any given time. Therefore, once a problem is found with one component, the troubleshooting process should continue to ensure the entire mechanism is functioning. Some devices (Nucleus 22, Nucleus 24 and Med El) provide a test wand that enables the teacher or parent to perform a quick check of the system without having to remove the device from the child's head. Minor problems can be easily solved when educational programs keep extra batteries and cords available to assist the child during the school day.

PEARL

When children stop responding to auditory input with their cochlear implants, the problem is most likely caused by low battery power. Replacing batteries is the most common form of troubleshooting to be performed on the implant system.

If the processor stops functioning entirely, it should be left on the child in the "off" position. This will prevent the unit from being lost or exposed to other damaging situations. (For example, removing the unit and placing it in the child's backpack might subject it to abuse from other materials in the backpack.) As long as the speech processor is in the "off" position, the child can continue to wear the nonfunctioning unit with no possibility of danger to the child or the unit.

In some instances, the external equipment is operating appropriately, but the child's auditory responsiveness deteriorates or is suddenly inconsistent. Although a number of circumstances might account for this behavior (e.g., a map change), a slight possibility also exists that there may be a problem with the function of the internal receiver. Therefore, it is important for the teacher to be aware of some of the red flags that may indicate a problem with the internal receiver. These red flags include behaviors such as sudden inconsistent auditory responses to sounds previously a part of the child's repertoire, deterioration in speech production, frequent equipment changes, or general lack of progress for no apparent reason. The presence of telemetry systems now make it much easier to troubleshoot internal receiver malfunctions and all of the newer devices have incorporated software that assesses device functionality each time the child is remapped. However, children with the Nucleus 22 channel system do not have access to this type of technology and cannot be routinely tested. Devices that are intermittent are extremely difficult to asses even with telemetry. Ongoing communication between the school and the implant center will assist in identifying any potential internal or external equipment problems.

A number of situations, both medical and environmental, should be avoided after implantation. Medically, implant recipients may not be evaluated using MRI because the internal receiver contains a magnet and physical damage may result. As noted previously, the Nucleus 24 device is MRI compatible because the internal magnet can be removed through a small skin incision. Once a child completes the MRI procedure, the magnet can be replaced through the same incision. Any other type of x-ray procedure will not be problematic. Implant patients should always inform physicians that they have a cochlear implant. Should the individual require any other type of surgery, it is important that the implanting surgeon be advised.

Implant users should be aware of possible interference from two-way radios or cellular telephones that may operate on the same frequency. Airport security systems may be activated because of the presence of the implant magnet. If security personnel require that the speech processor be placed through the x-ray system, it will not cause any damage. As a general rule, the implant center should be contacted when questions about implant integrity arise.

Auditory Learning with a Cochlear Implant

Traditional approaches to teaching deaf children focused on training children to listen. This type of activity required listening practice in small group activities using nonspeech stimuli such as musical instruments or environmental sounds. Exposure to speech occurred only after success was achieved with these gross stimuli. These training paradigms were seldom successful because children were not exposed to everyday spoken language (Ling, 1986). More recently, emphasis has been placed on the child's ability to learn through listening and incorporates a more natural intervention that exposes the child to speech on an appropriate cognitive level using common, daily experiences (Mischook & Cole, 1986).

PEARL

Because implant systems' processors are uniquely designed to process speech, meaningful spoken language is preferred over musical instruments or environmental sounds as input in developing listening skills.

Habilitation for the Young Child

The precise method used to develop listening skills will vary depending on the age at the time of implantation and the level of linguistic sophistication that the child exhibits. For children implanted at very young ages, there will likely be greater benefit in placing them in an environment in which listening has meaning and is required for completing tasks of interest. Language that is referenced to a preschool activity or a household routine, such as having a snack or getting ready for bed, provides the child with a consistent activity using vocabulary and language that is meaningful and predictable. The overall habilitation goal for children in this

group is the development of language. These activities can be adapted using new vocabulary and expanded language as the age of the child increases. Listening skills should be developed in a naturalistic manner by surrounding the child with speech appropriate to his or her level and sounds naturally occurring in their environment. However, there is also merit in providing these same youngsters with some opportunity to participate in activities in which listening is the focus of the language-driven task. Nursery rhymes, songs, and finger plays that incorporate body movements can also accomplish a great deal with respect to auditory and linguistic input for the young child. Moog et al (1994) note that auditory lessons require a high level of concentration, and effort and should be scheduled for only about 15 minutes each day. Auditory lessons can be constructed to practice discrete listening skills such as discrimination between words differing either in duration or initial consonant depending on the child's skill and language level.

The ultimate goal of auditory learning activities is auditory comprehension or understanding through listening. The development of auditory skills is always framed in a language context. Erber (1982) identified four levels of auditory processing that result in auditory comprehension. These include detection, discrimination, identification, and comprehension.

Detection requires that the listener indicate that a sound has been heard. It is unnecessary for the sound to be identified, but to demonstrate this skill the response of the child must occur with a certain time limit. Children may indicate detection ability by turning to a sound in the environment or in a more structured task such as placing beads on a string.

Discrimination requires the child to indicate that two sounds were either the same or different. These tasks are planned by the teacher and require the use of closed-set of responses. Children can be presented with alternatives that vary depending on a variety of acoustical features. These can be related to duration or intensity or can be segmental in nature. Initially, opportunities should be provided to the child to discriminate differences using both auditory and visual cues. Once the child has demonstrated ability in the task on this level, the visual signal can be removed and the child can be presented with the auditory signal alone.

In tasks of auditory *identification*, a child is asked to listen to one item presented from a group of similar items and choose the one presented. Once again, children should be provided with visual input before progressing to auditory-alone presentation of the stimuli. Linguistic levels of input should always be varied commensurate with the age and ability of the child and should not be restricted to single word items. Not only is the activity itself driven by the language level of the child, but the directions for participating in the activity must be within the child's language capability as well.

The level of auditory skill referred to as "thinking while listening" (Robbins et al, 1994) demonstrates the auditory *comprehension* of language. This skill requires the child to process the auditory stimuli and produce a verbal response that is more than a repetition of the signal. Auditory comprehension tasks can also be created at a variety of linguistic levels and professionals are encouraged to consider the linguistic environment of any auditory task (Nevins & Chute, 1996). As the age of the implant recipient increases, opportunities for listening at various levels can be incorporated into classroom routines and curriculum. Auditory lessons can be designed using content lessons from the standard curriculum, thereby offering the child information that is educational and meaningful. Nevins and Chute (1996) describe a method of adapting classroom curriculum for this purpose.

Rehabilitation for the Teenage Recipient

The adolescent implant recipient presents certain challenges that must be addressed to ensure continued implant use. For successful interaction with all adolescents some evaluation of identity, self-concept, and self-esteem must be obtained (Knoff, 1987). These issues become extremely important when addressing both the decision to implant and the rehabilitative needs of the teenage implant recipient. Traditional auditory training and speech production therapy should include a strong counseling component that addresses the teenager's ability to cope with change on a daily basis. Teenagers must be able to view their hearing loss as something that may be limiting but not devaluing. Training should include the acquisition of new social and coping skills that may help to minimize the effect of the hearing loss.

PITFALL
Boredom with traditional adult therapy materials, adapted for use with the teenage population, may result in disinterest and disillusionment with the cochlear implant.

Postimplant habilitation should begin with the subject or aspect of sound that holds the most interest for the teenager. It may be advisable to begin with half-hour sessions to avoid the possibility of boredom. Oftentimes, despite their deafness, teenagers enjoy watching programs on music video television stations. Sessions that compare different musical styles in a listening-only task can be fun and teach pattern recognition with material of interest to the student. Subject information from class assignments can be introduced as well. The key to working with the adolescent is to maintain interest and a willingness to return to and participate in habilitation activities.

Because speech-reading enhancement is one of the major benefits from use of a cochlear implant in the adolescent population, speech-tracking (DeFillipo & Scott, 1978) may be useful. Speech-tracking, a speech-reading technique that requires the individual to repeat verbatim a paragraph that is being read, is probably the best technique to use with this population because it will maintain interest (as long as the materials are chosen carefully) and provides a speech model that uses continuous discourse.

Interestingly, speech production is one of the single most important skills in which the adolescent wishes to acquire some improvement. The data available at this time indicate that little change exists with respect to the productive aspect of speech for this age group (Parisier & Chute, 1994). More long-term follow-up of this population is necessary to determine whether longer duration of implant use will be effec-

tive for adolescent users. Because the adolescent population represents the largest group of nonusers and the smallest group of implant recipients, it will take much longer periods of study before a definitive answer is available. With the miniaturization of implants creating a more cosmetically appealing device, renewed interest in implants may occur in this age group.

Role of Parents

Regardless of which age group in which the implanted child fits, the parents' role in the (re)habilitation process is critical to success (Tye-Murray et al, 1996). Parents must be active participants in the entire implantation process and act as the interface between the school and the implant facility. They are responsible for monitoring the child's performance with individual maps and coordinating input to the programming audiologist. In addition, parents must adhere to the follow-up schedule recommended by the implant center and make adjustments in that schedule, depending on the child's response. Archbold (1994) reported that the child spends only 1% of his or her time at the implant center; most of his or her remaining time is split between his or her home and school. If parents do not take responsibility for monitoring a child's implant use, the device will not be capable of allowing the child to reach his or her full potential.

PEARL
Encouraging a strong parent, implant center, and school network increases the likelihood that a child will experience success with his or her implant and habilitation program.

The consistent use of speech and voice by parents of deaf children who receive implants is a critical aspect of communicating in the home. Parents are urged to speak to their children in full-voice even if they are using simultaneous communication or cued speech. Cochlear implantation in children need not result in an alteration of whatever linguistic approach has been chosen by the family. Instead, the implant appears to supplement existing communication strategies. Robbins et al (1994) studied the language abilities of children who used total versus oral communication and found that children who used speech and sign performed as well as and in some areas better than the oral children. Speech production abilities of the children who used total communication appeared to lag somewhat; it was suggested that this was due to the tendency by parents and educators not to challenge these children productively. Regardless of which mode of communication is adopted, good auditory input by the parents and heightened expectation for spoken language are crucial for success.

Parents also need to cooperate with the school or private therapist who is providing the child's auditory and speech training. Families who offer their children an enriched listening and language environment encouraging the use of speaking and listening skills generally support some of the most successful implant users (Boothroyd, 1987). When parents are detached from the process and view children as the responsibility of the school and the therapist, the likelihood of the child maximizing his potential decreases. Conversely, when parents support the teachers and therapists by reinforcing skills that have been introduced, children appear to respond in a more positive fashion.

Role of the School

The school program can contribute substantially to a child's ability to develop good listening and speaking behaviors. Educational environments that value the role of audition and use it as an integral part of teaching and learning can provide the proper support for the developing auditory and speech skills of implant recipients. Conversely, classrooms cannot support children with cochlear implants when no voice is used and American Sign Language (ASL) is the designated language of instruction. To maximize school involvement, some facilities use an educational consultant model (Nevins et al, 1991) to maintain communication with the individual educational setting. These educational consultants offer guidance to the teacher/therapist regarding the importance of providing an environment that facilitates auditory learning while simultaneously acknowledging the demands and realities of a school day.

> ### PITFALL
>
> Implant centers that do not include local school professionals as extended members of the implant team may lose a valuable resource for ensuring implant success.

As noted earlier, school personnel should be well versed in the care and maintenance of the cochlear implant equipment so that any malfunction can be assessed and remediated as soon as possible. Liaison with the implant facility through a team educator can easily provide this information to the school members. In addition, with the introduction of multiple storage capacity speech processors, educational facilities can now become active participants in the remapping process by providing input about the child's performance with a particular program.

Finally, school professionals should also work in a cooperative effort with the parent to ensure good follow-up of the child's speech, language, and auditory program. A proactive communication philosophy will drive teacher reports of progress, plateaus, or equipment problems that can assist the parent in decisions regarding returns to the implant center or the direction that home training should take. Issues of educational management of the child with an implant do not end at any specified time after the child receives the device. Rather, new management concerns surface as the child moves through the educational system (Lutman et al, 1994).

PERFORMANCE OF CHILDREN WITH COCHLEAR IMPLANTS

Most of the published reports of performance of children with cochlear implants reflect the population of children who were implanted with the Nucleus 22 channel device using either the F0, F1, F2 extractor or the MPEAK strategy (Geers & Moog, 1989; Osberger et al, 1991; Staller et al, 1991; Tyler, 1993). More recently, studies by Skinner et al (1994) and Holden et al (1997) have reported performance of the Nucleus 22 channel SPEAK processing strategy. Because the Clarion device became available for use in the pediatric population in 1995, only recently has data concerning the follow-up of these children been reported. Although the study of the Med El implant has just begun in this country, preliminary data are available for a small subset of children from Europe.

Speech perception measures for the pediatric population generally assess children's ability to discriminate envelope and stress patterns, closed-set word recognition, open-set word recognition, sentence recognition, and, in some cases, vowel and consonant recognition. Over the years, test stimuli, patient demographics, and processing strategies have changed with a clear trend toward younger children and better performance. Because a great deal of published data already exist for the Nucleus 22 device, the results of the Nucleus 22 will be reviewed briefly with the reader being directed to the original sources for more information. Greater emphasis will be placed on the Nucleus 24, Clarion, and Med El devices and some of the early results reported for these devices.

Speech Perception

Assessing the degree of benefit from any sensory aid requires outcome measures that reflect changes in performance over time. The special considerations for testing speech perception in deaf children include the type of stimuli, the vocabulary and linguistic level of the child, the motoric and attentional abilities of the child, the test-retest reliability of the materials, and the need for stimuli that provide analytic information (Tyler, 1993). As the age of children being implanted decreases, it becomes more challenging to measure early changes in perception because these children most often lack the linguistic sophistication necessary to assess benefit. As a result of implantation, there has been a new emphasis on developing methods to assess changes in auditory perception in young children. These tests fall into two basic categories: standardized measures and questionnaires.

Tests of Speech Perception

In developing tests that can be used for the pediatric population, researchers must address certain issues that can affect performance and inadvertently provide misinformation. Boothroyd (1991) emphasizes the use of speech stimuli to measure performance in this population. Although some studies use nonspeech or synthetic speech-like stimuli (Dorman, 1993) for young children, speech is more meaningful and can be attended to for longer periods of time.

Speech perception measures for children can be classified in a manner similar to that used for adults (i.e., open and closed-set tasks). Closed-set tests of speech perception assess environmental sound awareness, timing, and intensity cues or segmental discrimination. Tests administered must be within the language and vocabulary level of the child to obtain a proper assessment of auditory ability. In addition, to maintain the attention of the child, tests for very young children often use brightly colored pictures or actual toys (Geers & Moog, 1989; Ross & Lerman, 1971), video games are now also available (Boothroyd, 1998).

A complete speech perception battery that evaluates the perception of phonemes, words, and phrases known as Evaluation of Auditory Responses to Speech (EARS) (Allum, 1997) was developed in Europe to be used with children of various countries and is available in 14 languages. Closed-set tests like the Word Intellgibility by Picture Identfication (WIPI) (Ross & Lerman, 1971) or the Northwestern University Children's Perception of Speech (NU-Chips) (Elliot & Katz, 1980) provide clinicians with information regarding an individual child's ability to identify words that have similar phonetic content. For the youngest implant users, the Early Speech Perception Test (ESP) (Geers & Moog, 1989), which also has a low verbal version, can begin to assess some of the earlier detection and pattern recognition abilities in younger children. In most cases young children require a live-voice presentation for testing because recorded speech does not hold their attention. Generally, tests using recorded speech are preferred; monitored live-voice (MLV) presentation using an unfamiliar speaker is acceptable. In all cases a number of speech perception measures are required for each child to obtain a more complete picture of his or her abilities. When possible, these tests should reflect a variety of stimuli and performance levels.

Tests of open-set speech recognition should be used for children who have some functional vocabulary. Traditional single word open-set tests, such as the Phonetically Balanced Kindergarten Test (PBK's) (Haskins, 1949), may be too difficult for this population because of the lack of vocabulary. For this reason, two tests, the Multisyllabic Lexical Neighborhood Test (MLNT) and the Lexical Neighborhood Test (LNT) were developed (Kirk et al, 1995) using vocabulary more likely to be in the repertoire of the deaf or language-impaired child. The Glendonald Auditory Screening Procedure (GASP) (Erber, 1982), a closed-set test has been adapted, in part, as an open-set test because much of the vocabulary was deemed to be familiar to the child.

For older children, assessment of conversational speech is recommended. Sentence material for this population includes measures such as the Common Phrases Test (Osberger et al, 1991), the Bamford-Kowal-Bench Sentences (BKB) (Bench & Bamford, 1979), and the Pediatric Speech Intelligibiliy test (PSI) (Jerger et al, 1980). Tests using single sentences have high validity because we communicate in sentences; however, the effects of vocabulary, syntax, grammar, and coarticulation must be considered (Tyler, 1993).

When possible, assessment of vowel and consonant feature perception should also be performed. These tests use a series of pictures that vary, depending on the feature being evaluated. Information from these tests can assist in remapping decisions by identifying frequency areas that may need to be adjusted. Instruments include the Audiovisual Feature Extraction Test, the Minimal Pairs Test, the Speech Patterns Contrast Test (SPAC) (Boothroyd, 1984), and the Three Interval Forced Choice Test (THRIFT) (Boothroyd, 1986). Recently, a video version of the SPAC for young children known as the

VIDSPAC has been developed (Boothroyd, 1998). For an extensive listing and description of speech perception measures used in the pediatric population the reader is directed to Tyler (1993).

For the very young implant recipient formal assessment is limited. In an attempt to obtain information regarding this group's use of audition and speech, a series of questionnaires was developed. Robbins et al (1991) devised the Meaningful Auditory Integration Scale (MAIS) and the Meaningful Use of Speech Scale (MUSS), which obtain information through parental report regarding a child's ability to use auditory and speech stimuli. An interviewer administers the questionnaires by providing a sequence of prompts and examples with respect to specific auditory or speech activities. Parents are asked to scale ability on a continuum from "never" to "always." These tests are administered at various intervals before and after implantation.

Results of Speech Perception Testing

Nucleus 22 channel studies demonstrated that within 1 year postimplantation children averaged 64% (standard deviation (SD = 24) correct on stress identification (Staller et al, 1991). Osberger et al, (1991) reported a similar finding (74%, SD = 14). These groups were composed of children who were considered prelinguistically and postlinguistically deaf. Word recognition after 1 year of implant use averaged 39%. However, this score included both prelinguistically and postlinguistically deaf children. The congenitally deaf children performed poorer than the postlinguistically deaf children on this test. It should be noted that the mean age at time of implantation of the congenitally deaf children was older than the mean age of this same group today (personal communication, Staller, 1998). Osberger et al (1991) noted that 28 children with the Nucleus device averaged 50% (SD = 31) on age-appropriate tests of word recognition. Open-set word recognition on the PBK words was reported for a subset of children and averaged 12% correct (SD = 23) (Staller et al, 1991). Similar findings were observed by Osberger et al (1991) and Geers and Moog (1994). Sentence recognition was very limited after 1 year of implant use; however, a small subset of children was able to score over 20% correct after 2 years of implant use. It is once again important to note that the patient population at that time consisted of children whose age at implantation was older and the duration of implant use was relatively short.

Geers and Moog (1994) compared cochlear implant recipients' performance with children who were "good" hearing aid users and a group who used a Tactaid vibrotactile device. Children who used vibrotactile aids showed performance increases over a 3-year period, but these results were similar to their hearing aid performance. Data comparing single-channel cochlear implants and tactile aids showed no significant difference (Roeser, 1989); however, the performance of single-channel versus multichannel stimulation demonstrated the superiority of the latter type of implant (Chute et al, 1990).

In 1994, Cochlear Corporation introduced a new speech processing strategy compatible with existing hardware. This strategy known as SPEAK (Spectral Peak) has been studied in a group of subjects who were initially fit with the MPEAK (Multi Peak) strategy and also in a group of subjects who began with the SPEAK strategy. Cowan et al (1995) reported on a small group of children ($N = 12$) and noted better performance in noise for SPEAK than MPEAK in that group.

In 1997 Cochlear Corporation introduced the Nucleus 24, which used a variation of the SPEAK strategy. The data (Staller et al, 1998) are reported on the basis of a small sample ($N = 24$) and is representative of only the first 6 months postimplantation. Children less than 5 years of age are analyzed separately because these children are unable to perform on many of the test procedures because of limited linguistic skills. Tables 16–2 and 16–3 list the various scores obtained for these two groups of children. Overall, the younger group demonstrated marked increases in their ability to perceive speech patterns within 6 months of implantation. Children in this group scored on the average of 46% after only 6 months of implant use as opposed to 25.4% at the preimplant interval. Older children demonstrated an average score of 50.4% on the Common Phrases Test (preimplant = 12.6%) after only 6 months of implantation. Pattern perception for this group was at 88.4% for the same time period. It should also be noted that children less than 5 years old were evaluated with

monitored live voice; the older children were evaluated using recorded speech.

Performance of children using the Clarion Multi-Strategy cochlear implant system (Tables 16–4 and 16–5) were reported by Osberger et al (1997). Children in this study were subdivided according to age and linguistic ability. Children less than 3 years old were evaluated using a lower verbal test battery than children older than 7. Children whose ages were between 3 and 7 years were given a screening test to determine which battery should be administered. All data were obtained using monitored live voice. Tables 16–4 and 16–5 display the results of a small subgroup of children ($N = 39$) after 1 year of implantation. The Level 1 children represent those children who were younger and/or had limited language capacity. Average scores on tests of closed-set recognition were at 67% after 12 months of use. A smaller group of children were able to obtain some open-set recognition and scored 13% on PBKs after 1 year. These children all used the CIS speech-processing strategy that was programmed in a monopolar mode. (NOTE: monopolar stimulation occurs when each active electrode is reference to a remote ground.)

TABLE 16–2 **Speech perception test results for younger children using the Nucleus 24 (18 mo–4 y, 11 mo)**

Test	Preoperative (%)	6 Mo Postoperative (%)
ESP-Pattern	25.4	46.0
ESP-Spondee	23.8	36.3
ESP-Monosyllable	24.2	30.6
GASP Words	2.8	12.0
MLNT-Words	0.5	5.2
MLNT-Phonemes	0.4	6.4

TABLE 16–3 **Speech perception test results for older children using the Nucleus 24 (5 y–17 y, 11 mo)**

Test	Preoperative (%)	6 Mo Postoperative (%)
ESP-Pattern	64.5	88.4
ESP-Spondee	47.3	76.3
GASP Words	27.4	66.3
MLNT-Words	8.5	37.5
MLNT-Phonemes	11.4	41.3
LNT Words	3.8	28.2
LNT Phonemes	10.3	39.5
PBK Words	4.1	22.9
PBK Phonemes	14.8	36.9
Common Phrases	12.6	50.4
BKB Sentences	8.3	38.6

TABLE 16–4   Speech perception test results for Level 1 children using the Clarion

Test	Preoperative (%)	12 Mo Postoperative (%)
MAIS	20	70
ESP-Monosyllable	25	67
GASP Words	2	37
GASP Sentences	1	14
PBK-Words	0	13
PBK-Phonemes	3	23

TABLE 16–5   Speech perception test results for Level 2 children using the Clarion

Test	Preoperative (%)	12 Mo Postoperative (%)
MAIS	38	72
ESP-Monosyllable	20	69
GASP Words	12	55
GASP Sentences	7	53
PBK-Words	0	22
PBK-Phonemes	9	45

Finally, the Med El Combi 40+ implant study in the pediatric population has just begun in the United States, but data from Europe have yielded the following results. Allum (1997) has reported on 37 children who were administered the EARS battery. These children were given a variety of the subtests depending on their age and level of vocabulary. On closed-set tasks that presented six word stimuli, pattern perception was 61% after 6 months of implant use. For monosyllabic word identification, a smaller group of subjects ($N = 7$) demonstrated an average score of 17% after 3 months of implant use. It should be noted that these data were collected using MLV and represent a number of different languages used throughout Europe.

Speech and Language Performance

Although a great deal has been published concerning the auditory perceptual changes that occur after implantation, fewer studies have measured the speech and language abilities of these children. A variety of methods have been used to measure speech production changes in this population. These include batteries typically used with hearing-impaired or normal-hearing children (Geers & Moog, 1991; Tobey & Hasenstab, 1991) in which children respond to spontaneous or imitated stimuli. The second method of assessment elicits speech samples from the children before and after implantation and analyzes these into certain categories (Osberger et al, 1991; Tait, 1993). As with many of the assessment tools with young children, a segment of the population is always incapable of performing some of the tasks because of

cognitive and linguistic constraints. Most recently, a test has been developed for use with very young children to obtain a measure of their recognition and production of simple speech contours. The Suprasegmental Recognition and Production Test (SRAPT) (Bollard et al, 1999) has been successfully used in children as young as 2 years of age with good results.

Speech Production

Most studies published in speech production area have measured these changes in children who used the Nucleus 22 channel device with the F0, F1, F2 strategy. A general finding is that speech production changes for the greater majority of implanted children progress at much slower rates than auditory perceptual changes (Tobey et al, 1994). Speech production measures for imitated speech suggests that the implant may assist children in beginning to develop phonemic elements and refine the articulatory gestures necessary to produce the elements (Tobey, 1993). More accurate vowel and diphthong production occurs with increased experience with multichannel implants (Geers & Tobey, 1992). Also, a greater repertoire of consonants is observed in the spontaneous speech of children with cochlear implants (Tobey et al, 1991). Tobey et al (1994) also reported that children with cochlear implants were more accurate on some of the less visible place features such as velars, manner features such as glides, and some voicing features of stops than were children with hearing aids or vibrotactile aids.

Osberger et al (1993) measured speech intelligibility in a group of children who used total communication versus a group that used oral communication. On the average, scores of children using oral communication were 27% higher than children using total communication. The authors also noted that some of the children in the oral group still had poor speech intelligibility and suggested that factors other than communication mode may influence the acquisition of speech production skills. Svirsky, (1997) reported a similar finding with respect to prelingually deaf children with cochlear implants and hearing aids. Conversely, Connor et al (1997) reported no significant difference between the oral and total communication groups of children on measure of speech intelligibility, receptive vocabulary, and reading comprehension. In fact, the children in total communication programs demonstrated greater expressive vocabularies.

Language Development

Language development in children with cochlear implants has received even less attention than speech production during the initial years of implant research. Studies of this nature are difficult to design because variables such as mode of communication and school placement often confound results. In addition, measures of implanted children's linguistic competence can be compared with normal-hearing children, hearing-impaired children, or deaf children. Depending on which population is used as a comparison group, results can be misleading. Now that there is better understanding of the effect of cochlear implants on audition, attention can turn to measuring outcomes in other areas such as language and education.

Despite some of the problems associated with assessing language achievement of children with cochlear implants, a number of studies have documented gains in language growth that can be attributed to implant use. Robbins et al (1997) reported on a group of children who were followed using the Reynell Developmental Language Scales and measured language growth as a function of implant use versus maturation. The results indicated that children with implants demonstrated a delay in language skills compared with normal-hearing children; however, they were progressing at faster rates than deaf unimplanted children. Similar findings were reported by Bollard et al (1999). Schopmeyer et al (1997) used video analysis to measure expressive vocabulary in a group of 20 implanted children. They reported positive influence on the rate of language development for this group of children. Likewise, Tait (1993) reported on video analysis of very young implant recipients and found a marked increase in conversational skills such as turn taking and initiation after implantation. Tyler et al (1997) also reported that expressive and receptive language typically increases over a 5-year period for children who received cochlear implants and especially for those who received them at early ages.

Regardless of the type of outcome measured to assess implant effectiveness, the performance capabilities of children who use cochlear implants will be affected by the age at implantation and duration of deafness (Boothroyd, 1993; Tyler, 1993). Younger children who have a shorter duration of deafness are able to take advantage of exposure to language in the first 2 to 3 years of life. Electrical stimulation at this early juncture may also prevent further deterioration and increase survival of spiral ganglia. Leake et al (1999) reported that in neonatally deafened cats, electrical stimulation maintains increased survival of spiral ganglion neurons and that normal temporal resolution is maintained by chronic stimulation with low-frequency signals. Thus there appears to be physiologic evidence supporting trends toward early implantation.

SPECIAL CONSIDERATION

Performance with a cochlear implant is most sensitive to age at implantation and duration of deafness. Children who are implanted at early ages are likely to show greater and more rapid auditory, speech, and language benefit than children implanted later with longer duration of deafness. However, progress of the latter group, although occurring at a slower rate, may still be impressive over time.

The performance of children who use cochlear implants can vary widely across subjects and devices. The magnitude of the change in both speech perception and speech production may vary according to physiologic and environmental factors. Long-term follow-up is required to determine the impact these devices will have on implanted children's educational achievements and lifestyle.

Educational Achievements of Children with Cochlear Implants

A continuum of school placements is available for deaf children driven by historical and political ideals. Children can be placed in residential schools for the deaf, self-contained classrooms, resource rooms, included classrooms, or in the mainstream. Residential schools for the deaf that embrace auditory/oral goals have proven to be effective placements for children with cochlear implants (Geers & Moog, 1994). Conversely, schools using ASL and de-emphasizing speaking and listening will be poor environments for children with implants and often lead to nonuse (Rose, 1995).

Self-contained classrooms may be found in local school districts and educate children in separate classes within the confines of a normal-hearing school environment. This situation allows social mainstreaming of deaf/hard-of-hearing children by providing them with exposure to normal-hearing children during nonacademic periods. Academic mainstreaming is also available for children whose skills and abilities warrant access to curriculum and instruction in regular classrooms. Resource rooms may be the first step in accessing the mainstream by providing small group, replacement instruction for particular academic areas such as language arts and reading, subjects traditionally challenging for children with hearing loss. The recent trend toward inclusion has resulted in small groups of children with hearing loss placed in regular classrooms. There, they receive instruction from a teacher of the deaf who collaborates with the classroom teacher. Full mainstreaming represents the ability of deaf children to achieve academically alongside their hearing peers. Most often a secondary goal of implantation for many parents is the desire for the integration of their child into a regular classroom.

Paul and Quigley (1984) and Ross et al (1991) note that mainstream placement may be the most appropriate setting for the hard-of-hearing child. Because children with implants appear to be achieving at levels that are similar to the moderately or severely impaired child (Boothroyd, 1993), it is a logical conclusion that these children be considered for mainstream placement. Pflaster (1980) and Allen and Osborn (1984) suggest that students in the mainstream attain higher levels of performance on standardized tests of achievement than do their nonmainstreamed peers. Therefore, in an effort to provide children with cochlear implants the opportunity to perform at levels near their hearing-age-mates, mainstream placement is considered an important decision for the child's academic career.

PITFALL

The use of a cochlear implant does not necessarily guarantee readiness for mainstream education. The decision to mainstream a child with an implant must be made using a number of criteria, only one of which is auditory perceptual ability.

Nevins and Chute (1996) suggest a "whole-child" approach in recommending children for the mainstream. Both formal and informal measures can be used to assist in this decision. Formal measures should include assessment in the areas of language and reading in addition to audition and speech production. Academically, children being considered for mainstream placement should be at the top of their self-contained class in their present school setting and, of course, have the desire to be mainstreamed.

The school receiving the child must also share some responsibilities by providing the appropriate educational and support services that will be needed for success. Modification of teaching style and physical setting may be necessary to ensure the best acoustic environment for the child (Berg, 1987). A commitment by the classroom teacher to communicate with the implant center and the parents regarding the child's progress is also necessary.

Chute and Nevins (1995) followed the school placements of 92 children with implants and found that experienced users all reached the mainstream within 7 years of implantation. In addition, they reported that more than half of the children implanted between 2 and 4 years of age were able to be placed in the mainstream within 2 years of implantation. Francis et al (1997) tracked 24 school-aged children with implants and observed progress toward educational independence starting at 20 months postimplantation. Hasenstab et al (1997) surveyed 26 parents of children who received the Nucleus 22 channel implant. Although only 30% of the questionnaires were returned, parents reported that most of these children were at least partially mainstreamed. Tyler et al (1997) followed 30 prelinguistically deafened children who were using total communication and were implanted with the Nucleus device for 3 to 5 years. They reported only a "few" children who experienced changes in educational placement and noted that these children demonstrated the largest gains in language and the highest speech perception scores.

Monitoring childrens' performance once they are in the mainstream has received very little attention. It is important to recognize that once placed in the mainstream, children require constant monitoring to ensure success. Nevins and Chute (1996) developed the mainstream checklist in conjunction with the Clarke School for the Deaf in an attempt to operationally define some of the classroom behaviors that contribute to success. This checklist provides quantitative data and identifies behaviors believed to be indicators of mainstream success. (For a copy of the checklist the reader is directed to the source by Nevins and Chute [1996].) Summerfield et al (1997) has adapted this checklist for use with children in the United Kingdom to assist in demonstrating how cochlear implants can alleviate some of the financial burden on the educational system.

The final analysis of the success of children with cochlear implants in educational settings will require years of monitoring and necessitate that large groups of children progress through the entire educational sequence. Certainly, there will always be a group of children who are academically unsuccessful. However, it is believed that children who receive implants at early ages can begin their academic careers in regular school settings and achieve at levels similar to their normal-hearing peers. Data collected on a small subgroup of children who were implanted for more than 5 years and in mainstream settings yielded standard reading scores approximating those of their hearing age-mates (Chute & Nevins, 1995). Although the number in this group is relatively small ($N = 8$), the demographics of these children are also very different from the children who are being implanted today. For this reason, it is believed that children who are implanted now at young ages should respond in a similar fashion. Further study in the area of the educational impact of the implant will serve to document its efficacy.

Performance of Special Populations

The number of implants performed in children has grown steadily through the years as devices have changed and performance has improved. For this reason, implants are now being used in children who previously may not have been considered ideal candidates for implantation. These are children with abnormal cochleas, secondary noncognitive handicaps, cognitive handicaps, and "soft" neurological signs.

Abnormal Cochleas

Although children with abnormal cochleas have received implants throughout the period of device investigation, performance has not been predictable or consistent. Children with either Mondini deformities or ossified cochleas are part of this group to receive implants in the past. Performance studies of these children vary depending on a number of factors. These may include variables such as the depth of insertion, the overall current levels required for stimulation, the age at implantation, and the duration of deafness. For children with Mondini malformations, the degree of the malformation has an impact on the number of electrodes that can be inserted. Novak et al (1990) note that even as the degree of malformation increases, children are still capable of using the signal from the implant to obtain an enhancement in speechreading ability. If a full insertion is possible, these children should perform similarly to other children with the same age at time of implant and duration of deafness.

Children with ossified cochleas demonstrate much more variability, and no consensus with regard to performance has emerged (Geier et al, 1993; Kemink et al, 1992; Kirk et al, 1997; Parisier & Chute, 1993). Some researchers report poorer performance, whereas others report equivalent performance. All studies note, however, that children with ossified cochleas often require longer periods of device use before substantial changes in performance are observed.

Noncognitive and Cognitive Handicaps

The effect of noncognitive secondary handicaps such as blindness, mild cerebral palsy, or spina bifida in children who receive cochlear implants has been studied in very small numbers of children. Results would indicate the primacy of factors that are related to the age of implantation and duration of deafness in predicting performance and not the nature of the additional handicap (Chute & Nevins, 1995; Garabedian et al, 1997). In contrast, children with secondary handicaps that are cognitive in nature tend to achieve at the lower end of the performance continuum, with most obtaining only sound detection and a smaller number obtaining pattern perception (Bellman, 1994; Lesinski et al, 1994). The poorest group of performers were the autistic children, and Lesinski et al (1994) suggest that these children do not perform well enough to warrant implantation. Hasenstab (1996) reported on a group of children who were diagnosed as learning disabled and received cochlear implants. These children demonstrated changes in performance over time but at a much slower rate than the general pediatric population.

Soft Neurologic Signs

The final group represents a population that is difficult to diagnose because they are being implanted at early ages. These children demonstrate "soft" neurological signs in that they have an inability to maintain eye contact, have poor or immature play skills, and also exhibit underdeveloped motor control. Because these children are receiving implants at early ages and represent some of the more recent implant recipients, it is unclear as to how this device will impact on their overall growth and development.

COCHLEAR IMPLANTS AND OTHER ASSISTIVE DEVICES

To expand the capabilities of implants and provide better SNRs in classrooms that might present an acoustical challenge, each of the manufacturers has developed patch cords allowing implants to be interfaced with conventional FM systems. Because this process requires a great deal of commentary and feedback from the user, this system setup is not recommended for very young children or children who are incapable of communicating about their auditory experiences. When children are fit with FM systems to be used with their cochlear implant, a school professional should be responsible for monitoring both pieces of equipment. However, in devices such as the Nucleus 22, it should be noted that as one plugs into the external input socket, the user's microphone is no longer functional. This effectively withdraws the child from responding to anything other than what is being fed directly into the unit by the teacher. Functionally, children will not be able to hear the discussion or interaction with other children in the class when the FM is activated. For this reason and because of the excessive bulk of wearing both devices, most parents have not chosen this option.

However, in some cases, FM use is necessary and recommended. Observations by trained teachers of the deaf and/or an educational consultant from the Implant Center should assist parents and school personnel in deciding if this is an option for a particular child. Although the benefits of traditional FM systems are well known, no organized research supports or refutes their use with a cochlear implant, and they represent a very small percentage of the pediatric population.

On the contrary, there has been a recent trend in classrooms of children with implants to provide sound field amplification systems to enhance the auditory signal. These systems are more cost-effective, service the entire class of schoolchildren and do not require any special attachments for the implanted child. A variety of systems are available, and the reader is directed to Chapter 21 in this volume on this topic.

PEARL

The use of sound field amplification systems for children with implants in mainstream settings provides enhanced auditory input for *all* children in the class, not just the implanted child.

Finally, older children, experienced in implant use, often discover that they can enjoy music through cassette or compact disc (CD) players more clearly when using a direct input through a patch cord. (The reader is referred to Chapter 20 in this volume.) In some cases individuals have also used these patch cords to obtain direct input from the television. Precautions are necessary when interfacing cochlear implant equipment into a source that is plugged directly into an electrical outlet. In these circumstances users are required to have a surge protector in-line with the outlet and the equipment. This is not a recommended use of the implant, and, as noted earlier, interfacing the Nucleus 22 disengages the standard microphone so that no other input can be heard.

Some implant manufacturers may provide telephone adapters that offer direct input into the telephone and deliver a slightly enhanced signal for many users. Experienced implant recipients who are capable of telephone use often find this accommodation helpful because it provides better speech recognition for some. Implant recipients are cautioned again about using this adaptor during electrical storms because they are connected directly into the telephone line. Generally speaking, children should not be interfaced with any additional external equipment unless they are sophisticated users of the implant, can provide appropriate feedback, and take responsibility for their actions.

FUTURE DIRECTIONS

Numerous technological changes on the horizon will affect the number and the profile of children who receive implants.

With the trend toward miniaturization, more parents of young children and older children themselves will be seeking this device because the cosmetics will be similar to conventional BTE hearing aids. Cochlear Corporation presently has a working BTE model available and both Advanced Bionics and Med El will be introducing their own models by the end of 1999. The number and variations of processing strategies that will be available within and among devices is also changing. Cochlear Corporation presently uses the SPEAK coding strategy but is introducing the newer ACE and CIS strategy in the adult population before the end of 1998. Advanced Bionics has redeveloped the compressed analog strategy into the present SAS and also plans to introduce hybrid strategies that use a combination of SAS and CIS. Med El is investigating the N of M strategy in addition to a high-speed CIS.

As implants change, the candidates for these devices will also change. Children with some residual hearing are already being implanted. It is conceivable that as more information becomes available, the degree of hearing loss that will be required to obtain an implant will decrease. In addition, as changes in performance after implantation in younger children become more precise, the age of implantation may be lowered to less than 18 months. Already a number of children less than this age have received implants for medical reasons and have performed well. Finally, bilateral implantation may not be far behind. Recently, Gantz (1998) has implanted one adult with bilateral implants. Results are forthcoming and may begin to answer questions about the usefulness of this procedure for both ears and provide information about which ear to implant.

In addition to all the technological and candidacy changes that will occur, one of the greatest impacts on the industry may come from the healthcare system itself. Cochlear implants are currently financed through private third-party insurers and managed care systems. Oftentimes restrictions exist by some carriers with regard to the type of device and investigational status with the FDA. Although it is hoped that financing of implants by insurers will continue, it is worrisome if the industry decides to view these devices as hearing aids and designate them as exclusionary. Even now, there are often problems obtaining funding for follow-up visits to the implant center. Managed care providers may not pay for services at a center outside their network even though it may have more experience and is the patient's choice. In addition to making decisions regarding which implant facility a patient must use, there may come a time when the decision regarding which device is implanted will be made by the managed care company and not the patient or his or her parents. Despite these concerns surrounding managed care, the future for implantation remains exciting and promises to surpass the impact that hearing aid technology had in the field of deafness and hearing loss in the 1950s.

REFERENCES

ABBAS, P.J., & BROWN, C.J. (1991). Electrically evoked auditory brain stem response: Growth of response with current level. *Hearing Research, 51;*123–138.

ALLEN, T., & OSBORN, T. (1984). Academic integration of hearing-impaired students: Demographic, handicapping and achievement factors. *American Annals of the Deaf, 129;* 100–113.

ALLUM, D.J. (1997). *Experience in evaluating children with cochlear implants using a multi-language test battery (EARS).* Paper presented at the meeting of the Fifth International Cochlear Implant Conference, New York, New York.

ARCHBOLD, S. (1994). Implementing a paediatric cochlear implant programme: Theory and practice. In: B. McCormick, S. Archbold, & S. Sheppard (Eds.), *Cochlear implants for young children* (pp. 25–59). London: Whurr.

BELLMAN, S. (1994). *Assessing multiply-handicapped children for cochlear implantation.* Paper presented at the meeting of the European Symposium on Paediatric Cochlear Implantation, Montpelier, France.

BENCH, J., & BAMFORD, J. (1979). *Speech-hearing tests and the spoken language of hearing-impaired children.* London: Academic Press.

BERG, F. (1987). *Facilitating classroom listening: A handbook for teachers of normal and hard-of-hearing children.* Boston: College Hill Press/Little, Brown.

BERTRAM, B., MEYER, V., & LENARZ, T. (1996). *Cochlear implantation in a 7 month old baby.* Paper presented at the Third European Symposium on Paediatric Cochlear Implantation, Hanover, Germany.

BILGER, R.C., BLACK, F.O., HOPKINSON, N.T., MYERS, E.N., PAYNE, J.L., STENSON, N.R., VEGA, A., & WOLF, R.V. (1977). Evaluation of subjects presently fitted with implanted auditory prostheses. *Annals of Otology, Rhinology, and Laryngology, 86,*(suppl. 38).

BOLLARD, P.M., CHUTE, P.M., POPP, A.L., & PARISIER, S.C. (1999). Specific language growth in young children using the Clarion cochlear implant. *Annals of Otology, Rhinology, and Larynogology, 108;*119–123.

BOOTHROYD, A. (1984). Auditory perception of speech contrasts by subjects with sensorineural hearing loss. *Journal of Speech and Hearing Research, 27;*134–144.

BOOTHROYD, A. (1985). Auditory capacity and the generalization of speech skills. In: J. Lauter (Ed.), *Speech planning and production in normal and hearing-impaired children.* Rockville, MD: American Speech-Language-Hearing Association, (ASHA Reports No. #15, pp. 8–14).

BOOTHROYD, A. (1986). *SPAC test version II: A test of the perception of speech pattern contrasts.* New York: City University.

BOOTHROYD, A. (1987). Perception of speech pattern contrasts via cochlear implants and limited hearing. *Annals of Otology, Rhinology, and Laryngology, 96,*(suppl. 128);58–62.

BOOTHROYD, A. (1991). Assessment of speech perception capacity in profoundly deaf children. *American Journal of Otology, 12*(suppl.);67–72.

BOOTHROYD, A. (1993). Profound deafness. In: R.S. Tyler (Ed.), *Cochlear implants* (pp. 1–34). San Diego: Singular Publishing Group, Inc.

BOOTHROYD, A. (1998). *Speech perception in pediatric implantees.* City University of New York, Graduate Program Research.

BRACKETT, D., & ZARA, C.V. (1997). *Re-examining cochlear implant candidacy: communicative outcomes of children implanted early and those with some residual hearing.* Paper presented at the Fifth International Cochlear Implant Conference, New York, New York.

CHUTE, P.M. (1997). Timing and trials of hearing aids and assistive devices. *Archives of Otolarynogology–Head and Neck Surgery, 117;*208–213.

CHUTE, P.M., & NEVINS, M.E (1994). *Educational placements of children with multichannel cochlear implants.* Paper presented at the meeting of the European Symposium on Paediatric Cochlear Implantation, Montpelier, France.

CHUTE, P.M., & NEVINS, M.E. (1995). Cochlear implants in people who are deaf/blind. *Journal of Visual Impairment and Blindness, 89;*297–300.

CHUTE, P.M., POPP, A.L., MORTON, S., & PARISIER, S.C. (1997). *The use of the Electroacoustic Reflex Threshold (EART) with the Clarion Cochlear Implant System.* Poster presentation at the meeting of the American Academy of Audiology, Los Angeles, CA.

COCHLEAR CORPORATION. (1996). *Static electricity and cochlear implants,* Englewood, CO: The Corporation.

CONNOR, C.M., ZWOLAN, T., HIEBER, S., & ARTS, H.A. (1997). *The education of children using cochlear implants: Oral or total communication.* Paper presented at the Vth International Cochlear Implant Conference, New York, NY, May.

COWAN, R.S.C., BROWN, C., WHITFORD, L.A., et al (1995). Speech Perception in children using the SPEAK speech processing strategy. *Annals of Otology, Rhinology, and Laryngology (Suppl.), 166;*318–321.

CRAIG, W. & CRAIG, H. (Eds.) (1975). Directory of services for the Deaf, *American Annals of the Deaf, 120;*118.

DEFILLIPO, C., & SCOTT, B. (1978). A method for training and evaluating the reception of ongoing speech. *Journal of the Acoustical Society of America, 63;*1186–1192.

DORMAN, M. (1993). Speech perception in adults. In: R.S. Tyler (Ed.), *Cochlear implants: Audiological foundations* (pp.145–190). San Diego: Singular Publishing Group, Inc.

DOWELL, R.C., BLAMEY, P.J., & CLARK, G.M. (1995) Potential and limitations of cochlear implants in children. *Annals of Otology, Rhinology and Laryngology, 104(9)(suppl. 166);* 324–327.

DOWELL, R.C., BROWN, A.M., & MECKLENBURG, D.J. (1990). Clinical assessment of implanted deaf adults. In: G.M. Clark, Y.C. Tong, & J.F. Patrick (Eds.), *Cochlear prostheses* (pp. 193–205). Edinburgh, Scotland: Churchill Livingstone.

ELLIOT, L., & KATZ, D. (1980). *Development of a new children's test of speech discrimination.* St. Louis, MO: Auditec.

ERBER, N. (1982). *Auditory training.* Washington, DC: Alexander Graham Bell Association for the Deaf.

FRANCIS, H.W., KOCH, M.E., DOBAJ, H., WYATT, J.R., & NIPARKO, J.K. (1997). *Trends in educational placement and cost benefit considerations in children with cochlear implants.* Paper presented at the meeting of the Fifth International Cochlear Implant Conference, New York, New York.

FRASER, G. (1991). The cochlear implant team. In: H. Cooper (Ed.), *Cochlear implants: A practical guide* (pp. 84–91). London, England: Whurr.

FRYAUF-BERTSCHY, H. (1992). Getting started at home. In: N. Tye-Murray (Ed.), *Cochlear implants and children: A handbook for parents, teachers and speech and hearing professionals.* Washington, DC: AG Bell Association for the Deaf.

GALLAUDET UNIVERSITY. (1994). Center for assessment and demographic studies. *Annual survey of deaf and hard of hearing children and youth.* Washington, DC.

GANTZ, B. (1998). *Bilateral cochlear implantation in adults.* Paper presented at the meeting of the Seventh Symposium on Cochlear Implants in Children, Iowa City, Iowa.

GARABEDIAN, E.N., BEUST, L., DENOYELLE, F., BUSQUET, D., MEATTI, L., & ROGER, G. (1997). *The value of pediatric cochlear implants in Usher's syndrome.* Paper presented at the Fifth International Cochlear Implant Conference, New York, New York.

GEERS, A.E., & MOOG, J.S. (1987). Predicting spoken language acquisition in profoundly deaf children. *Journal of Speech and Hearing Disorders, 52(1);*84–94.

GEERS, A.E., & MOOG, J.S. (1989). Evaluating speech perception skills: Tools for measuring benefits of cochlear implants, tactile aids, and hearing aids. In: E. Owen, & D. K. Kessler (Eds.), *Cochlear implants in young deaf children* (pp. 227–256). Boston: College-Hill Press.

GEERS, A.E., & MOOG, J.S. (1991). Evaluating the benefits of cochlear implants in an educational setting. *American Journal of Otology, 12* (Suppl.);116–125.

GEERS, A.E., & MOOG, J.S. (Eds.). (1994). The effectiveness of cochlear implants and tactile aids for deaf children: A report of the sensory aids study at Central Institute for the Deaf. *Volta Review, 96.*

GEERS, A.E. & TOBEY, E.A. (1992). Effects of cochlear implants and tactile aids on the development of speech production skills in profoundly hearing-impaired children. *Volta Review 94;*135–165.

GEIER, L., GILDEN, J., LUETJE, C.M., & MADDOX, H.E. (1993). Delayed perception of cochlear implant stimulation in children with postmeningitic ossified cochleae. *American Journal of Otology, 14;*556–561.

HASENSTAB, S. (1996). Learning disabilities in children with post meningitic cochlear implants. *Archives of Otolaryngology–Head and Neck Surgery, 122;*929–936.

HASENSTAB, S., KASTETTER, S., & VANDERARK, W. (1997). *Parent report of support services for their children using cochlear implants.* Paper presented at the Fifth International Cochlear Implant Conference, New York, New York.

HASKINS, H.A. (1949). *A phonetically balanced test of speech discrimination for children.* Unpublished masters thesis, Northwestern University, Evanston, IL.

HELLMAN, S.A., CHUTE, P.M., KRETSCHMER, R.E., NEVINS, M.E., PARISIER, S.C. & THURSTIN, L.C. (1991). The development of a children's implant profile. *American Annals of the Deaf, 136;*77–81.

HIEBER, S., CONNER, C., ASHBAUGH, C., & ZWOLAN, T. (1997) *Comparison of speech recognition abilities of children with cochlear implants enrolled in oral and total communication programs.* Paper presented at the meeting of the Fifth International Cochlear Implant Conference, New York, New York.

HODGES, A., RUTH, R., THOMAS, J.F., & BLINCOE, C.S. (1991). *Electrically evoked ABRs and ARs in cochlear implant users.* Paper presented at the meeting of the American Speech-Language-Hearing Association Convention, Atlanta, GA.

HOLDEN, L.K., SKINNER, M.W., & HOLDEN, T.A. (1997). Speech recognition with the MPEAK and SPEAK speech-coding strategies of the Nucleus Cochlear Implant. *Archives of Otolaryngology–Head and Neck Surgery, 116;*163–167.

KEMINK, J.L., ZIMMERMAN-PHILLIPS, S., KILENY, P.R., FIRSZT, J.B., & NOVAK, M.A. (1992). Auditory performance of children with cochlear ossification and partial implant insertion. *Laryngoscope, 102;*1001–1005.

KESSLER, D., & SCHINDLER, R. (1994). Progress with a multistrategy cochlear implant system: The Clarion. In: I.J. Hochmair, & E.S. Hochmair (Eds.), *Advances in cochlear implants* (pp. 354–362). Wien, Austria: Manz.

KILENY, P.R. (1991). Use of electrophysiologic measures in the management of children with cochlear implant: Brainstem, middle latency and cognitive (P300) responses. *The American Journal of Otology, 12;*37–42.

KIRK, K.I., PISONI, D.B., & OSBERGER, M.J. (1995). Lexical effects on spoken word recognition by pediatric cochlear implant users. *Ear and Hearing, 16;*470–481.

KIRK, K.I., SEHGAL, M., & MIYAMOTO, R.T. (1997). Speech perception performance of Nucleus multichannel cochlear implant users with partial electrode insertions. *Ear and Hearing, 6;*41–52.

KNOFF, H.M. (1983). Personality assessment in the schools: Issues and procedures for school psychologists. *School Psychology Review, 12;*391–398.

KNOFF, H.M. (1987). Assessing adolescent identity, self-concept and self-identity. In: R.G. Harrington (Ed.), *Testing adolescents: A reference guide for comprehensive psychological assessments* (pp. 51–81). St. Louis, MO: Westport Publishers.

LANE, H. (1992). *The mask of benevolence.* New York: Alfred A. Knopf.

LEAKE, P.A., HRADEK, G.T., & SNYDER, R.L. (1999). Chronic electrical stimulation by a cochlear implant promotes survival of spiral ganglion neurons after neonatal deafness. *Journal of Comparative Neurology, 12;* 543–562.

LESINSKI, A., HARTRAMPF, R., DAHM, M.C., BERTRAM, B., STRAUB-SCHEIR, A., & LENARZ, T. (1994). *Cochlear implantation in a population of multihandicapped children.* Presented at the International Cochlear Implant Speech and Hearing Symposium, Melbourne, Australia.

LING, D. (1986). Devices and procedures for auditory learning. *Volta Review, 88;*19–28.

LUTMAN, M., ARCHBOLD, S., GIBBIN, K., MCCORMICK, B., & O'DONOGHUE, G. (1994). Monitoring progress in young children with cochlear implants. In: D.J. Allum (Ed.), *Cochlear implant rehabilitation in children and adults* (pp. 31–51). London, England: Whurr.

MCKAY, C.M., & MCDERMOTT, H.J. (1991). Speech perception ability of adults with multiple-channel cochlear implants, using the spectral maxima sound processor. *Journal of Acoustical Society of America, 89*(suppl. 1);1959.

MISCHOOK, M., & COLE, E. (1986). Auditory learning and teaching of hearing-impaired infants. *Volta Review, 88;* 67–81.

MOOG, J., BIEDENSTEIN, J., DAVIDSON,L., & BRENNER, C. (1994). Instruction for developing speech perception skills. *Volta Review, 96*(5);61–74.

MOORES, D.F. (1987). *Educating the deaf: Psychology, principles and practices* (3rd ed.). Boston, MA: Houghton Mifflin.

MYRES, W., & KESSLER, K. (1992). Understanding the map. *NECCI News, 3;*1.

NEVINS, M.E., KRETSCHMER, R.E., CHUTE, P.E., HELLMAN, S.A., & PARISIER, S.C. (1991). The role of an educational consultant in a pediatric cochlear implant program. *Volta Review, 93;*197–204.

NEVINS, M.E., & CHUTE, P.M. (1996). *Children with cochlear implants in educational settings.* San Diego: Singular Publishing Group, Inc.

NIPARKO, J.K., CHANG, A.L., & GOODMAN, S.N. (1997). *Meta-Analysis of the pediatric cochlear implant literature.* Paper presented at the meeting of the Fifth International Cochlear Implant Conference, New York, New York.

NOVAK, M., FIRSZT, J.B., BROWN, C., & REEDER, R. (1990). *Cochlear implantation in severe cochlear deformities.* Paper presented at the meeting of the Second International Cochlear Implant Symposium, Iowa City, Iowa.

OSBERGER, M.J., CHUTE, P.M., POPE, M., KESSLER, K.S., CAROTTA, C.C., FIRSZT, J.B., & ZIMMERMAN-PHILLIPS, S. (1991). Pediatric cochlear implant candidacy issues. *American Journal of Otology, 12,*(suppl.);80–88.

OSBERGER, M.J., FISHER, L., & MURAD, C. (1997). Clinical results with the Clarion multi-strategy cochlear implant in children. *Proceedings from the Sixteenth World Congress of Otorhinolaryngology Head and Neck Surgery* (pp. 291–295). Sydney, Australia.

OSBERGER, M.J., MASO, M., SAM, L.K. (1993). Speech intelligibility of children with cochlear implants, tactile aids or hearing aids. *Journal of Speech and Hearing Research, 36;*186–203.

OSBERGER, M.J., ROBBINS, A.M., MIYAMOTO, R.T., BERRY, S.W., MYRES, W.A., KESSLER, K.S., & POPE, M.L. (1991). Speech perception abilities of children with cochlear implants, tactile aids or hearing aids. *American Journal of Otology, 12*(suppl 4);66–80.

PARISIER, S.C., & CHUTE, P.M. (1993). Mulitchannel implants in postmeningitic ossified cochleas. In: B. Fraysse, & O. Deguine (Eds.), *Cochlear implants: New perspectives* (pp. 49–58). Basel: Karger.

PARISIER, S.C., & CHUTE, P.M. (1994). *Speech production changes in children using multichannel cochlear implant.* Paper presented at the meeting of the European Symposium on Paediatric Cochlear Implants, Montpelier, France.

PATRICK, J.F., & CLARK, G.M. (1991). The Nucleus 22-channel cochlear implant system. *Ear and Hearing, 12*(suppl. 1);35–95.

PAUL, P., & QUIGLEY, S. (1984). Language and deafness. San Diego: College-Hill Press.

PFLASTER, G. (1980). A factor analysis of variables related to the academic performance of hearing-impaired children in regular classes. *Volta Review, 82;*71–84.

QUIGLEY, S.P., & KRETSCHMER, R.E. (1982). *The education of deaf children.* Baltimore, MD: University Park Press.

ROBBINS, A.M., & OSBERGER, M.J. (1991). *Meaningful use of speech scales.* Indianapolis, IN: University of Indiana School of Medicine.

ROBBINS, A.M., OSBERGER, M.J., MIYAMOTO, R., & KESSLER, K. (1994). Language development in young children with cochlear implants. *Advances in Otorhinolaryngology, 50;*160–166.

ROBBINS, A.M., RENSHAW, J.J., & BERRY, S.W. (1991). Evaluating meaningful auditory integration in profoundly hearing impaired children. *American Journal Otology, 12*(suppl.); 144–150.

ROBBINS, A.M., SVIRSKY, M., & KIRK, K.I. (1997). Children with implant can speak but can they communicate? *Archives of Otolaryngology–Head and Neck Surgery, 117;*155–160.

ROESER, R.J. (1989). Tactile aids: Development issues and current status. In: E. Ownes, & D.K. Kessler (Eds.), *Cochlear implant in young deaf children* (pp. 101–136). Boston, MA: College Hill.

ROSE, D.E., VERNON, M., & POOL, A. (1996). Cochlear implants in prelingually deaf children. *American Annals of the Deaf, 141;*258–261.

ROSS, M., BRACKETT, D., & MAXON, A. (1991). Assessment and management of mainstreamed hearing-impaired children. Austin, TX: Pro-Ed.

ROSS, R., & LERMAN, J. (1971). *Word intelligibility by picture identification.* Pittsburgh, PA: Stanwix House, Inc.

SCHOPMEYER, B., DOBAJ, H., & NIPARKO, J. (1997). *Emergence of spontaneous expressive vocabulary in children with cochlear implants.* Paper presented at the Fifth International Cochlear Implant Conference, New York, New York.

SCHOW, R.L., & NERBONNE, M.A. (1995). *Introduction to audiologic rehabilitation.* Old Tappan, NJ: Allyn & Bacon.

SHALLOP, J.K., GOIN, D.N., VAN DYKE, L., & MISCHKE, R.E. (1991). Prediction of behavioral threshold and comfort values for Nucleus 22-channel implant patients from electrical auditory brain stem response test results. *Annals of Otology, Rhinology and Layrngology, 100;*896–898.

SKINNER, M.W. (1994). *The borderline child.* Paper presented at the meeting of the Fifth Symposium on Cochlear Implants in Children, New York, New York.

SKINNER, M.W., CLARK, G.M., WHITFORD, L.A., et al. (1994). Evaluation of a new spectral peak coding strategy for the Nucleus 22 Channel Cochlear Implant System. *American Journal of Otology, 15*(2);15–27.

SKINNER, M.W., HOLDEN, L.K., HOLDEN, T.A., DOWELL, R.C., SELIGMAN, P.M., BRIMACOMBE, J.A., & BEITER, A.L. (1991). Performance of postlinguistically deaf adults with the Wearable Speech Processor (WSPIII) and Mini Speech Processor (MSP) of the Nucleus multi-electrode cochlear implant. *Ear and Hearing, 12;*3–22.

SPIVAK, L.G., & CHUTE, P.M. (1994). The relationship between electrical acoustic reflex thresholds and behavioral comfort levels in children and adult cochlar implant patients. *Ear and Hearing, 15;*184–192.

STALLER, S.J., BEITER, A.L., BRIMACOMBE, J.A., MECKLENBURG, D.J., & ARNDT, P. (1991). Pediatric performance with the Nucleus 22-channel cochlear implant system. *American Journal of Otology, 12*(suppl.);126–136.

STALLER, S.J., ZWOLAN, T.A., & ARNDT, P.L. (1998). *Clinical trial of the Nucleus 24 cochlear implant system.* Paper presented at the meeting of the American Academy of Audiology, Los Angeles, CA.

SUMMERFIELD, A.Q., & MARSHALL, D. (1995). Cochlear implantation: demand costs and utility. *Annals of Otology, Rhinology, and Laryngology, 104,9*(suppl. 166);245–248.

SUMMERFIELD, A.Q., MARSHALL, D.H., & ARCHBOLD, S. (1997). Cost-effectiveness consideration in pediatric cochlear implantation. *American Journal of Otology, 18;*166–168.

SVIRSKY, M. (1997). *Intelligibility of prelingually deaf children with cochlear implants and with hearing aids.* Paper presented at the Fifth International Cochlear Implant Conference, New York, New York.

TOBEY, E.A. (1993). Speech production. In: E.S. Tyle (Ed.), *Cochlear implants: Audiological foundations* (pp. 257–316). San Diego, CA: Singular Publishing.

TOBEY, E.A., GEERS, A.E., & BRENNER, C. (1994). Speech production results: Speech feature acquisition. *Volta Review, 96;* 109–129.

TOBEY, E.A., & HASENSTAB, S. (1991). Effects of Nucleus multichannel cochlear implant upon speech production in children. *Ear and Hearing, 12;* 48–54.

TOBEY, E.A., ANGELETTE, S., MURCHISON, C., NICOSIA, J., SPRAGUE, S., STALLER, S.J., BRIMACOMBE, J.A., & BEITER, A.L. (1991). Speech production performance in children with multichannel cochlear implants. *American Journal of Otology. 12;* 165–173.

TAIT, M. (1993). Video analysis: A method of assessing changes in preverbal and early linguistic communication after cochlear implantation. *Ear and Hearing, 14;*378–389.

TYE-MURRAY, N., SPENCER, L., WITT, S., & GILBERT-BEDIA, E. (1994). Parent and patient centered aural rehabilitation. In: D.J. Allum (Ed.), *Cochlear implant rehabilitation in children and adults* (pp. 65–82). London: Whurr.

TYE-MURRAY, N., SPENCER, L., WITT, S., & BEDIA, E. (1996) Parent and patient centred aural rehabilitation. In: D.J. Allum (Ed.), *Cochlear implant rehabilitation in children and adults* (pp. 65–82). London: Whurr.

TYLER, R. (1993). *Cochlear implants: Audiological foundations.* San Diego: Singular Publishing Group, Inc.

TYLER, R., FRYAUF-BERTSCHY, H., KELSAY, D.M., GANTZ, B.J., WOODWORTH, G.P., & PARKINSON, A. (1997). Speech perception by prelingually deaf children using cochlear implants. *Archives of Otorynoglogy–Head Neck Surgery, 117;*180–187.

TYLER, R., TOMBLIN, J.B., SPENCER, L., KELSAY, D., & FRYAUF-BERTSCHY, H. (1997). *How speech perception through a cochlear implant affects language and education.* Paper presented at the Fifth International Cochlear Implant Conference, New York, New York.

WALTZMAN, S.B., COHEN, N.L., SHAPIRO, W.H. (1986). Long-term effects of multichannel cochlear implant usage. *Laryngoscope, 6;*1083–1087.

ZIERHOFER, C.M., HOCHMAIR-DESOYER, I.J., & HOCHMAIR, E.S. (1995). Electronic design of a cochlear implant for multi-channel high-rate pulsatile stimulation strategies. *IEEE Transactions in Rehabilitation Engineering, 3;*112–116.

ZILBERMAN, Y., & SANTOGROSSI, T. (1995). Back telemetry in the cochlear implant prosthesis. *Annals of Otology, Rhinology and Laryngology, 104*(suppl. 166);146–147.

ZWOLAN, T.A., ZIMMERMAN-PHILLIPS, S., ASHBAUGH, C.J., HIEBER, S.J., KILENY, P.R., & TELIAN, S.A. (1997). Cochlear implantation of children with minimal open-set speech recognition skills. *Ear and Hearing, 18;*240–244.

PREFERRED PRACTICE GUIDELINES

For centers involved with, or contemplating involvement with, cochlear implants, "preferred practice guidelines" outlined by the American Speech-Language and Hearing Association emphasize the role of the audiologist.

Professionals Who Perform the Procedures

▼ Audiologists

Expected Outcomes

▼ Assessment is conducted to determine the appropriateness, type, and configuration of sensory prosthetic devices (e.g., tactile aids, cochlear implants, and other implantable devices) other than conventional amplification (i.e., hearing aids or assistive listening systems/devices).

Clinical Indications

▼ Individuals of all ages are assessed on the basis of audiological or hearing aid assessments.

▼ Assessment is recommended when patient/clients do not demonstrate benefit from conventional amplification.

Clinical Process

▼ Assessment includes additional trials or training with conventional amplification to determine benefit, assessment of before and after device performance on speech and nonspeech tasks, assessment of speechreading performance with and without the sensory device, administration of communication inventories, and counseling.9000000

▼ Assessment includes repeated testing with electrical and acoustic stimuli for cochlear implants and with vibrotactile and acoustic stimuli for tactile aids.

▼ Audiolgists may perform sensory aids assessment in conjunction with speech-language pathologists.

Documentation

▼ Documentation containing pertinent background information, assessment results, prognosis, and specific recommendations. Recommendations may address the need for further assessment, follow-up, or referral. When treatment is recommended, information is provided concerning the frequency, estimated duration, and type of service required.

▼ Documentation includes a record of compliance with state and federal guidelines/laws/regulations for hearing aids (ASHA, 1997).

Chapter 17

Cochlear Implants in Adults

Susan B. Waltzman and William H. Shapiro

Outline

Cochlear implants have developed into an accepted treatment for severe-to-profound deafness in those patients who derive minimal benefit from conventional amplification. The implants consist of an internally implanted electrode array and a receiver/stimulator. The external portion of the device consists of a microphone, speech processor and transmitter coil. Although a hearing aid amplifies incoming sound, a cochlear implant replaces the function of the damaged hair cells by converting mechanical energy into electrical pulses that enervate the remaining fibers of the eighth nerve. The microphone changes incoming sound into electrical signals that are shaped and amplified by the processor. The signal is then transmitted to the coil and transferred to the internal receiver/stimulator through a transcutaneous system. The electrodes are then stimulated in a manner that is determined by the processing strategy available in a particular prosthesis. Despite the fact that the basic structure of cochlear implants has remained relatively stable over a 30-year development period, significant changes and modifications have been made to both the design and information transfer schemes. The devices had either single or multiple electrodes and channels, and the electrode array could either be placed intracochlear or extracochlear. The processing schemes vary according to several factors, including analog versus pulsatile stimulation, simultaneous or sequential stimulation, and the pattern of speech representation and conversion. In addition to the evolution of the prostheses themselves, criteria for candidacy of hearing-impaired adults has also changed over the years. The history and nature of cochlear implants in adults has been well documented in previous publications. The intent of this chapter is to describe the current main variables and available devices and their effect on speech perception and production in adults with cochlear implants.

DEVICES

In the United States three multichannel devices are currently approved by the Food and Drug Administration (FDA) for use in adults: The Clarion, manufactured by Advanced Bionics, was approved for use in adults in 1995, the Nucleus 22 was approved by the FDA in 1985, and the newer Nucleus 24 was approved in 1998. The Clarion is a multistrategy cochlear implant that incorporates two distinct signal processing techniques: continuous interleaved sampling (CIS) strategy and simultaneous analog system (SAS). CIS uses a nonsimultaneous pulsatile pattern in which the stimuli, although interleaved, are not overlapping and can be delivered at very rapid rates and sequentially to minimize electrode interaction while maximizing data transmission (Wilson et al, 1990). The second available processing scheme in the Clarion device, SAS, is an analog system in which the signals are transferred simultaneously to electrodes with a bipolar configuration (Figs. 17–1 through 17–3).

When the Nucleus 22 device was initially introduced, it used a speech feature encoding strategy in which fundamental and formant frequency information was conveyed. Initially, F0F2 and then F0F1F2 information was extracted from the incoming speech signal and transmitted to the electrodes with pulsatile, nonsimultaneous bipolar stimulation. In 1990 the Multi Peak (MPEAK) strategy was introduced in which a filter bank circuit was added to the existing speech feature coding allowing three electrodes to be dedicated to high-frequency bands ranging from 2000 Hz to 6000 Hz. In 1994 the spectral peak coding strategy (SPEAK) superseded MPEAK. With SPEAK, 20 bandpass filters with center frequencies between 250 Hz and 10,000 Hz were the basis for coding. Six electrodes are selected and stimulated on the basis of the highest spectral peaks of the incoming stimulus. In addition, the rate at which the electrodes could be stimulated was both faster and more variable than with previous strategies. In 1996 the Nucleus 24 device was unveiled. For the first time, the CI24M incorporated modifications to the internal electronics package to accommodate newer processing strategies. The device implements three encoding modes: SPEAK, CIS, and ACE (advanced combined encoders). The ACE strategy incorporates elements of both the SPEAK and CIS coding

537

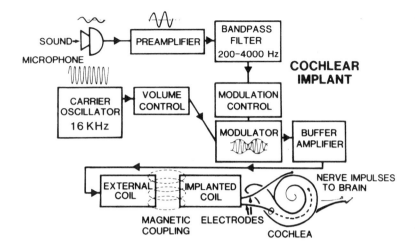

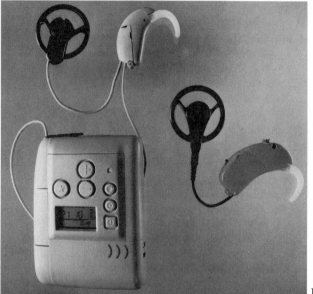

Figure 17–1 Schematic of a cochlear implant.

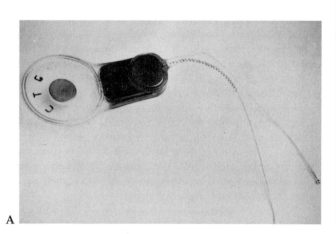

Figure 17–2 **(A)** Nucleus 24 internal receiver/stimulator and electrode array. **(B)** Nucleus 24 external system.

schemes by assigning electrodes on the basis of the stimulus and allowing for more variable and rapid stimulation to increase efficient transmission of timing cues.

The Med El Combi 40+ multichannel cochlear prosthesis, although not approved, is undergoing FDA-sponsored clinical trials. The implant offers the choice of two strategies: the CIS and an implementation of the number of maxima (n of m) coding system, which is the basis of the above-described SPEAK strategy (Fig. 17–4).

CRITERIA FOR IMPLANTATION

The criteria for implantation of adults has changed substantially since adults began receiving cochlear implants as a treatment for deafness. Initially, in the late 1970s and early to mid-1980s, the clinical trials required that only adults who were postlingually bilaterally profoundly deafened and received no benefit from appropriate hearing aids would be candidates for implantation. "No benefit from amplification" was most often defined as a score of 0% on monosyllabic words in the best aided condition. Several factors contributed to the relatively conservative criteria for implantation. First, too few published data were available that could confirm substantial benefit with an implant. Basically, nobody knew what was either realistic in terms of expectations or what the upper limits of the expectations could be. It was wise, then, to begin by implanting those individuals who would be most likely to gain; that is, adults who heard before and whose onset of deafness occurred after the development of speech and language. Second, to ensure that no loss of functional hearing was occurring, only those adults who had no measurable benefit from a hearing aid were deemed to be candidates. As the numbers of patients increased, along with more advanced speech processing strategies, the level of auditory-only speech perception that was being reported in adults was

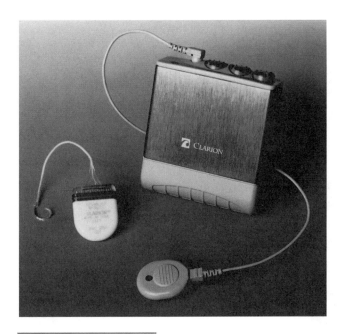

Figure 17–3 Clarion S-Series speech processor and enhanced bipolar electrode array.

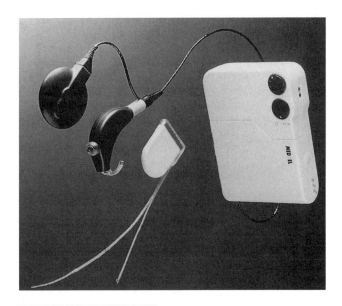

Figure 17–4 Med El Combi 40+ cochlear implant system.

quite good and exceeded expectations. This led to expanding the criteria for implantation in adults with some residual hearing and/or preoperative speech perception skills and prelingual or congenital deafness.

As previously mentioned, three devices are FDA approved for implantation in adults 18 years of age and older. The Clarion device, manufactured by Advanced Bionics, was approved in 1996 for implantation of postlingually deafened adults. Candidates are required to have bilateral profound deafness and minimum benefit from hearing aids as defined as a score of 20% or less on the CID sentence test. In 1997 the Clarion began clinical trials in the severely-to-profoundly hearing-impaired adult population. The adults in this group could

display borderline benefit from appropriate amplification as defined by a score of 40% or less on the Hearing in Noise Test (HINT) and a score of 20% or less on the CNC word test in the ear to be implanted and 30% or less in the nonimplant ear.

The Nucleus 22 implant was FDA approved for use in postlingually deafened adults in 1985, for severely hearing impaired adults in 1995, and for prelinguistically- and peri-linguistically deafened adults in 1995. Candidates are not permitted to have more than 30% speech recognition with appropriate hearing aids. In 1998 the newer Nucleus 24 device was approved for use in postlingually, perilinguistically, and prelinguistically deafened adults who obtain limited-to-no benefit from appropriate amplification. Lack of benefit from hearing aids is defined as a score of 40% or less on open-set sentence tests. Please remember that although this chapter is addressing the adult population, these devices are approved for children as well.

The Med El Combi 40+ is currently undergoing FDA clinical trials in adults in the United States. The major criteria for implantation include a postlinguistic bilateral profound sensorineural hearing loss and no significant benefit from conventional amplification as defined by an auditory-only score of no more than 20% on HINT sentences. In addition, they require that the candidates have an onset of deafness of age 6 years or more in the ear to be implanted.

It is important to point out that once a device receives post-market approval (PMA) from the FDA, the indications for use often serve only as guidelines, and individual practitioners frequently implant people outside of the recommended criteria.

New developments in hearing aid technology for the severe-to-profound hearing loss are currently in research trials. Although it is difficult to predict the effect these new hearing aids will have on potential implant candidates, at this time it is hard to envision a hearing aid producing equivalent levels of speech understanding and sound quality in the population that qualifies for a cochlear implant.

ASSESSMENT

The preoperative assessment determines whether the patient is both medically and audiologically appropriate for implantation and, if so, assists in the choice of ear to be implanted. Furthermore, the preoperative results serve as a baseline to which postoperative performance is compared; therefore the postoperative audiological assessment is virtually identical to the preoperative test battery.

The medical evaluation includes a physical examination and clearance for surgery and radiological studies. The cause of the hearing loss is determined and treatment options are discussed based on the results. Computed tomography (CT) scans and/or magnetic resonance imaging are a routine part of the preoperative assessment. The results are used to view anatomical abnormalities that might affect ear choice and to determine whether modifications to the surgical technique are necessary to ensure proper placement of the electrode array. Intraoperatively, a plain film is advisable to confirm proper placement of the internal device. Postoperatively, if a change is noted in the performance of the implant recipient, radiological studies are sometimes needed to determine whether electrode migration or damage has occurred. Under

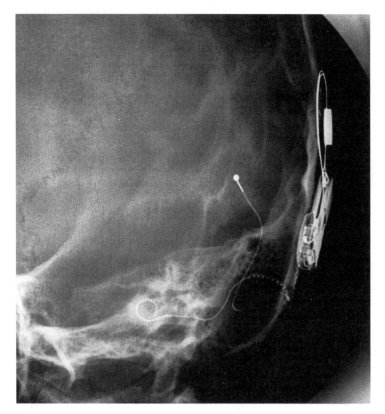

Figure 17–5 Stenvers view of Nucleus 24 taken at time of surgery.

these conditions, preoperative and intraoperative radiological studies are particularly helpful for comparison purposes (Fig. 17–5).

PEARL

All else being equal, vestibular function testing can sometimes be helpful in choosing the ear to be implanted or predicting short-term postoperative dizziness.

The audiological test battery is designed to determine the type and degree of hearing loss and the speech perception capabilities of the person unaided, aided (preoperatively), and with the implant postoperatively. Audiological testing includes unaided and aided pure tone air and bone thresholds, speech reception thresholds, and speech discrimination scores where possible. These measurements should be obtained both under earphones and in the sound field, preoperatively and postoperatively. Impedance measurements, otoacoustic emissions, and electrophysiological testing are often used to further confirm the extent of the hearing loss and provide additional diagnostic information. On occasion, the person may present with inappropriate amplification because of an increase in the degree of hearing loss and the use of outdated technology. This requires prescribing new hearing aids (usually on loan) before administration of the test battery to determine implant candidacy.

The measurement of speech perception and the acoustic cues that determine the level of recognition is central to the

---

PEARL

Preoperative promontory stimulation can be helpful in determining whether an ear responds to electrical stimulation.

---

preoperative and postoperative assessments. Preoperatively, the information is used to determine whether the individual fulfils the predetermined guidelines for implantation; that is, would this person be likely to perform better with an implant than with a hearing aid(s)? The results also serve as a baseline to which postoperative results are compared to determine device efficacy. Postoperatively, speech perception measures not only provide data on absolute performance but also assist in determining the signal processing scheme most beneficial to the person, the setting of the best "program" within a given strategy, and the perceptual areas most in need of auditory rehabilitation. It is important to note that over time and with listening experience, significant changes occur in the auditory percepts defined by the implant. Although one expects to see increases in auditory recognition with increased length of implant use, a decrease in perceptual skills could indicate the need for adjustments, and so forth.

Speech recognition depends on the ability to integrate a variety of acoustic cues, which are dynamic in nature, including frequency and time/intensity information. As an example, vowel identification is predicated on the presence of the first three formant frequencies, yet the same formant frequencies can allow for the recognition of several various speech sounds because the range of frequencies necessary for the identification of one vowel overlaps the range necessary for the determination of several other vowels (Denes & Pinson, 1963). The same applies to the identification of consonants: recognition depends on a variety of cues. For example, fricative sounds are distinguished from other consonants by virtue of the turbulent sound that is produced, but sounds within that category are distinguished from one another by virtue of intensity and spectral cues. The "s" and "sh" sounds can be differentiated from other fricative sounds such as "f" or "v" by the fact that they are more intense, but they can be differentiated from one another because of the difference in spectral composition: most of the energy of the "s" sound is in the area of 4000 Hz, whereas the concentration of energy for the "sh" sound is in the vicinity of 2000 to 3000 Hz (Denes & Pinson, 1963; Dorman, 1993). Although the importance of these varying acoustic cues is undeniable, the identification of speech is accomplished by incorporating the acoustic cues with the linguistic cues attached to a given language. It is our knowledge of the language, semantics, and other nonlinguistic cues that assist us in recognizing speech and deciphering the message. This is true whether the hearing is through the normal auditory channels or a cochlear implant. The assessment of speech perception preimplantation and postimplantation is based on the concept of characterizing the ability of the individual to recognize speech at the phoneme, word, and sentence levels.

Before the onset of cochlear implants as a treatment for profound deafness, few standardized tests were available to assess all levels of speech perception preimplantation and postimplantation. In 1981 Owens et al developed the minimum auditory capabilities battery (MAC). The battery included tests that evaluate suprasegmental and segmental aspects of the speech signal in both closed and open-set configurations. Tests of prosodic characteristics included accent, noise/voice, and question/statement, in which the subject was not required to identify the stimulus but merely to address whether it was a noise or a human voice or a question or statement, and so on. Closed-set tests assessed vowel recognition and spondee identification. Open-set tests included NU-6 monosyllabic words and CID sentences presented in an auditory-only condition. The battery also included measures to assess speech reading and speech reading plus audition skills. In 1983 Tyler et al developed a battery that added certain features to the MAC battery. It added an assessment of speech in noise and, in 1986, became available on laser disc to eliminate speaker bias on the visual and audiovisual segments of the battery.

In 1984, Boothroyd proposed a different concept for the assessment of acoustic cues delivered by means of a cochlear implant. He was concerned that any stimulus that had linguistic content could potentially enhance the perception of acoustic cues being transmitted by the implant. He developed the Speech Pattern Contrast Test (SPAC), which concentrated on assessing the ability of the implant to transmit the prosodic and phonemic features of the speech signal. The SPAC subtests included the following: rise/fall, roving stress, initial consonant manner, final consonant manner, vowel place, vowel height, initial consonant place, final consonant place, and phoneme recognition. Although the battery appeared to provide useful speech feature information that was potentially beneficial for both adjusting an implant and providing useful data regarding the development of processing strategies

(Filson et al, 1992; Waltzman & Hochberg, 1990), the test was lengthy and cumbersome to administer and, therefore, not widely used clinically. The SPAC was part of a larger battery of 26 audiological tests that were used in a study to differentiate between cochlear implants (Cohen et al, 1993; Waltzman & Cohen, 1992). Analyzing the results from this study, Filson and colleagues showed that a shorter battery of tests could describe individual patient performance, document improvement over time, and distinguish between devices and subjects. This further discouraged widespread clinical use of the SPAC.

As devices became more technologically sophisticated and patient performance improved dramatically after implantation, the speech perception test battery was condensed to include only measures of open-set phoneme, word and sentence recognition presented in the auditory-only condition. Still patients exist, however, whose postoperative performance requires a lower level of data accumulation. Longterm deafened adults often obtain only minimal benefit from an implant or require an extended period of use to demonstrate open-set speech discrimination. In this situation it is important to use closed-set or speech reading plus audition ability to show communication benefit.

At present, the more common clinically used measures include a monosyllabic word test scored as both words and phonemes correct and a sentence recognition test (Table 17–1). The more frequently used monosyllabic tests include the NU-6 test (Tillman & Carhart, 1966) and the Consonant-Nucleus-Consonant (CNC) test (Peterson & Lehiste, 1962). Sentence recognition tests include the CID Everyday Sentence test (Silverman & Hirsh, 1955), the Bench-Kowal-Bamford (BKB) (Bench et al, 1979) sentence test, and the HINT (Nilsson et al, 1994). Both tests have versions that allow for presentation in quiet and noise. As cochlear implant use became increasingly widespread and additional processing strategies became available, further standardization of a clinical test battery became necessary to allow for data comparison across centers, patients, devices, and strategies. Luxford (in press) convened a group of professionals representing implant

TABLE 17–1 Commonly used adult speech perception tests

Phoneme level
Vowel confusion test
Consonant confusion test
Word recognition level
NU-6 monosyllabic word test
CNC test
Sentence recognition level
CID sentence test
BKB sentence test
HINT sentences in quiet and in noise

centers and manufacturers who drafted a Minimum Speech Test Battery for Adult Cochlear Implant Patients. The battery included CNC word lists and HINT sentences. It was designed not to exclude other tests but to ensure that all implant centers are, at the very least, administering a given monosyllabic word test and sentence test. The manufacturers split the cost of creating CD versions of the test and the discs were made available to implant centers nationwide.

Vowel and consonant confusion tests provide yet another avenue for assessing perception at the phonemic level (Tyler et al, 1986). They were designed to isolate the ability of the individual to obtain manner, place of articulation, and voicing information through the implant itself. Theoretically, one could adjust processor programs that might facilitate the auditory percept of these cues. Although often lengthy to administer, consonant confusion measures provide valuable information and are the tools of choice for those involved with signal processing development.

Standardization of stimuli presentation level has also been attempted. Although test stimuli were routinely presented at a level of 70 dB SPL, in 1997 Skinner et al recommended that the presentation level be reduced to 60 dB SPL to better simulate conversational speech. They believed that the higher presentation level artificially inflated the speech perception capabilities, preoperatively and postoperatively, of implant recipients. Although not yet in widespread use, the need to specify the level at which a test is administered was reinforced.

SPEECH PERCEPTION WITH COCHLEAR IMPLANTS

Because the 3M House single-channel implant provided little in the way of time/intensity and frequency information, open-set speech recognition was rarely achieved (Gantz et al, 1988). Performance with the Vienna single-channel implant, however, was more equivocal in that some patients implanted with the device were reported to have open-set speech understanding (Hochmair et al, 1985; Tyler et al, 1989). In 1984 clinical trials with the Nucleus multichannel cochlear prosthesis using an F0F2 processing strategy began in the United States. Shortly thereafter the first formant frequency was added to provide additional information. Concurrently, the Ineraid multichannel cochlear prosthesis with a percutaneous transmitter was available. Although wide variability existed in performance, all patients showed improvement in perception when audition was combined with lipreading and some patients had significant amounts of closed-set and open-set speech discrimination with both devices (Cohen et al, 1985; Dorman et al, 1989; Dowell et al, 1986; Gantz et al, 1987, 1988). Open-set word and sentence recognition scores for these multichannel devices ranged from 0 to 100%.

PITFALL

Postimplantation sound field audiometric results are not necessarily indicative of speech understanding.

In 1986 in an attempt to clarify issues surrounding multichannel versus single-channel use and the possible differences between devices, a prospective randomized cooperative study was funded by the Department of Veterans Affairs. The study was designed to compare the efficacy of the three devices, which at the time had been shown to produce a range of open-set speech discrimination in adults. Eighty-two patients were randomly assigned to receive one of three cochlear implants: the Ineraid or Nucleus multichannel devices or the Vienna single-channel implant. Results showed a significant difference between the single-channel and multichannel devices: 60% of the patients who were randomized to either the Ineraid or Nucleus multichannel systems had varying degrees of open-set word and sentence recognition, whereas none of the single-channel users had any significant amount of open-set discrimination. When the study was initiated, the encoding scheme used in the Nucleus device was F0F1F2.

During the course of the study, the MPEAK strategy was implemented and incorporated into the study design. The results obtained with the Nucleus F0F1F2 and Ineraid devices were not significantly different from one another; however, when the Nucleus patients switched from the F0F1F2 strategy to the MPEAK strategy, they exhibited considerable improvement in performance. The mean open-set word recognition score increased from 15 to 25% and the mean open-set sentence score improved from 32 to 58%, scores that were significantly better than those obtained with the Ineraid device (Cohen et al, 1993; Waltzman et al, 1992). Similar results were reported by Skinner et al in 1991 when patients were switched from the F0F1F2 strategy to MPEAK.

In 1994, a filter bank encoding strategy, SPEAK, replaced MPEAK. Although the processor continued to extract formant information, information from three high-frequency bands were relayed to three fixed basal electrodes. In 1994, Clark reported on a series of 65 adults who were MPEAK users and switched to the SPEAK strategy. Mean percent correct scores showed an improvement in open-set word and sentence recognition, particularly when the stimuli were delivered in noise. Skinner et al (1994) conducted a multicenter study of subjects who obtained open-set speech recognition by use of the MPEAK strategy and were switched to SPEAK. Results were similar to those obtained by Clark in that the greatest improvement was noted for speech-in-noise conditions. Six-month data for 72 adult subjects who participated in the U.S. clinical trials for the SPEAK showed a mean percent correct score of 35% (median = 36%) for CNC words and a mean percent correct score of 78% (median = 88%) for CID sentences in quiet. Thirty-six of the patients met the criteria for testing in noise and achieved an average score of 44% (median = 35%) when CID sentences were presented in noise. In 1997 Cohen and colleagues, in an extension of the Veterans Affairs Cooperative Study, upgraded 21 of the original participants who had randomized to the Nucleus device from MPEAK to SPEAK. Closed-set and open-set phoneme, word, and sentence recognition were assessed in quiet and in noise in an audition-only condition. After three months of SPEAK use, statistically significant improvements in mean percent correct scores were found on all tests administered, but improvements were greatest in the speech-in-noise conditions. Average scores on the NU-6 word test increased from 14 to 22%, and the BKB sentence score in quiet improved from 38 to 46%. In the +15 and +10 signal-to-noise conditions the mean percent correct scores rose from 22 to 42% and 16 to 32%, respectively. Interestingly, however, subjects who had no open-set speech understanding with MPEAK did not improve after the switch to SPEAK.

A slightly different implementation of the SPEAK strategy was introduced in 1996 in the Nucleus CI24M cochlear prosthesis, and a study was initiated to compare the short-term (3 to 6 months) development of open-set speech recognition between the two versions. Results showed that both groups of users had significant open-set phoneme, word, and sentence recognition after short-term use. Although better absolute scores were obtained for users of the N24 device, a multivariate analysis revealed no significant difference between the two groups when the younger age at time of implantation and shorter length of deafness of the N24 subjects were taken into account (Waltzman et al, in press). Although the N24 is capable of delivering CIS and ACE processing in addition to SPEAK, comparative studies are currently ongoing and data have not yet become available.

The Clarion cochlear implant began clinical trials in the United States in 1994. The currently available device offers a choice of two signal processing strategies: CIS and SAS. Kessler (personal communication, 1997) reported a mean percent correct CID sentence score of 75%, with a median of 87% after 6 months use for 44 adult patients who received the Clarion 1.2 device as part of the FDA clinical trials; the NU-6 word score was 41% with a median of 44%. The MEDEL multichannel cochlear prosthesis is currently undergoing clinical trials in the United States and data are not yet published. Dorman (in press), however, reported an average score of 48% (median = 50%) on monosyllabic word recognition tests administered on patients implanted with the MEDEL device in Europe.

Comparisons between devices on the basis of data collected across institutions, however, remains problematic. Different patient selection criteria, test measures, methodology and data analysis make analogies extremely difficult. However, one recurrent theme occurs: most adult cochlear implant patients do extremely well with cochlear implants. In fact, as Dorman correctly pointed out, more than half of the adults score between 80 and 100% on open-set sentence recognition tests, enabling them to communicate well in a variety of situations including telephone use (Cohen et al, 1989). Although these results are very impressive, there still remains a large segment of the population who does not derive substantial benefit from implantation: the factors that might account for the variable performance need to be explored.

FACTORS AFFECTING PERFORMANCE

Despite the numerous advances in cochlear implant technology, one circumstance has remained constant: the variability of performance within and between devices. Open-set

perception scores continue to range between 0 and 100%, although, as technology has improved, the number of patients achieving higher end scores has most certainly increased over time. What are some of the variables that might account for this heterogeneity?

Surviving Neural Population

Undoubtedly, the number and place of surviving ganglion cells and how they are clustered plays a significant role in outcome. Despite the pervasive logic of this assertion, a preliminary histopathological account of temporal bones from four Nucleus multichannel cochlear implant users provided conflicting reports. In 1997 Linthicum and Otto reported that the subject with the second lowest cell count had the highest performance score, whereas the person with the highest cell count had the poorest score. However, complicating issues were present: the patient with the most remaining fibers had the shortest electrode array insertion. Morphological studies are continuing that will hopefully provide meaningful correlations between neural element survival and performance. Clinically, the capability of guesstimating cell survival has been elusive. It is conceivable that the development of neural response telemetry, the use of auditory evoked potentials as a method for assessing neural integrity, as a feature in commercially available implants will ultimately allow the clinician to obtain this information. (Neural response telemetry allows for the measurement of the whole nerve action potential. The response is characterized by a negative peak followed by a positive peak, the amplitude of which is depends on the stimulus level.)

Length of Deafness and Age at Implantation

Numerous reports have shown that adults with congenital and/or prelingual deafness obtained no measurable open-set speech recognition after implantation (Brimacombe et al, 1989; Waltzman et al, 1992; Zwolan et al, 1996). These studies, however, reflected performance with older speech-processing strategies rather than currently available more technologically advanced coding schemes. More recently, Waltzman and Cohen (in press) found that prelingually and/or congenitally long-term deafened adults showed postoperative improvement in speech understanding when the CIS strategy was used.

Despite the promise of new technology, a study by Waltzman et al (in press) revealed that length of deafness continues to be a significant contributor to performance. Results showed that adult Nucleus 22 and Nucleus 24 users programmed with the SPEAK strategy had significant open-set speech understanding; however, the absolute scores obtained by the N24 patients were notably better. This apparently enhanced performance was negated when the younger age at time of implantation and the shorter length of deafness of the N24 group was taken into account. The length of deafness was the stronger of the correlations and age was a factor when coupled with length of deafness. These results confirmed the finding reported in earlier studies using older processing strategies that the longer the time of deafness and the older the age at time of implantation, the poorer the prognosis for development of auditory-only open-set speech recognition (Gantz et al, 1988; Kileny et al, 1991; Waltzman et al, 1995).

Preoperative Hearing and Speech Perception Levels

Most recent work on the effects of residual hearing on postoperative performance has been conducted on children who have received either Nucleus or Clarion cochlear implants. The results uniformly show that children with better preoperative hearing levels and/or speech perception skills appear to achieve higher levels of performance postoperatively (Cowan et al, 1997; Gantz et al, in press; Osberger & Fisher, 1997; Seghal et al, 1997). It stands to reason although remains to be seen whether the trend will hold true in the adult population. Undoubtedly, the criteria for implanting adults has expanded to include those individuals with greater amounts of preoperative hearing and word and sentence recognition abilities (Brimacombe et al, 1995).

Depth of Electrode Array Insertion

Several studies have been performed that have attempted to correlate the depth of insertion of a multichannel electrode array to postoperative performance. Studies by Blamey et al in 1992, Marsh et al in 1993, and Ketten (personal communication, 1997) have all shown a correlation between depth of insertion of the electrode array and open-set auditory only scores obtained on either CID sentences or monosyllabic words. Because the configuration of electrode arrays is dynamic, it is unknown what affect this variable will ultimately have on results.

Other Factors

Additional potential contributors to outcome include cause of deafness (although to date this has not been shown to be significant), frequency and effectiveness of programming, psychological factors, family support, and expectations. As time goes on, we will no doubt learn more about the level of contribution of all possible variables. It is most important to remember, however, that as technology evolves, the influence of the many variables on results will no doubt change and what may have considerable effect under the current scheme of things may be reduced to insignificance in the future.

PEARL

Psychological evaluations can be helpful if the stability of a prospective candidate is in question.

PITFALL

Unrealistic expectations on the part of the patient can lead to disappointment and nonuse of the implant. It is vital that the candidate and family understand the range of postoperative performance.

CONCLUSIONS

Cochlear implants in adults have come a long way in 30 years. They have evolved from single-channel devices providing little or no speech understanding to multichannel implants using advanced signal processing strategies. The hearing-impaired adult has truly benefitted from the cooperative efforts of researchers and clinicians who have collaborated on numerous investigative endeavors in all areas of cochlear implantation: the results have been remarkable. Adults who have either lost their hearing or never heard have been provided with varying degrees of hearing that has enabled them to communicate with family and friends, resume or begin education and professional careers, enjoy music and other forms of entertainment, and maintain more independent lifestyles. Gratifying as these results may be, the task is not complete. There still remains a segment of the hearing-impaired adult population that does not benefit from the current technology. Nor have we reached the maximum capability for existing and future implant users. The field is extremely dynamic and the future very promising.

REFERENCES

BENCH, J., KOWAL A., & BAMFORD, J. (1979). The BKB sentence lists for partially-hearing children. *British Journal of Audiology, 13;*108–112.

BLAMEY, P., PYMAN, B., & GORDON, M. (1992). Factors predicting postoperative sentence scores in postlingually deaf adult cochlear implant patients. *Annals of Otology, Rhinology, and Laryngology, 101;*342–348.

BOOTHROYD, A. (1984). Auditory perception of speech contrasts by subjects with sensorineural hearing loss. *Journal of Speech and Hearing Research, 27;*338–352.

BRIMACOMBE, J., ARNDT, P., STALLER, S., & MENAPACE, C. (1995). *Multichannel cochlear implants in adults with residual hearing.* Presented at the 100th NIH Consensus Development Conference, Washington, DC.

BRIMACOMBE, J., BEITER, A., & BARKER, M. (1989). *Cochlear implant results in pre/perilinguistically deafened adults.* Presented at the 92nd Annual Meeting of the American Academy of Otolaryngology–Head and Neck Surgery, Washington, DC.

CLARK, G. (1994). *Evaluation of a new spectral peak coding strategy (SPEAK) for the Nucleus 22 channel cochlear implant system.* Presented at the meeting of the American Otological Society, Palm Beach, FL.

COHEN, N., WALTZMAN, S., ROLAND, J., BROMBERG, B., CAMBRON, N., GIBBS, L., PARKINSON, W., & SNEAD, C. (1997). Results of speech processor upgrade in a population of Veterans Affairs cochlear implant recipients. *American Journal of Otology, 18;*462–465.

COHEN, N., WALTZMAN, S., & FISHER, S. (1993). A prospective, randomized study of cochlear implants. *New England Journal of Medicine, 328;*233–237.

COHEN, N., WALTZMAN, S., & SHAPIRO, W. (1985). Clinical trials with a 22-channel cochlear prosthesis. *Laryngoscope, 95;* 1448–1454.

COHEN, N., WALTZMAN, S., & SHAPIRO, W. (1989). Telephone speech comprehension with use of the Nucleus cochlear implant. *Annals of Otology, Rhinology, and Laryngology, 98;*8–11.

COWAN, R., DETTMAN, S., PEGG, P., & BARKER. E. (1997). *Preoperative residual hearing as an indicator of postoperative benefit from multichannel cochlear implants.* Paper presented at the Fifth International Cochlear Implant Conference, New York, NY.

DENES, P., & PINSON, E. (1963). Speech recognition. In: P. Denes, & E. Pinson (Eds.), *The speech chain* (pp. 124–146). Murray Hill, NJ: Bell Telephone Laboratories.

DORMAN, M., (1993). Speech perception in adults. In: R. Tyler (Ed.), *Cochlear implants* (pp. 145–190). San Diego: Singular Publishing Group, Inc.

DORMAN, M. (In press). Cochlear implants in adults. In: S. Waltzman, & N. Cohen (Eds.), *Cochlear implants.* New York: Thieme Medical Publishers, Inc.

DORMAN, M., HANNLEY, M., DANKOWSKI, K., SMITH, L., & McCANDLESS, G. (1989). Word recognition by 50 patients fitted with the Symbion multichannel cochlear implant. *Ear and Hearing, 10;*40–43.

DOWELL, R., MECKLENBURG, D., & CLARK, G. (1986). Speech recognition for 40 patients receiving multi-channel cochlear implants. *Acta Otolaryngologia, 12;*1054–1059.

FILSON, K., FISHER, S., WESTON, S., & SHAPIRO, W. (1992). Evaluation and adaptation of a cochlear implant test battery. *Seminars in Hearing, 13;*208–217.

GANTZ, B., McCABE, B., TYLER, R., & PREECE, J. (1987). Evaluation of four cochlear implant designs. *Annals of Otology, Rhinology, and Laryngology, 96;*145–147.

GANTZ, B., RUBENSTEIN, J., TYLER, R., TEAGLE, H., COHEN, N., WALTZMAN, S., MIYAMOTO, R., & KIRK, K. (In press). Long term results of cochlear implants in children with residual hearing. *Annals of Otology, Rhinology, and Laryngology.*

GANTZ, B., TYLER, R., KNUTSON, J., WOODWORTH, G., ABBAS, P., McCABE, B., HINRICHS, J., TYE-MURRAY, N., LANSING, C., KUK, F., & BROWN, C. (1988). Evaluation of five different cochlear implant designs: Audiologic assessment and prediction of performance. *Laryngoscope, 98;*1100–1106.

HOCHMAIR, E., HOCHMAIR-DESOYER, I. (1985). Aspects of sound signal processing using the Vienna intra- and extracochlear implants. In: R. Schindler, & M. Merzenich (Eds.), *Cochlear implants* (pp. 101–110). New York: Raven Press.

KILENY, P., ZIMMERMAN-PHILLIPS, S., KEMINK, J., & SCHMALTZ, S. (1991). Effects of preoperative electrical stimulability and historical factors on performance with multichannel cochlear implants. *Annals of Otology, Rhinology and Laryngology, 100;*563–568.

LINTHICUM, F., & OTTO, S. (1997). *Functional histopathology of four 22-electrode cochlear implant temporal bones.* Presented at the Association for Research in Otolaryngology, St. Petersburg Beach, FL.

MARSH, M., XU, J., BLAMEY, P., WHITFORD, L., XU, S., SILVERMAN, J., & CLARK, G. (1993). Radiologic evaluation of multichannel intracochlear implant insertion depth. *American Journal of Otology, 14;*386–391.

NILSSON, M., SOLI, S., & SULLIVAN, J. (1994). Development of the Hearing in Noise Test for the measurement of speech reception thresholds in quiet and in noise. *Journal of the Acoustical Society of America, 95;*1085–1099.

OSBERGER, M., & FISHER, L. (1997). *Relationship between pre- and post-implant speech perception skills in pediatric Clarion patients.* Presented at the Fifth International Cochlear Implant Conference, New York, NY.

OWENS, E., KESSLER, D., & SCHUBERT, E. (1981). The minimum auditory capabilities (MAC) battery. *Hearing Aid Journal, 34;*9–34.

PETERSON, G., & LEHISTE, I. (1962). Revised CNC lists for auditory tests. *Journal of Speech and Hearing Disorders, 27;*62–70.

SEGHAL, S., KIRK, K., PISONI, D., & MIYAMOTO, R. (1997). *Effect of residual hearing on children's speech perception abilities with a cochlear implant.* Presented at the Fifth International Cochlear Implant Conference, New York, NY.

SILVERMAN, S., & HIRSH, I. (1955). Problems related to the use of speech in clinical audiometry. *Annals of Otology, Rhinology, and Laryngology, 64;*44–53.

SKINNER, M., CLARK, G., WHITFORD, L., et al. (1994). Evaluation of a new spectral peak coding strategy for the Nucleus 22 channel cochlear implant system. *American Journal of Otology, 15;*15–27.

SKINNER, M., HOLDEN, L., HOLDEN, T., Demorest, M., & Fourakis, M. (1997). Speech recognition at simulated soft, conversational and raised-to-loud vocal efforts by adults with cochlear implants. *Journal of the Acoustical Society of America, 101;*3766–3782.

SKINNER, M., HOLDEN, L., HOLDEN, T., DOWELL, R., SELIGMAN, P., BRIMACOMBE, J., & BEITER, A. (1991). Performance of postlingually deaf adults with the wearable speech processor (WSP III) and mini speech processor (MSP) of the Nucleus multi-channel cochlear implant. *Ear and Hearing, 12;*3–22.

TILLMAN, T., & CARHART, R. (1966). *An expanded test for speech discrimination utilizing CNC monosyllabic words.* Northwestern University Auditory Test No. 6 (USAF School of Aerospace Medicine Technical Report). Brooks Air Force Base, TX.

TYLER, R., MOORE, B., & KUK, F. (1989). Performance of some of the better cochlear implant patients. *Journal of Speech and Hearing Research, 32;*887–911.

TYLER, R., PREECE, J., & LOWDER, M. (1983). *Iowa cochlear implant tests.* Iowa City, IA: The University of Iowa.

TYLER, R., PREECE, J., & TYE-MURRAY, N. (1986). *The Iowa phoneme and sentence tests* (laser videodisc). Iowa City, IA: Department of Otolaryngology–Head and Neck Surgery (University of Iowa).

WALTZMAN, S., & COHEN, N. (In press). Implantation of patients with prelingual long term deafness. *Annals of Otology, Rhinology, and Laryngology.*

WALTZMAN, S., COHEN, N., FISHER, S. (1992). An experimental comparison of cochlear implant systems. *Seminars in Hearing, 13;*195–207.

WALTZMAN, S., COHEN, N., & ROLAND, J. (In press). A comparison of the growth of open set speech perception between the Nucleus 22 and Nucleus 24 cochlear implant systems. *American Journal of Otology.*

WALTZMAN, S., COHEN, N., & SHAPIRO, W. (1992). Use of a multichannel cochlear implant in the congenitally and prelingually deaf population. *Laryngoscope, 102;*395–399.

Waltzman, S., Fisher, S., Niparko, J., & Cohen, N. (1995). Predictors of postoperative performance with cochlear implants. *Annals of Otology, Rhinology, and Laryngology, 104*;15–18.

Waltzman, S., & Hochberg, I. (1990). Perception of speech pattern contrasts using a multichannel cochlear implant. *Ear and Hearing, 11*;50–55.

Wilson, B., Lawson, D., & Finley, C. (1990). *Speech processors for auditory prostheses.* Fourth Quarterly Progress Report on NIH Project N01-DC-9-2401: 4–24.

Zwolan, T., Kileny, P., & Telian, S. (1996). Self-report of cochlear implant use and satisfaction by prelingually deafened adults. *Ear and Hearing, 17*;199–210.

Chapter 18

Audiological Rehabilitation Intervention Services for Adults with Acquired Hearing Impairment

Jean-Pierre Gagné and Mary Beth Jennings

Outline

Audiological rehabilitation has been recognized as a domain of audiology ever since the emergence of audiology as an allied health discipline. Since its beginnings, the importance

of audiological rehabilitation services within the discipline of audiology and the types of services provided by rehabilitative audiologists and the service delivery models used to organize and define the scope of practice in rehabilitative audiology have been in constant evolution. At present, the scope of practice in rehabilitative audiology and the panoply of services provided by rehabilitative audiologists are more diversified than they have been at any time in the past. In recent years, conceptual models of rehabilitation have been developed and proposed. Those models have served to (re)define the goals of audiological rehabilitation and to organize the manner in which rehabilitative services are provided to patients.

This chapter focuses on audiological rehabilitative services for adults and elderly persons with acquired hearing loss. The intervention activities available and most frequently provided to this population are described. Then a conceptual framework of audiological rehabilitation is proposed. The framework serves to (re)define the goals and the organization of rehabilitation services and to place the various intervention strategies within a context of a comprehensive intervention program. The application of the framework to one specific model of intervention, defined as a solution-centered problem-solving intervention process, is presented. A case presentation that illustrates the application of this model of intervention is provided.

OVERVIEW OF AUDIOLOGICAL REHABILITATION

The Origins and Development of Audiological Rehabilitation Services

It is widely recognized that the field of audiological rehabilitation for persons with acquired hearing impairment emerged as a formal professional discipline after World War II. Army and Navy Veteran Administration (VA) services developed extensive rehabilitative programs for military personnel who had acquired hearing loss during the war. Intensive audiological rehabilitation services, provided over a period of several weeks, included hearing aid fitting, hearing aid orientation, information counseling, auditory and speech-reading training (provided individually or in groups), speech correction, and, when required, occupational and vocational

Audiology: Treatment. Edited by Valente, Hosford-Dunn, and Roeser. Thieme Medical Publishers, Inc., New York © 2000

training (Ross, 1987, 1997). Despite the reported success of those programs, audiological rehabilitation services failed to expand in a significant way beyond the VA settings. This is primarily because during the same period, major breakthroughs occurred in hearing measurement techniques and diagnostic audiology. The market economy and career opportunities encouraged many professionals (and professional training programs) to specialize in the area of medical (diagnostic) audiology rather than in rehabilitative services. Also, provisions in the professional Code of Ethics prevented audiologists from dispensing hearing aids (with the exception of audiologists employed by the VA services). This constituted a major obstacle to professionals interested in audiological rehabilitation because it excluded them from being directly involved in the provision of an important component of rehabilitation services designed for persons with hearing impairment (Schow & Nerbonne, 1982). Over the years, the high cost of providing comprehensive audiological rehabilitative services (particularly compared with diagnostic services) combined with the inability of audiologists to bill third parties (e.g., insurance companies) for the rehabilitation services they provide and the lack of experimental data to demonstrate the effectiveness of rehabilitation services, contributed to a general decline in interest in audiological rehabilitation.

Services Related to Amplification and other Technological Devices

At present, few public institutions offer comprehensive audiological rehabilitation services. Where they are available, audiological rehabilitation services are often limited to activities related to the recommendation of hearing aids and post-hearing-aid-fitting evaluation. In some settings hearing aid orientation services are provided to individuals who acquire those devices (see Chapter 14 in this volume).

Technological advances in the field of electronics in the mid-1960s (i.e., the miniaturization of electronic components used in hearing aids and the development of aids with flexible electroacoustic characteristics) and the development of programmable and digital hearing aids in the 1980s made it possible to design hearing aids that allowed customized adjustments of the devices provided to people with hearing loss. The expertise of audiologists was sought to select appropriate models and types of hearing aids and to adjust the amplification devices according to the characteristics of the patient's hearing loss. Thus, at present, a major focus of the activities provided by rehabilitative audiologists centers around various technical aspects of the hearing aid fitting process (see Chapters 4 and 5 in this volume). Also, particularly in the United States, a major milestone in the organization of audiological rehabilitation services occurred in 1979 when ASHA removed its restriction on allowing audiologists to dispense hearing aids (ASHA, 1978, 1979). At present, audiologists are recognized as the professionals who have the competency to provide all aspects of the rehabilitation services required by persons with hearing loss.

Since the last decade, the development and availability of *auxiliary aids* (frequently referred to as assistive listening devices—ALDs) have provided rehabilitative audiologists with additional armamentaria to respond to some of the

---

PITFALL

For many audiologists, the focus of audiological rehabilitation begins and ends with the prescription and fitting of hearing aids. The hearing aid fitting process is an important intervention strategy. However, the scope of audiological rehabilitation extends beyond hearing aid fitting.

---

needs expressed by persons with hearing loss (see Chapter 19 in this volume). Audiologists are often consulted for the selection, evaluation, and instruction on how to install, operate, and use auxiliary devices. The introduction of Public Law No. 101-336 (American Disabilities Act—ADA, 1991) constitutes another major milestone in the development of rehabilitative audiology. This law was enacted to provide a national mandate to eliminate discrimination against all persons with disabilities (including those with hearing disabilities) in the areas of employment, access to public accommodations, transportation, state and local government services, and telecommunications (see Fox-Grimm, 1991-92; Garstecki, 1994). In each of those areas the availability and use of auxiliary aids can provide important solutions to many of the difficulties encountered by individuals with hearing loss (DeWine, 1992). However, at present, audiologists are still not fully recognized as the professionals most competent to provide expert advice and consultation concerning the selection, installation, and use of services related to auxiliary aids that are required by the law. This aspect of rehabilitative audiology has yet to be fully exploited by audiologists. Yet, it represents an opportunity for the growth of the profession.

SPEECH-PERCEPTION TRAINING

Since the establishment of audiological rehabilitation as a discipline it has been recognized that amplification systems alone do not provide solutions to all the speech-perception difficulties encountered by persons with hearing loss. Speech-perception training programs have always been considered a cornerstone of audiological rehabilitation programs for adults with acquired hearing loss. Generally, these services are grouped under three different categories: auditory training, speechreading (lipreading) training, and auditory-visual speech-perception training. Several types of programs have been developed and proposed. Regardless of the sensory modality in which they are dispensed, the goal of speech-perception training programs is to overcome the speech-perception deficits that result from permanent hearing loss.

Initially, the programs developed by the Veteran's Administration services served as a model for many of the speech-perception training programs incorporated into rehabilitation services for individuals with acquired hearing loss. The introduction of commercially available tactile devices and cochlear implants for persons with profound hearing loss in the 1980s spawned a renewed interest in many of the initial activities traditionally associated with audiological rehabilitation. Specifically, clinical procedures were developed to assess the auditory, visual, and auditory-visual speech-perception performances of persons who were potential candidates for those devices (see Chapters 16 and 17 in this volume). Post-fitting training programs have been modified and redesigned to optimize the receptive speech-perception performances of persons with profound hearing loss. Some of the rehabilitative procedures developed primarily for tactile aid and cochlear implant users were redesigned for patients with a less severe degree of hearing loss. Also, several studies were designed to evaluate the effectiveness of speech-perception training programs provided to persons who sought these rehabilitative services (Alcantara et al, 1990; Danz & Binnie, 1983; Gagné et al, 1991b; Lansing & Davis, 1988; Lesner et al, 1987; Montgomery et al, 1984; Rubenstein and Boothroyd, 1987; Walden et al, 1977; Walden et al, 1981).

PEARL

Excellent auditory, visual, and auditory-visual speech-perception testing protocols have been developed for persons who are candidates for, or users of, cochlear implants and tactile aids. Also, several speech-perception training programs were developed for the same patients. Those materials can easily be adapted to testing and training speech-perception among persons with less severe acquired hearing impairment.

Recently, computer applications to speech-perception training have been developed. Examples of these programs include the Dynamic Audio Video Interactive Device (DAVID: Sims et al, 1979); Computer Assisted Speech Perception Evaluation and Training (CASPER: Boothroyd, 1987); Auditory-Visual Laser Videodisc Interactive System (ALVIS: Kopra et al, 1987); Computerized Laser Videodisc Programs for Training Speechreading and Assertive Communication Behaviors (Tye-Murray et al, 1988); Computer-Aided Speechreading Training system (CAST: Gagné et al, 1991a; Pichora-Fuller & Benguerel, 1991); and the Computer-Assisted Tracking Simulation (CATS: Dempsey et al, 1992). Table 18–1 provides a listing of some of the interactive speech-perception training programs that have been developed and the names and addresses of the persons who can be contacted for additional information. These programs make it possible to provide intensive speech-perception training to patients while minimizing the amount of preparation and direct-intervention time (and their related costs) normally required by the clinician.

Several issues must be considered when designing or selecting a speech-perception training program. Among them are decisions concerning the implementation of analytic-based or synthetic (global)-based training programs, the selection of the sensory modality in which to provide training, and decisions on whether the intervention program should be provided on an individual (one-to-one) basis or in a group setting.

CONTROVERSIAL POINT

Several computerized programs have been developed to provide intensive speech-perception training opportunities for persons with hearing impairment. In general, those programs have not provided the panacea that was expected in terms of significantly improving the speech-perception competencies of their intended patients. In our opinion computerized training programs have not (and will not) replaced the role of an experienced clinician in speech-perception training. However, an appropriate use of those programs may be the provision of additional training for individuals who are both familiar with computer technology and highly motivated to improve their speech-perception performances.

Analytic versus Synthetic Speech-Perception Training

Erber (1996) described a general framework that can be applied to speech-perception training (see Fig. 18–1). The matrix considers two aspects of speech-perception training: the type of stimuli used and the type of responses required to perform the task. Each cell of the matrix corresponds to a different speech-perception task. All possible speech-perception training tasks are incorporated into the matrix. However, some cells are more commonly applied than others (refer to Fig. 18–1).

Traditionally, speech-perception training has been considered under two broad categories: analytic and synthetic (or global). *Analytic* training programs involve breaking the speech signal into small components and training these components separately (Blamey & Alcantara, 1994). Typically, the types of activities grouped under analytic speech-perception training tasks include the detection of vowels; the discrimination of consonants; and the identification of various elements of speech, including suprasegmental features of speech sounds (e.g. prosody, accent), and speech elements (e.g., vowels, consonants, words) (see Fig. 18–1). Examples of analytic speech-perception training activities are described in Table 18–2. Slight changes in test procedures or changes in the test stimuli used can modify the level of difficulty of a speech-perception task. Suggestions of ways to modify an analytic speech-perception task to vary the level of difficulty associated with the activity are provided in Table 18–3. Over the years, several authors have described speech-perception training activities on the basis of an analytic approach. Examples of some of those programs include Jeffers and Barley (1971), Ordman and Ralli (1976), Haug and Haug (1977), Jeffers and Barley (1979), Erber (1982), Feehan et al (1982), Walther (1982), Auerback (1984), Greenwald (1984), Plant (1984), Whitehurst (1986), Spitzer et al (1993), Jennings (1994), Plant (1994; 1996c), and Tye-Murray (1997).

Synthetic speech-perception training focuses on bringing the patient to apply one's implicit knowledge of linguistics and one's "knowledge of the world" to the interpretation

TABLE 18–1 Information on computer applications to speech-perception training

Program	Additional Information Available From:
Dynamic Audio Video Interactive Device (DAVID)	Donald G. Sims Dept. of Communication Research National Technical Institute for the Deaf Rochester Institute of Technology Rochester, NY 14623-0887
Computer-Assissted Speech Perception Evaluation and Training (CASPER)	Nancy Plant c/o Arthur Boothroyd City University Graduate Center Dept. of Speech and Hearing Sciences 33 West 42nd St. New York, NY 10036
Auditory-Visual Laser Videodisc Interactive System (ALVIS)	Lennart L. Kopra c/o Dept. of Communication Sciences and Disorders The University of Texas at Austin CMA 7.202 Austin, TX 78712
Computerized Laser Videodisc Programs for Training Speechreading and Assertive Communication Behaviors	Richard S. Tyler Dept. of Otolaryngology, Head and Neck Surgery The University of Iowa Hospitals Iowa City, IA 52242
Computer-Aided Speechreading (CAST)	M.-K. Pichora-Fuller, School of Audiology and Speech Sciences University of British Columbia 5804 Fairview Ave. Vancouver, B.C. V6T 1W5 Canada
Computer-Assisted Tracking Simulation (CATS)	James J. Dempsey Dept. of Communication Disorders Southern Connecticut State University 501 Crescent St. New Haven, CT 06515-1355

and understanding of the speech message (Butler, 1984; Duncan & Katz, 1983; Gagné, 1994). Generally, synthetic programs are designed to teach patients to make optimal use of the linguistic redundancies available in ongoing speech. Boothroyd (1988) described several levels of linguistic redundancies that are available in speech. They include phonological constraints, lexical constraints, syntactic constraints, semantic constraints, topical constraints, and pragmatic constraints (Table 18–4). Knowledge and use of the linguistic rules that govern a spoken language can improve one's ability to understand a spoken message (Erber, 1996). Training activities may be designed to foster the use of any of those sources of linguistic redundancies. However, synthetic speech-perception activities typically include the identification or comprehension of phrases, sentences, and continuous discourse (i.e., narrative) (see Fig. 18–1). Examples of activities that have been designed to train synthetic speech-perception skills are described in Table 18–5. Examples of ways to modify the level of difficulty of synthetic training activities are provided in Table 18–6.

Training activities based on continuous discourse material have been developed by DeFilippo and Scott (1978) and Erber (1996). Speech tracking is a procedure developed by DeFilippo and Scott (1978) as a method for training and evaluating the reception of ongoing speech. Speech tracking requires that the patient (e.g., the receiver) listen to a segment of ongoing speech, usually taken from a written passage, spoken by a communication partner (e.g., the sender), and then repeat the utterance verbatim (Table 18–7). DeFilippo (1988) provides a detailed account of how speech tracking can be applied to speech-perception training in any sensory modality. Modifications to the original tracking procedure have been suggested by Fenn and Smith (1987), Owens and Raggio (1987), Matthies and Carney (1988), and Spens (1995).

Erber (1996) described a procedure entitled QUEST?AR. This activity is a conversational-based training procedure that provides interactive practice with common question-answer sequences. The patient asks a communication partner (e.g., the clinician) a series of 30 prepared questions (Table 18–8).

	Speech unit	Syllable	Word	Phrase	Sentence	Narrative
Detection	A	A				
Discrimination	A	A	A			
Identification	A	A	A	A/S	S	
Comprehension				S	S	S

Figure 18–1 Stimulus-response matrix summarizing various speech perception comptencies (adapted from Erber, 1996). Each cell represents a specific type of speech perception training task. The cells with a symbol indicate tasks most often incorporated into speech perception training programs for persons with an acquired hearing impairment. The cells containing the symbol "A" describe primarily analytic speech perception tasks, whereas those containing the symbol "S" describe primarily synthetic speech perception tasks.

The patient must either repeat the answer or indicate in some fashion that the response was understood. When a communication breakdown occurs, the patient and/or the communication partner must find ways to resolve the communication breakdown before they proceed to the next question. One advantage of this activity is that it is the patient who initiates each new question. Thus that person has some insights into the possible responses that can be provided. This procedure is an effective approach to developing synthetic speech-perception abilities. Erber (1996) provides a detailed account of the different ways that the QUEST?AR procedure can be adapted to practice various aspects of synthetic speech-perception skills.

In addition to the two clinical procedures presented previously, several other authors have described speech-perception training activities that can be used to practice synthetic abilities. Examples of those programs include Jeffers and Barley (1971), Ordman and Ralli (1976), Haug and Haug (1977), Fisher (1978), Jeffers and Barley (1979), Feehan et al (1982), Walther (1982), Auerback (1984), Broberg (1984), Plant, (1984), Kaplan et al (1985), Whitehurst (1986), Greenwald (1984), Marcus (1985), Spitzer et al (1993), Jennings (1994), Kleeman (1995), Erber (1996), Plant (1996a; 1996b; 1996c), Strachan et al (1997), and Tye-Murray (1997).

It is important to note that a speech-perception training program designed for an individual is seldom limited to one training approach. Typically, during one individual session, a person may complete both analytic and synthetic training activities and activities designed to develop conversational fluency and communication-management skills (see section following). Also, analytic and synthetic speech-perception training activities can be conducted in any sensory modality (auditory-only, visual-only, audiovisual). In some instances the stimuli used to conduct the activity may be degraded in some fashion to make the task more difficult for the patient. Several strategies can be used to degrade the audio signal in a clinical setting. They include low-pass filtering the signal, reducing the overall level of the signal, and introducing background noise so that the task is conducted at a poor signal-to-noise-ratio. Depending on the objectives of the program, the task can be conducted with or without the patient's personal speech-perception aid (e.g., hearing aid). Similarly, some strategies can be used to degrade the quality of the visual-speech signal during a visual or an audiovisual speech-perception training activity. For example, the distance and the

TABLE 18–2 Examples of analytic speech-perception training activities. All of these activities can be completed auditorily-alone, visually-alone, or audiovisually.

Syllables in Words

    Words are contrasted by a number of syllables. A stimulus word is presented by the clinician. The patient is asked to identify the stimulus word within a closed-set response format (e.g., beach vs. baseball vs. telephone).

Sentences Varying in Syllabic Pattern

    Sentences that differ in the number of syllables they contain are presented in a closed-set format (e.g., "The boy is crying," vs. "The kangaroo is jumping"). The clinician produces one of the sentences and the patient is asked to identify the stimulus-sentence.

Discrimination of Vowels

    Words or nonsense syllables (C-V-C) that differ only in their vowel content are contrasted (e.g., beet, bit, bat, but, boot). The clinician presents sequences of two test stimuli. The patient is asked whether the two stimuli were the same or different.

Identification of Vowels, Consonants, Words, or Syllabic Pattern

    Selected stimuli are presented in a closed-set format with a minimum number of two foils presented (e.g., bite vs. kite vs. fight). One of the stimuli is presented by the clinician. The patient must indicate which stimulus was presented from the set of possible responses.

TABLE 18–3 Examples of ways to modify the level of difficulty in analytic training activities

- Training can begin with a detection task, followed by a discrimination task, and finally move to an identification task.

- In any identification task the level of difficulty can be decreased by reducing the number of alternatives available in the response foils. The level of difficulty can be increased by increasing the number of alternatives available in the response foils.

- Initially, within a given task, the stimuli used should include the speech elements that are the most distinctive. Gradually, the task can be modified to include speech elements that are more similar in the sensory modality in which the activity is conducted (e.g., in an auditory training activity begin with "beet" vs. "bat" contrasts, later include "beet" vs. "bit" contrasts).

- Text support can be provided to decrease the difficulty of the task. Text support can be removed to increase the difficulty of the task.

- Initially, a slightly exaggerated production of the test stimulus can be presented to emphasize the speech element targeted. Later, a more natural production of the test stimulus can be presented.

- Initially, the test stimuli can be presented in isolation. Later, the test stimuli can be presented in a carrier phrase or in a sentence context. For example, the stimulus word "pepper" could be presented in isolation or in the context of a facilitating phrase such as: "Please pass the salt and _____".

TABLE 18–4 Levels at which linguistic rules that can be applied to enhance speech perception

Phonological constraints: Refers to the fact that rules govern how speech acts (e.g., phonemes) can be grouped together to produce words. For example, within any English word, the phoneme /z/ is not likely to be preceded by the phoneme /t/.

Lexical constraints: Refers to the fact that in any given language, the number of words that exist is finite. Moreover, some words are more familiar than others and some words are used more frequently than others. For example, during a conversation the word *telephone* is more likely to be uttered than the word *xylophone*.

Syntactic constraints: Refers to the fact that every language is governed by a set of grammatical rules that specifies the relationship between words used to communicate. For example, adjectives may be used to qualify nouns (as in "the *blue* shoes"); adjectives are not used to qualify verbs (as in "he *blue* ran").

Semantic constraints: Refers to the fact that the words used in a sentence are usually related to each other in a meaningful way. For example, although the sentence "Put the salt on the cloud" is syntactically correct, semantically, it is highly improbable.

Topical constraints: Refers to the fact that language usually takes place within a physical and social context. Generally, the use of language bears some relationship with the context in which it is used. For example, in a stadium, during a football game, it is more likely that the topic of discussion will center around sports-related activities than around religious beliefs and values.

Pragmatic constraints: Refers to the fact that language is governed by social norms that determine how it is used within a given community or situation. These rules are used to make the use of language more efficient for the purpose of exchanging ideas and to avoid confusion. For example, during a conversation, generally only one person talks at a time and there are rules that govern turn-taking.

Definitions and examples inspired by the work of Boothroyd (1988) and Erber (1996).

TABLE 18–5 Examples of synthetic speech-perception training activities. These activities can be accomplished auditorily-alone, visually-alone, or audiovisually.

Category Activities

A semantic category is selected (e.g., animals). The clinician presents words from the category and the patient is asked to recognize the items.

Fill-in-the-Blank Activities

Sentences are presented to the patient with text support. In each written sentence one or two words are replaced by a blank. The clinician presents the entire sentence (including the missing word[s]) and the patient is asked to identify the missing word[s]).

Question-Answer Activities

The patient is provided with a series of questions related to a topic of conversation. The patient presents the questions to the clinician, who then provides the answer. The patient must repeat the answer to the question before moving to the next question (see QUEST?AR: Erber, 1996).

Topic-Sentence Activities

The patient is presented with a topic. The clinician then presents sentences related to the topic and the patient is asked to repeat the sentences.

Direction-Following Activities

The patient is presented with directions and is required to carry out the actions requested by the clinician.

Speech-Tracking Activities

The clinician presents a phrase from a written passage. The patient is asked to repeat the utterance of speech verbatim (see DeFilippo, 1988).

Conversation Activities

The patient and the clinician carry out a conversation. The clinician assesses the fluency of the conversation and the patient and clinician discuss the general success of the conversation, identifying difficulties and possible solutions (see TOPICON: Erber, 1996).

viewing angle between the clinician and the patient can be increased, the overall illumination of the room can be reduced, and the lighting contrast between the background visual-field and the clinician's face can be increased.

Sensory Modalities

When designing a speech-perception training program for a patient, it is important to determine under which sensory modality(ies) to conduct the training activities. Traditionally, speech-perception training was conducted in a unisensory modality: either auditory training or visual speech-perception training (lipreading or speechreading). In recent years, it has been recognized that in most instances speech-perception is a multisensory activity. That is, except for some rare instances where the visual signal is not available (e.g., communicating by telephone or conversing with someone who is in another room) the persons involved in a conversation have access to both the auditory and the visual signals provided by the interlocutor. Thus, in most instances, the ultimate goal of speech-perception training for persons with acquired hearing loss should be to improve their auditory-visual speech-perception competencies. However, the question remains: In which sensory modality should training be conducted to optimize audiovisual speech perception performances? This question is particularly relevant because recent investigations

have shown that auditory-visual speech-perception does not necessarily involve the simple addition of cues extracted from the visual signal with the cues extracted from the auditory signal (for a detailed discussion of this issue, see Gagné, 1994). At present, for adults with acquired hearing loss, no clear evidence in the literature indicates whether training should be conducted in a unisensory modality (auditory or visually) or in a multisensory modality (audiovisual) (Gagné, 1994; Walden & Grant, 1993).

One way to determine in which sensory modality to focus training is to assess the patient's speech-perception competency in each of the unisensory modalities (auditory and visual). An analysis of the results of auditory-speech perception tests and the results of visual-speech perception tests will indicate whether the patient is functioning optimally in each of those two sensory modalities. Training should focus on practicing speech-perception in the sensory modality in which the patient is least proficient. For example, the results of an assessment test battery may indicate that in quiet, with his speech-perception aid, the patient performs as would be expected (considering the person's hearing loss) in the auditory-only modality. However, the results of visual-speech perception evaluation procedures may reveal that the patient fails to use visual cues optimally. For this person, speech-perception training should focus on speechreading activities.

TABLE 18–6   Examples of ways to modify the level of difficulty in synthetic training activities

- Selecting topics that are familiar to the patient will make the task easier; selecting topics that are less familiar to the patient will make the task more difficult.

- The use of test material that is written in simple language (in terms of vocabulary words, syntactic structure, semantic contents) will reduce the level of difficulty of the task; the use of linguistically more complex test material will increase the level of difficulty of the task.

- Informing the patient of the topic to be discussed before completing an activity will make the task easier; discussing the topic with the patient before completing the task (e.g., identifying key words and concepts) will further facilitate the task.

- The use of partly scripted (i.e., written) test materials during an activity will make the task easier; removing the text support will increase the level of difficulty of the task.

- Increasing the number of test items or the length of the utterances that the patient must attend to will increase the level of difficulty of a task; decreasing the number of test items or length of the utterances that the patient must attend to will decrease the level of difficulty of a task.

- Practicing the task under ideal environmental conditions (e.g., in quiet and under good lighting conditions) and presenting the stimuli in an audiovisual mode will facilitate the task; degrading the quality of the environmental conditions (e.g., adding background noise, increasing the distance between clinician and patient, degrading the lighting conditions in the room) will make the task more difficult.

- The use of clear speech and emphasis on keywords or phrases will facilitate the task; the use of conversational (natural) speech without any special emphasis will make the task more difficult.

At present, the tendency is to emphasize training in the patient's nondominant sensory modality (Erber, 1969, 1979; Gagné, 1994; Garstecki, 1981). For most persons with acquired moderately severe hearing loss, audition remains the primary sensory modality for speech-perception (especially after they have been fitted with an appropriate amplification system and once they have fully acclimatized to using the device). For those individuals, speech-perception training programs should be designed to help them fully exploit the visual information available in the speech signal. Training programs may be conducted in a visual-only mode. Alternately, speech-perception activities may be conducted audiovisually but under conditions in which the auditory signal is degraded to foster the integration of the available visual cues and the degraded audio signal. The following example will serve to illustrate this latter training condition. First, a speech-perception activity is initiated in an auditory-only mode. Second, a masking noise, such as speech-babble, is introduced and the level of the noise is adjusted until the patient's performance declines substantially (i.e., above chance level). Then, under that acoustic condition (audition in noise), visual speech cues are provided and the same training activity is completed. Under this latter condition, the patient will have access to some auditory cues but that information will be insufficient to perform the task optimally. Providing visual information will train the patient to combine the degraded audio signal with the available visual-speech cues. This training paradigm can be incorporated into analytic and synthetic training activities.

Group versus Individual Speech-Perception Training

Many of the training activities described previously can be conducted with patients on an individual basis (one-to-one) or with a small group of patients. Individual speech-perception training provides the clinician with the opportunity to tailor the programs to the specific skills, goals, and interests of the individual. Group speech-perception training may be carried out in small groups of individuals who are closely matched in their speech-perception competencies and for whom similar rehabilitative goals have been established. According to Blamey and Alcantara (1994), costs can be reduced through the use of group training, but it may be at the expense of the effectiveness of the training program. Moreover, in a group setting the clinician must be aware of (and able to cater to) the program objectives of each of the individuals in the group. Effective group training programs usually require that the clinician be very alert and experienced at coordinating speech-perception training activities.

A patient may be involved in both group and individual sessions. Individualized intervention programs constitute an efficient approach for the practice and development of specific speech-perception competencies. Group intervention programs provide the participants with an opportunity to practice their communication skills in a more realistic (yet somewhat controlled or safe) environment. Groups also provide comraderie and an opportunity for the participants to share their experience and expertise. In general, individual

TABLE 18–7   Example of the speech-tracking procedure developed by DeFilippo and Scott

Clinician:	(reading from a written text) He lit the lamp on the secretary… and began to write to his wife.*
Patient:	He bit the lamp . . .
Clinician:	He . . . *LIT* . . . the lamp (emphasizing the word in italics)
Patient:	He lit? . . .
Clinician:	He lit the lamp . . .
Patient:	He lit the lamp.
Clinician:	(nodding in approval) . . . on the secretary . . .
Patient:	and he was lazy?
Clinician:	ON THE SECRETARY (repeated slowly using clear speech)
Patient:	He lit the lamp on the . . .
Clinician:	SE-CRE-TARY (repeated with emphasis)
Patient:	secretion
Clinician:	SE-CRE-TARY . . . a table to write on . . . a desk . . . a SE-CRE-TARY . . . (using paraphrase and synonym).
Patient:	A table to write on?
Clinician:	Yes, a SE-CRE-TARY . . . (a confirmation and a repetition of the misperceived word with emphasis)
Patient:	A secretary?
Clinician:	(nodding to approve of the response) . . . He lit the lamp on the secretary . . .
Patient:	He lit the lamp on the secretary
Clinician:	and began to write to his wife
Patient:	and began to write his life
Clinician:	(facial expression indicating that the response was a close approximation) . . . and began to write TO his WIFE. . .
Patient:	and began to write to his wife!
Clinician:	(nods to indicate a correct response and then proceeds with the next sentence).

*Passage taken from Below, S. (1947). *The victim*. New York: Vanguard Press.

intervention programs are best suited for training analytic skills. On the other hand, group intervention programs are most appropriate for practicing communication-management skills (see following section).

Ideally, when group intervention programs are carried out, the minimum number of group members should be approximately five persons and the maximum number of participants should not exceed 10. Groups should consist of participants with similar functional skills and for whom the objectives retained as part of their rehabilitation program are compatible with each other rather than constituted strictly on the basis of their audiometric characteristics. Also, when possible, efforts should be made to regroup participants who share a similar socioeconomic status and educational level and who have similar work-related responsibilities. This will ensure that the discussions held within the group will be more homogeneous and of interest to all the group members. It is recommended that patients who have difficulty communicating in the language in which the group will be conducted, who are not cognitively intact, or who display

behaviors that might be disruptive within a group setting should not be invited to take part in a group intervention program. Those individuals will be better served within an individually based intervention program.

Group and individual training programs vary in their duration and in the length of each session. Typically, programs extend over a period of 8 to 12 sessions. Sessions, 60 to 90 minutes long, are usually held once or twice a week over this period of time, with assignments for home practice to be carried out between sessions. In a program that combines analytic, synthetic, and communication-management training, the analytic portion of the training program would rarely exceed 25% of a total time within a given session. Intensive group-intervention programs may also be provided. For example, participants may attend daily sessions over a period of 1 or 2 weeks (Bally & Kaplan, 1988; Jennings & Sheppard, 1992). In this case, daily sessions may include several 45- to 60-minute training activities, separated by coffee breaks and meals. Patient progress can be more easily monitored when the clinician uses work sheets for each exercise.

Telephone Training

The telephone has become an important means of communication for most people. However, communicating over the telephone can prove to be a challenge for persons with hearing loss. The acoustic signal received over the telephone will not be the same as a live-voice signal. The telephone may degrade the signal by narrowing the audio-frequency range available to the listener and by introducing background noise and distortion. Also, visual information is not available to supplement the auditory information in the speech signal. Thus communication by telephone may constitute an important rehabilitative need for many individuals with acquired hearing loss.

Telephone training may be provided to individuals with hearing loss who use hearing aids, cochlear implants, and tactile devices. The goal of the training program may be different, depending on the device used and the benefit the person receives from the device in auditory-only communication. The goal of telephone training will vary according to the individual. For some persons with acquired hearing loss the goal of an intervention program may be to allow them to carry out a conversation for business or personal purposes. For others, the goal of an intervention program may be limited to the transmission of essential information.

An important component of all telephone training programs will focus on the identification of the most appropriate coupling system to use for telephone communication. This will be determined by the types of telephones most often used by the patient and by the person's hearing loss and his or her personal hearing amplification system. For more information on telephone compatibility, refer to Chapter 19 in this volume. Also, some patients will require information on how to use a teletypewriter (TTY) and operator-assisted services. However, in most cases, the provision of information on these forms of telephone communication will not be sufficient. Instructions and systematic practice on how to use a TTY and operator-assisted services will be required (see Table 18–9).

Erber (1985) developed an intervention program for telephone use that consists of three phases. Initially, information concerning the individual's auditory abilities and

TABLE 18–8   Topics and questions from QUESTions for Aural Rehabilitation (QUEST?AR)

Where did you go?	*Museum, restaurant, post office, shopping, camping, doctor, zoo, beach, airport, swimming, mountains, picnic, music lesson, Mars, supermarket, and so forth*

Questions:

1. Why did you go there?
2. When did you go there?
3. How many people went with you?
4. Who were they (names)?
5. What did you take with you?
6. Where is (the place where you went)?
7. How did you get there?
8. What did you see on the way?
9. What time did you get there?
10. What did you do first?
11. What did you see?
12. How many? What color? etc.
13. What happened at (the place where you went)?
14. What else did you do?
15. What were other people doing at (the place where you went)?
16. What was the most interesting thing that you saw?
17. What was the most interesting thing that you did?
18. What did you buy?
19. What kind? What flavor? What color? etc.
20. How much did it cost?
21. Did anything unusual happen? What?
22. How long did you stay?
23. What did you do just before you came home?
24. When did you leave?
25. How did you get home?
26. What happened on the way home?
27. What time did you get home?
28. How did you feel then?
29. When are you going back?
30. Do you think that I should go sometime? Why?

Taken from Erber, (1996). QUEST?AR is published and distributed by Clavis Publishing, P.O. Box 233, Clifton Hill, Victoria 3068, Australia.

communication goals is collected. This information is obtained from case-history questionnaires and audiological test results. Also, interviews are used to assess the individual's auditory abilities/difficulties, and the person's need for telephone communication, and the person's goal in seeking this type of rehabilitative service. The second stage involves practicing simulated conversations. The results of this activity serve to define the specific goals for the intervention program. On the basis of this information, training exercises are designed to develop specific skills. Finally, the individual participates in conversations in practical, real-life situations over the telephone. Examples of training activities that may be incorporated into a telephone training program are outlined in Table 18–9. Few published comprehensive telephone training programs exist for persons with hearing loss. Two noteworthy exceptions are Erber (1985) and Castle (1988).

SPECIAL CONSIDERATION

Many persons with hearing impairment, particularly elderly individuals, may require assistance in learning how adjust and use the coupling system that they acquire to communicate by telephone. Furthermore, some individuals may benefit from training in the use of communication management strategies that can be applied during telephone conversations. Comprehensive rehabilitation programs should include the provision of all the services related to the use of the telephone by persons with hearing impairment.

TABLE 18–9 Activities that can be included in rehabilitation programs designed to improve communication by telephone

Orientation to Telephone Devices

The clinician provides information concerning auxiliary devices that are commercially available for use with the telephone (e.g., built-in amplifiers, in-line amplifiers, portable amplifiers, use of hardwired and wireless auxiliary devices that can be used with a telephone and telephones specifically designed for individuals with hearing loss). The patient may be oriented to other systems used for telephone communication such as devices that provide visual information (e.g., teletypewriter and voice carryover, fax, E-mail). Also, information may be provided on the existence and use of telephone relay services.

Hearing Aids and Telephones

The clinician would provide information on the different ways to couple telephones and hearing aids (i.e., hearing aid microphone, hearing aid telecoil, hearing aid hooked up to other types of assistive devices). For more information on this topic, the reader is referred to Chapter 19 in this volume. Practice sessions would be conducted to teach the patient how to use the telephone with the coupling system that is most suitable for the patient.

Development of Strategies

The clinician would provide an orientation to, and practice in, the use of anticipatory and repair strategies that can be used during telephone conversations. Some repair strategies that may be particularly applicable to telephone conversations include the use of spelling, code words, alphabet, numbers, counting, and key words (Castle, 1988). For those individuals who have great receptive difficulties over the telephone, training activities may focus on the use of code systems such as speech codes, number codes, International Morse Code, and touch-tone telephone code (Castle, 1988).

Conversational Practice

Role-playing activities may be carried out to simulate various conversations that might be held over the telephone (e.g., calling to make an appointment, calling to obtain information about schedules for plays or movies). At first, fully scripted scenarios can be used. Later, the scenarios may be modified so that the conversations are only partially scripted. Finally, the scenarios may include open-ended conversations (Erber, 1985). At each stage, the level of difficulty of the activities can be gradually increased. For example, initially the participants may conduct a face-to-face conversation. Then, the visual cues provided by the communication partner (often the clinician) can be gradually obscured (e.g., increasing the distance between the two partners or decreasing the amount of lighting in the room). Eventually, one of the communication partners can move to a different room. Finally, conversations can be held from remote locations by means of commercially-available telephones (Erber, 1985).

Carrying Out Real Conversations

Patients can also carry out real conversations within the clinical setting. At first, they would call persons with whom they are familiar such as friends or family members. Later, patients can carry out conversations with unknown individuals. For example, they can call the local transit company to ask for schedule or fare information.

COMMUNICATION-MANAGEMENT TRAINING

Over the years, expert clinicians observed that some persons with limited speech-perception competencies were proficient communicators, whereas others with better speech-perception competencies experienced communication difficulties in many situations. Also, experimental data showed that speech-perception training programs often produced benefits that were not measured by speech-perception tests (Binnie, 1977). Beginning in the early 1980s, interest was renewed in designing audiological rehabilitation programs that extended beyond speech-perception training. Those programs centered on the development of strategies aimed at facilitating *communication*, rather than focusing strictly on speech-perception competencies. They incorporated many aspects of linguistic and sociolinguistic models of communication such as the pragmatics of verbal exchanges. Also, these programs were based on a broader conception of communication that considered the effects of the type of information exchanged during conversations and the effects of the physical and social environment in which communication takes place (see Fig. 18–2). An important dimension of those programs was a recognition that communication is an interactive process between individuals and that communication partners are an integral part of this process. The attitudes and behaviors of individuals who communicate with persons who have hearing loss can have an impact on the success (or failure) of a conversational exchange. On the basis of this knowledge many rehabilitation programs were designed to help persons with hearing loss and their communication partners manage communication more effectively. Components of communication-management training programs include communication strategies, conversational fluency, assertiveness training, stress management, and personal adjustment.

Communication Strategies

Broadly defined, communication strategies include any verbal or nonverbal behaviors that can be used to improve the effectiveness of communication (Gagné et al, 1991c). Tye-Murray (1994) grouped communication strategies under two general categories: *facilitation strategies* and *repair strategies*. According to the author, facilitation strategies include behaviors used to prepare for and manage an ongoing conversation. Repair strategies are behaviors that are applied when a breakdown in communication occurs.

Facilitation strategies such as *anticipatory* strategies and *attending* strategies are used to optimize the recognition and comprehension of the verbal message. For example, preparing a list of potential vocabulary words, phrases, or sentences that may be used during an upcoming conversation (e.g., with a bank teller) would constitute a form of anticipatory strategy. Attending to the facial characteristics of a talker to obtain information concerning the emotional state of the person (e.g., anxious, happy, sad) constitutes a form of attending strategy because facial expressions are almost always consistent with the content of message.

Managing the physical environment in which a conversation takes place is another form of facilitation strategy. Patients can be taught to recognize physical properties of a given environment (e.g., living-room, kitchen, restaurant, meeting room) that are not ideal for communication (e.g., noise, reverberation, poor lighting). Moreover, patients can be informed of, and taught, strategies that can be used to manage or modify environmental conditions to maximize their speech-recognition performance. Instructional strategies are used to inform the communication partner of speaking behaviors that will facilitate speech understanding. For example, it has been shown that the use of clear speech can significantly improve a person's auditory-speech and visual-speech intelligibility (Gagné & Boutin, 1997; Gagné & Rochette, 1996;

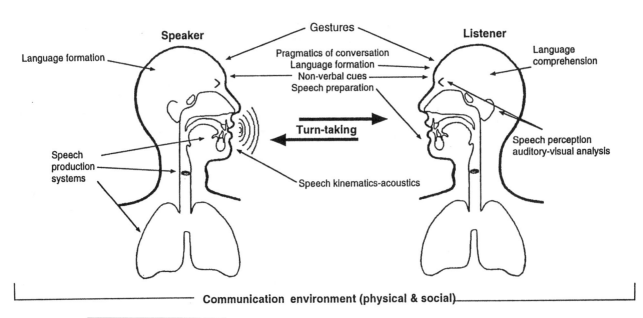

Figure 18–2   Simplified model of the communication process. (Adapted from an unpublished figure by McFarland and Gagné, personal communication, September 1998.)

Gagné et al, 1994; Gagné et al, 1995; Helfer, 1998; Picheny et al, 1985, 1986; Uchanski et al, 1996). Communication partners can improve their ability to be understood by persons with hearing loss if they use clear speech (Gagné & Paradis, 1995). In some cases communication partners might benefit from training in the production of clear speech. According to Schum (1997), the production of clear speech simply requires that the person talk naturally slower and louder, articulate accurately, use voice inflection to stress key words, and use pauses between phrases and sentences. Clinical experience has shown that even without extensive instructions or training almost everybody can modify their speech articulation pattern to produce clear speech that will improve their speech intelligibility. However, most persons without training in the use of clear speech will tend to revert to their usual speaking patterns after a short period of time. During a conversation, patients may need to periodically remind their communication partners to use clear speech.

Message-tailoring strategies are also effective facilitation strategies. For example, Erber (1988) has shown that persons with hearing loss have less difficulty answering questions that require a closed-set response than general open-ended questions (e.g., "Should we walk or take a bus to the concert?" rather than "How do we get there?"). Teaching persons with hearing loss to use and solicit these types of facilitation strategies constitutes an effective way of preventing or minimizing the number of communication breakdowns that may occur during a conversation.

Repair strategies are behaviors used to overcome a communication breakdown between communication partners. A communication breakdown occurs when one of the communication partners fails to understand a message that was intended for that person (Gagné et al, 1991c). Repair strategies can be used by the person who is providing the information (expressive strategies) or by the person for whom the message is intended (receptive strategies). The most frequently used repair strategy consists of asking the talker to repeat the message (Tye-Murray et al, 1992). Yet, indications show that other types of strategies may be more effective in repairing a communication breakdown (Gagné & Wyllie, 1989). Other types of repair strategies include asking the talker to rephrase the statement, simplifying the message, elaborating the message, providing the topic of the message, using natural gestures, and spelling or writing the misperceived message (Kaplan et al, 1987; Tye-Murray, 1994). Studies have shown that with some training, persons with hearing loss can be taught to request a wider range of repair strategies (Erber, 1996; Owens & Telleen, 1991; Tye-Murray, 1991).

Examples of programs that include activities designed to optimize the use of appropriate communication strategies include Kaplan et al (1987), Trychin (1987), Erber (1988), Jennings et al (1991), Jennings (1993), Spitzer et al (1993), Trychin (1993), Trychin and Albright (1993), Tye-Murray (1994, 1997), Tye-Murray and Schum (1994), Wayner and Abrahamson (1996), and Erber (1996).

Conversational Fluency

Conversation constitutes an important social behavior that involves more than the simple exchange of information between two or more individuals. During a conversation several factors influence the degree of satisfaction experienced by the participants. Erber (1988, 1996) identified several factors that contribute to the degree of satisfaction experienced by the participants during a conversation. They include temporal aspects/rhythm of interchange, meta-communication/ clarification, topic, intimacy/sensitivity, information, time/ direction/fantasy, attitude, honesty, power/control. These factors may differ in their importance to various communication partners. Other issues identified include the relationship between communication partners, the expectations of the communication partners, the purpose of the conversation, and the outcomes of the conversation. For a detailed discussion of the factors that influence conversational fluency and satisfaction and a description of clinical procedures that can be used to assess and train conversational fluency, the reader is referred to Erber (1996, especially Chapter 9, pp. 203-223). When one of the communication partners has hearing loss, the general fluency of a conversation is often affected. This can cause dissatisfaction for all the persons participating in the conversation (Gagné et al, 1991c).

PITFALL

Many communication-management intervention programs focus exclusively on the elimination (or minimization) of communication breakdowns that occur during conversations. Other factors related to the goal and the process of verbal communication are neglected. At best, those programs will increase the amount of information exchanged during a conversation. However, the motivation of the communication partners to communicate and their degree of satisfaction related to the conversation may be severely compromised. As Erber (1996) pointed out, several relevant variables must be considered when training conversational fluency.

Erber (1988; 1996) identified three basic correlates of conversational fluency. They are clarification ratio (the proportion of time devoted to successful exchanges of information), turn rate (the speaking turn-per-minute rate), and time sharing (the proportion of time each communication partner talks during a conversation). On the basis of this information he proposed two procedures that can be used to analyze aspects of conversational fluency (Erber, 1988, 1996; Erber & Yelland, 1998). CONAN (Erber and Yelland, 1998) consists of a procedure that can be used to collect, store, and analyze temporal aspects of a communication exchange while a conversation is in progress. DYALOG (Erber, 1996, 1998) is a computer-based program devised to measure the occurrences of communication breakdowns and the amount of time devoted to repairing those breakdowns during a conversation.

Erber and his collaborators (Erber, 1988, 1996; Erber & Lind, 1994; Erber & Yelland, 1998) have proposed several activities that can be used to train conversational fluency. Among them is an activity named TOPICON (Erber, 1988, 1996). In this activity the patient or clinician chooses a topic of interest from a prepared list. Then, the patient and clinician carry out a conversation. The clinician assesses the fluency of the conversation on the basis of a number of preselected variables known to influence conversational fluency and satisfaction. For example, the clinician may count the number of conversational turns between the dyad, the amount of speaking time taken by each person involved in the conversation, and the number of communication breakdowns that occur within a predetermined period. After the conversation is completed, the patient and clinician discuss the success of the conversation, identify the sources of difficulties encountered, and identify possible solutions that might be implemented to overcome those difficulties. Other activities include viewing and analyzing specific segments of videotaped conversations, identifying the global characteristics of the conversation, and judging the level of satisfaction experienced by the participants. In addition, Erber (1988, 1996) described conversational activities such as speech-tracking procedures, question-answer activities, and topic-centered conversations that can be used to improve conversational fluency. During those activities, initially the participants take part in controlled (scripted) conversations. Later, the participants take part in conversations that involve an increasing number of topic changes. Other training programs that may be used to assess and train conversational fluency include Kaplan et al (1985), Spitzer et al (1993), Jennings (1994), and Plant (1996a,b,c).

Assertiveness Training

Many persons with hearing loss learn to use appropriate communication strategies in a clinical environment where they feel secure. However, they may feel uncomfortable using those same strategies when they interact with persons with whom they communicate on an everyday basis outside the clinical setting. In such cases assertiveness training may be provided to overcome these obstacles. According to Tye-Murray (1994) and Trychin and his colleagues (Fortgatch & Trychin, 1989; Trychin, 1987, 1988; Trychin & Wright, 1989), the goal of assertiveness training is to increase the cooperation of communication partners while maintaining an equality among all the participants in a conversation (Erber & Lind, 1994). Patients can learn to use effective (neutral, nonaggressive) strategies that will enable them to solicit assistance from their communication partners without diminishing their own self-esteem (or the esteem others have of them) and maintain an appropriate role within a conversational framework. Important aspects of assertiveness training include requesting modifications in the physical environment and informing the communication partner of some difficulties experienced and the reason for those difficulties (e.g., "I have a hearing loss that makes it very difficult for me to follow a conversation when there is a lot of noise in the background. Would you mind if we continue our conversation in the living room where it is more quiet?"). Providing communication partners with appropriate (positive and constructive) feedback is also an important component of assertiveness training. Such behaviors will lead the patient and his or her communication partners to use and (over time) maintain good communication practices. Examples of programs that include assertiveness training include Trychin (1987), Jennings (1993), Trychin and Albright (1993), and Wayner and Abrahamson (1996).

Stress Management

In industrialized societies, almost every individual experiences stress at some point because of situations that occur in their work settings or in their personal lives. Some individuals may have difficulty adapting to prolonged stressful situations. Training in stress management has become popular among the general population. Most persons with an acquired hearing loss will experience the added stress of having to function in a hearing society. For example, they worry that they will not be able to detect, recognize, and react appropriately to warning signals (e.g., alarm-clock, microwave oven, doorbell, fax machine), that they will not know when someone speaks to them, or that they will not correctly understand the information provided by their communication partners.

The effects of stress may manifest themselves in several different ways. Stress may be the cause of headaches, upset stomach, disturbed sleep pattern (including nightmares), decreased productivity at work, disorganization, anxiety, depression, excessive worrying, withdrawal (Trychin, 1986b). Typical physiological responses to stress include an increase in muscle tension, pulse rate, blood pressure, perspiration, and shallow breathing (McCay, 1984; Trychin, 1986b). Stress management training programs have been developed for persons with hearing loss. In those programs participants are shown how to recognize stressful situations related to their hearing loss and identify their physical and psychological reactions to these situations. They are taught strategies to manage stressful situations. Furthermore, they are taught relaxation procedures to cope with the physical and psychological responses they exhibit. Examples of programs that include training in stress management are Trychin (1986b), Jennings (1993) and Wayner and Abrahamson (1996).

SPECIAL CONSIDERATION

Patients who report many symptoms of stress attributable to their hearing impairment may benefit from a stress management course. Ideally, courses should be adapted to the specific needs of persons with hearing impairment. However, if such courses are not available, patients may be referred to any reputable stress management course offered in the community.

Personal Adjustment

Persons with hearing loss must learn to adapt and cope with their hearing loss in all aspects of their lives, including their physical safety, basic communication needs, affective and social relationships, work or vocational performances, and sporting and other leisure activities. The process of adaptation to hearing loss is still not well understood (Hyde & Riko, 1994). However, it is recognized that it may take several years before a person with an acquired hearing loss is able to adapt completely to the effects of their hearing loss and (re)develop functional life habits (Getty et al, 1995; Hétu, 1996; Hétu et al, 1990; Hyde & Riko, 1994; Jones et al, 1987).

Hearing loss is not simply a physical impairment. A comprehensive rehabilitative program must cater to all the consequences of hearing loss on the person's life. Persons with hearing loss may request help from their rehabilitative audiologist regarding various aspects of the adjustment process. Intervention in this area of rehabilitation may address many different domains of personal adjustment, including the person's behavioral, emotional, cognitive, physical, and interpersonal reactions to the hearing loss (Schum, 1994; Trychin, 1993). Interventions centered on issues related to aspects of personal adjustment should not be considered different (or distinct) from any other forms of rehabilitation services provided to persons with hearing loss.

A panoply of intervention approaches exists to address personal adjustment difficulties. Counseling, a term used to describe strategies designed to help patients adjust to specific or situational problems, is often used when referring to intervention approaches designed to address personal adjustment difficulties. Erdman (1993) provides an excellent review of counseling approaches that can be applied to rehabilitative audiology. Programs that specifically explore aspects of intervention related to personal adjustment among persons with hearing loss include Trychin (1986a, 1993), Jennings (1993), Trychin and Albright (1993), and Wayner and Abrahamson (1996).

Individual versus Group Intervention Programs

An important issue that has yet to be resolved empirically is whether audiological rehabilitation services are more effective when they are provided on an individual basis or when they are incorporated into a group intervention program. Current clinical practice favors the use of group intervention programs for services related to communication strategies, conversational fluency, assertiveness training, stress management, and personal adjustment. Several reasons may account for this tendency. First, group intervention programs are more time efficient because several participants receive services at once. Second, some intervention activities are more easily conducted within a group setting. For example, role-playing activities involving several participants can be easily completed in a group setting. Third, group sessions provide a relatively secure environment in which participants can practice newly acquired skills. An individual can practice a specific intervention strategy with other group members and with the audiologist. Fourth, groups provide excellent opportunities for discussions. They allow the participants to describe difficulties that they and other group members may encounter or that other members of the group may not have recognized as difficult situations. For example, a participant with hearing loss may express a feeling of insecurity when he or she is alone because of not always being able to hear the doorbell. Other participants with hearing loss may express a similar feeling, whereas still others, including participants without hearing loss (e.g., accompanying persons), may become aware that this situation is truly problematic for someone with hearing loss. Participants without hearing loss may learn that this difficulty is not unique to their communication partner. Another example would be a participant with normal

hearing who reports that he or she feels lonely because his or her social life has been severely curtailed on account of the partner's unwillingness to attend social gatherings because of his or her hearing loss. Again, participants with hearing loss and those without hearing loss may be able to relate this experience to their own situation.

In many societies a negative stigma is attached to persons who have a hearing impairment (e.g., cognitive limitations, old age, senility). The complex process of stigmatization associated with hearing loss is beyond the scope of the present chapter. Interested readers should refer to Hétu's (1996) excellent treatment of this topic. For the purpose of this discussion, suffice it to say that on learning (or acknowledging) that they have hearing loss, a person must reconstruct the image that one has of himself or herself. Hearing loss brings about changes in one's physiological system. More importantly, it changes one's perception of self and social identity. This process invariably leads to a diminishment of one's self-image and self-esteem. This is due not only to the stereotype that society holds of hearing loss but also because often the person's own view of hearing impairment, before learning of their hearing loss, is in many respects consistent with the negative image that society in general holds of hearing impairment. This often leads to feelings of guilt and shame. In some cases this process may lead to the development of maladaptive behaviors (e.g., denial, withdrawal, isolation, aggression) and it almost always, at least for some period of time, constitutes an obstacle to the person's ability to manage his or her rehabilitative needs.

The psychological literature has shown that group intervention programs constitute an effective approach to reconstructing one's self-image (de Gaulejac, 1996). Groups help the participants realize that they are not the only person to experience specific hearing disabilities and that their situation is not unique. Groups provide a forum to discuss feelings, behaviors, and problematic situations attributable to hearing impairment. Group discussions and activities can serve to explain and describe the causes and consequences of hearing impairment for the persons with hearing loss and for their communication partners. Also, groups offer opportunities to overcome one's feelings of ineptness in dealing with the problems they experience (initiate a process of normalization of one's social identity). For those reasons alone, group programs constitute an important intervention approach to certain aspects of rehabilitative audiology. That is not to say that in certain cases a person's rehabilitative needs may not be better served by an individual (one-to-one) or combined individual and group intervention program.

Group intervention programs should include a small number of persons (usually less than 12 participants) who share similar predicaments and rehabilitative needs. The participants with hearing loss do not necessarily need to be matched in degree or type of hearing loss. Groups should also involve the participation of persons who interact with the participants that have hearing impairment (i.e., accompanying persons including spouse and other family members, friends, relatives, coworkers). Activities should involve both the persons with hearing loss and their communication partners. In some cases activities can involve separating the participants into two groups, one consisting of persons with hearing loss, and the other consisting of the persons who accompany them. However, such activities should be kept to a minimum given that an important objective of group intervention programs is to allow both groups of participants to mutually inform each other of their experiences.

Group intervention programs typically run for 8 to 12 sessions in a term. Sessions are typically held once or twice a week, with assignments for home practice to be carried out between sessions. Each session would be approximately 60 to 90 minutes. Group programs may also be provided on a more intensive basis, such as in full-day or half-day sessions over a period of 1 or 2 weeks.

Group intervention programs may be organized in a comprehensive manner to provide a wide range of information and training to the participants. These programs may include information regarding hearing loss and devices, speechreading training, and communication-management training. Examples of this type of program include Getty and Hétu (1991), Hétu and Getty (1991), Jennings et al (1991), Spitzer et al (1993), and Wayner and Abrahamson (1996).

Communication Partners

In the audiological rehabilitation literature the term *communication partners* usually refers to all individuals who communicate on a regular basis with persons who have hearing loss (e.g., spouses, other family members, close friends, relatives, and colleagues). In recent years interest in involving communication partners in audiological rehabilitation programs has increased. This is equally so for individual and group intervention programs.

Many of the intervention programs designed for adults and elderly persons with acquired hearing loss address issues related to communication difficulties experienced in certain situations. Communication necessarily involves the participation of more than one person. Communication breakdowns attributable to hearing loss result in an experience that is less than satisfactory for all the persons involved in the exchange (i.e., the person with hearing loss and his or her communication partners) (Erber, 1996). As discussed in previous sections, strategies to avoid or overcome communication breakdowns can be used by both persons with hearing loss and their communication partners (e.g., expressive communication repair strategies).

Communication partners play an important role throughout the personal and emotional adjustment processes that persons with acquired hearing loss undergo as they adapt to their new life situation. In addition to being empathetic and supportive of their companion, communication partners may be invited to play an active role in the intervention program. For example, they may be asked to complete exercises or activities designed to improve communication between persons with hearing loss and the persons with whom they interact (see Erber, 1996; Tye-Murray & Schum, 1994). The participation of communication partners in an intervention program may facilitate the rehabilitation of their partners with hearing loss. Moreover, their involvement in an intervention program will make them (communication partners) more aware of some of the difficulties experienced by persons with hearing loss.

It has been documented that spouses and other communication partners may experience their own difficulties because of their interactions with persons who have hearing loss (Hétu et al, 1987; Hétu et al, 1993). For example, the fact that the person with hearing loss has to listen to the television at a very high volume may be very annoying to the other members of the household who do not have hearing loss. Or, always having to act as the "unofficial interpreter" at social gatherings may be burdensome for the spouse of a person with hearing loss. A couple's intimate and sexual relationship can suffer when one of the partners has hearing loss (Hétu et al, 1993). In sum, communication partners also experience difficulties associated with the fact that they interact with a person who has hearing loss. Those problems are legitimate and should not be neglected. Intervention programs in rehabilitative audiology should cater to the needs of those persons.

CONTROVERSIAL POINT

The contribution of communication partners in group intervention programs for persons with hearing impairment is unclear. In some settings communication partners are viewed mainly as a resource person to assist individuals with hearing impairment overcome difficulties they experience. However, the literature has shown that communication partners may be candidates for rehabilitation services in their own right. Comprehensive rehabilitation programs should cater to the specific needs of communication partners.

FOUNDATIONS OF AUDIOLOGICAL REHABILITATION

Definitions

Many definitions of rehabilitative audiology exist (Table 18–10). Some of those definitions describe the activities that comprise intervention (treatment) programs associated with rehabilitative audiology (see ASHA, 1984). Others define audiological rehabilitation as a process that aims primarily to resolve the communication disabilities experienced by persons with hearing loss (Hull, 1982; McCarthy & Culpepper, 1987). Still others define the goal of rehabilitative audiology as the alleviation (or minimization) of handicaps created by hearing impairment (Erdman, 1993; Gagné, 1998; McKenna, 1987; Ross, 1997). Generally, those definitions are based on the respective authors' theoretical orientation toward rehabilitation. Since the 1970s dramatic changes have taken place in the way rehabilitation in general (and rehabilitative audiology in particular) has been conceptualized. This section will outline a contemporary conceptual model of audiological rehabilitation.

Models of Rehabilitative Audiology

In all disciplines that involve the use and application of knowledge, the way in which a concept is conceived has an influence on how the available information is applied to the

TABLE 18–10 Examples of definitions of rehabilitative audiology

Hull (1982, p. 6):

"Aural rehabilitation is an attempt at reducing the barriers to communication resulting from hearing impairment, and facilitating adjustment relative to the possible psychosocial, occupational and educational impact of that auditory deficit."

ASHA (1984, p. 37):

"Aural rehabilitation refers to services and procedures for facilitating adequate receptive and expressive communication in individuals with hearing impairment."

Erdman (1993, p. 374):

"The ultimate goal of rehabilitative audiology is to facilitate adjustment to the auditory and nonauditory consequences of hearing impairment."

McKenna (1987, p. 5):

"Ultimately the aim of rehabilitation must be the restoration of the individual to as high a level of functioning as possible."

McCarthy and Culpepper (1987, p. 305):

"The purpose of an aural rehabilitation program is to focus on assisting hearing-impaired individuals in the realization of their optimal potential in communication, which is needed in educational, vocational, or social settings."

Ross (1997, p. 19):

Aural rehabilitation … "it includes, …, any device, procedure, information interaction, or therapy which lessens the communicative and psychosocial consequences of a hearing loss."

Gagné (1999, p. 70):

"The goal of audiological rehabilitation is to eliminate or reduce the situations of handicap experienced by individuals who have a hearing impairment and by persons with normal hearing who interact with those individuals."

discipline. A conceptual model provides a framework that is used to organize, describe, and investigate various elements of knowledge and factors related to a concept of interest. Hyde and Riko (1994) argue that one important function of conceptual models is to provide precise and comprehensive definitions of concepts and domains. They state that, "terminology is more than labels; it reflects and affects its underlying constructs and it provides the vehicle for debate and research" (Hyde & Riko, 1994, p. 347). Moreover, models guide the way clinical services are dispensed to persons who seek these services. Conceptual models are rarely static; they evolve over time. As elements of the concept are investigated, a better understanding of the general model is developed and refinements are made to the original model or the model is rejected and replaced by other more comprehensive models.

Not unlike other disciplines, research and clinical services in audiological rehabilitation are model-driven. Over the years, our conception of rehabilitation has evolved and the practice of audiological rehabilitation has been greatly influenced by this evolution. It has been recognized (the pioneers of our discipline might say "rediscovered") that audiological rehabilitation must involve more than fitting patients with appropriate amplification devices, in some cases complemented by hearing aid orientation information and sometimes supplemented by speechreading and auditory training sessions.

Professionals and academics recognize the need to provide more comprehensive (global) services to their patients. A greater awareness exists of the effects of hearing impairment on communication and on other aspects of life (including the impacts made on persons with normal hearing who interact with individuals who have hearing loss). Since the early 1970s, several models of service delivery in rehabilitative audiology have been proposed. Most noteworthy for their contribution to the development of rehabilitation services provided to persons with acquired hearing loss are the models proposed by Sanders (1971), Goldstein and Stephens (1981), Giolas (1982), Sanders (1982), Alpiner (1987), McKenna (1987), Hyde and Riko (1994), and Erber (1996). Each of these authors presents a model of service delivery that is unique and consistent with their views of rehabilitative audiology. All these models are similar in that they insist on the need for a systematic approach to the delivery of services in audiological rehabilitation. In general, the approaches consist of a process that includes procedures to evaluate the patient's competencies and needs, the selection of an intervention strategy designed to respond to those needs, an implementation of the intervention program retained, and a postintervention evaluation. On the basis of the results of the postintervention evaluation, patients are either discharged or encouraged to pursue the same or different rehabilitation objectives. One important contribution of those service delivery models is that they differentiate the acts of intervention (treatment services, such as the use of amplification, speech-perception training, or communication management training) from the process of rehabilitation programs (assessment, intervention, evaluation). Conceptually, this was an important advancement in the evolution of the profession.

The WHO Classification System

In the 1980s a concerted effort was begun to develop a generic conceptual model of rehabilitation that would be accepted internationally and that would apply to all forms of rehabilitation services, regardless of the discipline. A main objective of the World Health Organization Classification (WHO, 1980) scheme was to propose definitions for concepts that could be used by all professionals involved in rehabilitation. Specifically, the WHO (1980) classification scheme of rehabilitation is based on the concepts of impairment, disability, and handicap. These concepts are well defined and have guided our interpretation of what rehabilitation is; what the goal of rehabilitation services ought to be; and how rehabilitation services should be conceived, organized and dispensed.

Table 18–11 provides a definition of impairment, disability, and handicap provided by WHO (1980). The following example illustrates how these three concepts apply to audiological rehabilitation. A loss of external hair cells in the cochlea is an example of an *auditory impairment*. A person's inability to hear speech normally because of an auditory impairment would constitute a *hearing disability*. The person's inability to perform activities considered normal for the society (such as communicating by telephone) would be considered a *handicap*. It is important to recognize that the progression from impairment to disability and handicap is not always simple. An impairment may not always cause a disability, and a disability does not necessarily cause a handicap (Hyde & Riko, 1994). The types and extent of the handicaps experienced by two persons with the same type and degree of hearing loss and similar hearing disabilities may differ. For example, reduced sound localization abilities in noise (a disability) may be very handicapping for a person who works outdoors on noisy construction sites and who must attend appropriately to the warning signals placed on mobile equipment. The same disability (reduced sound localization) may not constitute a handicap for another person who works in a quiet business office and whose responsibilities do not require the localization of sounds. Also, two persons with different degrees of disability may experience a similar handicap. For example, the construction worker cited above may have a moderately severe hearing loss and his colleague may have a

severe hearing loss. Yet, both workers may experience a similar handicap on the construction site. Stephens and Hétu (1991) described how the concepts of impairment, disability, and handicap apply to rehabilitative audiology.

CONTROVERSIAL POINT

As it relates to audiological rehabilitation, at present, a universal consensus on the definition of the terms disability and handicap does not exist. Professionals in Europe tend to rely on the WHO (1980) classification system. In the United States some professionals adhere to definitions provided by WHO, whereas others prefer the definitions recognized by AHSA (1981). The differences in the definitions proposed by those two bodies are not trivial. We favor the WHO classification system (and its recently adopted revisions—WHO, 1997) especially as it relates to the elaboration of conceptual models of rehabilitation.

The WHO classification system and its adaptation to audiological rehabilitation is helpful in defining the goal of audiological rehabilitation. Audiological rehabilitation rarely addresses the domain of hearing impairment. That is, audiological rehabilitation services for a person with a sensorineural hearing loss do not focus on eliminating or reducing that person's hearing impairment (i.e., the person's hearing loss will not change as a result of rehabilitation services). Some aspects of rehabilitation programs are designed to reduce or eliminate hearing disabilities. For example, wearing hearing aids may help the person understand speech under several communicative conditions (i.e., in quiet and noisy environments). Speechreading training programs are designed to enhance audiovisual speech-perception performance in a variety of communicative settings. In some instances intervention programs in audiological rehabilitation address specific situations of handicap. For example, some patients consult an audiologist because they experience difficulties in performing certain specific activities that have a direct impact on their everyday living activities (e.g., responding appropriately when the doorbell rings, conversing with clients on the

---

TABLE 18–11 WHO (1980) definition of impairment, disability, and handicap

> An *impairment* refers to:
> "any loss or an abnormality of a psychological, or anatomical structure or function."
>
> A *disability* refers to:
> "any restriction or inability (resulting from an impairment) to perform an activity in the manner or within the range considered normal for a human being."
>
> A *handicap* refers to:
> "any disadvantage for a given individual, resulting from an impairment or a disability, that limits or prevents the fulfillment of a role that is normal (depending on age, sex, and social and cultural factors) for that individual."

telephone). In those cases the intervention program may focus on addressing the patient's specific handicaps that are attributable to hearing loss. Also, professionals may choose to focus an intervention program on certain specific activities that are deemed important by their patient. For example, a person may report having difficulty adapting to a new work environment. Hence, the intervention program may be designed to solve specific problems that manifest themselves in that particular environment.

Recently, the Canadian Society for the International Classification of Impairment, Disabilities and Handicaps (CSI-CIDH, 1991) proposed a refinement to the WHO's (1980) definition of handicap. This was done to clarify the distinction between the concepts of disability and handicap. The revised definition clearly identifies the role of the environment in the production of a handicap. As illustrated by Figure 18–3, a *handicap* is the situational result of an interactive process between two sets of causes: (1) the characteristics of the person's impairments and disabilities resulting from disease or trauma, and (2) the characteristics of the environment that create social or physical obstacles in a given situation. According to this definition, depending on the environmental obstacles they face, persons with an impairment may or may not experience a situation of handicap. Recently, the WHO (1997) revised their classification system for impairments, disabilities, and handicaps. The revised model (WHO, 1997) is consistent with the framework proposed by the CSICIDH (1991).

Noble and Hétu (1994) described an ecological model of hearing disability and handicap. Within this framework, a handicap occurs as the result of an interaction between a person's reduced hearing abilities and the auditory demands of a given situation. According to these authors, it is inappropriate to use the term *hearing handicap*. Rather, it is important to refer to certain difficulties that are experienced because of hearing disability as a *situation of handicap*. That is, a handicap must always be defined as a function of the context (the environment) in which a disability manifests itself. Within an ecological framework, a person with hearing loss may (or may not) experience a handicap, depending on the auditory abilities required for a given task and the environment (physical and sociocultural context) in which those auditory abilities are required. For example, a person with hearing impairment and his or her spouse may have no difficulty conversing when they are alone in their living room and the room is quiet and well lit. However, those two persons may experience difficulty conversing during dinner when they, and their three children, are at the dinner table and there is a lot of interefering noise from the clanging of cutlery and dishes or other ongoing conversations among the children. Thus *a situation of handicap is always defined as a function of the characteristics of the persons involved and a given context*.

Individuals with normal hearing may also experience situations of handicap because of the hearing disabilities of the persons with whom they interact in certain situations. For example, a person with hearing loss may choose to increase the volume of the television to understand it adequately. In some regards, this action may constitute an effective strategy to overcome the difficulties experienced by that person in that situation. However, that solution may create a situation of handicap for the persons that share the same living quarters (e.g., the spouse). Specifically, the normal hearing spouse may experience a situation of handicap because the increased

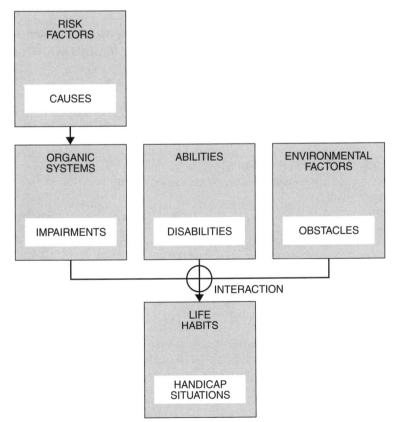

Figure 18–3 The handicap creation process as defined by the Canadian Society for the International Classification of Impairments, Disabilities and Handicaps. (Reprinted from CSICDH [1991], p.13, with permission.)

---

volume level of the television prevents that person from conversing with a friend in the adjoining dining room. However, under similar circumstances, the spouse may not experience a situation of handicap if he (or she) is engaged in an activity that is not perturbed by the sound of the television (i.e., completing a puzzle in a room that is located at the other end of the house). In sum, it is more appropriate to refer to problems associated with hearing loss as situations of handicap than to refer to them as a hearing handicap.

The concept of *situation of handicap* derived from the WHO (1980) conceptual framework of rehabilitation (and modifications thereof) has important ramifications on how audiological rehabilitation services are conceived and organized. The goal of rehabilitative audiology may be defined *as the provision of services designed to reduce or eliminate situations of handicap that are attributable to hearing disabilities experienced by one of the persons involved in the problematic situation.*

The Influence of a Person's Predicament and the Environment in Defining Situations of Handicap

As defined by CSICIDH (1991), several factors may be involved in creating a situation of handicap. Those factors can be grouped under two broad categories: factors related to the individual and his or her characteristics (predicament) and factors related to the environment and its characteristics. According to Hyde and Riko (1994) a *predicament* can be defined as the sum of all pertinent aspects of patient state, including disorders, impairments and disabilities, and the person's resources, beliefs, perceptions, attitudes, aptitudes, lifestyle, and behaviors. Two persons with the same hearing impairment and hearing disabilities may experience a different situation of handicap in the same environment. This implies that factors associated with the individual, beyond those related to hearing impairment and hearing disabilities, have an influence on the production of a situation of handicap. For example, in a given situation a person who is shy and introverted may experience difficulties that are quantitatively and qualitatively different from a person who is outspoken and self-confident. The important point being made here is that every individual is unique. The sum of all the personal factors related to that individual contributes to determining whether a problem exists because of hearing loss

and the extent to which the problem will have a deleterious effect on the individual.

The difficulties experienced by a person with hearing loss may also vary according to the environment. A person with hearing loss may experience difficulties conversing with a partner in a noisy restaurant but not experience any difficulty when conversing with the same person in a quiet, well-lit living room. Thus the physical environment is a key factor in defining what constitutes a situation of handicap. Excessive background noise levels, reverberation, and poor lighting conditions are examples of environmental conditions that have been identified as factors that can contribute to the creation of a situation of handicap. However, within the context of an ecological model of rehabilitation, the social and cultural milieu are also considered environmental factors that may contribute to the production of a situation of handicap. That is, the shared beliefs, attitudes, norms, and behaviors that are held by a group of individuals will also have an influence on the creation of a situation of handicap. A simple example will serve to demonstrate this point. In most American religious communities, asking a Pastor to repeat a misunderstood statement may be acceptable during an informal conversation on the staircase of the church. However, the same repair strategy (asking for a repetition) would not be acceptable during a formal worship ceremony held inside the church. Thus defining the environment (physical and sociocultural) in which difficulties occur is also a key concept in identifying a situation of handicap. Moreover, it is a key step in identifying solutions that can be applied and would be acceptable to resolve specific situations of handicap. The important point to be made here is that the context in which a problem exists will depend not only on the individuals involved and their predicaments but also on the environment in which those problems are experienced. To truly capture the impact of a handicap experienced by a person it is necessary to describe and to define the specific environment in which a problem manifests itself.

A recognition that the goal of audiological rehabilitation is to alleviate situations of handicap and that intervention programs based on this premise must consider all the relevant aspects of the patient's predicament and the specific context in which a handicapping situation is experienced, has many implications for the way that rehabilitation services should be conceived, organized, and provided. Some of those implications are presented in Table 18–12.

Rehabilitation as a Process

It is recognized that rehabilitation is a process that takes place over a long time (Erdman, 1993; Gagné et al, 1995; Hétu & Getty, 1991; Hyde & Riko, 1994; Sanders, 1982; Schum, 1994). Rehabilitation does not occur only during the limited period of time during which the patient takes part in a structured audiological rehabilitation program. Recent investigations have shown that a person's awareness of having hearing difficulties and the impact of the impairment on the person's life is part of a process that evolves from the time the hearing impairment is acknowledged to the time when the individual has reached an optimal restoration of his or her normal life habits (Getty et al, 1995; Hétu, 1996; Hyde & Riko, 1994). This process may extend over a period of several years. During

TABLE 18–12 **Implications for intervention programs on the basis of the premise that the goal of audiological rehabilitation is to alleviate situations of handicap**

- An important component of all intervention programs should be to identify and describe, in a precise manner, the situations in which specific difficulties arise because one of the individuals involved in that situation has hearing loss.

- All the factors that may contribute to the production of a situation of handicap must be identified, including the factors related to the predicaments of the persons involved and the factors related to the environment in which the situation of handicap occurs.

- Persons who have normal hearing may also experience situations of handicap because someone in their environment has hearing loss. Those individuals may be candidates for audiological rehabilitation services.

- A very personal and "subjective" dimension is present in what constitutes a situation of handicap. Thus a situation of handicap can only be described and defined by the persons who are involved in that situation. That is, *capturing the individuals' perspective and perception of the problem is essential to the intervention process.*

- The major focus of intervention services must be placed *on real-life situations.* Accordingly, *objectives of intervention programs must be individualized and contextualized.*

- Each situation of handicap is unique. Hence, the solution to each problem must also be unique and adapted to the persons and the context in which difficulties are experienced.

- Solutions to hearing difficulties generally include more than the individual with hearing impairment. Hence, the participants in an intervention program should include all the persons who are involved in, and committed to, resolving the targeted situation of handicap. That is, the description of the situation of handicap and the possible solutions to the difficulties experienced must take into account the perspectives of all the persons involved in the intervention program.

- Possible solutions to problems must to take into account the uniqueness of each situation of handicap and identify solutions that are possible, and acceptable, for all the persons involved in the intervention program.

- The clinician and the other participants must be involved in identifying and selecting the intervention strategy that is most likely to succeed in resolving the targeted situation of handicap. The intervention strategy retained must take into account the predicaments of all the participants and the context in which the situation of handicap occurs. Furthermore, only those solutions that are acceptable to all the participants should be considered as possible intervention strategies. This implies that for each intervention program, the solution retained as an intervention strategy must be negotiated with the participants.

- Generic intervention programs (such as wearing hearing aids or participation in a communication-management training program) constitute potential intervention strategies that may be applied to resolve targeted situations of handicap. However, the goal of an intervention program must center on resolving the situations of handicap experienced by the participants and not on the application of (or compliance with) the intervention strategy per se.

- Only the persons who experience a targeted situation of handicap are able to describe what would constitute a satisfactory outcome (for them!) as a result of taking part in an intervention program.

that period of time, a person's perception and description of the problems encountered because of the hearing loss, and their reactions to those problems, evolve (Hétu, 1996). Moreover, a person's predicament (including auditory demands, beliefs, resources, attitudes, aptitudes, behaviors, perceptions, and lifestyle) also changes as a function of time. Intervention programs must recognize this evolutionary process of rehabilitation. Moreover, those programs must cater to the

specific problems expressed by the individual at a given point in time during this process of rehabilitation.

A recognition that rehabilitation is a process implies that solutions to problems associated with hearing loss are not likely to be solved by a one-shot intervention program such as wearing hearing aids or participating in a communication management program. The rehabilitation needs of patients change as a function of time. Their ability to manage problematic situations also changes as a function of time. At any given time during the process of rehabilitation, a proposed intervention strategy may or may not be acceptable to a patient. The acceptability of an intervention strategy is closely linked to the patient's predisposition in terms of the process of rehabilitation. Typically, early in the process of rehabilitation patients will more readily comply with intervention strategies that are not intrusive to their communication partners (e.g., they will agree to wear a hearing aid, use auxiliary aids at home, use visual cues (speechreading) to optimize their speech-perception competencies, use receptive communication strategies). Later on, sometimes years later, the patient may be able and willing to apply intervention strategies that require the cooperation of others (i.e., informing the communication partner that he or she has hearing loss and asking others to use clear speech or other specific expressive communication repair strategies; requesting preferential seating at a restaurant or theater).

PITFALL

Both for the clinician and the patient, it is unrealistic to imagine that all the rehabilitative needs of a person with acquired hearing loss can be met within one intervention program. Rehabilitation is a process that extends over a long period of time and the rehabilitative needs of patients evolve as a function of time. Every intervention program should be confined to resolving specific situations of handicap that are reported by the patients at the time they consult for rehabilitation services.

In selecting an intervention strategy to resolve a situation of handicap, consideration must be given to solutions that are possible and acceptable to the patient. That is, professionals must take into account the patient's predisposition in terms of the process of rehabilitation. To comply with this principle of rehabilitation, all the components of an intervention program must be openly discussed and negotiated with the patient. Intervention programs that fail to respect this condition of intervention are not likely to succeed. Experimental data or clinical experience may suggest that a given intervention strategy is well suited to overcome specific hearing disabilities. However, if the patient is not able or willing to implement this strategy to address the situation of handicap under consideration, that strategy should not be incorporated into the intervention program. Patients are not likely to participate in an intervention program that does not cater to their specific needs. Also, they are unlikely to implement solutions that are retained as intervention strategies if they are not comfortable with those strategies. A failure to respect these conditions of intervention may lead the patient to withdraw from the rehabilitation program altogether.

Rehabilitation as a Solution-Centered Intervention Process

In an earlier section it was stated that the goal of rehabilitative audiology is to reduce or eliminate situations of handicap that are attributable to hearing disabilities experienced by one of the persons involved in the problematic situations. The implication of this perspective on intervention programs was discussed. Given this perspective and consistent with the acknowledgment that rehabilitation is a process, intervention programs in rehabilitative audiology can be viewed as a solution-centered problem-solving process (Erdman, 1993; Gagné, 1998; Gagné et al, 1995; Gagné et al, 1998; Hyde & Riko, 1994; McKenna, 1987). As it relates to intervention programs in rehabilitative audiology, the general sequence of events involved in problem-solving are outlined in Table 18–13.

For this problem-solving process to be successful and relevant, it is essential that the patient participate in all aspects of the intervention program. Specifically, the patient must be involved in the recognition, identification, and description of the situations of handicap encountered; the negotiation and definition of the objectives of the intervention program; the identification, selection, and implementation of the intervention strategy; the definition of the desired outcome (including the criteria used to evaluate the success of the intervention program); the identification of the factors (positive and negative) that contributed to the outcome; and the evaluation of the effects, impacts, and consequences of the intervention program.

A solution-centered problem-solving approach to intervention incorporates a phenomenological dimension (Erdman, 1993; Gagné et al, 1995). Consideration of the patient's *perspective* is essential to capture the personal meaning of the experience of hearing difficulties, identify potential ways to solve the problems, and evaluate the process and success of the negotiated intervention program. The procedures used to obtain this information must make it possible for the patient to provide his or her perception of all the facets of the intervention program. The most effective method to achieve these goals is to use open-ended interviews.

PEARL

The more a person is involved in the definition of the objective, the implementation, and the evaluation of his or her intervention program, the more likely it is that the program will correspond to the person's rehabilitative needs. Also, increasing a person's involvement in all aspects of the management of his or her intervention program will increase the likelihood that the intervention program will be successful.

Perhaps the most critical components of a solution-centered problem-solving approach to intervention consist of identifying as precisely as possible the situation of handicap to be addressed by the intervention program and defining the specific objectives of the program. A thorough understanding

TABLE 18–13 General sequence of events that apply to problem solving in audiological rehabilitation

1. Recognize that a problem exists.

2. Identify the problem.

3. Describe the problem (analyze the situation).

4. Set objectives and define desired outcome taking into account:

   - The problem (i.e., the situation of handicap)
   - The predicament of the person with hearing loss
   - The predicaments of the other persons involved in the situation of handicap
   - The environment (physical and social context) in which the situation of handicap occurs

5. Identify possible solutions.

6. For each solution identified, analyze and evaluate the implications of choosing that solution (in terms of potential benefits, feasibility, and acceptability).

7. Select one (or more) acceptable solution(s).

8. Implement the solution(s).

9. Evaluate the effects of applying the solution(s) (regarding outcome, impacts, and consequences).

10. Identify the factors that facilitated, or constituted an impediment to, the implementation of the solution(s).

Adapted from Gagné et al (1998).

of the problem encountered by the patient(s) in a given environment (i.e., a situation of handicap) will enable the clinician and all the other participants to clearly identify the objective of the intervention program. As mentioned previously, the description of a situation of handicap can only be provided by the persons involved in that situation. The clinician's role is to ensure that all the dimensions of the situation of handicap have been identified. On the basis of this information the specific objective of the intervention program can be formulated. McKenna (1987) provided a useful framework for defining the objectives of an intervention program in audiological rehabilitation. According to the author, each specific objective should state clearly (in an unambiguous fashion and in quantifiable terms) how the participants will behave if the intervention program is successful. Some essential components of defining the objective of an intervention program are provided in Table 18–14.

Once defined, the objective of the intervention program constitutes a form of agreement (i.e., a contract) among the clinician and the participants. The objective states who will do what and under what circumstance. Also, it specifies the time frame for the implementation of the intervention strategy. Objectives that are well defined will help the participants (including the clinician) identify possible solutions that could

TABLE 18–14 Defining the objective of an intervention program (based on McKenna, 1987)

The process of defining a specific objective should:

1. Include all the individuals involved in the pursuit of the objective.

2. Define the role and responsibilities of each person involved in the intervention program.

3. Describe the conditions under which the stated objective will be accomplished (personalized and customized according to the expressed needs, willingness, and capabilities of each participant).

4. Specify the criteria that will be used to evaluate whether the objective has been reached (i.e., the outcome measure).

5. Provide a time frame within which the objective should be reached.

TABLE 18–15   Example of an intervention objective according to the criteria described by McKenna (1987)

> Mr. King and his poker partners will use appropriate repair strategies whenever a communication breakdown occurs during their weekly card-playing evening. As a result of an 8-week communication management program, in which Mr. King and all of his partners will participate, Mr. King will be able to understand the messages intended for him after no more than two repair strategies have been provided to him.

be implemented to attain the objectives. An example of an objective formulated according to the criteria specified by McKenna (1987) is provided in Table 18–15.

Evaluating the outcome of the intervention program is a critical component of a problem-solving approach to rehabilitation. That is, once the intervention component of the program has been completed, it is important to evaluate whether the objective of the program has been met. Clearly defined objectives will greatly facilitate outcome evaluation. A component of problem solving that is often overlooked is the evaluation of the process, impacts, and consequences of the intervention program. Throughout an intervention program, and especially at the conclusion of the program, time should be taken to evaluate the process of the intervention program. For example, the clinician and the participants should discuss the frequency and the duration of individual sessions, the length of the intervention program, and the nature of the activities included in the program. Information regarding these and other aspects of the intervention process may provide the clinician and the participants with useful insights concerning the application of specific intervention strategies. Also, it may suggest modifications that could be implemented to existing intervention strategies to make them more effective and appropriate for solving certain situations of handicap.

Almost always, participation in an intervention program has some impacts and consequences that are not directly related to the objective or the outcome of the program. The impacts and consequences of taking part in an intervention program may be positive or negative. For example, Mrs. Smith may participate in an intervention program to learn communication strategies that could be used to solve problems she encounters during family gatherings. Later, she may report having used those same strategies (successfully) in other settings (e.g., during business meetings). Mr. Jones reports that he has difficulty understanding coworkers in the lunch room. The negotiated intervention strategy (i.e., asking his colleagues to face him when they speak to him) has proven to be very successful in terms of the stated objective of the program (i.e., when he applies the strategy, he does not have any difficulty understanding his coworkers). However, the implementation of this strategy has had a negative impact (e.g., revealing to his colleagues that he has difficulty understanding speech because of hearing loss). As a consequence, he has to bear the brunt of all the jokes about persons with hearing loss (deaf persons), and he finds this very demeaning. The important point to be retained from these examples is that the evaluation of an intervention program should extend beyond the measurement of outcome. An evaluation of the impacts and consequences of an intervention program is essential to evaluate the patient's satisfaction with the treatment.

This information also provides a more comprehensive evaluation of the effectiveness of an intervention program. Data concerning the possible impacts and consequences of an intervention program can be used by the clinician and the patient to evaluate the advantages and disadvantages of implementing a given intervention strategy. This information may serve to modify or adapt intervention programs for other patients who experience similar situations of handicap.

The implementation of a solution-centered problem-solving approach to rehabilitation represents a major change from traditional approaches to rehabilitation. First, the relationship between the clinician and the participants is altered. In traditional rehabilitation programs the clinician assumes the role of the "expert." The "expert" diagnoses the problems, informs the patient of the causes and the consequences of the problems, selects an intervention strategy judged to be appropriate to "fix the patient's problem," and informs and trains the patient in the application of the intervention strategy retained. Often, the clinician decides when to terminate the intervention program (of course the preceding description of the clinician is a complete caricature). In a solution-centered problem-solving approach to rehabilitation, during the course of an intervention program, the role of the expert is often assumed by the patient (who else can truly describe the situation of handicap, express the desired outcome, determine which of the possible intervention strategies is acceptable, and evaluate the success of the intervention program?). Throughout most of the intervention program the clinician and the participants are equal partners with a common goal: identifying solutions to situations of handicap. As mentioned earlier, the involvement of the participants is essential in all phases of the intervention program. Second, the selection of an intervention strategy is negotiated between the clinician and the participants, and it is always guided by the objective of the program. That is, the intervention strategy retained, whether novel or generic, must always be tailored to the specific objective of the program.

Third, and perhaps most important, the focus of the intervention program is shifted. Often, the implicit goal of many rehabilitation programs is to solve the problems experienced by the person with hearing loss. The source of the problem is deemed to be the hearing loss. The focus of the rehabilitation program is on the disabilities of the patient and the responsibility of overcoming the problems rests with the person with hearing loss. In a solution-centered problem-solving approach to rehabilitation the focus is placed on resolving a situation of handicap (it is the situation that is problematic, not the person with hearing loss). This change in perspective has implications for intervention. Solutions to problems must consider changes that can be made to the environment in which the situation of handicap occurs. Also, possible solutions should consider all the persons, including those individuals with no hearing disabilities, who are involved in the production of a situation of a handicap. Changing the perception of the rehabilitation process will serve to reestablish the role and responsibility of all the persons involved in a situation of handicap. It recognizes that the burden of solving a problem does not rest solely on the person with hearing loss (the consequences of this change in perception will most likely have a positive impact on the person's self-esteem). Also, it clearly indicates that other persons involved in that situation have a role in the production of a situation of handicap. Moreover, it offers those individuals an opportunity to participate in the resolution of problems that they may themselves experience in that situation.

Finally, two additional issues concerning the implementation of a solution-centered problem-solving approach will be addressed briefly. First, an intervention program will rarely include only one objective. Generally, patients will be able to identify several situations of handicap that they encounter in their daily lives. A given intervention program may include more than one objective. However, to attend appropriately to each of the objectives selected, the number of objectives retained should be limited. Typically, an intervention program will be comprised of two or three objectives. However, this may vary considerably depending on the patient's predicament, the nature of the situations of handicap, the clinician's competency and motivation, and the amount of time available to provide rehabilitation services. The negotiated objectives must be realistic and there should be indications that those objectives can be reached within the time period established for the intervention program. In this regard the clinician's role in negotiating objectives for an intervention program is critical.

It is best to select objectives that can be attained within a period of 3 months. Objectives that would require a longer period of intervention should be broken down into smaller components that can be evaluated within this time frame. Once the period of time negotiated to attain an objective has been reached, an evaluation of the process, outcome, impacts, and consequences of the intervention program should be conducted. On the basis of the results of the evaluation, the initial objective may be redefined (if the goal was not reached), other objectives may be pursued, or the patient may decide to suspend his participation in a structured intervention program.

Second, patients should learn to implement the problem-solving process independently. This could be included as one of the negotiated objectives of an intervention program (with the approval of the patient, of course). The process of problem solving is systematic, fairly simple to learn, and it can be applied to all problematic situations. Patients can be taught the different steps and the sequence involved in problem solving. They can be trained on how to address each component of this process. Initially, the clinician may play a more active role in the implementation of the process. Gradually, patients should be encouraged to implement the sequence of problem solving themselves, first with the support of the clinician and eventually independently. With some guidance and training most patients will be able to apply the problem-solving process by themselves. In doing so, they will become much more independent in managing their own rehabilitation process.

PEARL

The principles and application of a problem-solving process are simple and can be applied to all problematic situations. Most patients can learn to apply the process of problem solving to resolve problems they encounter in their everyday lives. In doing so, they will become more proficient at managing their rehabilitative needs.

CASE PRESENTATION

The final section of this chapter will illustrate how a solution-centered problem-solving process can be applied to rehabilitative audiology. This will be accomplished in the form of a fictitious case presentation.

Background Information

Five years ago, C.D., a 50-year-old man, had bilateral hearing loss develop over a period of approximately 6 weeks. His hearing loss was attributed to a virus. Initially, the hearing loss was profound. Gradually, over a period of 6 months, his hearing sensitivity improved slightly. Since then, C.D.'s audiograms have been stable and indicate that he has severe hearing loss bilaterally. Audiological test results indicate that he has poor auditory-word recognition abilities in quiet in both ears. Within 2 months of acquiring his hearing loss, C.D. was fitted binaurally with behind-the-ear hearing aids. Both aids are equipped with a t-coil and a direct audio input. Also, he owns an FM system that he uses primarily for meetings at work. C.D. has not been able to use a telephone successfully, even with auxiliary devices. He relies on the use of a TTY, E-mail, and fax for distance communication, both at home and at work.

C.D. actively participated in audiological rehabilitation programs for a period of 2 years after the onset of his hearing loss. Those programs consisted of hearing aid orientation, individualized speech-perception training, and communication-management training. C.D.'s wife has been very supportive throughout the process of rehabilitation. She was actively involved in the rehabilitation programs. Also, since the onset of his hearing loss, C.D. participates in a support group for individuals with sudden hearing loss.

C.D. is employed by a large consulting firm in computer applications. His employer and coworkers are aware of C.D.'s hearing loss. In fact, he was given a 1-year disability leave at the time he acquired his hearing loss. When he returned to work, his ability to perform his regular duties were reassessed and he was informed that he could resume his previous position within the company. Primarily, his responsibilities involved debugging commercial software application programs.

C.D. contacted his rehabilitation audiologist 3 years after he had completed his previous intervention program. He reported that he had recently been promoted to a new position within the company. The position involved working in a team of six professionals, serving clients both on-site and off-site.

Description of the Situation of Handicap

Discussions with the clinician revealed that C.D.'s new position involved regular team meetings both with and without clients. Those meetings often centered around very technical aspects of computer applications and the information discussed was essential for C.D. to do his work. C.D. was concerned because frequently he was not able to follow the discussion in those meetings. Recently, he failed to complete work that was given to him because he was unaware that he had been assigned those tasks. When asked to describe specific instances in which he experienced problems because of his hearing difficulties, C.D. identified two different situations in which he had problems: (1) during the team's weekly meeting, and (2) when he met with clients in their workplace. It was decided that initially the intervention program would focus on resolving the situation of handicap experienced during the team's weekly meetings.

C.D. was asked to identify the possible causes for the difficulties experienced during the weekly meetings. Specifically, he was asked to consider (1) factors related to himself, (2) factors related to the other members of the team who took part in the meetings, and (3) factors related to the environment in which the meetings were held. During discussions with the clinician, several possible causes for the difficulties experienced were identified for each of the three factors. With regard to himself, C.D. reported that his speechreading abilities had "slipped" somewhat over the years. He found it difficult to speechread in a group that involved six or more participants. Also, he observed that the meetings were held late in the afternoon when he was tired. He believed that this made it more difficult for him to concentrate and follow the discussions.

Concerning the other members of the team, C.D. noted that his coworkers empathized with his situation. He remarked that they tried to be helpful because they realized that "a team's accomplishments are only as good as the sum of its members." However, he reported that they often forgot that he has hearing loss. Frequently, several persons would talk at the same time; most of the individuals forgot to let him know when they were the one talking; and some of the team members had weak voices yet didn't make an effort to speak up. C.D. stated that he used his FM system during the meetings, but he observed that his lapel microphone failed to pick up the voices of all the participants.

Concerning factors related to the environment, C.D. reported that the conference room was equipped with a long rectangular table. He sat on one side of the table, which made it difficult for him to see everyone around the table. He was aware that sitting at the end of the table would offer better speechreading opportunities but that place was taken by the team leader. C.D. also reported that there was a coffee machine in the conference room. Periodically, the machine generated noise, but the frequency of occurrence and the duration of the noise was unpredictable.

Negotiated Objective and Structure of the Intervention Program

When asked what his objective was in seeking rehabilitative services, C.D. reported that he would like to be able to follow the discussions perfectly during the meetings but stated that this was not a realistic goal. He added, "I guess my goal would be to communicate to my optimum level during the meetings." Discussions with the clinician focused on identifying a tangible indicator that could be used to measure whether he was communicating optimally during the meetings. The indicator retained was that C.D. would no longer miss completing tasks that were assigned to him during the meetings.

It was agreed that the first part of the intervention program would concentrate on identifying possible solutions for the difficulties C.D. encountered during the meetings. The second part of the program would be devoted to exploring and implementing the solutions retained. Furthermore, it was agreed that for those two components of the intervention program, C.D. and the clinician would meet twice weekly over a period of 1 month. Also, it was agreed that once the intervention strategies had been implemented, the overall success of the intervention program would be evaluated over a period of 3 months.

Intervention Program

C.D. was asked to identify possible strategies that could be used to improve his ability to understand conversations during the team meetings. The strategies identified by the clinician and C.D. are listed in Table 18–16. Discussions ensued on the potential benefit, feasibility, and acceptability of each of the strategies identified. Two strategies were discarded. First, the possibility of requesting that the meetings be held in another (more quiet) conference room was discussed. However, according to C.D., this request was not realistic because no other room was available for meetings in the building. Likewise, C.D. stated that no oval or round conference table was available. He rejected the idea of requesting that the company purchase a new conference table.

C.D. stated that he would continue to use his FM system during the meetings. Also, C.D. agreed that he would meet with his team leader to discuss the implementation of some of the other strategies identified. Specifically, he would (1) request that strategies involving the participation of the other team members be discussed during a team meeting, (2) request that he sit at the end of the conference table so that he could more easily speechread all the team members, (3) suggest that the coffee machine be moved to a different room, (4) investigate the possibility that the company would purchase a conference microphone for his FM system, (5) investigate the possibility that the company would purchase a computerized note-taking system.

Several sessions were devoted to preparing C.D. for his upcoming meetings with his team leader and his coworkers. For example, activities were designed to enable C.D. to describe to his coworkers the types of hearing disabilities and difficulties he experienced during team meetings. Ways of presenting this information in a factual, nonaccusatory fashion and without appearing to rely on self-pity or somehow diminishing his contribution to the group were discussed and practiced during sessions. Other activities were designed to identify approaches that could be used to solicit the active participation of his coworkers in implementing strategies that could be used by all team members during the weekly meetings (without appearing to be aggressive or accusatory and

TABLE 18–16 List of possible strategies identified to resolve the situation of handicap

Strategies related to the patient
- Sharpen speechreading skills
- Increase level of self-confidence and not hesitate to request a clarification when he has not understood
- Inform and remind other team members of his communication needs*
- Re-establish a set of communication rules that should be followed during the meetings*
- Always use his FM system during the meetings*
- Select/request a better place to sit in the conference room*

Strategies that involve the cooperation/participation of the other team members
- Follow the established communication rules
    - Only one person speaks at a time*
    - Talker signals that he is talking
- Use appropriate communication strategies
    - Look at C.D. when they talk*
    - Provide cueing for C.D. when necessary
    - Use clear-speech*
- Holding the meetings at an earlier time of the day when C.D. is less tired and it is easier for him to concentrate on the discussion at hand*

Strategies related to the physical environment
- Hold the meetings in a different (more quiet) conference room
- Alternately, remove the coffee machine from the conference room*
- Change present rectangular table for an oval or round table

Other possible solutions
- Replace the existing FM system microphone with a conference microphone*
- Make use of a computerized note-taking system

The asterisk (*) indicates strategies that were incorporated into the intervention program.

taking into account the personality of the team members and the dynamics of the group). Different communication-management strategies were identified. Ways that they could be integrated into the weekly team meetings were discussed. Also, approaches to providing feedback to his coworkers to reinforce their use of facilitating strategies were discussed and practiced. Many of the activities incorporated into this part of the intervention program were accomplished through role-playing activities; first with the clinician, and then with his spouse assuming the role of the team members. Also, the clinician guided C.D. on where to obtain information on a conference microphone for his FM system and a computerized note-taking system (addresses, costs, advantages/disadvantages of each system). Practice sessions were devoted to finding ways to present this information to his superiors at work.

After approximately 1 month of attending his rehabilitation sessions on a regular basis, C.D. met with his team leader. As a result of this meeting, the following actions were agreed on and initiated: (1) The team leader agreed to change seating positions with C.D. during the weekly meetings (he didn't see this as a big issue and he was unaware that sitting at the end of the conference table would be advantageous for C.D.). (2) Ways to improve the flow of information that would enable C.D. to understand better and participate more actively in the meetings would be discussed during an upcoming team meeting. The team leader would include an item on the meeting agenda that would be entitled *Optimizing communication flow within the group*. Furthermore, the team

leader would introduce the topic to the team members and ask C.D. to preside the discussion on this topic. (3) The team leader and C.D. agreed that the option of scheduling the meetings at an earlier time of the day would be discussed with the other group members. (4) The team leader would inquire about the possibility of relocating the coffee machine. This was done and within a week the coffee machine was moved to another room. (5) The team leader set up a meeting with the company's budget director, C.D., and himself. The purpose of the meeting was to discuss the possibility of acquiring a computerized note-taking system and a conference microphone for the FM system. The budget for the computerized note-taking system was not granted, but funds were made available to purchase a conference microphone. C.D. was responsible for ordering the microphone.

The group discussion on how to optimize communication during team meetings was held approximately 3 weeks after C.D. met with the team leader. During the meeting C.D. described to his coworkers some of the difficulties he encountered during team meetings because of his hearing loss. Many of the team members reported that they were aware that C.D. had hearing loss but that they did not realize that he had difficulty following group discussions, especially because he did so well during one-to-one conversations. According to them, overall, C.D.'s participation and performance during the team meetings did not seem to present any problems ("You seem to be doing so well!"). C.D. described the conference microphone and showed how it could be used during team meetings. It was agreed that team members would face C.D. when they spoke during meetings, they would speak clearly without overexaggerating their pronunciation, and only one person would speak at a time. Whenever those rules were not followed, it would be every team member's responsibility (including C.D.) to remind the group of the communication rules that were agreed on.

The team members agreed to hold the meetings in the morning rather than late in the afternoon. Also, everybody agreed that it would be helpful to have a written record of the topics discussed during the meetings. Those notes would specifically include a list of *actions* to be completed by each team member. It was decided that, on a rotating basis (excluding C.D.), one team member would take notes on a laptop computer. Immediately after the meeting, the notes would be sent to all team members via E-mail. Finally, it was agreed that this agenda item (optimizing communication during team meetings) would be rediscussed by the group in approximately 2 months.

After the initial series of regular sessions that took place during the first month of the intervention program, C.D. and the rehabilitation audiologist met on four different occasions. For each of those meetings, the primary topics of discussion were as follows: Session 1, postmortem of C.D.'s meeting with his team leader; Session 2, postmortem of C.D.'s meeting with the team members; Session 3, preparation for review meeting with team members that was held 2 months after the implementation of strategies to improve communication during team meetings; Session 4, postintervention evaluation of the intervention program with the rehabilitation audiologist.

Outcome, Impacts, and Consequences of the Intervention Program

Three months after the intervention program was initiated, C.D. met with the rehabilitation audiologist to evaluate the outcome, impacts, and consequences of the program. C.D. reported that overall the action plan established with his team members was beneficial. Related to the objective of the program, C.D. reported that he had not missed any assignments since the intervention program had been implemented. On the basis of those results, both C.D. and the rehabilitation audiologist agreed that the intervention program was successful. According to C.D., removing the coffee machine from the conference room, changing his seating position during meetings, and the fact that the meetings were changed to an earlier time during the day all contributed to the success of the program. The implementation of communication rules negotiated with his team members was somewhat successful. However, C.D. reported that not everybody always followed the rules. Also, the other team members did not always remind the "culprits" that they were contravening the established procedures. C.D. did not feel that he should be the only person to remind others of the agreement so he was not consistent in asking his teammates to follow the established procedures. C.D. always used his FM system and the conference microphone during the meetings. This proved to be of some help during the meetings.

C.D. reported that the single most beneficial component of the intervention program was the fact that a note-taking system was implemented. This strategy was extremely useful for C.D. because it provided him (in writing) with some of the important information he had missed during the meeting (in fact, it made C.D. realize how much information he missed during the meetings). During the team meeting devoted to evaluate the success of the communication rules established within the team, all the team members reported that they benefited personally from the note-taking system. The notes served as an archive for the discussions and decisions made during the meetings. Notes from previous meetings were often retrieved and used to remind the team members of past decisions and the rationale underlying those decisions. The team leader reported that the note-taking strategy had significantly improved the efficacy of the group meetings. As a result, he had incorporated this strategy with other groups that he coordinated.

Based on C.D.'s own admission, one negative impact of implementing the note-taking system was that he played a less active role during the meetings. Specifically, he was less attentive to the group discussions because he knew he could rely on the notes to obtain the important information. However, by doing so, he felt that he missed out on some of the details that were discussed during the meetings. Also, because he could rely on the notes, C.D. was not consistent in requesting that his coworkers use the communication rules whenever he did not follow what was being discussed during the meetings.

On the basis of the post-intervention evaluation, C.D. and the rehabilitation audiologist agreed that the intervention program would be pursued further. One aspect of the program would focus on improving the use of communication strategies during team meetings. Another aspect of the program would consider solutions to difficulties that C.D. encountered when he met with clients in their own offices.

CONCLUSIONS

The process of adapting to hearing loss is long, complex, and yet to be fully understood. Most adults and elderly persons with acquired hearing impairment could benefit from the expertise of rehabilitation audiologists to help facilitate this process of adaptation. In this chapter we have described some of the tools of rehabilitation (intervention strategies) that can be integrated into a comprehensive rehabilitation program (e.g., speech-perception training, communication-management training). Special consideration was given to the process of intervention (e.g., identifying situations of handicap, defining objectives, implementing intervention strategies, and evaluating the success of the program).

A solution-centered problem-solving approach to intervention was described. The approach is on the basis of a conceptual model of rehabilitation that is rooted in a belief that the goal of rehabilitative audiology is to assist patients in solving specific situations of their handicap that are attributable to hearing disabilities experienced by one of the persons involved in the problematic situations. This approach to rehabilitation differs from traditional paradigms of rehabilitative audiology. It clearly defines the goal and the process of intervention in rehabilitative audiology. Moreover, it redefines the role of the clinician and the patient(s) in the intervention process. More importantly, it provides concrete solutions to real problems experienced by patients in their everyday lives. It has been shown that the successful application of a solution-centered problem-solving approach to rehabilitative audiology is not only beneficial to patients but also gratifying to clinicians (Dillon et al, 1991a,b, 1997).

REFERENCES

ALCANTARA, J.I., COWAN, R.S.C., BLAMEY, P.J., & CLARK, G.M. (1990). A comparison of two training strategies for speech recognition with an electrotactile speech processor. *Journal of Speech and Hearing Research, 33*;195–204.

ALPINER, J. (1987). Rehabilitative audiology: an overview. In: J.G. Alpiner, & P.A. McCarthy (Eds.), *Rehabilitative audiology: Children and adults* (pp. 3–17). Baltimore: Williams & Wilkins.

AMERICAN SPEECH-LANGUAGE-HEARING ASSOCIATION. (1978). Board moves to change dispensing rules. *AHSA, 16*;68–70.

AMERICAN SPEECH-LANGUAGE-HEARING ASSOCIATION. (1979). Legislative council changes ASHA's name, ratifies ERA motion, adopts code changes. *ASHA, 21*;33–35.

AMERICAN SPEECH-LANGUAGE-HEARING ASSOCIATION. (1981). Task force on the definition of hearing handicap. *ASHA, 23*;293–297.

AMERICAN SPEECH-LANGUAGE-HEARING ASSOCIATION. (1984). Committee on Rehabilitative Audiology: definition of and competencies for aural rehabilitation. *ASHA, 26*;37–41.

AUERBACK, J. (1984). *One-to-one lipreading lessons for adults.* Springfield, Il: Charles C. Thomas.

BALLY, S.J., & KAPLAN, H. (1988). The Gallaudet University aural rehabilitation elder hostels. *Journal of the Academy of Rehabilitative Audiology, 21*;99–112.

BELOW, S. (1947). *The victim.* New York: Vanguard Press.

BINNIE, C.A. (1977). Attitude changes following speechreading training. *Scandinavian Audiology, 6*;13–19.

BLAMEY, P., & ALCANTARA, J.I. (1994) Research in auditory training. In: J.P. Gagné, & N. Tye-Murray (Eds.), *Research in audiological rehabilitation: Current trends and future directions* [Monograph]. *Journal of the Academy of Rehabilitative Audiology, 27*;161–191.

BOOTHROYD, A. (1987). CASPER, computer-assisted speech-perception evaluation and training. In: *Proceeding of the 10th Annual Conference of the Rehabilitation Society of North America* (pp. 734–736). Washington, DC: Association for Advancement of Rehabilitation Technology.

BOOTHROYD, A. (1988). Linguistic factors in speechreading. In: C.L. DeFilippo, & D. Sims (Eds.), *New reflections on speechreading.* Special Monograph of the *Volta Rev, 90*(5);77–88.

BROBERG, R.F. (1984). *The lipreaders' calendar.* Washington, DC: Alexander Graham Bell Association for the Deaf.

BUTLER, K. (1984). Language processing and halfway up the down staircase. In: G. Wallach, & K. Butler (Eds.), *Language learning disabilities in school age children* (pp. 60–81). Baltimore: Williams & Wilkins.

CANADIAN SOCIETY FOR THE ICIDH. (1991). The handicaps creation process: Analysis of the consultation, new full proposals. *ICIDH International Network, 4* (1–2).

CASTLE, D.L. (1988). *Telephone strategies.* Bethesda, MD: Self Help for Hard of Hearing People, Inc.

DANZ, A.D., & BINNIE, C.A. (1983). Quantification of the effects of training the auditory-visual reception of connected speech. *Ear and Hearing, 4*;146–151.

DEFILIPPO, C.L. (1988). Tracking for speechreading training. In: C.L. DeFilippo, & D. Sims (Eds.), *New reflections on speechreading.* Special Monograph of the *Volta Review, 90* (5);215–239.

DEFILIPPO, C.L., & SCOTT, B.L. (1978). A method for training and evaluating the reception of ongoing speech. *Journal of the Acoustical Society of America, 63*;1186–1192.

DE GAULEJAC, V. (1996). *Les sources de la honte.* Paris: Desclée de Brouwer.

DEMPSEY, J.J., LEVITT, H., JOSEPHSON, J., & PORRAZZO, J. (1992). Computer-assisted tracking simulation (CATS). *Journal of the Acoustical Society of America, 92*;701–710.

DEWINE, L. (1992). Americans with Disabilities Act: A declaration of opportunities. *Audecibel,* July-August-September; 7–10.

DILLON, H., JAMES, A., & GINIS, J. (1997). Client Oriented Scale of Improvement (COSI) and its relationship to several other measurements of benefit and satisfaction provided by hearing aids. *Journal of the American Academy of Audiology, 8*;27–43.

DILLON, H., KORITSCHONER, E., BATTAGLIA, J., LOVEGROVE, R., GINIS, J., MAVRIAS, G., CARNIE, L., RAY, P., FORSYTHE, L., TOWERS, E., GOULIAS, H., & MACASKILL, F. (1991a). Rehabilitation effectiveness I: Assessing the needs of clients entering a national hearing rehabilitation program. *Australian Journal of Audiology, 13*;55–65.

DILLON, H., KORITSCHONER, E., BATTAGLIA, J., LOVEGROVE, R., GINIS, J., MAVRIAS, G., CARNIE, L., RAY, P., FORSYTHE, L., TOWERS, E., GOULIAS, H., & MACASKILL, F. (1991b). Rehabilitation effectiveness II: Assessing the outcomes for clients of a national hearing rehabilitation program. *Australian Journal of Audiology, 13*;68–82.

DUNCAN, J.F., & KATZ, J. (1983). Language and auditory processing: Top-down and bottom-up. In: E.Z. Laskey, & J. Katz (Eds.). *Central auditory processing problems of speech-language and hearing disorders* (pp. 31–45). Austin, TX: Pro-Ed.

ERBER, N.P. (1969). Interaction of audition and vision in the recognition of oral speech stimuli. *Journal of Speech and Hearing Research, 12*;423–425.

ERBER, N.P. (1979). Auditory-visual perception of speech with reduced optical clarity. *Journal of Speech and Hearing Research, 22*;212–223.

ERBER, N.P. (1982). *Auditory training.* Washington, DC: Alexander Graham Bell Association for the Deaf.

ERBER, N.P. (1985). *Telephone communication and hearing impairment.* San Diego, CA: College-Hill Press.

ERBER, N.P. (1988). *Communication therapy for hearing-impaired adults.* Melbourne, Australia: Clavis Publishing.

ERBER, N.P. (1996). *Communication therapy for hearing-impaired adults* (2nd ed.). Melbourne, Australia: Clavis Publishing.

ERBER, N.P. (1998). DYALOG: A computer-based measure of conversational performance. *Journal of the Academy of Rehabilitative Audiology.* In press.

ERBER, N.P., & LIND, C. (1994). Communication therapy: Theory and practice. In: J.P. Gagné, & N. Tye-Murray (Eds.), *Research in audiological rehabilitation: Current trends and future directions* [Monograph]. *Journal of the Academy of Rehabilitative Audiology, 27;* 267–287.

ERBER, N.P., & YELLAND, J. (1998). CONAN: A system for analysis of temporal factors in conversation. *Journal of the Academy of Rehabilitative Audiology.* In press.

ERDMAN, S.A. (1993). Counseling hearing-impaired adults. In: J.G. Alpiner, & P.A. McCarthy (Eds.), *Rehabilitative audiology: Children and adults* (2nd ed.) (pp. 374–413). Baltimore: Williams & Wilkins.

FEEHAN, P.J., SAMUELSON, R.A., & SEYMOUR, D.T. (1982). *CLUES: Speechreading for adults.* Austin, TX: Pro-ed.

FENN, G., & SMITH, B.Z.D. (1987). The assessment of lipreading ability: Some practical considerations in the use of the tracking procedure. *British Journal of Audiology, 21;*253–258.

FISHER, M. (1978). *Lively lipreading lessons.* Washington, DC: Alexander Graham Bell Association for the Deaf.

FORTGATCH, M., & TRYCHIN, S. (1989). *Getting along* [Manual and Videotape]. Washington, DC: Gallaudet University Press.

FOX-GRIMM, M.E. (1991–1992). The Americans with Disabilities Act: An overview. *National Student Speech Language and Hearing Association Journal, 19;*49–54.

GAGNÉ, J.P. (1994). Visual and audiovisual speech perception training: Basic and applied research needs. In: J.P. Gagné, & N. Tye-Murray (Eds.), *Research in audiological rehabilitation: Current trends and future directions* [Monograph]. *Journal of the Academy of Rehabilitative Audiology, 27;*133–159.

GAGNÉ, J.P. (1998). Reflections on evaluative research in audiological rehabilitation. *Scandinavian Audiology* (Suppl.), *27*(49); 69–79.

GAGNÉ, J.P., & BOUTIN, L. (1997). The effect of speaking rate on visual speech intelligibility. In: C. Benoît, & R. Campbell (Eds.), *Proceedings of the ESCA workshop on audio-visual processing: Cognitive and computational approaches.* Genoble, (France): Presses de l'Université de Grenoble.

GAGNÉ, J.P., DINON, D., & PARSONS, J. (1991a). An evaluation of CAST: A computer-aided speech-reading training program. *Journal of Speech and Hearing Research, 34;*213–221.

GAGNÉ, J.P., HÉTU, R., GETTY, L., & MCDUFF, S. (1995). Towards the development of paradigms to conduct functional evaluative research in audiological rehabilitation. *Journal of the Academy of Rehabilitative Audiology, 28;*7–25.

GAGNÉ, J.P., MASTERSON, V., MUNHALL, K.G., BILIDA, N., QUERENGESSER, C. (1994). Across talker variability in auditory, visual, and audiovisual speech intelligibility for conversational and clear speech. *Journal of the Academy of Rehabilitative Audiology, 27;*135–158.

GAGNÉ, J.P., MCDUFF, S., GETTY, L. (1999). Some limitations of evaluative investigations based solely on normed outcome measures. *Journal of the American Academy of Audiology, 10;*46–62.

GAGNÉ, J.P., & PARADIS, M.J. (1995). *Within and across talker differences in visual speech intelligibility.* Paper presented at the International Collegium of Rehabilitative Audiology, Göteborg, Sweden.

GAGNÉ, J.P., PARNES, L.S., LAROQUE, M., HASSAN, R., VIDAS, S. (1991b). Effectiveness of an intensive speech perception training program for adult cochlear implant recipients. *Annals of Otology, Rhinology, and Laryngology, 100;*700–707.

GAGNÉ, J.P., & ROCHETTE, A.J. (1996). Auditory, visual and audiovisual speech intelligibility: A comparison of conversational and clear speech. In: *Proceedings of the 1st ESCA tutorial and research workshop on speech production modelling: From control strategies to acoustics* (pp. 233–236). France: Presses de l'Université de Grenoble.

GAGNÉ, J.P., STELMACHOWICZ, P., & YOVETICH, W.S. (1991c). Reactions of normal hearing subjects to requests for clarifications used by hearing-impaired individuals. *Volta Review, 93;*921–928.

GAGNÉ, J.P., & WYLLIE, K.A. (1989). The relative effectiveness of three communication strategies on the visual-identification of misperceived words. *Ear and Hearing, 10;*368–374.

GARSTECKI, D.C. (1981). Auditory-visual training program for hearing-impaired adults. *Journal of the Academy of Rehabilitative Audiology, 14;*223–238.

GARSTECKI, D.C. (1994). Assistive devices for the hearing-impaired. In: J.P. Gagné, & N. Tye-Murray (Eds.), *Research in audiological rehabilitation: Current trends and future directions* [Monograph]. *Journal of the Academy of Rehabilitative Audiology, 27;*113–132.

GETTY, L., & HÉTU, R. (1991). Development of a rehabilitation program for people affected with occupational hearing loss: 2. Results from group intervention with 48 workers and their spouses. *Audiology, 30;*317–329.

GETTY, L., HÉTU, R., & WARIDEL, S. (1995). Étude du processus de réadaptation chez des travailleurs atteints de surdité professionnelle. *Final Report: CQRS Grant #EA 319/092.*

GIOLAS, T.G. (1982). Aural rehabilitation: An orientation. In: T.G. Giolas. *Hearing handicapped adults* (pp. 78–105). Englewood Cliffs, NJ: Prentice Hall.

GOLDSTEIN, D.P., & STEPHENS, S.D.G. (1981). Audiological rehabilitation: Management model I. *Audiology, 20;*432–452.

GREENWALD, A.B. (1984). *Lipreading made easy.* Washington, DC: Alexander Graham Bell Association for the Deaf.

HAUG, O., & HAUG, S. (1977). *Help for the hard-of-hearing.* Springfield, Il: Charles C. Thomas.

HELFER, K.S. (1998). Auditory and auditory-visual recognition of clear and conversational speech by older adults. *Journal of the American Academy of Audiology, 9;*234–242.

HÉTU, R. (1996). The stigma attached to hearing impairment. *Scandinavian Audiology* (Suppl.), *25*(43);12–24.

HÉTU, R., & GETTY, L. (1991). Development of a rehabilitation program for people affected with occupational hearing loss: 1. A new paradigm. *Audiology, 30;*305–316.

HÉTU, R., JONES, L., & GETTY, L. (1993). The impact of acquired hearing impairment on intimate relationships: implications for rehabilitation. *Audiology, 32;*363–381.

HÉTU, R., LALONDE, M., & GETTY, L. (1987). Psychosocial disadvantages associated with occupational hearing loss as experienced in the family. *Audiology, 26;*141–152.

HÉTU, R., RIVERIN, L., GETTY, L., LALANDE, N.M., & ST-CYR, C. (1990). The reluctance to acknowledge hearing difficulties among hearing-impaired workers. *British Journal of Audiology, 24;*265–276.

HULL, R.H. (1982). What is aural rehabilitation? In: R.H. Hull (Ed.), *Rehabilitative audiology* (pp. 3–11). New York: Grune and Stratton.

HYDE, M.L., & RIKO, K. (1994). A decision-analytic approach to audiological rehabilitation. In: J.P. Gagné, & N. Tye-Murray (Eds.), *Research in audiological rehabilitation: Current trends and future directions* [Monograph]. *Journal of the Academy of Rehabilitative Audiology, 27*;337–374.

JEFFERS, J., & BARLEY, M. (1971). *Speechreading (lipreading)*. Springfield, Il: Charles C. Thomas.

JEFFERS, J., & BARLEY, M. (1979). *Look, now hear this*. Springfield, Il: Charles C. Thomas.

JENNINGS, M.B. (1993). *Aural rehabilitation curriculum series: Hearing help class II: Coping with hearing loss*. Toronto: Canadian Hearing Society.

JENNINGS, M.B. (1994). Service delivery models for older adults with hearing impairments: Individual sessions. In: P.B. Kricos, & S.A. Lesner (Eds.), *Hearing care for the older adult: Audiologic rehabilitation* (pp. 227–265). Boston, MA: Butterworth-Heinemann.

JENNINGS, M.B., & SHEPPARD, A. (1992). *Introducing adult aural rehabilitation programs into the mainstream*. Paper presented at the Summer Institute of the Academy of Rehabilitative Audiology, Austin, TX.

JENNINGS, M.B., SHEPPARD, A., & SUTHERLAND, G. (1991). *Aural rehabilitation curriculum series: Hearing help class I: Help for hearing aid users*. Toronto: Canadian Hearing Society.

JONES, L., KYLE, J., & WOOD, P. (1987). *Words apart: Losing your hearing as an adult*. London: Tavistock Publications.

KAPLAN, H., BALLY, S.J., & GARRETSON, C. (1985). *Speechreading: A way to improve understanding*. Washington, DC: Gallaudet University Press.

KAPLAN, H., BALLY, S., & GARRETSON, C. (1987). *Speechreading: A way to improve understanding* (2nd ed.). Washington, DC: Gallaudet University Press.

KLEEMAN, M. (1995). *I see what you say: Self help lipreading program*. Washington, DC: Alexander Graham Bell Association for the Deaf.

KOPRA, L., KOPRA, M., ABRAHAMSON, J., & DUNLOP, R. (1987). Lipreading drill and practice software for an auditory-visual interactive system. *Journal of Comprehensive Users Speech Hearing, 3*;58–68.

LANSING, C.R., & DAVIS, J.M. (1988). Early versus delayed speech perception training for adult cochlear implant users: Initial results. *Journal of the Academy of Rehabilitative Audiology, 21*;11–28.

LESNER, S., SANDRIDGE, S., & KRICOS, P. (1987). Training influences on visual consonant and sentence reognition. *Ear and Hearing, 8*;283–287.

MARCUS, I. (1985). *Your eyes hear for you: A self-help course in speechreading*. Bethesda, MD: Self-Help for Hard of Hearing People, Inc.

MATTHIES, M.L., & CARNEY, A.E. (1988). A modified speech tracking procedure as a communicative performance measure. *Journal of Speech and Hearing Research, 31*; 394–404.

MCCARTHY, P., & CULPEPPER, B. (1987). The adult remediation process. In: J.G. Alpiner, & P.A. McCarthy (Eds.), *Rehabilitative audiology: Children and adults*. (pp. 305–342). Baltimore, MD: Williams and Wilkins.

McCAY, V. (1984). Psychological stress and hearing loss. *Self Help for Hard of Hearing People, July/August; 3–6.*

MCKENNA, L. (1987). Goal planning in audiological rehabilitation. *British Journal of Audiology, 21*;5–11.

MONTGOMERY, A.A., WALDEN, B.E., SCHWARTZ, D.M., & PROSEK, R.A. (1984). Training auditory-visual speech reception in adults with moderate sensorineural hearing loss. *Ear and Hearing, 5*;30–36.

NOBLE, W., & HÉTU, R. (1994). An ecological approach to disability and handicap in relation to impaired hearing. *Audiology, 33*;117–126.

ORDMAN, K.A., & RALLI, M.P. (1976). *What people say* (5th ed.). Washington, DC: Alexander Graham Bell Association for the Deaf.

OWENS, E., & RAGGIO, M. (1987). The UCSF tracking procedure for evaluation training in speech reception by hearing-impaired adults. *Journal of Speech and Hearing Disorders, 52*;120–128.

OWENS, E., & TELLEEN, C.C. (1991). Tracking as an aural rehabilitative process. *Journal of the Academy of Rehabilitative Audiology, 24*;207–216.

PICHENY, M., DURLACH, N., & BRAIDA, L. (1985). Speaking clearly for the hard of hearing I: Intelligibility differences between clear and conversational speech. *Journal of Speech and Hearing Research, 28*:96–103.

PICHENY, M., DURLACH, N., & BRAIDA, L. (1986). Speaking clearly for the hard of hearing II: Acoustic characteristics of clear and conversational speech. *Journal of Speech and Hearing Research, 29*;434–446.

PICHORA-FULLER, M.K., & BENGUEREL, A. (1991). The design of CAST (Computer-aided speechreading training). *Journal of Speech and Hearing Research, 34*;202–212.

PLANT, G. (1984). *COMMTRAM: A communication training program for profoundly deaf adults*. Sydney: National Acoustics Laboratories.

PLANT, G. (1994). *ANALYTIKA: Analytical testing and training lists*. Somerville, MA: Hearing Rehabilitation Foundation.

PLANT, G. (1996a). *COMMTRAC: Modified connected discourse tracking exercises for hearing-impaired adults*. Somerville, MA: Hearing Rehabilitation Foundation.

PLANT, G. (1996b). *SYNTREX: Synthetic training exercises for hearing-impaired adults*. Somerville, MA: Hearing Rehabilitation Foundation.

PLANT, G. (1996c). *TACTRAIN: Tactaid VII training program for hearing impaired adults*. Somerville, MA: Hearing Rehabilitation Foundation.

ROSS, M. (1987). Aural rehabilitation revisited. *Journal of the Academy of Rehabilitative Audiology, 20*;13–23.

ROSS, M. (1997). A retrospective look at the future of aural rehabilitation. *Journal of the Academy of Rehabilitative Audiology, 30*;11–28.

RUBENSTEIN, A., & BOOTHROYD, A. (1987). Effect of two approaches to auditory training on speech recognition by hearing-impaired adults. *Journal of Speech and Hearing Research, 30*;153–160.

SANDERS, D.A. (1971). *Aural rehabilitation*. Englewood Cliffs, NJ: Prentice Hall.

SANDERS, D.A. (1982). *Aural rehabilitation* (2nd ed.). Englewood Cliffs, NJ: Prentice Hall.

SCHOW, R.L., & NERBONNE, M.A. (1982). Communication screening profile: Use with elderly clients. *Ear and Hearing, 3*;135–147.

SCHUM, R.L. (1994). Personal adjustment counseling. In: J.P. Gagné, & N. Tye-Murray (Eds.), *Research in audiological rehabilitation: Current trends and future directions* [Monograph]. *Journal of the Academy of Rehabilitative Audiology, 27;*223–236.

SCHUM, D. (1997). Beyond hearing aids: Clear speech training as an intervention strategy. *Hearing Journal, 50;*10,36–40.

SIMS, D., VON FELDT, J., DOWALIBY, F., HUTCHINSON, K., & MYERS, T. (1979). A pilot experiment in computer assisted speechreading instruction utilizing the data analysis video interactive device (DAVID). *American Annals of Deafness, 124;*618–623.

SPENS, K.E. (1995). Evaluation of speech tracking results: Some numerical considerations and examples. In: G. Plant, & K.E. Spens (Eds.), *Profound deafness and speech communication* (pp. 417–437). London: Whurr Publishers Ltd.

SPITZER, J.B., LEDER, S.B., & GIOLAS, T.G. (1993). *Rehabilitation of late-deafened adults: Modular program manual.* St. Louis: Mosby.

STEPHENS, D., & HÉTU, R. (1991). Impairment, disability and handicap in audiology: Towards a consensus. *Audiology, 30;*185–200.

STRACHAN, S., SCULLINO, M.L., & JENNINGS, M.B. (1997). *Aural rehabilitation curriculum series: Hearing help class III & IV: Speechreading.* Toronto, ON: Canadian Hearing Society.

TRYCHIN, S. (1986a). Stress management—III. *Self Help for Hard of Hearing People, January/February;* 12–13.

TRYCHIN, S. (1986b). *Relaxation procedures for hard of hearing people.* [Manual for Practitioners, Manual for Trainees, Videotapes]. Washington, DC: Gallaudet University Press.

TRYCHIN, S. (1987). *Did I do that?* [Manual and Videotape]. Washington, DC: Gallaudet University Press.

TRYCHIN, S. (1988). *So that's the problem!* Washington, DC: Gallaudet University Press.

TRYCHIN, S. (1993). *Communication issues related to hearing loss.* Washington, DC: Gallaudet University Press.

TRYCHIN, S., & ALBRIGHT, J. (1993). *Staying in touch: Suggestions for solving communication problems for hard of hearing people and those who live and work with them.* Bethesda, MD: Self Help for Hard of Hearing People, Inc.

TRYCHIN, S., & WRIGHT, F. (1989). *Is that what you think?* Washington, DC: Gallaudet University Press.

TYE-MURRAY, N. (1991). Repair strategy usage by hearing-impaired adults and changes following communication therapy. *Journal of Speech and Hearing Research, 34;*921–928.

TYE-MURRAY, N. (1994). Communication strategies training. In: J.P. Gagné, & N. Tye-Murray (Eds.), *Research in audiological rehabilitation: Current trends and future directions* [Monograph]. *Journal of the Academy of Rehabilitative Audiology, 27;*193–207.

TYE-MURRAY, N. (1997). *Communication training for older teenagers and adults: Listening, speechreading and using conversational strategies.* Austin, TX: Pro-ed.

TYE-MURRAY, N., PURDY, S.C., & WOODWORTH, G. (1992). The reported use of communication strategies by members of SHHH and its relationship to client, talker, and situational variables. *Journal of Speech and Hearing Research, 35;*708–717.

TYE-MURRAY, N., & SCHUM, L. (1994). Conversation training for frequent communication partners. In: J.P. Gagné, & N. Tye-Murray (Eds.), *Research in audiological rehabilitation: Current trends and future directions* [Monograph]. *Journal of the Academy of Rehabilitative Audiology, 27;*209–222.

TYE-MURRAY, N., TYLER, R., BONG, B., & NARES, T. (1988). Using laser videodisc technology to train speechreading and assertive listening skills. *Journal of the Academy of Rehabilitative Audiology, 21;*143–152.

UCHANSKI, R.M., CHOI, S.S., BRAIDA, L.D., REED, C.M., & DURLACH, N.I. (1996). Speaking clearly for the hard of hearing IV: Further studies of the role of speaking rate. *Journal of Speech and Hearing Research, 39;*494–509.

UNITED STATES ARCHITECTURAL & TRANSPORTATION BARRIERS COMPLIANCE BOARD. (1991). Americans with Disabilities Act (ADA): Accessibility guidelines for buildings and facilities. *Federal Register, 56;*144.

WALDEN, B.E., ERDMAN, S.A., MONTGOMERY, A.A., SCHWARTZ, D.M., & PROSEK, R.A. (1981). Some effects of training on speech recognition by hearing-impaired adults. *Journal of Speech and Hearing Research, 24;*207–216.

WALDEN, B.E., & GRANT, K.W. (1993). Research needs in rehabilitative audiology. In: J.G. Alpiner, & P.A. McCarthy (Eds.), *Rehabilitative audiology: Children and adults.* (2nd ed.). (pp. 501–528). Baltimore, MD: Williams and Wilkins.

WALDEN, B.E., MONTGOMERY, A.A., SCHERR, C.K., & JONES, C.J. (1977). Effects of training on the visual recognition of consonants. *Journal of Speech and Hearing Research, 20;*130–145.

WALTHER, E.F. (1982). *Lip reading.* Chicago, Il: Nelson-Hall.

WAYNER, D.S., & ABRAHAMSON, M.A. (1996). *Learning to hear again: An audiologic rehabilitation curriculum guide.* Austin, TX: Hear Again.

WHITEHURST, M.W. (1986). *Listen to me: Auditory exercises for adults.* Washington, DC: Alexander Graham Bell Association for the Deaf.

WORLD HEALTH ORGANIZATION. (1980). *International classification of impairments, disabilities and handicaps.* Geneva: Author.

WORLD HEALTH ORGANIZATION. (1997). *ICIDH—2. International classification of impairments, activities and participation: A manual of dimensions of disablement and Functioning.* [On-line]. Available: http://www.who.int/msa/mnh/ems/icidh/index.htm.

PREFERRED PRACTICE GUIDELINES

Professionals Who Provide Rehabilitation Services

▼ Rehabilitation audiologists

Expected Outcomes

▼ The objectives of the intervention program negotiated with the patient have been attained.

▼ The participants report that the situations of handicap addressed by the intervention program have been resolved in a satisfactory manner.

▼ Any negative impacts and consequences that may arise as a result of the intervention program do not constitute an obstacle to the implementation of the program for any of the participants.

▼ The participants report that they are able and willing to implement the intervention strategies on a regular and consistent basis whenever the situation of handicap occurs.

Clinical Indications

▼ The participants are able to report specific situations of handicap that they experience in their everyday lives because at least one of the persons involved in that situation has hearing impairment.

▼ The participants agree to take part in an intervention program designed to resolve the specific situations of handicap identified.

Clinical Process

▼ The participants are able to describe the factors related to their predicaments and the environmental context that contribute to the production of a situation of handicap.

▼ The participants play an active role in defining the specific objectives of the intervention program.

▼ The participants are involved in identifying potential solutions to the situation of handicap.

▼ The participants are able (and agree) to implement the intervention strategies that were retained to resolve the situation of handicap identified.

▼ The participants are able to evaluate the outcome of the intervention program (as it relates to the specific objective of the program).

▼ The participants are able to report the impacts and consequences (positive and negative) of implementing the intervention strategies.

▼ The participants are able to identify the factors that contributed to the success of the intervention program.

▼ The participants are able to identify the factors that constituted an impediment to the attainment of the stated objective of the intervention program.

Documentation

▼ A detailed description of each situation of handicap experienced by the participants.

▼ A clear statement of the objective negotiated for each situation of handicap addressed in the intervention program.

▼ A detailed description of the intervention strategies retained for each situation of handicap.

▼ A report of the outcome of the program that includes the elements of the intervention program that were successful and the elements that were not successfully implemented.

▼ A description of the impacts and the consequences of the intervention program.

Chapter 19

When Hearing Aids Are Not Enough
The Need for Assistive Devices

Peter O. Bengtsson and Preben B. Brunved

Outline

WHY ASSISTIVE LISTENING DEVICES?

Many people with hearing loss who benefit from the use of hearing aid(s) can function in quiet, close, or person-to-person situations. However, background noise, long distances to the sound source, and reverberation degrade intelligibility much faster for people with hearing loss whether they wear hearing aids or not. Thus people with hearing loss are often prevented from participating on equal terms with normal-hearing people in group conversations or in larger assembly areas that are not equipped with an assistive listening system (ALS). Even the best in sound systems technology combined with the best in hearing aid technology cannot solve the intelligibility problems faced by people with hearing loss. In recognition of this, requirements for assistive listening systems were included in the Americans with Disabilities Act (ADA) of 1990 (ADA, 1990). Although many assistive listening

Audiology: Treatment. Edited by Valente, Hosford-Dunn, and Roeser. Thieme Medical Publishers, Inc., New York © 2000

(ALDs) devices may also be obtained for personal use, it is important to understand the rights of people with hearing loss and the Americans with Disabilities Accessibility Guidelines (ADAAG, 1994).

THE AMERICANS WITH DISABILITIES ACT

The ADA is essentially a civil rights law that guarantees equal opportunity for services in the private and public sector and employment for individuals with disabilities. Generally, the ADA prohibits discrimination on the basis of disability. The ADA was modeled after the Civil Rights Act of 1964 and the Rehabilitation Act of 1973. Signed into law by President Bush on July 26, 1990, the specific requirements of the ADA will be phased in through the year 2010. The ADA covers five separate titles. It is important to be familiar with all five titles, although interest may be limited to sections pertaining to ALDs. The following is a brief summary of the five titles.

Title I: Employment

Under the law, employers must not refuse employment to a qualified person with a disability on the basis of that person's disability, who, with or without reasonable accommodations, can perform the essential functions of the job. Therefore employers must ensure their employment practices do not discriminate against qualified persons with disabilities in the application and recruitment processes, hiring, advancement, training, compensation, or discharge of an employee, or in any other terms, conditions, and privileges of employment. Reasonable accommodation need not be required if it creates an undue hardship on the employer.

Title II: Public Sector Services

State and local governments are prohibited from discriminating against persons with disabilities or from excluding participation or denying benefits of programs, services, or activities to persons with disabilities. Title II also covers transportation services by requiring that all public transportation systems be accessible to all people, including individuals with disabilities.

Title III: Private Sector Services

Places of public accommodation are required to be accessible to and usable by people with disabilities. Places of public accommodation include motels, restaurants, bars, movie theaters, convention centers, grocery stores, clothing stores, malls, museums, libraries, gyms, bowling alleys, amusement parks, or just about any other facility commonly used by the general public. Private businesses must not discriminate in the "goods, services, facilities, procedures, and privileges, advantages, and accommodations" offered to the public."Readily achievable" alterations must be made to existing buildings, and new construction must be barrier free. Reasonable modifications must be made to policies and auxiliary aids provided as long as they do not create an undue burden on the business or fundamentally alter the nature of the goods and services provided. Businesses cannot discriminate by excluding people with disabilities, by treating them separately, or by requiring them to participate in separate programs.

Title IV: Telecommunications

Common carriers offering telephone services to the general public are required to increase the availability of interstate and intrastate telecommunications relay services to individuals with hearing and speech impairments. All common carriers of telephone services must offer nonvoice relay services that interface with voice services.

Title V: Miscellaneous Provisions

This title includes several miscellaneous provisions such as (1) The ADA cannot be construed to apply a lesser standard of compliance than does the Rehabilitation Act of 1973. (2) The ADA does not limit or invalidate other federal or state laws that provide equal or greater protection. (3) Title V explicitly prohibits coercion, intimidation, or threats against persons exercising their rights under the ADA.

Enforcement

Enforcement of the ADA is divided among several federal agencies. General enforcement is by the Department of Justice including Title II, state and local governments, and Title III, public accommodations and commercial facilities. Design, construction, and alteration of public transportation facilities and specifications for public and private transportation vehicles are covered by the Department of Transportation (DOT) regulation. The provision of complementary paratransit and general service requirements for public transit agencies is also regulated by DOT. The Federal Transit Administration (FTA) has general oversight with respect to compliance and provides technical assistance. The ADA Title I employment provisions are enforced by the Equal Employment Opportunities Commission (EEOC). Finally, the ADA Title IV requirement for relay services and the requirements of section 225 of the Telecommunications Act of 1934 (ADA Amendment, 1996) are regulated by the Federal Communications Commission (FCC). The ADA also provides for a "private right of action" so that individuals can file lawsuits to enforce the act. The Telecommunications Act does not provide a private right of action and complaints must be filed with the FCC.

AUXILIARY AIDS AND SERVICES

The ADA, in its entirety, is very comprehensive, with the bulk of it covering aspects not related to the subject of assistive listening devices. Of particular interest to this chapter is the paragraph pertaining to Auxiliary Aids and Services (28 CFR Part 36).

General

A public accommodation shall take those steps that may be necessary to ensure that no individual with a disability is excluded, denied services, segregated, or otherwise treated differently than other individuals because of the absence of auxiliary aids and services, unless the public accommodation can demonstrate that taking those steps would fundamentally alter the nature of the goods, services, facilities, privileges, advantages, or accommodations being offered or would result in an undue burden (i.e., significant difficulty or expense).

Examples

The term "auxiliary aids and services" includes the following:

1. Qualified interpreters, notetakers, computer-aided transcription services, written materials, telephone handset amplifiers, assistive listening devices, telephones compatible with hearing aids, closed caption decoders, open and closed captioning, telecommunication devices for the deaf (TDD's), videotext displays, or other effective methods of making aurally delivered materials available to individuals with hearing impairments

2. Qualified readers, taped texts, audio recordings, Brailled materials, large print materials, or other effective methods of making visually delivered materials available to individuals with visual impairments

3. Acquisition or modification of equipment or devices

4. Other similar services and actions

Effective Communication

A public accommodation shall furnish appropriate auxiliary aids and services where necessary to ensure effective communication with individuals with disabilities.

Telecommunication Devices for the Deaf

1. A public accommodation that offers a customer, client, patient, or participant the opportunity to make outgoing telephone calls on more than an incidental convenience basis shall make available, upon request, a TDD for the use of an individual who has impaired hearing or a communication disorder.

2. This part does not require a public accommodation to use a TDD for receiving or making telephone calls incident to its operations.

Closed Caption Decoders

Places of lodging that provide televisions in five or more guest rooms and hospitals that provide televisions for patient use shall provide, on request, a means for decoding captions for use by an individual with impaired hearing.

Alternatives

If provision of a particular auxiliary aid or service by a public accommodation would result in a fundamental alteration in the nature of the goods, services, facilities, privileges, advantages, or accommodations being offered or in an undue burden (i.e., significant difficulty or expense), the public accommodation shall provide an alternative auxiliary aid or service, if one exists, that would not result in an alteration or such burden but would nevertheless ensure that, to the maximum extent possible, individuals with disabilities receive the goods, services, facilities, privileges, advantages, or accommodations offered by the public accommodation.

ADA ACCESSIBILITY GUIDELINES (ADAAG)

The intent of this section is to provide basic information about requirements as they relate to assistive listening systems (ALSs) and to bring about an understanding of how the law is formulated. ADAAG are updated on a regular basis. Therefore do not use this section to provide legal advice as it pertains to specific cases or particular legal matters.

Types of Listening Systems (Ref. ADAAG 4.33.7)

ALSs are intended to augment standard public address and audio systems by providing signals that can be received directly by persons with special receivers or by their own hearing aids and eliminate or filter background noise. The type of ALS appropriate for a particular application depends on the characteristics of the setting, the nature of the program, and the intended audience. Magnetic induction loops, infrared systems, and radiofrequency systems are types of listening systems that are appropriate for various applications. These systems are described later in this chapter.

Assembly Areas (Ref. ADAAG 4.1.3 [19] [b])

This paragraph applies to assembly areas where audible communications are integral to the use of the space (e.g., concert and lecture halls, playhouses and movie theaters, meeting rooms). Such assembly areas, if (1) they accommodate at least 50 persons or if they have audio-amplification systems, and (2) if they have fixed seating shall have a permanently installed ALS. For other assembly areas, a permanently installed ALS, or an adequate number of electrical outlets or other supplementary wiring necessary to support a portable ALS shall be provided. The minimum number of receivers to be provided shall be equal to 4% of the total number of seats, but in no case less than two. Signage shall be installed to notify patrons of the availability of a listening system.

Placement of Listening Systems (Ref. ADAAG 4.33.6)

If the provided listening system serves individual fixed seats, such seats shall be located within a 50 ft (15 m) viewing distance of the stage or playing area and shall have a complete view of the stage or playing area.

Symbols of Accessibility (Ref. ADAAG 4.30.7 [4])

In assembly areas where permanently installed ALS are required, the availability of such systems shall be identified with signage that includes the international symbol of access for hearing loss (Fig. 19–1).

Equivalent Facilitation (Ref. ADAAG 2.2)

Departures from particular technical and scoping requirements of this guideline by the use of other designs and technologies are permitted where the alternative designs and technologies used will provide substantially equivalent or greater access to and usability of the facility.

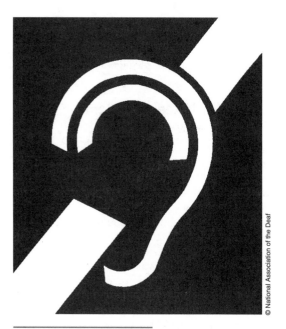

© National Association of the Deaf

Figure 19–1 International symbol of access for hearing loss.

ASSISTIVE LISTENING DEVICES AND SYSTEMS

The purpose of an ALD is to transmit signals from a sound source as directly as possible to a sound-generating transducer in the ear(s) of people with hearing loss, thereby bypassing poor room acoustics or distance to the sound source. All ALDs have three common basics: a *sound pickup,* a *signal transfer method,* and a *sound-generating transducer/coupler.* Within each of these elements are several options that must be carefully considered to provide the most effective solution for a given application. Figure 19–2 shows the most common components that apply to ALDs. As illustrated, any one signal transfer method may be combined with any one sound pickup method or source. Likewise, any one sound-generating transducer or coupler can be combined with any one signal transfer method (some restrictions may apply with direct cable). In general, systems are separated into two major categories: portable, body-worn devices often referred to as *"personal ALDs,"* and *"installed systems"* for residential and commercial applications.

SOUND PICKUP

No matter what signal transfer method is used, sound pickup is the single most important factor. For installed systems, the electrical signal is routed directly from an output connector on the sound system, TV, radio, or other electronic device. The wire connecting the sound source to the ALD is referred to as a "patch cord." When no direct connection can be made, the only method of sound pickup is through a microphone. For person-to-person communication, a microphone is always required for sound pickup. Depending on the nature of the problem, different applications require microphones with different acoustic characteristics.

Omnidirectional and Unidirectional Microphones

Every microphone has a characteristic polar pattern that determines how well it accepts or rejects signals coming from various directions around the microphone. An omnidirectional microphone treats all signals equally, regardless of where those signals originate (in front, behind, or to the side). In contrast, unidirectional microphones, commonly referred to as directional microphones, are specifically designed to accept mostly signals coming directly from the front and reject signals coming from behind or the sides. Because the amount of directionality is frequency dependent, the directional pattern for microphones are shown as polar pattern diagrams. Figure 19–3 illustrates a typical polar pattern for a directional microphone.

Microphone manufacturers use terminology such as cardioid, supercardioid, and hypercardioid polar patterns to describe the characteristic properties of their individual microphone models. The most extreme variation of cardioid is the hypercardioid pattern. The hypercardioid is very effective for rejecting signals arriving from the sides at back (~110 degrees and 230 degrees) but is less effective than the cardioid in rejecting signals from behind. The polar pattern also determines how prone a particular microphone is to inducing acoustic feedback. The greater rejection of signals not coming directly from the front of the microphone, the less risk of feedback.

From an acoustic point of view, the directional microphones would always be preferred because most of the problems are related to background noise and reverberation. However, situations occur in which omnidirectional microphones are required even at the cost of reduced signal-to-noise ratio (SNR). This would typically be in rooms where several people have to share the same microphone (i.e., a conference room). Also, in lecture rooms where people in the audience may ask questions, the directional microphone would not pick up very well from certain directions. Thus the people with hearing loss would not be able to understand the questions or conversation between the lecturer and other members of the audience. An omnidirectional microphone is often preferred in classroom settings. The directional characteristic of the directional microphones varies greatly from model to model and from manufacturer to manufacturer. But whatever the front-to-back or front-to-side relationship is in dB, the SNR will be improved by that amount. Both types of microphones are available in a variety of shapes and sizes depending on the application.

Microphone Designs for Assistive Listening Devices

Practically all microphones used with ALS are *electret*-type or *condenser*-type microphones. These have the advantage over the conventional *dynamic* microphones in that they are small and very lightweight. Electret microphones incorporate a small field effect transistor (FET) amplifier; thus a power source, often referred to as phantom power, is required for them to operate. Electret microphones used with ALDs typically operate on voltages between 1 and 10 volts. Most devices are designed to provide phantom power to the micro-

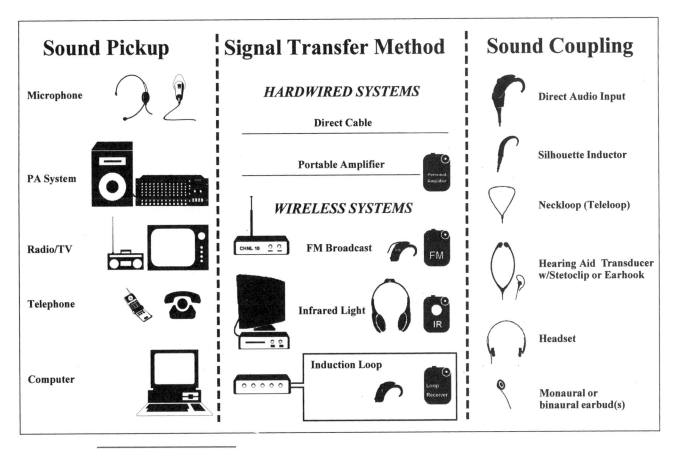

Figure 19–2 Sound pickup sources, signal transfer methods, and sound couplings for ALDs. (Reprinted with permission of Centrum Sound Systems.)

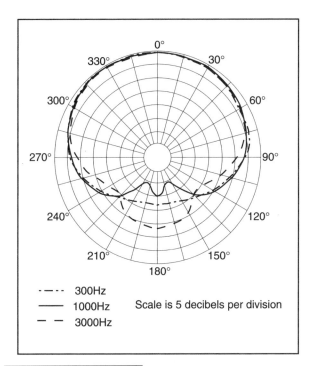

Figure 19–3 Directional microphone polar patterns at three different frequencies. (Courtesy Samson Technologies Corporation.)

phone through the microphone jack, eliminating the need for additional batteries. Commercial electret microphones may have in-line battery compartments or require phantom power as high as 48 volts from a microphone mixer.

Lapel/Handheld Microphones

The most common microphone for use with portable systems is the *lapel*-type microphone. Available in omnidirectional and directional versions, its small size makes it convenient and inconspicuous to attach to clothing near the speaker's mouth. Some microphones may be designed as a combination *lapel/handheld* style. Other manufacturers may include a small desk stand so they also can be used as podium or desktop microphones.

Head-Worn Microphones

In environments with continuous high noise levels, it may become necessary for the speaker to use a *boom-style microphone*. Two mechanically different designs exist: an over-the-head style and a behind-the-neck style. From an acoustic point of view, the two different designs perform alike, but the individual speaker may prefer one design to another. However, the over-the-head style may be combined with a headphone for some applications. The concept with either design is to bring the microphone as close to the mouth as possible to avoid surrounding noise from masking the speaker's voice. The microphone can be omnidirectional, directional, or a "noise-canceling" type. The noise-canceling microphone is designed for use in environments where the ambient noise level is 80 dB or greater and is most effective for frequencies above 2000 Hz. The noise-canceling characteristics are achieved by designing the microphone with a rear opening. Unwanted sounds arrive behind the microphone diaphragm out of phase and at the same time with sounds arriving from the front, thereby canceling each other out. Only speech originating very close to the microphone opening is fully reproduced. The noise-canceling concept may also be found in other microphone styles.

Conference Microphones

At roundtable discussions in conference rooms or around larger dinner tables, the lapel microphone is not a convenient option. Such a microphone would need to be passed around from person to person, causing disturbances to other people. Often, it would not get to the other person in time for the person with hearing loss to hear the full sentence. Special conference (boundary) microphones are available for such applications. Figure 19–4 shows a small portable conference microphone. The basic principle in a boundary microphone is that the direct sound and the reflected sound from a hard surface below the microphone arrive at the microphone's diaphragm at the same time and in phase. This doubles the sound pressure and increases the electrical output of the microphone by 6 dB without increasing the microphone's internal noise level. Some manufacturers claim the effective pickup range of conference microphones to be up to 20 feet. However, the realized range varies greatly, depending on environmental conditions and the individual user's discrimination ability. Five to 15 feet is more realistic. Conference microphones designed for ALD applications are omnidirectional. However, commercial boundary microphones are also available with a directional polar pattern.

Other Microphone Styles

The variety of microphone designs for commercial applications is practically endless. It is usually up to a sound contractor, user, or facilities manager to select the most adequate type of microphone for a given application. One of the most interesting microphones that can be successfully used with

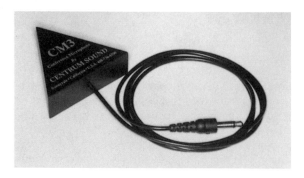

Figure 19–4 Multipurpose conference microphone. (Courtesy Centrum Sound Systems.)

ALDs is the *shotgun* microphone. This is the only type of microphone that can be aimed at, and clearly pick up, different speaker's voices in a highly reverberant room from more than 20 feet away. A shotgun microphone has a special hypercardioid polar pattern that is achieved by its mechanical design. The drawback of conventional shotgun microphones is their high cost and their large physical size, (i.e., 1 inch in diameter and usually between 15 and 20 inches long). However, recent developments in microphones that use two microphone elements and electronic filtering promises smaller and less expensive shotgun microphones in the future.

Public Address Systems

On commercial public address (PA) systems, the ALD is often connected to the sound system's mixer through the tape output, line output, or monitor/headphone output. Many different types of output connectors exist for commercial sound equipment. The most typical for "tape output" is the phono (RCA) jack often used on home stereos and TVs. Line output signals may use male XLR (Cannon) or ¼-inch phone jacks. A monitor headphone output usually uses a ¼-inch phone jack. Unlike phone jacks, XLR connectors can be male or female. As a general rule, input connectors are female and output connectors are male. However, to make installations more cost-effective for sound contractors, some equipment manufacturers provide screw-type terminals only. Many sound systems are rack mounted and not always accessible without tools. It is usually up to the installer to select an appropriate patch cord. Most common patch cords are available from ALD manufacturers, but it is often necessary to convert from one type of connector to another by means of adaptors and gender (male-to-female or female-to-male) changers. When no electrical output is available, a microphone can be placed close to the loudspeaker. Connections to personal devices such as tape decks and TVs are described in the Direct Audio Input section later in this chapter.

SIGNAL TRANSFER METHOD

Two principal methods of routing the signal from the source pickup to the sound-generating transducer/coupler exist: hardwired or wireless transmission. Because most sound-generating transducers are low-impedance devices and require a stronger signal than that of the output of a microphone, an amplifier is required. Most amplifying devices have a volume control, allowing the signal to be adjusted by or for the individual person's needs. Some device manufacturers also incorporate tone controls and balance controls to better accommodate the individual user's needs.

Hardwired Systems

As the name indicates, the hardwired devices make the connection between the sound source and the output by means of a wire or cable. The terms *wire* or *cable* are usually associated with commercial installations. Because of the relative small size of the cables associated with personal ALDs, these are referred to as cords. The cord connecting the source signal to the amplifier is shielded to avoid inductive interference caused by other electrical installations. The cord connecting the output transducer to the amplifier does not need to be shielded because of the low output impedance of an amplifier.

In the past, facilities, particularly churches, provided assistive listening by means of hardwired headset connections. Therefore people with hearing loss were limited to designated seats, usually within the first five rows. Large bulky headphones were the most common listening option, thus these systems were never popular among people with hearing loss. But the development of cost-effective wireless systems in recent years has eliminated the need for commercial fixed-hardwired systems. However, a personal portable amplifier is an economical solution for person-to-person conversations in noisy environments. The basic system consists of a pocket-sized amplifier, a microphone, and an appropriate sound-generating output transducer (see Fig. 19–2). The microphone is often designed as a plug-in unit that eliminates the need for the microphone cord. In noisy environments the microphone/amplifier is held close to the speaker's mouth, thereby improving the SNR substantially. The plug-in microphone can also be attached to a short cord or simply replaced with a wired lapel microphone. This provides the user the option to use it as a handheld microphone or as a lapel microphone.

PEARL

A person with hearing loss is having difficulty understanding in even close person-to-person conversations in situations where the background noise level is unusually high (i.e., at restaurants, parties, and conferences). The person has hearing aids with t-coils but no direct audio input (DAI) (described later in this chapter). A personal amplifier with plug-in microphone and a neckloop is a sensible solution.

For TV or radio listening, a microphone extension cord can be inserted, allowing the microphone to be placed close to the loudspeaker. Most newer TVs, VCRs, and other audio equipment also have "audio output" jacks. The patch cord may be connected directly to such an output jack, thereby eliminating the need for the microphone as the pickup source. Despite the high portability of these devices, the user has limited mobility to move around once the system is in place.

Wireless Technologies

The optimal solution to provide full mobility to the ALD user is by routing the signal from the sound source to the user by means of wireless transmission. Three basic wireless technologies are available today that provide different methods of transmission: *Teleloop* (induction loop) *technology, FM broadcast technology,* and *infrared light technology.* No single technology is best for all applications. Each type has its own advantages and disadvantages. All three types of ALSs can successfully be applied, as long as their individual limitations are observed.

INDUCTION LOOP SYSTEMS (TELELOOP)

The induction loop technology is the oldest and perhaps the most popular (among people with hearing loss) of the three wireless technologies. It is based on electromagnetic or inductive transmission and has the unique advantage that the signal is received directly by the user's personal t-coil on the hearing aid without the need for an additional receiver as is required by all other wireless technologies. Induction loop receivers are available for people with hearing loss without hearing aids or without the t-coil feature. The most common loop receiver is a pocket-sized beltclip device with headset or earphone. However, loop receivers are also available in a wandlike style or as a standard canal instrument (no microphone or volume control). Typical applications for induction loop systems include home radio/TV listening, small to medium size auditoriums, houses of worship, senior centers, council chambers, automobiles, and an endless number of counterapplications where a physical barrier separates service personnel and individual customers or where environmental noise may be excessive.

The Concept of the Induction Loop

The transmission component of an induction loop (room loop) system consists of an amplifier and a discrete wire (the loop) that runs along the perimeter of a room or designated area. The audio signal from the sound source is routed to the input of the amplifier and the amplifier's output is connected to the room loop. When an audio signal is delivered to the input of the amplifier, an alternating current (AC) flows through the loop. This current generates an inductive field inside the loop that is being picked up by the t-coil in the hearing aid or by a special loop receiver as illustrated in Figure 19–2. Conceptually it works like a transformer, where the loop simply is the primary coil of a transformer, and the t-coil is the secondary coil of the transformer.

Electromagnetic Field Strength and Frequency Response of Room Loops

To take advantage of using personal hearing aids as receivers with room loops, the magnetic field strength must be chosen so that it is high enough to produce an acceptable SNR, but not so high as to cause overloading of the hearing aid. The international standard (IEC Standard 118-4) recommended magnetic field strength for a loop system is 100 mA/m, or −20 dB (± 3 dB) re 1 A/m, created with a 1000 Hz sinusoidal input signal of level equal to the long-time average of the speech signal applied to the input of the system. This value generates an acoustic output from the hearing aid equivalent to the output of the hearing aid with normal speech level input to the microphone. The maximum recommended field strength is 400 mA/m, or −8 dB re 1A/m, derived on the basis that the difference of the peak short-time average level between a speech signal (approximately 125 ms) and the long-time average level is approximately 12 dB. The recommended frequency response of the magnetic field with an electrical input signal is 100 Hz to 5000 Hz ± 3 dB of the value at 1000 Hz. Although the standard does not specify a fixed value for SNR, installation of a loop system can generally not be recommended if an ambient electromagnetic interference greater than 10 mA/m, or −40 dB re 1 A/m, can be measured.

Loop Amplifiers

Two types of amplifiers are used for conventional room loop applications: *constant current* and *constant voltage*. Both can be very effective, but are not equally easy to install. Although it is not necessary for an installer to be able to calculate wire sizes and output currents required for specific applications, it is important to understand the difference between the two amplifier concepts. Also, it is important to understand that it is the amount of current flowing through the loop, not the power rating of the amplifier, that produces the strength of the inductive field. The constant current amplifier, also referred to as an *impedance matching amplifier*, is designed to keep the output current constant regardless of the load impedance. Figure 19–5 shows a constant current amplifier designed for commercial applications. Similar but smaller loop amplifiers are also available for radio or TV listening.

PEARL

A person with hearing loss has been fitted with two power BTE hearing aids and is doing very well in person-to-person conversations but is having difficulty understanding when watching TV. Turning up the TV volume does not help. A personal radio or TV induction loop system is recommended. The user needs only to switch the hearing aids to t-coil position to receive intelligible speech from the TV set. Once installed, the system is completely maintenance free.

For loop applications the load impedance is the resistance in the loop wire. The output voltage will change by whatever amount is required for the current to remain constant. The

advantage of this design is that the loop wire typically can be a single 14- to 18-AWG hookup wire, which is easy to install and conceal. For a room size, for example 40 by 60 ft., the total loop length would typically be close to 250 ft. long. The resistance in the loop wire with a 16 AWG hookup wire would be 1.0 ohm. With 14 AWG wire and same length loop, the resistance or load impedance would be 0.5 ohm. The output current would be the same with either loop, which eliminates the need for complex calculations as may be required by its counterpart, the constant voltage amplifier.

In the constant voltage amplifier the output voltage will remain constant irrespective of the load impedance. This type of amplifier is used for practically any loudspeaker application, commercial or residential. These amplifiers are typically designed to drive loudspeakers with impedances between 4 and 16 ohms (8 ohms being standard). Therefore when using this type of amplifier for loop applications, the resistance in the loop wire must be equivalent to or greater than the manufacturer's stated minimum impedance for loudspeakers. To "build up" the resistance with a wire size commensurate with the current required, the loop wire may have to encircle the room three to five times. In large rooms this causes an increase in inductive impedance, resulting in loss of higher frequencies. The only way of correcting for this loss is by means of equalization. Some amplifiers are equipped with graphic equalizers that can compensate for such loss.

Although manufacturers offering constant voltage amplifiers for loop applications may perform the necessary calculations and provide loop wire or multiconductor cables, these may be difficult to install and to conceal. However, despite the many drawbacks of the constant voltage amplifier, it still remains very popular for portable meeting room applications, simply because of low cost and general availability.

Installation Limitations and Considerations

Room loops for residential applications such as radio and TV listening do not require any special considerations. However, before recommending room loops for commercial applications, it is important to ensure that a uniform field strength throughout the designated listening area can be achieved. A field strength variation over the covered area of ± 3 dB would be a reasonable criterion. The best way to achieve this is to install the loop at floor level or approximately 8 ft. above the floor. It is important to be sure that the loop wire can be routed along the perimeter at one of those levels. Installing the loop on a wall at normal listening height (4 ft. above the floor for an adult person sitting down) will result in an intensive field strength increase closer to the wall and should be avoided. It is equally important to provide manufacturers of loop systems information about room size and layout and building materials (i.e., steel-reinforced concrete floor, wooden floor, crawl space) to ensure selection of an adequate loop amplifier. The crawl space or basement, if any, immediately underneath the room often offers the easiest and best place for loop wire installation. To verify systems performance the magnetic field strength can be measured with a field strength meter.

Although most room loops are designed to encircle the entire, or part of, designated seating area, the inductive field is not limited to within the loop. A certain amount of

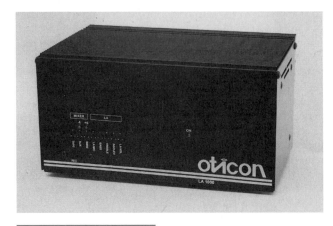

Figure 19–5 Large area constant current loop amplifier. (Courtesy Centrum Sound Systems.)

"spillover" will always be present outside of the physical layout of the loop wire. The amount of spillover varies with loop size and building materials. The loop signal may be picked up as far away as one half the width of the loop (i.e., with a loop size 40 by 40 ft., the signal may be heard up to 20 feet outside the loop). Therefore multiple room loop installations cannot be recommended where signals may interfere with adjacent rooms or facilities.

FREQUENCY MODULATED BROADCAST SYSTEMS

The frequency modulated (FM) radio broadcast systems offer people with hearing loss the greatest versatility of any of the wireless technologies. In principle, FM systems designed for hearing assistance applications work just like commercial FM broadcast systems operating in the 88 to 108 MHz range. However, in the United States, the FM hearing enhancement systems operate at FCC-designated frequency bands in the range from 72 to 76 MHz and from 216 to 217 MHz. Manufacturers of transmitters are required to have their designs FCC approved, but no licence is required to operate such systems. The transmitting power is restricted by FCC to a maximum

field strength of 8 mV/m at 30 m in the 72 to 76 MHz band and 100 mW effective radiated output power in the 216 to 217 MHz band. The 216 to 217 MHz band is intended for auditory assistance applications only. However, licenced users share the same band. An FM hearing enhancement system consists of a transmitter and one or more receivers. With current technology, transmitters and receivers can be designed for portable battery-operated applications, permanent installation, or a combination of the two. Therefore FM systems may be used in a broad scope of applications ranging from small personal systems for indoor/outdoor use (Fig. 19–6) to educational and commercial large area applications. Transmission ranges vary depending on the equipment and antenna used but are typically up to 100 ft. for personal systems and up to 1000 ft. or more for commercial large area systems.

Frequency Modulation Technology

An FM transmitter is designed to oscillate at a given radio frequency (RF) called the carrier or center frequency. When an audio signal is applied to a circuit within the transmitter called a modulator, the carrier frequency will change up and down in frequency in tune with the audio signal. The amount of deviation from the center of the carrier frequency is an expression of the intensity or volume of the audio signal, whereas the speed with which it changes its frequency is an expression of the audio frequency applied. The FM receiver detects these deviations and converts (demodulate) the RF signal back to an audio frequency (AF) signal.

Wide-Band and Narrow-Band Frequencies

The frequency range from 72 to 76 MHz can be divided into 10 wide-band channels or 40 usable narrow-band channels. In the past, most systems manufactured were wide-band systems, but with increased demand for more channels and interference-free channels and for rejection of near-frequency

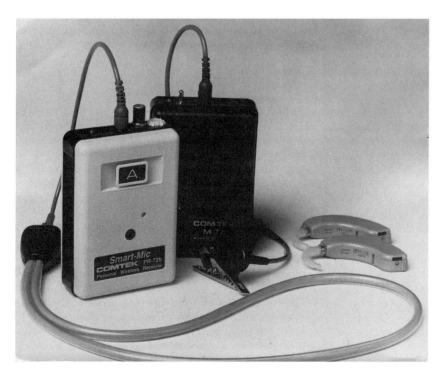

Figure 19–6 Personal FM system with neckloop. (Courtesy Comtek Inc.)

signals, newer designs are based on narrow-band technology. Channelization of this band was dropped in 1989, thus no standards exist for assignment of carrier frequencies and bandwidths. However, most wide-band frequencies are spaced 200 kHz apart with an allowed maximum frequency deviation of $\pm$ 75 kHz. Narrow-band systems in the 72 to 76 MHz band are typically spaced only 50 kHz apart, with a typical maximum allowed frequency deviation $\pm$10 kHz. The maximum allowed occupied bandwidth in the 216 to 217 MHz band is 50 kHz. Some manufacturers have chosen to divide the band into 20 channels spaced 50 kHz apart, whereas others may have chosen 40 channels spaced 25 kHz apart.

PITFALL

The terminologies *narrow-band* and *wide-band* are not expressions for audio performance but terms describing RF bandwidth technology for a specific product line. The transmitted and received frequency responses with either one of the two bandwidth technologies are wider than the frequency bandwidth of a hearing aid anyway.

Wide-Band Systems

In conventional wide-band systems the selection of a carrier frequency is made by tuning a coil (oscillator) inside the transmitter to the desired frequency. The receiver is then tuned to the same frequency. The tuning coils are often made "field-tunable" so individual users can make necessary adjustments for the purpose of avoiding outside radio interference or simply to listen in on another channel. However, the electronic components are often voltage or temperature sensitive, causing the transmitter or receiver to "drift" in frequency. To compensate for this drift, receivers are usually equipped with an electronic frequency control circuit—automatic frequency control (AFC).

Another method of stabilizing the carrier frequency is by crystal control. In these systems, both the transmitter and receiver incorporate a crystal that oscillates at a specific frequency practically unaffected by change in operating voltage or temperature. The transmitting/receiving frequencies of such systems can only be changed by replacing the crystals. In some systems the crystals are made as plug-in modules that can easily be exchanged by the user. Because channels for wide-band systems were standardized before the channelization was dropped in 1989, most wide-band systems use the same 10 carrier frequencies irrespective of manufacture. Each of the 10 frequencies or channels have been assigned a letter between A and H. Systems that are field-tunable are normally factory tuned to operate on a specific channel identified by a letter. Crystal-controlled devices are usually labeled on the crystal plug-in module or on the front face of the unit of nonreplaceable crystal-controlled devices. Generally full compatibility exists between different manufacturers' devices using this letter coding.

Narrow-Band Systems

The advantages of being able to offer 40 channels as opposed to only 10 are obvious, particularly at educational institutions or in multiplex movie houses, and so forth where more than 10 systems may be operating simultaneously. Other advantages are present with the narrow-band systems. To use all 40 channels, the bandwidth of the receivers must be narrow so as not to pick up signals transmitted on adjacent channels. The bandwidth of "true" narrow-band receivers must therefore always be less than 50 kHz as opposed to 200 kHz for the wide-band receivers. In practical terms this means that narrow-band systems are substantially less susceptible to radio interference than wide-band systems.

Narrow-band and wide-band systems are not compatible with one another. Also, narrow-band systems are available that are not "true" narrow-band systems. The transmitters may use narrow-band technology, but the filters in the receivers are not steep enough to reject adjacent channels. Thus such systems can at best use up to 20 of the 40 available channels.

The demands in terms of frequency stability and selectivity are far greater than for wide-band systems. Because the maximum deviation may only be up to $\pm$ 10,000 Hz and on some systems only up to 3000 to 4000 Hz, the transmitting frequency must remain stable within a few hundred hertz. Subsequently, these devices are always crystal controlled. Narrow-band systems are available with fixed crystals, interchangeable crystals, and channel selector switches. Channel selector systems are based on crystal-controlled digital frequency synthesis technology or so-called phase-lock loop. From a theoretical point of view no limit exists as to how many channels can be squeezed into a band, but attempts to make bandwidths less than 25 kHz may have a high price tag in terms of degraded SNR or substantially higher acquisition cost.

Narrow-band systems use two-digit channel numbering or a color-code system. Because manufacturers' selected carrier frequencies and bandwidths may not be the same, compatibility does not necessarily exist between two systems labeled with the same channel number.

Transmitter Types

FM transmitters are generally available in two basic configurations, *commercial large area* transmitters and *portable battery-operated* transmitters for personal or educational use. Whether they are designed for wide-band or narrow-band operation does not alter the mechanical or electrical configuration in terms of how they may be used for a specific application.

The large-area transmitter is commonly referred to as a base station. The type of antenna used determines to a high degree the transmission range. Some manufacturers supply a "rubber-duck" type antenna with their base station. Others provide pullout telescopic-type antennas. The transmission range is also influenced by building materials, but typical range is about 300 feet with the rubber-duck antenna and up to 1000 feet with the telescopic antenna. To cover arenas and sport stadium–size facilities, manufacturers offer large area or rooftop antennas to increase the transmission range. A connector for remote location of the antenna is provided on most systems. Rack-mount kits for installation in standard 19-inch racks are also available. When installing a transmitter in a metal rack cabinet, it is always necessary to remotely locate the antenna outside the cabinet.

Base stations have at least two input connections: one microphone input used for stand alone operation and one line level input used for hookup to PA systems (public address or sound reinforcement systems). Some base stations may also have a separate input for speaker level. When the base station is used with a PA system, a line-level signal is fed from the sound system's mixer to the line-level input on the base station. This is always the best method, but at times, it may be required to hook up to the loudspeaker output of the system. This should be the last resort because the sound system's intensity to the general audience should have no impact on the signal to the people with hearing loss. Newer designs may have an automatic level control to ensure that the input signal always will be optimal for that particular system. Older designs usually have user adjustable input controls and some kind of visual level control in form of a peak indicator or volume unit (VU) meter.

Personal body-worn transmitters are designed for use with electret microphones. The actual microphone can be any one of the electret microphones described in the microphone section earlier in this chapter. The microphone cord is used as the antenna; therefore it is important that the cord be fully extended. A curled-up microphone cord will result in substantially reduced transmission range. The microphone input can also be hooked up to other sound sources but may require an attenuated patch cord (see DAI later this chapter). Some manufacturers also offer a separate auxiliary input (AUX) for use with high-level output devices. If the microphone is removed while using the AUX input, a special antenna may have to be connected to maintain maximum transmission range. For most personal systems this is approximately 100 ft.

FM Receiver Types

Unlike the transmitters, FM receivers may have different physical and electrical designs based on user preference or applications. Several specialty receivers are available, one of which is the auditory trainer (ATE). This type of FM receiver incorporates all the necessary electronic circuitry to simulate a hearing aid or binaural hearing aids. The ATE can therefore be fitted by an audiologist to an individual student in much the same fashion as the student's personal hearing aid. ATE equipment of future designs will all be narrow-band systems incorporating digital frequency synthesis for ease of channel selection.

A smaller more personal version is the BTE FM hearing aid illustrated in Figure 19–2. In this design, the FM receiver and hearing aid are combined in a BTE case. Because of space limitations, the antenna is located outside the case. The antenna is made of pliable material so it can be moved away from the case for better reception. Some FM hearing aids are narrow-band systems operating on frequencies in the 72 to 76 MHz band. Channel selection, if applicable, is made with interchangeable crystals. The user can choose to operate it in FM mode only, hearing aid only, or a combination of the two. Combined with a personal transmitter, it offers an ideal solution for many students of middle school age or older. Because of the inconspicuous design, adults may also prefer this system to the more conventional belt-clip–style receiver. However, there are limitations in terms of hearing losses to which they can be fitted and to receiving distance.

To overcome fitting-related problems and to offer a more economical and cosmetic solution, some hearing aid manufacturers offer an FM receiver boot. The FM boot is a separate module that fits onto the hearing aid in the same fashion as a DAI boot (see the DAI section later in this chapter). Like the FM hearing aids, the FM boots are based on either narrowband technology, usually designed to operate in the 216 to 217 MHz band, or wide-band technology, operating in the 72 to 76 MHz band. The only method of channel selection is through boot exchange. Major drawbacks with this design is short receiving distance and that the FM boot is powered by the hearing aid's battery; therefore battery life is relatively short.

A unique boot receiver is the so-called TMX TeleMagnetix boot attachment. This attachment is designed to receive a pulse-width–modulated 40 kHz signal from a neckloop attached to a special FM receiver as part of the ATE. The system has several advantages over conventional FM boot systems and neckloop/t-coil systems, such as no inductive disturbances (hum), broad audio frequency range (10,000 Hz), SNR as good as with DAI input, not sensitive to head position and movements, low current consumption, and long receiving distance.

A belt-clip–style receiver is the most common style for personal use and the only style recommended for commercial use. Used with appropriate sound coupling methods (i.e., DAI cord, neckloop, hearing aid transducer or so-called button receiver, headset) in combination with the user's personal hearing aid, practically all degrees of hearing loss can be helped. Belt-clip–style receivers are available with all previously mentioned technologies, such as wide-band and narrowband, field-tunable or crystal-controlled, digitally synthesized, or crystal interchangeable.

Some FM receivers are offered with a built-in environmental microphone. This version gives the user the flexibility to use it as an FM receiver or as a personal amplifier previously described under hardwired systems. They may be equipped with a dual volume control system or a balancing control, permitting the user to mix the environmental microphone signal with the FM signal. This is an important feature particularly in lecture or classroom-type settings, where questions from the general audience otherwise may not be understood. The environmental microphone feature may not be important to hearing aid users whose hearing aids can combine DAI with the hearing aid's internal microphone. Other features offered by some manufacturers include fitteradjustable or user-adjustable tone controls or stereo output with left or right balance control.

INFRARED LIGHT SYSTEMS

Infrared (IR) light can be used for signal transmission in the same fashion as with FM transmission. However, unlike FM transmission and induction loop technology, IR cannot pass through walls. Therefore, IR transmission is ideal for facilities operating several systems simultaneously in different rooms in that all receivers can be identical with no need for frequency coordination. Typical applications in which the advantages of the IR technologies are best used, include performing arts and multiplex theaters, courtrooms, and numerous applications where confidentiality is important. It is also an economical solution for home TV listening for people with hearing loss who do not have t-coil hearing aids or no hearing aids at all. Like other wireless technologies used for ALD purposes, no licensing is required to operate an IR system. The disadvantage of IR systems is that the receivers are susceptible to sunlight interference. This may limit use to shady areas or for some systems to indoor applications only. Also, because of the relative high power consumption of transmitters, most systems require hookup to a main outlet that limits portability.

Infrared Technology

An IR system consists of three basic components: a transmitter (base station), an emitter, and a receiver. The audio signal is conveyed onto a subcarrier in the base station, which in turn is converted into IR light by the emitter. The receiver detects the IR signal and converts it back into the original audio signal.

IR systems used for ALD purposes are wide-band–type systems implying a frequency modulation of the subcarrier of approximately ±40 kHz. Narrow-band systems generally do not provide an adequate frequency response for people with hearing loss and are typically used for simultaneous language translation and other communication purposes.

Early IR ALD systems primarily used the 95 kHz subcarrier with 250 kHz as an option for stereo or language translation. Until the mid-90s, the IR technology appeared to be interference free. FM systems are susceptible to outside radio interference and loop systems to inductive interference caused by electrical installations and in particular the magnetic ballasts used with flourescent lights. However, with the introduction of the electronic ballast for fluorescent lights, severe interference problems started to occur with the 95 kHz systems. The electronic ballasts generate a 30 kHz square

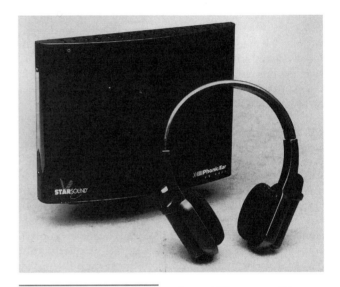

Figure 19–7 Large area two-channel IR system. (Courtesy Phonic Ear, Inc.)

wave signal that is picked up by the IR receiver. The interference can be heard as a loud howling sound that renders the entire system useless. Therefore manufacturers of 95 kHz systems also offer 250 kHz systems as standard or on a conversion basis. Because the electronic ballasts are used in new construction and for retrofit of older facilities, manufacturers of two-channel or stereo systems have switched to 2.3- and 2.8-MHz subcarriers. Figure 19–7 shows a 2.3/2.8 MHz two-channel large area system with headset. To date no sources of interference (other than direct sunlight) are known with systems operating at those frequencies. General compatibility exists between manufacturer's equipment using same subcarrier and frequency modulation.

Transmitters and Emitters

The audio signal is routed to the IR base station in the same way as for FM and induction loop systems. Home TV systems are usually supplied with patch cord for direct hookup or with a TV microphone. Likewise, the commercial systems can hook up to PA systems or operate as stand-alone systems when PA systems are not required. The input connectors and input level controls are the same as for FM systems and part of the base station section.

The emitter section may be combined with the base station or it may be a separate unit referred to as an emitter panel (also called a repeater). Whether separate or not, an emitter consists of an array of special light-emitting diodes (LED). The number of LEDs determines how large an area can be irradiated. Home TV systems typically only require five LEDs, whereas large area systems may require between 50 and 144 per channel, depending on the desired coverage area. Coverage information provided by manufacturers for a specific product should be used only as a guideline. Some of the more powerful IR panels offered for ALD applications can cover areas of 12,000 ft or more in an oblong-shaped room. It is a common belief that IR systems are line-of-sight only. This is not necessarily so. Although invisible to the eye, IR light behaves similar to visible light. It is reflected off light-colored walls and ceilings and absorbed by dark surfaces. To avoid shadow effects or simply to increase coverage area, most emitter panels are designed with daisy-chain capability (in a daisy-chain the signal is routed from one unit to the next in a continuous chain, with only one unit actually connected to the source). Therefore IR systems can consist of a single base station with several emitter panels. The emitter panels should be installed 10 ft. or higher and angled downward. The best method of avoiding shadow effects is to install a panel on each side and point them diagonally across the room. Two low-powered emitter panels (i.e., each 5000 ft specified coverage) will usually provide far better coverage than one high-powered panel (i.e., specified at 10,000 ft).

Two basic methods of transferring the signal from the base station to the IR panel(s) exist. Each method has its advantages and disadvantages. One method is to transfer the sub-carrier from the base station by means of standard coaxial cable with BNC-type connectors to the emitter panel. With this method, any number of emitter panels can be daisy chained to a base station. The disadvantage is that each emitter panel requires power from a main AC outlet. The other method is to send both audio signal and a low-voltage DC to the emitter panels along a three-conductor cable. Such systems are simple to install, but limitations exist in terms of how many emitter panels can be added.

Most emitter panels are designed for wall mounting. Supplied with pivoting brackets, they are easy to install and can be aimed for best possible coverage. Although not portable in the same fashion as the FM belt-clip–style transmitter, even large venue IR systems can be set up in a short time. When mounted on floor stands, they can quickly be brought into a room and connected to the sound system. Portable battery-operated systems are also available. The sound pickup is through a builtin boundary microphone. The LEDs are positioned in the dome for 360-degree IR radiation.

Infrared Receivers

One of the reasons that IR systems have become very popular is the high-quality sound reproduction through IR headsets. Available in two versions, over-the-head and under-the-chin–style, they provide unsurpassed fidelity for people with mild-to-moderate hearing losses. Both types are available in mono and stereo versions.

The more conventional lavalier-style receiver is used mostly for commercial applications. It can be fitted with any

---

PEARL

A person is fitted with two canal instruments and is doing very well. However, when watching TV at home, the TV's volume control is set so loud that it is a nuisance to other family members and neighbors. A personal IR TV system with an under-the-chin–style headset solves the problem.

---

sound-coupling method (see Fig. 19–2) from direct audio input to neckloops as described later this chapter. Most over-the-head style receivers radiate an inductive field compatible with the t-coil sensitivity of hearing aids. Some of the under-the-chin-style receivers are also available with output jacks for use with neckloops, silhouette inductors, and DAI to hearing aid(s).

The critical element for good reception is positioning of the optical lens capturing the IR signal in combination with the amount of power radiated. The over-the-head style receivers provide 360-degree reception because the receiving lens (or lenses) is positioned so it can "see" the emitter panel from all directions. On lavalier-style and under-the-chin-style receivers, the lens is located so as to receive signals coming from the front. Wide-angle lenses offered by some manufacturers may have receiving angles up to 160 degrees. Shadow effects from people moving in front of the listener may result in occasional poor SNR or, at times, for the receiver to completely drop out if equipped with a squelch. Squelch is a circuit that mutes the receiver function when no signal is present or when the signal is too weak to provide an adequate SNR. Units without a squelch circuit would generate a loud unpleasant hissing sound when no IR signal is present. As mentioned earlier, the best method of avoiding shadow effects is to install two emitter panels and point them diagonally across the room.

BATTERIES AND CHARGING SYSTEMS

Most older designs of personal amplifiers, FM transmitters/receivers, and loop receivers operate on 9 V disposable and/or rechargeable batteries. Operation time with this battery is relatively short (less than 8 hr. for some systems), especially with rechargeable nicad batteries.

PITFALL

It should be noted that two types of 9 V nicad batteries exist. The nicad batteries offered by the ALD manufacturers are a 7-cell type (8.4 V), whereas commercial over-the-counter types are only 6-cell (7.2 V). The operation time between recharges may be severely reduced with the 7.2 V battery.

Most of the newer the belt-clip designs, regardless of technology and application, operate on two AA size disposable or rechargeable batteries as the most economical power source. Disposable AA batteries are inexpensive and rechargeable nicad batteries (1.2 V cells) have sufficient capacity to last through the day in even the most current consuming systems.

Irrespective of battery type, manufacturers offer two methods of charging the batteries without physically having to remove them. The output jack on receivers/amplifiers or Mic/AUX-INPUT jack on transmitters are often designed to also accommodate charging of battery. The charge cord is simply connected to the jack and the unit is left on charge overnight ready for use the next day. The charger can be a wall-type AC adaptor with a single charge cord for personal amplifiers, or it may have a double cord for a transmitter/receiver combination. Multichargers accommodating between 10 and 20 units are also available.

Other ALDs are designed with external contacts, so the unit may be "dropped" into the charger instead of connected to a cord. Drop-in chargers are usually available as two-unit chargers. Some chargers, especially for ATE, are designed to be expandable by adding additional two-unit modules, yet others may be designed as multichargers accommodating between 10 and 20 units. Some devices are designed to accommodate both charging methods.

Whatever the design, most devices are equipped with a charge indicator to ensure the user that the unit is being charged and not just merely plugged in. As a general rule, all rechargeable systems using nicad batteries may be left on charge even if the units are not to be used for days. The expected lifetime of a nicad battery, claimed by manufacturers, may vary, but they all pretty much last between 1 and 3 years.

Some devices are not designed for use with rechargeable batteries. Most over-the-head–style IR headsets operate on disposable AAA size batteries. Yet others may be designed with nonstandard rechargeable battery packs or nonreplaceable rechargeable batteries.

SOUND COUPLINGS AND FITTING OPTIONS

The sound-generating transducer is usually the internal receiver in a hearing aid. The signal from the output of the amplifier or wireless receiver can be routed to the hearing aid's amplifier by means of a DAI connection if the hearing aid is equipped for this. An alternative routing method is through an inductive transducer to a t-coil in the hearing aid. Neckloops and silhouettes are the two types of inductive couplers used with ALD receivers. When the signal transfer method is a room loop, the hearing aid user only needs to set the hearing aid's input selector to "T" position. If the hearing aid is not equipped with a DAI connector or a t-coil or if the person with hearing loss does not have hearing aids at all, the only alternative is to provide the user with an external hearing aid receiver/transducer, earbuds, or headset that is driven directly by the ALD's receiver.

Direct Audio Input

The usual input to hearing aids are acoustic through the microphone or electromagnetic through the induction pickup coil.

However, a need exists (e.g., for educational purposes) for an electrical connection from sound sources, such as a radio, tape/CD player, IR system, external microphone, or computer. The electrical audio signal is routed from the source directly to a socket on the hearing aid through a cord. The connection inside the hearing aid is usually made to the same point as that of the microphone. The above-mentioned is referred to as DAI. An alternative name, often used in Europe, is AUX.

Physical and Electrical Standardization of Direct Audio Input

Efforts to use a common DAI plug and socket and compatible input/output signals were initiated by European dispensers and manufacturers in 1982. The consequence was a tacit understanding that a DAI system must consist of "Euro" compatible elements. The "Euro-Audio-Input System" was adopted by the International Electrotechnical Commission in Switzerland in 1984 as IEC standard 118-6. This standard calls for the BTE plug of the DAI cord to be a three-pin polarized plug of specific dimensions and signal polarity. The socket on the hearing aid must, obviously, be designed to accept the plug. Furthermore, the standard specifies that the input sensitivity required to produce a specific output shall be stated. This output is defined as being equal to the output generated with 70-dB SPL acoustic input to the microphone. It is typically on the order of 1 mV. Today most hearing aid–producing countries have adopted the IEC 118-6 Standard.

The Direct Audio Input "Boot"

The DAI plug is a physically large plug, and most hearing aids cannot accommodate its socket. Most hearing aid manufacturers therefore offer an adaptor—commonly called a boot. The boot is slipped onto the bottom of the hearing aid where it connects with the hearing aid's dedicated (small) DAI contacts. The DAI plug is then inserted into the boot (Fig. 19–8). Because the boot is dedicated to individual manufacturer's hearing aids (physically as well as electrically), it must be obtained from the manufacturer of the hearing aid with which DAI is to be used.

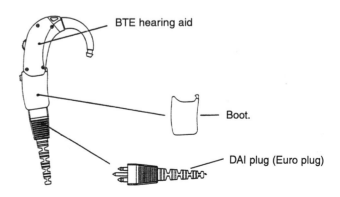

Figure 19–8 The DAI boot shown as adaptor between the hearing aid and the DAI plug. (Courtesy Oticon, Inc.)

Attenuation of Direct Audio Input Cords or Boots

The signal level of most audio sources is too high to be connected to the hearing aid without a certain level of attenuation. The signal levels can be categorized as follows:

1. *Microphone level (.5 to 5 mV)*—needs no attenuation
2. *Low line-level (100 to 500 mV)*—needs some attenuation
3. *High line-level and headset level (500 to 1500 mV)*—needs more attenuation
4. *Loudspeaker and high-output headset level (1.5 to several volts)*—needs maximum attenuation

The amount of attenuation depends largely on the setting of the audio source's volume control and on its impedance. Some manufacturers have chosen to provide the attenuation in the boot and to even allow it to be adjustable. Others offer attenuated DAI cords.

PITFALL
It is important to avoid using attenuated cords with attenuated boots. Such "double" attenuation will result in very weak output from the hearing aid.

The end opposite the DAI plug must terminate with a plug that fits into the output connection of the audio source. Commonly used are two-pin plugs, three-pin plugs, and mini (3.5 mm) plugs.

Direct Audio Input Sources and Connections

The list of audio sources that can be used with DAI is virtually endless. Figure 19–9 shows an external microphone directly connected to a hearing aid through the DAI cord. As mentioned earlier, no attenuation should be used with external microphones as the sound source. Figure 19–10 shows the connection from a monitor-type TV. The jacks marked Audio Out (L and R) must be used for this type of TV. The volume control of the TV usually has no influence on the signal from

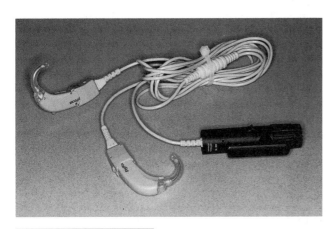

Figure 19–9   External microphone connected to hearing aid. (Courtesy Oticon, Inc.)

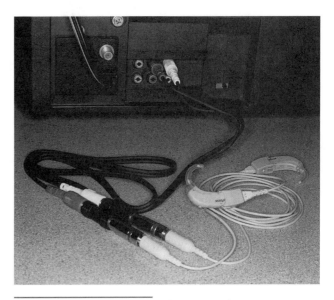

Figure 19–10   DAI hearing aids connected to a monitor-type TV. (Courtesy Oticon, Inc.)

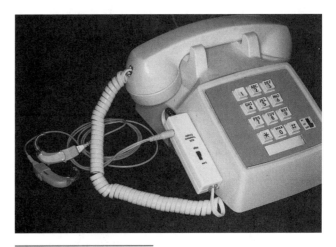

Figure 19–11   Telephone coupler connected to hearing aids. (Courtesy Oticon, Inc.)

these jacks, and 40- to 50-dB of attenuation is needed. It may be difficult to obtain a DAI cord that terminates with a phono (RCA) plug (monitor-type TVs use phono jacks). A DAI cord terminating with a mini (3.5 mm) plug can be used with a mini-plug-to-phono-plug adaptor as shown in Figure 19–10. Figure 19–11 shows a coupler that fits in between the handset cord and the base of a telephone. The signal from the telephone is then picked up by a mini-plug DAI cord that is inserted into the jack on the coupler. This setup can give disturbance-free binaural listening, which may not be possible if the t-coil of the hearing aid is used. Some 35- to 45-dB attenuation is needed in position High of the coupler and 15- to 25-dB is needed in position Low. The handset can be substituted by a hand-free headset if preferred.

ATE is perhaps the most common use of DAI (Fig. 19–12). The signal is picked up from the earphone connection of the ATE receiver and routed to the hearing aids. The amount of

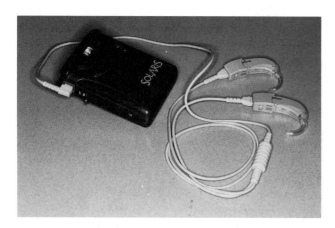

Figure 19–12 Typical DAI use with an auditory trainer. (Courtesy Oticon, Inc.)

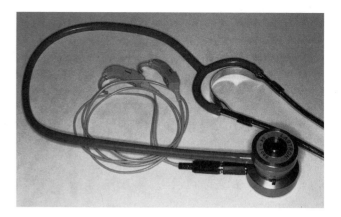

Figure 19–13 DAI from an amplified medical stethoscope. (Courtesy Oticon, Inc.)

attenuation ranges from between 20- and 50-dB and depends largely on the position of the ATE receiver's volume control.

PITFALL

The DAI cord doubles as an antenna for the ATE receiver. It should be kept long (at least 15 inches) and not coiled up, which would shorten the transmitting range of the ATE.

Figure 19–13 shows DAI from an amplified medical stethoscope. The signal is routed from the output connection on the transducer part of the stethoscope and routed into the hearing aids. The volume control on the hearing aids, if any, should be left as for everyday use. The signal level from the stethoscope is adjusted by the volume control on the transducer part until the loudness is satisfactory. The tubings to the ear (stethoscope part) are not used. Heart sounds are primarily composed of low frequencies. Hence, hearing aids with good low-frequency reproduction will work best with this setup. About 5- to 10-dB of attenuation is required.

Other common DAI sources are IR systems, walkaround stereos, tape players, CD players, computer sound cards, dictaphones, and so on.

PEARL

A student has been issued an FM system with a neckloop and has been very pleased with the performance. However, after starting a class where a computer is required, the inductive interference from the monitor renders the system useless. The student is issued a DAI boot and a cord for direct coupling to the receiver. When inserting the boot, the t-coil is automatically switched off so only the FM signal is picked up.

Control Settings of the Hearing Aid

The main switch of the hearing aid is normally kept in M (microphone) position during DAI use. That way, the environmental microphone remains active during delivery of the DAI signal. In addition, most manufacturers offer a "DAI-only" option that disables the environmental microphone, allowing only the DAI signal to be present. This can be achieved several different ways: one boot for DAI-only mode and another for DAI plus environmental microphone; a switch on the boot or hearing aid or a special design where the t-coil setting is used. In this design when the boot is attached, an electronic switch disables the induction coil and allows the DAI signal to pass. The volume control, if any, is normally left in its everyday position. In a classroom using ATE with DAI and the environmental microphone simultaneously, the attenuation may be adjusted to make the DAI signal (teachers voice) override 5- to 10-dB the signal from the environmental microphone.

Inductive Transfer of Signals

As an alternative to electrical input, inductive transfer may be used. This requires that the hearing aid is equipped with a t-coil. The most typical use of inductive transfer is with a telephone. Surrounding the receiver end of the handset is a magnetic induction field that radiates the audio signal from the receiver. The induction field is picked up by the t-coil within the hearing aid. Not all t-coils are compatible with all telephones, stationary and mobile ones. In cases of poor compatibility an induction amplifier (Fig. 19–14) can be used. The one pictured has a small microphone facing the receiver of the telephone handset. The audio signal from the receiver is picked up by the microphone, amplified, and converted into a strong induction field that is received by the hearing aid's induction coil. The strap-on amplifier shown has an electrical output connection allowing it to be used (e. g., with DAI to hearing aids). The connection may alternately be used to drive two inductors, sometimes referred to as silhouettes (see Fig. 19–14). The inductors are placed behind the ears together with either BTE or in-the-ear (ITE) type hearing aids. The inductors emit a strong inductive field that is picked up by the induction coil in the hearing aids. This is one way to receive a binaural induction signal from a telephone. The

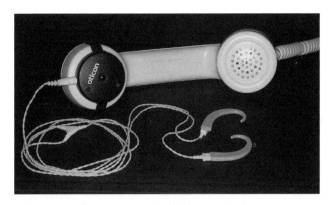

Figure 19–14 Strap-on type induction amplifier with binaural silhouette inductors attached. (Courtesy Oticon, Inc.)

strap-on amplifier can also be used as a "close-talk" microphone. In a noisy place it can be held close to a speaker's mouth and the signal routed by means of DAI to the hearing aid(s). On a TV that has no electrical output connections it can be mounted on or close to the loudspeaker and used with an extension cord to the hearing aid(s). The same holds true for other audio sources that have no electrical connections.

Some hearing aid users, in particular adults, prefer a neckloop as an alternative to silhouette inductors. This is because it fits around the neck and can easily be concealed. Also, binaural listening is possible without the need for attachments to the hearing aids if the user has two t-coil equipped hearing aids. However, because of the neckloop's very low impedance, an amplifier is required to provide a strong enough induction field for the hearing aid's t-coils. Induction (telephone) amplifiers such as the one shown in Figure 19–14 does not have sufficient power to drive a neckloop. Neckloops are most often used in connection with ALD and ATE receivers but may also be hooked up directly to the headphone jack of TVs and walkaround-type devices.

Limitations and Drawbacks with Inductive Transfer

Although no serious drawbacks or limitations exist with electrical DAI (other than limited mobility), some disadvantages and limitations may be experienced with inductive transfer. A humming sound is present in most environments. The hum may be perceived at an annoying level by people with milder hearing losses but may be inaudible for people with more severe hearing losses. It is worse around equipment that radiates strong magnetic induction fields such as computers and monitors, fluorescent lights, microwave ovens, and large electrical installations. Hearing aid manufacturers are often asked to shield the induction coil for hum. This is not feasible because such a shield would render the t-coil useless. A good low-frequency notch filter would relieve most of the hum, but such a filter requires several additional space-consuming components in an analog hearing aid. An effective notch filter, however, is possible in a fully digital hearing aid without adding extra components.

If a neckloop is used, positioning of the loop relative to the head is critical. Head positioning and movements can cause noticeable changes in output from the hearing aid. Telephones, induction loops, and neck loops do not radiate their inductive field in the same direction. However, many hearing aid's induction coils can be physically positioned inside the hearing aid to optimize the inductive transfer (e.g., a horizontal position when worn works best with telephones and a vertical position is the only position that is compatible with room induction loops). Neither position is optimal with neckloops. Dual induction coils in both horizontal and vertical positions are often limited in effectiveness because of reduced sensitivity to avoid internal magnetic coupling (instability).

Electromagnetic Compatibility

Electromagnetic compatibility (EMC) is the most commonly used terminology when describing inductive compatibility or interference from cellular telephones. Not all cellular phones produce sufficient inductive radiation to provide acceptable output from the hearing aid. Worse yet, most digital cellular phones transmit a signal that is picked up by the hearing aid as an annoying—often very loud—distorted buzzing sound. Worst interference can be expected from systems such as Time Division Multiple Access (TDMA) and Global System Mobile (GSM). Less interference can be expected from Code Division Multiple Access (CDMA). No hearing aids are immune for this type of interference, which is caused by wires and component leads in the hearing aid acting as miniature antennas. Generally speaking, the smaller the hearing aid the less the interference. Fully digital hearing aids are most "immune" because of their few analog components and pathways.

The problem has no easy solutions. Tiny capacitors mounted in the early signal path may be able to partially shorten the interference signal, thereby rendering some alleviation. Metalizing the hearing aid casing is more effective but may result in allergenic reactions. In addition to the hearing aid manufacturers, the telephone companies are searching for solutions as described by H. Stephen Berger (1997).

Induction Coil Sensitivity

Induction coils are tested according to ANSI S3.22 in an electromagnetic field of 31.5 mA/m at 200 to 500 Hz. The hearing aid is positioned manually for best inductive transfer, and the acoustic output sound pressure level (SPL) is recorded. ANSI S3.22 does not specify any requirement for sensitivity. In general, if the output SPL in a 31.5 mA/m field is equivalent to, or greater than, the output SPL obtained with 60 dB SPL acoustic input, the coil sensitivity is very acceptable.

CONTROVERSIAL POINT

31.5 mA/m is for testing and comparing only. In real life the hearing aid is normally subjected to at least 100 mA/m, being 10 dB more than the 31.5 mA/m.

External Hearing Aid Transducers, Headsets, and Earbuds

When the user's hearing aid(s) is not equipped with DAI or a t-coil, the only option is to use an appropriate sound-generating transducer and, if necessary, remove one or both hearing aids. Obviously, this option also applies to people with hearing loss who do not wear hearing aids. When considering the number of hearing aid users and the number of hearing aids equipped with DAI or t-coils versus the total number people with hearing loss who can benefit from the use an ALD, the number of people falling into this category is rather large. Therefore it is important to select a transducer type that can provide a high acoustic output to better use the residual hearing of the individual user.

The external hearing aid receiver (transducer) commonly supplied by ALD manufacturers offers several advantages over conventional headsets and earbuds. When fitted with a stetoclip for binaural or nylon hook for monaural listening as shown in Figure 19–15, the maximum output is close to 120 dB SPL. Some manufacturers offer the stetoclip with washable mushroom tips in place of the replaceable foam pads shown in the picture, thereby increasing the overall output to approximately 125 dB SPL. This type transducer can also be fitted with a standard size canal tip for individuals (monaural and binaural fittings possible), thereby increasing the output to more than 130 dB SPL.

Conventional nonoccluding headsets generally do not exceed 115 dB SPL, whereas earbuds may be closer to 120 dB SPL. Only few manufacturers make technical specifications (ANSI S3.22) available for their products. Also, when headsets and earbuds are used with personal amplifiers or with ALD receivers equipped with environmental microphones, severe feedback problems may occur as a result of acoustic leakage. In addition, there are sanitary concerns with earbuds and headsets at public facilities and some reluctance by users to use the over-the-head–style headsets.

PEARL

A city purchasing manager needs ALSs for some of the city's public facilities, which include the council chamber, the senior center, the community center, a small auditorium for employee training, and some courtrooms. Because no single technology is best for all applications, each facility is evaluated as a separate entity.

A loop system with wand-style loop receivers is recommended for the council chamber because of the low maintenance and administration factor. A loop system is also recommended for the senior center because several patrons have t-coil hearing aids. However, the loop receivers are the belt-clip–style equipped with hearing aid transducers and stetoclips to provide the greatest possible dynamic range.

Because of the large size and ever-changing floorplan layout at the community center, an FM system is recommended. The transmitter is installed in the existing PA systems rack and the antenna remote located inside the auditorium. The receivers are supplied with hearing aid transducers and stetoclips. In addition, a supply of neckloops is provided (half the quantity of receivers). The employee training facility is also equipped with an FM system. However, the facility is not equipped with a PA system. Thus the transmitter is of the belt-clip style equipped with an omnidirectional lapel microphone.

The courtrooms are equipped with IR systems to ensure full confidentiality. At the same time, receivers can be handed out from a central point, regardless of which courtroom they will be used in. The chosen style is the over-the-head type because of their 360 degree reception capability.

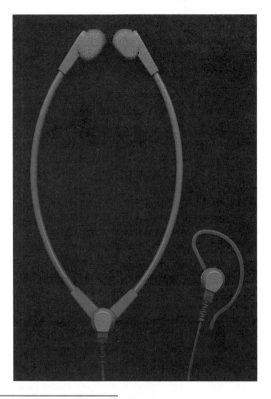

Figure 19–15 100 Ohm hearing aid transducer fitted with stetoclip and monaural earhook. (Courtesy Centrum Sound Systems).

CONCLUSIONS

When recommending an ALD or ALS, one must understand the nature of the problem to which the solution has to be applied. The optimum solution for same type of problem will differ on the basis of whether an ALD is for an individual person wishing to obtain a personal system as opposed to a place of public accommodation. Many people with hearing loss share information about their hearing aids or ALDs with each other. Likewise, facilities managers of public or commercial facilities also share information with one another. Just because one type of system works well for one individual or in one facility that does not mean it is the optimal solution for another. Thus it is very important to recognize and explain the advantages and disadvantages of the individual ALD components because they relate to sound pickup, signal transfer method, and sound couplings/fitting options for each application.

The use of ALDs has greatly improved the communication abilities of hearing aid users and nonusers as well. The availability and innovation of these devices will continue to improve and so will public awareness and education.

REFERENCES

AMERICAN NATIONAL STANDARD INSTITUTE. Specifications of hearing aid characteristics (ANSI S3.22 1996) New York: ANSI.

AMERICANS WITH DISABILITIES ACT OF 1990. (ADA, 1990). 42 USC 12101, Equal Opportunity for the Disabled, Washington, DC.

AMERICANS WITH DISABILITIES ACT. (ADA 1991). 28 CFR Part 36, Nondiscrimination on the Basis of Disability by Public Accommodations and in Commercial Facilities, *Federal Register,* Washington, DC.

AMERICANS WITH DISABILITIES ACT ACCESSIBILITY GUIDELINES. (ADAAG 1994). 36 CFR Part 1191, Accessibility Guidelines for Buildings and Facilities, *Federal Register,* Washington, DC.

BERGER, H.S. (1997). *Hearing aid and cellular phone compatability—Working toward solutions.* Paper presented at Gallaudet University, May 1997. Wireless telephones and hearing aids: New challenges for audiology.

CIVIL RIGHTS ACT OF 1964. 42 USC 2000e, Public Health & Welfare. Washington, DC.

FEDERAL COMMUNICATION COMMISSION (FCC) 47 CFR part 0 to 19. *Federal Register,* Washington, DC.

INTERNATIONAL ELECTROTECHNICAL COMMISSION. *Magnetic field strength in audio-frequency induction loop for hearing aid purposes (IEC 118–4 1981).* Geneva, Switzerland: Bureau Central de la Commission Electrotechnique Internationale.

INTERNATIONAL ELECTROTECHNICAL COMMISSION. *Characteristics of electrical input circuits for hearing aids (IEC 118–6 1984).* Geneva, Switzerland: Bureau Central de la Commission Electrotechnique Internationale.

REHABILITATION ACT OF 1973. 29 USC 791, Employment of Individuals with Disabilities. Washington, DC.

TELECOMMUNICATIONS ACT OF 1934. (ADA Amendment, 1996). 47 USC 225, Telecommunications Services for Hearing-Impaired and Speech-Impaired Individuals, Washington, DC.

PREFERRED PRACTICE GUIDELINES

Professionals Who Perform The Procedure(s)

▼ Audiologists

Expected Outcomes

▼ The ALSs provide user(s) mobility to perform all assigned job functions, or to participate in public events on equal terms with people without hearing loss.

▼ Facilities have proper signage for hearing accessibility.

▼ Facilities have procedures for proper maintenance of equipment and training of designated personnel.

▼ The ALS can be handed out and operated with little or no instructions. In public facilities where several output couplings are offered, coupling options are clearly posted so individual users can identify which option is most suitable for their particular needs.

▼ The ALS is hardwired directly from the sound source and properly attenuated or a microphone(s) with proper directional characteristics has been or can be placed in a position alleviating appropriate acoustic problems.

▼ The ALS can provide (1) an inductive output that is compatible with the sensitivity of the hearing aid's t-coil, or (2) an electrical output that is compatible with the sensitivity of the hearing aid's DAI circuit, or (3) an acoustic output level sufficient to maximize the dynamic range of a non-hearing-aid user.

Clinical Process

▼ Evaluation of an individual person's intelligibility problems at home, in the workplace, and on the go.

▼ Selection and/or recommendation of ALS that will overcome identified problems in a simple, unobtrusive, and cost-effective way.

▼ Counseling on the care of batteries and recharging of batteries when applicable.

▼ Evaluation of public facilities as they relate to advantages and disadvantages of various types of ALSs.

▼ Recommend type of ALS that will comply with minimum requirements of the ADA and provide a source for obtaining the system(s).

▼ Advice on maintenance procedures and other practical administrative aspects as they relate to handling of receivers and related accessories.

Documentation

▼ Documentation contains pertinent background information for selection/recommendation of ALS.

▼ Documentation includes all information related to ALS in terms of transmission type, frequency, receiver style, and related output couplings (i.e., neckloop[s], silhouette inductor[s], DAI cord, type of boot).

Chapter 20

Room Acoustics for Listeners with Normal-Hearing and Hearing Impairment

Carl C. Crandell and Joseph J. Smaldino

Beginning in 1975 with the Education of All Handicapped Children Act and proceeding through 1997 with amendments to the Individuals with Disabilities Education Act (IDEA), and the Americans with Disabilities Act (ADA), interest has been sustained in removing acoustic barriers to individuals with hearing loss, particularly in our nation's classrooms (Access Board Web site, 1998; Bess et al, 1996; Crandell, 1991b, 1992a; Crandell & Smaldino, 1994, 1995; Crandell et al, 1995; Education of Handicapped Children, P.L. 94–142 Regulations, 1977; Education of Handicapped Act Amendments, P.L. 99–457 Regulations, 1986; Education of Handicapped Act Amendments, P.L. 101–476 Regulations, 1990; Flexer, 1992; Individuals with Disabilities Education Act Web site, 1998; Smaldino, 1997). Because classroom learning occurs primarily through the teacher verbally communicating with the students, accurate recognition of the teacher's speech signal by the students is an obvious prerequisite for learning to take place. To the extent that the acoustic characteristics of the classroom listening environment interfere with accurate speech recognition, the acoustics are barriers to learning in a classroom. Acoustic barriers to listening and learning have been extensively studied over the past 20 years (see Crandell et al, 1995, for a review). From this research it is clear that the acoustic factors that most often affect accurate speech recognition in a room include (1) the relative intensity of the information-carrying components of the speech signal to a noninformation-carrying signal or noise (i.e., signal-to-noise ratio) (SNR); (2) the degree to which the temporal aspects of the information-carrying components of the speech signal are preserved; (3) the distance from the speaker to the listener; and (4) the interaction among these variables. In addition, speech recognition in a room can be influenced by linguistic and/or articulatory factors. Linguistic factors include word familiarity and vocabulary of the listener, context, the number of syllables in the word, and linguistic competency of the listener. Articulatory factors include the gender of the speaker and the articulatory abilities and dialect of the speaker. This chapter will focus on the acoustic factors that influence speech recognition in rooms, with a primary emphasis on classrooms. For discussions of the linguistic or articulatory variables that influence speech recognition, the reader is directed to Godfrey (1984), Sanders (1993), Kent (1997), and McLaughlin (1998).

INTENSITY OF THE SPEAKER'S VOICE

For optimal speech recognition to occur in a room, the speaker's voice must be heard clearly above (1) the individual listener's threshold of audibility and (2) the background

601

noise level of the enclosure. The intensity of a speaker's voice varies with the amount of pressure developed by the lung, the length of time the vocal folds are closed, and the resonances of the vocal tract (which change with the position of the tongue). The degree of mouth opening is also an important factor for appropriate projection of the voice. The human voice has relatively limited acoustic power. The vowels are the strongest components of speech, whereas consonants are the weakest. The average sound pressure level (SPL) that is produced by a speaker (at 1 m) during quiet, normal, and loud speech is 45 dB, 65 dB, and 85 dB, respectively (Denes & Pinson, 1993; Hawkins & Yacullo, 1984). The range of speech is approximately 30 dB (+12 dB to −18 dB).

Because of the limited power of the human voice and the acoustic environment in an enclosure (noise, reverberation, and distance), many rooms will require the use of an amplification device to ensure a high level of speech recognition. Speaking loudly in many rooms will not improve speech recognition because loud speech generally increases the intensity of the vowel phonemes not the consonant phonemes. As will be discussed in a later section, most cues important for accurate speech recognition are carried by consonant phonemes, not vowels (French & Steinberg, 1947; Licklider & Miller, 1951; Sher & Owens, 1974; Wang et al, 1978). Moreover, speaking with a high vocal output for extended periods can often lead to various forms of vocal pathosis, such as chronic hoarseness and vocal nodules. Gotaas and Starr (1995) showed that 80% of public school teachers, who often have to speak loudly during an entire school day, reported vocal fatigue compared with 5% in the general population. In addition, it appears that many speakers cannot sustain loud levels of speech for extended periods. Ottring et al (1992) investigated the potential of training teachers to increase their speaking levels behaviorally in the classroom. Results indicated that it was possible to train teachers to increase their speaking level from 3- to 5-dB, but continual training was necessary to sustain the level enhancement. It was concluded that classroom amplification is the most consistent means to increase teacher's voice levels over their normal speaking level.

BACKGROUND ROOM NOISE

In addition to the power of the speaker's voice, background (or ambient) noise in a room may also compromise speech recognition. Background noise refers to any auditory disturbance that interferes with what a listener wants or needs to hear (Crandell et al, 1995). Background noise in a room can emanate from several possible sources. These sources include *external noise* (noise that is generated from outside the building, such as airplane traffic, local construction, automobile traffic, and playgrounds), *internal noise* (noise that originates from within the building but outside the room, such as rooms adjacent to cafeterias, lecture rooms, gymnasiums, and/or busy hallways), and *room noise* (noise that is generated within the room) (Crandell & Smaldino, 1994, 1995, 1996b; Johns & Thomas, 1957; Olsen, 1977, 1981). Sources of room noise include individuals talking, sliding chairs or tables, and shuffling hard-soled shoes on noncarpeted floors. Heating, ventilation, and air-conditioning systems may also significantly contribute to room noise levels.

Measurement of Room Noise

The acoustic characteristics of background noise often vary considerably in a room as a function of time because of the changing activities taking place in that room. This variability often makes it difficult to reliably measure room noise and its effects in a simple manner. Despite this difficulty, most measures of room noise continue to be single number descriptions. One of the most common single number descriptors of room noise is the measurement of the relative SPL of the noise at a specific point or points in time on an A-weighting scale. A device called a *sound level meter* is usually used for this measurement. A sound level meter is an instrument that measures the amplitude of sound. Sound level meters range from compact, inexpensive, battery-operated units to computer-based devices that can measure and record numerous properties of a signal. Sound level meters are classified according to standards set forth in ANSI S1.14 (1983). Type I sound level meters meet the most rigorous standards, whereas type II is for general purpose, and type III is for hobby use. Most serious measurement of room noise would require at least a type II meter, and preferably a type I instrument. Many sound level meters incorporate weighting filter networks. The A-weighting network is designed to simulate the sensitivity of the average human ear under conditions of low sound loudness (40 phons). The B-weighting simulates loud sound (70 phons), and the C-weighting approximates how the ear would respond to very loud sound. The convention for room and factory noise measurements is the use of the A-weighting network.

The single number obtained from a sound pressure measurement performed with the A-weighting scale can be obtained with a number of very different spectra. A more thorough manner to measure noise in an enclosure is to conduct a spectral analysis of the noise. Spectral analyses of the noise (usually from 63 Hz to 8000 Hz) requires an octave band, or one-third octave band, filter network associated with the sound level meter. Another procedure of evaluating the effects of noise on speech communication is through the use of *noise criteria (NC) curves* (Beranek, 1954). NC curves are a family of frequency/intensity curves based on octave band sound pressure across a 20 to 10,000 Hz band and have been related to successful use of an acoustic space for a variety of activities. When using NC curves (see Fig. 20–1), sound levels are plotted across eight standard frequencies. The NC value that characterizes a room is determined by the highest octave band SPL that intersects the NC family of curves. Thus, in Figure 20–1, the NC curve would be 50 dB. The NC rating is generally 8 to 10 dB below the dB(A) level of that room. To illustrate the advantages of this procedure over a single number descriptor, assume that a great deal of low-frequency noise was present in an enclosure. This noise would have a great effect on the NC unit assigned to the room; however, a single number measure such as dB(A) would not provide enough detail to identify and reduce offending frequency bands. It is recommended therefore that whenever possible, background noise levels in rooms be measured by means of NC curves because this procedure gives the examiner additional information regarding the spectral characteristics of the noise. Specifically, with this information the audiologist or acoustic engineer can isolate and modify sources of excessive noise in the room. Appropriate NC units for various rooms are found in Table 20–1. Table 20–2 presents the effects of different NC units on communicative efficiency. A similar concept to NC curves are *room criteria (RC) curves*. In the development of RC curves, NC

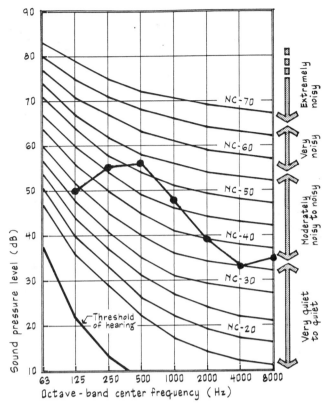

Figure 20–1 Example of NC curves. (Adapted from Egan [1987].)

curves were modified at very low and very high frequencies to include frequencies commonly associated with mechanical noises, such as heating or air-conditioning units. The reader is directed to Beranek (1954), Borrild (1978), Knudsen and Harris (1978), Hassall and Zaveri (1979), Cremer and Muller (1982), Egan (1987), and Harris (1991) for further details concerning the measurement of noise.

Background Noise Levels in Rooms

Background noise levels have been reported in many enclosures, such as classrooms, department stores, transportation settings, and homes (Bess et al, 1984; Blair, 1977; Crandell, 1992a; Crandell & Smaldino, 1994, 1995; Finitzo-Hieber, 1988; Markides, 1986; McCroskey & Devens, 1975; Nober & Nober,

TABLE 20–1 Appropriate NC units, and computed equivalent dB(A) readings, for various environments

Type of Space	NC Units	Computer Equivalent dB(A) Readings
Broadcast studios	15–20	25–30
Concert halls	15–20	25–30
Theaters (500 seats, no amplification)	20–25	30–35
Music rooms	25	35
Schoolrooms (no amplification)	25	35
Television studios	25	35
Apartments and hotels	25–30	35–40
Assembly halls (amplification)	25–35	35–40
Homes (sleeping areas)	25–35	35–45
Motion-picture theaters	30	40
Hospitals	30	40
Churches (no amplification)	25	35
Courtrooms (no amplification)	25	30–35
Libraries	30	40–45
Restaurants	45	55
Coliseums for sports only (amplification)	50	60

From Berg (1993), with permission.

TABLE 20–2   Effects of different NC units on communicative efficiency

NC Units	Communication Environment	Typical Applications
20–30	Very quiet office, telephone use satisfactory, suitable for large conferences	Executive offices and conference rooms for 50 people
30–35	"Quiet" office, satisfactory for conferences at a 15-ft table, normal voice 10 to 30 ft, telephone use satisfactory	Private or semiprivate offices, reception rooms, and conference rooms for 20 people
35–40	Satisfactory for conferences at a 6-ft to 8-ft table, telephone use satisfactory, normal voice 6 ft to 12 ft	Medium-sized offices and industrial business offices
40–50	Satisfactory for conferences at a 4-ft to 5-ft table, telephone use occasionally slightly difficult, normal voice 3 ft to 6 ft, raised voice 6 ft to 12 ft	Large engineering and drafting rooms
50–55	Unsatisfactory for conferences of more than two or three people, telephone use slightly difficult, normal voice 1 ft to 2 ft, raised voice 3 ft to 6 ft	Secretarial areas (typing), accounting areas (business machines), blueprint rooms, etc.
Above 55	Very noisy, office environment unsatisfactory	Not recommended for any type of room

From Berg (1993), with permission.

1975; Paul, 1967; Pearsons et al, 1977; Ross, 1978; Ross & Giolas, 1971; Sanders, 1965). Sanders (1965) measured the noise levels in 47 occupied and unoccupied classrooms in 15 different school buildings. Mean occupied noise levels ranged from an average of 69 dB(B) in kindergarten classrooms to 52 dB(B) in classrooms for the hearing impaired. Unoccupied classroom noise levels were approximately 10 dB lower than the occupied classroom settings, ranging from 58 dB(B) for kindergarten classrooms to 42 dB(B) in classrooms used for the hearing-impaired. Pearsons et al (1977) reported that noise levels averaged 45 dB(A) for suburban residential settings and 55 dB(A) for urban dwellings. Mean outdoor noise levels were 2 to 10 dB more intense than indoor settings. Noise levels were measured at 54 dB(A) for department store environments and 77 dB(A) in transportation locales (train and aircraft noise). Bess et al (1984) measured background noise levels in 19 classrooms for children with hearing impairment. Median unoccupied noise levels were 41 dB(A), 50 dB(B), and 58 dB(C). When the classroom was occupied with students, background noise levels increased approximately 15 dB to 56 dB(A), 60 dB(B), and 63 dB(C). Crandell and Smaldino (1995) reported that background noise levels in 32 unoccupied classroom settings were 51 dB(A) and 67 dB(C). As will be shown later, noise levels of the magnitude measured in many rooms make accurate speech recognition difficult, if not impossible, particularly for listeners with hearing impairment.

General Effects of Noise on Speech Recognition

Background noise in a room deleteriously affects a listener's speech recognition by reducing, or *masking*, the highly redundant acoustic and linguistic cues available in the speaker's voice. Masking refers to a phenomena in which the threshold of a signal, such as speech, is raised by the presence of another sound, such as room noise. For example, a listener may be able to understand a speaker who is speaking at normal conversational levels comfortably in a quiet room. However, if other persons begin to talk, the slide projector is turned on and/or the ventilation system begins to generate noise, the speaker will now have to raise the level of his or her voice for the listener to still perceive what is being discussed. If the speaker does not raise his or her voice, the noise in the room will mask much of the important acoustic information presented by the speaker.

In general, because the spectral energy of consonant phonemes is considerably less intense than vowel phonemes, background noise in a room often masks the consonants more than the vowels. Loss of consonant information has a great effect on speech recognition because most of the cues important for accurate speech recognition are carried by the consonants (French & Steinberg, 1947; Licklider & Miller, 1951; Sher & Owens, 1974; Wang et al, 1978). Several variables affect the ability of a noise to mask speech. These variables include (1) the long-term acoustic spectrum of the noise, (2) the average intensity of the noise relative to the intensity of speech, and (3) fluctuations in the intensity of the noise over time (e.g., Beranek, 1954; Crandell et al, 1995; Knudsen & Harris, 1978; Miller, 1974; Miller & Nicely, 1955; Nabelek, 1982; Nabelek & Pickett, 1974a,b). Low-frequency noise in a listening environment tends to be a more effective masker of speech than high-frequency noise because of *upward spread of masking*. Upward spread of masking is a phenomenon in which a masking noise produces greater masking at frequencies above the frequency of the masker than at frequencies below the masker.

For example, a 500 Hz noise would more effectively mask a 1000 Hz signal than a 4000 Hz masker would. The fact that low-frequency noise has a greater effect on speech recognition than high-frequency noise is important because the predominant spectra of noise found in typical listening environments are low frequency (Crandell & Smaldino, 1995: Crandell et al, 1995). The most effective masking noises are commonly those with a spectra similar to the speech spectrum because all speech frequencies are masked to some degree. Room noises that are continuous in nature are generally more effective maskers than interrupted or impulse noises. These differences in masking occur because continuous noises more effectively reduce the spectral-temporal information available in the speech signal. Continuous noises in the room include the hum of air-conditioning or heating systems, faulty fluorescent lighting, and the long-term spectra of individuals talking.

In most listening environments the fundamental determinant for speech recognition is not the overall level of the room noise but rather the relationship between the intensity of the signal and the intensity of the background noise at the listener's ear. This relationship is referred to as the *SNR*, or *message-to-competition ratio (MCR)*. To illustrate, if a speech signal is presented at 75 dB (Ls) and a noise is 70 dB (Ln), the SNR (or MCR) is 75 dB minus 70 dB or +5 dB. For listeners with normal-hearing and listeners with hearing impairment, speech recognition ability tends to be the highest at favorable SNRs and decreases as the SNR of the listening environment is reduced (Cooper & Cutts, 1971; Crandell et al, 1995; Crum, 1974; Finitzo-Hieber & Tillman, 1978; Miller, 1974; Nabelek & Pickett, 1974a,b). For example, Crum (1974) examined the word recognition of adult normal hearers at various SNRs (SNR = +12 dB, +6 dB, and 0 dB). Word recognition scores reached a plateau at high SNRs (95% at a +12 dB SNR) but diminished as the SNR became less favorable (80% and 46% at +6 dB SNR and 0 dB SNR, respectively). Generally speaking, speech recognition in adults with normal-hearing is not severely degraded until the SNR approximates 0 dB (speech and noise are at equal intensities). As discussed in the *"Criteria for Appropriate Signal-to-Noise Levels"* section following, this SNR depends on many factors, such as the type of noise, type of speech stimuli, and articulatory abilities/dialect of the speaker.

Signal-to-Noise Ratios in Various Enclosures

Because of high background noise levels, relatively poor SNRs have been reported in many settings. Pearsons et al (1977) reported that average SNRs were +14 to +9 dB in suburban and urban residential settings, respectively. In outdoor settings SNRs decreased to approximately +8 to +5 dB. Additional measurements indicated that in department store settings the average SNR was +7 dB, whereas transportation settings yielded an average SNR of −2 dB. Plomp (1986) reported that the average SNR found at cocktail parties ranged from +1 dB to −2 dB. In classroom environments (Table 20–3) the range of SNRs has been reported to be from +5 dB to −7 dB (e.g., Blair, 1977; Crandell et al, 1995; Finitzo-Hieber, 1988; Markides, 1986; Paul, 1967; Sanders, 1965).

TABLE 20–3 A summary of studies examining classroom signal-to-noise ratios (SNRs)

Investigator/Year	Signal-to-Noise Ratio (SNR)
Sanders (1965)	+1 to +5
Blair (1977)	−7 to 0
Markides (1986)	+3
Finitzo-Hieber (1988)	+1 to +4

SPECIAL CONSIDERATION

Background noise and speaker levels in occupied rooms can fluctuate immensely as a function of time. To obtain a meaningful estimate of the SNR in an occupied room, multiple measurements should be taken primarily during the informational-carrying time epochs.

Effects of Noise on Speech Recognition in Listeners with Hearing Impairment and "Normal-Hearing"

It has been amply demonstrated that the speech recognition performance of listeners with sensorineural hearing loss (SNHL) is reduced in noise when compared with listeners with normal-hearing (Crandell, 1991a; Dirks et al, 1982; Finitzo-Hieber & Tillman, 1978; Keith & Talis, 1972; Killion, 1997; Nabelek & Pickett, 1974a,b; Plomp, 1978; Ross, 1978; Suter, 1985). For example, Suter (1985) reported that at a SNR of −6 dB, listeners with SNHL obtained monosyllabic recognition scores of 27% correct compared with 63% correct for normal hearers. In general, it appears that listeners with SNHL require the SNR to be improved by 4 to 12 dB (Crandell et al, 1995; Killion, 1997; Moore, 1997) and by an additional 3 to 6 dB in rooms with moderate levels of reverberation (Hawkins & Yacullo, 1984) to obtain recognition scores equal to normal hearers. The degree of SNHL apparently influences the SNR required by the individual with hearing impairment. Killion (1997) reported that a listener with a 30 dB SNHL requires a +4 dB greater SNR than a normal hearer to maintain equivalent speech recognition. With a 90 dB SNHL, the required SNR is +12 dB. Despite the speech recognition deficits seen in the hearing impaired, the specific auditory, cochlear, central, and/or cognitive mechanism(s) to explain these difficulties remain unclear. The reader is directed to Crandell (1991a), Humes (1991), Sammeth and Ochs (1991), Crandell et al (1992), Needleman and Crandell (1996a,b), and Killion (1997) for reviews of possible hypotheses to explain speech recognition difficulties in the hearing-impaired.

Although it is recognized that listeners with SNHL experience greater speech recognition deficits in noise than normal hearers, a number of populations of children with "normal-hearing" sensitivity also experience significant difficulties recognizing speech in noise (Bess, 1985; Bess &

TABLE 20–4 Children with "normal-hearing" who may experience difficulty recognizing speech in noise

- Young children (< 15 y old)
- Conductive hearing loss
- History or recurrent otitis media
- Language disorder
- Articulation disorder
- Dyslexia
- Learning disabilities
- Non-native English
- Central auditory processing deficit
- Minimal degree of bilaterial SNHL
- Unilateral SNHL
- Developmental delays
- Attentional deficits

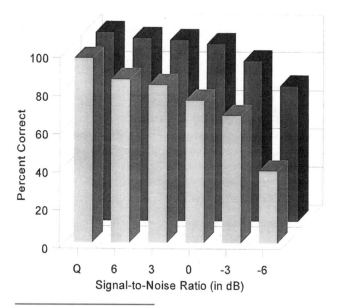

Figure 20–2 Mean speech recognition scores (in % correct) of children with normal-hearing (*dark shaded bars*) and children with minimal degrees of SNHL (*light shaded bars*) in quiet and at various SNRs. (Adapted from Crandell et al [1995].)

Tharpe, 1986; Boney & Bess, 1984; Crandell, 1991b, 1992a, 1993, Crandell & Smaldino, 1992, 1994, 1995, 1996a,b; Crandell et al, 1995; Nabelek & Nabelek, 1994). These listeners, as shown in Table 20–4, adapted from Crandell (1995), include children with fluctuating conductive hearing loss (or a history of recurrent otitis media with effusion), learning disabilities, articulation, language, and/or reading (dyslexia) disabilities, central auditory processing deficits, minimal degrees of SNHL (pure tone sensitivity from 15- to 25-dB HL), unilateral SNHL, developmental delays, attention deficit disorders, and children for whom English is a second language (ESL). For example, Crandell (1993) examined the speech recognition abilities of children with minimal degrees of SNHL at commonly reported classroom SNRs ranging from +6 to −6 dB. The minimally hearing-impaired children exhibited pure tone averages (500 to 2000 Hz) from 15- to 25-dB HL. Speech recognition was assessed with the Bamford-Koval-Bench (BKB) Standard Sentence test (Bench et al, 1979), and the multitalker babble from the Speech Perception in Noise (SPIN) test was used as the noise competition. Results from this investigation are presented in Figure 20–2 and indicate that children with minimal degrees of SNHL performed poorer than normal hearers across most listening conditions. Moreover, the differences in recognition scores between the two groups increased as the listening environment became more unfavorable. For example, at a SNR of +6 dB, both groups obtained recognition scores in excess of 80%. At a SNR of −6 dB, however, the minimally hearing-impaired group was able to obtain less than 50% correct recognition compared with approximately 75% recognition ability for the normal hearers.

SPECIAL CONSIDERATION

Removing acoustic barriers to listening and learning extends the scope of practice of the audiologist to include not only individuals with hearing impairment but also "normal-hearing" populations.

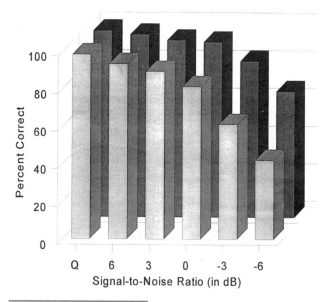

Figure 20–3 Mean speech recognition scores (in % correct) of native English children (*dark shaded bars*) and nonnative English children (*light shaded bars*) in quiet and at various SNRs. (Adapted from Crandell et al [1995].)

Crandell and Smaldino (1996a) examined the speech recognition of 20 native English-speaking children and 20 nonnative English-speaking children under classroom SNRs of +6, +3, 0, −3, and −6 dB. Speech recognition was assessed by BKB sentences, and the SPIN multitalker babble was used as the noise competition. The same trends in speech recognition as demonstrated for the minimally hearing-impaired children were shown for these populations (see Fig. 20–3).

That is, although both groups obtained essentially equivalent speech recognition scores in quiet, the non-native English-speaking group performed significantly poorer as the listening environment became less favorable. Similar findings have been reported for adult ESL listeners (Bergman, 1980; Buus et al, 1986; Florentine, 1985; Nabelek & Donahue, 1984). Bergman (1980), for example, examined the speech perception of adult native-Hebraic listeners under various conditions of acoustic degradations, including noise (SNR = +3 dB), reverberation (RT = 2.5 s), and split-band dichotic listening. Results indicated that the ESL subjects obtained significantly poorer perception scores than the native-English speakers across all listening conditions. Interestingly, these results were obtained, although the native-Hebraic listeners had been speaking English for more than 50 years.

Another group of "normal-hearing" children is young listeners. Prior research has indicated that children require higher SNRs than adult listeners to achieve equivalent speech recognition scores (Crandell & Bess, 1986, 1987; Elliott, 1979; 1982; Elliott et al, 1979; Nabelek & Robinson, 1982). Elliott (1982) and Nabelek and Robinson (1982) reported that young listeners require an additional 10 dB of signal strength to produce equivalent recognition scores to those of adults. Moreover, adultlike ability to recognize speech in noise is not reached until approximately 13 to 15 years of age (Crandell & Bess, 1986, 1987; Elliott, 1979, 1982; Elliott et al, 1979; Nabelek & Robinson, 1982). Presumably, the additional signal strength is necessary to provide adequate acoustic cues to the immature auditory and linguistic system. On the basis of the aforementioned data, it is reasonable to assume that commonly reported levels of classroom noise have the potential of adversely affecting speech recognition in all pediatric listeners. To examine this assumption, let us inspect speech recognition data from the germinal article by Finitzo-Hieber and Tillman (1978). In their study they compared the word recognition ability of 12 normal-hearing and 12 children with mild-to-moderate binaurally symmetrical SNHL under varying conditions of SNR and reverberation time (RT). The results of the speech recognition in noise aspect of this study are summarized in Table 20–5. The word recognition scores for the children with normal-hearing decreased to 60% at a SNR of 0 dB (a commonly reported SNR in the classroom). At the same SNR, word recognition scores for the children with SNHL were only 42%. Certainly, it is reasonable to assume that

learning, attention, and behavior could be adversely affected if such reduced amounts of the acoustic signal were available to either child (particularly the child with hearing loss).

Criteria for Appropriate Signal-to-Noise Levels

A number of acoustic, linguistic, and articulatory factors influence the determination of appropriate SNRs in a room. Acoustic factors include the spectrum of the noise, fluctuations in the noise over time, the type of signal that is being presented (sentences, words, nonsense syllables, vowels, consonants) and/or the power of the speaker's voice. Linguistic factors include word familiarity and/or vocabulary size of the listener, context, the number of syllables in a word and linguistic competency. Articulatory factors incorporate the gender of the speaker and the articulatory abilities and/or dialect of the speaker or listener. Unfortunately, to date, no federal standard (only suggested guidelines) exists for appropriate SNRs or background noise levels in rooms for listeners with SNHL (see Table 20–6 for suggested guidelines for classroom noise levels). Only the state of Washington has a legal requirement for background noise levels in classrooms (NC = 35 dB). The Los Angeles County Unified School District (the largest school district in the world) has recently established a similar NC rating for the output of HVAC equipment in the classroom (Access Board Web site, 1998). As noted previously, speech recognition in adults with normal-hearing is not severely compromised until the SNR of the listening environment is approximately 0 dB. For listeners with SNHL, investigators have suggested that SNRs in learning environments should exceed a minimum of +15 dB (ASHA, 1995; Crandell, 1991b, 1992a,b; Crandell & Smaldino, 1992, 1994, 1995, 1996a,b; Crandell et al, 1995, 1997; Finitzo-Hieber, 1988; Finitzo-Hieber and Tillman, 1978; Fourcin et al., 1980; Gengel, 1971; Niemoeller, 1968; Olsen, 1988). This recommendation is based on the finding that the speech recognition of listeners with hearing impairment tends to remain relatively constant at SNRs in excess of +15 dB but deteriorate at poorer SNRs. In addition, when the SNR decreases below +15, persons with hearing loss have to spend so much attentional effort in listening to the message that they often prefer to communicate through other modalities (e.g., sign language/written materials). To accomplish this SNR in most settings, it appears that unoccupied room noise levels cannot

TABLE 20–5 Mean speech recognition scores (% correct) by children with normal-hearing (*n* = 12) and children with SNHL (*n* = 12) for monosyllabic words in quiet and at various SNRs

SNR	Groups	
	Normal-Hearing	Hearing Impaired
Quiet	94.5	87.5
+ 12 dB	89.2	77.8
+ 6 dB	79.7	65.7
0 dB	60.2	42.2

Adapted from Finitzo-Hieber and Tillman (1978).

TABLE 20–6   Recommended unoccupied classroom noise levels in dB (A) to achieve optimum speech recognition for children with normal-hearing and children with hearing impairment

Investigator/Year	Unoccupied Noise Level	Population
Niemoeller (1968)	30 dB(A)	Hearing-impaired
Gengel (1971)	30 dB(A)	Hearing-impaired
Ross (1978)	35 dB(A)	Hearing-impaired
Knudsen & Harris (1978)	35 dB(A)	Normal-hearing
Borrild (1978)	35 dB(A) 25 dB(A)	Normal-hearing/ hearing-impaired
Fourcin et al (1980)	35 dB(A)	Hearing-impaired
Bradley (19686)	30 dB(A)	Normal-hearing
Finitzo-Hieber (1988)	35 dB(A)	Hearing-impaired
Portuguese School Standard (1988)	35 dB(A)	Normal-hearing/ hearing-impaired
German Performance/ Design Standard (1989)	30 dB(A)	Normal-hearing/ hearing-impaired
Swedish Board of Housing, Building, and Planning (1994)	30 dB(A)	Normal-hearing/ hearing-impaired
Berg (1993)	35- to 40-dB(A)	Normal-hearing
ASHA (1995)	30 dB(A)	Normal-hearing/ hearing-impaired
Crandell et al (1995)	30- to 35-dB(A)	Normal-hearing/ hearing-impaired
Crandell & Smaldino (1996b)	30- to 35-dB(A)	Normal-hearing/ hearing-impaired

Adapted from the Access Board Web site (1988).

exceed 30- to 35-dB(A) or approximately a NC 25 dB curve (ASHA, 1995; Bess & McConnell, 1981; Crandell, 1991b; 1992a; Crandell and Smaldino, 1992, 1994, 1995, 1996a,b; Crandell et al, 1995; Finitzo-Hieber, 1988; Finitzo-Hieber & Tillman, 1978; Fourcin et al, 1980; Gengel, 1971; Niemoeller, 1968; Olsen, 1988). Disparagingly, a review of studies that have measured acoustic characteristics of typical classrooms indicate that these noise standards are infrequently achieved in the academic setting (Crandell, 1992a,b; Crandell & Smaldino, 1995; Crum & Matkin, 1976; McCroskey & Devens, 1975). McCroskey and Devens (1975) demonstrated that only one of nine elementary classrooms actually met these acoustical recommendations. Crandell and Smaldino (1995) reported that none of 32 classrooms met recommended criteria for noise. Acoustical guidelines for SNRs and background noise levels have not been developed for "normal-hearing" children. Until such standards are clarified, it has been recommended that SNRs in learning environments should follow those recommended for listeners with SNHL (i.e., room noise levels cannot exceed 30- to 35-dB(A) or a NC 20- to 25-dB curve, whereas SNRs should surpass +15 dB) (ASHA, 1995; Crandell & Smaldino, 1995, 1996a,b; Crandell et al, 1995, 1998).

Noise Effects on Academic and Teacher Performance

In addition to deleteriously affecting speech recognition, background noise can also compromise academic performance, reading and spelling skills, concentration, attention, and behavior in children (Ando & Nakane, 1975; Crook & Langdon, 1974; Dixon, 1976; Green et al, 1982; Ko, 1979; Koszarny, 1978; Lehman & Gratiot, 1983; Sargent et al, 1980). Koszarny (1978) reported that noise levels tend to more seriously affect concentration and attention in children with lower IQs and/or high anxiety levels. Green et al (1982) found that classroom noise alone accounted for approximately 50% to 75% of the variance in reading delays of 1 year or more in elementary school children. Lehman and Gratiot (1983) reported that reductions in classroom noise (by means of acoustical modification) had a significant effect of increasing concentration, attention, and participatory behavior in children. Interestingly, the noise levels were reduced from typically reported noise levels of 35- to 45-dB(A) to the suggested guideline of 30 dB(A). Classroom noise has also been shown to affect teacher performance (Crook & Langdon,

1974; Ko, 1979; Sargent et al, 1980). For example, Ko (1979) obtained information from more than 1200 teachers concerning the effects of noise in the classroom. Results indicated that noise related to classroom activities and traffic and/or airplane noise was correlated with teacher fatigue, increased tension and discomfort, and an interference with teaching and speech recognition. In a recent survey of school administrators, the General Accounting Office found that inappropriate classroom acoustics was the most commonly cited problem that affected the learning environment (Access Board Web site, 1998). Additional studies (Crandell et al, 1996; Sapienza et al, 1998) have reported that teachers exhibit a significantly higher incidence of vocal problems than the general population. It is reasonable to assume that these vocal difficulties are caused, at least in part, by having to increase vocal output to overcome the effects of classroom noise during the school day.

REVERBERATION

Reverberation refers to the prolongation or persistence of sound within an enclosure as sound waves reflect off hard surfaces (bare walls, ceilings, windows, floor) in the room. Operationally, RT refers to the amount of time it takes for a sound, at a specific frequency, to decay 60 dB (or one millionth of its original intensity) after termination of the signal. For example, if a 110 dB SPL signal at 1000 Hz took 1 second to decrease to 50 dB SPL, the RT of that enclosure at 1000 Hz would be 1 s. A common formula used to estimate RT was suggested by Sabine (1964):

$$RT_{60} = \frac{0.049V}{\Sigma S\alpha}$$

where RT_{60} = reverberation time in seconds; *0.049* is a constant (use 0.161 if room volume is stated in meters); V = room volume in cubic feet; and $\Sigma S\alpha$ = the sum of the surface areas of the various materials in the room multiplied by their respective absorption coefficients at a given frequency. If one reviews the variables in the RT formula just described, it is apparent that two basic factors effect the RT in a room. The first is the room volume. The larger the room volume, the longer the RT will be. The second variable is the amount of sound absorption in the room. The greater the area and sound absorptive characteristics of such materials, the shorter the RT. Although not apparent in the formula, room shape may also effect the level of reverberation. Rooms with irregular shapes, such as oblong, often exhibit higher RTs than rooms with more traditional quadrilateral dimensions.

Measurement of Reverberation

RT is usually measured by presenting a high-intensity, broadband stimulus, such as white or pink noise, into an unoccupied room and measuring the amount of time required for that signal to decay 60 dB at various frequencies (Davis & Jones, 1989; Harris, 1991; Nabelek & Nabelek, 1994; Sabine, 1964; Siebein et al, 1997). Commercially available instruments for the recording RT vary from inexpensive, compact, battery units that allow the audiologist to do rudimentary measures of RT to highly technological, computer-based devices that

can measure and record numerous aspects of the decay properties of an environment. RT can also be estimated from formulas similar to the one presented earlier by means of commercially available software programs that calculate the dimensions, volume, and absorption characteristics of an enclosure. Because the primary energy of speech is between 500 and 2000 Hz, RT is often reported as the mean decay time at 500, 1000, and 2000 Hz. Unfortunately, such a measurement paradigm may not adequately describe the reverberant characteristics of a room because high RTs may exist at additional frequencies. Room reverberation varies as a function of frequency and should therefore be measured at discrete frequencies. Generally, because most materials do not absorb low frequencies well, room reverberation is shorter at higher frequencies and longer in lower frequency regions. It is recommended that RT be measured at discrete frequencies from 125 to 8000 Hz whenever possible. Such information could significantly aid the audiologist in determining the appropriate degree and type of absorptive materials needed for reduction of RT in that environment. The reader is directed to Beranek (1954), Knudsen and Harris (1978), Hassall and Zaveri (1979), Harris (1991), Cremer and Muller (1982), Egan (1987), Siebein (1994), and Siebein et al (1997) for further details concerning the measurement of reverberation.

Reverberation Times in Rooms

Essentially all rooms exhibit some degree of reverberation. Audiometric test booths usually exhibit RTs of approximately 0.2 s. Living rooms and offices often have RTs between 0.4 and 0.8 s (Knudsen & Harris, 1978; Nabelek & Nabelek, 1994). As can be seen in Table 20–7, RTs for classrooms are usually reported to range from 0.4 to 1.2 seconds (Bradley, 1986; Crandell, 1992a; Crandell & Smaldino, 1995; Crandell et al, 1995; Finitzo-Hieber, 1988; Kodaras, 1960; McCroskey & Devens, 1975; Nabelek & Pickett, 1974a,b; Olsen, 1988; Ross, 1978). Auditoriums, churches, and assembly halls often have RTs in excess of 3.0 s (Crandell, 1992a; Knudsen & Harris, 1978; Nabelek & Nabelek, 1994; Siebein et al, 1997).

General Effects of Reverberation on Speech Recognition

It is well documented that excessive reverberation can adversely effect speech recognition (see Nabelek & Nabelek,

TABLE 20–7 A summary of studies examining classroom RTs

Investigator/Year	RT (seconds)
Kodaras (1960)	0.40–1.10
Nabelek & Pickett (1974a)	0.50–1.00
McCroskey & Devens (1975)	0.60–1.00
Bradley (1986)	0.39–1.20
Crandell & Smaldino (1994)	0.35–1.20

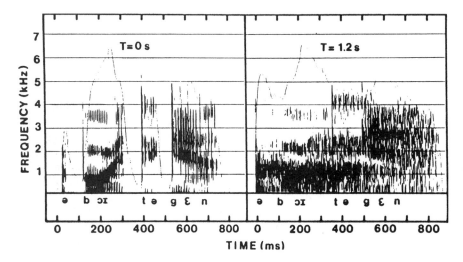

Figure 20–4   A spectrograph of the phrase "the beet again" in nonreverberant (RT = 0.0 s) and reverberant (RT = 1.2 s) conditions. (From Nabelek & Nabelek [1994], with permission.)

1994). Reverberation degrades speech recognition through the masking of direct and early reflected energy by reverberant energy (Bolt & McDonald, 1949; Kurtovic, 1975; Lochner & Burger, 1964; Nabelek, 1982; Nabelek & Pickett, 1974a,b). The reverberant speech energy reaches the listener after the direct sound and overlaps with that direct signal, resulting in a "smearing" or masking of speech. Figure 20–4 presents a spectrograph of the phrase "the beet again" in reverberant (RT = 1.2 s) and nonreverberant (RT = 0.0 s) listening environments. In this figure, time (in milliseconds) is presented on the abscissa, whereas frequency (in kilohertz) is shown on the ordinate. Amplitude, or intensity, of the speech sample is indicated by the relative density or darkness of the pattern. As can be seen, reverberation causes a prolongation or "spread" of the spectral energy of the vowel sounds, which tends to mask succeeding consonant phonemes, particularly those consonants in word final positions. It is reasonable to expect that the masking effect for reverberation would be greater for vowels than for consonants because vowels exhibit greater overall power and are of longer duration than consonants. Note that in Figure 20–4, the reverberant sound energy of the /i/ phoneme in the word *beet* has extended over the energy of the final /t/ consonant, making recognition of that consonant (and consequently the entire word) more difficult. In highly reverberant environments, words may actually overlap with one another, thus causing reverberant sound energy to fill in temporal pauses between words. Moreover, in highly reverberant environments, such as auditoriums or gymnasiums, temporal pauses between sentences may be lost, causing difficulty in distinguishing where one sentence ends and another sentence begins.

Effects of Reverberation on Speech Recognition in Listeners with Hearing Impairment and "Normal-Hearing"

Speech recognition tends to decrease as the RT of the environment increases (Crandell et al, 1995; Finitzo-Hieber & Tillman, 1978; Gelfand & Silman, 1979; Houtgast, 1981; Kurtovic, 1975; Lochner & Burger, 1964; Moncur & Dirks, 1967; Nabelek &

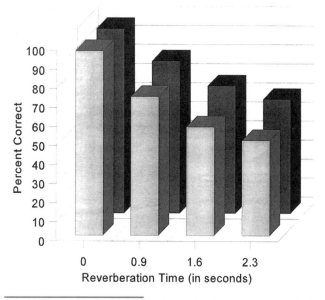

Figure 20–5   Monaural (*light shaded bars*) and binaural (*dark shaded bars*) speech recognition at various RTs. (Adapted from Moncur & Dirks [1967].)

Pickett, 1974a,b; Neuman & Hochberg, 1983). Moncur and Dirks (1967) examined the monosyllabic word recognition of adult listeners with normal-hearing at four different RTs (RT = 0.0, 0.9, 1.6, and 2.3 s) in monaural (near ear) and binaural listening conditions. Results indicted that speech recognition ability was markedly reduced as RT increased (see Fig. 20–5). In addition, results indicated that binaural recognition scores were significantly higher than monaural perceptual abilities. Improved binaural speech recognition in reverberation with and without hearing aids has been documented in other studies as well (Berkley & Allen, 1993; Houtgast, 1981; Nabelek & Mason, 1981; Nabelek & Pickett, 1974a,b; Nabelek & Robinson, 1982; Neuman & Hochberg, 1983).

Speech recognition in adults with normal-hearing is often not compromised until the RT exceeds approximately 1.0 s (Crum, 1974; Gelfand & Silman, 1979; Moncur & Dirks, 1967;

Nabelek & Pickett, 1974a,b). As with background noise, however, a number of acoustic, linguistic, and articulatory factors determine the degree to which reverberation affects speech recognition. Listeners with SNHL, however, need considerably shorter RTs (i.e., 0.4 to 0.5 s) for maximum speech recognition (Crandell, 1991b, 1992a; Crandell & Bess, 1986; Crandell et al, 1995; Finitzo-Hieber, 1988; Finitzo-Hieber & Tillman, 1978; Niemoeller, 1968; Olsen, 1988). Additional studies have also indicated that the populations of "normal-hearing" children discussed previously also have greater speech recognition difficulties in reverberation than do young adults with normal-hearing. Boney and Bess (1984), for example, demonstrated that children with minimal degrees of SNHL (pure tone thresholds from 15- to 30-dB HL at 500 to 2000 Hz) experience greater difficulty understanding speech degraded by reverberation than children with normal-hearing sensitivity. Specifically, speech recognition scores were obtained in nonreverberant (RT = 0.0 s) and reverberant environments (RT = 0.8 s). Results from this investigation indicated that the children with minimal hearing loss performed significantly poorer than the control group, particularly within the reverberant listening condition (Fig. 20–6).

Reverberation and Subjective Sound Quality

In addition to speech recognition, excessive reverberation can also affect subjective sound quality. For example, the subjective quality of music has been shown to improve with the addition of reverberation. Formulas to derive optimum RTs, as a function of room characteristics and various forms of music, have been developed for theaters and auditoriums (Barron, 1993; Berkley & Allen, 1993; Harris, 1991;

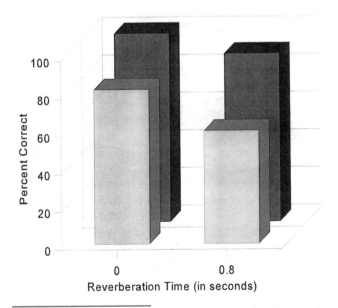

Figure 20–6 Mean speech recognition scores (in % correct) of children with normal-hearing *(dark shaded bars)* and children with minimal degrees of SNHL *(light shaded bars)* in a nonreverberant (RT = 0.0 s) and reverberant (RT = 0.8 s) listening condition.

Knudsen & Harris; 1978; Siebein, 1994; Siebein et al, 1997). Often, these formulas suggest RTs of 2 or 3 s to add "liveness" or "coloration" to music. The effect of reverberation on speech quality, however, tends to not be as well recognized. Haas (1972) indicated that early reflections and some reverberation enhance the quality of speech, causing an increase in loudness, "liveliness," and "growth in body." Overall, it appears that short to moderate RTs increase the subjective quality of speech, whereas excessive reverberation causes speech to sound muffled and less understandable.

Recommended Criteria for Reverberation Time

As previously discussed, speech recognition in adults with normal-hearing is not significantly affected until the RT exceeds approximately 1.0 s. For listeners with SNHL, most investigators have recommended that listening environments should not exceed approximately 0.4 s (through the speech frequency range: 500, 1000, and 2000 Hz) to provide optimum communicative efficiency. A summary of suggested guidelines for RTs in the classroom can be found in Table 20–8. As with background noise levels, federal standards for appropriate classroom RTs for children with SNHL do not currently exist. A review of the literature suggests that appropriate RTs for the hearing impaired are rarely achieved (Crandell, 1991a, 1992a,b; Crandell & Smaldino, 1995; Crum & Matkin, 1976; McCroskey & Devens, 1975). Crandell & Smaldino (1995) reported that only 9 of 32 classrooms (27%) displayed RTs of 0.4 s or less. As with background noise levels, acoustic criteria for appropriate RTs have not been well established for the diverse populations of "normal-hearing" children previously discussed. Until additional research is conducted, a conservative standard for RTs in listening environments for "normal-hearing" children seems appropriate. Specifically, the RT of such enclosures should follow the same acoustic recommendations used for listeners with hearing loss (RT = 0.4 s). At the time of this writing, no federal or state standards exist for reverberation in classrooms.

Effects of Noise and Reverberation on Speech Recognition

Thus far, the isolated effects of background noise and reverberation have been discussed, However, these acoustic events do not occur separately in a room. In most enclosures noise and reverberation combine in a *synergistic* manner to adversely effect speech recognition (Crandell & Bess, 1986; Crandell & Smaldino, 1995; Crandell et al, 1995; Crum, 1974; Finitzo-Hieber & Tillman, 1978; Nabelek & Pickett, 1974a,b). Synergetic suggests that the sum of the two variables is greater than one would expect by simply adding the two variables together. For example, let us imagine that we have two specially designed test rooms that have only noise *or* reverberation. If we test an individual in the noisy room, we may see recognition scores diminish 10% (from scores obtained in quiet). In the reverberant room let us assume that we see a similar 10% decrease in recognition. If, however, we now place this individual in a room that contains *both* noise

TABLE 20–8   Recommended classroom RT, in seconds, to achieve optimum speech recognition for children with normal-hearing and children with hearing impairment

Investigator/Year	RT (seconds)	Population
Niemoeller (1968)	0.4–0.6	Hearing-impaired
Gengel (1971)	0.7	Hearing-impaired
Knudsen & Harris (1978)	0.75	Normal-hearing
Ross (1978)	0.4	Hearing-impaired
Borrild (1978)	0.9 0.4	Normal-hearing/ hearing-impaired
Fourcin et al (1980)	0.5	Hearing-impaired
Bess & McConnell (1981)	0.4	Hearing-impaired
Bradley (1986)	0.4	Normal-hearing
Egan (1987)	0.5	Hearing-impaired
Finitzo-Hieber (1988)	0.4	Hearing-impaired
Portuguese School Standard (1988)	0.6–0.8 0.4–0.6	Normal-hearing/ hearing-impaired
ASHA (1995)	0.4	Normal-hearing/ hearing-impaired
Crandell et al (1995)	0.4	Normal-hearing/ hearing-impaired
Crandell & Smaldino (1996b)	0.4	Normal-hearing/ hearing-impaired

Adapted from the Access Board Web site (1998).

and reverberation, we would not see a 20% decrease in recognition (i.e., 10% for noise; 10% for reverberation), but perhaps a 30 or 40% reduction. It appears that this synergism occurs because reverberation fills in the temporal gaps in the noise, making the noise more steady state in nature and a more effective masker. As with noise and reverberation in isolation, research indicates that listeners with hearing impairment and "normal-hearing " children experience greater speech recognition difficulties in noise and reverberation than adult normal listeners (Crandell & Bess, 1986; Crandell & Smaldino, 1994, 1995, 1996a,b; Crandell et al, 1995; Finitzo-Hieber & Tillman, 1978; Nabelek & Pickett, 1974a,b).

An example of the synergetic effect of noise and reverberation on the monosyllabic word recognition of children with normal-hearing and SNHL is shown in Table 20–9. Note that even at the best SNR and RT (SNR = +12 dB, RT = 0.4 s), children with normal-hearing do not recognize speech perfectly (83%) and children with hearing impairment perform even more poorly (60%). As the SNR becomes poorer or as RT gets longer, speech recognition decreases to the worse case studied (SNR = +0 dB; RT = 1.2 s), where children with normal-hearing achieve a 30% score and children with hearing loss recognize virtually none of the speech (11%). It should be noted that each of these listening conditions has been commonly reported in classroom environments. Imagine trying

to succeed in school, perceiving only 11% of what is presented by the teacher.

SPEAKER-LISTENER DISTANCE

In most rooms the acoustics of a speaker's speech signal changes as it travels to the listener. Figure 20–7 shows some of the paths of *direct* and *reflected sounds* from a speaker to a listener in a room. The direct sound is that sound that travels from the speaker to a listener without striking other surfaces within the room. The direct sound is usually the first sound to arrive at the listeners' ears because it travels the shortest path between the speaker and the listener. The power of the direct sound decreases with distance because the acoustic energy is spreading over a larger area as it travels from the source. Specifically, the direct sound decreases 6 dB in SPL with every doubling of distance from the sound source. This phenomenon, called the *inverse square law*, occurs because of the geometric divergence of sound from the source. According to the inverse square law, if a speaker's SPL is 65 dB at 1 m (average conversational levels), then his or her voice will be 59 dB at 2 m, 53 dB at 4 m, and so on. Because the direct sound energy decreases so quickly, only those listeners who are seated close to the speaker will be hearing direct sound energy.

TABLE 20–9 Mean speech recognition scores (% correct) by children with normal-hearing (*n* = 12) and children with SNHL (*n* = 12) for monosyllabic words across various SNRs and RT

Testing Condition	Groups	
	Normal-Hearing	Hearing-Impaired
RT = 0.0 s		
Quiet	94.5	83.0
+12 dB	89.2	70.0
+6 dB	79.7	59.5
0 dB	60.2	39.0
RT = 0.4 s		
Quiet	92.5	74.0
+12 dB	82.8	60.2
+6 dB	71.3	52.2
0 dB	47.7	27.8
RT = 1.2 s		
Quiet	76.5	45.0
+12 dB	68.8	41.2
+6 dB	54.2	27.0
0 dB	29.7	11.2

Adapted from Finitzo-Hieber and Tillman (1978).

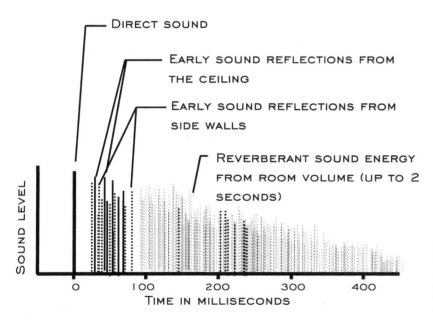

Figure 20–7 Components of sound (direct sound, early reflections, and late reflections) in a room. (From Siebein et al [1997], with permission.)

At slightly farther distances from the speaker, *early sound reflections* will reach the listener. Early sound reflections are those sound waves that arrive at a listener within very short time periods (approximately 50 ms) after the arrival of the direct sound. Early sound reflections are often combined with the direct sound and may actually increase the perceived loudness of the sound (Bradley, 1986; Lochner & Burger, 1964; Nabelek & Nabelek, 1994; Thiele, 1953). This increase in loudness may actually improve speech recognition in listeners with normal-hearing. In a typical room most of the early

reflections strike minimal room surfaces on their path from speaker to listener.

As a listener moves farther away from a speaker, *reverberation* dominates the listening environment. As discussed in an earlier section, reverberation consists of the sound waves that strike multiple room surfaces as they move from speaker to listener. As sound waves strike multiple room surfaces, they are generally decreased in loudness as a result of the increased path length they travel and the partial absorption that occurs at each reflection with the room surfaces. Some

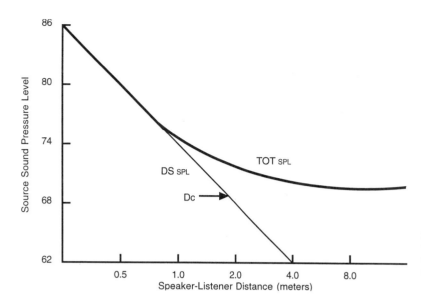

Figure 20–8 The distribution of sound within a room as a function of speaker-to-listener distance (Adapted from Nabelek & Nabelek [1994].)

reverberation is necessary to reinforce the direct sound and to enrich the quality of the sound. However, reverberation can lead to acoustic distortions of the speech signal, including temporal smearing and masking of important perceptual cues.

Another way of looking at sound distribution in an enclosure is shown in Figure 20–8. In this figure, line DS_{SPL} represents the relative SPL of the direct sound in the room. Curve TOT_{SPL} depicts the total sound pressure in the room. The total sound pressure is the summation of reflected and direct sound energy in the enclosure. Stated otherwise, the total sound pressure is that sound energy that a listener will hear in a room at various distances. Curve TOT_{SPL} shows that sound decay in accordance with the inverse square law *only* occurs in free field environments because no surfaces reflect sound and reinforce that sound wave. Point D_c shows the "critical distance" of the room, which refers to that point in a room in which the intensity of the direct sound is equal to the intensity of the reverberant sound (Klein, 1971; Puetz, 1971). Within the critical distance the effects of reverberation on the speech signal would be minimized. Operationally, critical distance (D_c) is defined by the following formula:

$$D_c{}^x = 0.20\sqrt{VQ/nRT}$$

where V = volume of the room in m^3, Q = directivity factor of the source (the human voice is approximately 2.5), n = number of sources, and RT = reverberation time of the enclosure at 1400 Hz. In an average-sized classroom with a commonly reported level of reverberation, the critical distance of the room would be approximately 3 m.

As noted previously, the inverse square law does not apply to enclosures such as classrooms or theaters. Thus one cannot determine the SPL of the speaker's voice by simply deducting 6 dB for every doubling of distance from the source. To estimate the SPL (and thus the SNR) at any given location in a room (in meters), the following formula can be used:

$$SPL = Ps + 10\,Log\,[(1/4\pi r^2) + (4/A)]$$

where Ps = the sound power of the source and A = the total sound absorption of the room.

Effects of Distance on Speech Recognition

Speech recognition in many rooms depends on the distance of the listener from the speaker (Crandell, 1991a,b; Crandell & Bess, 1986; Crandell & Smaldino, 1995; Klein, 1971; Leavitt & Flexer, 1991; Puetz, 1971). If the listener is within the critical distance of the room (relatively close to the speaker), reflected sound waves have minimal effects on speech recognition. Beyond the critical distance, however, the reflections can compromise speech recognition if enough of a spectrum and/or intensity change in the reflected sound is present to interfere with the recognition of the direct sound. Overall, speech recognition scores tend to decrease until the critical distance of the room is reached. Beyond the critical distance, recognition ability tends to remain essentially constant unless the room is very large (such as an auditorium). In such environments speech recognition may continue to decrease as a function of increased distance. These findings suggest that speech recognition ability can be maximized by decreasing the distance between a speaker and listener within the critical distance of the room.

PEARL

Preferential seating may not significantly aid speech recognition in many rooms. To improve speech recognition, the listener must be within the critical distance of the room at all times. In classrooms the critical distance is often no more than 6 to 8 ft from the teacher. To keep listeners within the critical distance, hearing assistive technologies, such as an FM system is often required.

In a series of studies Crandell and Bess (1986, 1987) examined the effects of distance on the speech recognition of children with normal-hearing in "typical" classroom environments (SNR = +6 dB; RT = 0.45 seconds). Crandell and Bess (1986) recorded Phonetically Balanced Kindergarten

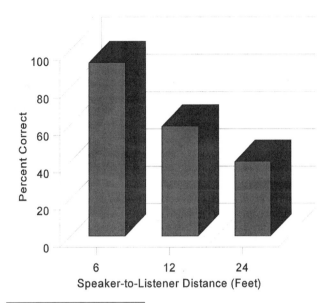

Figure 20–9 Mean speech recognition scores (in % correct) of children with normal-hearing in a "typical" classroom environment (SNR = +6 dB; RT = 0.6 seconds) as a function of speaker-to-listener distance. (Adapted from Crandell et al [1995].)

(PBK) monosyllabic words through a Knowles Electronics Manikin for Acoustical Research (KEMAR) at speaker-listener distances often encountered in the classroom (6, 12, and 24 ft). The multitalker babble derived from the SPIN test was used as the noise competition (Kalikow et al, 1977). Subjects consisted of children 5 to 7 years of age. Results from this investigation, shown in Figure 20–9, indicate a decrease in speech recognition ability as the speaker-listener distance was increased. Specifically, mean word recognition scores of 89%, 55%, and 36% were obtained at 6, 12, and 24 ft, respectively. These results suggest that children with normal-hearing who are seated in the middle to rear of a typical classroom setting have greater difficulty understanding speech than is commonly suspected.

Before concluding this section, it is important to note that a number of theoretical considerations and resulting acoustic formulas have been developed to estimate speech recognition in rooms of varying acoustical qualities at different locations with the room. These formulas include the (1) articulation index (AI); (2) speech transmission index (STI); (3) early-to-late ratios (ELR); (4) early decay time (EDT$_{10}$); (5) early-to-late energy ratios (EL$_t$); (6) useful-to-detrimental energy ratio (U$_{80}$); (7) early energy fraction (D$_{50}$); (8) relative loudness or relative strength; and (9) articulation loss of consonants. Unfortunately, most of these indices were developed for adult listeners with normal-hearing and may not be applicable for children or listeners with SNHL. For a review of these formulas the reader is directed to Harris (1991), Berg (1993), and Siebein et al (1997).

METHODS TO IMPROVE ROOM ACOUSTICS

The remaining sections of this chapter will address procedures for reducing the effects of noise, reverberation, and distance in rooms. These procedures include (1) acoustic

modifications of the room, (2) using "clear" speech procedures, (3) reduction of speaker-listener distance, (4) optimizing visual communication, and (5) personal and group amplification systems.

Acoustical Modifications of the Room

The speech recognition difficulties experienced by listeners with hearing impairment and children with "normal-hearing" highlight the need to provide an appropriate listening environment for these populations. Recall that acoustic guidelines for such populations indicate that SNRs should exceed +15 dB; unoccupied noise levels should not exceed 30 to 35 dB(A), and RTs should not surpass 0.4 s (through the speech frequency range). These acoustic recommendations, however, are rarely achieved in most listening environments. Recall also that background room noise can originate from external and/or internal sources. Background noise can also originate from within the room itself. To conduct the most appropriate modification of the room, it must first be determined which specific noise source or sources need to be reduced. Following are common procedures for reducing various types of noise in rooms, such as classrooms. For more complete discussions on acoustic modifications and noise reduction the reader is directed to Knudsen and Harris (1978), Egan (1987), Harris (1991), Barron (1993), and Crandell et al (1995).

SPECIAL CONSIDERATION

Background noise levels and RTs are constantly interacting in a room. Although improving one often improves the other, this is not always true. Both noise and reverberation must be thoroughly evaluated when establishing the adequacy of a room for communication. This evaluation includes a spectral analysis of both the background noise (such as NC or RC curves) and the reverberant characteristics of the room.

Reduction of External Noise Levels

1. Rooms used for the hearing-impaired or "normal hearers" must be located away from high-noise sources, such as busy automobile traffic, railroads, construction sites, airports, and furnace/air-conditioning units. The most effective procedure for achieving this goal is through appropriate planning with contractors, school officials, architects, architectural engineers, audiologists, and teachers for the hearing impaired *before* the design and construction of the school building. Such consultation should include strategies for locating rooms away from high external noise sources. Moreover, acoustic modifications such as the placement of vibration reduction pads underneath the supporting beams of the building to reduce structure-borne sounds can be implemented. Unfortunately, acoustic planning before building construction is rare (Crandell & Smaldino, 1995; Crandell et al, 1995).

2. *A sound transmission loss (STL)* of at least 45- to 50-dB is often required for external walls. STL refers to the amount of noise that is attenuated as it passes through a material. If an external noise of 100 dB SPL was reduced to 60 dB SPL in the room, the exterior wall of that room would have an STL of 40 dB SPL. A 7-inch concrete wall provides approximately 53 dB attenuation of outside noise, whereas windows and doors provide only 24 dB and 20 dB attenuation, respectively. Therefore doors and/or windows on the external wall should be avoided in situations of high external noise levels. Average STL values for different structures can be found in most books published on acoustics. Procedures to increase the STL of an external wall include (1) the placement of absorptive materials (such as fiberglass material) between the wall studs, (2) thick or double-concrete construction on the exterior wall, and (3) the addition of several layers of gypsum board (at least 5/8 inch) or plywood material.

3. All exterior walls must be free of cracks or openings that would allow extraneous noises into the room. Even small openings in external walls can significantly reduce the STL.

4. If windows are located on the external wall, they must be properly installed, heavy weighted, or double-paned (such as storm windows) and remain closed (whenever possible) if high external noise sources exist. In addition, existing windows can be sealed with nonhardening caulk to increase the STL. Of course, safety regulations must be checked before sealing outside windows.

5. Landscaping strategies can also attenuate external noise sources. These strategies include the placement of trees or shrubs (that bloom all year long) and earthen banks around the school building.

6. Solid concrete barriers with an STL of 30- to 35-dB can be placed between the school building and the noise source to reduce external noise entering into the room.

Reduction of Internal Noise Levels

1. Often, the most cost-effective procedure for reducing internal noise levels in the room is to relocate the children in that room to a quieter area of the building. Rooms used for communication must not be located next to a high-noise source such as the gymnasium, metal shop, cafeteria, or bandroom. At least one quiet environment, such as a storage area or closet, should separate rooms from each other or from high-noise sources in the school building.

2. If suspended ceilings separate the room from another room, sound-absorbing materials should be placed in the plenum space above the wall.

3. Double-wall or thick-wall construction should be used for the interior walls, particularly those walls that face noisy hallways or rooms. Additional layers of gypsum board, plywood, and/or the placement of absorptive materials between wall studding can also increase the attenuation characteristics of interior wall surfaces. Moreover, all cracks between rooms should be sealed.

4. Acoustic ceiling tile and/or carpeting can be used in hallways outside the room.

5. All rooms should contain acoustically treated or well-fitting (preferably with rubber or gasket seals) high-mass-per-unit-area doors. Hollow-core doors between rooms, and facing the hallway, should not be used. Doors (or interior walls) should not contain ventilation ducts that lead into the hallways.

6. Heating or cooling ducts that serve more than one room can be lined with acoustic materials or furnished with baffles to decrease noise emitting from one room to another.

7. Permanently mounted blackboards can be backed with absorptive materials to reduce sound transmission from adjacent rooms.

Reduction of Room Noise Levels

1. The simplest procedure to reduce the effects of room noise is to position children away from high-noise sources, such as fans, air conditioners, heating ducts, faulty lighting fixtures, and doors or windows adjacent to sources of noise. Often, however, room-noise sources are so intense that no location in the room is appropriate for communication. In these cases acoustic modification of the room must be conducted.

2. Malfunctioning air conduction/heating units and ducts should be replaced or acoustically treated. Heating ducts, for example, can be lined with acoustic materials or fit with silencers to reduce both vibratory and airborne noise. In addition, rubber supports and flexible sleeves or joints should be used to reduce the transmission of structural-borne noise through the ductwork system. Moreover, all fans and electrical motors in air conditioning/heating units must be lubricated and maintained on a regular basis.

3. Installation of thick, wall-to-wall carpeting (with adequate padding) to dampen the noise of shuffling of hard-soled shoes, the movement of desks/chairs, and so forth can reduce room noise levels.

4. Acoustic paneling can be placed on the walls and ceiling. Wall paneling typically should be placed partly down the wall and not on walls parallel to one another.

5. The placement of some form of rubber tips on the legs of desks and chairs can decrease room noise. This recommendation is particularly important if the room is not carpeted.

6. Acoustically treated furniture can be purchased for rooms. It must be noted that such furniture can be expensive and may present hygiene problems.

7. Hanging of thick curtains or acoustically treated venetian blinds over window areas to dampen room noise levels can be effective.

8. Avoid open-plan rooms for children because it is well recognized that such rooms are considerably noisier than regular rooms.

9. Instruction should not take place in areas separated from other teaching areas by sliding doors, thin partitions, or temporary walls. Walls between instruction areas must be of sufficient thickness and continuous between the solid ceiling and floor. Walls that are not continuous allow for significant sound transmission between rooms.

10. Fluorescent lighting systems, including the ballast, need to be regularly maintained and replaced if faulty.

11. Typewriter or computer keyboard noise can be lowered by the placement of rubber pads or carpet remnants under such instruments. Whenever possible, such instruments

(and any other office equipment) should be located in separate rooms. Rubber pads to reduce vibratory noise should be placed under all office equipment in the school.

12. Children can be encouraged to wear soft-soled shoes.

Reduction of Room Reverberation

The presence or absence of absorptive surfaces within a room will affect the reverberant characteristics of that environment. Materials with hard, smooth surfaces such as concrete, cinder block, and hard plaster are poor absorbers, whereas materials with soft, rough-surfaced, and/or porous surfaces (cloth, fiberglass, corkboard) tend to be good absorbers of sound. Hence, rooms with bare cement walls, floors, and ceilings tend to exhibit higher RTs than rooms that contain absorptive surfaces such as carpeting, draperies, and acoustic ceiling tile. A useful index in determining the reverberant characteristics of a room is the *absorption coefficient*. Absorption coefficient (α) refers to the ratio of unreflected energy to incident energy present in a room. A surface with an absorption coefficient of 1.00 would technically absorb 100% of all reflections, whereas a surface structure with an absorption coefficient of 0.00 would reflect all of the incident sound. A summary of absorption coefficients for different materials is found in Table 20–10. Note that the absorption coefficients, which are typically indicated from 125 to 4000 Hz, are frequency dependent.

Specifically, most surface materials in a room do not absorb low-frequency sounds as effectively as higher frequencies. Because of these absorption characteristics, room reverberation is often shorter at higher frequencies than in lower frequency regions. Generally, surfaces are not considered absorptive until they reach an absorption coefficient of 0.20. When excessive reverberation occurs, the tendency is to treat most or all of the surfaces in a room with sound-absorbing materials. If all of the surfaces become sound absorbent, then the speaker is effectively speaking in an anechoic or nonreverberant environment. The speaker will have to raise his or her voice or use an amplification system to overcome the lack of reflected sounds that would normally be present in a room. Several procedures to reduce reverberation in a room include the following:

1. Reverberation can be reduced by covering the hard reflective surfaces in a room with absorptive materials, such as acoustic paneling. To reduce reverberation, ceilings should

PITFALL

When making modifications to reduce the reverberation in a room, care must be taken to avoid overapplication of acoustic materials that absorb the low-intensity, high-frequency components of speech. Overapplication may reduce speech recognition and affect sound quality.

TABLE 20–10 An example of absorption coefficients for various materials

Material	Frequency (Hz)					
	125	250	500	1000	2000	4000
Ceilings						
Plaster or gypsum	0.14	0.10	0.06	0.05	0.04	0.03
Acoustic tiles, 2/3 inch (suspended 16 inches from ceiling)	0.25	0.28	0.46	0.71	0.86	0.93
Acoustic tiles, 1/2 inch (suspended 16 inches from ceiling)	0.52	0.37	0.50	0.69	0.79	0.78
Acoustic tiles, 1/2 inch (cemented directly to ceiling)	0.10	0.22	0.61	0.56	0.74	0.72
High-absorbent panels, 1 inch (suspended 16 inches from ceiling)	0.58	0.88	0.75	0.99	1.00	0.96
Walls						
Brick	0.03	0.03	0.03	0.04	0.05	0.07
Concrete painted	0.10	0.05	0.06	0.07	0.09	0.08
Window glass	0.35	0.25	0.18	0.12	0.07	0.04
Marble	0.01	0.01	0.01	0.02	0.02	0.00
Plaster or concrete	0.12	0.09	0.07	0.05	0.05	0.04
Plywood	0.28	0.22	0.17	0.09	0.10	0.11
Concrete block, (coarse)	0.36	0.44	0.31	0.29	0.39	0.25
Heavyweight drapery	0.14	0.35	0.55	0.72	0.70	0.65
Fiberglass wall treatment, 1 inch	0.08	0.32	0.99	0.76	0.34	0.12
Fiberglass wall treatmnet, 7 inches	0.86	0.99	0.99	0.99	0.99	0.99
Wood paneling on glass fiber blanket	0.40	0.99	0.80	0.50	0.40	0.30
Floors						
Wood parquet on concrete	0.04	0.04	0.07	0.60	0.06	0.07
Linoleum	0.02	0.03	0.03	0.03	0.03	0.02
Carpet on concrete	0.02	0.06	0.14	0.37	0.60	0.65
Carpet on foam rubber padding	0.08	0.24	0.57	0.69	0.71	0.73

be covered with acoustic paneling. The ceiling should contain an acoustic tile ceiling. The acoustic tile should be suspended from the structural deck and have an absorption coefficient of at least 0.65. This will absorb multiple order sound reflections from the corners of the room and reduce the RT to acceptable levels. Acoustic panels may also be placed on walls but typically not on walls parallel to one another. Cork bulletin boards, carpeting, and bookcases can also be strategically placed on the walls; however, such materials are not as absorptive as acoustic paneling. Interestingly, the installation of absorptive materials will not only reduce reverberation in the environment but also will decrease the noise level in the room by 5- to 8-dB.

2. Thick carpeting on the floors can also significantly reduce reverberation and noise in a room. Rooms that contain both ceiling tile and carpets have approximately 60% of room surfaces covered with absorptive material. However, rooms with just the ceiling and floor covered are prone to acoustic defects such as flutter echoes. *Flutter echoes* are the continued reflection of sound waves between two opposite parallel surfaces. This is a particular problem in small rooms, such as classrooms. It can be heard as a distinctive "slapping" or "ringing" sound. Absorbing materials can be placed on the walls or the walls can be splayed slightly to reduce this problem. Sound-absorbent acoustic panels (1-inch thick minimum) can be placed on the sidewalls at the front of the room to reduce flutter in the area where the teacher speaks.

3. Curtains or thick draperies can be placed to cover the hard reflective surfaces of windows. Even when the curtains are open, they will serve to minimally reduce the RT of the enclosure.

4. Positioning of mobile bulletin boards and blackboards at angles other than parallel to opposite walls will also reduce the reflected sound in an enclosure.

5. Some teachers have used creative artwork from egg cartons or carpet scraps attached to walls or suspended from ceilings to help absorb noise and reduce reverberation. Safety regulations must be checked before placing potentially non-fire-retardant materials in the room.

6. Recall that as room size increases, so does RT. Therefore keeping classrooms small and designing rooms with moderate ceiling heights is an important consideration. A ceiling height of approximately 10 ft to 13 ft is usually acceptable.

7. In rooms where greater teacher-to-student distances are encountered, such as middle schools and high schools, it is useful to provide a surface to reflect sound waves to the students. This becomes relatively easy in rooms that are used for conventional lecture-style teaching. An area of the room can be designated as the "teaching" area. This is the location from which the teacher will speak. The acoustic design issue is to provide early sound reflections from the ceiling to seats in the room. The front part of the ceiling should be gypsum board, plaster, or other sound-reflecting material. This will allow early sound reflections from the teacher's voice as she or he speaks to reinforce the direct sound and increase the loudness of sound reaching students in the room.

Present Status of Acoustical Modification in Classrooms

Despite the numerous strategies for treating the acoustic environment, classrooms often exhibit minimum degrees of acoustic modifications. Bess et al (1984) reported that although 100% of rooms had acoustic ceiling tiles, only 68% had carpeting, and only 13% had draperies. None of the classrooms contained any form of acoustic furniture treatment. Crandell and Smaldino (1995) reported that although all the 32 classrooms examined had acoustic ceiling tiles, only 14 (54%) contained carpeting. Moreover, only one of the classrooms (3%) had drapes, whereas none of the rooms had acoustic furniture treatments.

"Clear" Speech

"Clear" speech procedures may also facilitate speech recognition in many enclosures. "Clear" speech refers to a process in which the speaker focuses attention on a clearer pronunciation of speech while using a slightly reduced rate of speaking and a slightly higher intensity (Picheny et al, 1985a,b). Several investigations have demonstrated that "clear" speech can significantly augment speech recognition in noisy and reverberant environments (Crandell et al, 1998; Payton et al, 1994; Picheny et al, 1985a,b; Schum, 1996). Payton et al (1994), for example, demonstrated that the average improvement in speech recognition when using "clear" speech was 20% for listeners with normal-hearing and 26% for listeners with SNHL. Crandell et al (1998) found that recognition scores in a typical classroom environment (SNR = 0 dB; RT = 0.6 s) improved 18% when using "clear" speech procedures. It is not unreasonable to expect speakers, such as teachers, to learn "clear" speech procedures because talkers can be trained to continuously produce "clear" speech after a minimal amount of instruction and practice (Schum, 1996).

PEARL

Meeting acoustic guidelines in a room does not necessarily ensure high speech recognition for all listeners in that room. To ensure optimal speech recognition, the speaker may still need to decrease speaker-listener distance (physically or through room amplification systems), provide ample visual information, and/or use speaking techniques such as "clear" speech.

Reducing Speaker-to-Listener Distance

Another consideration in reducing the adverse effects of noise and reverberation is to ensure that the listener receives the speaker's voice at the most favorable speaker-listener distance possible. That is, for optimum speech recognition to occur, the listener needs to be in a face-to-face situation and in the direct soundfield of the speaker. Recall that speech recognition can only be improved within the critical distance of the room. Beyond the critical distance, recognition ability tends to remain essentially constant. Therefore in any listening environment, the speaker-listener distance should not exceed the critical distance of the room. Unfortunately, the critical distance in many rooms is present only at speaker-listener distances relatively close to the speaker. Thus the simple recommendation of preferential seating is often not adequate to ensure an appropriate listening environment. Rather, to remain within the critical distance of a room, restructuring of the room may need to be considered. For example, whenever possible, small group instruction (where the speaker addresses one small group at a time) should be recommended over more "traditional" room settings (where the speaker instructs in front of numerous rows of listeners). Crandell et al (1997) showed that recognition scores for children in normal classroom settings were 92% when they were instructed in small group settings.

Optimizing Visual Communication

Proximity to the speaker and face-to-face contact will also aid the listener with hearing impairment in maximizing speechreading skills. Optimal speaker-listener distance for maximum speech reading has been shown to be approximately 5 ft (Schow & Nerbonne, 1996). Speechreading ability tends to decrease significantly at 20 ft. Several investigators have reported that speechreading benefit increases as a function of decreasing SNR (Erber, 1979; Middleweerd & Plomp, 1987; Rosenblum et al, 1996). That is, listeners often obtain significantly more information visually as the acoustical environment becomes more adverse. In a recent investigation Rosenblum et al (1996) noted that speechreading can improve the SNR in typical classroom noise levels by more than 17 dB.

Personal and Group Amplification Systems

Another potential procedure for reducing speaker-listener distance is through the use of a personal or group amplification system. Before any amplification system is recommended in a room, physical modifications of the room must be always be first conducted. Unfortunately, it is often the case that significant acoustic modifications of a room cannot be accomplished because of excessive cost. A variety of personal and group amplification systems have been used to improve speech recognition in rooms. These systems include (1) personal hearing aids and (2) room amplification systems.

Hearing Aids

Hearing aids often offer little to no benefit in noisy or reverberant environments (Boothroyd, 1991; Crandell, 1991; Crandell et al, 1995; Duquesnoy & Plomp, 1983; Festen & Plomp, 1983; Moore, 1997; Plomp, 1987, 1986; Van Tassell, 1993). Simple amplification in and of itself often does little to improve the SNR of the listening environment. Plomp (1986) reported that hearing aids offered limited speech recognition benefit when background noise level exceeded 50 dB(A). Duquesnoy and Plomp (1983) indicated that minimum benefit occurred from personal amplification when background noise levels reached 60 dB(A). Certainly, a review of everyday background noise levels (see "Background Noise Levels in Rooms" section) would suggest that most environments exhibit background noise level in excess of 50- to 60-dB(A). Clearly, these data suggest that children should not use *just* a hearing aid in the classroom setting. Several potential SNR-enhancing options for hearing aids, however, may help the listener separate the signal from noise. The following section overviews several of these strategies. For more complete discussions of these technologies, the reader is directed to Chapters 12 and 13 in this volume.

Use of Directional Microphones

Because of the design of directional microphones, specific frequency spectra coming from various azimuths around the head (usually the front) are amplified more than other spectra coming from different azimuths (usually the sides and back). Thus if a speaker is in front of the listener, the hearing aid microphone will pick up much of the speech from the speaker while not amplifying the background noise. This differential sensitivity to sound, if used wisely by the hearing aid wearer, can improve the SNR in a particular situation as much as 3- to 4-dB (Hawkins & Yacullo, 1984). Directional microphones appear to be the single most effective option available in hearing aids today to improve the SNR if the signal is coming from the front of the listener and the noise from the rear of the listener. It must be noted, however, that in a classroom the technology must be used cautiously because if the wearer is not well schooled in how to position the directional microphones, the wanted signal may be attenuated in favor of background noise. In addition, with an environment such as a classroom, situations exist in which reception of signals all around the child's head is desirable, such as during classroom discussion. In a highly reverberant room the advantages offered by the microphone may be reduced or negated (Hawkins & Yacullo, 1984; Studebaker et al, 1980). Improvements in directional microphone technology are ongoing. Recently, dual microphone designs coupled with digital signal processing technology appear to be able to offer even greater improvements in SNR than conventional dual microphone designs. In the future multiple microphone arrays of up to five microphones, working in concert with digital algorithms may theoretically be able to improve the SNR by 11- to 13-dB.

Binaural Amplification

The advantages of listening to speech in noise through two ears (as opposed to one) or binaural amplification (compared to one hearing aid) are well recognized (Libby, 1980; Nabelek & Nabelek, 1994; Zurek, 1993). The advantages stem primarily from head shadow effects and binaural interaction factors. *Head shadow effects* refer to the acoustic effects of the head on speech and noise when these sources are at different locations in a room. Specifically, the listener with two ears, or two hearing aids, has the capability of favorably placing one ear toward the desirable sound (speech) and positioning the head to partially block the acoustics of an undesirable signal (noise). *Binaural interaction* refers to the various central auditory processing phenomena known to exist when listening with two ears. These phenomena include analysis of time and intensity cures arriving at the ears (*localization*), *binaural summation*, and *binaural release from masking* (masking level differences). Head shadow effects and binaural interaction are believed to be the basis (at least partially) for a listener with binaural hearing (or binaural hearing aids) to demonstrate greater abilities to localize, focus attention, and perceive speech in a background of noise (*cocktail party effect*).

Modification of Frequency Response

One of the earliest strategies for reducing the upward spread of masking effects of low-frequency noise is shaping the frequency response of the hearing aid so that the high frequencies (encompassing the consonants) are emphasized and the low frequencies are de-emphasized. In a room with abundant steady-state low-frequency noise, such as air-conditioning/ventilator noise, the ability to shift the frequency response of the amplification system in this way can effectively improve the SNR. As the interfering noise spectrum becomes more speechlike, the effectiveness of this strategy is diminished because important speech frequencies are removed. Modification of the frequency response has been available for many years in hearing aids through the nonadaptive high-pass filter setting. In recent years digitally programmable instruments have been made available that offer up to eight programs or memories, which are user selectable through a remote control unit.

Adaptive Signal Processing Strategies

Many of the hearing aids available today use some form of adaptive signal processing in an attempt to enhance the SNR of the listening environment. Adaptive signal processing strategies are those strategies that alter the electroacoustic characteristic(s) of the hearing aid in response to the specific environment the individual is in. These adaptive signal processing strategies include (1) conventional single channel automatic gain control; (2) adaptive compression; (3) multichannel compression; (4) bass increases at low levels (BILL) strategies, such as the Manhattan circuitry; and (5) treble increases at low levels (TILL) strategies, such as the K-Amp. A review of the speech recognition data concerning these strategies has been equivocal. That is, research has demonstrated that these strategies benefit some listeners in noise, but not others. The reader is directed to Sammeth and Ochs (1991) and Valente (1996a,b) for a review of these investigations and Chapters 1, 5, and 6 in this volume.

Digital Noise Reduction

Considerable research has been conducted to develop digital signal processing methods that can enhance a desired speech signal while reducing the background noise. Many of the methods require a great deal of computing power to implement, which has not been feasible in a wearable device. The recent development and implementation of digital signal processing in a form that can be placed in a wearable device has rekindled research interest in digital noise reduction methods. For example, strategies that use both one and multiple microphones are currently being researched. Single microphone designs attempt to identify the speech spectrum versus the noise spectrum and to selectively filter the noise spectrum, thus improving the SNR. Typical multiple microphone designs are of two general types. One type involves a scheme to adaptively subtract a noise (received from one microphone) from a noise + signal (received by another microphone) to derive a signal minus most of the noise component. The second type (referred to as adaptive beam forming) involves adaptively changing the sensitivity of an array of multiple microphones, so that the sensitivity pattern of the microphones is maximum for a forward occurring speech signal and minimal for surrounding noise (Dillon & Lovegrove, 1993; Levitt, 1993; Weiss & Newman, 1993).

Use of FM, Direct Audio Input, and Inductance Coupling

Certainly, the most effective procedure for improving the SNR for a hearing aid user is through an assistive listening device, such as direct audio input (DAI), inductance coupling, or frequency modulation (FM) technology. These technologies will be briefly discussed in the next section. For a more complete discussion of these technologies, please see Chapter 19 in this volume.

Room Amplification Systems

If placed correctly, room amplification systems can significantly enhance the SNR of the listening environment. Studies concerning room amplification systems in classrooms have shown that such systems can improve speech recognition, listening, attention, academic performance, and on-task behaviors (see Lewis, 1991; Crandell et al, 1995; Ross et al, 1991, for reviews). Several forms of room amplification systems are commonly used. These systems include (1) personal FM amplification, (2) sound field FM amplification, (3) induction loop, and (4) infrared.

Personal FM Amplification

With a personal FM system (often called an *auditory trainer*), the teacher's voice is picked up through an FM wireless microphone located near his or her mouth (thus decreasing the speaker-listener distance), where the detrimental effects of reverberation and noise are minimal. The acoustic signal is then converted to an electrical waveform and transmitted by an FM signal to a receiver. The electrical signal is then amplified, converted back to an acoustic waveform, and conveyed to one or more listeners in the room. The listeners can receive the signal through headphones, earbuds, or directly through their hearing aids through induction loop or DAI technology. Because of the high SNR provided by this arrangement (often 15- to 25-dB), personal FM systems are an essential recommendation for students with hearing loss or children with "normal-hearing," who exhibit significant speech recognition difficulties in classroom settings. Personal FM systems have recently become available for both children with SNHL and children with normal-hearing in behind-the-ear models. Such models have been shown to be particularly useful for students in junior or senior high school who may not want to use personal FM systems because of the potential stigma traditionally associated with such devices. Currently, FM systems on the market permit a personal FM receiver to be added to, and become part of, a regular hearing aid. It is likely that FM systems of this type will be widely available as options on more hearing aids in the future.

Sound Field Frequency Modulation Amplification

A recent form of FM technology is sound field FM amplification. A sound field FM system is similar to a personal FM system; however, the speaker's voice is conveyed to listeners in the room through one or more strategically placed loudspeakers. Sound field FM systems are generally used to assist "normal-hearing" children in the classroom. The objectives when placing a sound field FM system in a classroom are twofold: (1) to amplify the speaker's voice by approximately 8- to 10-dB, thus improving the SNR of the listening environment and (2) to provide amplification uniformly throughout the classroom regardless of teacher or student position. Sound field systems vary from compact, portable, battery-powered single-speaker units to more permanently placed, alternating-current (AC) powered speaker systems that use multiple (usually four) loudspeakers. Numerous investigations have shown that when sound field amplification systems are positioned within the classroom, psychoeducational and psychosocial improvements occur for children with normal-hearing sensitivity (see Berg, 1993; Crandell & Smaldino, 1996b; Crandell et al, 1995, for a review of these studies). In what is often considered the original investigation on sound field amplification, the Mainstream Amplification Resource Room Study (MARRS) examined the following educational strategies on academic achievement: (1) children receiving regular classroom instruction supplemented by resource room instruction and (2) children educated in the regular classroom with sound field amplification (Sarff, 1981; Sarff et al, 1981). Students consisted of children with normal-hearing and children with minimal degrees of SNHL. Results indicated that both groups of children, particularly the minimally hearing-impaired children, demonstrated significant improvements in academic achievement, particularly in reading, when receiving amplified instruction. Younger children tended to demonstrate greater academic improvements than older children. Furthermore, academic gains in the amplified group were obtained at a faster rate, to a higher level, and with reduced cost, when compared with the unamplified group. A number of studies have reported similar findings (see Crandell et al [1995] for a review of these studies).

CONTROVERSIAL POINT

When using sound field FM amplification in a classroom, the number of loudspeakers (one or multiple) and location of the loudspeakers (ear level, ceiling, on the walls, in front of the room, in the corners, etc.) can be a confusing decision to make. Although no consensus exists in the literature, the goal of uniformly enhancing the SNR approximately 8- to 10-dB can be accomplished by a number of speaker configurations.

It is reasonable to assume that these academic improvements were the result of the improved listening environment offered by the sound field FM amplification system. Crandell and Bess (1987) examined the effects of sound field FM amplification on the speech recognition of children with normal-hearing in a classroom environment (SNR = +6 dB; RT = 0.45 s). BKB sentences were recorded in amplified and unamplified listening conditions at speaker-listener distances of 6, 12, and 24 ft. The SPIN multitalker babble was used as the noise competition, and subjects consisted of 20 children, aged 5 to 7 years. Results from this investigation (Fig. 20–10) showed that

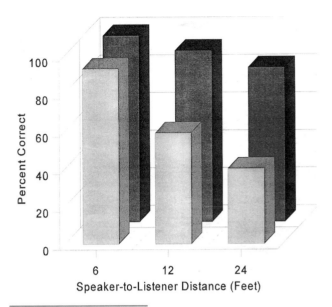

Figure 20–10 Mean speech recognition scores (in % correct) of children with normal-hearing in a "typical" classroom environment (SNR = +6 dB; RT = 0.6 s) with *(dark shaded bars)* and without *(light shaded bars)* sound field FM amplification. (Adapted from Crandell et al [1995].)

sound field FM amplification improved speech recognition at every speaker-listener distance, particularly at 12 ft and 24 ft. Numerous studies have reported similar improvements in speech recognition with the use of sound field technology (see Crandell et al [1995] for a review of these studies).

Sound field amplification systems in the classroom have been shown to be extremely cost-effective for several reasons. First, such systems are typically the most inexpensive of all the available classroom amplification systems. Second, sound field systems provide benefit for every child in the classroom, whereas personal FM systems or personal hearing aids only offer benefit to the individual user. In addition, because sound field systems provide amplification for all children in the classroom, these systems do not stigmatize certain children, which can be the situation with auditory trainers or hearing aids. Third, sound field systems are often the most inexpensive procedure of improving classroom acoustics. Acoustic modifications, such as acoustic ceiling tile, wall panels, or acoustically modified furniture, can be cost-prohibitive for some schools. As noted, however, essentially all classrooms will require at least a minimal degree of acoustic modification before the installation of sound field amplification. Finally, the use of sound field amplification systems has been shown to reduce the number of children requiring resource room assistance (Crandell et al, 1995; Flexer, 1989, 1992). If it is estimated that the average cost of a sound field system is $700 and the cost is divided by all of the children in the classroom (because it will benefit all children in the room), this equates to approximately $28 per child (considering a class size of 25 students). If this cost per student is computed over a 10-year period (the estimated life span of a sound field system), the unit cost per child is only $2.80. Because sound field systems significantly improve the classroom listening environment, additional cost-effectiveness may be obtained by reducing the number of children requiring resource room assistance. For selection procedures to determine whether a child is a candidate for personal or sound field FM technology the reader is directed to Feigin and Stelmachowicz (1991); Crandell et al (1995); and Bess et al (1996) for a thorough discussion of amplification options in the pediatric population.

CONTROVERSIAL POINT

Numerous investigations have demonstrated that sound field FM amplification improves academic, psychoeducational, and psychosocial achievement in "normal-hearing" children. To date, there remains limited information to support the use of this technology for children with mild-to-profound degrees of SNHL. Because of this paucity of data and because personal FM systems offer a substantially better SNR (15- to 25-dB) than sound field FM systems (8- to 10-dB), it is recommended that personal FM systems be used by children with SNHL whenever possible. It is also important to remember that hearing aids alone will often offer limited benefit to the child within a classroom.

Electromagnetic Induction Loop System

An induction loop system consists of a microphone connected by means of a cord or an FM radio signal to an amplifier. A length of wire, which is wound around a magnetic core under its installation, extends from the amplifier. This wire is placed either around the head of an individual (neckloop) or around a designated area, such as a classroom or theater. When an electrical current flows through the wire loop, it creates a magnetic field, which can be picked up through the telecoil of a hearing aid. Generally speaking, induction loop systems require a hearing aid to have a telecoil that is sensitive enough to pick up the magnetic field throughout the classroom for good speech recognition to occur. Moreover, speech recognition tends to decrease as the listener moves away from the induction loop.

Infrared Light Wave Systems

Infrared systems consist of a wireless microphone, infrared converter, and infrared receiver. The microphone converts the acoustic signal to an electrical signal, which is then transmitted to the converter. The converter transduces the electrical signal to an invisible infrared signal and transmits it to a receiver that is worn by the listener. The receiver then transduces the infrared signal back into electrical energy. The electrical signal is then changed into acoustic energy and routed to the listener through an induction loop/hearing aid telecoil setup or through headphones. For optimum sound quality with such systems, the listener must be in a direct line with the transmitter. For large

rooms, such as theaters and auditoriums, arrays of transmitters must be used to ensure that all listeners are appropriately placed with the infrared light beam. Infrared systems cannot be used outside, or in highly lit rooms, because they are susceptible to interference from sunlight.

EFFICACY MEASURES FOR INTERVENTIONS TO IMPROVE ROOM ACOUSTICS

On the basis of an evaluation of the acoustic status of a room (see Crandell et al [1995] for a step-by-step protocol), a decision may be made to improve the acoustic situation. No matter how the improvement is attempted, whether it is through physical modifications or the use of assistive technology, a measurable outcome of the intervention will be required in order to prove that the intervention was effective. Conversely, outcome measures can also show that the intervention was not effective and that a different intervention may be more appropriate.

PEARL

Whenever acoustical modifications or room amplification systems are implemented, it is imperative that efficacy of that procedure be established. Moreover, when establishing efficacy, it is important to obtain data from as many sources as possible. For example, within the classroom setting, information (speech recognition, academic improvements behavior, listening, attention, etc.) should be obtained from both the teacher and students (and parents if possible).

Many rooms, such as classrooms, are a difficult place to conduct efficiency studies. Not only are teachers often reluctant to conduct intrusive and lengthy test procedures, but measures must often be conducted during the school day with all of the students occupying the classroom. The logistics can frequently be intimidating. Despite this, a number of different approaches have been used to document the effects of intervention to improve acoustics on speech recognition, listening, and learning in the classroom. Some of the earliest efforts involved observing global changes in academic achievement or "on task" behavior. Because these measures were so global and possibly influenced by factors unrelated to the acoustic interventions, it is difficult to use these measures to establish unambiguous cause-and-effect relationships in the classroom. In an attempt to resolve the ambiguities, researchers have used a variety of speech recognition measures with stimuli ranging from nonsense syllables, words, and sentences to establish efficacy of acoustic interventions. Some of the more analytical speech test materials even allowed researchers to pinpoint specific problems not only with the acoustics of the room but also with perceptual differences between students in the classroom. Although speech recognition materials are intuitively pleasing, the linkage between speech recognition, listening, and learning is not well established. In addition, speech recognition testing is awkward to do in the confines of the school day and many of the test protocols are simply too complex or too lengthy to be practical in the classroom setting. Because of these difficulties, researchers have turned to subjective report questionnaires to obtain specific information concerning variables known to directly influence learning in the classroom. The trend toward the use of report inventories parallels the increased use of hearing handicap inventories by audiologists as a primary vehicle to document successful hearing aid fittings in adults. Several of these subjective questionnaires can be completed by the teacher. The most prominent of these questionnaires is the *Screening Instrument for Targeting Educational Risk (SIFTER)* (Anderson, 1989), wherein the teacher observes and rates each student (or classroom of students) in five content areas: academics, attention, communication, class participation, and school behavior. The total score in each content area is then categorized as pass, marginal, or fail. A preschool version of the SIFTER has also developed to evaluate younger children (3 years through kindergarten) (Anderson & Matkin, 1996). Although originally intended as a tool to help identify students at risk for listening problems, it has proven to be useful in establishing efficacy of intervention in the classroom. When used in a pretest/posttest experimental design, any change in student performance as a result of classroom acoustic intervention can be documented. An extension of the SIFTER called the *Listening Inventories for Education (LIFE)* (Anderson & Smaldino, 1998) retains a teacher self-report questionnaire but also adds a self-report questionnaire that is completed by the student. By obtaining direct input from the student regarding listening difficulties in the classroom, the overall validity of the subjective approach to efficacy should be improved. Samples of the SIFTER, Preschool-SIFTER, and LIFE are provided in the Appendix.

CONCLUSIONS

Audiologists have a significant role to play in ensuring that acoustic barriers to communication are minimized. With that consideration in mind, the purpose of this chapter was to review known acoustic barriers to listening and learning in rooms, particularly classrooms. SNR, RT, speaker-listener distance, and combination effects were discussed in light of their effects on accurate speech recognition for children with "normal-hearing" and children with hearing impairment. On the basis of considerable research, it was concluded that a prudent acoustic standard for listening and learning in many rooms for such listeners would be an unoccupied noise level of no more than 30- to 35-dB(A) (or an NC curve of 20 to 25), a SNR of + 15 dB or better, an RT of 0.4 s. Methods were suggested to improve room acoustics, including acoustic modifications of the room, reduction of speaker-listener distance, enhancing visual communication, and use of "clear" speech procedures. Technological suggestions included personal and sound field FM, induction loop, and infrared room amplification devices. Finally, approaches were outlined that have been used for documenting the efficacy of acoustic modifications or room amplification in an acoustic environment.

CONTROVERSIAL POINT

At present, no federal standards exist for background noise levels, SNRs, or RTs in classrooms. We suggest that federal standards be developed that are similar to acoustical guidelines proposed by ASHA. The ASHA proposal is the only current guideline that (on the basis of a vast amount of scientific literature) sets acoustical criteria for both listeners with SNHL and listeners with "normal-hearing."

Appendix

1. Listening Inventory For Education (L.I.F.E.): Teacher Appraisal of Listening Difficulty

2. Listening Inventory For Education (L.I.F.E.): Student Appraisal of Listening Difficulty

3. Screening Instrument for Targeting Educational Risk (S.I.F.T.E.R.)

4. Screening Instrument for Targeting Educational Risk in Preschool Children (age 3–Kindergarten) (Preschool S.I.F.T.E.R.)

L.I.F.E.
Listening Inventory For Education
Teacher Appraisal of Listening Difficulty
An Efficacy Tool by Karen L. Anderson, Ed.S. & Joseph J. Smaldino, Ph.D.

Name _____ **Grade** _____ **Date** _____
(Complete only for trial periods with individuals)

School _____ **Teacher** _____

Whole Classroom Sound Field Amplification Trial Period **Y / N**   Class Trial Period Length ___ Weeks
Individual Amplification Trial Period **Y / N**   Hearing Aid User **Y / N**   Trial Period Length ___ Weeks
Type of Hearing Technology Used With Individual: _____

Instructions: Circle the number which best describes student listening and learning behaviors.
See reverse for suggestions to aid students in listening and understanding classroom instruction.

The student's:	AGREE	NO CHANGE	Not Observed		DISAGREE
1. Focus on instruction has improved (more tuned in to instruction).	(2)	(1)	(0)	(-1)	(-2)
2. Appears to understand class instruction better.	(2)	(1)	(0)	(-1)	(-2)
3. Overall attention span has improved (less fidgety and/or less distracted).	(2)	(1)	(0)	(-1)	(-2)
4. Attention has improved when listening to directions presented to whole class.	(2)	(1)	(0)	(-1)	(-2)
5. Stays on task longer with less need for redirection.	(2)	(1)	(0)	(-1)	(-2)
6. Follows directions more quickly or easily (less hesitation before beginning work).	(2)	(1)	(0)	(-1)	(-2)
7. Answers questions in a more appropriate way or answers appropriately more often.	(2)	(1)	(0)	(-1)	(-2)
8. Improved understanding of instructional videos and/or morning announcements.	(2)	(1)	(0)	(-1)	(-2)
9. More involved in class discussions (volunteer more, follow better).	(2)	(1)	(0)	(-1)	(-2)
10. Improved understanding of answers or comments by peers during discussions.	(2)	(1)	(0)	(-1)	(-2)
11. Improved attention and understanding when noise is present (ventilator fan, transitions).	(2)	(1)	(0)	(-1)	(-2)
12. Improved ability to discriminate similar words or sounds (bat vs back, page 11 vs page 7).	(2)	(1)	(0)	(-1)	(-2)
13. Attention improved when listening in groups (small group/cooperative learning activities).	(2)	(1)	(0)	(-1)	(-2)
14. Socially more confident with other children or more comfortable in peer conversations.	(2)	(1)	(0)	(-1)	(-2)
15. Rate of learning seems to have improved (quicker to comprehend instruction).	(2)	(1)	(0)	(-1)	(-2)
16. Based on my knowledge and observations I believe that the amplification system is beneficial to the student's overall attention, listening and learning in the classroom.	(5)	(2)	(0)	(-2)	(-5)

Comments: (e.g., absences, equipment use problems)

Total Appraisal Score _____

APPRAISAL SUMMARY (circle one)

Highly Successful   26 - 35

Successful   16 - 25

Minimally Successful   5 - 15

Distributed by the Educational Audiology Association
4319 Ehrlich Rd, Tampa FL 33624 1-800-460-7322

LISTENING INVENTORY FOR EDUCATION
SUGGESTIONS FOR ACCOMMODATING STUDENTS WITH AUDITORY DIFFICULTIES

Students with auditory problems face extra challenges learning in a typical classroom setting. Typically, they can hear the teacher talk, but miss parts of speech or do not hear clearly, especially if noise is present. Students usually do not know what they didn't hear because they didn't hear it. They often may not know that they "misheard" a message unless they have already had experience with the language and topic under discussion. Use of amplification, having fluctuating hearing ability, hearing loss in just one ear, permanent hearing loss of any degree or central auditory processing disorders all compromise a student's ability to focus on verbal instruction and comprehend the fragments of speech information that are heard. The following items are suggestions for accomodating these student's special auditory needs and helping them learn their best in your classroom.

1. **Seat the student close to where you customarily teach.**
Sound weakens as it crosses distance. If a student has any auditory difficulties, how close you are to him/her will make a big difference on how well the student can hear and understand you.
   - Can the student be moved to the front of the room?
   - Can the student be allowed flexible seating so they can move to a better vantage point as classroom activities change? (e.g. move close to TV during movies)
   - If your teaching style causes you to move around the room when you talk, is it possible to stay in close proximity to the student with auditory problems?
   - When giving test directions, can you see the student's face clearly? Are you standing near the student's desk? Is the lighting on your face and not from a window behind you? Be sure the student is watching you.
   - Develop a signal the student can use if he or she does not understand or has missed critical information.

2. **Be aware of the benefits and limitations of lipreading.**
   - Only about 30-40% of speech sounds are visible on the lips. Lipreading supplements a student's hearing but is most helpful when the topic of conversation and vocabulary are known. New concepts and new vocabulary words have little meaning using lipreading.
   - Is the student seated so they can see your face clearly? Too close and they view your face from a skewed angle, too far and the quick, tiny mouth movements are imperceptible.
   - Lipreading is only possible if you are facing the student. If you use the chalkboard, do not provide verbal instruction while writing or be prepared to summarize or repeat that information for the student.
   - Reading aloud to the class with your face downward makes lipreading very difficult. Hold the book below your chin so your face is easily visualized.
   - Students cannot lipread and take notes at the same time. Classroom notetakers can use carbonized (NCR) paper and share notes easily. The student can use these notes from other students to fill in gaps in understanding.
   - The extra demands of trying to understand using only speech fragments and of constantly trying to lipread can be very fatiguing. Listening breaks are natural, especially after rapid class discussions, lectures or new information.

3. **Noise is a barrier to learning.**
   - Adults and children with normal hearing usually can tolerate a small amount of background noise without having their speech understanding compromised. Students with auditory problems are already missing fragments of what is said, especially if a message is spoken farther than from 3-6 feet away. Noise covers up word endings and brief words, reverberation smears the word fragments that are perceived.
   - Can the student be allowed flexible seating so they can move away from noise sources? (e.g. lawn mower)
   - Overhead projectors allow the student to clearly view the teacher's face, however, their fan noise interferes with understanding. If the student has a poorer hearing ear, face that one toward the overhead projector (or noisy ventilator, etc.) and seat close, but not next to the projector.
   - If possible, eliminate or dampen unnecessary noise sources. Sometimes apsorbtive material, such as styrofoam or a thick bathtowel placed under an aquarium heater or animal cage will absorb some noise. Seat the student away from animal distractions.
   - Keep your classroom door closed, especially when classes pass in the hall, gym or lunchroom activities are audible.
   - One of the main causes of noise in the classroom is due to the activity of students. Seat away from peers who are very active or habitually noisy. Allow student's time to search their desks so that the noise generated will not occur during verbal instruction. Inform the custodian of especially squeaky desks.

4. **Control or allow for distance.**
   - During group discussion, students with auditory problems typically can understand the students seated next to them but cannot understand students who are answering from more distant seats.
   - Use a student's name when calling on them to answer a question. This will allow the student with hearing needs a chance to turn to face the answering student and to lipread if at all possible.
   - Summarize key points given by classmates, especially brief messages like numeric answers, yes/no, etc.
   - Allow or assign a student buddy that the student with auditory problems can ask for clarification or cueing.

L.I.F.E.

Listening Inventory For Education
An Efficacy Tool
Student Appraisal of Listening Difficulty
By Karen L. Anderson, Ed.S. & Joseph J. Smaldino, Ph.D.

Name _____ Grade _____ Date _____

School _____ Teacher _____

Hearing Aid User Y / N   Trial Period   Type of Classroom

Trial Period Y / N   Length ____Weeks   Hearing Technology _____

Instructions: Circle the item which best describes the student's difficulty listening in the situations shown on picture card items 1-10. Optional items 11-16 can be scored if these situations are encountered in the listening environment. See reverse for intervention suggestions to improve listening and understanding.

Classroom Listening Situations	ALWAYS		SOMETIMES		NEVER
1. Teacher talking in front of room Comments:	(10)	(7)	(5)	(2)	(0)
2. Teacher talking during transition time Comments:	(10)	(7)	(5)	(2)	(0)
3. Teacher talking with back turned Comments:	(10)		(5)	(2)	(0)
4. Listening with hallway noise present Comments:		(7)		(2)	(0)
5. Other students making noise Comments:	(10)	(7)	(5)	(2)	(0)
6. Student answering during discussion Comments:	(10)	(7)	(5)	(2)	(0)
7. Listening with overhead projector fan on Comments:	(10)	(7)	(5)	(2)	(0)
8. Teacher talking while moving Comments:	(10)	(7)	(5)	(2)	(0)
9. Word recognition during a test or directions Comments:	(10)	(77)	(5)	(2)	(0)
10. Watching a video movie in classroom Comments:	(10)	(7)	(5)	(2)	(0)

Additional Listening Situations					
11. Cooperative small group learning	(20)	(15)	(10)	(5)	(0)
12. Listening in gym (inside & outside)	(20)	(15)	(10)	(5)	(0)
13. Listening in school assembly	(20)	(15)	(10)	(5)	(0)
14. Listening to students during lunch	(20)	(15)	(10)	(5)	(0)
15. Students talking while coats are hung up	(20)	(15)	(10)	(5)	(0)

Scoring

		PRE-TEST		POST-TEST
Sum of Items 1 - 10	(100 possible)	_____	CLASSROOM LISTENING SCORE	_____
Sum of Items 11-16	(100 possible)	_____	ADDITIONAL SITUATIONS SCORE	_____
Total Score of Items	(200 possible)			

The LIFE Student Appraisal was inspired by the Hearing Performance Inventory for Children. The authors recognize T. Giolas, A. Brancia Maxon & A. Riordan Kessler for their work in developing the HPIC.

LISTENING INVENTORY FOR EDUCATION
SUGGESTIONS FOR IMPROVING CLASSROOM LISTENING

Mark an X next to each statement that corresponds with the situations indicated on the reverse side in which the student is experiencing any difficulty.

Classroom Difficult Listening Situations

_X_ 1. Let the teacher know that you cannot understand. Develop a signal system with your teacher.

_X_ 1. Be sure that you are seated near the teacher. Ask to move if needed.

_____ 2. Ask a student buddy to explain the directions ("Did she say page 191?).

_____ 2. Before the teacher hands out a test to the class, ask what kind of test it is and how you take it (fill in all blanks, true/false, multiple choice).

_____ 3. Have another student or two in your class that will share their class notes with you, the teacher can help to arrange this and provide carbonized paper. It is still your job to listen very carefully as your teacher talks. Notes can help you fill in gaps you may have missed as you study later.

_____ 3. Be sure that the teacher is aware of how important it is for you to see his/her face. Ask your parent to send a note to the teacher. Ask for the teacher to repeat information, ask a neighbor, use your signal.

_____ 4. If there is noise in the hall, ask for door to be closed. Arrange with your teacher ahead of time to have permission to get up and close the door whenever it's noisy.

_____ 5. Let your teacher know that noise from classmates is interfering with your understanding; use your signal system to alert your teacher that it's too noisy.

_____ 6. Ask your teacher to say student's names when calling on them to answer questions. Watch her face and listen carefully for names so you can quickly turn to face the talking student.

_____ 6. If you miss information from student answers or discussion: 1) ask answering student to repeat the information, 2) ask the teacher to repeat, 3) ask a neighbor

_____ 7. If you did not hear all of the announcements, ask the teacher or a neighbor what they were about.

_____ 8. If you cannot understand what the teacher is saying as he or she talks when the class is getting out books or papers it is important to be sure you are ready and watching the teacher during these times. If you miss a page number or other information be sure to raise your hand and ask - you are probably not the only one who didn't hear the teacher clearly in all the noise of changing activities.

_____ 9. Spelling tests are easiest if you really know the word list and can tell the difference between similar words (e.g., champion and trampoline have similar sounds but have different endings). Sit close and watch the teacher's face carefully. If you are not sure you clearly heard a word, let the teacher know immediately (you could use your signal).

_____ 10. Hearing speech clearly in a movie can be hard because of the background music on some videos. Sit close to the TV even if it means sitting in a different seat. If used, ask the teacher to put the FM microphone next to the TV. Have a note taker. Request closed captioned videos be used.

Additional Difficult Listening Situations

_____ 11. In small group work, be sure to sit close to other students and try to be able to see all of their faces. If used, pass the FM microphone from student to student. Ask students to repeat what you missed. It helps if your group could meet in a quieter spot of the class or in the hall while you work.

_____ 12. While in the gym, stand close to the teacher for directions and ask other children for directions you may have missed. Ask the teacher to repeat what you missed. Use a signal system to let your teacher know you didn't understand.

_____ 13. To hear in an assembly it is important to be near the front. If you have a personal FM the person speaking should wear the transmitter.

_____ 14. Ask your friends to repeat or clarify when something is missed (Did you say tomorrow night?"). Sit where you can easily see their faces and try to sit away from noisier children or noisy areas of your classroom. Remind your friends they may need to tap you to get your attention when it's really noisy and if you are not watching their faces.

_____ 15. You need to depend on your friends to catch your eye, tap you or for them to wait until they see you looking at them before they talk to you. Ask them to repeat what you have missed (Practice is at what time? You called Suzy when?).

S.I.F.T.E.R.

SCREENING INSTRUMENT FOR TARGETING EDUCATIONAL RISK

by Karen L. Anderson, Ed.S., CCC-A

STUDENT _____ TEACHER _____ GRADE _____

DATE COMPLETED _____ SCHOOL _____ DISTRICT _____

The above child is suspect for hearing problems which may or may not be affecting his/her school performance. This rating scale has been designed to sift out students who are educationally at risk possibly as a result of hearing problems.

Based on your knowledge from observations of this student, circle the number best representing his/her behavior. After answering the questions, please record any comments about the student in the space provided on the reverse side.

1. What is your estimate of the student's class standing in comparison of that of his/her classmates?	UPPER 5 4	MIDDLE 3 2	LOWER 1
2. How does the student's achievement compare to your estimation of her/her potential?	EQUAL 5 4	LOWER 3 2	MUCH LOWER 1
3. What is the student's reading level, reading ability group or reading readiness group in the classroom (e.g., a student with average reading ability performs in the middle group)?	UPPER 5 4	MIDDLE 3 2	LOWER 1

ACADEMICS ☐

4. How distractible is the student in comparison to his/her classmates?	NOT VERY 5 4	AVERAGE 3 2	VERY 1
5. What is the student's attention span in comparison to that of his/her classmates?	LONGER 5 4	AVERAGE 3 2	SHORTER 1
6. How often does the student hesitate or become confused when responding to oral directions (e.g., "Turn to page . . .")?	NEVER 5 4	OCCASIONALLY 3 2	FREQUENTLY 1

ATTENTION ☐

7. How does the student's comprehension compare to the average understanding ability of her/her classmates?	ABOVE 5 4	AVERAGE 3 2	BELOW 1
8. How does the student's vocabulary and word usage skills compare with those of other students in his/her age group?	ABOVE 5 4	AVERAGE 3 2	BELOW 1
9. How proficient is the student at telling a story or relating happenings from home when compared to classmates?	ABOVE 5 4	AVERAGE 3 2	BELOW 1

COMMUNICATION ☐

10. How often does the student volunteer information to class discussions or in answer to teacher questions?	FREQUENTLY 5 4	OCCASIONALLY 3 2	NEVER 1
11. With what frequency does the student complete his/her class and homework assignments within the time allocated?	ALWAYS 5 4	USUALLY 3 2	SELDOM 1
12. After instruction, does the student have difficulty starting to work (looks at other students working or asks for help)?	NEVER 5 4	OCCASIONALLY 3 2	FREQUENTLY 1

CLASS PARTICIPATION ☐

13. Does the student demonstrate any behaviors that seem unusual or inappropriate when compared to other students?	NEVER 5 4	OCCASIONALLY 3 2	FREQUENTLY 1
14. Does the student become frustrated easily, sometimes to the point of losing emotional control?	NEVER 5 4	OCCASIONALLY 3 2	FREQUENTLY 1
15. In general, how would you rank the student's relationship with peers (ability to get along with others)?	GOOD 5 4	AVERAGE 3 2	POOR 1

SCHOOL BEHAVIOR ☐

Additional copies of this form are available in pads of 100 each from
The Educational Audiology Association
4319 Ehrlich Road, Tampa, FL 33624
ISBN 0-8134-2845-9

TEACHER COMMENTS

Has this child repeated a grade, had frequent absences or experienced health problems (including ear infections and colds)? Has the student received, or is he/she now receiving, special support services? Does the child have any other health problems that may be pertinent to his/her educational functioning?

The S.I.F.T.E.R. is a SCREENING TOOL ONLY

Any student failing this screening in a content area as determined on the scoring grid below should be considered for further assessment, depending on his/her individual needs as per school district criteria. For example, failing in the Academics area suggests an educational assessment, in the Communication area a speech-language assessment, and in the School Behavior area an assessment by a psychologist or a social worker. Failing in the Attention and/or Class Participation area in combination with other areas may suggest an evaluation by an educational audiologist. Children placed in the marginal area are at risk for failing and should be monitored or considered for assessment depending upon additional information.

SCORING

Sum the responses to the three questions in each content area and record in the appropriate box on the reverse side and under Total Score below. Place an **X** on the number that corresponds most closely with the content area score (e.g., if a teacher circled 3, 4 and 2 for the questions in the Academics area, an **X** would be placed on the number 9 across from the Academics content area). Connect the **X**'s to make a profile.

CONTENT AREA	TOTAL SCORE	PASS						MARGINAL		FAIL				
ACADEMICS		15	14	13	12	11	10	9	8	7	6	5	4	3
ATTENTION		15	14	13	12	11	10	9	8	7	6	5	4	3
COMMUNICATION		15	14	13	12	11		10	9	8	7	6	5	4	3
CLASS PARTICIPATION		15	14	13	12	11	10	9	8	7	6	5	4	3
SOCIAL BEHAVIOR		15	14	13	12	11	10	9	8	7	6	5	4	3

PRESCHOOL S.I.F.T.E.R.

Screening Instrument for Targeting Educational Risk
in Preschool Children (age 3-Kindergarten)
by Karen L. Anderson, Ed.S. & Noel Matkin, Ph.D.

Child _____ Teacher _____ Age _____

Date Completed ____/____/____ School _____ District _____

The above child is suspect for hearing problems which may affect his/her ability to listen, pay attention, develop language, follow teacher instruction and learn normally. This rating scale has been designed to sift out children who are at risk for educational delay and who may need further evaluation. Based on your knowledge of this child, circle the number that best represents his/her behavior. If the child is a member of a class that has students with special needs, comparisons should be made to normal learning classmates or normal developmental milestones. Please share additional comments about the child on the reverse side of this form.

PRE-ACADEMICS

1. How well does the child understand basic concepts when compared to classmates (e.g., colors, shapes, etc.)?
   ABOVE 5 AVERAGE 4 3 2 BELOW 1

2. How often is the child able to follow two-part directions?
   ALWAYS 5 FREQUENTLY 3 SELDOM 2 1

3. How well does the child participate in group activities when compared to classmates (e.g., calendar, sharing)?
   ABOVE 5 AVERAGE 4 3 2 BELOW 1

ATTENTION

4. How distractible is the child in comparison to his/her classmates during large group activities?
   SELDOM OCCASIONAL 4 2 FREQUENT 1

5. What is the child's attention span in comparison to classmates?
   LONG 5 AVERAGE 3 2 SHORTER 1

6. How well does the child pay attention during a small group activity or circle time?
   ABOVE 5 AVERAGE 4 3 2 BELOW 1

COMMUNICATION

7. How does the child's vocabulary and word usage skills compare to classmates?
   ABOVE 5 AVERAGE 4 3 2 BELOW 1

8. How proficient is the child at relating an event when compared to classmates?
   ABOVE 5 AVERAGE 4 3 2 BELOW 1

9. How does the child's overall speech intelligibility compare to classmates (i.e., production of speech sounds)?
   ABOVE 5 AVERAGE 4 3 2 BELOW 1

CLASS PARTICIPATION

10. How often does the child answer questions appropriately (verbal or signed)?
    ALMOST ALWAYS 5 FREQUENTLY 4 3 SELDOM 2 1

11. How often does the child volunteer information during group discussions?
    ALMOST ALWAYS 5 FREQUENTLY 4 3 SELDOM 2 1

12. How often does the child participate with classmates in group activities or group play?
    ALMOST ALWAYS 5 FREQUENTLY 4 3 SELDOM 2 1

SOCIAL BEHAVIOR

13. Does the child play in socially acceptable ways (i.e., turn taking, sharing)?
    ALMOST ALWAYS 5 FREQUENTLY 4 3 SELDOM 2 1

14. How proficient is the child at using verbal language or sign language to communicate effectively with classmates (e.g., asking to play with another child's toy)?
    ABOVE 5 AVERAGE 4 3 2 BELOW 1

15. How often does the child become frustrated, sometimes to the point of losing emotional control?
    NEVER 5 4 SELDOM 3 FREQUENTLY 2 1

Copyright ©1996 by Karen Anderson & Noel Matkin

Additional Copies of this form are available in pads of 100 each from
The Educational Audiology Association 1-800-460-7322
4319 Ehrlich Road, Tampa, FL 33624

TEACHER COMMENTS: (frequent absences, health problems, other problems or handicaps in addition to hearing?)

The Preschool S.I.F.T.E.R. is a SCREENING TOOL ONLY. The primary goal of the Preschool S.I.F.T.E.R. is to identify those children who are at-risk for developmental or educational problems due to hearing problems and who merit further observation and investigation. Analysis has revealed that two factors, expressive communication and socially appropriate behavior, discriminate children who are normal from those who are at-risk. The greater the degree of hearing problem, the greater the impact on these two factors and the higher the validity of this screening measure. If a child is found to be at-risk then the examiner is encouraged to calculate the total score in each of the five content areas. Analysis of the content area score may assist in developing a profile of the child's strengths and special needs. The profile may prove beneficial in determining appropriate areas for evaluation and developing an individual program for the child.

SCORING

There are two steps to the scoring process. First, enter scores for each of the indicated questions in the spaces provided and sum the total of the 6 questions for the expressive communication factor and then the 4 questions for the socially appropriate behavior factor. If the child's scores fall into the At-Risk category for either or both of these factors, then sum the 3 questions in each content area to develop a profile of the child's strengths and potential areas of need.

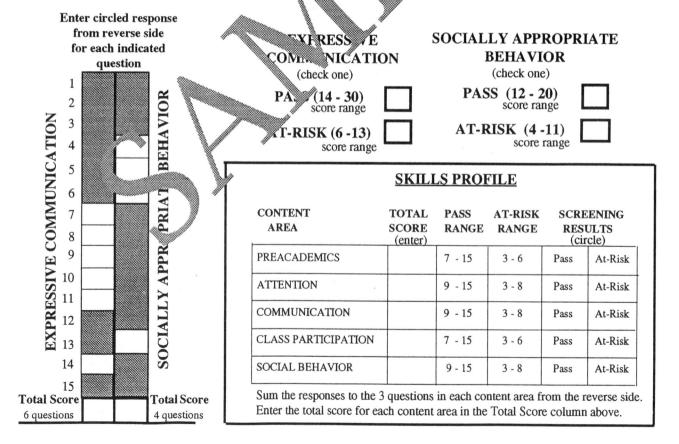

REFERENCES

ACCESS BOARD WEB SITE. (1998). http:www.access-board.gov

AMERICAN NATIONAL STANDARDS INSTITUTE. (1983). *Specifications for sound-level meters (ANSI S1.14–1983).* New York: ANSI.

AMERICAN SPEECH-LANGUAGE-HEARING ASSOCIATION. (1995). Guidelines for acoustics in educational environments. *ASHA, 37*(Suppl. 14);15–19.

ANDERSON, K. (1989). *Screening instrument for targeting education risk (SIFTER).* Tampa, FL: Educational Audiology Association.

ANDERSON, K., & MATKIN, N. (1996). *The preschool screening instrument for targeting education risk.* Tampa, FL: Educational Audiology Association.

ANDERSON, K., & SMALDINO, J. (1998). *The listening inventories for education (LIFE).* Tampa, FL: Education Audiology Association.

ANDO, Y., & NAKANE, Y. (1975). Effects of aircraft noise on the mental work of pupils. *Journal of Sound Vibration, 43*(4);683–691.

BARRON, M. (1993). *Auditorium acoustics and architectural design.* London: E & FN Spon.

BENCH, J., KOVAL, A., & BAMFORD, J. (1979). The BKB sentence lists for partially-hearing children. *British Journal of Audiology, 13*;108–112.

BERANEK, L. (1954). *Acoustics.* New York: McGraw-Hill.

BERG, F. (1993). *Acoustics and sound systems in schools.* Boston: College-Hill Press.

BERGMAN, M. (1980). *Aging and the perception of speech.* Baltimore:University Park Press.

BERKLEY, D., & ALLEN, J. (1993). Normal listening in typical rooms: The physical and psychophysical correlates of reverberation. In: G. Studebaker, & I. Hochberg (Eds.), *Acoustical factors affecting hearing aid performance* (pp. 3–14). Boston: Allyn & Bacon.

BESS, F. (1985). The minimally hearing-impaired child. *Ear and Hearing, 6*;43–47.

BESS, F., GRAVEL, J., & THARPE, A. (1996). *Amplification for children with auditory deficits.* Nashville: Bill Wilkerson Center Press.

BESS, F., & MCCONNELL, F. (1981). *Audiology, education and the hearing-impaired child.* St. Louis: Mosby.

BESS, F., SINCLAIR, J., & RIGGS, D. (1984). Group amplification in schools for the hearing-impaired. *Ear and Hearing, 5*;138–144.

BESS, F., & THARPE, A. (1986). An introduction to unilateral sensorineural hearing loss in children. *Ear and Hearing, 7*(1); 3–13.

BLAIR, J. (1977). Effects of amplification, speechreading, and classroom environment on reception of speech. *Volta Review, 79*;443–449.

BOLT, R., & MACDONALD, A. (1949). Theory of speech masking by reverberation. *Journal of the Acoustical Society of America, 21*;577–580.

BONEY, S., & BESS, F. (1984). *Noise and reverberation effects in minimal bilateral sensorineural hearing loss.* Paper presented at the American Speech-Language- and Hearing Association Convention, San Francisco, CA.

BOOTHROYD, A. (1991). Speech perception measures and their role in the evaluation of hearing aid performance in a pediatric population. In: J. Feigin, & P. Stelmachowicz (Eds.), *Pediatric amplification* (pp. 77–91). Omaha, NE: Boys Town National Research Hospital.

BORRID, K. (1978). Classroom acoustics. In: M. Ross, & T. Giolas (Eds.), *Auditory management of hearing-impaired children* (pp. 145–179). Baltimore: University Park Press.

BRADLEY, J. (1986). Speech intelligibility studies in classrooms. *Journal of the Acoustical Society of America, 80*(3);846–854.

BUUS, S., FLORENTINE, M., SCHARF, B., & CANEVET, G. (1986). Native French listeners perception of American English in Noise. *Proceedings of Inter-Noise, 1986*;895–899.

COOPER, J., & CUTTS, B. (1971). Speech discrimination in noise. *Journal of Speech and Hearing Research, 14*;332–337.

CRANDELL, C. (1991a). Individual differences in speech-recognition ability: Implications for hearing aid selection. *Ear and Hearing, 12*(6);100–108.

CRANDELL, C. (1991b). Classroom acoustics for normal-hearing children: Implications for rehabilitation. *Educational Audiology Monographs, 2*;18–38.

CRANDELL, C. (1992a). Classroom acoustics for hearing-impaired children. *Journal of the Acoustical Society of America, 92*(4);2470.

CRANDELL, C. (1992b). Speech recognition in the elderly listener: The importance of the acoustical environment. *Texas Journal of Audiology and Speech Pathology, 17*;25–30.

CRANDELL, C. (1993). Noise effects on the speech recognition of children with minimal hearing loss. *Ear and Hearing, 7*;210–217.

CRANDELL, C., & BESS, F. (1986). Speech recognition of children in a "typical" classroom setting. *ASHA, 29*;87.

CRANDELL, C., & BESS, F. (1987). Sound field amplification in the classroom setting. *ASHA, 29*;87.

CRANDELL, C., HENOCH, M., & DUNKERSON, K. (1992). A review of speech perception and aging: some implications for aural rehabilitation. *Journal of the Academy of Rehabilitative Audiology, 24*;121–132.

CRANDELL, C., SAPIENZA, C., & CURTIS, B. (1996). *Effects of sound-field amplification on vocal pathology.* Paper presented at the American Academy of Audiology, Salt Lake City, UT.

CRANDELL, C., SIEBEIN, G., GOLD, M., HASSELL, M., ABBOT, P., HERR, C., LEE, H., & LEHDE, M. (1998). Classroom acoustics IV: Speech perception of normal- and hearing-impaired children. *Journal of the Acoustical Society of America, 103*(5); 3063.

CRANDELL, C., SIEBEIN, G., HASSELL, M., ABBOT, P., GOLD, M., HERR, C., LEE, H., & LEHDE, M. (1997). Pilot studies of speech communication in elementary school classrooms: Literature review and methods. *Journal of the Acoustical Society of America, 101*(5);3069.

CRANDELL, C., & SMALDINO, J. (1992). Sound field amplification in the classroom. *American Journal of Audiology, 1*(4);16–18.

CRANDELL, C., & SMALDINO, J. (1994). The importance of room acoustics. In: R. Tyler, & D. Schum (Eds.), *Assistive listening devices for the hearing-impaired* (pp. 142–164). Baltimore: Williams & Wilkins.

CRANDELL, C., & SMALDINO, J. (1995). An update of classroom acoustics for children with hearing impairment. *Volta Reviews, 1*;4–12.

CRANDELL, C., & SMALDINO, J. (1996a). The effects of noise on the speech perception of non-native English children. *American Journal of Audiology; 5;*47–51.

CRANDELL, C., & SMALDINO, J. (1996b). Sound field amplification in the classroom: Applied and theoretical issues. In: F. Bess, J. Gravel, & A. Tharpe (Eds.), *Amplification for children with auditory deficits* (pp. 229–250). Nashville: Bill Wilkerson Center Press.

CRANDELL, C., SMALDINO, J., & FLEXER, C. (1995). *Sound field FM amplification: Theory and practical applications.* San Diego: Singular Press.

CREMER, L., & MULLER, H. (1982). *Principles and applications of room acoustics.* (Vols. 1 and 2). English Translation with Additions by T.J. Schultz. New York: Applied Science Publishers.

CROOK, M., & LANGDON, F. (1974). The effects of aircraft noise in schools around London airport. *Journal of Sound Vibration, 34;*221–232.

CRUM, D. (1974). *The effects of noise, reverberation, and speaker-to-listener distance on speech understanding,* Doctoral dissertation. Chicago: Northwestern University.

CRUM, D., & MATKIN, N. (1976). Room acoustics: The forgotten variable. *Language Speech and Hearing Service Schools, 7;*106–110.

DAVIS, G., & JONES, R. (1989). *Sound reinforcement handbook.* Milwaukee: Hal Leonard Publishing.

DENES, P., & PINSON, E. (1993). *The speech chain.* New York: W.H. Freeman.

DILLION, H., & LOVEGROVE, R. (1993). Single microphone noise reduction systems for hearing aids: A review and evaluation. In: G. Studebaker, & I. Hochberg (Eds.), *Acoustical factors affecting hearing aid performance* (pp. 353–372). Boston: Allyn & Bacon.

DIRKS, D., MORGAN, D., & DUBNO, J. (1982). A procedure for quantifying the effects of noise on speech recognition. *Journal of Speech and Hearing Disorders, 47;*114–123.

DIXON, P. (1976). *The effects of noise on children's psychomotor, perceptual, and cognitive performance,* Doctoral dissertation. Ann Arbor: University of Michigan.

DUQUESNOY, A., & PLOMP, R. (1983). The effect of a hearing aid on the speech-reception threshold of hearing-impaired listeners in quiet and in noise. *Journal of the Acoustical Society of America, 73;*2166–2173.

EDUCATION OF HANDICAPPED CHILDREN, P.L. 94–142 Regulations. (1977, August, 23). *Federal Register, 42(163);*42474–42518.

EDUCATION OF HANDICAPPED ACT AMENDMENTS OF 1986, P.L. 94–457 Regulations. (1986, October 8). *United States Statutes at Large, 100,*1145–1177.

EDUCATION OF HANDICAPPED ACT AMENDMENTS OF 1990, P.L. 101–476 Regulations. (1990, October 30). *United States Statutes at Large, 104,*1103–1151.

EGAN, M. (1987). *Architectural acoustics.* New York: McGraw-Hill.

ELLIOTT, L. (1979). Performance of children aged 9 to 17 years on a test of speech intelligibility in noise using sentence material with controlled word predictability. *Journal of the Acoustical Society of America, 66;*651–653.

ELLIOT, L. (1982.) Effects of noise on perception of speech by children and certain handicapped individuals. *Sound Vibration, Dec.;*9–14.

ELLIOTT, L., CONNORS, S., KILLE, E., LEVIN, S., BALL, K., & KATZ, D. (1979). Children's understanding of monosyllabic nouns in quiet and in noise. *Journal of the Acoustical Society of America, 66;*12–21.

ERBER, N. (1979). Auditory-visual perception of speech with reduced optical clarity. *Journal of Speech and Hearing Research, 22;*213–223.

FEIGIN, J., & STELMACHOWICZ, P. (1991). *Pediatric amplification.* Omaha: Boys Town National Research Hospital.

FESTEN, J., PLOMP, R. (1983). Relations between auditory functions in impaired hearing. *Journal of the Acoustical Society of America, 73;*652–661.

FINITZO-HIEBER T. (1988). Classroom acoustics. In: R. Roeser (Ed.), *Auditory disorders in school children* (2nd ed.) (pp. 221–233). New York: Thieme-Stratton.

FINITZO-HIEBER, T., & TILLMAN, T. (1978). Room acoustics effects on monosyllabic word discrimination ability for normal and hearing-impaired children. *Journal of Speech and Hearing Research, 21;*440–458.

FLEXER, C. (1989). Turn on sound: An odyssey of sound field amplification. *Educational Audiology Association News, 5;* 6–7.

FLEXER, C. (1992). Classroom public address systems. In: M. Ross (Ed.), *FM auditory training systems: Characteristics, selection and use* (pp. 189–209). Timonium, MD: York Press.

FLORENTINE, M. (1985). Non-native listener's perception of American English in noise. *Proceedings of Inter-Noise 1985;* 1021–1024.

FOURCIN, A., JOY, D., KENNEDY, M., KNIGHT, J., KNOWLES, S., KNOX, E., MARTIN, M., MORT, M., PENTON, J., POOLE, D., POWELL, C., & WATSON, T. (1980). Design of educational facilities for deaf children. *British Journal of Audiology,* Suppl. 3.

FRENCH, N., & STEINBERG, J. (1947). Factors governing the intelligibility of speech sounds. *Journal of the Acoustical Society of America, 19;*90–119.

GELFAND, S., & SILMAN, S. (1979). Effects of small room reverberation upon the recognition of some consonant features. *Journal of the Acoustical Society of America, 66(1);*22–29.

GENGEL, R. (1971). Acceptable signal-to-noise ratios for aided speech discrimination by the hearing-impaired. *Journal of Audiological Research, 11;*219–222.

GODFREY, J. (1984). Linguistic structure in clinical and experimental tests of speech recognition. In: E. Elkins (Ed.), *ASHA report 14: Speech recognition by the hearing-impaired* (pp. 52–56). Rockville, MD: ASHA.

GOTASS, C., & STARR, C. (1995). Vocal fatigue among teachers. *Folia Phoniatrica, 45;*120–129.

GREEN, K., PASTERNAK, B., & SHORE, B. (1982). Effects of aircraft noise on reading ability of school age children. *Archives of Environmental Health, 37;*24–31.

HAAS, H. (1972). The influence of a single echo on the audible speech. *Journal of the Audiological Engineering Society, 20* (2);146–159.

HARRIS, C. (1991). *Handbook of acoustical measurements and noise control.* New York: McGraw-Hill.

HASSALL, J., & ZAVERI, K. (1979). *Acoustic noise measurements.* Naerum, Denmark: Bruel & Kjaer.

HAWKINS, D., & YACULLO, W. (1984). Signal-to-noise ratio advantage of binaural hearing aids and directional microphones under different levels of reverberation. *Journal of Speech and Hearing Disorders, 49;*278–286.

HOUTGAST, T. (1981). The effect of ambient noise on speech intelligibility in classrooms. *Applied Acoustics, 14;*15–25.

HUMES, L. (1991). Understanding the speech-understanding problems of the hearing-impaired. *Journal of the American Academy of Audiology, 2;*59–69.

INDIVIDUALS WITH DISABILITY EDUCATION ACT WEB SITE. (1998). http://www.edlaw.net/ptabcont.htm

JOHNS, J., & THOMAS, H. (1957). Design and construction of schools for the deaf. In: A. Ewing (Ed.), *Educational guidance and the deaf child* (pp. 176–187). Washington, DC: Volta Review.

KALIKOW, D., STEVENS, K., & ELLIOTT, L. (1977). Development of a test of speech intelligibility in noise using sentence materials with controlled word predictability. *Journal of the Acoustical Society of America, 61;*1337–1351.

KEITH, R., & TALLIS, H. (1972). The effects of white noise on PB scores of normal-hearing and hearing-impaired listeners. *Audiology, 11;*177–186.

KENT, R. (1997). *The speech sciences.* San Diego: Singular Publishing Group.

KILLION, M. (1997). SNR loss: I can hear what people say, but I can't understand them. *Hearing Review, 4*(12);8,10,12,14.

KLEIN, W. (1971). Articulation loss of consonants as a criterion for speech transmission in a room. *Journal of the Audiological Engineering Society, 19;*920–922.

KNUDSEN, V., & HARRIS, C. (1978). *Acoustical designing in architecture.* Washington, DC: The American Institute of Physics for the Acoustical Society of America.

KO, N. (1979). Response of teachers to aircraft noise. *Journal of Sound Vibration, 62;*277–292.

KODARAS, M. (1960). Reverberation times of typical elementary school settings. *Noise Control, 6;*17–19.

KOSZARNY, Z. (1978). Effects of aircraft noise on the mental functions of school children. *Archives of Acoustics, 3;*85–86.

KURTOVIC, H. (1975). The influence of reflected sound upon speech intelligibility. *Acustica, 33;*32–39.

LEAVITT, R., & FLEXER, C. (1991). Speech degradation as measured by the rapid speech transmission index (RASTI). *Ear and Hearing, 12;*115–118.

LEHMAN, A., & GRATIOT, A. (1983). Effects du bruit sur les enfants à l'école. *Proceedings of the 4th congress on noise as a public health problem* (pp. 859–862). Milano: Centro Ricerche e Studi Amplifon.

LEVITT, H. (1993). Digital hearing aids. In: G. Studebaker, & I. Hochberg (Eds.), *Acoustical factors affecting hearing aid performance* (pp. 317–335). Boston: Allyn & Bacon.

LEWIS, D. (1991). FM systems and assistive devices: Selection and evaluation. In: J. Feigin, & N. Stelmachowicz (Eds.), *Pediatric amplification* (pp. 115–138). Omaha: Boys Town National Research Hospital.

LIBBY, R. (1980). *Binaural hearing and amplification.* (Vol. 1 and 2). Chicago: Zenetron.

LICKLIDER, J., & MILLER, G. (1951). The perception of speech. In: S. Stevens (Ed.), *Handbook of experimental psychology.* New York: John Wiley & Sons.

LOCHNER, J., & BURGER, J. (1964). The influence of reflections in auditorium acoustics. *Journal of Sound and Vibration, 4;* 426–454.

MARKIDES, A. (1986). Speech levels and speech-to-noise ratios. *British Journal of Audiology, 20;*115–120.

MCCROSKEY, F., & DEVENS, J. (1975). Acoustic characteristics of public school classrooms constructed between 1890 and 1960. *NOISEXPO Proceedings;* 101–103.

MCLAUGHLIN, S. (1998). *Introduction to language development.* San Diego: Singular Publishing Group.

MIDDLEWEERD, M., & PLOMP, R. (1987). The effect of speechreading on the speech reception threshold of sentences in noise. *Journal of the Acoustical Society of America, 82;*2145–2146.

MILLER, G. (1974). Effects of noise on people. *Journal of the Acoustical Society of America, 56;*724–764.

MILLER, G., & NICELY, P. (1955). An analysis of perceptual confusions among some English consonants. *Journal of the Acoustical Society of America, 27;*338–352.

MONCUR, J., & DIRKS, D. (1967). Binaural and monaural speech intelligibility in reverberation. *Journal of Speech and Hearing Research, 10;*186–195.

MOORE, B. (1997). *An introduction to the psychology of hearing.* San Diego: Academic Press.

NABELEK, A. (1982). Temporal distortions and noise considerations. In: G. Studebaker, & F. Bess (Eds.), *The Vanderbilt hearing-aid report: State of the art-research needs* (pp. 51–59). Upper Darby, PA: Monographs in Contemporary Audiology.

NABELEK, A., & DONAHUE, A. (1984). Perception of consonants in reverberation by native and non-native listeners. *Journal of the Acoustical Society of America, 75;*632–634.

NABELEK, A., & MASON, D. (1981). Effect of noise and reverberation on binaural and monaural word identification by subjects with various audiograms. *Journal of Speech and Hearing Research, 24;*375–383.

NABELEK, A., & NABELEK, I. (1994). Room acoustics and speech perception. In: J. Katz (Ed.), *Handbook of clinical audiology* (4th ed.) (pp. 624–637). Baltimore: Williams & Wilkins.

NABELEK, A., & PICKETT, J. (1974a). Monaural and binaural speech perception through hearing aids under noise and reverberation with normal and hearing-impaired listeners. *Journal of Speech and Hearing Research, 17;*724–739.

NABELEK, A., & PICKETT, J. (1974b). Reception of consonants in a classroom as affected by monaural and binaural listening, noise, reverberation, and hearing aids. *Journal of the Acoustical Society of America, 56;*628–639.

NABELEK, A., & ROBINSON, P. (1982). Monaural and binaural speech perception in reverberation for listeners of various ages. *Journal of the Acoustical Society of America, 71*(5); 1242–1248.

NEEDLEMAN, A., & CRANDELL, C. (1996a). Speech perception in noise by hearing-impaired and masked normal-hearing listeners. *Journal of the American Academy of Audiology, 2;* 65–72.

NEEDLEMAN, A., & CRANDELL, C. (1996b). Simulation of sensorineural hearing loss. In: M. Jestadt (Ed.), *Modeling sensorineural hearing loss* (pp. 461–474). Boston: Allyn & Bacon.

NEUMAN, A., & HOCHBERG, I. (1983). Children's perception of speech in reverberation. *Journal of the Acoustical Society of America, 73*(6);2145–2149.

NIEMOELLER, A. (1968). Acoustical design of classrooms for the deaf. *American Annals of Deafness, 113;*1040–1045.

NOBER, L., & NOBER, E. (1975). Auditory discrimination of learning disabled children in quiet and classroom noise. *Journal of Learning Disorders, 8;*656–773.

OLSEN, W. (1977). Acoustics and amplification in classrooms for the hearing impaired. In: F. Bess (Ed.), *Childhood deafness: Causation, assessment and management* (pp. 251–264). New York: Grune & Stratton.

OLSEN, W. (1981). The effects of noise and reverberation on speech intelligibility. In: F. Bess., B. Freeman, & J. Sinclair

(Eds.), *Amplification in education* (pp. 225–236). Washington, DC: Alexander Graham Bell Association for the Deaf.

OLSEN, W. (1988). Classroom acoustics for hearing-impaired children. In: F. Bess (Ed.), *Hearing impairment in children* (pp. 266–277). Parkton, MD: York Press.

OTTRING, S., SMALDINO, J., PLAKKE, B., & BOZIK, M. (1992). *Comparison of two methods of improving classroom S/N ratio.* Paper presented at the American Speech- Language- and Hearing Association Convention, San Antonio, TX.

PAUL, R. (1967). *An investigation of the effectiveness of hearing aid amplification in regular and special classrooms under instructional conditions,* Doctoral dissertation. Detroit: Wayne State University.

PAYTON, K., UCHANSKI, R., & BRAIDA L. (1994). Intelligibility of conversational and clear speech in noise and reverberation for listeners with normal and impaired hearing. *Journal of the Acoustical Society of America, 95*(3);1581–1592.

PEARSONS, K., BENNETT, R., & FIDELL, S. (1977). Speech levels in various noise environments. *EPA 600/1-77-025,* Office of Health & Ecological Effects, Washington, DC

PICHENY, M., DURLACH, N., & BRAIDA, L. (1985a). Speaking clearly for the hard of hearing. I. Intelligibility differences between clear and conversational speech. *Journal of Speech and Hearing Research, 28*;96–103.

PICHENY, M., DURLACH, N., & BRAIDA, L. (1985b). Speaking clearly for the hard of hearing II. Acoustical characteristics of clear and conversational speech. *Journal of Speech and Hearing Research, 29*;434–446.

PLOMP, R. (1987). Auditory handicap of hearing impairment and the limited benefit of hearing aids. *Journal of the Acoustical Society of America, 75*;1253–1258.

PLOMP, R. (1986). A signal-to-noise ratio model for the speech reception threshold for the hearing impaired. *Journal of Speech and Hearing Research, 29*;146–154.

PUETZ, V. (1971). Articulation loss of consonants as a criterion for speech transmission in a room. *Journal of the Audiological Engineering Society, 19*;915–929.

ROSENBLUM, L., JOHNSON, J., & SALDANA, H. (1996). Point-light facial displays enhance comprehension of speech. *Journal of Speech and Hearing Research, 39*;1159–1170.

ROSS, M. (1978). Classroom acoustics and speech intelligibility. In: J. Katz (Ed.), *Handbook of clinical audiology* (pp. 756–771). Baltimore: Williams & Wilkins.

ROSS, M., BRACKETT, D., & MAXON, A. (1991). *Assessment and management of mainstreamed hearing-impaired children.* Austin: Pro-Ed.

ROSS, M., & GIOLAS, T. (1971). Effects of three classroom listening conditions on speech intelligibility. *American Annals of Deafness,* December; 580–584.

SABINE, W. (1964). *Collected papers on acoustics.* Cambridge: Harvard University Press, 1927. (Reprinted by Dover Publications.)

SAMMETH, C., & OCHS, M. (1991). A review of current "noise reduction" hearing aids: Rationale, assumptions, and efficacy. *Ear and Hearing, 12*(6);116–124.

SANDERS, D. (1965). Noise conditions in normal school classrooms. *Exceptional Children, 31*;344–353.

SANDERS, D. (1993). *Management of hearing handicap.* Englewood Cliffs, NJ: Prentice Hall.

SAPIENZA, C., CRANDELL, C., & CURTIS, B. (1999). Effect of sound field FM amplification on vocal intensity in teachers. *Journal of Voice, 13*(3);375–381.

SARFF, L. (1981). An innovative use of free field amplification in regular classrooms. In: R. Roeser, & M. Downs (Eds.), *Auditory disorders in school children* (pp. 263–272). New York: Thieme-Stratton.

SARFF, L., RAY, H., & BAGWELL, C. (1981). Why not amplification in every classroom? *Hearing Aid Journal, 11*;44,47–48,50,52.

SARGENT, J., GIDMAN, M., HUMPHREYS, M., & UTLEY, W. (1980). The disturbance caused by school teachers to noise. *Journal of Sound Vibration, 62*;277–292.

SCHOW, R., & NERBONNE, M. (1996). *Introduction to audiologic rehabilitation* (3rd ed.). Boston: Allyn & Bacon.

SCHUM, D. (1996). Intelligibility of clear and conversational speech of young and elderly listeners. *Journal of the American Academy of Audiology, 7*(3);212–218.

SHER, A., & OWENS, E. (1974). Consonants phonemic errors associated with hearing loss above 2000 Hz. *Journal of Speech and Hearing Research, 17*;656–668.

SIEBEIN, G. (1994). *Acoustics in buildings: A tutorial on architectural acoustics.* New York: Acoustical Society of America.

SIEBEIN, G., CRANDELL, C., & GOLD, M. (1997). Principles of classroom acoustics: Reverberation. *Educational Audiology Monographs, 5*;32–43.

SMALDINO, J. (1997). *Room acoustics.* Paper presented at the Acoustical Society of America Conference on Acoustical Barriers to Listening and Learning, Los Angeles, CA.

STUDEBAKER, G., COX, R., & FORMBY, C. (1980). The effect of environment on the directional performance of head-worn hearing aids. In: G. Studebaker, & I. Hochberg (Eds.), *Acoustical factors affecting hearing aid performance* (pp. 81–105). Boston: Allyn & Bacon.

SUTER, A. (1985). Speech recognition in noise by individuals with mild hearing impairments. *Journal of the Acoustical Society of America, 68*;887–900.

THIELE, R. (1953). Richtungsverteilung und Zeitfolge der Schallruckewerfe in Raumen. *Acustica, 3*;291–302.

VALENTE, M. (1996a). *Hearing aid standards, options, and limitations.* New York: Thieme Medical Publishers.

VALENTE, M. (1996b). *Strategies for selecting and verifying hearing aid fittings.* New York: Thieme Medical Publishers.

VAN TASSELL, D. (1993). Hearing loss, speech, and hearing aids. *Journal of Speech and Hearing Research, 36*;228–244.

WANG, M., REED, C., & BILGER, R. (1978). A comparison of the effects of filtering and sensorineural hearing loss on patterns of consonant confusions. *Journal of Speech and Hearing Research, 24*;32–43.

WEISS, M., & NEUMAN, A. (1993). Noise reduction in hearing aids. In: G. Studebaker, & I. Hochberg (Eds.), *Acoustical factors affecting hearing aid performance* (pp. 337–352). Boston: Allyn & Bacon.

ZUREK, P. (1993). Binaural advantages and directional effects in speech intelligibility. In: G. Studebaker, & I. Hochberg (Eds.), *Acoustical factors affecting hearing aid performance* (pp. 337–352). Boston: Allyn & Bacon.

PREFERRED PRACTICE GUIDELINES

Professionals Who Perform the Procedure(s)

▼ Audiologists
▼ Architects
▼ Acoustic engineers

Expected Outcomes

▼ Optimum speech recognition (and subjective clarity) in a room for all listeners, particularly those individuals with SNHL or "normal-hearing." To meet this goal, acoustic guidelines must be met as closely as possible. The American Speech-Language-and Hearing Association (ASHA) suggests the following acoustic guidelines:

1. Unoccupied background noise level of 30 to 35 dB(A) or an NC curve of approximately 25
2. SNR of +15 dB or better
3. RT not exceeding 0.4 seconds

▼ If acoustic guidelines cannot be met (and even in some cases when they can), installation of a room amplification system should be considered. Room amplification systems include personal FM, sound field FM, induction loop, and infrared systems. The room amplification system should provide high speech recognition and speech clarity, while being comfortable for the listener to use. The amplificaiton system should also provide minimal negative stigma to the user.

Clinical Indications

▼ Rooms that have acoustic characteristics that act as barriers to speech recognition, listening, and learning

▼ Rooms that are used by individuals who have SNHL or "normal-hearing"

Clinical Process

▼ Observation of room, including major sources of noise, speaker style, and seating arrangements
▼ Comprehensive measurement of background noise, RT, and SNR in the room
▼ Identification of individuals who have SNHL or "normal-hearing" in room
▼ Determination of appropriate acoustic modifications and/or room amplification system
▼ Acoustic modifications and/or fitting/installation of room amplification system
▼ If room amplification system is installed, speaker (teacher) training is imperative
▼ If room amplification system is installed, regular monitoring of the equipment is needed

Documentation

▼ Schematic of room with acoustic characteristics noted at various listener locations
▼ Notation of acoustic characteristics of room after acoustic modification and/or installation of room amplification system
▼ Preintervention and postintervention measures of efficacy

Chapter 21

Vestibular Rehabilitation

Alan L. Desmond

Outline

Vestibular disorders, responsible for complaints of vertigo and dysequilibrium, are a common complaint in the adult and geriatric population. In 1994 these complaints accounted for 11 million doctor visits in the United States (Nashner, undated). Various studies indicate that "dizziness" is among the three most common complaints encountered in the primary care setting, sharing equal time with headaches and low back pain (Watson & Sinclair, 1992). After the age of 65, it is one of the most frequent reasons for an office visit and hospital admission (Sloane, 1989; Weindruch et al, 1989). As the elderly population increases, so will the total number of complaints regarding balance disorders. The world population of citizens older than 60 will double between 1990 and 2030 (Strom, 1996). The need and opportunity for audiologists trained in the assessment and treatment of vestibular disorders is obvious.

The audiology "Scope of Practice" includes "the conduct and interpretation of behavioral, electroacoustic, or electrophysiologic methods used to assess hearing, balance and neural system function," and "consultation and provision of rehabilitation to persons with balance disorders using habituation, exercise therapy and balance retraining" (ASHA, 1996).

DEFINITIONS

Although terms such as *vestibular rehabilitation, vestibular adaptation, compensation,* and *habituation* seem to be used interchangeably in the literature, important distinctions need to be made. For the purposes of this chapter, we will use the following definitions.

Vestibular rehabilitation refers to the process of training the patient in the techniques for recovery from vestibular weakness. Rehabilitation, in general, is defined as the process of "putting back in good condition, bringing or restoring to a normal or optimal state of health by medical treatment and … therapy"(*Websters*, 1976).

Vestibular adaptation refers to the response of the central nervous system to asymmetrical peripheral vestibular afferent activity and resulting sensory conflicts. This implies a gradual decrease in neuronal response to a constant abnormal stimuli (Curthoys & Halmagyi, 1996).

Vestibular compensation encompasses the entire repertoire of strategies used by the patient to reduce symptoms and improve overall balance function and stabilize gaze. This includes neuronal adaptation of the vestibular ocular reflex (VOR), sensory substitution, and alternative predictive and cognitive strategies used to overcome the symptoms of vestibular deficit (Zee, 1994).

Vestibular habituation is "the long term reduction in a neurologic response to a particular stimulus that is facilitated by repeated exposure to the stimulus. In the vestibular system, the unpleasant response is usually a vertiginous sensation,

639

often associated with nausea, in response to certain head movements" (Shepard & Telian, 1996). In this context, vestibular rehabilitation involves maximizing vestibular compensation and promoting the learning and formation of habits (habituation) to promote reduction of symptoms and enhance postural and gaze stability.

PAST APPROACHES TO THE PATIENT WITH DIZZINESS

Treatment for vestibular disorders has historically fallen in to three categories: (1) medical treatment of symptoms and underlying pathological conditions; (2) surgical stabilization of the end organ or vestibular nerve through reparative or ablative techniques; and (3) observation, reassurance, and counseling to "learn to live with it."

Medical treatment most often involves prescribing vestibular or central nervous system (CNS) sedating medications. The most common medication prescribed is meclizine (Antivert). It has been reported that 61% to 70% of patients complaining of "dizziness" to a primary care physician receive meclizine (Burke, 1995; Sloane et al, 1994). The use of vestibular suppressant and CNS sedative medications has been questioned because evidence suggests that vestibular compensation and rehabilitation are delayed by these medications (Brandt, 1991; Shepard et al, 1990; Zee, 1985). Kroenke et al (1990) report that only 31% of patients treated with prescription medication believed this therapy to be helpful. In addition, side effects of CNS sedative and vestibular suppressant medications include drowsiness and slowing of reaction time, leading to an increased risk of falling (Manning et al, 1992; Tideiksarr, 1989).

Surgical approaches to vestibular pathological conditions are applicable only to unstable or progressive peripheral lesions. Conditions such as endolymphatic hydrops, Meniere's disease, and perilymphatic fistula are sometimes treatable through reparative surgeries. Ablative procedures may be recommended for intractable benign paroxysmal positional vertigo (BPPV) or Meniere's disease. Conditions such as acoustic neuroma or vestibular schwannoma frequently require surgical intervention and often result in permanent loss of vestibular input from the affected side. These conditions represent a minority of patients with vestibular complaints (see Chapter 11 in this volume).

Observation, reassurance, and counseling that the condition is not life threatening may be appropriate and helpful in many cases but do not address the needs of symptomatic patients seeking some relief from their symptoms. Physicians tend to focus more on potential mortality as opposed to the patient's quality of life (Sloane et al, 1994). Many patients cannot or do not wish to "learn to live with it," and most patients seen by a primary care physician with complaints of dizziness report experiencing these symptoms for more than 3 months (Kroenke et al, 1992). Quality of life rating is significantly lower for elderly people complaining of dizziness than their counterparts without dizziness (Clark et al; 1993, Grimby & Rosenhall, 1995). Vestibular loss often leads to restriction and disability, and patients with chronic balance disorders often persist in seeking diagnosis and treatment. It is not uncommon for a patient with a chronic balance problem to see several different specialists with little or no coordination between specialists, often resulting in duplication of tests (Internet survey, *Coping with Dizziness*).

Vestibular rehabilitation offers an alternative form of treatment to many patients previously falling into one of the three aforementioned categories. Treatment of vestibular disorders through exercise and repositioning techniques has gained popularity within the last decade, and recent literature supports the efficacy of these approaches. The concept of an exercise or rehabilitation approach to dizziness and balance disorders is not new. British otolaryngologist Terrance Cawthorne is the earliest documented proponent of an exercise approach in treating patients with vestibular symptoms. Cawthorne (1945a,b) published articles describing the complexity of the balance system and the relationship between the vestibular system and visual and somatosensory inputs. In his early writings Cawthorne discussed the benefits of activity and exercise in recovery from "vestibular injuries." He noted that after unilateral labyrinthectomy, active patients seemed to recover faster and more completely than more sedate patients.

Cawthorne, along with physiologist, Dr. F.S. Cooksey, developed a series of exercises, currently known as "Cawthorne-Cooksey Exercises," thought to promote central compensation and habituation through repetition of symptom-provoking maneuvers. These exercises laid the basic framework of current vestibular rehabilitation programs. Concepts such as critical periods of compensation after injury, the need to provide the patient with progressively more difficult exercises, and the need to reduce functional disability are all addressed (Cooksey, 1945).

Very little progress occurred in the acceptance of exercise as a treatment option over the 25 years after Cawthorne (1945a,b) and Cooksey's (1945) original articles. During the 1970s and early 1980s, a flurry of activity produced several articles expanding on the theories of the vestibular compensation process and reintroducing the concept of vestibular exercises (Hood, 1970; Pfaltz, 1983; Pfaltz & Kamath, 1971).

McCabe, in 1970, expanded on Cawthorne's ideas and described "labryinthine exercises" as "our most useful single tool in the alleviation of protracted recurrent vertigo." He advocated the importance of patient education and the need for proper stimulus to allow the brain to "get over" vestibular losses. McCabe described the two peripheral vestibular apparatus as "partners" and his explanation regarding vestibular exercises is worth repeating.

1. Exclude, through careful investigation, progressive neurological, otological, or other disease.
2. Explain to the patient the nature of his disorder. He has a disease of the balance center, and:
   a. The two balance centers are partners, and they work not against but with each other.
   b. In his disorder, one partner cannot carry his share of the load.
   c. At certain times a comparison of partners occurs, and one is found wanting—then trouble (vertigo) ensues.
   d. The longer the two partners ignore each other, the more major the trouble is going to be when they meet.
   e. The closer and more often the two partners confront each other with the problem they mutually want to solve (dysequilibrium), the more quickly it will be solved.
   f. When the partners reach an agreement which is mutual, balance results.

3. Give to the patient on the basis of the above rationale a series of instructions, which he can carry out pertinent to the nature, and severity of his symptoms and his disease.
4. You do not have a life-threatening process. Your symptoms are only as important to the degree to which they annoy you. You will in time master them: when you do, they will be gone."

McCabe goes on to note that medications strong enough to suppress symptoms might also "prevent or delay the reparative process."

Hecker et al (1974) reported the results of Cawthorne-Cooksey exercises on a group of patients they believed to be "vestibular types." However, they included patients believed to have vertigo from vascular insufficiency and those with "Hallpike-type vertigo." They found that 84% of these patients treated with such exercises reported improvement. In this study the authors believed that the failures were due to lack of patient compliance and emotional distress.

Norre and DeWeert (1980) also proposed a therapy program for patients with peripheral vestibular disorders on the basis of the concept of habituation. They selected only patients with what they described as "provoked" vertigo or vertigo elicited only by movement. These patients were instructed to repetitively perform maneuvers that elicited vertigo. It is noted that more than 50% of patients in this study were believed to have paroxysmal positional vertigo (described later in this chapter). Ninety-one percent of their cases reported "some improvement," whereas 64% reported more than a 75% reduction in symptoms. A small control group demonstrated lack of improvement from "sham" exercises, but after changing their program to include habituation or provoking movement, improvement was noted. Failure to correctly perform the prescribed exercises was considered a major factor in patients showing little improvement. They found no significant effect related to delaying initiation of therapy after onset of symptoms.

Margaret Dix (1984) promoted the concept of vestibular rehabilitation in the United Kingdom with numerous publications during the 1980s. She emphasized encouragement, motivation, and patient education as critical factors for success. She based her therapy program on the original Cawthorne-Cooksey exercises, but adds, "The rationale, then, of head exercises in vestibular disorders is to provoke deliberately and systematically as many spells of vertigo as can be tolerated."

A common bond between most of the published reports of this era is the emphasis on intentionally provoking symptoms by creating an error signal or sensory conflict (Pfaltz, 1983). In theory, cerebellar or "adaptive" plasticity works to integrate what is initially perceived as abnormal and through repetition and motor learning (habituation) interprets the vestibular signals as normal. Adaptive plasticity refers to the brain's ability to modify the amount (or gain) of the vestibular ocular reflex to minimize visual-vestibular conflict. Sensory conflicts occur when disagreement exists between incoming (afferent) information regarding movement, balance, and orientation. This can occur when an asymmetrical response occurs between the two labyrinths in response to head movement or when a disagreement (or conflict) exists between vestibular, visual, or proprioceptive input. An example of sensory conflict would be the frequently described sensation of movement or disorientation that occurs while sitting in a car next to a large truck or bus. The size of the truck or

bus allows for full-field stimulation. When the truck or bus moves forward, a brief illusory sensation that one is moving backwards occurs. Those with a healthy vestibular system quickly prioritize the incoming information and rely on the vestibular response, indicating lack of movement. Patients with vestibular weakness may not react quickly or appropriately and lose balance or orientation.

PHYSIOLOGICAL BASIS FOR RECOVERY

Static Symptoms

The tonic or resting state of the paired vestibular labyrinths is a delicate balance that can be disrupted by a sudden injury to one or both labyrinths. Conditions responsible for unilateral vestibular injury include vestibular neuronitis, labyrinthitis, or surgical procedures such as eighth nerve section or labyrinthectomy. After a sudden loss or reduction in the function of one labyrinth, a predictable set of clinical signs and symptoms occurs. These "static" symptoms include spontaneous nystagmus after Alexander's law, a subjective sensation of vertigo, postural instability, ataxia, and ocular tilt reaction. (Curthoys & Halmagyi, 1996; Halmagyi et al, 1979; Leigh & Zee, 1991; Robinson et al, 1984). These symptoms result from a sudden profound asymmetry in resting activity between the two vestibular nuclei. Whenever an imbalance exists in the output of the vestibular nuclei, a sense of rotation toward the vestibular nuclei with the higher resting potential is perceived. Alexander's law refers to the pattern of nystagmus typically seen during the acute phase of peripheral vestibular asymmetry. The intensity of nystagmus increases when gaze is directed toward the fast phase of nystagmus (away from the lesioned side) and decreases when gaze is directed toward the slow phase (toward the lesioned side). Ocular tilt reaction indicates tonic imbalance of the activity of the VOR* and consists of skew deviation (vertical misalignment) and ocular counterrolling (fixed torsion) of the eyes and head tilt toward the lower eye. The reader is referred to Leigh and Zee (1991) for a complete review.

Over a period of hours to days, these symptoms diminish considerably through the process of vestibular adaptation. Because evidence suggests that labyrinthine receptors and peripheral neurons do not regenerate, the process of adaptation is thought to be a result of plasticity within the CNS. The exact mechanism is not understood, but most researchers believe that the process of vestibular adaptation is a function of alterations in activity of the vestibular nuclei. Smith and Curthoys (1989) and Curthoys and Halmagyi (1996) offer thorough reviews of studies pertaining to "tonic rebalancing" after unilateral labyrinthine loss.

It is estimated that human peripheral vestibular afferent fibers have resting potentials of up to 100 spikes per second. Considering that approximately 18,000 vestibular afferents are in each labyrinth, the resting activity being received by each vestibular nucleus may be more than 1 million spikes per second (Curthoys & Halmagyi, 1996). Any head movement results in a change in this resting potential, and the vestibular nuclei receive asymmetrical inputs from the two

---

*The VOR may be defined as reflexive eye movement in response to head movement.

vestibular labyrinths. Earlier reports of vestibular physiology described a simple "push-pull" arrangement, in which a head movement would cause an excitatory response in one vestibular nucleus and a corresponding, but not necessarily equal, inhibitory response in the contralateral vestibular nucleus. It is now believed that for each head movement, both inhibitory and excitatory responses occur in both vestibular nuclei and that the inhibitory responses are the result of inhibitory commissural connections from the contralateral vestibular nucleus (Curthoys & Halmagyi, 1996). It is these commissural connections that help explain the process of tonic rebalancing.

After the sudden loss of or reduction in function of one labyrinth, an immediate dramatic *decrease* occurs in the resting activity of the ipsilateral vestibular nucleus. An immediate *increase* in resting activity also occurs in the contralateral vestibular nucleus, which is likely the result of the loss of inhibitory commissural connections normally received from the lesioned side (Smith & Curthoys, 1989; Igarashi, 1984). Simply stated, the two vestibular nuclei are interactive and depend on each other to maintain equal resting outputs. Each exerts some inhibitory influence on the other. When the function of one is lost, the other temporarily responds with an increase in activity over and above its normal resting level of activity. This creates a sudden profound asymmetry in the two vestibular nuclei and leads to the above-mentioned signs and symptoms of sudden unilateral vestibular deafferentation (UVD).

The CNS responds by reducing the resting level of the intact side (a process known as "cerebellar clamp") and gradually restores activity in the vestibular nucleus on the lesioned side. This process leads to tonic rebalancing and a reduction in static symptoms. Restoration of activity in the vestibular nucleus on the lesioned side should not be confused with restoration of response from the lesioned peripheral labyrinth. This process of tonic rebalancing and the time course for reduction of static symptoms such as spontaneous nystagmus and ocular tilt do not appear to depend on visual or physical exercise stimulation (Zee, 1994).

The rebalancing of neural activity between the two vestibular nuclei becomes evident when a subject with previous unilateral vestibular loss, after a period of adaptation, has a loss in the contralateral labyrinth. Because the symptoms of sudden unilateral vestibular loss as described previously are believed to be a result of sudden asymmetry in the resting potentials of the vestibular nuclei, common sense would dictate that a loss of function in the remaining labyrinth would result in the absence of, but symmetrical output from, the two vestibular labyrinths. However, in such a case the subject responds behaviorally as if the loss of the remaining labyrinth results in a sudden asymmetry, with the well-known pattern of static symptoms of acute unilateral loss (Precht et al, 1966). This *Bechterews phenomonon* provides evidence of restoration of activity in the vestibular nucleus on the lesioned side. The role of the commisural connections has been described by Beinhold and Flor (1978). To determine the role of these connections in vestibular compensation, they surgically destroyed commisural connections in the frog at various stages of compensation after unilateral labyrinthectomy. They noted (1) an immediate return of symptoms of unilateral labyrinthectomy, (2) that the level of symptoms was independent of the time allowed and level of compensation, and (3) that no

recompensation could be observed. This indicates that without these commisural connections allowing for information from the contralateral labyrinth to be received by the lesioned side vestibular nucleus, vestibular adaptation could not take place. The restoration of activity in the vestibular nucleus of the lesioned side may play an important role in the recovery from static symptoms but does not appear to contribute significantly to the reduction of dynamic symptoms (Smith & Curthoys, 1989).

CONTROVERSIAL POINT

Fetter and Zee (1988) report the findings of a contradictory study in which they suggest that changes in commissural gain play little or no role "in the restoration of static vestibular balance" in the rhesus monkey.

Dynamic Symptoms

Dynamic symptoms would include those symptoms that occur as a result of head movement resulting from dysfunction of the VOR. The role of the VOR is to allow for stable gaze or focus while the head is moving. The VOR performs this function by causing eye movements that are equal and opposite of head movements, in effect visually canceling out head movement (see Fig. 21–1). Although the static symptoms of acute unilateral vestibular loss are quite predictable and easily identified, dynamic symptoms of VOR dysfunction are more subtle, and recovery of VOR function is more dependent on external influences.

Symptoms of VOR dysfunction typically do not include complaints of vertigo but rather visual blurring with head movement (oscillopsia) and visual-provoked and motion-provoked dysequilibrium. Brandt (1991) defines oscillopsia as "apparent movement of the visual scene due to involuntary retinal slip in acquired ocular oscillations or deficient VOR." In this context, "acquired ocular oscillations" would be nystagmus, which should be evident to the examiner. Nystagmus is involuntary eye movement associated with tonic imbalance within the peripheral or central vestibular system. When nystagmus is present, this eye movement may prohibit accurate visual fixation or visual following, leading to oscillopsia without head movement. Patients without nystagmus but with a "deficient VOR" will typically experience oscillopsia only when they are moving. Some patients with confirmed (by calorics) bilateral vestibular loss experience no more than mild dysequilibrium, whereas others complain of blurred vision and "bouncing" of their visual world with any head movement. J.C., a physician treated with vestibulotoxic aminoglycosides, reports (1952) that to read he had to hold his head steady by bracing it through the rails of his bed. Otherwise, his heartbeat and pulse caused too much head movement to allow for gaze stability. Patients with oscillopsia tend to be asymptomatic when they are not moving. To varying degrees, head movement causes a decrease in visual acuity, which can be easily documented with a standard Snellen eye chart (Longridge & Mallinson, 1984).

The basis for these complaints is termed "retinal slip" or the inability to maintain focused, centered vision (foveal

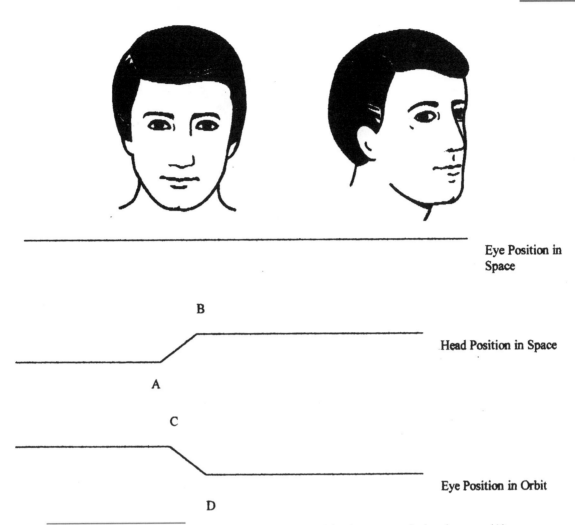

Figure 21–1 The role of the VOR is to maintain eye position in space as the head moves. **(A)** represents onset of head movement, whereas **(C)** represents onset of reflexive eye movement in the orbit (typically less than 16 ms after **A**). This minimal duration of retinal slip accounts for maintenance of gaze stability with head movement. **(B)** and **(D)** represent a 30-degree excursion of head movement and eye movement in opposite directions, demonstrating a gain of one, and in effect visually canceling out the effect of head movement. (Adapted from Leigh and Zee [1991], with permission.)

vision) with head movements. Retinal slip occurs when the VOR cannot adequately compensate for head movement and images do not remain stable on the retina. Visual acuity is best when an image is centered and stable on the retina. A gradual decline in visual acuity is noted as visual images move across the retina at increasing speeds. No significant decrease is noted when images move across the retina at speeds of 2 to 3 degrees per second, but at 4 to 5 degrees per second and above gaze stability and visual acuity are compromised (Demer et al, 1994; Leigh & Zee, 1991). Gaze stability may be defined as the ability to maintain foveal vision during head movements.

It is estimated that the range of head speeds encountered in real life is from 0.5 to 5 Hz, and the VOR normally responds efficiently up to head speeds of 8 Hz (Gresty et al, 1977; Sawyer et al, 1994). A variety of voluntary cerebellar-generated eye movements may allow for gaze stability at speeds less than 1 Hz, but only the VOR can allow for gaze stability and clear vision to head movements greater than

2 Hz. It is impossible to voluntarily move the eyes at speeds needed to maintain visual acuity during typical head movements. The latency of response for the VOR is less than 16 ms, whereas the latency for a voluntary eye movement is approximately 76 ms for a predictable target, and 150 to 250 ms for an unpredictable target (Hain, 1993; Leigh & Zee, 1991).

When retinal slip occurs and visual acuity is compromised, a sensory conflict between perceived visual, vestibular, and somatosensory information can occur. Patients with vestibular deficits tend to become more reliant on accurate visual and somatosensory feedback for maintenance of equilibrium, orientation, and balance. In the early stages after vestibular injury, a noted greater reliance on visual information is noted (Keshner, 1994). Gaze instability leads to inaccurate visual feedback, affecting appropriate sensory integration of the incoming information.

Recovery of the VOR is believed to occur primarily as a result of CNS and cerebellar plasticity and is possibly part of the process of cerebellar clamp. The retinal slip caused by

VOR dysfunction leads to an "error signal" in that images would be blurred during locomotion. CNS plasticity uses this error signal and gradually recalibrates the output (or gain*) of the VOR in an effort to enhance stable and clear vision. Several investigators have demonstrated that VOR gain and direction can be modified by subjecting patients with normal vestibular function to error signals (Demer et al, 1989; Gonshor & Melvill-Jones, 1976; Khater et al, 1990). It is believed that the error signal induced by VOR dysfunction triggers an adaptive response from the CNS. Several investigators report that visual and somatosensory deprivation delays or may ultimately limit vestibular compensation, although these effects appear to be species dependent and have yet to be satisfactorily determined in humans (Courjon et al, 1977; Lacour et al, 1976; Smith et al, 1986).

Some authors have described the short latency neuronal connections between the peripheral vestibular sensory receptors and the extraocular muscles that control eye movements as a simple three-neuron arc (Shepard & Telian, 1996). Discussions of this short latency network responsible for the VOR do not explain its adaptive capabilities when faced with an error signal.

Lisberger (1988) reports that the primitive nature of the three-neuron arc appears to allow for such short latencies in eye movement response to head movement. Any adaptation or recalibration in response to reduced visual acuity appears to take place higher in the brain stem. In other words, one part of the neural network is responsible for short latencies, whereas another part is responsible for accurate eye movements. (See Chapter 4 in *Diagnosis* for a comprehensive overview of the vestibular system.)

As noted earlier, a gradual reduction in resting activity in the vestibular nuclei occurs on both sides after unilateral vestibular deafferentation. Regarding dynamic symptoms, a noted reduction in gain of the VOR also occurs in both directions immediately after unilateral labyrinthectomy. Over a period of days to weeks, a gradual increase in the gain of the VOR in response to head movements toward the *lesioned* side occurs. The gain of the VOR for head movements toward the *intact* labyrinth remains reduced compared with its preoperative level. This increase of gain on the lesioned side and reduction in gain on the intact side results in a reduction in asymmetrical response to horizontal head movements (Smith & Curthoys, 1989).

Restoration of VOR function plays a large role in the recovery of dynamic visual acuity after unilateral vestibular injury. For slow-to-moderate head movements, the intact labyrinth can provide sufficient stimulation to both vestibular nuclei to allow for adequate VOR response (therefore clear vision). The inhibitory response from the intact labyrinth provides the necessary stimulus for these slow-to-moderate head movements. Because of the nonlinearity of the excitatory versus inhibitory responses of the sensory receptors (cristae) on the intact side, the faster the head movement, the less useful the inhibitory information from the intact side becomes when the head moves away from the intact side. There does

---

*Gain may be defined as the ratio of eye movement amplitude to head amplitude. A 10-degree head movement should result in a 10-degree eye movement in the opposite direction, for a perfect gain of 1.

not appear to be a measurable limit to the range of excitatory response, and the VOR responds normally to head movements toward the intact side up to 8 Hz. The inhibitory response saturates at zero spikes per second at moderate speed head movements, which prohibits the intact labyrinth from accurately responding to faster head movements away from the intact side. This deficit appears to be permanent and results in retinal slip with faster head movements toward the lesioned side (Curthoys & Halmagyi, 1996).

CONTROVERSIES IN VESTIBULAR REHABILITATION

The science of vestibular testing and treatment is still in a relative infancy stage. Many areas of disagreement and controversy exist. At this time, no "gold standard" test provides a conclusive diagnosis in many vestibular patients. As a result, sensitivity and specificity of various vestibular tests cannot be determined. Past studies on the effectiveness of various treatment techniques often combined patients with stable vestibular insufficiency with patients experiencing only provoked vertigo (see section on BPPV). Despite evidence suggesting that vestibular rehabilitation is effective and medication is not effective for most patients with dizziness, most patients with dizziness are still treated with medication. The following section reviews literature pertaining to some of these areas of controversy.

Critical Periods of Compensation

The existence of critical periods of compensation for vestibular compensation is unresolved. Animal studies have been focused on the effects of physical activity and visual stimulation on the rate and extent of recovery after vestibular deafferentation. Lacour et al (1976) performed unilateral vestibular neurectomy on a population of baboons. The legs of one group were restrained by a plaster cast for 4 days, whereas a second group was allowed freedom of movement. Rate of recovery measured by locomotor ataxia (difficulty walking) was significantly delayed in the restrained group. Mathog and Peppard (1982) reported a 58% to 70% faster rate of recovery after unilateral labyrinthectomy in cats forced into exercise than cats without exercise. Exercise in this study essentially involved allowing the cats freedom to walk about the laboratory as opposed to being restricted to their cage. Squirrel monkeys forced into activity by means of a motor-driven rotating cage recovered from unilateral labyrinthectomy significantly faster than monkeys left to recover naturally (Igarashi et al, 1981).

Cats kept in the dark after unilateral labyrinthectomy showed reduced gain of the VOR and persistence of spontaneous nystagmus (representing a tonic imbalance in the vestibular system) compared with a control group exposed to light. Gain increased and spontaneous nystagmus quickly diminished when the same cats were allowed exposure to light (Courjon et al, 1977). Although this effectively demonstrates the role of vision in vestibular adaptation, it does not support the concept of critical periods of compensation. A similar study performed on guinea pigs showed that total visual deprivation had no effect on spontaneous nystagmus after labyrinthectomy (Smith et al, 1986). This indicates the possibility of species-specific patterns of compensation and casts some caution toward the use of animal studies to predict the mechanisms of vestibular adaptation in humans. Human studies have been contradictory on the subject. Several investigators found that the final outcomes were similar when delaying therapy to a specific group of patients (Norre & DeWeert, 1980; Szturm et al, 1994).

Rehabilitation versus Repositioning

Brandt and Daroff (1980), on the basis of the principles of habituation, promoted the use of provocative movements for the treatment of BPPV. Although reporting dramatic benefits from the prescribed exercise, they believed that the rate of recovery was too fast to be the result of centrally mediated habituation or "CNS compensation." They speculated that the exercises "provided a mechanical means to promote loosening and ultimate dispersion of the otolithic debris from the cupula." The movements recommended are strikingly similar to those recommended by Semont et al (1988) as they describe their technique for the liberatory maneuver. Norre et al (1987) and Norre and Beckers (1987) compared the relative effectiveness of medications, vestibular habituation therapy (VHT), and what they described as the "brisk method" in treating patients with diagnosed BPPV. The brisk method is similar to the Semont maneuver and the authors refer to the work of Toupet and Semont (1985) in describing the maneuver. They found VHT to be significantly more effective than vestibular suppressant medication in reducing the complaints and nystagmus response of BPPV. In addition, they found the "brisk method" to result in a reduction of positional vertigo in 52% of patients, whereas 32% of VHT patients had similar improvement at 1 week after treatment. This study demonstrates that patients with BPPV benefit from single treatment procedures more quickly than from traditional habituation therapy. Improvement was based on both the patient's subjective sensation of vertigo and the presence of nystagmus typically associated with BPPV. Single treatment approaches to BPPV will be discussed later in this chapter.

In contrast to some earlier research, which include patients with BPPV in studies thought to be measuring adaptation and habituation, most of the more recent research has excluded these patients, limiting subjects to patients believed to have chronic peripheral vestibulopathy (stable and permanent vestibular dysfunction).

Vestibular Rehabilitation versus Medication

Three recent studies demonstrate the efficacy of exercises versus medication in improving postural control in patients with vestibular deficiency. Horak et al (1992) compared "relative effectiveness of vestibular rehabilitation, general conditioning exercises, and vestibular suppressant medication" on subjective dizziness and postural control. Postural control was measured by sensory organization testing (SOT) (see Chapter 24 in *Diagnosis* for a review of SOT) and timed one-leg standing, eyes open, and eyes closed. Vestibular rehabilitation consisted of intensive (twice per week) sessions with a physical therapist, performing exercises customized to the patient's specific complaints. General conditioning consisted of similar intensive therapy sessions with strength, range of motion, and cardiac fitness as the therapy goals. These exercises were nonspecific to the patient's complaints. The medication group was treated with diazepam (Valium) or meclizine, both centrally sedating medications. Over a 6-week treatment period, all groups reported a reduction in symptoms, but only the vestibular rehabilitation group showed significant objective improvement in scores obtained from SOT and standing balance tests.

Fujino et al (1996) reported differences in subjective improvement in clinical signs and symptoms in two groups. One group was treated with medication only (histamine—believed to stimulate circulation in the inner ear), with instructions to "take a rest" during the study period. The medication, betahistine, had previously been shown to reduce severity of dizziness in patients with peripheral vestibular-induced vertigo. A second group was treated with the same medication but concurrently treated with a modified version of Cawthorne-Cooksey exercises. Over an 8-week period Fujino et al (1996) noted significantly greater improvement in the exercise group.

The use of centrally sedating medication may, in fact, impede the benefits of vestibular rehabilitation therapy. Shepard et al (1990) reported that patients taking vestibular suppressants, antidepressants, tranquilizers, and anticonvulsants ultimately achieve the same level of compensation as patients not taking similar medications, but the length of therapy is significantly longer.

Generic versus Customized Exercise

Cawthorne-Cooksey exercises had been used as the standard treatment for vestibular patients and had been used in most studies designed to demonstrate the efficacy of an exercise approach to treating these patients. Recently, investigators have examined the relative benefits of a more customized approach, designing specific exercises for each patient on the basis of complaints and diagnosis.

Szturm at al (1994) reported findings of a study comparing two groups. One group was treated with an intensive customized exercise program designed to produce retinal slip and increase postural control. The second group received Cawthorne-Cooksey exercises on a home program basis. Performance was measured before and after therapy by SOT and rotary chair testing. The customized group showed a significant improvement in standing balance performance and in reducing VOR asymmetry. The home-based program group showed no significant improvement in either test. Patients originally placed in the home-based group, eventually provided with the customized exercises, ultimately displayed improvement similar to that of the original custom exercise group. This study demonstrates the efficacy of intensive customized treatment using objective measures and demonstrates the benefit of customized versus generic vestibular exercises.

Shepard and Telian (1995) performed a similar study and found that 84% of chronic vestibular patients treated with an exercise program customized to the patients needs reported complete or dramatic improvement, whereas 64% of patients treated with generic exercise reported similar improvement. Objectively, the customized exercise group demonstrated significantly improved performance on a number of balance function measures, whereas the generic group only showed significant improvement in standing balance tests.

ADAPTIVE STRATEGIES

Patients with loss of vestibular function, either unilateral or bilateral, adopt a number of strategies to increase gaze stability with head movement. In addition to the described recovery of the VOR through plasticity of the CNS, some behavioral changes and substitutions of vestibular responses take place.

Cervical-Ocular Reflex Input

The input of the cervical-ocular reflex (COR) has been recognized since Robert Barany's work in the early 1900s. The COR is thought to be a compensatory reflexive eye movement in response to stimulation from the ligaments, muscles, and joints in the neck. The COR's input for gaze stabilization in patients with normal vestibular function is insignificant (Barlow & Freedman, 1980; Bronstein & Hood, 1986; Sawyer et al, 1994). This is probably also true of patients with unilateral vestibular loss. In patients with bilateral loss of labyrinthine function the COR has been shown to provide a small contribution to eye-head coordination at very low speeds of head movement.

Bronstein and Hood (1986) reported that, "in the absence of vestibular function, the COR appears to take on the role of the vestibulo-ocular reflex in head-eye coordination in a) the initiation of the anti-compensatory saccade which takes the eyes in the direction of the target, and b) the generation of the subsequent slow compensatory eye movements." Kasai and Zee (1978) concluded that central preprogramming played a large role in COR functioning. The COR operates only at very low frequencies in normal subjects (maximum gain at 0.025 Hz, negligible at 0.4 Hz); however, significant contribution from the COR is noted in patients with vestibular loss up to 0.5 Hz (Barlow & Freedman, 1980; Kasai & Zee, 1978). The COR may also contribute to postural stability in normal patients as "injections of local anesthetics into the neck in humans produces temporary dysequilibrium and ataxia" (de Jonge et al, 1977).

Modification of Saccades

Saccades are the fastest eye movements and may be voluntary or involuntary (as in the fast phase of nystagmus). Saccades allow us to refixate our gaze with minimal duration of retinal slip. The speed of initiation of a saccade is 150 to 250 ms when the target is unpredictable and approximately 76 ms with a predictable target (Leigh & Zee, 1991). Research indicates that saccades are amenable to increased efficiency through practice. Fischer and Ramsperger (1986) report that daily practice results in a small but significant reduction in response latency and an increase in accuracy. Because response latency is significantly decreased when the target is predictable, it is likely that some *central preprogramming* of eye movements occurs when a patient with vestibular loss moves his head. These patients may make a voluntary saccade contralateral to the direction of head movement to compensate for the inefficient VOR response (Kasai & Zee, 1978). Through repetitive conditioning and feedback, patients tend to predict the necessary

saccade in response to head movement. Modification of saccades is noted in both unilateral and bilateral patients.

Modification of Smooth Pursuit

Smooth pursuit tracking, or visual following, allows for gaze stability on objects moving through the field of vision. This type of eye movement is generated in the cerebellum and can either function alone while the head is still or can interact with the VOR to assist in gaze stability while moving. Smooth pursuit tracking ability does not appear to improve in well-compensated individuals with adult-onset vestibular loss. Smooth pursuit abilities tend to break down around 1 Hz in both normal individuals and labyrinthine-deficient patients (Gresty et al, 1977; Leigh at al, 1987). The increased plasticity of the CNS in children may be evident in two reports: Chambers et al (1985) report that subjects with onset of bilateral vestibular loss before adulthood did not complain of oscillopsia, whereas those with adult-onset loss did complain. Gresty et al (1977) report on a patient with bilateral labyrinthine dysfunction since childhood, demonstrating accurate smooth pursuit after up to 3 Hz.

Substitution of Sensory Inputs and Decreased Head Movements

After the loss of vestibular function bilaterally, a "reweighting" of priority and dependency on visual and somatosensory inputs occurs for the maintenance of balance and postural control (Herdman, 1994). Initially, a shift toward visual dependency occurs. While walking, patients may visually lock on to targets and use this to provide information regarding relative motion. Gradually, these patients learn to more equally distribute their dependency on proprioceptive and visual information.

A deficient VOR is not an issue when the head is not moving; therefore some patients develop a strategy of avoiding any rapid head movements to avoid the symptoms of retinal slip. This strategy does not allow for the natural compensation process to take place and does not alter the fact that when the head is inevitably moved quickly, symptoms will ensue.

PLANNING, GOAL WRITING, AND DOCUMENTATION

In establishing reasonable goals and planning a therapy program suitable for a patient, the therapist must take into consideration a number of variables that include the following:

1. The patient's specific complaints and concerns regarding lifestyle limitations
2. Any permanent impairments not amenable to therapy
3. A realistic expected level of improvement
4. The therapist's concern regarding patient safety and the risk of falling

Following formal vestibular, audiological, otological, and/or neurological evaluation, an initial pretherapy assessment will help the therapist design a specific treatment plan and will provide data for comparative outcome measures during and after therapy. The pretherapy assessment usually consists of a combination of objective and subjective tests. Objective tests may include the following:

1. *SOT:* Numeric sway data may be obtained by a variety of methods and techniques, including computerized platform posturography.
2. Timed one-leg standing.
3. Dynamic visual acuity can be measured with a standard Snellen chart, comparing visual acuity with and without head movement.

Subjective rating scales frequently used include the following:

1. *Dizziness handicap inventory* (DHI): The DHI consists of 25 questions designed to elicit the patient's response to the "functional, emotional and physical impact of balance system disease" (Jacobson & Newman, 1990).
2. *Motion sensitivity quotient* (MSQ): The MSQ includes a subjective rating of severity of symptoms related to 16 different preselected positions (Shepard & Telian, 1996).

In addition, the therapist may perform rating scales of the patient's performance during various activities.

The data obtained in the pretherapy assessment is crucial in obtaining *outcome measures*. These objective and subjective measures can be obtained during and after the course of therapy and comparisons made. Cowand et al (1998) recently reported that VR provided significant improvement in the functional and physical subtests of the DHI but did not significantly alter the emotional subtest scores.

PEARL

Videotaping all therapy sessions not only provides documentation of therapy activities but can also dramatically demonstrate improvement (if any) when, at the end of the therapy program, the therapist allows the patient to comparatively view his or her performance on specific tasks before and after therapy.

The format for constructing an individual therapy session will seem familiar to many audiologists trained in the basics of speech and language pathological conditions. The plan for each session should include (1) objectives, (2) methods and materials, (3) results, and (4) plans for the next session (Table 21–1).

1. *Objectives* include a description of the activity the patient will perform, including conditions, criteria for acceptable performance, and goal and functional outcome to be achieved.
2. *Methods and materials* include the name of the exercise(s) to be performed, including specific conditions under which the patient is to perform (i.e., speed, time, position, range of movement). Also included would be any materials needed (i.e., physioball, mirror, targets, foam pad).
3. *Results* include documentation of patient's performance, including any dizziness, nausea, or inability to perform the task to completion. This can also include a statement regarding the patient's perception of performance using a numeric rating scale.
4. *Plans for the next session* include any progression or modification of the exercises to challenge or help the patient's performance. Exercises may be discontinued, added to the patient's home program, or modified for the next session.

Each therapy session should be planned on the basis of the results of the patient's vestibular evaluation, pretherapy assessment, and/or performance in the previous therapy session. Each therapy session should begin with a review of the patient's status as of the previous session and any perceived progress since that time. The therapist must be prepared to make modifications to the plan when indicated. If exercises are provoking symptoms to the point of frustration or nausea, the difficulty level may need to be reduced. If the patient can complete the exercises with no symptoms, the therapist must move on to another exercise or add another component to the exercise (i.e., standing with eyes closed can be changed to standing with eyes closed on a compliant surface).

Therapy can, and in most cases should, be performed in the home between scheduled sessions with the therapist. Frequent exercise sessions are necessary to promote learning and carryover.

SPECIAL CONSIDERATION

It is my experience that frequent phone and personal contact between patient and therapist increases compliance in vestibular therapy.

The therapist must base his or her recommendation of home-based exercises on the patient's risk of falling. In many

---

TABLE 21–1 Example of a "lesson plan" for a vestibular therapy session. The numbers noted in the *results* column indicate a numeric rating of the patients' perceived performance or level of subjective symptoms associated with this particular exercise.

Objectives	Methods	Results	Plan
While walking forward, the patient will turn his or her head from side to side and up and down to show VOR and gait stability for fall prevention.	Walking with head turns • Bring patient to hallway. • 5 minutes in each condition. 1. Side to side 2. Up and down 3. Alternating	1. [2] Minimal dizziness. 2. [2] Moderate dizziness. Good stability. 3. [4] Patient was very disoriented. Slow movement.	Patient will perform side to side and up and down only at home. Repeat alternating in next therapy session.

cases a family member can be trained to assist the patient while he or she exercises at home. Younger, healthier patients may not be at risk for falling and can complete most of the therapy program at home. It is my practice to have younger healthy patients attend one or two in-office sessions to learn proper technique for appropriate exercises then have them return at 1 or 2 weeks to perform a therapy session while being observed by the therapist. It is not uncommon for patients to modify their exercise (usually by slowing down required movement) to avoid symptoms. The therapist then makes suggestions and appropriate additions or deletions to the therapy program. To ensure that the patient has improved satisfactorily and to obtain outcome data, the patient is asked to attend one follow-up session several weeks later.

PITFALL

Many patients beginning therapy, as in any exercise program, feel worse before they begin to feel better. It is our practice to ask patients to commit to 4 weeks of therapy before judging its effectiveness.

TREATMENT STRATEGIES

The goals of vestibular rehabilitation (VR) are as follows:

1. To minimize symptoms and functional disability
2. To increase mobility and independence
3. To reduce the risk of falls and injury

Treatment strategies are determined by the results of the vestibular evaluation, patient symptoms and complaints, pretherapy assessment, and the general health and physical abilities of the patient. Patients may have specific functional limitations that they wish to focus on. The patient's general health and residual vestibular function may dictate reasonable therapy goals. In designing a program for VR, it is important to keep in mind that each patient will compensate in a different way. The exercises described in the following will assist the patient in developing compensatory strategies, but the specific compensatory technique each patient develops is unpredictable. Equipment needed to perform most of the exercises, along with suppliers, is listed in Appendix B.

General guidelines to optimize the benefits of VR are as follows:

1. Make every effort to have the patient decrease the use of centrally sedating or vestibular-suppressant medications.
2. Exercises must provoke symptoms and create an "error signal." Adopt a "no pain, no gain" approach, educating the patient that the VOR will only modify its gain and symmetry when the brain recognizes a conflict or error signal situation.
3. Extensive counseling before initiating therapy may enhance patient compliance. Patients who understand their condition and its limitations and understand how their symptoms are provoked may be less fearful and more willing to continue therapy.
4. Therapy should be initiated as soon as possible. It appears that delaying therapy may not negatively affect final

outcomes but appears to result in a longer period of therapy for similar results.
5. Therapy sessions should be performed frequently to foster carryover and motor learning.
6. Exercises should be varied in speed and direction and should simulate real-life conditions when possible.
7. Once therapy goals have been reached, a general conditioning program and maintenance exercises are necessary to prevent a return of symptoms.
8. Patients should be counseled that they may experience periods of decompensation and may require further intensive therapy.

Treatment of Unilateral Vestibular Loss

Therapy designed to treat the patient with one normal functioning labyrinth and a loss or reduction in function in the other labyrinth is frequently termed *adaptation therapy*. The goal of adaptation therapy is the following:

1. To promote tonic rebalancing of the vestibular nuclei
2. To decrease symptoms associated with head movements through habituation therapy
3. To increase gaze stability through modification and enhancement of oculomotor abilities
4. To increase postural stability through sensory integration training

Exercises to promote recovery from unilateral vestibular loss are listed in Table 21–2, and an alphabetical listing and description of each of these exercises can be found in Appendix A.

Treatment of Bilateral Vestibular Loss

Therapy designed for the patient with bilateral vestibular loss is based on the premise that no remaining peripheral vestibular response to head movement exists and therefore no VOR function exists. Appropriate therapy for the patient with absence of VOR function is termed *substitution therapy*.

The goal of substitution therapy is as follows:

1. To promote the use of alternative sensory inputs, such as visual and somatosensory information, when vestibular function is lost
2. To promote alternative gaze stabilization strategies through enhancing oculomotor abilities and potentiating the COR
3. To teach the patient to recognize situations where alternative sensory information is unavailable or unreliable
4. To provide information regarding fall hazards and techniques to minimize the risk of falling

Exercises to promote recovery from bilateral vestibular loss are listed in Table 21–3, and a description of these exercises can be found in Appendix A.

Another category of patients may not appear to fall into one of the two preceding groups. These patients will generally have normal vestibular evaluations if evaluated by the standard test protocol that does not address VOR deficits to head speeds above the range tested by ENG and rotational chair tests. Many of these patients have unilateral vestibular

TABLE 21–2   Exercises to promote recovery from unilateral vestibular loss

Saccades—To promote accuracy and decrease latency of saccadic eye movements

Tracking—To promote smooth pursuit tracking ability and increase dynamic visual acuity with moving objects

Head movements—To promote habituation and VOR stability

Head movements with targets—To promote visual suppression of the VOR through a combination of saccadic and smooth pursuit tracking

Focus head turns—To modify VOR gain and increase stability of the VOR

Focus head turns (two times)—To modify VOR gain and to promote VOR stability and interaction with the smooth pursuit system

Ankle sways—To promote appropriate use of ankle strategy for fall prevention, increase limits of stability, increase leg strength, and increase translational VOR stability and COG control

Circle sways—Same as ankle sways

Balance ball bounce—To promote vertical VOR stability and hip strategy

Balance board—To promote proper use of ankle and hip strategies for fall prevention, increase awareness of proprioceptive input, increase VOR stability and COG control

Ball circles—To promote VOR stability, postural stability, and habituation

Ball kick—To promote eye/foot coordination; COG training for fall prevention (weight shifting) and visual tracking ability

Ball toss—To promote eye/hand coordination, COG training, and visual tracking

Bend and reach—To promote VOR stability and habituation to vertical movements

Ball sitting—To promote vertical VOR stability and proper use of hip strategy

Crossover step—To promote gait control and one-legged balance for walking or climbing stairs

Face to knee—To promote habituation of movement and position-induced vertigo

Foam walk—To promote gait control on an uneven surface

Obstacle course—To promote gait stability in real-life situations

Roll against wall—To promote VOR stability and habituation

Sit to stand—To promote habituation of movement-related dizziness and increase VOR stability and leg strength

Standing—To promote static postural stability and COG control

Trampoline ankle sway—To promote use of ankle strategy on a compliant or uneven surface

Trampoline circle sway—Same as above

Trampoline walk—To promote gait stability on a compliant or uneven surface

Walk stop—To promote gait stability and standing balance when walking is interrupted

Walking with head turns—To promote habituation, VOR stability, sensory integration, and gait stability

Walking turns—To promote habituation, VOR stability, and gait stability

---

hypofunction and may only demonstrate abnormalities on high-frequency rotational testing (Leigh & Brandt, 1993; Leigh et al, 1992). These patients have been labeled "high frequency non-compensated vestibular loss" (Gans, 1996). They typically do not complain of dizziness, vertigo, or postural instability, but rather a sense of visual blurring or "after-motion" with rapid head movements, particularly toward the side of a mostly compensated lesion. These patients are believed to have achieved a large degree of central adaptation and compensation but have not developed optimal alternative gaze-stabilizing strategies. Exercises geared toward reducing symptoms in these patients are referred to as *gaze stabilization exercises* or eye-head coordination exercises. These exercises (see Table 21–4) are also useful for patients with confirmed unilateral or bilateral vestibular loss and patients with resolved BPPV complaining of residual dysequilibrium.

The exercises listed in Tables 21–2 through 21–4 and described in Appendix A are a combination of exercises used in the vestibular rehabilitation programs at the American Institute of Balance (St. Petersburg, FL), University of Michigan Vestibular Laboratory, Johns Hopkins University Hospital, and those modified and developed at the authors vestibular rehabilitation facility.

Limits of Vestibular Rehabilitation

In designing a vestibular therapy program the therapist must keep in mind that balance is a multisensory function, and impairments in any of the sensory systems involved in balance can limit the potential benefits of vestibular rehabilitation. As noted in the section on dynamic symptoms, a permanent impairment in the VOR response to rapid head movements in the direction of the damaged labyrinth exists. Fetter and Zee (1988) report that years after labyrinthectomy horizontal VOR gain to rapid impulsive head movement toward the lesioned side remains significantly less than normal. At head speeds greater than 2 Hz, no efficient strategies for correcting retinal slip exist, and in many well-compensated patients this accounts for their only lasting complaint.

Unstable lesions do not respond well to VR. Unstable lesions include conditions such as Meniere's disease and perilymph fistula. CNS adaptation depends on a stable asymmetry in the vestibular nuclei (Herdman, 1997). VR may be

TABLE 21–3   Exercises to promote recovery from bilateral vestibular loss

Walk stop—See Table 21–2
Ankle sways—See Table 21–2
Balance board—See Table 21–2
Balance beam—To promote increase in awareness of proprioceptive input and use of hip strategy
Ball circles—See Table 21–2
Ball toss and kick—See Table 21–2
Bend and reach—See Table 21–2
Crossover step—See Table 21–2
Foam walk—See Table 21–2
Focus head turns two times—See Table 21–2
Hand to hand ball toss—To promote smooth pursuit and interaction with the VOR
Imaginary targets—To potentiate the cervical-ocular reflex
Head movements—See Table 21–2
Moving saccades—To promote alternative gaze stability strategies
Standing—See Table 21–2
Obstacle course—See Table 21–2
One-leg stand—To promote postural stability through weight shifting
Roll against wall—See Table 21–2
Sit to stand—See Table 21–2
Stepping patterns—To promote eye/foot coordination and one-legged standing
Trace the alphabet—Same as above
Targets—See Table 21–2
Walking with head turns—See Table 21–2
Walking turns—See Table 21–2

TABLE 21–4   Exercises to promote gaze stability

Hand to hand ball toss—See Table 21–2
Saccades—See Table 21–2
Tracking—See Table 21-2
Head movements—See Table 21–2
Targets—See Table 21-2
Focus head turns—See Table 21-2
Head circles—See Table 21–2
Moving saccades—See Table 21-2
Imaginary targets—See Table 21-2
Ball circles—See Table 21–2
Ball toss and kick—See Table 21–2
Gait with head moves—To promote VOR and gait stability
Balance ball bounce—See Table 21–2
Crossover steps—See Table 21–2

helpful in patients with Meniere's disease if their episodes are infrequent (i.e., several weeks minimum between episodes), but intensive therapy would need to be reinstituted after each episode (Shepard & Telian, 1996). Ablative procedures are sometimes recommended to create a stable asymmetry. In these cases VR should be started as soon as possible after the procedure.

Cerebellar dysfunction as the result of stroke or degeneration inhibits VR. Tonic rebalancing and modifications to the gain of the VOR are believed to depend on plasticity within the cerebellum. If the cerebellum is dysfunctional, the adaptation process may be slower and limited. CNS abnormalities (i.e., cerebrovascular accident [CVA]) do not necessarily inhibit vestibular compensation if the lesion is not located within the vestibular pathways, although historically these patients require longer therapy programs. It is important to keep in mind that cerebellar dysfunction can be caused by vestibular or centrally sedating medications, because the goal of these medications is to reduce the asymmetry in activity by inhibiting the cerebellar response and activity within the vestibular nuclei. It is this same asymmetry that serves as a stimulus for adaptation and compensation.

Vestibular Therapy and "Central" Lesions

Patients with persistent complaints regarding postural stability of "central" origin have long been considered to have limited potential benefit from vestibular therapy and have been eliminated from most studies of vestibular rehabilitation. Because the actual process of adaptation is believed to take place in the cerebellum and brain stem, injuries to the central region might reasonably limit vestibular adaptation and ultimately impair overall compensation from vestibular injury.

Cass et al (1996) demonstrated significant improvement in postural stability after customized vestibular therapy in patients exhibiting a "vestibular loss" pattern on SOT. Patients exhibiting a "nonspecific" pattern on SOT, most of whom had previously been classified as having "central vestibular dysfunction," did not demonstrate significant improvement after similar vestibular therapy.

Conversely, Fiebert and Brown (1979) report that patients who have had recent CVA demonstrated greater ability to ambulate after a 2-week program of vestibular stimulation than did patients who had a CVA who did not receive this program. Shepard et al (1993) report on an observational study indicating that although patients with central or mixed central peripheral lesions require longer periods of vestibular therapy, their prognosis for improvement is good. Gill-Body at al (1997) report two case studies of the effects of vestibular rehabilitation on patients with confirmed cerebellar lesions. After a 6-week course of vestibular therapy, both patients exhibited increased performance in postural and gaze stability and in self-perception of balance.

Compromised visual or somatosensory inputs are not uncommon in the elderly population. The potential then for sensory substitution is limited if a patient has decreased vision or proprioception. Normal visual changes with aging include reduced night vision resulting from yellowing of the cornea and a slowing of pupillary reaction to lighting changes (Tideiksaar, 1989). Binocular vision plays a role in depth perception and visual feedback of relative motion. Patients with monocular or asymmetrical vision are not uncommon, particularly those in the process of having cataract surgery. Patients relying on visual feedback can be hampered by bifocal lenses. It is well known that magnifying lenses induce changes in VOR gain. Each time the patient changes their gaze through different lenses, they experience a change in magnification, which can lead to oscillopsia and visual disturbance (Demer et al, 1989). The constant alterations in spectacle magnification experienced with use of bifocals may inhibit appropriate changes in VOR gain.

To maximize recovery of the VOR, a visual stimulus for retinal slip is needed. If the patient is *visually impaired*, he or she may not be able to adequately see targets during therapy. Visual deprivation has been demonstrated to impede recovery of horizontal VOR function (Fetter & Zee, 1988). Admittedly, these patients most likely do not relate visual blurring only in response to head movements.

Patients with *peripheral sensory neuropathy* or decreased leg strength as a result of injury may have limited use of proprioceptive feedback. Muscle mass is reduced by as much as 50% in the elderly, and leg strength is necessary for efficient use of ankle strategy (Tideiksaar, 1989).

Patient compliance is the key to a successful VR program and is noted as a factor in many published studies (Hecker et al, 1974, Norre & DeWeert, 1980). Desmond and Touchette (1998) report that 35% of patients for whom VR was recommended elected not to participate in a therapy program. They report that most of these patients stated that they were "not interested" even though they apparently believed the need to undergo vestibular evaluation. The authors interpreted this as a lack of motivation or confidence that they could benefit from therapy. Physicians who do not understand, or accept, the concept of VR may reinforce this attitude. Sloane et al (1994) report that when dealing with a patient with the complaint of "dizziness," primary care physicians prescribed treatment as follows:

- 61%: Medication (most commonly meclizine) was prescribed
- 72%: Observed (with or without prescribing medication)
- 42%: Received reassurance

Primary care physicians appear to be focused on potential mortality as opposed to the patient's quality of life. Even though the study showed a higher reported suspicion of "inner ear disorder" than other suspected diagnoses such as brain tumor or transient ischemic attack, less than 1% of patients were referred for vestibular evaluation, whereas 13% were referred for imaging or vascular studies. A quote from that article may give insight as to primary care physician's approach to the patient with dizziness: "Physicians tend to treat conservatively the more classic symptoms of vertigo, which often have self-limited causes and to conduct more investigation when a neurologic or cardiologic diagnosis was suspected."

Fall Prevention

Even with VR, patients with vestibular loss are at higher risk for falling, particularly in situations in which visual and somatosensory information is absent or unreliable. Falls are one of the most serious problems associated with aging. The statistics are startling. It is estimated that one third to one half of all people older than 65 fall at least once (Coogler, 1992). In fact, falls are the leading cause of injury in older adults and account for more than 200,000 hip fractures annually in the United States alone (Haupt & Graves, 1982). Of these, 25% will never regain full mobility (Coogler, 1992). In essence, a fall leading to a hip fracture may forever change a patient's life.

From the perspective of the elderly patient, these statistics make it clear that fall prevention programs are important and worthwhile. Healthcare providers also need to recognize that fall prevention planning can significantly reduce health care costs. The cost of direct care alone for patients with hip fracture is in the billions of dollars annually (Allison, undated). In addition, many of these elderly fallers are admitted to chronic care institutions (Tinetti & Williams, 1997).

A number of contributing factors may put someone at a higher risk for falling. These are mostly associated with decreased efficiency of the visual, vestibular, and proprioceptive inputs, which are a common part of aging. A variety of medical conditions including peripheral neuropathy, postural hypotension, and transient ischemic attacks may contribute to an increased risk for falling. As mentioned earlier in the section on limits of vestibular rehabilitation, some patients with vestibular loss may be susceptible to falling under certain conditions. For these patients, education as to potential fall hazards and environmental modifications to minimize fall hazards is indicated. For a thorough review of fall prevention environmental assessments and appropriate modifications, the reader is referred to *Falling in Old Age: Its Prevention and Treatment* (Tideiksaar, 1989).

BENIGN PAROXYSMAL POSITIONAL VERTIGO

BPPV represents the single most likely diagnosis in a patient complaining of vertigo and accounts for up to 30% of patients with peripheral vestibular dysfunction (Epley, 1992a; Herdman, 1997). Diagnosis and treatment of BPPV does not require sophisticated or expensive equipment. The treatment of BPPV falls into the scope of VR as its most effective treatment involves "treatment and therapy" designed "to bring or restore to a normal or optimum state of health…"(*Webster's*, 1976). The theory behind treating BPPV is unlike that of other vestibular pathological conditions. Whereas most VR strategies use repetition, motor learning and CNS plasticity in hopes of relieving symptoms, treatment for BPPV typically includes none of these. In fact, recent evidence regarding the pathophysiology of BPPV and the success of single treatment procedures sheds some speculation on the conclusions of many previous VR studies using BPPV patients as subjects. Some researchers (Hecker et al, 1974; Norre & DeWeert, 1980) concluded that patients with positional vertigo improved as a result of habituation and adaptive plasticity. More recent findings regarding the natural remitting course of BPPV, and the speed at which recent repositioning techniques result in resolution of symptoms, would indicate that at least some of the patients noting improvement in these earlier studies did not improve for the reasons described by the authors.

Pathophysiology of Benign Paroxysmal Postional Vertigo

General agreement exists that the site of lesion in BPPV is the ampulla of the offending semicircular canal, with the posterior canal of one labyrinth involved in 90% of cases (Fife, 1995):
Typical diagnostic signs include the following.

1. A provoking position (lying supine with affected ear down)
2. A short latency before vertigo and nystagmus occur (usually 3 to 15 seconds)
3. Severe subjective vertigo accompanied by nystagmus (typically geotropic rotary nystagmus when the posterior canal is involved)
4. A short duration of symptoms (usually less than 1 minute)
5. Fatigability (repeated provocation results in a reduced response)
6. A reversal in the direction of nystagmus on rising (sometimes)

Many patients with BPPV will also complain of associated dysequilibrium and postural instability. Black and Nashner (1984) and Baloh et al (1987) report a significant correlation between BPPV and abnormal posturography scores. Some speculation exists that there may be abnormal responses from the affected semicircular canal or that the otolith structures (particularly the utricles) are no longer functioning symmetrically as a result of displaced otoconia. In addition, a high incidence (32% to 47%) of abnormal caloric responses occurs in patients with BPPV (Baloh et al, 1987; Norre et al, 1987).

Schuknecht (1969) first proposed the theory of *cupulolithiasis* in which he suggested that BPPV was the result of otoconial debris attached to the cupula of the offending posterior semicircular canal. Epley (1992a) offered an alternative theory of *canalithiasis* that more thoroughly explains the source of the above-mentioned typical signs and symptoms of BPPV. The theory of canalithiasis proposes that there are free-floating particles (otoconia) that have gravitated from the utricle and collect near the cupula of the posterior canal. When the head is moved into a position that causes the particles to move away from the cupula, the resulting hydrodynamic drag causes cupular deflection (and asymmetrical stimulation), resulting in vertigo and nystagmus until the particles

come to rest in the now gravitationally dependent section of the canal. It is likely that both of these conditions exist (Herdman et al, 1993; Steddin & Brandt, 1996) and treatments have been proposed for both.

Treatment for Cupulolithiasis

As noted earlier, Brandt and Daroff (1980) found that the symptoms of BPPV were quickly relieved by repeatedly provoking symptoms through head-positioning exercises. They speculated that the noted rapid improvement was not a result of habituation, but rather a means of "dispersion of otolithic debri from the cupula." Toupet and Semont (1985) took this a step further and proposed the first single treatment approach for BPPV. Norre and Beckers (1987) report that this "brisk method" effectively resolved the symptoms of BPPV in 52% of patients within 1 week. Currently known as the *Liberatory* or *Semont* maneuver, it was described in detail by Semont et al (1988) (Fig. 21–2). Semont and his colleagues, over an 8-year period involving 711 cases, report an 84% success rate after one maneuver and a 93% success rate after two maneuvers. More recently, Serafini et al (1996) report that complete resolution of symptoms was achieved within one treatment in more than 50% of cases; whereas more than 90% of cases were resolved within five treatment sessions. Theoretically, the movement required to displace otoconia from the cupula must be relatively rapid and may be contraindicated in elderly patients or patients with a history of back or neck problems.

Treatment for Canalithiasis

The canalith repositioning procedure for canalithiasis was introduced by John Epley of the Portland Otologic Clinic (1980). This procedure has undergone several modifications and is known by a variety of names:

1. CRP (*c*analith *r*epositioning *p*rocedure)
2. CRM (*c*analith *r*epositioning *m*aneuver)
3. Particle repositioning maneuver
4. Epley maneuver

All these procedures are based on the belief that free-floating otoconia in the posterior canal are responsible for BPPV. The goal of each maneuver is to cause the otoconia debris to migrate out of the posterior canal, through the common crus, and into the vestibule where it is believed that the otoconia harmlessly dissolves in the endolymph (Mira et al, 1996) (Fig. 21–3).

The efficacy of canalith repositioning procedures has been detailed in a number of studies, with success rates typically around 90% (Desmond & Touchette, 1998; Epley, 1992b; Lynn et al, 1995; Parnes & Robichaud, 1997). Lynn et al (1995) performed CRP on one group of patients with BPPV, and a "placebo" procedure on a second group. Eighty-nine percent of those treated with CRP were symptom free 1 month after treatment, whereas 27% treated with the "placebo" procedure were improved. The natural course of BPPV, with frequent spontaneous remission within a few weeks, may be a confounding factor in determining precisely the success rate of CRP. Steenerson and Cronin (1996) compared the relative efficacy of vestibular habituation therapy and CRP. They found that after 3 months, 63% of patients treated with habituation therapy were symptom free, whereas 82% treated with CRP

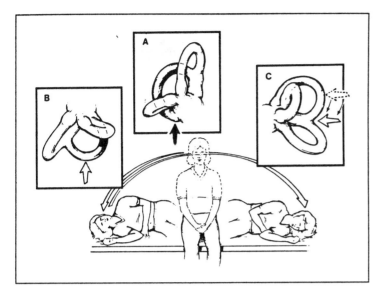

Figure 21–2 The Semont maneuver. The patient is moved quickly from sitting (**A**) into the position that provokes vertigo (**B**) and is kept in that position for 2 to 3 minutes. He is then turned rapidly to the opposite ear-down position (**C**), with the therapist maintaining the alignment of the neck and head on the body. The patient must stay in this position for 5 minutes. The patient is then slowly taken into a seated position. He must remain in the vertical position for 48 hours and avoid the provoking position for 1 week. The position of the right labyrinth is shown in each head position and the posterior canal is shaded. The solid arrow indicates the location of the cupula of the posterior canal; the open arrow indicates the location of debris free-floating in the long arm of the posterior canal during the different stages of the treatment. (Reprinted with permission from Herdman SJ, Tusa RJ, Zee DS, Proctor LR, Mattox DE. [1993]. Single treatment approaches to benign paroxysmal positional vertigo. *Archives of Otolaryngology–Head and Neck Surgery, 119;*450-454. Copyright 1993; American Medical Association.)

were symptom free. Only 25% of a control group receiving no treatment reported resolution of symptoms. In addition, these authors suggest that CRP results in faster resolution of symptoms and may be better tolerated by patients than habituation therapy, which repeatedly provokes symptoms.

Epleys original description of the CRP is as follows:

1. *Preliminary:* Identification of offending canal and noted latency and duration of nystagmus response.

2. *Preparation:* Premedication with transdermal scopolomine or diazepam.

3. *Maneuvers:* Commencement of maneuvers as described in Figure 21–3, changing head positions when the nystagmus response has ceased. If no nystagmus is appreciated, an estimate of latency plus duration of previous response (typically "6 to 13 seconds") dictates when the head is moved to the next position. Complete cycles are performed until no nystagmus response is present.

4. *Oscillation:* A handheld oscillator with a frequency of approximately 80 Hz is applied to the mastoid process of the affected side.

5. *Follow-up:* Patients are advised to keep their head upright for 48 hours after the procedure. The CRP may be repeated weekly until the patient is asymptomatic and no nystagmus is noted in the Hallpike position (Epley, 1992b).

Subsequent reports have offered modifications of the CRP. Many investigators and practicing clinicians do not use any type of oscillation (Herdman et al, 1993, Parnes & Robichaud, 1997; Steenerson & Cronin, 1996), and have reported results similar to those of Epley (1992b). Li (1995) noted a significantly reduced rate of resolution of symptoms after one treatment with CRP in patients *not* treated with oscillation during the procedure.

The length of time that the patient needs to remain upright after treatment has also been modified. Some period of time is recommended to keep the free-floating otoconia from gravitating back into the posterior canal. Although most published reports recommend 48 hours, it is the author's practice to require the use of a neck collar and that the patient remain upright for only 24 hours after treatment. The success rate for this procedure is similar to previous reports of efficacy.

PEARL

Many patients are reluctant to spend a night sitting up in a chair. For these patients, the author has performed the CRP early in the morning and asked the patient to remain upright as long as possible. Our experience has been that this technique is quite effective both in obtaining consent for the procedure and in resolving symptoms in most patients. This is only recommended if the patient objects to the standard follow-up period.

Variant Forms of BPPV

In the last several years BPPV of the anterior and horizontal semicircular canals has been reported (Fife, 1995; Lempert & Tiel-Wilck; 1996, Stockwell, 1996). Fife (1995) estimates that anterior canal BPPV accounts for 4% of all cases, with horizontal canal involvement in 6% of cases. The remaining 90% are believed to involve the posterior canal. Both canalithiasis and cupulolithiasis have been implicated as causative factors and may be the determining factor in the direction of nystagmus noted. Anterior canal BPPV is most typically provoked by a Hallpike manuever with the affected ear on the up side. Because the same position can trigger posterior canal BPPV of the down side ear, differentiating canal involvement is done

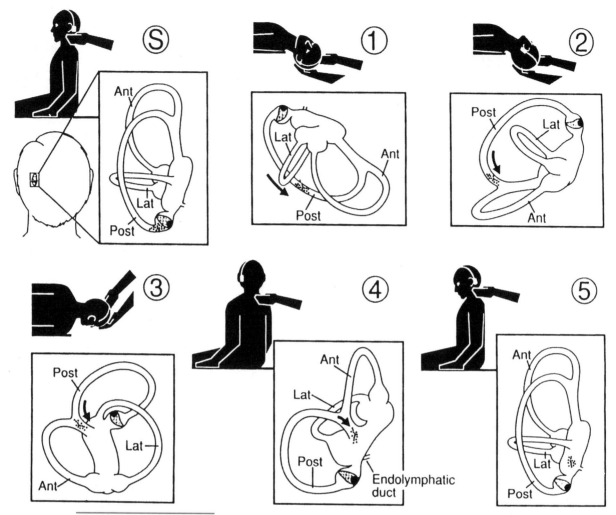

Figure 21–3 Positions of the left posterior semicircular canal (PSC). 1. Patient is brought into the offending left Hallpike position, causing flow of debris away from cupula of the left PSC. 2. While the patient remains in the supine position, the head is rotated to the right side. 3. With the orientation of the head to the right shoulder unchanged, the patient is rolled over onto his right shoulder and hip, looking down toward the floor. 4. The head remains to the right, tilted down, the patient rises to the sitting position. 5. The head is rotated forward, chin tilted down. NOTE: Patient should be kept in each of these positions until nystagmus has ceased or for a time period at least equal to the duration of time from initiation of provoking (Hallpike) maneuver to the cessation of nystagmus. Nystagmus should be viewed in all positions because a change in the direction of nystagmus indicates possible failure to deposit all the debris in the vestibule. (Reprinted and adapted with permission from Epley J. [1992]. The canalith repositioning procedure: for treatment of benign paroxysmal positional vertigo. *Otolaryngology–Head and Neck Surgery, 107*(3);399–404.)

by observing the direction of nystagmus while the patient experiences vertigo. As noted earlier, posterior canal BPPV is marked by *geotropic* (beating *toward* the earth) rotary nystagmus; in anterior canal BPPV, the nystagmus is primarily *ageotropic* (beating *away* from the earth) (Stockwell, 1996). Treatment of anterior canal BPPV may be accomplished by performing CRP as if treating posterior canal BPPV in the opposite ear.

Horizontal canal BPPV may be elicited during the Hall-pike maneuver but is best provoked by having the patient lie flat in the supine position and then move the head quickly to the ear-down position, both to the right and the left. Horizontal canal BPPV may be diagnosed by observing horizontal

geotropic nystagmus while the patient is vertiginous. The patient is typically more vertiginous, and the intensity of the nystagmus is greater, when the affected ear is down. As in other forms of BPPV, there is a short latency and a transient response with a duration typically longer than that observed in BPPV of the other two canals. Repositioning technique for horizontal canal BPPV involves having the patient, starting in the supine position, rotate 360 degrees in the direction away from the affected canal.

Although success rates of CRP are impressive, a number of patients with intractable positional vertigo do not respond to repositioning procedures. These patients may be candidates for surgical intervention. Surgical procedures to relieve the symptoms of BPPV include sectioning of the posterior nerve (singular neurectomy) to eliminate response from the ampulla of the posterior canal and occlusion of the posterior canal (canal plugging) to preclude loose otoconia from entering the posterior canal (Gacek, 1991; Parnes & McClure; 1990).

VESTIBULAR DISORDERS AND PANIC DISORDER

Numerous investigators and authors have noted a correlation between vestibular symptoms and anxiety or panic disorder. Whether vestibular disorders may lead to panic disorder or whether vestibular complaints are a consequence of panic disorder is a subject of much speculation and research. Alvord (1991) noted that "dizzy" patients scheduled for ENG had a much higher self-assessment of anxiety than did either non-dizzy patients scheduled for auditory-evoked potential tests or subjects with no medical complaints. Hoffman et al (1994) reported abnormal scores on the vestibular autorotation test on all patients seen in a panic disorder clinic. These patients were not selected or excluded on the basis of a complaint of dizziness. Jacob (1988) offers a historical perspective and proposes possible theories as to the cause-and-effect relationship of panic disorder and the vestibular system. Jacob performed vestibular evaluations on 21 patients with a history of panic disorder and/or agoraphobia. He reports that 71% of patients with panic disorder had abnormal calorics and 75% had abnormal posturography. These figures were somewhat lower (45% had abnormal calorics, 62% had abnormal posturography) in patients with both panic disorder and agoraphobia. Sklare et al (1990) reported 71% of patients with a history of panic disorder had some abnormality on ENG testing.

It is possible that a connection exists between agoraphobia* and/or "supermarket syndrome" and subtle or undiagnosed vestibular abnormalities. Patients with vestibular weakness are subject to an optokinetic effect when walking down the aisle of a store.

Optokinetic tracking is, to some degree, involuntary. Different colored objects on the shelves can create an optokinetic effect similar to that perceived during sustained horizontal rotation, and a sense of dysequilibrium or spatial disorientation will ensue. Many patients with vestibular weakness will describe a sensation of disorientation and anxiety when walking in a crowded area such as a shopping mall, particularly when walking against traffic. It is well known that patients with vestibular loss become very reliant on visual information for postural stability in the early stages of compensation. In this situation the patient's visual field is moving, making it unreliable for judging relative motion. A sense of disorientation or fear may overcome the uncompensated patient. This can easily be misinterpreted as, or may eventually become, an anxiety-producing event leading to agoraphobia. The common denominator of these situations is the "decreased visual input for orientation in space" (Jacob, 1988).

Treatment for these individuals involves a combination of vestibular training to increase gaze stability and "lock on" to stable visual targets for orientation and counseling to reduce

the anxiety component. This anxiety component usually presents itself either as a panic disorder, agoraphobia, or generalized anxiety disorder.

It is interesting that *The Anxiety and Phobia Workbook* (Bourne, 1995) includes the following quote: "It is common for the agoraphobic to avoid a variety of situations. Some of the more common ones include: (1) Crowded public places such as grocery stores, department stores, restaurants; (2) Enclosed or confined places such as tunnels, bridges, or the hairdressers chair; (3) Public transportation such as trains, buses, subways, planes; (4) Being home alone." Many of these situations sound strikingly familiar to complaints of vestibular loss patients, particularly "fear of crowded spaces" (moving visual fields?), tunnels (optokinetic effect?), and the hairdressers chair (BPPV?).

Hyperventilation is more of an anxiety disorder than a vestibular disorder. However, many of these patients' primary complaints are of dizziness or light-headedness, which they feel is unprovoked. Many are unaware of any coexisting symptoms until questioned by a clinician. Drachman and Hart (1972) reported that hyperventilation contributed to complaints of dizziness in 25 of 104 patients evaluated and was the sole cause in four patients. Sama et al (1995) report similar results stating that hyperventilation caused dizziness in 5% of subjects and was a contributing factor in another 21%. Hyperventilation occurs when "ventilatory effort exceeds metabolic need" and causes constriction of the cerebral blood vessels and reduction of cerebral blood flow. Typical signs and symptoms include complaints of light-headedness, frequent sighing, chest pain, and numbness and tingling around the mouth. Some of these symptoms can be reproduced during examination in affected individuals. Anxiety can lead to increased heart rate and respirations, which can lead to hyperventilation. Sama et al (1995) estimate that 65% of cases of hyperventilation are psychogenic, 31% mixed organic and psychogenic, and only 3% are pure organic. Treatment for hyperventilation may be out of the scope of practice for most audiologists, and referral to a psychiatrist or psychologist may be indicated. In some cases simply making the patient aware of the anxiety/hyperventilation cycle may resolve symptoms, whereas some patients may benefit from brown bag breathing at the onset of symptoms. Counseling and therapy for breathing and relaxation exercises may be recommended by the appropriate specialist.

BILLING CODES

Because reimbursement and coding guidelines may change depending on the specific insurance carrier, the reader is advised to investigate local and current guidelines individually. Most patients requiring vestibular rehabilitation are elderly, so it is fair to assume that Medicare guidelines would be most applicable to explore. Medicare regulations may vary from state to state, but the guidelines for VR would generally fall under the heading of "physical medicine." Physical medicine codes most applicable to VR are as follows:

97530—"Therapeutic activities ... directed at loss or restriction of mobility, strength, balance and coordination."

*Agoraphobia—an abnormal fear of being in open or public places (*Websters*, 1976).

97112—"Therapeutic procedure…to improve balance coordination, kinesthetic sense, posture and proprioception."

Physical medicine codes can be billed by physical therapists, occupational therapists, or any employee (including audiologists) under the direct supervision of a physician. Independent practicing audiologists cannot be reimbursed for the provision of VR services. An audiologist may be reimbursed if he or she meets the criteria for "incident to" services. To meet these requirements the audiologist must be working, either part time or full time, as an employee of the physician billing for the service. The supervising physician must be:

1. Involved in the initial evaluation
2. Physically present in the same office suite when therapy is taking place
3. Involved in the course of treatment enough to reflect "his/her continuing active participation in and management of the course of treatment"

Medicare allows "12 to 18 visits within a 4 to 6 week period," and "the usual treatment session in the office or home setting is from 30 to 45 minutes." Additional therapy "beyond this frequency and duration may require documentation supporting the medical necessity of continued treatment."

Diagnosis codes (ICD-9) for specific vestibular complaints such as vertigo and dysequilibrium and for specific vestibular pathological conditions such as labyrinthitis and BPPV will not be accepted as appropriate diagnosis codes for billing

---

PITFALL

At the time of printing, Medicare does not allow for independent practicing audiologists to be reimbursed for vestibular therapy.

---

the aforementioned codes applicable to VR. Covered diagnosis codes that are applicable to balance disorders and may benefit from VR include 719.77—difficulty walking, 781.2—gait abnormality, 781.9—abnormal posture (Medicare Newsletter, 1997).

CONCLUSIONS

Research and clinical experience indicate that a large number of patients with vestibular dysfunction can benefit from vestibular therapy. Past approaches to treating patients with dizziness have been shown to be less effective than a customized intensive therapy program. However, acceptance of vestibular rehabilitation is still in its early stages. The goal of this chapter is to review the clinical evidence, explain the basis for vestibular adaptation and compensation, and give the reader some practical tools to begin a vestibular rehabilitation program.

Appendix A
Rehabilitation Exercises

Ankle Sways

1. Have the patient stand on a firm surface with the feet shoulder distance apart, equal weight on both feet, and arms relaxed at the sides while looking straight ahead. This exercise may be performed with a target or in front of a mirror for extra visual reinforcement.
2. While the patient looks straight ahead, have the patient slowly shift the weight forward (toes) and backward (heels). Keep the amount of movement forward and back restricted to prevent bending at the hips. All movement should be at the ankles.
3. Next, have the patient shift the weight from side to side, placing more weight first to the right side, then on the left. Again, prevent bending at the hips.
4. This exercise can be done with the eyes open, then closed. This exercise can also be done with the patient standing on a compliant surface such as a foam pad or cushion. Manipulation of these variables allows for sensory organization training.

Balance Ball Bounce—Eyes Fixed on Target

1. Assist the patient to a sitting position on large physio ball. The patient's feet should be touching the floor and the hands placed on the side of the ball.
2. Once the patient feels comfortable sitting on the ball, have the patient slowly bounce on the ball while continuing to focus on the target.
3. After the patient is comfortable with this activity, hold a small object approximately 18 inches in front of the patient's eyes and tell the patient to focus on this object while he or she resumes the bouncing action.

Balance Beam

1. Patient is to place the right foot onto the beam while instructor provides assistance.
2. Assist patient onto the beam and have the patient place the left foot in front of the right in a heel-to-toe pattern. The patient's eyes should be directed forward at all times.
3. Have patient follow the path of the beam, keeping one foot in front of the other.

4. If needed, allow the patient to extend arms out to the side for balance.
5. This exercise can begin with the patient walking a tape line on the floor.

Balance Board Exercise

1. Make sure that the patient's feet are placed in the center of the board, assist the patient to a standing position on the balance board.
2. While the patient's body is kept erect and bending at the hips is prevented, have the patient gradually lean forward. (The board will move forward with the patient.)
3. Have the patient gradually lean back on the heels and come back to the center position. Have the patient continue leaning back further on the heels while the front of the board comes up. Have the patient lean forward without bending at the hips and come back to the center position.
4. Perform the exercise with movement from side to side.
5. Repeat the exercise but allow bending at the hips.

Ball Circles

1. Have the patient stand with feet shoulder width apart, weight equal on both feet. Instruct the patient to hold a ball (or other soft object) with both hands, arms straight out from the body, and to keep the eyes on the ball at all times.
2. While keeping arms straight, the patient moves the ball in a complete, smooth, and continuous circle. The patient is instructed to move the head and eyes in this activity but is at all times to keep the eyes on the ball and continue circling for a minimum of 1 minute in each direction.
3. The patient can also move the ball from side to side and up and down while keeping the eyes focused at all times.
- **If dizziness increases with this activity, the patient should stop movement until the feeling subsides, then begin again.**
4. If the patient becomes very dizzy during this activity or is unsafe standing, this exercise can be done sitting in a chair, preferably one without arms.

Ball Kicking

1. Instruct the patient that a ball will be slowly rolled toward him or her and that on approach of the ball the patient should kick it back with the side or top of the foot, whichever is most comfortable. Advise the patient that it is important that a wide stance is maintained and the center of gravity is found before attempting to kick the ball.
2. Once the patient is standing comfortably and well balanced, gently roll the ball toward him or her. Alternate the foot used for kicking.
3. When this action is successfully completed and the patient feels comfortable, instruct the patient to try taking two steps to the side before kicking the ball back.

Ball Sitting

1. Carefully assist the patient into a sitting position on a physio ball. The patient's feet should comfortably reach the floor.
2. Allow the patient to get his or her balance and to become as comfortable as possible.
3. The patient is to perform a rolling motion, first to the front and back, then side to side.
4. After the patient is comfortable with the ball, have the patient lift the legs off the ground while maintaining balance.

Ball Toss

1. Instruct the patient that he or she is to attempt to catch the ball as it passes before him or her.
2. Stand to the side, a moderate distance from the patient, and gently toss a ball across the patient's front.
3. As the patient gains success in catching, toss the ball to different positions so that the patient must take additional action before catching the ball (i.e., taking a step, bending, stepping side to side).

Bend and Reach

1. Have the patient begin by standing in a wide balanced position. Using proper lifting technique, the patient should pick up a ball from the floor and stand up. Then the patient should reach over his or her head to put the ball in the hands of the assistant.
2. This same procedure should be repeated for 1 minute, increasing in speed when possible.
3. The exercise should be repeated for 1 minute in the reverse order. The patient reaches up to take the ball from the assistant's hands and bends down to place the ball on the floor.
4. The patient should breath appropriately and not hold his or her breath at any time.

Circle Sways

1. Have the patient stand with the feet shoulder distance apart, arms resting at the sides.
2. The patient should breath deeply and be encouraged to relax. The patient is to focus thoughts on the feeling of the feet in contact with the floor.
3. Without bending at the hips, the patient is to practice swaying the body in a small circle. The patient is to repeatedly sway forward, to the right side, to the rear, to the left side, and forward again. A mirror may be used for extra visual reinforcement.
4. Have the patient gradually increase the size of the circle by moving the body further each way but without bending the hips or taking a step.
5. This exercise can be done with the eyes open and closed.

Crossover Step

1. Have the patient stand near a wall with the feet slightly apart.
2. Instruct the patient to cross the right foot in front of the left, hold it there for 5 seconds, then return the foot to its starting position.
3. Repeat this action with the left foot.
4. Have the patient repeat steps two and three repetitively for a specified number of times.
5. This exercise can be done with the eyes open and closed or in front of a mirror.

Face to Knee

1. Have the patient start by sitting in an upright and comfortable position. Place each hand in a fist on each knee.
2. Slowly at first, have the patient bend over until the patient's face touches his or her fist. Bend down to the right, sweep over to the left, then sit up. Repeat bending down to the left, moving right, then sitting up.
3. Repeat, alternating, for a minimum of 1 minute, making movements progressively faster if possible.

Foam Sideways

1. Position the patient so that he or she is standing on one end of a foam floor mat and facing a wall that will be used as a guide.
2. Making sure that the feet are pointing straight ahead (toward the wall), have the patient begin stepping sideways to the end of the mat and then return to the starting position.
3. Once the patient feels comfortable with this procedure, have him or her perform the same action with eyes closed, first touching the wall, then without (increase use of proprioceptive input).

Foam Walk

1. Position the patient so that he or she is standing at one end of a foam floor mat and facing the other end.
2. Have the patient walk at a comfortable pace using the stepping patterns and paths: forward, toe-toe, heel-heel, heel-heel to toe-toe, diagonal, and backward.
3. Instruct the patient to repeat each pattern a specified number of times.
4. This exercise can be done with the eyes open and closed, with one hand on the wall.

Focus While Turning Head

1. Have the patient bring the index finger or a target to approximately 18 inches from the front of his or her nose (this can be done by taping a target to the wall).
2. While focusing on the target, have the patient turn his or her head from side to side for a minimum of 1 minute. Repeat the exercise moving the head up and down.
3. Gradually have the patient increase the speed of the head turns.

NOTE: This exercise can be done sitting if needed. When performed standing, the patient can initially assume a wide-based stance. With improvements in standing balance, the base of support is gradually shortened.

Focus While Turning Head Two Times

1. Have the patient hold a business card in front of him or her so that it can be read. The patient should move the head and the card side to side *in opposite directions* while keeping eyes on the card.
2. The head should be moved as quickly as possible, keeping the words or letter in focus. Continue this for 1 to 2 minutes without stopping.
3. Repeat this exercise moving the head up and down.

NOTE: This exercise can be done sitting if needed. When performed standing, the patient can initially assume a wide-based stance. With improvements in standing balance, the base of support is gradually shortened.

Foot Work

1. This exercise can be performed sitting or standing, whichever is more comfortable and safe for the patient. A collection of objects of different size and texture should be presented to the patient.
2. The patient is instructed to feel the object with his or her foot and describe the texture and size. If the object can be picked up, the patient should attempt to do so with his or her foot.
3. It is important that the patient concentrate on the sensation and location of the object on the foot. Each foot should be presented several objects.

Hand-to-Hand Ball Toss

1. Have the patient sit in a chair, preferably without arms.
2. Have the patient toss a tennis or other small rubber ball from hand to hand above eye level.
3. As the patient feels comfortable with this activity while sitting, have him or her do the same ball tossing while standing in a stable, centered stance.

Head Circles

1. Have the patient begin moving his or her head in a circular motion with their eyes open.
2. Specifically, the patient is to first place his or her chin on the chest, then left ear on left shoulder, move head directly across to, right ear on right shoulder, and finally return chin to chest. Do not have the patient bend his or her head backwards.
3. Assist the patient in making this motion as fluid as possible for a minimum of 1 minute.
4. After the patient becomes comfortable with this activity, have the patient reverse the direction of rotation.
5. Have the patient repeat the exercise in both directions with eyes closed.

NOTE: This exercise can be done sitting if needed. When performed standing, the patient can initially assume a wide-based stance. With improvements in standing balance, the base of support is gradually shortened.

Head Movements

1. While keeping the trunk still, have the patient quickly turn his or her head and look to the right, then turn and look to the left, then return to center, returning to the forward-looking position. Have the patient maintain this forward-looking position for 5 seconds. Repeat for 1 minute.
2. Have the patient perform the exercise, moving his or her head up and down.
3. This exercise can also be done with the eyes closed.

NOTE: This exercise can be done sitting if needed. When performed standing, the patient can initially assume a wide-based stance. With improvements in standing balance, the base of support is gradually shortened.

Imaginary Target

1. Have the patient fixate on a visual target directly in front of him or her, close the eyes, and rotate the head in one direction imagining that he or she is still looking directly at the target. After the head rotation has stopped, the eyes are opened. The eyes should still be held on the target.
2. Repeat in the opposite direction. The patient should be as accurate as possible. Vary the speed and the amount (stopping point) of head rotation.
3. Repeat the exercise but move the head up and down.
4. Practice for 5 minutes, stopping if necessary.

Moving Saccades

1. The patient can start this exercise sitting if necessary but should advance to a standing progression as soon as possible. Place two targets at eye level, arm's length away, and slightly greater than shoulder width apart.

2. The patient starts with the head rotated approximately 40 degrees to the right with the gaze directed at the right visual target. With the head stationary, gaze is shifted with a saccade to fixate on the visual target on the left, followed by the patient rotating the head to face the left target.

3. The movements are then repeated in the opposite direction. The individuals are instructed to perform these movements as quickly as possible, while keeping the visual target in focus. The exercise should be performed for a minimum of 1 minute.

Obstacle Course

1. Set up an obstacle course using chairs, pillows, trash can, and whatever else might be readily available. Some of the objects should be small enough so that the patient can step over them and still see them so that they can be walked around.

2. The patient is then instructed to walk the obstacle course in a specified route or pattern.

3. As the patient progresses, have him or her pick up and carry the smaller objects.

4. In time, change the course so that it does not become routine; to add difficulty, you may toss a ball to the patient for the patient to catch as he or she walks.

One-Leg Stand

1. Have the patient stand on one leg, with the back to a padded corner for safety, for 30 seconds.

2. This activity should be done 10 times on each leg.

3. This exercise can be done with the eyes open and closed.

Roll Body Against Wall

1. Have the patient stand with the back against a wall. Instruct the patient to take his or her right shoulder off the wall and turn to the left until the front of the body is against the wall.

2. In a similar manner have the patient take the left shoulder off the wall and turn to the left until the back is again against the wall.

3. Have the patient continue steps 1 and 2 until he or she has moved down the wall to its end. At this point, instruct the patient to stop and regain the balance.

4. Have the patient return to the starting position and repeat this activity for a specified number of times.

5. This exercise can be done with the eyes open and closed.

Saccades

1. Have the patient hold a small index card in each hand, level with the eyes, at arm's length, about 18 inches apart.

2. Keeping the head still and without stopping between cards, have the patient look quickly from one card to the other. Have the patient perform this action for 1 to 2 minutes.

3. Repeat the exercise having the patient perform the same action but in a vertical direction.

NOTE: *This exercise can be done sitting if needed. When performed standing, the patient can initially assume a wide-based stance. With improvements in standing balance, the base of support is gradually shortened.*

Sit to Stand

1. Have the patient begin by sitting in an chair without arms (arms can be used if needed).

2. The patient should rise quickly, using only the legs, looking straight ahead. The patient should remain standing for 5 seconds or until any dizziness is gone.

3. Next, the patient should sit back down into the chair in a controlled but rapid manner. Do not let the patient just drop into the chair. The patient should use his or her legs to control the descent. The patient should remain sitting for 5 seconds or until any dizziness is gone.

4. This exercise can be done with two chairs facing each other. The patient would stand, turn around, and sit in the opposite chair.

5. This exercise can be repeated with eyes closed.

6. This exercise should not be performed on patients with postural or orthostatic hypotension.

Sit to Supine

1. Have the patient sit on foam or a padded platform that he or she can fully recline on and place a pillow under the patient's knees.

2. Instruct the patient to turn the head to the desired side.

3. Have the patient lay down as rapidly as possible so that he or she is flat and keeping the head turned.

4. Have the patient stay in this position for as long as symptoms last (or for 15 seconds if no symptoms).

5. Have the patient sit up as rapidly as possible.

6. Once sitting, wait until symptoms again subside (or 30 seconds if no symptoms).

7. Repeat the exercises with patient for the desired number of times.

Sitting on a Chair/Stool

1. Have the patient sit quietly and without moving on a firm surface, such as a chair or stool, breathing deeply a few times and then relaxing.

2. Instruct the patient to concentrate on the sensation of sitting in the chair or stool. A mirror may be used for extra visual reinforcement.

3. Next, have the patient close the eyes for 10 seconds and again concentrate on the sensation of his or her body sitting.

Standing

1. Have the patient stand in front of a long mirror with hands at the sides, feet shoulder-width apart, head up, shoulders back, and looking straight ahead. Have the patient notice his or her posture and instruct the patient to maintain this posture throughout the exercise. Ask the patient to concentrate on not swaying and to stand still for 1 minute.

2. Have the patient maintain this same stance but look straight ahead at a target on the wall. Maintain this position for 1 minute.

3. Progressively narrow the base of support (move feet closer 1 inch at a time) from feet apart to feet together to a semi-heel-to-toe position to heel-to-toe (one foot in front of the other). Do the exercises first with arms outstretched, then with arms close to the body, then with arms folded across the chest. Hold each position for 30 seconds, then move to the next most difficult position. Alternate between mirror and target.

4. Repeat above with head bent forward 30 degrees, then back 30 degrees.

5. Repeat basic standing exercise with eyes closed, at first intermittently and then continuously, instructing the patient to make an effort to mentally visualize his or her surroundings.

6. All these exercises can also be performed while standing on a foam mat or other uneven surface.

7. Be sure to maintain a position near the patient to assist him or her if needed, especially during the time when the patient has the eyes closed. Some patients may need these instructions given in sections because they will try to do too much too soon if not directed. They should only move on when they can successfully complete the previous section.

Stepping Patterns

1. This exercise uses numbered squares arranged in a pattern on the floor.

2. Instruct the patient to stand behind a base line, to tap the designated foot on the specified card as its number is called forth, then return the foot to the starting position.

3. Tell the patient which foot to use and call out 2, 3, or 4 numbers in a row.

Targets

1. Choose three targets that are at eye level, one directly in front of the patient, one to the extreme right, and the other to the extreme left.

2. Have the patient, turning only his or her head, look at the target to the left, then the one at center, then to the target located to the right. Focus on each target.

3. Have the patient repeat this activity for 1 minute without stopping.

4. When the patient is ready, have him or her repeat the same exercise except to stop at each target to focus.

5. This exercise can also be done horizontally and/or vertically.

NOTE: *This exercise can be done sitting if needed. When performed standing, the patient can initially assume a wide-based stance. With improvements in standing balance, the base of support is gradually shortened.*

Trace the Alphabet

1. Position the patient near a wall or counter so that he or she has something to hold on to if it becomes necessary.

2. Have the patient trace the first 10 letters of the alphabet on the floor with a foot. Once completed, have the patient repeat the tracing procedure with the other foot.

3. As the patient's proficiency improves with step 2, have him or her trace all the letters of the alphabet.

Tracking Exercise

1. Give the patient a small index card with several words written on it. Instruct the patient to hold the card about 18 inches in front of the eyes.

2. While keeping the head still and following the card only with the eyes, have the patient slowly move the card horizontally to the right, to the left, and back to center. Have the patient perform this action for a minimum of 1 minute.

3. As the patient progresses in ability, have him or her move the arm at faster and faster speeds until he or she can no longer read the words. Remember, the patient is to keep the head still during this exercise and follow the card only with the eyes.

4. This exercise should also be done with vertical and diagonal movement.

NOTE: *This exercise can be done sitting if needed. When performed standing, the patient can initially assume a wide-based stance. With improvements in standing balance, the base of support is gradually shortened.*

Tracking/VOR Interaction

1. While the patient is standing on an uneven or movable surface (e.g., trampoline, vestibular board, foam mat), have him or her focus on an object that you move in front of the field of vision. Instruct the patient to maintain balance while focusing on the object.

2. As the patient becomes proficient in this activity, vary the exercise by moving the object in a vertical or diagonal motion.

Trampoline Ankle Sway

1. Position the patient on the trampoline so that the feet are shoulder-width apart, with equal weight on both feet, arms relaxed at the side, and looking straight forward at a target.
2. Have the patient slowly and carefully shift the weight forward, then backward. All movement should be at the ankles, and the patient should not be allowed to bend at the hips.
3. Next, have the patient shift the weight from side to side, placing more weight first on the right side, then on the left. Again, do not permit the patient to bend at the hips.
4. This exercise can be repeated with the eyes closed.

Trampoline Circle Sway

1. Assist the patient to the center of the trampoline with the feet shoulder distance apart.
2. Relax the patient by having him or her breathe deeply and slowly expel the air.
3. Have the patient slowly sway the body in small circles. Instruct and help the patient sway forward, to the right side, to the rear, to the left side, and forward again. This should be performed without the patient bending at the hips.
4. As the patient progresses in ability, have the patient gradually increase the size of the circle while making sure not to bend at the hips or take a step.
5. This exercise can be performed with the eyes closed.

Trampoline Walk

1. Instruct the patient to slowly step up onto the trampoline, and provide assistance when necessary. The patient is to keep the head up and eyes focused on a specified, fixed object that is located at eye level.
2. Beginning with small steps at first, the patient is to gradually increase the stepping height and speed until almost marching.
3. Once the patient feels comfortable with the stepping motion, have the patient continue to step, then march with the eyes closed.

Walk-Stop

1. Have the patient begin walking approximately 10 steps at a good pace, then have the patient stop abruptly at your command. Allow the patient sufficient time to regain his or her balance.

2. Have the patient repeat this activity a specified number of times.

Walking with Eyes Closed

1. Before having the patient perform this exercise, have him or her walk the length of the room next to a wall with the eyes open. Ask the patient to pay attention and get used to the surface.
2. Standing a little away from the wall, have the patient extend the arms out so that the fingertips are lightly touching the wall.
3. Using the wall as a guide, have the patient begin walking along the wall with the eyes closed and head up. The patient should attempt to imagine a straight line as he or she walks.
4. If the patient at any time feels off balance or likely to fall, he or she is to open the eyes. Only after the patient feels that he or she has regained balance is the patient to begin again.

Walking with Head Turns

1. Instruct the patient to begin walking at a normal speed. (Walk next to the patient to ensure safety.)
2. Have the patient turn his or her head to the right and left while walking (about every three steps).
3. Instruct the patient to try to focus on different objects while walking.
4. Gradually the patient should move the head faster and more often.
5. Have the patient repeat this activity for a minimum of 2 minutes.

NOTE: This exercise should also be performed with head movements up and down and diagonal.

Walking with Turns

1. Have the patient walk in a large circle but gradually make smaller and smaller turns. Be sure to have the patient make circles in each direction.
2. When the circles are relatively small, have the patient take five steps and turn around to the right (180 degrees) and keep walking. Take five more steps, turn to the left (180 degrees), and keep walking. Repeat five times, rest, and repeat the entire sequence.

Appendix B
Equipping the Vestibular Rehabilitation Facility

The equipment needed for performing vestibular rehabilitation is relatively inexpensive when compared with the facilities required for most aspects of audiology. A larger room is preferable, but nearly all VR activities can be performed in a 10 ft by 10 ft space, as long as a long unobstructed hallway is available for walking exercises. The therapy room should be equipped with a monitoring camera and VCR to record all therapy sessions. Exercise equipment can be purchased from a number of vendors (one supplier offers a Vestibular Rehabilitation Kit), or many of the needed items can be made by the therapist or purchased from a local department store.

The following list is incomplete but is representative of the types of equipment that may be useful in performing VR therapy.

Balance beam—For hip strategies exercises

Large, thick foam mat (8 inches thick, 4 ft by 8 ft)—For compliant surface while walking and patient safety

Full-length lightweight movable wall mirror—To provide visual feedback

Minitrampoline—For compliant surface and vertical VOR stimulus

Physio balls (large and small)—For hip strategy and vertical VOR exercises

Lightweight 12-inch rubber ball—For ball toss and kick exercises

Safety belt—To support patient during exercises

Metronome—To time head and eye movements

Kitchen timer—To time exercises

Balance board—For hip strategy exercises

Examination table—For canalith repositioning procedures

Balance master—Includes a spring-loaded platform that measures center of gravity and sway from center, numeric data regarding sway, and visual feedback for improving postural control

A list of suppliers follows.

Abilations—Select Service and Supply Co., Inc., One Sportime Way, Atlanta GA 30340.

Flaghouse—150 North MacQueston Parkway, Mount Vernon, NY 10550

Fabrications—P.O. Box 1500, White Plains, NY 10602.

Neurocom International, Inc.—9570 SE Lawnfield Road, Clackamas, OR 97015-9943.

Smith & Nephew, Inc.—One Quality Drive, P.O. Box 1005, Germantown, WI 53022-8205.

REFERENCES

ALLISON, L. (undated). Identifying and managing elderly fallers. *Neurocommunication International, Inc. Literature*, 1–8.

ALVORD, L.S. (1991). Psychological status of patients undergoing electronystagmography. *Journal of the American Academy of Audiology, 2*;261–265.

AMERICAN SPEECH-LANGUAGE-HEARING ASSOCIATION. (1996). Scope of practice in audiology. *ASHA supplement 16*(38);2,12–15.

BALOH, R., HONRUBIA, V., & JACOBSON, K. (1987). Benign positional vertigo: Clinical and oculographic features in 240 cases. *Neurology, 37*;371–378.

BARLOW, D., & FREEDMAN, W. (1980). Cervico-ocular reflex in the normal adult. *Acta Otolaryngologica, 89*;487–496.

BIENHOLD, H., & FLOR, H. (1978). Role of commisural connections between vestibular nuclei in compensation after unilateral labyrinthectomy. *Journal of Physiology, 284*;178P.

BLACK, F.O., & NASHNER, L.M. (1984). Postural disturbances in patients with benign paroxysmal positional nystagmus. *Annals of Otology, Rhinology, and Laryngology, 93*;595–599.

BOURNE, E.J. (1995). *The anxiety and phobia workbook*. Oakland, CA: New Harbinger.

BRANDT, T. (1991). Medical and physical therapy. In: T. Brandt (Ed.), *Vertigo: It's multisensory syndromes* (pp.15–17). New York: Springer-Verlag.

BRANDT, T., & DAROFF, R. (1980). Physical therapy for benign paroxysmal positional vertigo. *Archives of Otolaryngology, 106*;484–485.

BRONSTEIN, A.M., & HOOD, D. (1986). The cervico-ocular reflex in normal subjects and patients with absent vestibular function. *Brain Research, 373*; 399–408.

BURKE, M. (1995). Dizziness in the elderly: Etiology and treatment. *Nurse Practitioner, 20*(12);28–35.

CASS, S.P., BORELLO-FRANCE, D., & FURMAN, J.M. (1996). Functional outcome of vestibular rehabilitation in patients with abnormal sensory-organization testing. *American Journal of Otology, 17*;581–594.

CAWTHORNE, T. (1945a). The physiological basis for head exercises. *Chart Social Physiotherapy, 30*;106–107.

CAWTHORNE, T. (1945b). Vestibular injuries. *Proceedings of the Royal Society of Medicine, 39*;270–273.

CHAMBERS, B.R., MAI, M., & BARBER, H.O. (1985). Bilateral vestibular loss, oscillopsia, and the cervico-ocular reflex. *Archives of Otolaryngology–Head and Neck Surgery, 93*;403–407.

CLARK, M.R., SULLIVAN, M.D., KATON, W.J., RUSSO, J.E., FISCHL, M., DOBIE, R.A., & VORHEES, R. (1993). Psychiatric and medical factors associated with disability in patients with dizziness. *Psychosomatics, 34*(5);409–415.

COOGLER, C.E. (1992). Falls and imbalance. *Rehabilitation Management*, April/May;53.

COOKSEY, F.S. (1945). Rehabilitation in vestibular injuries. *Proceedings of the Royal Society of Medicine: Section of Otology*; 273–278.

COURJON, J.H., JEANNEROD, M., OSSUZIO, I., & SCHMID, R. (1977). The role of vision in compensation of vestibulo ocular reflex after hemilabyrinthectomy in the cat. *Experiments in Brain Research, 28*;235–248.

COWAND, J., WRISLEY, D., WALKER, M., STRASNICK, B., & JACOBSON, J. (1998). Efficacy of vestibular rehabilitation. *Archives of Otolaryngology–Head and Neck Surgery, 118*(1);49–54.

CURTHOYS, I.S., & HALMAGYI, G.M. (1996). How does the brain compensate for vestibular lesions? In: R.W. Baloh & G.M. Halmagyi (Eds.), *Disorders of the vestibular system* (pp. 145–154). New York: Oxford University Press.

DE JONGE, P.T.V.M., DE JONGE, V.J.M.B., COHEN, B., & JONKEES, L.B.W. (1977). Ataxia and nystagmus induced by injection of local anesthetics in the neck. *Annals of Neurology, 1*;240–246.

DEMER, J.L., HONRUBIA, V., & BALOH, R.W. (1994). Dynamic visual acuity: A test for oscillopsia and vestibular-ocular reflex function. *American Journal of Otology, 15*;340–347.

DEMER, J.L., PORTER, F.I., GOLDBERG, J., JENKINS, H.A., & SCHMIDT, K. (1989). Adaptation to telescopic spectacles: Vestibulo-ocular reflex plasticity. *Investigative Opthalmology and Visual Science, 30*(1);159–170.

DESMOND, A.L., & TOUCHETTE, D.A. (1998). *Balance disorders: Evaluation and treatment; A short course for primary care physicians*. Micromedical Technologies.

DIX, M. (1984). Rehabilitation of vertigo. In M.R. Dix & J.D. Hood (Eds.), *Vertigo* (pp. 467–479). New York: John Wiley & Sons.

DRACHMAN, D.A., & HART, C.W. (1972). An approach to the dizzy patient. *Neurology, 22*;323–333.

EPLEY, J. (1992a). BPPV diagnosis and management. *Vestibular update: Micromedical Technologies, 8*;1–4.

EPLEY, J. (1992b). The canalith repositioning procedure: For treatment of benign paroxysmal positional vertigo. *Archives of Otolaryngology–Head and Neck Surgery, 107*(3);399–404.

EPLEY, J., & HUGHES, D.W. (1980). Positional vertigo: New methods of diagnosis and treatment [abstract]. *Archives of Otolaryngology– Head and Neck Surgery, 88*;49.

FETTER, M., & ZEE, D. (1988). Recovery from unilateral labyrinthectomy in rhesus monkey. *Neurophysiology, 59*(2); 370–393.

FIEBERT, I., & BROWN, E. (1979). Vestibular stimulation to improve ambulation after a cerebral vascular accident. *Physical Therapy, 59*(4);423–426.

FIFE, T.D. (1995). Horizontal canal benign positional vertigo. *ENG Report*, ICS Medical, August.

FISCHER, B., & RAMSPERGER, E. (1986). Human express saccades: Effects of randomization and daily practice. *Experiments in Brain Research, 64*;569–578.

FUJINO, A., TOKMASU, K., OKAMOTO, M., NAGANUMA, H., HISHINO, I., ARAI, M., & YONEDA, S. (1996). Vestibular training for acute unilateral vestibular disturbances: Its efficacy in comparison with an anti-vertigo drug. *Acta Otolaryngologica (Stockholm) Supplement, 524*;21–26.

GACEK, R.R. (1991). Singular neurectomy update. II. A review of 102 cases. *Laryngoscope, 101*;855–862.

GANS, R. (1996). *Vestibular rehabilitation: Protocols and programs*. San Diego: Singular Publishers.

GILL-BODY, K.M., POPAT, R.A., PARKER, S.W., & KREBS, D.E. (1997). Rehabilitation of balance function in patients with cerebellar dysfunction. *Physical Therapy, 77*(5); 534–551.

GONSHOR, A., & MELVILL-JONES, G. (1976). Extreme vestibular ocular adaptation induced by prolonged optical reversal of vision. *Journal of Physiology (London), 256*;381–414.

Gresty, M.A., Hess, K., & Leech, J. (1977). Disorders of the vestibulo-ocular reflex producing oscillopsia and mechanisms compensating for loss of labyrinthine function. *Brain, 100*;693–716.

Grimby, A., & Rosenhall, U. (1995). Health related quality of life in old age. *Gerontology, 41*;286–298.

Hain, T.C. (1993). Interpretation and usefulness of ocular motility testing. In: G.P. Jacobson, C.W. Newman, & J.M. Kartush (Eds.), *Handbook of balance function testing* (pp. 101–122). St. Louis, MO: Mosby.

Halmagyi, G.M., Gresty, M.A., & Gibson, W.P.R. (1979). Ocular tilt reaction with peripheral vestibular lesion. *Annals of Neurology, 6*;80–83.

Haupt, B.J., & Graves, E. (1982). *Detailed diagnosis and surgical procedures for patients discharged from short stay hospitals.* U.S. Dept. of Health and Human Services. DHHS Publication No. (PHS) 82–1274–1.

Hecker, H.C., Haug, C.O., & Herndon, J.W. (1974). Treatment of the vertiginous patient using cawthorne's vestibular exercises. *Laryngoscope, 84*;2065–2072.

Herdman, S.J. (1994). Assessment and management of bilateral vestibular loss. In: S.J. Herdman (Ed.), *Vestibular rehabilitation* (pp. 316–330). Philadelphia: FA Davis Co.

Herdman, S.J. (1997). Advances in the treatment of vestibular disorders. *Physical Therapy, 77*(6);602–617.

Herdman, S.J., Tusa, R.J., Zee, D.S., Proctor, L.R., & Mattox, D.E. (1993). Single treatment approaches to benign paroxysmal positional vertigo. *Archives of Otolaryngology–Head and Neck Surgery, 119*;450–454.

Hoffman, D., O'Leary, D., & Munjack, D. (1994). Autorotation tests abnormalities of the horizontal and vertical vestibulo-ocular reflex in panic disorder. *Archives of Otolaryngology–Head and Neck Surgery, 110*;259–269.

Hood, J.D. (1970). The clinical significance of vestibular rehabilitation. *Annals of Otology, Rhinology, and Laryngology, 17*;149–157.

Horak, F.B., Jones-Rycewicz, C., Black, F.O., & Shumway-Cook, A. (1992). Effects of vestibular rehabilitation on dizziness and imbalance. *Archives of Otolaryngology–Head and Neck Surgery, 106*;175–180.

Igarashi, M. (1984). Vestibular compensation: An overview. *Acta Otolaryngologica (Stockholm) Supplement, 406*;78–82.

Igarashi, M., Levy, J.K., O-Uchi, T., & Reschke, M.F. (1981). Further study of physical exercise and locomotor balance compensation after unilateral labyrinthectomy in squirrel monkeys. *Acta Otolaryngologica, 92*;101–105.

Jacob, R.G. (1988). Panic disorder and the vestibular system. *Psychiatric Clinics of North America, 11*(2);361–374.

Jacobson, G.P., & Newman, C.W. (1990). The development of the dizziness handicap inventory. *Archives of Otolaryngology–Head and Neck Surgery, 116*;424–427.

J.C. (1952). Living without a balancing mechanism. *New England Journal of Medicine, 246*;458–460.

Kasai, T., & Zee, D. (1978). Eye-head coordination in labyrinthine-defective human beings. *Brain Research, 144*;123–141.

Keshner, E.A. (1994). Postural abnormalities in vestibular disorders. In: S.J. Herdman (Ed.), *Vestibular rehabilitation* (pp. 47–67). Philadelphia: F.A. Davis Co.

Khater, T.T., Baker, J.F., & Peterson, B.W. (1990). Dynamics of adaptive change in human vestibulo-ocular reflex direction. *Journal of Vestibular Research, 1*;23–29.

Kroenke, K., Arrington, M.E., & Mangelsdorff, A.D. (1990). The prevalence of symptoms in medical outpatients and the adequacy of therapy. *Archives of Internal Medicine, 150*;1685–1689.

Kroenke, K., Lucas, C.A., Rosenberg, M.L., Scherokman, B., Herbers, J.E., Wehrle, P.A., & Boggi, J.O. (1992) Causes of persistent dizziness: A prospective study of 100 patients in ambulatory care. *Annals of Internal Medicine, 117*(11); 898–905.

Lacour, M., Roll, J.P., & Appaix, M. (1976). Modifications and development of spinal reflexes in the alert baboon (*Papio papio*) after a unilateral vestibular neurectomy. *Brain Research, 113*;255–269.

Leigh, R.J., & Brandt, T. (1993). A re-evaluation of the vestibulo-ocular reflex: New ideas of its purpose, properties, neural substrate, and disorders. *Neurology, 43*;1288–1295.

Leigh, R.J., Sawyer, R.N., Grant, M.P., & Seidman, S.H. (1992). High-frequency vestibuloocular reflex as a diagnostic tool. *Annals of the New York Academy of Science, 656*;305–314.

Leigh, R.J., Sharpe, J.A., Ranalli, P.J., Thurston, S.E., & Hamid, M.A. (1987). Comparison of smooth pursuit and combined eye-head tracking in human subjects with deficient labyrinthine function. *Experiments in Brain Research, 66*;458–464.

Leigh, R.J., & Zee, D.S. (1991). *The neurology of eye movements.* (2nd ed.). Philadelphia: F.A. Davis Co.

Lempert, T., & Tiel-Wilck, K. (1996). Positional maneuver for treatment of horizontal-canal benign positional vertigo. *Laryngoscope, 106*;476–478.

Li, J.C. (1995). Mastoid oscillation: A critical factor for success in the canalith repositioning procedure. *Otolaryngology–Head and Neck Surgery, 112*;670–675.

Lisberger, S. (1988). The neural basis for learning of simple motor skills. *Science, 242*;728–735.

Longridge, N.S., & Mallinson, A.I. (1984) A discussion of the dynamic illegible "E" test: A new method of screening aminoglycoside vestibulotoxicity. *Archives of Otolaryngology–Head and Neck Surgery, 92*;671–677

Lynn, S., Pool, A., Rose, D., Brey, R., & Suman, V. (1995). Randomized trial of the canalith repositioning procedure. *Archives of Otolaryngology–Head and Neck Surgery, 113*(6);712–719.

Manning, C., Scandale, L., Manning, E.J., & Gengo, F.M. (1992). Central nervous system effects of meclizine and dimenhydrate: Evidence of acute tolerance to antihistimines. *Journal of Clinical Pharmacology, 32*;996–1002.

Mathog, R.H., & Peppard, S.B. (1982). Exercise and recovery from vestibular injury. *American Journal of Otolaryngology, 3*;397–407.

McCabe, B.F. (1970). Labyrinthine exercises in the treatment of diseases characterized by vertigo: Their physiologic basis and methodology. *Laryngoscope, 80*;1429–1433.

Medicare Newsletter. (1997). Physical medicine and rehabilitation (pp. 13–22). Ohio: Nationwide Insurance.

Mira, E., Valli, S., Zucca, G., & Valli, P. (1996). Why do episodes of benign paroxysmal positioning vertigo recover spontaneously? *Journal of Vestibular Research-Equil Orient, 6*(4s);S49.

Nashner, L. (undated) The case for balance centers. *Neurocommunication International Literature.*

Norre, M.E., & Beckers, A. (1987). Exercise treatment for paroxysmal positional vertigo: Comparison of two types of exercise. *Annals of Otology, Rhinology, and Laryngology, 244*;291–294.

NORRE, M.E., & BECKERS, A. (1988). Comparative study of two types of exercise treatment for paroxysmal positioning vertigo. *Annals of Otology, Rhinology, and Laryngology, 42;*287–289.

NORRE, M.E., & DeWEERDT, W. (1980). Treatment of vertigo based on habituation: Technique and results for habituatuion training. *Journal of Laryngology and Otology, 94;* 971–977.

NORRE, M.E., FORREZ, G., & BECKERS, A. (1987). Vestibular habituation training and posturography in benign paroxysmal positioning vertigo. *Archives of Otology, Rhinology, and Laryngology, 49;*22–25.

PARNES, L.S., & McCLURE, J.A. (1990). Posterior semicircular canal occlusion for intractable benign positional vertigo. *Annals of Otology, Rhinology, and Laryngology, 99;*330–333.

PARNES, L.S., & ROBICHAUD, J. (1997). Further observations during the particle repositioning maneuver for benign paroxysmal positional vertigo. *Archives of Otolaryngology–Head and Neck Surgery, 116*(2);238–243.

PFALTZ, C.R. (1983). Vestibular compensation. *Acta Otolaryngologica, 95;*402–406.

PFALTZ, C.R., & KAMATH, R. (1971). The problem of central compensation of peripheral vestibular disorders. *Acta Otolaryngologica, 71:*266–272.

PRECHT, W., SHIMAZU, H., & MARKHAM, C. (1966). A mechanism of central compensation of vestibular function after hemilabyrinthectomy. *Journal of Neurophysiology, 29;*996–1010.

ROBINSON, D., ZEE, D.S., HAIN, T.C., HOLMES, A., & ROSENBUG, L. (1984). Alexander's law: Its behavior and origin in the human vestibulo-ocular reflex. *Annals of Neurology, 16*(6);714–722.

SAMA, A., MEIKLE, J.C.E., & JONES, N.S. (1995). Hyperventilation and dizziness: Case reports and management. *British Journal of Clinical Psychology, 49*(2):79–82.

SAWYER, R.M., THURSTON, S.E., BECKER, K.R., ACKLEY, C.V., SEIDMAN, S.H., & LEIGH, J.R. (1994). The cervico-ocular reflex of normal human subjects in response to transient and sinusoidal trunk rotations. *Journal of Vestibular Research, 4*(3);245–249.

SCHUKNECHT, H.F. (1969). Cupulolithiasis. *Archives of Otolaryngology—Head and Neck Surgery, 90;*765–778.

SEMONT, A., FREYSS, G., VITTE, E. (1988). Curing the BPPV with a liberatory maneuver. *Annals of Otology, Rhinology, and Laryngology, 42;*290–293.

SERAFINI, G., PALMIERI, A.M.R., & SIMONCELLI, C. (1996). Benign paroxysmal positional vertigo of posterior semicircular canal: Results in 160 cases treated with Semont's maneuver. *Annals of Otology, Rhinology, and Laryngology, 105;*770–774.

SHEPARD, N.T., & TELIAN, S.A. (1995). Programmatic vestibular rehabilitation. *Archives of Otolaryngology–Head and Neck Surgery, 112*(1);173–182.

SHEPARD, N.T., & TELIAN, S.A. (1996). *Practical management of the balance disorder patient.* San Diego: Singular Publishing Group.

SHEPARD, N.T., TELIAN, S.A., & SMITH-WEELOCK, M. (1990). Habituation and balance retraining therapy: A retrospective review. *Neurology Clinics, 8*(2);459–475.

SHEPARD, N.T., TELIAN, S.A., & SMITH-WHEELOCK, M. (1993). Vestibular and balance rehabilitation therapy. *Annals of Otology, Rhinology, and Laryngology, 102;*198–205.

SKLARE, D.A., STEIN, M.B., PIKUS, A.M., & UHDE, T.W. (1990). Dysequilibrium and audiovestibular function in panic disorder: Symptom profiles and test findings. *American Journal of Otology, 11*(5);338–341.

SLOANE, P.D. (1989). Dizziness in primary care: Results from the national ambulatory medical care survey. *Journal of Family Practice, 29*(1); 33–38.

SLOANE, P.D., DALLARA, J., ROACH, C., BAILEY, K.E., MITCHELL, M., & McNUTT, R. (1994). Management of dizziness in primary care. *Journal of the American Board of Family Practitioners, 7;*1–8.

SMITH, P.F., & CURTHOYS, I.S. (1989). Mechanisms of recovery after unilateral labyrinthectomy: A review. *Brain Research Review, 14;*155–180.

SMITH, P.F., DARLINGTON, C.L., & CURTHOYS, I.S. (1986). The effect of visual deprivation on vestibular compensation in the guinea pig. *Brain Research, 364;*195–198.

STEDDIN, S., & BRANDT, T. (1996). Horizontal canal benign paroxysmal positéioning vertigo (h-bppv): Transition of canalithiasis to cupulolithiasis. *Annals of Neurology, 40;*918–922.

STEENERSON, R., & CRONIN, G. (1996). Comparison of the canalith repositioning procedure and vestibular habituation training in forty patients with benign paroxysmal positional vertigo. *Archives of Otolaryngology–Head and Neck Surgery, 114*(1);61–64.

STOCKWELL, C. (1996). Tutorial on the three forms of benign positional vertigo. *(BPV) ICS Tutorial,* April.

STROM, K. (1996). Understanding the senior market: A statistical profile. *Hearing Review, 3*(10);8–66.

SZTURM, T., IRELAND, D.J., & LESSING-TURNER, M. (1994). Comparison of different exercise programs in the rehabilitation of patients with chronic peripheral vestibular dysfunction. *Journal of Vestibular Research, 4*(6);461–479.

TIDEIKSAAR, R. (1989). Medical causes of falling. In: R. Tideiksaar (Ed.), *Falling in old age: Its prevention and treatment* (pp. 21–47). New York: Springer Publishing Co.

TINETTI, M.E., & WILLIAMS, C.S. (1997). Falls, injuries due to falls, and risk of admission to a nursing home. *New England Journal of Medicine, 337*(18);1279–1284.

TOUPET, M., & SEMONT, A. (1985). La physiotherapie du vertige paroxystique bénin. In: R. Hausler (Ed.), *Les vertiges d'origine périphérique et centrale* (pp. 21–27). Paris: Ipsen.

WATSON, M.A., & SINCLAIR, H. (1992). *Balancing act.* Portland, OR: Vestibular Disorders Association.

WEBSTER'S NEW WORLD DICTIONARY. (1976). Cleveland: William Collins & World Publishing Co.

WEINDRUCH, R., KROPER, S., & HADLEY, E. (1989). The prevalence of dysequilibrium and related disorders in older persons. *Ear Nose and Throat Journal, 68*(12);925–929.

ZEE, D. (1985). Perspectives on the pharmocotherapy of vertigo. *Archives of Otolaryngology—Head and Neck Surgery, 111;*609–612.

ZEE, D.S. (1994). Vestibular adaptation. In: S.J. Herdman (Ed.), *Vestibular rehabilitation* (pp. 68–79). Philadelphia: F.A. Davis Co.

PREFERRED PRACTICE GUIDELINES

Professionals Who Perform the Procedure(s)

▼ Audiologists

▼ Physical therapists

▼ Occupational therapists

Expected Outcomes

▼ The patient understands the results of vestibular evaluation and balance assessment.

▼ The patient understands the potential and limitations of vestibular rehabilitation.

▼ The patient is given the tools, or exercises, to promote vestibular compensation, understanding that each patient will adapt in a unique manner.

▼ The patient will be given encouragement and guidance during and after the therapy program.

Clinical Indications

▼ Vestibular rehabilitation is appropriate for any patient with functional or physical limitations related to impairment of the peripheral or central vestibular system.

Clinical Process

▼ Vestibular evaluation and pretherapy assessment.

▼ Subjective self-assessment and self-rating scales before initiating therapy.

▼ Exercises designed to enhance recovery of the vestibular-ocular reflex, adaptive gaze stabilization strategies, and sensory substitution.

▼ Exercises should be made progressively more demanding throughout the therapy program.

▼ Objective and subjective outcome measures at the end of scheduled therapy program.

▼ Long-term use of conditioning exercises to maintain level of compensation.

▼ Counseling regarding the possibility and likely causes of periods of decompensation.

Documentation

▼ Include the patient's initial complaints, pertinent medical history, and results of formal vestibular evaluation.

▼ Include a therapy plan describing goals of therapy, specific exercises, patient's performance ratings and plans for future sessions.

▼ Include pretherapy and posttherapy objective and subjective ratings used for outcome measures.

Chapter 22

Hearing Protection Devices*

Elliott H. Berger and John G. Casali

Outline

A hearing protection device (HPD) is a personal safety product that is worn to reduce the harmful auditory or annoying effects of sound. Hearing protectors are often a method of last resort when other means, such as engineering controls or removal of the person from the noisy environment, are not practical or economical. To a large extent, research and development in hearing protection began during and after World War II in response to the tremendous hearing loss caused by military weapons. Hearing conservation programs and use of hearing protection in the military and industry followed in the early 1950s and proliferated in the early 1970s and then again in the 1980s (OSHA, 1983) in response to federal regulations mandating use of hearing protection in occupational settings.

This chapter, which begins by describing HPDs and how to dispense and use them, continues with the more technical issues of hearing protector physics, and measurement and performance assessment. It also includes guidance on how to estimate protection and the effects of HPDs on auditory perception, and concludes with mention of special types of HPDs and relevant standards and regulations.

TYPES OF HEARING PROTECTION DEVICES

HPDs may be broadly categorized into *earplugs*, which are placed into the earcanal to form a seal and block sound,

---

*This chapter is based on a prior work by E. H. Berger & J. G. Casali. (1997). Hearing protection devices. In: M. J. Crocker (Ed.), *Encyclopedia of acoustics* (pp. 967–981). New York: John Wiley & Sons. It also draws, for additional information, on a more comprehensive manuscript, Berger, E. H. (2000). Hearing protection devices. In: E. H. Berger, L. H. Royster, J. D. Royster, D. Driscoll, & M. Layne (Eds.), *The noise manual* (5th ed.). Fairfax, VA: American Industrial Hygiene Association.

Audiology: Treatment. Edited by Valente, Hosford-Dunn, and Roeser. Thieme Medical Publishers, Inc., New York © 2000

earmuffs, which fit over and around the ears (circumaural) to provide an acoustic seal against the head, and *helmets*, which normally encase the entire head. Although in special cases, acoustical concerns may dictate the selection of a particular type of HPD, normally ergonomic considerations, personal preference, or compatibility with other safety gear and job requirements, are the deciding factors.

Earplugs

Earplugs are made from materials such as slow-recovery closed-cell foam, vinyl, silicone, elastomer formulations, spun fiberglass, and cotton/wax combinations. They are available in a wide variety of types and styles, some of which are shown in Figure 22–1.

Foam earplugs, also called "roll-down" foam earplugs to emphasize the fact that such products must be rolled and compressed before insertion, are made from slow-recovery foam materials that expand, once inserted into the earcanal, to create an acoustic seal. *Premolded earplugs* are formed from flexible materials into conical, bulbous, or other shapes, often including flanges or sealing rings, which are typically affixed to or enshroud a flexible stem for handling and insertion. They usually are available in a range of sizes to fit most ears and are pushed into place in the earcanal, whereupon a seal is made against the canal walls. By contrast, *formable earplugs*, which are made from materials such as fiberglass and silicone putty, are pressed into the canal and forced to deform to seal the canal at its entrance. *Custom-molded earplugs* are manufactured from an individual impression of the earcanal, which must precisely match the shape of the canal to create a seal and block the noise.

A final type of earplug is the *semi-insert* (also called semi-aural, canal caps, or concha seated), which consists of soft pods held in place against or slightly inside the rim of the earcanal by a lightweight band. They are easily stored around the neck when not in use.

Earmuffs

Earmuffs normally consist of rigid molded plastic earcups that completely enclose and seal around the outer ear (also called the pinna) using foam-filled or fluid-filled cushions. The earcups are held in place by an adjustable headband or by short spring-loaded arms attached to a hard hat or other headgear. Headbands, which may be of plastic or metal construction, may function in only a single position or be "universal," suited for use over the head, behind the neck, or under the chin. The earcups are lined with acoustical material, typically foam, to absorb high-frequency (>2000 Hz) energy within the cup.

Helmets

Helmets enclose a substantial portion of the head and are usually designed primarily for impact protection. When they contain circumaural earcups or a dense liner to seal around the ears, they can also provide beneficial amounts of hearing protection. The most common applications of the dual function helmet for impact and hearing protection is in the military, an example being a flight crew helmet. Such devices also normally include two-way communication systems.

DISPENSING, FITTING, USE, AND CARE

Initial Dispensing or Purchase

Initial dispensing of HPDs within an occupational hearing conservation program has a substantial effect on the efficacy of the overall hearing conservation effort. It is best accomplished one-on-one or in small groups, with a student/instructor ratio of no more than 5:1 so that the compatibility and fit of protectors can be individually checked on each employee (Royster & Royster, 1985).

With the aid of a focused light source (such as an otoscope, earlight, or penlight), a visual inspection of the external ear and head should be made to identify medical or anatomical conditions that might interfere with or be aggravated by the hearing protector (e.g., inflammation, tenderness, excessive or impacted cerumen). When such conditions are present, medical consultation or corrective treatment should be obtained (Berger, 1985).

When consumers purchase HPDs for occasional nonoccupational use, it is usually neither feasible nor necessary to have an ear examination before purchase or use. However, if ear pain or other aural symptoms develop or if discomfort persists, use should be discontinued until audiological or medical advice is obtained. In addition, other brands or types of HPDs may need to be evaluated until the one best suited to the individual is found.

Fitting Tips

Earplugs generally require more skill and attention than earmuffs during the initial issue, but a common mistake is to presume that earmuffs are foolproof and to dispense them indiscriminately without assistance. Quite to the contrary, earmuffs must also be evaluated for fit when initially issued because not every wearer can be fit by all models or sometimes by any model. Circumaural irregularities may be so great that the cushions cannot properly seal to the head, heads may be so large or small that the bands cannot be extended or retracted sufficiently to accommodate, or pinnae may be so large that the cups cannot be comfortably fitted around them. Instructions for use must be reviewed and fitting must be demonstrated.

The wearer should be exposed to noise during the fitting procedure, when possible, so he or she can hear the noise diminish to the lowest perceived level while adjusting the HPD. A portable cassette player can be used to present recordings of broadband noise or representative industrial sounds. For all types of earplugs, insertion is easier when the pinna is pulled *outward* and *upward* with the hand opposite the ear that is being fitted as shown in Figure 22–2.

Earplugs should be inserted into the right ear using the right hand and into the left ear using the left hand. This allows the hand inserting the earplug to have the best line of approach to the earcanal.

Foam earplugs are prepared for insertion by rolling them into a *very thin* crease-free cylinder. This is accomplished by squeezing lightly as one begins rolling, and then applying progressively greater pressure as the plug becomes more tightly compressed. Unlike other types of earplugs, foam earplugs should not be readjusted while in the ear. If the

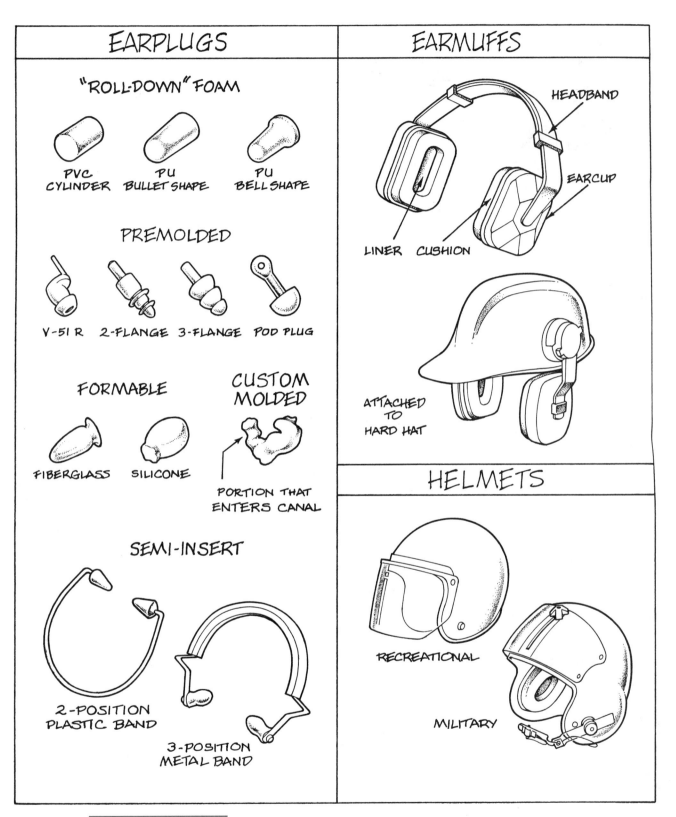

Figure 22–1 Personal hearing protection devices.

initial fit is unacceptable, they should be removed, rerolled, and reinserted.

A properly inserted premolded earplug will generally create a blocked-up feeling because of the requisite airtight seal. When the seal is present, suction should be felt if an attempt is made to withdraw the plug from the canal.

The Occlusion Effect and Its Use as a Test for Fit

The occlusion effect is the increase in efficiency with which bone-conducted sound is transmitted to the ear at frequencies less than 2000 Hz when the earcanal is occluded and sealed with an earplug or an earmuff. This effect causes wearers of HPDs to experience a change in the perceived loudness and quality of their own voice and other body-generated sounds or vibrations, such as chewing, breathing, and walking.

The effect is easily demonstrated by plugging one's ears with the fingers while reading aloud. The voice will appear to have added fullness or resonant bassness. Wearers also describe the change in quality as deeper, hollow, or muffled. The occlusion effect is often cited as an objectionable characteristic of wearing hearing protection. Its magnitude varies with the way in which the ear is occluded and may be reduced by adjusting earplugs toward a deeper insertion or selecting earmuffs with larger volume earcups. The maximum effect occurs for semi-inserts and supra-aural devices (those that rest on the pinna but do not enclose it).

Listening for the presence (*not* the magnitude) of the occlusion effect is a useful technique for fitting nearly all types of HPDs. A wearer conducts the fit test for either earplugs or earmuffs by humming or repeating loudly the words "boom beat," while listening for the change in voice quality, which results from creating an acoustical seal and generating the associated occlusion effect.

Comfort

Comfort is a critical feature of an HPD, equivalent in importance to the attenuation that the device can provide. Although comfort assessments are of necessity subjective in nature, research in recent years has been directed at quantifying the important parameters (Casali, 1992).

An HPD that is uncomfortable will not be worn consistently and correctly or perhaps will not be worn at all. Comfort can be improved by properly matching the device to the wearer and by providing instruction in its proper use. Common sources of discomfort include improperly sized or inserted earplugs, overly tight earmuff headbands, worn-out devices with hardened/cracked cushions or stiffened/ragged flanges, and the use of earmuffs in very hot environments.

HPDs are personal items that must be dispensed accordingly. Users should be involved in the selection process by allowing them to choose from a variety of suitable options, including a minimum of four different devices, consisting of at least one earmuff and two types of earplugs. It takes time for even seasoned HPD wearers to become accustomed to new devices, both how they feel and how they "sound." Novice users may require a week or two to fully adapt to the feeling of wearing HPDs and to appreciate the benefits that their use provides.

Hygiene and Maintenance

HPDs should be cleaned regularly according to manufacturers' instructions. Normally, warm water and mild soap are satisfactory cleansing agents. Earplugs should be washed and dried thoroughly before reuse or storage, although some earplugs, such as those made from putty, silicone resin, or spun fiberglass, are not designed for washing. Earmuff cushions should be periodically wiped or washed clean. When they cannot be adequately cleaned or no longer retain their original appearance or resiliency, earmuff cushions and earplugs should be replaced.

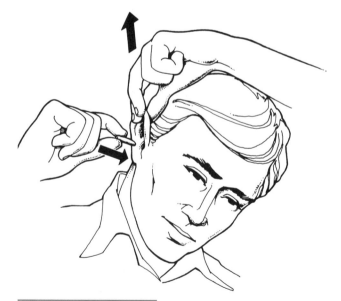

Figure 22–2 Method of pulling the outer ear (pinna) both outward (away from the head) and upward for easier and more effective insertion of earplugs. Note the pinna is grasped between thumb and opposing fingers.

Although the likelihood of hearing protection devices increasing the incidence of outer ear infections is minimal (Berger, 1985), such ear infections may occur. Earplugs or earmuffs that may be implicated are commonly found to be contaminated with caustic or irritating substances or are embedded with sharp or abrasive materials. Medically trained personnel should be consulted to determine whether persistent ear infections are associated with hearing protection devices or with other predisposing factors unrelated to the wearing of HPDs.

The headbands on earmuffs and semi-insert earplugs may lose their force with time or be purposely sprung to reduce force and increase comfort. This will degrade attenuation. Regular inspection of HPDs and proper instructions to the users are necessary to overcome this problem.

Safety

Commercially available HPDs are safe to wear as long as the manufacturers' recommendations are followed; however, some precautions are advisable. Earplugs that create an airtight seal, such as premolded inserts, should be removed with a slow twisting or rocking motion to gradually break the seal as they are withdrawn to ensure that removal does not cause pain or harm to the ear. When corded earplugs (two earplugs attached by a common cord for ease of handling) are worn, the cord must be draped in such a way that it does not hang loose where it might become caught or snagged. Smaller, lightweight earmuffs with lower profiles will normally be less likely to interfere with workers' activities than their larger counterparts.

SOUND PATHWAYS TO THE OCCLUDED EAR

In the *un*occluded ear, the dominant sound path for external sounds is along the earcanal to the eardrum. However, in the occluded ear four distinct and important paths by which sound can penetrate the HPD can be identified as described below.

Air Leaks

For maximum protection, HPDs must make a virtually airtight seal with the walls of the earcanal or the circumaural regions surrounding the pinna. Air-leakage paths can reduce attenuation by 5- to 15-dB over a broad range of frequencies, depending on the type of hearing protector and the size of the leak. Typically the loss is most noticeable at low frequencies.

Hearing Protector Vibration

Because of the flexibility of the earcanal flesh, earplugs can vibrate in a pistonlike manner, thus limiting their low-frequency attenuation. Earmuffs, too, vibrate as a mass/spring system, the stiffness of the spring depending on the dynamic characteristics of the earmuff cushion and the circumaural flesh, as well as the volume of the air entrapped inside the earcup. These actions limit low-frequency attenuation. Representative maximum values at 125 Hz for

earmuffs, premolded earplugs, and foam earplugs are 25 dB, 30 dB, and 40 dB, respectively.

Structural Transmission

In much the same way as sound will propagate through any barrier, so too will it pass through an HPD, albeit with diminished intensity. The transmission depends on the mass, stiffness, and internal damping of the HPD materials, including in the case of earmuffs the cushion liner and bladder, as well as the acoustical absorption within earcups. The limitations caused by this transmission path are most pronounced above 1000 Hz.

Bone and Tissue Conduction

Even if an HPD were completely effective in blocking the preceding pathways, the sound would still reach the inner ear by bone and tissue conduction, thus imposing a limit on the maximum real-ear attenuation that a device can provide. However, because that limit is 40- to 50-dB below the sound level reaching the ear through the open earcanal, it does not become important unless attenuation of the HPD itself approaches such values. This is not often the case unless dual HPDs are worn (see section "Dual Protection" and Fig. 22–3).

MEASURING ATTENUATION

In excess of a dozen different methods of measuring HPD attenuation have been described in the literature, but only a few have been found practical and reliable and are commonly used (Berger, 1986).

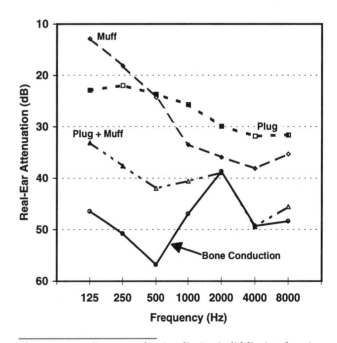

Figure 22–3 Bone-conduction limits *(solid line)* to hearing protector attenuation and an example of attenuation provided by an earplug, earmuff, and the two devices worn together.

Laboratory Procedures

Hearing protector research is usually conducted under laboratory conditions. This allows the experimenter to exert the most control over the relevant parameters of which he or she is aware and provides the best assurance of generating repeatable test data. However, even the most accurate of the laboratory methods will only provide data representative of field (real-world) protection to the extent that (a) the HPD is fit and worn by the subjects in the same manner as by wearers in practice, and (b) the test population is representative of the actual users.

Real-Ear Attenuation at Threshold

The most common, and also one of the most accurate, HPD attenuation test is the measurement of real-ear attenuation at threshold (REAT) as specified in numerous national and international standards (ANSI S3.19-1974; ANSI S12.6-1997; ISO 4869-1:1990). Virtually all available manufacturers' reported data have been derived by this method, and it is the procedure required by the Environmental Protection Agency (EPA) to obtain data for computation of the Noise Reduction Rating (NRR).

REAT is a measurement of the difference between the minimum level of sound that a subject can hear without wearing an HPD (open threshold) and the level needed when the HPD is worn (occluded threshold). The difference between the two thresholds, the threshold shift, is a measure of the real-ear attenuation provided by the device. This method accurately represents the performance of all conventional HPDs (those that provide constant attenuation regardless of sound level [i.e., level-*in*dependent HPDs]). For those HPDs whose attenuation increases with level (i.e., level-*de*pendent HPDs), REAT usually provides a lower-bound estimate. Application of REAT data to high-level impulsive sources is somewhat questionable (ANSI, 1997; see also section "Impulse and Weapon Noise"). The only procedural artifact that is known to distort REAT results is masking of the occluded thresholds by physiological noise. This spuriously elevates the low-frequency attenuation (below 500 Hz) by a few decibels, with the error increasing as frequency decreases (Berger, 1986; Schroeter & Poesselt, 1986).

Since promulgation of ANSI S3.19 in 1974, U.S. REAT standards have specified that measurements are to be conducted in a diffuse sound field (i.e., fields with uniform energy distribution and randomly distributed direction of propagation of sound) using 1/3-octave bands of noise and a minimum of 10 subjects whose open and occluded thresholds are measured three times each. This results in multiple data points at each frequency, from which a mean attenuation and a standard deviation (SD) are computed, the latter parameter providing an indication of the variability in attenuation across subjects and replications. The mean attenuation represents protection that approximately 50% of the test subjects meet or exceed. When it is appropriate to estimate the protection that a greater percentage of the subjects attain, adjustments to the mean may be computed by subtracting one or more standard deviations (see section "Using Attenuation Data to Estimate Protection").

Historically, hearing protector standards committees have been primarily concerned with the precision of HPD attenuation measurements (i.e., the repeatability of the data) both within and between laboratories. Although this is certainly an important issue, experience has shown that undue emphasis on precision and the attendant efforts to involve the experimenter to "control" the testing, with a consequent lack of regard for accuracy or "realism," may lead to data of questionable utility. By definition, "useful" data should predict with a reasonable accuracy the protection that can typically, or even optimally, be expected to be achieved in practice (Berger, 1992).

CONTROVERSIAL POINT

In the past it was argued that careful experimenter controls during REAT evaluations, with the intention of reducing the within-test standard deviations as much as possible, led to repeatable and useful data. Research in the past decade has demonstrated this is counterproductive and leads to data that are of little value in estimating field performance under typical real-world conditions.

Regardless of the attention of standards writing groups to issues of precision, the variability of test data across multiple measurements within a given facility ("repeatability") or across measurements made in different facilities ("reproducibility") has been a problem. The most recent interlaboratory study on this topic (Royster et al, 1996), which led to the development of the new HPD attenuation standard that includes a procedure with improved precision (ANSI, 1997; and see discussion of Method B, below) found a range of attenuation values for three different earplugs and one earmuff across four laboratories of about 5- to 8-dB in the octave-band data. In terms of the NRR the range was 3- to 8-dB for the earplugs and 2 dB for an earmuff. With this in mind, it is clearly absurd for purchasers of hearing protectors to place great emphasis on small differences in the NRRs of competing products.

The latest version of the U.S. standard provides a substantial departure from prior U.S. standards for measuring HPD attenuation in that it recognizes the importance of providing useful data (ANSI, 1997). This is accomplished by defining two testing procedures, Method A (experimenter-supervised fit) and Method B (subject fit). Method A corresponds most closely to tests using prior U.S. standards and is useful in the design of hearing protectors to provide a theoretical understanding of their performance limitations and for routine testing for quality assurance purposes. By contrast, Method B is intended to provide "an approximation of the upper limits to the attenuation that can be expected for groups of occupational users." The standard goes on to acknowledge that properly trained and motivated individuals can potentially attain larger amounts of protection. However, subject-fit values provide a closer correspondence to real-world performance for groups of users than do the experimenter-supervised fit data.

The 1997 ANSI standard is recent and has not yet been referenced in the now elderly EPA hearing protector labeling regulation (EPA, 1979). The regulation still calls for testing to the 1974 ANSI standard, which uses a fitting procedure even more artificially controlled than Method A of S12.6-1997, namely a strict experimenter-fit interpretation of ANSI S3.19 (ANSI, 1974). It will be some time before users are routinely able to access 1997 Method B data (see section "Attenuation Characteristics of Hearing Protection Devices").

Microphone in Real-Ear

The microphone in real-ear (MIRE) method uses physical (acoustical) measurements to determine either the difference between the sound pressure levels (SPLs) in the human earcanal, with and without the HPD in place, termed *insertion loss*, or the difference between the SPLs outside and underneath the HPD, termed *noise reduction*. Of necessity, insertion loss measurements must be recorded sequentially for the protected and unprotected conditions, but noise reduction data can be acquired with two simultaneous measurements. Hence, this method is ideally adapted for field use. For insertion loss, the levels are measured by means of a miniature or probe microphone at the entrance to, or sometimes in, the earcanal itself (ANSI, 1995), and the subject who wears the HPD is required to sit still and behave as an inanimate acoustic test fixture. With the noise-reduction approach, the exterior microphone is generally mounted on the earmuff itself.

The insertion-loss form of MIRE measurements can be viewed as an objective type of REAT because in both cases a difference in levels is measured at one point in the auditory system. MIRE data do not suffer from the physiological-noise contamination discussed previously with respect to REAT, and thus tend to show lower (more accurate) values of attenuation in the low frequencies. However, MIRE suffers some of its own artifactual errors in the higher frequencies (Berger, 1986).

MIRE can be used to measure attenuation for all types of hearing protectors, including those fitted with electronics; difficulties can arise with earplugs because of the problems of inserting both a microphone and an earplug simultaneously into the earcanal (Smoorenburg, 1996). The MIRE method is much less time consuming than REAT testing and provides an acceptable alternative, especially when measurements are required at high sound levels such as needed for investigation of the response of HPDs to weapons fire and explosions. Although MIRE values are objective and thus obviate inconsistencies in the subjects' threshold responses, they do include their own measurement error as a result of positioning of the microphones; MIRE derived SDs are less than or equal to those found with REAT procedures (Berger & Kerivan, 1983; Berger et al, 1996; Casali et al, 1995).

Acoustical Test Fixture

The acoustical test fixture (ATF) method is directly analogous to the MIRE method, except that an inanimate fixture is used in place of a test subject (ANSI, 1995). The ATF incorporates a microphone at the approximate eardrum location and, depending on its sophistication, may match the impedance of the eardrum (through a suitable acoustic coupler) and also include simulations of the circumaural and earcanal tissues.

ATF measurements provide a quick assessment for product development, quality control, and acceptance testing of earmuffs and helmets and have also been successfully used to explore the level-dependent response of passive and active types of HPDs (Dancer et al, 1996). Although substantial gains have been made in ATF modeling and design (Kunov et al, 1986; Schroeter, 1986), measurements of earplugs are still problematical, and for all devices the data are generally not suitable for direct prediction of real-ear attenuation values. In all cases modeling of the bone-conduction pathways is incorporated as a postmeasurement mathematical correction because the difficulties of physically incorporating the necessary mechanical elements to mimic the response of the human skull have not been overcome.

Field Procedures

Generally, the best of the laboratory procedures, modified to reduce cost and improve portability and ruggedness, are those that are used under field conditions. The purpose is to derive more accurate estimates of the attenuation provided by HPDs under actual use. The procedures that have been most successfully used are sound field REAT in a manner similar to that described in the existing standards (ANSI, 1997; ISO, 1990), REAT conducted using large circumaural cups for the stimulus presentation instead of loudspeakers in a defined acoustical space, and the MIRE approach with microphones simultaneously mounted on the inside and outside of earmuffs.

When the REAT-type procedures are implemented, workers are usually selected without warning from their place of work and accompanied to a test site with care taken to ensure they do not readjust their HPDs prior to testing. For the MIRE procedure, the instrumented earmuffs are used to simultaneously measure the protected and unprotected noise doses received by the exposed workers.

Audiometric Database Analysis

Audiometric database analysis (ADBA) refers to the analysis of the annual audiometric data, which are recorded by law as a part of U.S. occupational hearing conservation programs (OSHA, 1983). Although ADBA does not provide a direct estimation of the in-field attenuation of HPDs, it provides one of the best indicators of the adequacy of a company's hearing conservation effort and of the HPDs being used in their program (ANSI, 1991).

ATTENUATION CHARACTERISTICS OF HEARING PROTECTION DEVICES

The attenuation provided by a hearing protector is strongly controlled by the way in which the wearer or test subject fits the device, especially for insert-type devices (Casali & Lam, 1986). This leads to a wide variation in reported attenuation, even in the case of purportedly "optimum fit" data measured in the laboratory (Berger et al, 1982). Thus comparison of published NRRs and rank ordering of HPDs can be substantially influenced as a function of the data being compared. Precise rank ordering is meaningful only for data from a single laboratory. Sources of interlaboratory variability are (1) differences in interpretation and implementation of the standardized measurement method, (2) uncertainty of obtaining the proper fit to avoid acoustic leaks, (3) differences in subject selection and training, and (4) differences in data reduction techniques.

The repeatability of attenuation measurements in the same laboratory is also subject to variation (but to a lesser extent than between laboratories). Principal determinants of this variability are changes in (1) the laboratory's personnel or their experience, (2) the subject population, (3) subject selection criteria, (4) HPD fitting and sizing techniques, and (5) the instrumentation.

Optimum Laboratory Performance

The values reported in this section and in Table 22–1 are representative of those obtained in laboratory-based REAT measurements, wherein the HPDs are either fitted by, or under the close supervision of, the experimenter. Highly motivated and trained individual users can potentially achieve the upper end of the attenuation values listed for each device in Table 22–1, but average values for groups of users will fall near or below

> ### SPECIAL CONSIDERATION
>
> **Differences in the labeled NRRs of competing products of less than 3 dB have no practical importance, as a consequence of the interlaboratory and intralaboratory variability discussed previously, and even changes of 4- to 5-dB are of questionable significance unless closely controlled data are being compared.**

the lower end of the ranges and will be better approximated by the data in the section "Real-World Attenuation."

A wide degree of overlap exists in attenuation among the various types of earplugs, but in general, formable slow-recovery foam earplugs provide among the highest overall protection of any single device. Their attenuation can range from 30- to 45-dB at and above 2000 Hz, and depending on the depth of insertion from about 20- to 40-dB below 2000 Hz. For many users even the higher values of attenuation can be achieved while still retaining an excellent degree of comfort. Attenuation of custom-molded earplugs can vary widely due

TABLE 22–1   Representative minimum and maximum mean attenuation values of well-fitted hearing protectors under laboratory conditions, in decibels

Type of Hearing Protector	Octave-Band Center Frequency (Hz)						
	125	250	500	1000	2000	4000	8000
Foam earplugs (attenuation varies with depth of insertion)	20–40	20–40	25–45	25–45	30–40	40–45	35–45
Premolded earplugs	20–30	20–30	20–30	20–35	25–35	30–45	30–45
Formable (fiberglass)	20–30	20–30	20–30	25–30	25–30	35–40	35–40
Formable (wax or silicone)	20–25	20–25	20–25	25–30	30–35	40–45	40–45
Custom-molded earplugs	15–35	15–35	15–35	20–35	30–40	35–45	30–45
Semi-insert earplugs	15–30	15–30	10–30	15–30	25–35	25–45	30–45
Earmuffs (with or without communications components)	5–20	10–25	15–40	25–45	30–40	30–40	25–40
Military helmets	0–15	5–15	15–25	15–30	25–40	30–50	20–50
Dual protection (earplugs + earmuffs)	20–40	25–45	25–50	30–50	35–45	40–50	40–50
Active noise reduction (closed-cup systems; identical to conventional muffs above 1000 Hz)	15–25	15–30	20–45	25–40	30–40	30–40	25–40
Cotton balls	0–5	0–10	5–10	5–10	10–15	10–20	10–20
Motorcycle helmets	0–5	0–5	0–10	0–15	5–20	10–30	15–35
Air-fed shotblasting helmets	0–5	0–5	0–5	0–15	15–25	15–30	15–25
Fingertips in earcanals	25–30	25–30	25–30	25–30	25–30	30–35	30–35

Data are intended to account for brand and testing variability; however, not all manufacturers' reported data or values referenced in the literature will necessarily fall within the ranges cited. All data are from E·A·RCAL Laboratory, except for the shotblasting helmets (Price & Whitaker, 1986) and fingertips (Holland, 1967).

to impression-taking and manufacturing procedures and differences in impression materials. On average, the attenuation of these devices tends to be similar to premolded and formable earplugs.

The attenuation of earmuffs is substantially controlled by earcup volume and mass, the area of the cup opening, headband force, and the size, shape, and material of the cushion. The attenuation usually increases about 8- to 9-dB/octave from 125 Hz to 1000 Hz, and at 2000 Hz approaches the limit imposed by bone conduction of approximately 40 dB (see Fig. 22–3). Above that frequency, attenuation averages around 35 dB. In general, earplugs, especially the roll-down foam variety, provide better attenuation than earmuffs below 500 Hz and equivalent or greater protection above 2000 Hz. At 1000 Hz, larger volume earmuffs will usually provide attenuation that exceeds that of earplugs.

The loss in earmuff attenuation that eyeglass temples create, with cushions in good condition, is normally 3- to 7-dB. The effect varies widely among earmuffs and the fit and style of the eyeglasses, with the losses in attenuation being reduced by thinner, closer-fitting temple pieces.

Helmets, unless they seal well around the head or contain internal circumaural cups, provide very little attenuation, especially at the frequencies below 2000 Hz. As shown in Table 22–1, typical motorcycle helmets provide less than 10 dB of protection below 1000 Hz and only from 10- to 35-dB at the higher frequencies, and air-fed shotblasting helmets perform similarly. Some military helmets (e.g., flight helmets) which possess an effective acoustical design yield attenuation that is comparable to conventional earmuffs but still about 5- to 10-dB less at the frequencies below 2000 Hz. From 4000 to 8000 Hz, military helmets can actually surpass earmuff attenuation by about 5 dB if they fully enclose the head since this decreases bone-conduction transmission at high frequencies.

The data in Table 22–1 suggest that in a pinch, for brief exposures, fingers can provide high levels of protection equivalent to that of most hearing protectors.

Real-World Attenuation

HPD attenuation in the workplace is much less than that typically measured in the laboratory. Laboratory measurements reflect the maximum attenuation that can be expected with a device that is worn under ideal circumstances, evaluated by closely supervised experienced subjects who properly fit and wear correctly sized HPDs, which are new and in good condition. By contrast, many of these factors are not, or cannot be, implemented in the workplace. This is partly because of the emphasis in most laboratory testing on obtaining maximum attenuation, disregard of comfort during fitting of protectors (primarily earplugs), and the short time periods that the test subjects wear the devices (5 to 10 minutes).

The disparity between laboratory and workplace attenuation values is also due to the fact that workplace performance usually falls short of what could reasonably be expected to be achieved. Poor workplace performance arises because of factors such as lack of wearer indoctrination and training, poor motivation, incorrect protector size and fit, slippage of HPDs during use, deterioration of devices, and HPD modifications by employees that degrade attenuation.

Numerous studies have been conducted in the field to assess real-world performance. The data in the next section are drawn from 22 such studies spanning seven countries, greater than 90 different industrial sites, and approximately 3000 worker/subjects (Berger et al, 1996). The results provide an excellent indication of the real-world performance of HPDs, circa 1990, that can be anticipated in the better industrial and military hearing conservation programs.

Comparative One-Third Octave-Band Data

Attenuation measured in the workplace, with actual workers as subjects, shows lower mean attenuation values (most notably for earplugs) and higher standard deviations (by a factor of 2 to 3) than do manufacturers' reported laboratory data. For example, mean attenuation values in the workplace are lower than laboratory data by approximately 15- to 20-dB for premolded earplugs, 10- to 15-dB for foam earplugs, and 5- to 10-dB for earmuffs. Earmuff performance in the workplace is better relative to earplugs than would be predicted from laboratory data (Park & Casali, 1991), but regardless of the HPD that is selected, individual noise exposure can be substantially underestimated when it is computed from laboratory attenuation values (see Fig. 22–4).

Comparative Noise Reduction Rating Data

Whether attenuation is estimated using the laboratory octave-band data or by a single-number rating, such as the NRR (see section "Noise Reduction Rating"), which is computed therefrom, the discrepancies with respect to field data are the same. Figure 22–5 presents the published NRRs for a wide range of products (computed using a 2 SD correction) compared with the available field attenuation values achieved by 84% of the wearers in the workplace. If in fact the field data were shown with a comparable 2 SD (98th percentile) adjustment, many of the field NRRs would be negative numbers, simply indicating that some of the population receives an overall protection of approximately 0 dB.

The field NRRs attained by 84% of the wearers are less than or equal to 7 dB for all types of earplugs, except the foam variety, which yields about 13 dB, a value roughly comparable to that found for most earmuffs.

Attenuation versus Use Time

The effective protection of a device is substantially reduced when it is removed by an employee for even short periods of time during the workday as illustrated in Figure 22–6. An HPD with a nominal NRR of 25 dB that is removed by the user for 15 minutes during an 8-hour workday provides an effective NRR of only 20 dB, for a loss of 5 dB. Greater reductions in effectiveness are observed for higher NRRs. Little effect is observed for NRRs of less than 10 dB.

Dual Protection

Dual protection, such as earplugs worn in combination with earmuffs, helmets, or communications headsets, typically provides greater protection than either device alone (Berger, 1983b, Damongeot et al, 1989). However, the attenuation of the combination is not equal to the sum of the individual

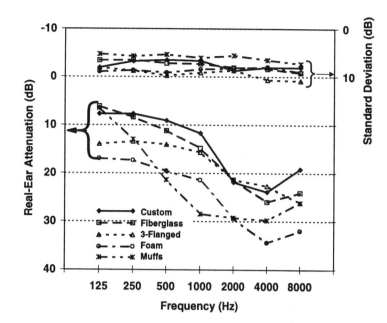

Figure 22–4   Summary of "real-world" data for hearing protectors separated into four earplug and one earmuff categories. (Adapted from Berger et al [1996].)

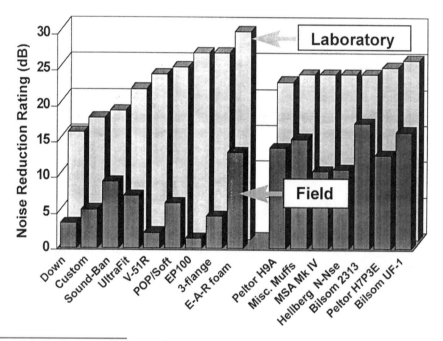

Figure 22–5   Comparison of manufacturers' laboratory Noise Reduction Ratings (NRRs) published in North America to "real-world" (field) data. Laboratory NRRs are computed with a 2 SD correction, whereas field NRRs include a 1 SD correction. (See text; adapted from Berger et al [1996].)

attenuation values, as illustrated in Figure 22–3. No empirical or theoretically derived equations are available that can predict the attenuation of an earplug and earmuff combination with sufficient accuracy to be useful. Dual protection is advisable when 8-hour time-weighted-average exposures exceed 105 dBA but is often problematical for exposures below that level because of interference with communication and the difficulty of motivating and enforcing use of HPDs in lower sound levels. The use of dual HPDs is especially recommended when high-intensity noise is dominated by energy at or below 500 Hz because it is in this frequency range that

the attenuation of single HPDs will be the least and the potential gains from dual protection are the greatest.

At individual frequencies the incremental gain in performance for dual hearing protection varies from approximately 0- to 15-dB over the better single device, but at 2000 Hz the gain is limited to only a few decibels. Attenuation changes very little when different earmuffs are used with the same earplug, but for a given earmuff the choice of earplug is critical for attenuation at frequencies below 2000 Hz. At and above 2000 Hz, all dual-protection combinations provide attenuation essentially equal to the limitations imposed by

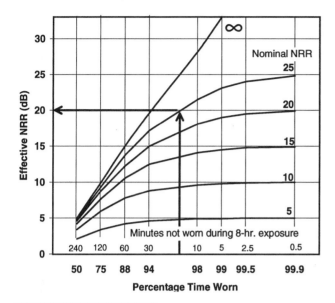

Figure 22–6 Corrections to nominal Noise Reduction Ratings (NRRs) as a function of the time during a workday that a hearing protection device is worn, based on a 5 dB trading relationship.

the bone-conduction pathways, approximately 40- to 50-dB, depending on frequency. As a rule of thumb, the OSHA procedure of computing the dual protection by adding 5 dB to the NRR of the more protective of the two devices is a reasonable approximation.

Infrasound/Ultrasound

REAT data are normally limited to the frequency range of 125 Hz to 8000 Hz, although some laboratories test to frequencies as low as 63 Hz, especially in Europe. However, a few published reports are available from which to draw conclusions. Well-fitted insert earplugs provide attenuation at infrasonic frequencies (i.e., below about 20 Hz) that is about equal to those in the 125 Hz one-third octave band (OB). However, at those same frequencies, earmuffs provide very little protection and may even amplify sound (Nixon et al, 1967; Paakkonen & Tikkanen, 1991). Conventional earplugs and earmuffs generally provide adequate protection at ultrasonic frequencies (i.e., above about 20,000 Hz), with attenuation exceeding 30 dB for frequencies from about 10,000 to 30,000 Hz (Behar & Crabtree, 1997; Berger, 1983a).

Impulse and Weapon Noise

Estimation of the attenuation provided by HPDs in the presence of impulsive noise is one of the most problematic issues in hearing protection. Not only are the damage risk criteria (DRC) for impulse noise being re-examined, but application of those criteria to hearing-protected ears is questionable because the time history of a waveform under an HPD is so different from the free-field conditions under which the DRC were derived. Under the HPD, especially under earmuffs, the waveform lacks the sharp rise time of the incident pulse and generally also exhibits substantial low-frequency components not present in the original (Dancer et al, 1996).

Although a number of studies have used MIRE techniques to measure either the noise reduction (NR) (i.e., the differences in SPLs between sound field and earcanal mounted mics) or the insertion loss (IL) (i.e., the difference in SPLs between the protected and unprotected conditions as measured in the concha or earcanal), the meaningfulness of the resultant measurements is in question in that such measurements significantly underestimate the actual protection provided in terms of reduction of temporary threshold shift (TTS) (Johnson & Patterson, 1992). MIRE measurements indicate attenuation of peak SPLs for typical earmuffs of about 30 dB for pistol fire, about 18 dB for rifle fire, and as little as 5 dB for cannons. Foam earplugs were found to provide similar attenuation to earmuffs against pistols, but substantially more noise reduction than earmuffs against cannons and bazookas, providing attenuation greater than 15 dB. Dual HPDs were found to afford extra protection especially for low-frequency impulses with attenuation values of 20- to 25-dB (Ylikoski et al, 1995). These values also correspond with predictions based on use of conventional REAT data applied to the OB spectrum of the impulses (Berger, 1990).

In a recent large-scale multilaboratory European study that examined earmuff performance in industrial impulse noise arising from pneumatic nailers, hammers, punch presses, and plastic explosives, it was concluded that for both active and passive earmuffs, the impulse noise attenuation tends to be larger than or equal to the attenuation found for steady broadband noise at lower levels (Smoorenburg, 1996). In a separate study Lloyd (1996) drew similar conclusions. The only exception that Smoorenburg observed to this finding was in the case of explosions that were of sufficient intensity to actually cause blast-induced movements of the earcups that would break the acoustic seal of the earmuff against the side of the head. Johnson and Patterson (1992) have documented similar cup motion in the presence of 190 dB SPL explosive impulses intended to mimic high-level military exposures.

A point of confusion has existed since 1979 as a result of mandated wording on the EPA hearing protector label, which states,

> Although hearing protectors can be recommended for protection against the harmful effects of impulsive noise, the NRR is based on the attenuation of continuous noise and may not be an accurate indicator of the protection attainable against impulsive noise such as gunfire.

Many misread this to suggest that HPDs cannot attenuate gunfire. To the contrary, HPDs can and do attenuate gunfire. The purpose of this caution, when drafted, was to suggest that certain HPDs, especially amplitude-sensitive devices (see section "Amplitude-Sensitive Hearing Protection Devices") might work better in gunfire than the REAT-derived NRR would suggest, and indeed, current research supports such a conclusion.

It would seem that the best estimates of HPD performance in impulse and weapon noise should be based on studies of TTS in the presence of actual impulses. Johnson and Patterson (1992) and Dancer at al (1996) have provided such data and they suggest that a variety of conventional hearing protectors, even with intentional acoustical leaks introduced, can provide sufficient protection for even high-intensity weapon noise. A cautionary note was voiced by Johnson for protection from very high-level impulses (above 180 dB SPL) using earplugs.

He observed that the earplug type that was most likely to ensure an acoustical seal in the earcanal was the safest choice, namely a foam earplug (Johnson, 1997). With respect to analytical predictions, application of REAT values to the peak of the impulse with the requirement that it be reduced below 140 dB peak SPL is overly conservative. Instead, Dancer et al (1996) have suggested use of attenuation values based on IL measurements that are applied to exposures assessed in terms of $L_{Aeq,8}$ values (i.e., 8-hour A-weighted equivalent continuous sound level using a 3 dB exchange rate) as the best conservative approximation at this time.

USING ATTENUATION DATA TO ESTIMATE PROTECTION

Either laboratory or real-world attenuation data (depending on the purpose of the predictions) may be used to estimate the protected noise exposures that a wearer receives in a given noise exposure. But first, a word of caution.

The accuracy with which the laboratory or real-world data can predict the protection for an individual, or group of users, is critically dependent on the correspondence between the test and actual use conditions. The accuracy can be very poor as is clearly shown when optimum laboratory data are used to estimate protection in a typical hearing conservation program (see section "Optimum Laboratory Performance"). Therefore, undue emphasis on protection estimates is unwarranted. Furthermore, because noise-exposure estimates also have limited precision, this has led some authors to recommend categorizing noise exposure estimates into ranges as wide as 5 dB (Royster & Royster, 1985). At time-weighted average levels (TWA as defined by OSHA [i.e., the A-weighted average sound level with a 5 dB exchange rate, normalized to 8 hours]) below about 95 dBA, it is more important to focus on the facilitation and enforcement of proper HPD use than on the precise determination of HPD attenuation or noise-exposure estimates.

Octave-Band Method

Potentially, the most accurate computational procedure for applying test data to estimate protected exposures is the OB method, as illustrated in Table 22–2. At each frequency, the HPD's mean attenuation less an SD correction is subtracted from the measured A-weighted OB SPLs. Two SDs are normally used in the United States, one SD in Europe and Australia. The protected levels are then logarithmically summed to determine the A-weighted sound level under the HPD. This computation requires that the user have OB noise data available and that the computations be made individually for each HPD/noise spectrum combination.

Noise Reduction Rating (NRR)

A single-number descriptor is convenient and often sufficiently accurate to estimate protected exposures. The descriptor that has been standardized in the United States since 1979, and hence precalculated by manufacturers and provided on their packaging, is the NRR (EPA, 1979). It is an attenuation index that represents the overall average noise reduction in decibels that an HPD will provide in an environment with a known C-weighted sound level. (See Fig. 22–7 for an explanation of C-weighting.) The NRR is identical (within 0.5 dB) to NIOSH method No. 2, from which it was adapted (Kroes et al, 1975).

The NRR is calculated in a manner analogous to the OB approach, except that a pink noise spectrum (equal energy in each OB) is used instead of the actual noise spectrum (line 1 in Table 22–2), the estimated protected A-weighted levels are subtracted from the C-weighted pink noise and not the A-weighted environmental noise, and an additional spectral safety factor of 3 dB is subtracted. The spectral factor accounts for errors arising from use of pink noise instead of the actual noise spectrum to which the wearer is exposed. As in the OB method, the computation incorporates a 2 SD adjustment for percentage of population protected (i.e., theoretically a 98% protection factor, sometimes explicitly denoted as NRR_{98}).

TABLE 22–2 Octave-band (OB) method of calculating HPD noise reduction

Octave-Band Center Frequency	125	250	500	1000	2000	4000	8000	dBA*
1. Measured SPLs	85	87	90	90	85	82	80	
2. A-weighting correction (see Fig. 22–7)	−16.1	−8.6	−3.2	0.0	+1.2	+1.0	−1.1	
3. A-weighted sound levels (step 1 + step 2)	68.9	78.4	86.8	90.0	86.2	83.0	78.9	93.5
4. Attenuation, typical premolded earplug	27.4	26.6	27.5	27.0	32.0	44.0[†]	42.2[‡]	
5. SD × 2	7.8	8.4	9.4	6.8	8.8	7.0[†]	10.4[‡]	
6. Estimated protected A-weighted sound levels (step 3 − step 4 + step 5)	49.3	60.2	68.7	69.8	63.0	46.0	47.1	73.0

The estimated protection for 98% of the users in the noise environment, assuming they wear the device in the same manner as did the test subjects and assuming they are accurately represented by the test subjects, is

93.5 − 73.0 = 20.5 dBA

*Logarithmic sum of the 7 OB levels in the row.
[†]Arithmetic average of 3150 and 4000 Hz data.
[‡]Arithmetic average of 6300 and 8000 Hz data.

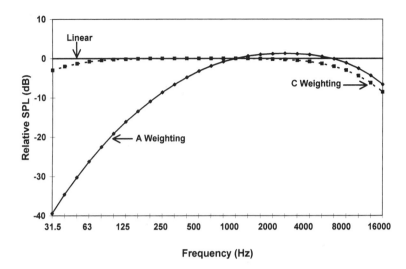

Figure 22–7 Relative frequency response of the standardized A-, C-, and linear-weighting characteristics used in sound measurements.

The NRR computed for the example in Table 22–2 is 20.7 dB. For the full computational details of the NRR see EPA (1979) or Berger (1988).

SPECIAL CONSIDERATION

A critical conceptual error that is often made is to presume that the SD correction adjusts laboratory data to estimate real-world values. The actual purpose of the SD is to adjust the mean test data to reflect the attenuation achieved by 84% (for a 1 SD correction) or 98% (for a 2 SD correction) of the test subjects.

The NRR is used to estimate wearer noise exposures by subtracting it from the C-weighted sound levels as shown in Equation 1.

Estimated exposure
(dBA) = Workplace noise level (dBC) − NRR   (1)

The practice of subtracting the NRR from the C-weighted sound level may seem illogical; however, it is justified on theoretical and empirical grounds (Berger, 1988). Considerable accuracy is lost when the NRR is subtracted from A-weighted sound levels, in which case an additional safety factor of 7 dB must be included, as shown in Equation 2. This method has been referred to as NIOSH method No. 3 (Kroes et al, 1975).

Estimated exposure
(dBA) = Workplace noise level (dBA) − (NRR − 7 dB)   (2)

The 7 dB safety factor in Equation 2 is a "worst-case" correction, which in most cases will overestimate actual C-A differences. As an alternative, one can correct the A-weighted time-weighted average (TWA) (obtained from dosimeters that are usually only capable of A-weighted measurements) by using a sound level meter to develop a C-A value for typical processes, areas, or job descriptions. This C-A value is added to the A-weighted TWA to calculate an estimated

C-weighted TWA or C-weighted workplace noise level, from which the NRR can be subtracted using the procedure of Equation 1. To the extent that an accurate C-A value can be estimated, this method will provide enhanced accuracy over use of Equation 2 for those situations in which C-weighted exposures are unavailable.

Comparison of Octave-Band and Noise Reduction Rating Estimates

Although errors may arise in using the NRR to estimate results computed using the OB method, the values are usually of sufficient accuracy considering the inaccuracies in the basic OB data from which both sets of computations are made. For the example shown in Table 22–2, with an exterior C-weighted sound level of 95.2 dB SPL (computed by applying C-weighting corrections to the OB SPLs shown in row 1 of the table) and an exterior A-weighted sound level of 93.5 dB SPL (see row 2 of the table), the OB-computed protected exposure level is 73.0 dBA compared with the NRR-computed values of

95.2 dBC − 20.7 = 74.5 dBA   (3)
or
93.5 dBA − (20.7 − 7) = 93.5 − 13.7 = 79.8 dBA   (4)

Note the substantially larger discrepancy between the estimate from Equation 4 and the OB value, than from Equation 3. This is due to the very conservative 7 dB adjustment required when only A-weighted sound levels are available.

The presumed increase in accuracy that should be provided by the OB method is not usually achieved because of the large discrepancies between laboratory and real-world data. The primary reason for using the OB data is to better match the attenuation curve of the device to the noise spectrum. For example, both laboratory and workplace data show that earmuffs are a poor choice for noises with significant low-frequency energy (125 to 250 Hz) but are preferred for strong mid-frequency energy (primarily around 1000 Hz). A foam or premolded earplug is the best for noises containing significant low-frequency energy.

Performing this type of HPD/noise spectrum matching may also be of limited value because of the difficulty of assigning particular protectors to specific jobs in a plant (based on spectrum shape). It is difficult enough to ensure that HPDs are worn and used correctly, without also trying to keep devices from shifting among work areas with different spectral characteristics, and also having to ensure that certain devices are worn only by employees exposed to specific noise spectra.

Derating Hearing Protection Device Attenuation Data and OSHA's 50% Factor

The NRR, or the laboratory data from which it is computed, must be reduced (derated) to provide attenuation values more realistic for the workplace. The most commonly cited derating factor in use today is an across-the-board value of 50%, although some authors have suggested that a percentage derating should be less for the easier-to-fit HPDs such as earmuffs than for the harder-to-fit devices such as earplugs (Park & Casali, 1991). A potentially more accurate approach is to base estimates on the type of real-world attenuation values cited earlier in the chapter (Figs. 22–4 and 22–5) and in the future to avoid the need for any deratings at all by using S12.6-1997 Method B data as the basis for field estimates.

Although no single derating scheme will be accurate for all HPDs, hearing conservationists must choose at least one approach if they wish to use currently available manufacturer's data to develop even rough estimates of workplace performance. Whatever derating is selected, it must also be applied to the OB calculations of attenuation (i.e., if a percentage derating is used for NRRs, that same percentage should also be taken from the OB attenuation values before they are entered in row 4 of Table 22–2).

OSHA (1983) specifies use of manufacturers' labeled data, derived from laboratory measurements, to assess adequacy of HPDs for the noise exposures in which they are worn. Subsequent to publication of the Hearing Conservation Amendment, OSHA (1987) recognized that laboratory data must be derated. They now recommend reducing published NRRs by 50% (e.g., an NRR of 24 dB would be reduced to 12 dB) but only for the purpose of evaluating the relative efficacy of HPDs and engineering noise controls (noise reduction through equipment design and modification). The derated NRRs are not applicable for determining compliance with the hearing protection requirements of the Hearing Conservation Amendment. The situation is confusing to both hearing conservationists and OSHA compliance officers alike. See Berger (1993) for details.

The 50% derating cited above has no relationship to the well-known 7 dB correction specified in Appendix B of the Amendment (OSHA, 1983). The 50% derating adjusts labeled values to better reflect real-world performance, whereas the 7 dB correction accounts for use of the NRR with A-weighted instead of C-weighted sound levels. When using both the derating and the correction together, 7 dB is subtracted before derating by 50%.

> ### PITFALL
>
> The 7 dB correction to the NRR is not a real-world correction. Rather, it accounts for "worst-case" differences between the A-weighted and C-weighted noise levels when the NRR is applied to A-weighted data.

EFFECTS OF HEARING PROTECTION DEVICES ON AUDITORY PERCEPTION AND INTELLIGIBILITY

Speech Communications

Conventional hearing protectors cannot differentiate and selectively pass speech versus noise energy at a given frequency, thus the devices do not improve the speech/noise ratio, which is the most important factor for achieving reliable intelligibility. However, hearing protectors sometimes do afford intelligibility improvements in intense noise by lowering the total energy of both speech and noise incident on the ear. Overload distortion in the cochlea is thereby reduced, establishing more favorable conditions for discrimination.

Prediction of the effects of protectors on speech intelligibility in noise is a complex issue that depends on a host of factors, including the listener's hearing abilities, absolute speech and noise levels, and speech-to-noise, whether the talker is occluded, HPD attenuation, reverberation time of the environment, facial cues, and content/complexity of the message set.

Several contradictions exist among the many empirical studies concerning speech communication for *normal hearers* with HPDs; however, a distillation of the evidence generally suggests that conventional passive HPDs have little or no degrading effect on intelligibility in noise above about 80 dBA but cause considerable misunderstanding at lower levels, for which the use of protection is not typically needed anyway. At ambient noise levels greater than about 85 dBA, several studies have reported slight intelligibility improvements with specific HPDs (e.g., Casali & Horylev, 1987), whereas others attempting to simulate on-the-job conditions have reported small intelligibility decrements, especially when the talker is occluded (Hormann et al, 1984). When wearing HPDs in noise, one tends to lower the voice level because the bone-conducted voice feedback inside the head is amplified by the presence of the protector, especially at low frequencies. In comparison, attenuation of the ambient noise occurs primarily through interruption of air-conduction by the HPD. Thus one's own voice is perceived as louder in relation to the noise than is actually true, causing a compensatory lowering of about 2- to 4-dB unless a conscious effort is made to "speak up" (Berger, 1988).

For individuals with high-frequency hearing losses, the effects of HPDs on communications are not clear-cut, although these persons are certainly at disadvantage because their already elevated thresholds for mid- to high-frequency speech sounds are further raised by the protector. As the amount of hearing loss increases, the chances of degrading communications with HPDs also increases. Although complete consensus does not exist among studies, it does appear that hearing-impaired individuals often experience no improvement or even reduced communications abilities with HPDs in noise environments from 80- to 95-dBA.

Auditory Warning Signals and Other Sounds

As with speech communication effects, the same HPD influences on signal/noise ratio and reduction of aural distortion apply to the detection and recognition of nonverbal signals, such as warnings, target annunciators, and machinery sounds. Due to the high-frequency bias in attenuation of conventional HPDs, coupled with the typically elevated high-frequency thresholds of the sensorineural hearing-impaired, signals above about 2000 Hz are the most likely to be missed. However, warning signal parameters, such as frequency, intensity, and temporal profile, may be designed to help alleviate detection problems and increase perceived urgency. For instance, low-frequency (i.e., below 500 Hz) warning signals more readily diffract around barriers and are less attenuated by HPDs, thereby aiding detection.

Although aural cues may sound spectrally different under an HPD, the bulk of empirical studies indicates that signal detection will not be compromised by HPDs for normal-hearing individuals. (Wilkins & Martin, 1987). Although the evidence is less extensive for hearing-impaired listeners, they can be expected to experience some detection and recognition difficulty, depending on the particular signal, ambient noise, and hearing protector worn. When an occluded/unoccluded detection disadvantage does occur, it is more common with earmuffs than earplugs, perhaps because of the muffs' stronger tendency to attenuate high-frequency signals and to pass more low-frequency noise, which effects an upward spread of masking.

Localization

Perceptual judgments of sound direction and distance may be influenced by HPDs, at least partially because some of the high-frequency binaural cues (above about 4000 Hz) that depend on the pinnae are lost or altered. Earmuffs and helmets, which completely obscure the pinnae, interfere most with localization in the vertical plane and also tend to cause contralateral (left-right) and ipsilateral (front-back) judgment errors. Earplugs may cause some ipsilateral (front-back) errors but generally induce fewer localization problems than muffs.

General Remarks

For most applications, even though the quality of the auditory experience may change under HPDs, detection and intelligibility performance is not hampered for individuals of normal-hearing. Although hearing-impaired individuals may exhibit a reduced communications ability under HPDs in noise, HPD use is not contraindicated; instead, it is essential that the remaining auditory sensitivity be preserved by proper protector use. All individuals may benefit from visually-presented or tactually presented cues to augment auditory information, or in certain situations from the use of HPDs incorporating special communications features as described next.

HEARING PROTECTION DEVICES WITH SPECIAL FEATURES

Special hearing protector designs have been developed to improve speech communication and auditory perception capabilities of the noise-exposed wearer. These devices may be categorized into passive (i.e., without electronics), active (i.e., incorporating electronics), and communications headsets (Casali & Berger, 1996).

Passive Hearing Protection Devices
Frequency-Sensitive Hearing Protection Devices

Efforts to improve communications under earplugs have involved the use of apertures or channels through an earplug body, sometimes opening into an air-filled cavity encapsulated by the earplug walls. For example, a small (~ 0.5 mm) longitudinal channel through a custom-molded earplug creates an air-leak that produces a low-pass filter characteristic. Attenuation is negligible below about 1000 Hz, increasing up to about 30 dB at 8000 Hz. Because most of the speech frequencies critical to intelligibility lie in the range from 1000 to 4000 Hz, the communications benefit potential of the low-pass feature may be relatively small, especially in low-frequency noise, which causes upward masking into the critical speech band. Furthermore, the attenuation may be insufficient for many industrial noise environments.

Amplitude-Sensitive Hearing Protection Devices

Because a conventional HPD provides a constant amount of attenuation that is independent of incident sound level, hearing ability is compromised during the quiet periods of intermittent sound exposures. Amplitude-sensitive or level-dependent HPDs address this problem by providing reduced attenuation at low sound levels, with increasing protection at high levels.

Passive HPDs use a nonlinear component, such as a valve, diaphragm, or sharp-edged orifice opening into a duct to effect the change in attenuation. The latter technique, used with success in both earmuffs and earplugs, takes advantage of the fact that low-intensity sound waves predominantly exhibit laminar airflow and pass relatively unimpeded through the aperture, whereas high-intensity waves involve more turbulent flow and are attenuated because of increasing acoustic resistance (Allen & Berger, 1990).

A critical performance parameter is the transition sound level, normally 110- to 120-dB SPL, above which insertion loss increases at a rate of about 1 dB for each 2- to 4-dB increase in sound level. Because this transition level is so high, passive amplitude-sensitive HPDs are best suited for outdoor impulsive blasts and gunfire exposures. At lower, but still hazardous sound levels, most passive devices exhibit vented earplug behavior, affording very weak protection at frequencies less than 1000 Hz. One exception is an orifice-type earmuff that provides approximately 25 dB attenuation from 400 to 8000 Hz (Allen & Berger, 1990).

PEARL

To protect workers in areas where noise exposures are sudden and unexpected, such as in a blasting region, amplitude-sensitive HPDs should be considered. They can alleviate the tendency to remove conventional HPDs during quiet periods and the unsafe practice of quickly donning the HPD when upcoming noise is anticipated.

Uniform-Attenuation Hearing Protection Devices

Because the attenuation of conventional HPDs increases with frequency, the wearer's perception of pitch is artificially imbalanced. Not only are sounds reduced in level, they are colored in a spectral sense. This problem contributes to protector nonuse when, for instance, a machine operator's auditory feedback from a cutting tool is distorted or a musician's pitch perception is compromised. To counter these problems, flat or uniform-attenuation HPDs are designed to impose attenuation that is nearly linear from about 100 to 8000 Hz. One successful technique establishes a Helmholtz resonator and a sound channel through a custom-molded or premolded earplug. With proper selection of channel diameter and length, as well as network components, a flat attenuation profile of about 15 dB has been obtained (Killion et al, 1988), and recently versions with approximately flat performance of 10 dB and 25 dB have also been introduced.

Properly fit uniform attenuation HPDs provide adequate protection and better hearing perception in low to moderate noise exposures of about 90 dBA or less. Workers with high-frequency hearing losses and professional musicians may find them particularly beneficial. However, for noises having substantial high-frequency energy, uniform-attenuation earplugs generally offer less protection than conventional earplugs.

Active Hearing Protection Devices

Amplitude-Sensitive Sound Transmission Hearing Protection Devices

Active sound transmission hearing protectors consist of modified conventional earmuffs or earplugs that incorporate microphone and limiting amplifier systems to transmit

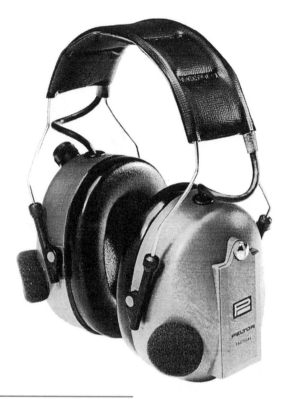

Figure 22–8   Example of an amplitude-sensitive sound transmission hearing protector (Peltor® Tactical™ 7 Stereo Electronic Earmuff) illustrating forward-facing microphones with windscreens on the lower portion of each cup, battery compartment on the outer face of the left cup, and volume control on the top outer face of the right cup. Earphones (not visible) are located within each earcup.

external sounds (often filtered to include the critical speech frequencies) to earphones mounted inside the earcups (see Fig. 22–8). Typically, the limiting amplifier maintains a predetermined (in some cases user-adjustable) earphone level, often at about 85 dBA, until the ambient noise is so intense that direct transmission through the earcup becomes the controlling factor. In comparison to both conventional and passive amplitude-sensitive earmuffs, sound-transmission earmuffs are more expensive (upwards of $100) but offer a viable alternative for use in intermittent noises, especially those with impulse-type (e.g., gunfire) or short-duration on-segments. However, in continuous, high-level noise, the distortion products of some systems may cause annoyance and compromise hearing ability.

Auditory perception and noise level under sound transmission earmuffs depend on electronic design factors such as cutoff sound level and sharpness of attenuation transition at this level, system response delay, frequency response and bandwidth, distortion and residual electronic noise, signal/noise ratio at sound levels below the cutoff, and sensitivity to wind effects. Microphone design may be diotic, wherein a single microphone in one earcup feeds both earphones, or dichotic, in which each earcup has an independent microphone. The latter approach provides better localization performance where wearers must rely on the placement and direction of environmental sounds.

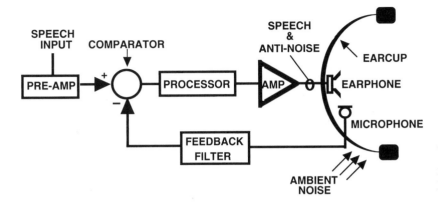

Figure 22–9 Block diagram of an active noise reduction (ANR) communications headset.

Active Noise Reduction Hearing Protection Devices

Recently integrated with conventional passive earmuffs, active noise reduction (ANR) electronics rely on the principle of destructive interference of sound waves in a common field to cancel noise. A microphone senses the sound inside the earcup, which is then fed back through a phase compensation filter to a processing circuit and drive amplifier (Fig. 22–9). The resultant "antinoise" signal is presented through an earphone at equal amplitude to, but 180 degrees out-of-phase with, the original noise, causing energy cancellation.

ANR is most effective against repetitive or continuous noises that are relatively invariant in spectrum or level, which allow the electronics to stabilize and fine-tune the phase and amplitude parameters needed for cancellation. Furthermore, ANR is limited to the reduction of low-frequency noises below about 1000 Hz, with maximum attenuation of 20- to 25-dB occurring below 300 Hz. Some ANR devices are particularly susceptible to leakage under the ear cushion, such as caused by eyeglass temples. This can result in a reduction in active attenuation, or even amplification at some frequencies (Nixon et al, 1992).

The low-frequency effectiveness of ANR is fortuitous in that it compensates the typically high-frequency biased protection of a passive earmuff. If the noise environment consists of only low-frequency energy, open-back ANR headphones may offer communications and perhaps comfort advantages over circumaural ANR earmuffs. Consisting of lightweight supra-aural earphones that rest on the pinnae, these devices have the disadvantage of offering no passive protection if the ANR circuit malfunctions.

Attenuation tests for ANR hearing protectors are as yet not standardized. A combination procedure may be required (i.e., real-ear tests [e.g., as per ANSI S12.6-1997]) to obtain the passive muff's attenuation and miniature microphone insertion-loss tests on a human head (e.g., as per ANSI S12.42-1995) to obtain active attenuation. The synergistic benefits of both passive and active attenuation in ANR devices currently come at a relatively high price of about $500 to $1000 per unit, although these costs are decreasing with technology improvements and volume manufacturing.

Hearing Protection Devices with Communications Features

For provision of communication or music signals at the ear, small loudspeakers have been integrated into HPDs.

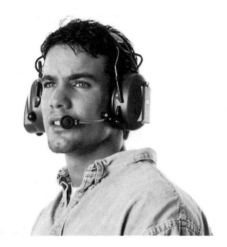

Figure 22–10 Example of self-contained communication headset (Peltor® PowerCom™ two-way UHF radio headset) with boom-mounted noise-canceling microphone.

Headsets (including ANR examples) consist of earphones housed in earmuff earcups or semi-insert pods, which support a directional microphone (often noise-canceling or voice-activated) in front of the mouth (see Fig. 22–10). Small receivers can also be remotely located on a hard hat or behind the pinna and coupled to the ear by means of tubing through earplugs. An alternative is an earplug-like unit, called an ear microphone, which consists of a receiver button and a microphone that picks up the wearer's voice as a result of sound radiation from the bone-conduction excited earcanal walls. Each of these approaches is available as one-way or two-way systems, using wireless (radiofrequency or infrared) or wired technology.

It is important that communications earphones and receiver buttons be output-limited so that amplified signal levels do not pose a hearing hazard. A reasonable and safe limit value is 85 dBA equivalent sound field. (Note that although the values are measured in the ear, they must be transformed to equivalent sound field values because those are the measurements on which damage risk criteria are based.) Furthermore, care must be exercised when selecting such a communications device that must double as a hearing protector. While some circumaural devices provide passive attenuation comparable to a standard earmuff, ear microphones typically provide less protection than comparable conventional earplugs (Mauney & Casali, 1990).

In cases where the attenuation afforded by a circumaural headset is inadequate such that communications signals are noise-masked, improvements can be realized by wearing an earplug under the headset. Although the earplug will reduce the communications signal and the noise, the signal/noise ratio in the earcanal can be improved if the earphone provides sufficient distortion-free gain to compensate for the insertion loss of the earplug. Other enhancements may be provided in the system electronics, such as peak-clipping and signal conditioning, to enhance the acoustic power of consonants that are critical to word discrimination.

PEARL

Although ANR-based HPDs provide excellent protection, especially in applications such as aircraft cockpits and tank crew compartments, equivalent or better passive protection can usually be obtained at much lower cost through the use of a well-fitted earplug under a conventional earmuff.

As diagrammed in Figure 22–9, ANR has been integrated into communications headsets. The sound (speech and noise) signal from the earcup microphone is fed back to a comparator through a filter that reverses the phase. The comparator's difference output is the undesirable noise component which is out-of-phase with the noise inside the earcup. Because the low-frequency components of the (desired) speech signal are also canceled by the ANR, a speech preamplifier is used for compensation. For certain noise situations, ANR headsets result in an improvement in speech intelligibility over the use of passive devices alone (Nixon et al, 1992).

HEARING PROTECTION DEVICE STANDARDS, REGULATIONS, AND GOVERNMENT LISTINGS

United States

Two current U.S. standards pertain specifically to hearing protectors, ANSI S12.6-1997, which specifies REAT evaluations of HPDs, and ANSI S12.42-1995, which specifies MIRE and ATF measurements of HPDs (see section "Laboratory Procedures"). A third standard, ANSI S3.19-1974, twice supplanted by newer REAT documents and currently withdrawn, is still specified in the U.S. EPA Hearing Protector Labeling Regulation and thus has substantial impact in the marketplace (see next section). Users often mistakenly presume ANSI REAT standards contain criteria for judging the acceptability of HPDs. In fact, these standards only describe methods for determining hearing protector attenuation. The methods in no way confer approval or attribute a particular degree of quality to the devices being tested.

A Department of Commerce accreditation process also exists and is managed by the National Voluntary Laboratory Accreditation Program (NVLAP). Laboratories, of which there are currently three in the United States, can be accredited by the program to test according to ANSI S3.19 and ANSI S12.6, and this indicates that they adhere to extensive and specific procedures. It does not, however, ensure the results on any particular test, nor does it certify the devices that are tested. At this time no federal or state agencies or U.S. standards-writing organizations approve or accredit particular HPDs for sale or use, although an existing EPA regulation requires the labeling of all HPD packaging.

OSHA specifies hearing protector use in the Hearing Conservation Amendment (OSHA, 1983), requiring that HPDs reduce an employee's TWA to 90 dBA or less and in the case of employees demonstrating standard threshold shifts to 85 dBA or less. No particular types or brands of HPDs are specifically recommended or proscribed. The method for assessing the amount of reduction to be expected is contained in Appendix B of the amendment (see section "Derating Hearing Protection Device Attenuation and OSHA's 50% Factor"). A related government agency, the Mine Safety and Health Administration (MSHA), issues a "Hearing Protector R & D Factor List." The only criterion for having a device placed on the list is that it be tested according to an ANSI REAT standard, and that the data be available in sales literature or on specification sheets.

EPA Labeling Regulation

The Noise Control Act of 1972 empowered the EPA to label all noise-producing and noise-reducing devices. The first and only standard that was promulgated for noise-reducing devices was the hearing protector labeling regulation (EPA, 1979). As with the preceding regulations that have been discussed, it did not specify criteria by which HPDs were to be deemed acceptable or unacceptable. It did, however, specify that the attenuation of any device or material capable of being worn on the head or in the earcanal that is sold wholly or in part on the basis of its ability to reduce the level of sound entering the ear was to be evaluated according to ANSI S3.19-1974. An NRR was to be computed and placed on a label whose size and configuration was specified.

In the early 1980s budget cuts at EPA led to elimination of the noise enforcement division. In recognition of their inability to enforce the regulation, EPA then revoked the product verification testing and the attendant reporting and recordkeeping requirements. However, the remainder of the regulation remains law, and in the 20 years since its promulgation it has clearly been recognized in the professional community as providing misleading guidance to potential purchasers of products. In 1995 a multiorganizational Task Force on Hearing Protector Effectiveness provided specific recommendations to improve the labeling regulation, including testing according to Method B, Subject Fit of ANSI S12.6-1997 and computation of a revised NRR (Berger & Royster, 1996). Although virtually all professional organizations involved in hearing conservation (including ASHA) endorse the recommendations, EPA has not acted, primarily because of lack of funds and staff to review the proposal.

SPECIAL CONSIDERATION

Because of inaction on the part of the EPA, the hearing protector labeling regulation of 1979 still calls for testing by a 25-year-old standard (ANSI, 1974) that yields estimates of NRRs that provide less usefulness than the agency's early and much-maligned fuel-economy ratings. Until data are routinely available from Method B of the new ANSI standard (S12.6-1997), deratings like the 50% value discussed in the text are recommended.

International Standards and Regulations

The International Organization for Standardization (ISO) maintains two working groups ISO/TC43/SC1/WG17 and ISO/TC94/SC12 that are responsible for standards on hearing protection.

WG17 developed the 4869 series, Part 1 on REAT measurements (ISO, 1990), Part 2 on number ratings systems (ISO, 1994), and Part 3 on use of an ATF (ISO, 1989). Part 1 corresponds to S12.6-1997 but differs in details of subject selection and HPD fitting. It currently lacks a procedure that would correspond with subject fit (Method B). No current U.S. counterpart exists to Part 2, although the NRR and ISO's single number rating (the SNR) are roughly equivalent. Part 3 is similar in some respects to the ATF portion of ANSI S12.42 in that both specify use of ATFs. In addition, WG17 is working on standards for the measurement of level-dependent hearing protectors and the assessment of the performance of HPDs in impulsive environments.

SC12 has produced three documents, two pertaining to approval of earplugs and earmuffs (ISO/DIS 10453 and ISO/DIS 10449), and a third one on selection and use of HPDs (ISO/DIS 10452). These documents closely correspond to European regulations on the approval of hearing protectors for sale in the European Community. The United States has no counterpart to this HPD approval process because the feeling has generally been that for devices of this nature, approvals are best left with the purchasing organizations so as not to burden inexpensive and readily replaceable products with potentially unnecessary testing.

CONCLUSIONS

This chapter provides a review and analysis of the design, selection, issuing, measurement, and performance of HPDs. It cannot be overemphasized that the greatest impact that the audiologist can have on long-term hearing conservation is in the areas of issuing and fitting, training and motivation, and enforcement. In fact, when TWAs are less than or equal to 95 dBA, most hearing protectors will suffice as long as they fit well and are worn correctly and consistently (Royster & Royster, 1985). It is only when daily exposures exceed 95 dBA that greater attention should be directed toward real-world attenuation and field estimates of performance, and when they approach and exceed 100 dBA that selection becomes a substantial concern. In such instances data would suggest that foam earplugs, or earmuffs, or for exposures above about 105 dBA, a combination of the two, should be required.

Hearing protectors are not a panacea and cannot be dispensed indiscriminately, but they can and do work when utilized within the context of a well-defined and properly implemented hearing conservation program (Bruhl & Ivarsson, 1994; Dobie, 1995). Effective implementation refers primarily to the human interaction and not the technical side of the equation. In fact, in one large-scale study that demonstrated hearing conservation effectiveness with a database of well over 100,000 audiograms, no relationship was observed between the changes in observed hearing levels between the groups wearing class A (most protective) and class B (less protective) devices (Gillis & Harrison, 1993). This was evident across all industries studied. Such findings support a widely quoted, but often unappreciated axiom—the best hearing protector is the one that is worn and worn correctly. And that protector will be the one that is matched to the noise, the environment, and especially to the person in need of protection.

REFERENCES

ALLEN, C.H., & BERGER, E.H. (1990). Development of a unique passive hearing protector with level-dependent and flat attenuation characteristics. *Noise Control Engineering Journal, 34*(3);97–105.

AMERICAN NATIONAL STANDARDS INSTITUTE. (1974). *Method for the measurement of real-ear protection of hearing protectors and physical attenuation of earmuffs* (ANSI S3.19-1974). New York: ANSI.

AMERICAN NATIONAL STANDARDS INSTITUTE. (1991). *Evaluating the effectiveness of hearing conservation programs* (Draft ANSI S12.13-1991). New York: ANSI.

AMERICAN NATIONAL STANDARDS INSTITUTE. (1995). *Microphone-in-real-ear and acoustic test fixture methods for the measurement of insertion loss of circumaural hearing protection devices* (ANSI S12.42-1995). New York: ANSI.

AMERICAN NATIONAL STANDARDS INSTITUTE. (1997). *Methods for measuring the real-ear attenuation of hearing protectors* (ANSI S12.6–1997). New York: ANSI

BEHAR, A., & CRABTREE, R.B. (1997). Measurement of hearing protector attenuation at ultrasonic frequencies. In: C.D. Burroughs (Ed.), *Proceedings of Noise-Congress 97* (pp. 97–102). Poughkeepsie, NY: Noise Control Foundation.

BERGER, E.H. (1983a). *Attenuation of hearing protectors at the frequency extremes*. 11th International Congress on Acoustics. Paris, Vol. 3:289–292.

BERGER, E.H. (1983b). Laboratory attenuation of earmuffs and earplugs both singly and in combination. *American Industrial Hygiene Association Journal, 44*(5);321–329.

BERGER, E.H. (1985). EARLog #17—Ear infection and the use of hearing protection. *Journal of Occupational Medicine, 27*(9);620–623.

BERGER, E.H. (1986). Review and tutorial—Methods of measuring the attenuation of hearing protection devices. *Journal of the Acoustical Society of America, 79*(6);1655–1687.

BERGER, E.H. (1988). Hearing protectors—Specifications, fitting, use, and performance. In: D.M. Lipscomb (Ed.), *Hearing conservation in industry, schools, and the military* (pp. 145–191). Boston, MA: College-Hill Press.

BERGER, E.H. (1990). Hearing protection—The state of the art (circa 1990) and research priorities for the coming decade. In: *Program and Abstracts of the NIH Consensus Development Conference on Noise and Hearing Loss* (pp. 91–96). Bethesda, MD: National Institutes of Health.

BERGER, E.H. (1992). Development of a laboratory procedure for estimation of the field performance of hearing protectors. In: *Proceedings of Hearing Conservation Conference.* (pp. 41–45). Lexington, KY: Office of Engineering Service, University of Kentucky.

BERGER, E.H. (1993). *EARLog #20—The naked truth about NRRs*. Indianapolis, IN: E•A•R/Aearo Co.

BERGER, E.H., FRANKS, J.R., & LINDGREN, F. (1996). International review of field studies of hearing protector attenuation. In A. Axlesson, H. Borchgrevink, R.P. Hamernik, P. Hellstrom, D. Henderson, & R.J. Salvi (Eds.), *Scientific basis of noise-induced hearing loss* (pp. 361–377). New York: Thieme Medical Publishers, Inc.

BERGER, E.H., & KERIVAN, J.E. (1983). Influence of physiological noise and the occlusion effect on the measurement of real-ear attenuation at threshold. *Journal of the Acoustical Society of America, 74*(1);1–94.

BERGER, E.H., KERIVAN, J.E., & MINTZ, F. (1982). Inter-laboratory variability in the measurement of hearing protector attenuation. *Sound and Vibration, 16*(1);14–19.

BERGER, E.H., & ROYSTER, L.H. (1996). In search of meaningful measures of hearing protector effectiveness. *Spectrum (Suppl. 1),13;*29.

BRUHL, P., & IVARSSON, A. (1994). Noise-exposed male sheet-metal workers using hearing protectors. *Scandinavian Audiology, 23*(2);123–128.

CASALI, J.G. (1992). Comfort: The "other" criterion for hearing protector design and selection. In: *Proceedings of Hearing Conservation Conference.* (pp. 47–53). Lexington, KY: Office of Engineering Services, University of Kentucky.

CASALI, J.G., & BERGER, E.H. (1996). Technology advancements in hearing protection circa 1995: Active noise reduction, frequency/amplitude-sensitivity, and uniform attenuation. *American Industrial Hygiene Association Journal, 57*(2);175–185.

CASALI, J.G., & HORYLEV, M.J. (1987). Speech discrimination in noise: The influence of hearing protection. In: *Proceedings of the Human Factors Society—31st Annual Meeting* (pp. 1246–1250). New York: Human Factors Society.

CASALI, J.G., & LAM, S.T. (1986). Effects of user instructions on earmuff/earcap sound attenuation. *Sound and Vibration, 20*(5);22–28.

CASALI, J.G., MAUNEY, D.W., & BURKS, J.A. (1995). Physical vs. psychophysical measurement of hearing protector attenuation—a.k.a. MIRE vs. REAT. *Sound and Vibration, 29*(7);20–27.

DAMONGEOT, A., LATAYE, R., & KUSY, A. (1989). An empirical formula for predicting the attenuation given by double hearing protection (earplugs and earmuffs). *Applied Acoustics, 28*(3);169–175.

DANCER, A.L., FRANKE, R., PARMENTIER, G., & BUCK, K. (1996). Hearing protector performance and NIHL in extreme environments: Actual performance of hearing protectors in impulse noise/nonlinear behavior. In: A. Axlesson, H. Borchgrevink, R.P. Hamernik, P. Hellstrom, D. Henderson, & R.J. Salvi (Eds.), *Scientific basis of noise-induced hearing loss*. (pp. 321–338). New York: Thieme Medical Publishers, Inc.

DOBIE, R.A. (1995). Prevention of noise-induced hearing loss. *Archives of Otolaryngology–Head and Neck Surgery, 121;*385–391.

EPA. (1979). Noise labeling requirements for hearing protectors. Environmental Protection Agency. *Federal Register, 44*(190),40CFR Part 211:56130–56147.

GILLIS, H.R., & HARRISON, C. (1993). Hearing protection—What is the best? *Spectrum (Suppl. 1),10;*20–21.

HOLLAND, H.H., JR. (1967). Attenuation provided by fingers, palms, tragi, and V-51R earplugs [Letter to the Editor], *Journal of the Acoustical Society of America, 41*(6);1545.

HORMANN, H., LAZARUS-MAINKA, G., SCHUBEIUS, M., & LAZARUS, H. (1984). The effect of noise and the wearing of ear protectors on verbal communication. *Noise Control Engineering Journal, 23*(2);69–77.

INTERNATIONAL ORGANIZATION FOR STANDARDIZATION. (1989). *Acoustics—Hearing protectors—Part 3: Simplified method for the measurement of insertion loss of ear-muff type protectors for quality inspection purposes* (ISO/TR 4869–3: 1989). Geneva, Switzerland: IOS.

INTERNATIONAL ORGANIZATION FOR STANDARDIZATION. (1990). *Acoustics—Hearing protectors—Part 1: Subjective method for the measurement of sound attenuation* [ISO 4869–1: 1990(E)]. Geneva, Switzerland: IOS.

INTERNATIONAL ORGANIZATION FOR STANDARDIZATION. (1994). *Acoustics—Hearing protectors—Part 2: Estimation of effective A-weighted sound pressure levels when hearing protectors are worn* [ISO 4869–2:1994(E)]. Geneva, Switzerland: IOS.

INTERNATIONAL ORGANIZATION FOR STANDARDIZATION. (1996a). *Hearing protectors—Safety requirements and testing—earmuffs* (ISO/DIS 10449). Geneva, Switzerland: IOS.

INTERNATIONAL ORGANIZATION FOR STANDARDIZATION. (1996b). *Hearing protectors—Recommendations for selection, use, care and maintenance—Guidance document* (ISO/DIS 10452). Geneva, Switzerland: IOS.

INTERNATIONAL ORGANIZATION FOR STANDARDIZATION. (1996c). *Hearing protectors—Safety requirements and testing—earplugs* (ISO/DIS 10453), Geneva, Switzerland: IOS.

JOHNSON, D.L. (1997). *Blast overpressure studies*. Albuquerque, NM: U.S. Army Medical Research and Materiel Command, DAMD 17-93-C-3101.

JOHNSON, D.L., & PATTERSON, J. JR. (1992). Rating of hearing protector performance for impulse noise. In: *Proceedings, Hearing Conservation Conference* (pp.103–106). Lexington, KY: Office of Engineering Services, University of Kentucky.

KILLION, M., DEVILBISS, E., & STEWART, J. (1988). An earplug with uniform 15 dB attenuation. *Hearing Journal, 41*(5):14–17.

KROES, P., FLEMING, R., & LEMPERT, B. (1975). *List of personal hearing protectors and attenuation data*. Cincinnati: National Institute for Occupational Safety and Health, U.S. Department of Health, Education and Welfare, Report No. 76-120.

KUNOV, H., ABEL, S.M., & GIGUERE, C. (1986). *An acoustic test fixture for use with hearing protective devices*. Toronto: Mount Sinai Hospital and University of Toronto, Final Report on Contract No. 8SE84-00241, Department of National Defence (DCIEM).

LLOYD, J.A. (1996). Assessing hearing protectors for use in impulsive noise. In: F.A. Hill, & R. Lawrence (Eds.), *Proceedings of Inter-Noise 96* (pp. 971–974). St. Albans, UK: Institute of Acoustics.

MAUNEY, D., & CASALI, J.G. (1990). *Preliminary noise attenuation assessment of AICOMM's AIMic: Current fitting device performance and improved ear couplers*. Blacksburg, VA: Virginia Polytechnical Institute and State University, Industrial Engineering and Operations Research, Technical Report 9001.

NIXON, C.W., HILLE, H.K., & KETTLER, L.K. (1967). *Attenuation characteristics of earmuffs at low audio and infrasonic frequencies*. Wright-Patterson, AFB: Report AMRL-TR-67–27.

NIXON, C.W., MCKINLEY, R.L., & STEUVER, J.W. (1992). Performance of active noise reduction headsets. In: A. Axlesson, H. Borchgrevink, R.P. Hamernik, P. Hellstrom, D. Henderson, & R.J. Salvi (Eds.), *Scientific basis of noise-induced hearing loss* (pp. 389–400). St. Louis, MO: Mosby–Year Book.

OSHA. (1983). Occupational noise exposure: Hearing conservation amendment. Occupational Safety and Health Administration, *Federal Register, 48*(46);9738–9785.

OSHA. (1987). OSHA Instruction CPL 2–2.20A, change 2, March 1. In: *Industrial hygiene technical manual* (pp. VI-13–VI-20). Washington, DC: U.S. Government Printing Office.

PAAKKONEN, R., & TIKKANEN, J. (1991). Attenuation of low-frequency noise by hearing protectors. *Annals of Occupational Hygiene, 35*(2);189–199.

PARK, M.Y., & CASALI, J.G. (1991). A controlled investigation of in-field attenuation performance of selected insert, earmuff, and canal cap hearing protectors. *Human Factors, 33*(6);693–714.

PRICE, I.R., & WHITAKER, G. (1986). Noise exposure during shotblasting and the acoustic properties of air-fed helmets. In: R. Lotz (Ed.), *Proceedings of Inter-Noise 86* (pp. 559–564). Poughkeepsie, NY: Noise Control Foundation.

ROYSTER, J.D., BERGER, E.H., MERRY, C.J., NIXON, C.W., FRANKS, J.R., BEHAR, A., CASALI, J.G., DIXON-ERNST, C., KIEPER, R.W., MOZO, B.T., OHLIN, D., & ROYSTER, L.H. (1996). Development of a new standard laboratory protocol for estimating the field attenuation of hearing protection devices. Part I. Research of Working Group 11, Accredited Standards Committee S12, Noise. *Journal of the Acoustical Society of America, 99*(3);1506–1526.

ROYSTER, L.H., & ROYSTER, J.D. (1985). Hearing protection devices. In: A.S. Feldman, & C.T. Grimes (Eds.), *Hearing conservation in industry* (pp. 103–150). Baltimore, MD: Williams & Wilkins.

SCHROETER, J. (1986). The use of acoustical test fixtures for the measurement of hearing protector attenuation. Part I. Review of previous work and the design of an improved test fixture. *Journal of the Acoustical Society of America, 79*(4);1065–1081.

SCHROETER, J., & POESSELT, C. (1986). The use of acoustical test fixtures for the measurement of hearing protector attenuation. Part II. Modeling the external ear, simulating bone conduction, and comparing test fixture and real-ear data. *Journal of the Acoustical Society of America, 80*(2);505–527.

SMOORENBURG, G.F. (1996). *Assessment of hearing protector performance in impulsive noise. Final Report*. Soesterberg: TNO Human Factors Research Inst., Rept. TM-96-CO42.

WILKINS, P., & MARTIN, A.M. (1987). Hearing protection and warning sounds in industry—A review. *Applied Acoustics, 21*(4);267–293.

YLIKOSKI, M.E., PEKKARINEN, J.O., STARCK, J.P., PAAKKONEN, R.J., & YLIKOSKI, J.S. (1995). Physical characteristics of gunfire impulse noise and its attenuation by hearing protectors. *Scandinavian Audiology, 24*(1);3–11

PREFERRED PRACTICE GUIDELINES

Professionals Who Perform the Procedure(s)

▼ Audiologists

▼ Nurses

▼ Industrial hygienists

▼ Physicians

▼ Occupational hearing conservationists

Expected Outcomes

▼ The HPD is comfortable and can be worn throughout all expected exposures.

▼ The HPD provides sufficient protection but does not overprotect.

▼ The wearer is properly trained in the use and care of the HPD.

▼ The wearer understands the hazards of noise exposure and is motivated to protect his or her hearing.

Clinical Indications

▼ Hearing protector issuing and training is conducted for all persons exposed to noise sufficient to cause hearing loss and also for those who find the noise objectionable.

Clinical Process

▼ Understands the occlusion effect and how to use it to demonstrate proper fit.

▼ Can train users how to properly pull the pinna to ease earplug insertion.

▼ Otologic inspection or examination to be sure no medical conditions of the earcanal or circumaural region contraindicate use of HPDs.

▼ Is aware of new hearing protection technology such as amplitude-sensitive and flat-attenuation HPDs and understands when such devices are applicable.

▼ The applications of laboratory versus real-world data are understood.

▼ The mechanics of using attenuation data, the NRR, and how these impact selection are properly applied.

Documentation

▼ Documentation of type and size (if appropriate) HPD issued.

▼ Documentation of training in use of hearing protection.

Chapter 23

Subjective Tinnitus: Its Mechanisms and Treatment

Robert E. Sandlin and Robert T. Olsson

Outline

Over the past 25 years the number of studies investigating *subjective tinnitus* has significantly increased. We mention subjective tinnitus because it is, by far, the most prevalent. Subjective tinnitus may be defined as the perception of an acoustic-like sensation for which no external generation exists. *Objective tinnitus* (vibratory tinnitus), on the other hand, is an acoustic-like sensation that can be heard by others and lends itself to physical measurement. Chronic myoclonus (chronic muscle spasms) involving the tensor tempani, stapedius, and palatine muscles; blood flow turbulence; and movement involved in the opening of the eustachian tube are representative of causes of objective tinnitus. Perhaps one

might also include otoacoustic emissions as a form of objective tinnitus. This chapter is primarily concerned with the mechanisms, evaluation, and treatment of subjective tinnitus.

For those contemplating the provision of clinical service to patients with subjective tinnitus four important messages exist. First, no consensus exists regarding the cause of this perplexing disorder. Second, no known "cure" exists for subjective tinnitus. Third, no single therapeutic modality is sufficiently compelling to warrant its use above all others. We are not suggesting individuals cannot be helped with some form of therapeutic intervention but rather that much is to be learned about the neurophysiological generation of subjective tinnitus and the psychodynamics of those who are suffering from it. Fourth, enough intellectual and clinical challenge in the treatment of subjective tinnitus is present to warrant the interest and active involvement of audiologists.

Those working with the patient who has tinnitus deal with the symptoms of the disorder. The clinician can control, to some extent, the patient's awareness of the ongoing tinnitus but can do nothing to effect a cure. To cure this perplexing problem, a way must be found to suppress the tinnitus generator(s), whatever it (they) may be, and thereby alter the abnormal neural activity that gives rise to the perception of subjective tinnitus.

Our task here is to review tinnitus as it relates to history, prevalence, cause (mechanisms), evaluation, and treatments. The understanding of tinnitus and its treatment has advanced to that point where it is no longer necessary or prudent for the physician or any other health practitioner to advise the patient to "learn to live with it."

HISTORICAL OVERVIEW OF TINNITUS

Throughout much of recorded history the disorder that we now refer to as subjective or objective tinnitus has been mentioned. Its explanation took many forms, including providential intervention. Several millennia ago, the Phoenicians mentioned a disorder that can be described as tinnitus. Egyptian hieroglyphics suggest that tinnitus was of concern during the Pharaonic period. The Ebers papyrus (about 1650–1532 B.C.) defines patients with tinnitus as those with "bewitched ears" (*Kamal's Dictionary of Pharaonic Medicine*).

We are grateful to Dr. Richard Nodar of the Cleveland Clinic, Cleveland, Ohio, for much of the information referenced in our historical review.

Audiology: Treatment. Edited by Valente, Hosford-Dunn, and Roeser. Thieme Medical Publishers, Inc., New York © 2000

Aristotle (384–322 B.C.) notes the phenomenon of tinnitus in his *Problemata Physica*. The physician Galen (129–199 B.C.) described tinnitus as echoes. Interestingly, Alexander of Tralles (A.D. 522–605) hypothesized that tinnitus may follow an emotional or physical crisis. In 1821 Jean Marie Gaspard Itard (1775–1838) mentioned true tinnitus and false tinnitus, suggesting perhaps that which we now refer to as objective and subjective tinnitus. Itard was among the first to mention that tinnitus could be masked by some external means. He suggested that a roaring fire might be effective in masking tinnitus sounds akin to rushing wind or rushing water. Tonal tinnitus may be masked by placing green wood on an active fire. For tinnitus described as a high whistling sound, the resonance generated by water dripping into a large metallic bowl may provide relief. In 1801 Grappengiesser (Staller, 1998) was among the first investigators to use direct electrical stimulation of the ear to treat tinnitus. His claims of success, however, have never been validated by other studies. However, his observation that current had to flow with the positive terminal in proximity of the ear is still a valid observation. In 1855 Duchenne de Boulogne (Staller, 1998) used an alternating current (AC) delivered by an electrode immersed in water in the external auditory meatus. He reported that 8 of 10 patients were "cured." Little documentation is available to back up such tales of clinical success. In 1941 Fowler suggested that tinnitus is vibratory or nonvibratory.

In terms of tinnitus management, Dr. Jack Vernon introduced a wearable masker device in 1975. He was instrumental also in defining *residual inhibition*, a term first coined by Feldman in Germany. In 1990 Jastreboff introduced his model for tinnitus and subsequently developed a therapeutic approach based on that model. His therapeutic approach is referred to as *tinnitus retraining therapy*. At about the same time, Jonathan Hazel in England introduced the Jastreboff approach in that country.

Among noted personalities who had tinnitus, one may include Smetana, Goethe, Martin Luther, Beethoven, and Van Gogh. In more recent times celebrities such as Barbra Streisand, William Shatner, and Tony Randall are among those having had extended experience with subjective tinnitus.

In *Merriam-Webster's Collegiate Dictionary* (tenth edition), both TINN-i-tus and tin-EYE-tis are acceptable pronunciations. The English word *tinnitus* derives from the Latin verb *tinnire*, to ring or tinkle. Because the first syllable is accented in the present infinitive form of this Latin verb, it would seem more logical to place the accent on the first syllable in the derived English noun. Balancing this logic is the natural tendency to treat the word as a medical term, which would cause the accent to be on the second syllable. At least in the United States, which pronunciation a speaker might use seems to be primarily a matter of geography. We have not been able to locate any firm data and so must rely on our own and others' reports. It seems the West Coast tends to prefer the accent on the second syllable, the middle portions of the country prefer to accent the first syllable, and those on the East Coast seem to be evenly divided.

CAUSE AND PREVALENCE OF TINNITUS

Because one does not know the cause of subjective tinnitus, one can only assume that something caused it or that some relationship exists between a specific incident, or a set of conditions, and the onset of tinnitus. Little doubt exists that disease, drugs, or trauma contribute to the onset of tinnitus, but its precise cause has yet to be revealed. Anecdotally, 25% reported that their tinnitus was due to noise exposure. Seven percent believed that the onset of tinnitus was due to some pathological condition of the hearing mechanism. An additional 6% believed that a positive correlation was present between head injury and the onset of tinnitus. Two percent reported that whiplash injury gave rise to their tinnitus. Fifteen percent reported a variety of other possible causes for their tinnitus. A striking 47% of those patients with severe tinnitus had no idea what caused it.

Estimates of the number of patients experiencing tinnitus vary. The American Tinnitus Association estimates that 50 million persons in the United States have some form of tinnitus. Of this number, 12 million have it in its severe form (Meikle et al, 1995). Whatever the actual number may be, it is evident that it represents a sizable group of individuals seeking or needing some kind of therapeutic intervention.

Tinnitus is not restricted to those with some degree of hearing impairment. Heller and Bergman (1953) conducted a study in which 70 subjects with normal-hearing were placed in an anechoic chamber for no more than 5 minutes. Of that population, 94% experienced some form of tinnitus consistent with that experienced by a control group of persons with impaired hearing. It is apparent for normal-hearing individuals that customary and everyday acoustic environments effectively mask low-level tinnitus.

The data presented here are taken from the Tinnitus Data Registry collected by the Oregon Hearing Research Lab (Meikle et al, 1995). Dr. Mary Meikle is to be given a great deal of credit for the development and management of this very important registry. The demographic data reported here represent only a very small segment of that which exists. It does reflect some of the more salient facts about tinnitus. For more information about the Tinnitus Registry, the reader should access its Internet Web page at http://www.ohus.edu/ohrc-otda/.

The phenomenon of loudness perception is not completely understood by those investigating the mysteries of tinnitus. When 1544 patients were rating loudness on a visual analog scale (VAS) from 0 to 10, those having "tonal" tinnitus gave an average rating of 7.5, whereas those with the "noise" type gave an average rating of 5.5. This is despite the fact that most patients, regardless of the sound of their tinnitus, can be masked at sensation levels (SLs) seldom exceeding 14 dB. It would therefore seem that "tonal" tinnitus seems to be louder than tinnitus that has a broader frequency spectrum. One might conjecture this is due to its contrast with the surrounding acoustic environment. In another sample of 1503 patients with severe tinnitus, 88% reported their loudness to be 11 dB SL or less. The average loudness level of this group was 5.7 dB SL (Vernon, 1998). In a broad historical review of studies of tinnitus loudness, Tyler and Stouffer (1989) found that 71% of patients had tinnitus whose perceived loudness was 10 dB SL or less, and 88% had a perceived loudness of 20 dB SL or less. A broad band of high-frequency noise of 2000 to 12,000 Hz presented at 8 dB SL could mask the tinnitus of yet another group of 818 patients with severe but maskable tinnitus. Fully 68% of the patients could be masked with 14 dB SL or less (Vernon, 1998).

One might assume that a lower loudness SL indicates that the patient does not have a severe problem. This assumption is incorrect. Our own long experience with tinnitus patients and the extensive data collected by the Oregon Tinnitus Data Registry (Vernon, 1998) shows no positive correlation between the perceived loudness of tinnitus and the psychological behavior or emotional response to it.

Clinicians studying the masking of tinnitus often observe another phenomenon, that of *residual inhibition*. Vernon (1998) describes residual inhibition as "a temporary period of suppressed tinnitus immediately following a period of masking" (p. xvi). The authors have observed patients who have reported only a few seconds of residual inhibition and those who report several days of inhibition after a period of use of a masker device. From a sample of 1445 tinnitus patients tested for residual inhibition, 91% evidenced some residual inhibition. Some of these patients had complete residual inhibition (a complete absence of the perception of tinnitus). Others evidenced some degree of partial residual inhibition (a lessening of the subjective loudness of the ongoing tinnitus after a defined period of noise stimulation).

Many patients with subjective tinnitus report some difficulty with sleep. They had trouble obtaining sleep or, if awakened, had difficulty regaining a sleep state. Again, reporting from the Tinnitus Data Registry, 78% of 1113 patients, when asked about sleep interference, reported some problem.

SOUNDS OF TINNITUS

The acoustic composition of tinnitus is not the same for every patient. When patients were asked to describe their ongoing tinnitus, the answers cover a wide range of sounds. Among the more common descriptions, one may include "buzzing," "roaring," "whistling" (teapot), "ringing" (usually described as a pure tone signal), "static" (radio and power lines), "crickets," "music," and "pulsing." Of a total population of 1664 patients, 54% reported their tinnitus was perceived as a single sound. For 26%, tinnitus was reported to consist of two sounds. Nine percent stated that their tinnitus had three distinct sounds, 6% estimated four or more sounds, and 5% were unable to determine how many sounds were present. In terms of the acoustic quality of tinnitus, 79% of 1544 patients indicated their tinnitus closely approximated a pure tone signal. Only 6% of this population described their tinnitus as some type of noise. The remaining 15% thought their tinnitus was a combination of both noise and tone. In terms of pitch perception, most patients in one particular study could match their ongoing tinnitus to an 8000 Hz tone (Meikle et al, 1995).

The perceived location of tinnitus appears to have a bilateral preponderance. The location of the tinnitus varied from right ear only, left ear only, both ears, at the ears, and outside the head. The Oregon Tinnitus Registry (Meikle et al, 1995) reports that of 1932 patients, 60% reported the tinnitus to be located in each ear. It was located in only one ear for 20% (9% for the right ear and 11% for the left). In 1% of this population the location of the tinnitus varied between ears. Seldom is tinnitus reported to have its location outside the head. Tinnitus sounds were reported to be either constant or intermittent.

Logically, it would seem that the description of tinnitus might contribute to its cause or support the mechanisms producing the sound. To date, no such association exists between the description and the mechanism(s) or the site(s) of lesion. A large number of patients reporting noise exposure as the probable cause of tinnitus tended to describe their tinnitus as having more of a pure tone, rather than a complex sound, quality.

Regardless of its description, tinnitus is not some weird manifestation of a psychiatric disorder or pronounced mental disturbance. A physical cause gives rise to all these manifested disturbances. Although an acoustic neuroma can be the cause (Levy & Arts, 1996; Valente et al, 1995), the incidence seems to be rare (Fisher et al, 1994).

MECHANISMS OF TINNITUS

One must agree with Feldman's (1995) statement that

> Tinnitus is a functional disorder of the auditory system that probably can originate from different lesions and at different sites. The auditory system, however, is so complex, involving highly complicated peripheral organs, a multitude of afferent and efferent pathways, and a great number of nuclei which form a meshwork capable of logistic processes of the highest order, such as habituation, recognition, [and] memory learning, that the aim to pinpoint a certain disorder in one structure, or to assign a certain malfunction to one defined lesion is questionable. Somehow, the whole system is always involved. (p. 43)

To define the mechanisms of tinnitus is not unlike four blind men attempting to describe an elephant by touching it. It depends on what part of the elephant's anatomy is being tactically examined as to the conclusions reached. Or it may be more akin to the actions of a select committee whose task it was to design a horse and, in reality, produced something more akin to a camel. Among the several possibilities for defining the mechanism of tinnitus, one may consider (1) vibratory tinnitus; (2) phase-locked spontaneous discharge of cells bodies, wherein the electrical activity normally present within neurons becomes synchronized with that of adjacent neurons, with a resulting signal strong enough to be detected; (3) aberrant behavior of the efferent system; (4) involvement of neurotransmitter substances, the chemicals the brain uses as the means of communications between its cells; (5) central origin; (6) vascular compression of the seventh nerve, plus several other possible mechanisms.

Clinicians simply do not know, with absolute certainty, where within the neurology of man lie the neurogenerators responsible for the production of subjective tinnitus. Furthermore, clinicians are not certain that tinnitus totally depends on the specific receptor or neural sites giving rise to its perception. The perpetuation of tinnitus may be a CNS phenomenon dictated by novel peripheral activity. For example, a body of information suggests that tinnitus is not unlike the phantom limb phenomenon (Jastreboff, 1990). An individual having had an amputation of a limb may still perceive pain associated with that limb long after surgery. One of the authors (R.S.) recalls a graduate fellow at the university who lost a leg during World War II and often experienced an incessant itching of his big toe, even though the amputation had taken place many months before. Although one may not know the mechanisms giving rise to tinnitus as a phantom sensation, little doubt exists that such mechanisms are active and are not dissimilar to the neural mechanisms responsible for the phantom limb response and other sensory sensations (Jastreboff, 1990, 1995a, 1995b; Melzack, 1992; Schultz & Melzack, 1991). A strong point is made for this argument when it is realized that patients with chronic, debilitating tinnitus who had surgical sectioning of the eighth nerve did not always find resolution to their tinnitus problem. Although some did experience complete absence of the tinnitus, a certain percentage of the surgical population found the tinnitus to be worse after surgery and others experienced little change (R. Johnson, personal communication, 1997). Peripheral and central neural mechanisms play different roles in the onset and perpetuation of tinnitus. The problem is one of trying to ferret out which is which. Even if such revelations came about, no assurance exists that an absolute therapeutic intervention would be developed. Probably several causes and mechanisms for the generation of tinnitus exist. The authors agree with Dr. Pawel Jastreboff (personal communication, 1998) and with other investigators, who state that tinnitus is a symptom of many causes and may be based on a number of different mechanisms.

Lockwood et al (1998) conducted an important experiment whose purpose was to help identify the neural mechanisms and loci of disabling tinnitus. Their tool was positron emission tomography (PET) scanning, a technique that maps, in real time, areas of the brain experiencing increased blood flow. The researchers cited numerous studies that had previously demonstrated that PET scans could isolate those areas of the brain responsible for the production of transient, subjective sensations. Lockwood and his team monaurally stimulated one ear of six normally hearing subjects with pure tones. They used PET scans to determine that blood flow increased in the bilateral auditory cortexes. They then repeated this experiment with four patients who had high-frequency sensorineural hearing losses, were quite bothered by tinnitus, and could increase their tinnitus through oral-facial movements. The pure tone stimulation again produced increased blood flow in the bilateral auditory cortexes. When the tinnitus patients created oral-facial movements that increased their tinnitus, the increased blood flow occurred only in the contralateral auditory cortex. In addition, blood flow increased in the left hippocampal area (the patients had right-sided tinnitus) and in the lenticular nuclei. These two latter brain areas are associated with emotional responses.

Were tinnitus a sound generated within the cochlea, Lockwood and his team reasoned, the responses in the auditory cortex would be the same for tinnitus and for an externally applied sound. This was not the case. On the basis of the abnormal response in the auditory cortex, they concluded that tinnitus arises in the central auditory system not in the cochlea. Furthermore, as shown by the involvement of the hippocampus and the lenticular nuclei, in persons who "suffer from," rather than merely "experience," tinnitus, the involved emotional centers of the brain prevent adaptation to tinnitus.

Whatever the tinnitus mechanisms are, they involve both the peripheral and central nervous systems (Meikle et al, 1995). Whatever the neural mechanisms are, the onset of tinnitus must depend, in part, on an alteration or change in the inhibition or excitation of neural activity in the auditory pathway or somewhere in the peripheral system. Two significant alterations in the function of the central auditory system are created by hearing impairment (Gerkin, 1995). First is the sensitivity of auditory neurons to selected electrical stimulation. Second is the auditory system's ability to process stimuli of different duration (temporal integration) when either acoustic stimuli are presented to the ear or electrical stimulation is applied directly to the auditory brain stem nuclei. Such changes in the function of the central auditory system may provide a theoretical basis for the onset and perpetuation of peripherally based tinnitus and for the generation of central tinnitus.

Alterations in the function of the inferior colliculus may give rise to the onset of subjective tinnitus. Jastreboff (1995b) holds that the mechanism for tinnitus may involve a discordant dysfunction of outer hair cell (OHC) and inner hair cell (IHC) systems. Type I myelinated afferent fibers innervate only IHC and unmyelinated type II fibers innervate the OHC. Any discordant function between the two may cause tinnitus. If one system becomes dsyfunctional because of loss of cell population and the other system remains healthy, a difference is created in the activity of type I and type II fibers. As reported by Stypulkowski (1989) and Jastreboff (1990), ototoxic drugs can damage the OHC without initially inflicting damage on the IHC. When damage to the OHC system has occurred, usually involving the basal end of the membrane in the early stages, the mechanical properties of the organ of Corti are altered. It may be the alternation of the functional efficiency of the organ of Corti that initiates tinnitus onset.

Whatever one's precept is of the mechanisms causing tinnitus, it must involve to some extent changes in neural activity involving peripheral and central systems. Or changes in the actions of neurotransmitter substances might be responsible for the onset and perpetuation of tinnitus. Some investigators (Brummett, 1995; Hindmarch et al, 1990) believe that gamma amino butyric acid (GABA), a neurotransmitter that acts on the inferior colliculus, plays a major role in tinnitus genesis.

Animal models have been proposed (Jastreboff, 1995a) to explain the origin and mechanisms underlying the onset and perpetuation of tinnitus. Although correlations have been observed between the animal model and human behaviors, much has yet to be accomplished before the total picture is complete.

It is not the purpose of this chapter to provide an exhaustive overview of theories relating to possible active mechanisms of tinnitus. Suffice it to say that subjective tinnitus is a neurophysiological reality for which understanding and solutions are being sought, but none has been found to date.

ASSESSMENT AND EVALUATION OF TINNITUS

Medical Evaluation and Case History

The assessment of tinnitus can be considered from two perspectives. First is the attempt to identify the source of tinnitus, to describe it qualitatively, and to quantify it numerically. Second is the assessment of how the tinnitus affects the patient.

A thorough medical evaluation is an essential, early component of tinnitus assessment. In a perfect world the medical evaluation would be performed by a neuro-otologist. In reality, a neuro-otological evaluation tends to be reserved for those cases that do not fall under an obvious cause. The medical evaluation would include a review of standard audiological data, including pure tone air and bone, speech, immittance measures, acoustic reflex patterns, and acoustic reflex decay tests. The last three tests should be deferred until loudness discomfort levels for both pure tones and speech are obtained. The physician would take a careful history, with questions seeking to uncover any symptoms or conditions that would lead him or her to suspect retrocochlear or neurological abnormalities. When appropriate, brain stem–evoked response audiometry, otoacouostic emission tests, electronystagmography (ENG), and magnetic resonance imaging (MRI) or computed tomography (CT) are ordered.

Perhaps to avoid the possibility of overlooking anything, the University of Maryland Tinnitus and Hyperacusis Center includes such a medical evaluation as part of its assessment of every patient (Jastreboff, personal observation and correspondence, 1995, 1997). This same center also universally administers an otoacoustic emission test. At the Sonus Center for Tinnitus, we do not provide a medical evaluation. It is our experience that by the time a patient sees the clinician, he or she has already had a multitude of medical workups for tinnitus. Nor have we, to date, found clinical usefulness in the otoacoustic emission test for tinnitus patients, although this is certainly subject to re-evaluation.

Audiometric Evaluation

Our test battery begins with the standard diagnostic audiological evaluation. Because clinicians are searching for subtle differences between ears, they need exact threshold measures for later comparison and for counseling purposes. The air conduction threshold frequencies used are 250, 500, 1000, 2000, 3000, 4000, 6000, 8000, and 12,000 Hz. Half-octaves are tested in the lower frequencies if a step of 15 dB or more is present between octaves. Word recognition testing uses full word lists. If the most comfortable level (MCL) is at a relatively low sensation level, such as 40 dB HL or lower, and the word recognition scores are less than 90%, and if discomfort is not a problem, the audiologist will use one or two more word lists at a higher presentation level.

Pitch Matching

Defining the patient's tinnitus numerically is the next step. One can use several individual pieces of equipment to achieve desired measurement goals. In the past a few researchers and clinicians have used a tinnitus synthesizer to come as close as possible to reproducing the tinnitus sound(s) that patients hear. A tinnitus synthesizer is a sophisticated electronic oscillator that produces a host of sounds, including pure tones and narrow noise bands. The width of the noise band can be set manually. The use of a tinnitus synthesizer provides a means of achieving a closer frequency match than does a conventional audiometer. The pitch of the tinnitus is clinically assessed by presenting a tone to the ear contralateral to the tinnitus. Various stimuli may be used, depending on the individual's description of the tinnitus. For example, if the tinnitus is reported to be high pitched, a pure tone stimulus may be the most appropriate. For persons reporting a hissing-like sensation, a high-frequency noise band may be used in the matching procedure. A number of different sounds might be selected if the patient reports the tinnitus to have a roaring sound quality to it.

Because most audiometers produce only octave or half-octave pure tones, its accuracy is less than desired in obtaining precise pitch matching. Yet because of the time involved

in training the patient to use a tinnitus synthesizer and the expense of the equipment itself, the use of this equipment is rare. The one manufacturer who was making a clinical tinnitus simulator (tinnitus synthesizer) has, as far as we know, stopped manufacturing them several years ago. At present, we usually use a clinical audiometer. The ability to produce a 12,000 Hz signal is again quite helpful for this purpose.

The audiologist instructs the patient to judge whether the pitch of the first or the second of two successive tones is closer to the tinnitus he hears. In case of unilateral tinnitus, the audiologist presents the tones to the unaffected ear. The audiologist brackets with successive approximations. Because the audiometer uses discrete steps, the final frequency recorded will be an approximation rather than an exact definition. Once the most dominant frequency has been identified, the patient chooses whether a pure tone, narrow band noise, speech noise, or white noise best matches the perceived tinnitus.

> ### PITFALL
>
> Experience has taught clinicians that the pitch match test is not always a simple procedure. Indeed, general consensus exists among most who treat the patient with tinnitus that pitch matching is more difficult and less precise than loudness matching. Some patients have a difficult time matching an external tone or sound to their ongoing tinnitus. We have observed what Vernon (personal correspondence, 1995) described as "octave confusion." A patient first decides that his tinnitus is best matched to a 3000 Hz tone. However, repeating the pitch-matching test often results in a more positive and consistent match an octave higher, at 6000 Hz. In some cases we have noticed patients who report that the dominant sound of their tinnitus may change from time to time. On one assessment session, the patient matches to a specific frequency. On a subsequent evaluation, however, the frequency match may be far different than that obtained on the initial assessment date.

Loudness Matching

The clinician and patient then repeat the process for the tinnitus' loudness. Although no universally accepted method of loudness judgment exists, it is a commonly used assessment tool. We believe it to be a clinically useful procedure in the diagnostic process. Although loudness judgments may vary from test to test, they do provide a useful piece of information during the initial evaluation process.

The loudness match uses the external sound previously identified during pitch matching. That external sound is presented to the ear contralateral to the tinnitus and is increased or decreased in intensity until the patient judges that the loudness is equal to that of his or her tinnitus. The test for the intensity match is delivered in 1 dB steps. Because hearing thresholds were tested in 5 dB steps, it is not rare to discover that the tinnitus has a negative sensation level. If the patient's actual threshold of the tinnitus' frequency is 21 dB HL, for example, his recorded threshold will be 25 dB HL. His tinnitus might have an intensity of 24 dB HL (i.e., −1 dB SL). As stated earlier, the equal loudness measure of the tinnitus seldom exceeds 11 dB SL.

Minimum Masking Level

The next step is to determine the minimum level of white noise needed to achieve masking of the ongoing tinnitus (i.e., the *minimum masking level*). This, too, is tested in 1 dB steps. Depending on the type of tinnitus the patient experiences, this subtest might be performed monaurally in the affected ear or binaurally if the tinnitus is present bilaterally. If the presentation is binaural, the starting point for each ear should be at the perceived level of the tinnitus in that particular ear. For example, the test might begin in one ear at 12 dB HL, whereas the opposite ear receives the stimulus at 17 dB HL. The second presentation would be at 13- and 18-dB, the third at 14- and 19-dB, and so on.

The patient must be admonished during the test for the minimum masking level that either the tinnitus might become louder or the test stimulus might become uncomfortably loud. The patient is directed to halt the test immediately if either event begins to occur.

Residual Inhibition

Next we test for *residual inhibition*. The audiologist first explains the test procedure, covering the points presented in this paragraph. The clinician then delivers 1 to 2 seconds of white noise to the affected ear, or to both ears if the tinnitus is binaural, at 10 dB above the minimum masking level. The patient verifies that the test stimulus is not traumatic or uncomfortably loud. If it is, the test for residual inhibition is not performed. If it is not, the white noise is presented for 60 seconds. At the end of 1 minute, the patient assesses whether the tinnitus is gone, diminished, unchanged, or louder. The time it takes for the tinnitus to return to its pretest state is recorded. If the tinnitus is completely absent after a 1-minute exposure to the white noise, it is referred to as *complete residual inhibition (CRI)*. If the tinnitus is reduced but not completely absent for a period of time, it is referred to as *partial residual inhibition (PRI)*.

Loudness Discomfort Level

Loudness discomfort levels are evaluated next. An ascending technique (Hawkins, 1987) with a seven-category loudness scale that ranges from "very soft" to "uncomfortably loud" is used. The safety given to patients who have *hyperacusis*, a disproportionate growth in the subjective loudness of sounds, more than compensates for the compromise in statistical validity that might occur from not using random presentations. Loudness discomfort is tested for both ears for speech,

using a spondee or a short sentence; pure tones of 1000, 2000, 4000, and 8000 Hz; and for the tinnitus frequency if it is not one of these tones. It is not until loudness discomfort levels have been assessed that immittance audiometry, acoustic reflex, and acoustic reflex decay testing are obtained. Deferring these tests until this time allows the clinician to be sure that the immittance probe tone, approximately 75 dB HL at 250 Hz, and the stimuli used for testing acoustic reflex thresholds will not violate the patient's loudness tolerance.

> ## PITFALL
>
> **We recommend that every audiologist warn every patient, before embarking on acoustic reflex decay testing, that the test stimuli will be quite loud and will last for a full 10 seconds. One of the authors' patients, who came from another facility, reported tinnitus caused by acoustic reflex decay testing. He already had a medical diagnosis for his unilateral hearing loss (Meniere's disease) and knew he was sensitive to loud sound in the affected ear. The audiologist who tested his acoustic reflexes did not give him any advance warning concerning the intensity of the test stimuli.**

Certainly, it is logical and straightforward to question the value of the time spent and of the information gleaned from the audiological tinnitus assessment. In response, one must keep in mind that the original audiological treatment for tinnitus is masking. The test data gathered will let the clinician know if the tinnitus reported by the patient can be masked. If the patient can benefit from masking, the frequency of the tinnitus must be known. If the patient's tinnitus cannot be effectively masked, it is essential for both clinician and patient to know this.

Often the value of the data obtained lies in its counseling contribution. For patients who have a hearing loss, tinnitus is most often at, or next to, the area of greatest nerve damage. This factoid, when combined with an explanation of tinnitus generation in language the patient can understand, usually reinforces Jastreboff's and Hazel's (1993) theory of tinnitus generation. Some patients, despite all the sophisticated testing they have had, are still not sure "the doctors didn't overlook something." The same type of counseling tends to reinforce in the patient's mind that the tinnitus is strictly an inner ear or auditory system problem and not a harbinger of deafness or disease.

The information is also very useful in counseling patients about the actual value of their tinnitus. We are able to tell most, although not all, patients, "If we could take your tinnitus out of your head and put it down here on the table, it would be a soft sound." This bit of information does two things. First, it reinforces the theory that *tinnitus is not bothersome because it is "objectively" loud, but rather because it is louder than surrounding environmental (ambient) sounds*. It seems to be loud for the same reason a single birthday candle on a cake seems to be bright if the room is dark. The data give ammunition to the clinician who counsels that the problem with tinnitus lies not in the sound but in one's reaction to the sound. Finally, the minimum masking level measure helps the clinician "ballpark" the volume control setting of tinnitus retraining therapy or masker therapy devices.

Subjective Assessment

We have just covered the first aspect of tinnitus assessment, its audiological measures. The second aspect is that of determining its effect on the patient. This second segment is, in our opinion, equally as important as the first segment. Generally, very little correlation exists between the two. That is, the data extracted from the audiological analysis provide little, if any, insight as to how the patient copes with tinnitus.

At the Sonus Center for Tinnitus, patient interviews include not only subjective descriptions of the tinnitus and its history but also 20 to 40 minutes of open-ended questioning. During this session, the clinician not only writes what the patient says, we also watch the face, hands, posture and gesture, and listen to the tone of voice. We want to get a feel for the *affect* of the tinnitus on the patient.

Two excellent psychometric tinnitus inventories that we use at our center (see Appendices A and B) are the *Tinnitus Severity Scale* and the *Tinnitus Handicap Inventory*. The latter is particularly useful in that it includes behavioral changes brought about by tinnitus. Each is self-explanatory and can be completed in a relatively short time.

To summarize, the evaluation of tinnitus is a time-consuming but critical aspect of the total patient management program. Although no general agreement exists as to what to assess, the authors have presented what is believed to be a reasonable clinical approach.

PEARL

The reader may have surmised at this point that the clinical assessment process is time consuming. A tinnitus treatment program requires a commitment to spend quite a bit of time with each patient. The program's fees must also reflect the time involved.

TREATMENT MODALITIES

Drug Therapy

Audiologists are not involved in the administration of drugs in the treatment of tinnitus, but understanding the rationale for their use and the characteristic response of various drugs is important. As suggested in other sections of this chapter, the intent is not to offer an extensive overview but rather a general assessment of the role of drug therapy in the treatment of this perplexing disorder.

Please note that drugs that are used to control tinnitus, as opposed to those that may cause tinnitus, are discussed here. For example, some drugs have a very positive correlation between use and tinnitus onset. Such agents as aminoglyco-

side antibiotics have been reported to produce tinnitus. Among this group we find gentamicin, kanamycin, neomycin, streptomycin, tobramycin, and a host of others. Other common steroidal anti-inflammatory drugs known, or thought, to give rise to tinnitus include aspirin, ibuprofen, and naproxen. Paradoxically, some drugs reported to cause tinnitus have been successful in the treatment of this disorder.

Any review of drug therapy should be prefaced with a statement from Dr. Robert Brummett (1998), nationally recognized pharmacologist at the Department of Otolaryngology, Oregon Hearing Research Center at the Oregon Health Sciences University. He states, "There are many reasons why we do not yet have a drug cure for tinnitus. We do not know the mechanism by which the many different agents, such as drugs, trauma, noise, and even different diseases can cause tinnitus. Because we do not know how, or even where, with any specificity, tinnitus is generated, it is very difficult to rationally design a drug that would be expected to remedy the malady" (p. 34).

A review of the literature clearly suggests that the purpose of drug therapy is not to effect a cure but rather to treat specific symptoms. Antianxiety and antidepressant medications are frequently prescribed by the physician as a means to lessen the psychological and behavioral consequences of relentless tinnitus. The actual dosages of these drugs may vary, depending on the physical or emotional state of the individual.

Antianxiety Drugs

Anxiety may be defined as a feeling of apprehension, uncertainty, and fear generated by known or unknown causes or events. Although definitions may vary, anxiety is a common disturbance that can alter the quality of life. The use of medicines to reduce or control the magnitude of anxiety is common practice. Many of the more common antianxiety drugs fall under the general classification of benzodiazepines. Some of them are alprazolam (Xanax), chlorodiazepoxide (Librium), clonazepam (Klonopin), flurazepam (Dalmane), and temazepam (Restoril).

Some data support the use of benzodiazepines for the management of the tinnitus patient. Johnson et al (1993) reported on a double-blind study in which alprazolam was the active drug and a sugar pill (lactose) served as the placebo. The initial dose of alprazolam was 0.5 mg taken at bedtime. After 7 days, subjects returned for an evaluation and the dosage was increased to 0.5 mg at night (bedtime) and 0.25 mg taken two times a day. After 21 days, subjects were given 0.5 mg three times a day. This regimen continued for 56 days. Each patient was gradually withdrawn from the use of alprazolam by reducing the dose by 0.5 mg over a 3-day period. Nineteen of the 20 subjects taking the placebo and 17 of those taking alprazolam completed the entire program.

Analysis of the data indicated no change in hearing thresholds for any subject. No significant changes occurred in the minimum masking levels (MML) for either the control or experimental group. Of interest were the changes in tinnitus loudness levels. Reductions in both tinnitus loudness levels and decreased loudness were measured on a 10-point scale for those receiving the alprazolam and no significant change was seen in the placebo group. We concluded that the perception of loudness decreased for some of the subjects as a result of taking alprazolam. However, a warning was issued, suggesting that alprazolam was similar to other benzodiazepine drugs and could be addicting (chemical dependency). As a result, it was recommended that tinnitus patients not take alprazolam for periods longer than 4 months. At the end of the 4-month period, a withdrawal schedule should be instituted.

It has occurred to some that if alprazolam reduces but does not eliminate tinnitus perception, other additional nonmedical therapeutic procedures may be instituted to gain further attenuation of the tinnitus. For example, the use of masker devices or other nonmedical management schemes may be of value to the patient.

Antidepression Drugs

Antidepression drugs are of the tricyclic family, such as nortriptyline. Antidepression drugs include such brand names as Elavil, Norpramin, Prozac, Zoloft, Adventyl, and Paelor.

Depression can be defined as a reduction or decrease in functional activity. Such definition may include the absence of hope and cheerfulness and a pronounced emotional dejection. However depression is defined, its presence can severely affect the ways in which one leads his or her life and can significantly influence activities of daily living.

Little doubt exists that for some patients the onset and perpetuation of relentless tinnitus can and does lead to depression. Because we as audiologists do not have effective clinical indicators to inform us what the emotional or psychological effects of subjective tinnitus may be, it is difficult to intervene early on with some treatment modality. Nevertheless, severe emotional disturbances can be a consequence of tinnitus and can be treated with antidepression medication. It is the responsibility of the physician to delineate between anxiety and depression and to select the appropriate medication. Medically, an emotional condition called major depression (MD) exists. When compared with other depression stages, MD is more severe and more prolonged and causes a greater disruption of life's activities.

Dobie and Sullivan (1998) reported that about 60% of their tinnitus patients had MD, which was about six times more frequent than that anticipated from an average outpatient load seen at most clinics. They made an interesting comment related to the period of MD. "Without treatment, MD usually runs its course over a period of six to eighteen months, although about 15 percent of depressed people get worse and eventually commit suicide" (p. 45).

When treating tinnitus patients with nortriptyline, several positive responses were noted, including improved sleep patterns, functioning at a higher level, and an improved feeling of well-being. They surmised that their observations did not prove necessarily that nortriptyline was responsible for the improvement. In a double-blind study, they used nortriptyline as the experimental drug and a milk sugar pill as the placebo. The physical appearance of the placebo was identical to the drug. Some of the results were predictable in that the experimental group showed improvement but so did some of the patients in the placebo group. The magnitude of improvement was derived from responses to the Beck Inventory, the short form of which is a questionnaire permitting an analysis of relative degrees of depression. Patients in each group showed improvement in tinnitus, but more patients in the experimental group reported improvement.

The authors concluded that nortriptyline is effective in reducing symptoms of tinnitus and depression. It is questionable what effect it has on tinnitus itself. That is, it may have a minor effect on the sensation of tinnitus. The placebo effect can be very instrumental in assisting the tinnitus patient to deal effectively with the tinnitus and the troublesome depression.

In general, tricyclic drugs do not have severe, adverse side effects. However, the following experiences have been reported: drowsiness, dizziness, confusion, blurred vision, dry mouth, constipation, and difficulty in urination. Some of the reported problems have been related to fatigue, headache, and an increase in appetite. Some of the effects are age related, and the older patient is subject to more potential side effects.

Drugs other than benzodiazepines and tricyclics have been investigated as to their effect on the perception of subjective tinnitus. A case in point is furosemide (Lasix). Furosemide is known to work primarily on the function of the kidney and the inner ear.

Lasix is a powerful diuretic and is frequently used for that purpose. Furosemide is also known to decrease the endocochlear potential. Only a few diuretics affect the inner ear as does furosemide. Chief among these are bumetanide and ethacrynic acid. To our knowledge, no serious side effects resulting from the use of furosemide have been reported.

The jury is still out as to whether tinnitus is generated as a result of an increase or decrease of endocochlear potential. It is known that the ingestion of aspirin will increase this potential. Animal studies have confirmed that an increased potential exists when substances such as aspirin are injected in controlled amounts. Given this fact, Guth (1998) asked a most interesting question: If tinnitus in humans is characterized by a similar increase in nerve activity, then might a drug suppress tinnitus by reducing the endocochlear potential? (p. 54)

Forty patients reporting tinnitus were injected with 80 mg of furosemide or used another diuretic known not to affect inner ear performance integrity. Of the 40 subjects, 20 patients injected with furosemide reported a suppression in the loudness of their tinnitus. Improvement was measured by using self-rating or subjective scales of improvement and by audiometric loudness scaling procedures. Knowing that injections of furosemide had some positive effect on tinnitus, the next step was to determine whether oral administration of furosemide would yield the same or similar results. Twelve of the 20 patients showing tinnitus suppression were given various doses of oral furosemide. These patients were each given 80 mg/day (two 40 mg tablets/day). Three of the patients yielded positive responses at this level. For the remaining number, the dosage was increased to 120 mg (three 40 mg tablets/day). Three patients showed positive response at this level, and the remaining six patients were given increased doses (160 mg [four 40 mg tablets/day for 5 days]). Four patients in this group responded at this level.

Since the completion of this study, more than 800 tinnitus patients have been seen at the Tinnitus Clinic at Tulane University. One hundred and eighty have received this "furosemide challenge." Of this number, 85 (47%) gave positive responses and were placed on oral furosemide.

Guth (1998) concluded that furosemide is known not to affect brain function. Hence, if a positive response occurs from the use of furosemide, it suggests that the cause lies within the cochlea. If no reduction in tinnitus loudness occurs after the furosemide challenge, the offending site lies elsewhere.

Although one is not certain of the action of various drugs in ameliorating the person's perception of tinnitus, drugs have proven to be of great clinical value in patient management. The reader is reminded that current use of various drugs is directed toward a reduction in one's perception, and negative behavior and is not to be construed as a means or method of cure. Furthermore, many drugs used in the management of the patient with tinnitus can induce chemical dependency. Therefore, medical guidance is a necessity if prolonged use is to be entertained.

Laser Therapy

Early on there was considerable interest in the usefulness of laser therapy for the treatment of tinnitus. Because lasers are known to produce heat, the rationale for their use has been that applying heat to the cochlea would promote healing. Witt and Felix (1989) investigated the use of a low-power laser in combination with ginkgo therapy. They reported a 60% improvement in or the elimination of chronic tinnitus.

However, these impressive results were never confirmed in other clinical studies. Walger et al (1995a) conducted a study in which 155 patients with tinnitus participated. These subjects were reported to have "therapy-resistant tinnitus" and ranged in age from 16 to 80 years. The study was designed so that subjects were randomly placed in one of four groups: group I: laser/ginkgo; group II: ginkgo; group III: laser; group IV: placebo. To assess the efficacy of treatment, audiometric and psychometric measures were used. The analysis of data suggested that no significant differences could be observed between the four groups in all the parameters investigated. In view of these findings, it was concluded that reported improvement was related to a placebo effect. They rejected the conclusion of Witt and Felix (1989) that laser therapy was beneficial in the relief of tinnitus.

Walger and his associates further showed that no healing effect in the cochlea from the application of laser-induced heat could be demonstrated (Walger et al, 1995b). By placing photodiodes in fixed human temporal bones, they proved that the He/Ne-laser rays were completely absorbed before reaching the cochlea. In addition, pulsed infrared rays were reduced to 9.995% of their primary output. On the basis of these findings, they concluded that "results do not support theories of laser activated repair mechanisms within the inner ear of tinnitus patients" (p. 99).

Witt's and Felix's (1989) patients might have experienced a placebo effect. Some clinicians tend to underestimate this effect, which can play such a strong role in the treatment of human disorders. The placebo effect is a potent ingredient to successful therapy. We have seen a number of patients presenting with similar tinnitus histories. One will respond positively to the selected treatment modality, whereas the other remains almost completely resistant. In other cases one patient will evidence a positive change in tinnitus control, whereas the other takes a considerable period of time to achieve the same level of improvement.

Psychological Intervention

Little doubt exists that for a number of patients with subjective tinnitus, psychologically based therapeutic programs are needed and have proven to be of benefit. The question not yet answered completely is what type of intervention best meets the needs of the patient. The basic question underlying psychological approaches is whether patients can resolve their problems or learn to cope more effectively with them. The general consensus is that the goal of some types of psychological intervention is that of having the patient think and react differently to the problem so that negative responses (i.e., maladaptive and nonproductive behaviors) can be greatly reduced or eliminated. Successful therapeutic intervention reduces the stresses caused by the disorder and significantly increases the ability of one to cope more effectively with it.

Because many psychologically based protocols are available for the treatment of tinnitus, it is impossible to review all of them in this chapter. We will concentrate on *cognitive therapy*. Cognitive therapy can best be defined as a process through which the patient changes the way in which life's events are interpreted so that the act of interpretation itself results in one's feeling better. Studies by Jakes et al (1985, 1988), Sweetow (1989), and Wayner (1998) all report on the usefulness of cognitive therapy as a positive adjunct to the counseling armamentarium of the clinician. Wayner (1998) suggests that the "cognitive approach attempts to modify individual's attitudes about the tinnitus by assisting them to adjust to their reaction to it. It cannot and does not alleviate the experience of tinnitus but has been useful in improving how persons perceive the tinnitus and in doing this provides relief" (p. 116).

The genesis of cognitive therapy was the creative thinking of Dr. David Burns (1980). As a psychiatrist, he formulated the principles underlying this particular therapeutic approach. His popular book, *Feeling Good: The New Mood Therapy*, has received wide acceptance among the professional community treating the patient with tinnitus. The following statement by Dr. Burns encapsulates the essence of cognitive therapy: "As you learn to master your moods, you will learn that personal growth can be an exhilarating experience. In the process you will develop a more meaningful set of personal values and adopt a philosophy of living that will make sense and bring you the results you want: increased effectiveness and greater joy" (p. 2).

There are four goals of cognitive therapy as follows:

- *Rapid symptomatic improvement:* This is finding relatively quick relief from troubling symptoms
- *Understanding:* A clear explanation why mood changes occur
- *Self control:* A means through which one uses safe and effective coping strategies
- *Prevention and personal growth:* A process by which mood changes can be avoided on the basis of reassessment of basic values and attitudes

To the extent that thought processes perpetuate negative, and oftentimes emotionally painful, behaviors, they are labeled *cognitive distortions. Cognitive distortions* are negative, unrealistic thoughts that produce a number of negative behaviors regarding a condition or problem. Cognitive therapy supports the belief that thoughts can and do create feelings. The clinician and the patient must work together to identify those cognitive distortions the patient has consciously or unconsciously accepted, after which the patient examines existing thoughts or behaviors in a different and more logical light. For example, the patient might manifest the cognitive distortion "overgeneralization," stating that "the tinnitus is *always* present." Yet the patient might not perceive the tinnitus when sleeping or when concentrating on a specific task. The clinician helps the patient realize moments exist when tinnitus is not at conscious awareness.

The group or workshop setting, based on the format developed by Dr. Richard Hallam (1989) and published in his book, *Living with Tinnitus*, may be an excellent way of changing attitudes and thoughts about tinnitus. Normally, the process of going from distress to acceptance is a prolonged process covering months if not years. In an intensive weekend setting the process of acceptance is accelerated and the participants often make remarkable strides in dealing more realistically with their tinnitus (Wayner, 1998). One cannot stress too strongly the need for organization and structure. The facilitator(s) must be strong leaders if the workshop is to have positive outcomes for the participants. Attention should not be drawn to the tinnitus without some method or organizational plan for alleviating stresses produced by the tinnitus. Otherwise the behaviors might only be intensified.

No magic time period exists in which one achieves success through cognitive therapy. After six to eight 1-hour sessions, one should be able to determine the effectiveness of this therapeutic approach. If progress has been minimal or the patient has not been willing to carry out the tasks assigned, some other therapeutic intervention should be considered. Cognitive therapy also serves as an effective adjunct to other methods of treatment, including masking.

As mentioned previously, a number of psychological treatments are available for tinnitus. It would be wise for the audiologist to become familiar with alternative methods of psychological intervention. We would admonish the reader to assess his or her own clinical competence and to avoid undertaking clinical tasks for which one may not be fully qualified by training or experience.

Biofeedback

Of interest is the fact that the principles underlying biofeedback stemmed from studies of transcendental meditation, cardiac physiology, and the studies of Eastern religions. It was realized by some scientists that animals could regulate to some extent their heart rate, temperature, blood pressure, and other physiological functions simply by offering them a reward for so doing. Even rats could learn to slow their heart rate to the point where death was imminent.

Relating to transcendental meditation, it was discovered that certain feats of relaxation were responsible for the generation of *alpha waves*. It was simple to confirm the presence of alpha waves by the simple expedient of an electroencephalogram. As a result, it was thought that many of the ills affecting mankind could be alleviated through relaxation. Because stress is the very antithesis of relaxation, methods to reduce or eliminate stress could be very beneficial to the feeling or "state" of well-being. It is generally accepted that in a

---

CONTROVERSIAL POINT

Should audiologists provide cognitive therapy?

The arguments against: Audiologists do not have specific training in the provision of cognitive therapy, which might well be considered a form of psychological counseling. They are not equipped to handle the emotional needs of tinnitus or of any other patients. They might be causing damage either by not giving a needed referral or by lulling the patient into believing he is getting as much from counseling as can be had. Audiologists might run a liability risk for these reasons.

The arguments for: An audiologist with proper training in tinnitus theory and therapy is more capable than anyone else to help the patient appreciate that the problem with tinnitus is not the sound of the tinnitus; rather, it is the reaction to that sound. Second, cognitive therapy for tinnitus does not seek to address underlying emotional issues. It restricts itself to behaviors caused directly by tinnitus. One might therefore argue that providing cognitive therapy for tinnitus does not require specific psychological training. Most importantly, audiologists already routinely engage in counseling of family members on effective communication strategies, parents on the effects of hearing loss, and hard-of-hearing patients on the effects of central presbycusis. Counseling about tinnitus-related behavior might therefore be seen as a logical extension of this existing skill.

---

state of relaxation, it is most difficult to experience moments of anxiety. For example, if one is basking in the sun and is in a relaxed state and muscle tension is absent, one can experience a lessening of tension and mental anxiety.

Clinically, it was a simple task to attach appropriate sensors to muscle groups and record changes in electromyographic activity as the person became more relaxed. For example, one could attach sensors to the frontalis muscle and train the individual to relax that muscle. Having achieved this state, the person could be taught to generalize this relaxation to other parts of the body. The only fly in the methodological ointment was that muscle relaxation and stress reduction do not always reduce the subjective loudness of the tinnitus.

Grossan (1989) reports the success of biofeedback experiments to reduce tension and stress, thus reducing anxiety. He states,

> Experiments have demonstrated that the effects of relaxation were long lasting. For example, migraine headaches are vascular in origin and people who suffer from them were trained to increase circulation of one or both hands by placing a thermistor on the hand. The individual was encouraged to relax

and warm that hand through mental processes. Various studies suggested that this could ward off migraine attacks. (p. 2)

One of the phenomenological results arising from various biofeedback studies was that once it was demonstrated that alpha waves could be produced through relaxation and mentally controlled through selected physiological functions, intentional alpha wave production became commonplace.

It is assumed that anxiety will reinforce the symptoms of whatever the physical or behavioral problem is. If stress induces anxiety and biofeedback assists in reducing stress, the anxiety should diminish as well. Putting it in a somewhat different context: If stress increases anxiety and anxiety increases the subjective loudness of the ongoing tinnitus, then any clinical intervention that reduces stress and anxiety should have a positive effect on the loudness judgment of the tinnitus. This statement is tempered with the realization that no therapeutic intervention, including biofeedback, is going to be successful in all cases.

During the process of biofeedback training, no direct or alternating current passes through the body, even though electrodes are normally attached to the forehead. The single purpose of the electrode(s) is to pick up electromyographic activity. Such instruction given to the patients often alleviates concern over the possibility of shock or pain.

A good deal of similarity exists between tinnitus and pain. Each is difficult to measure precisely or objectively, nor can one predict either's course. As an example, if a leg is amputated, the pain may linger long after the amputation. Similarly, if the hearing nerve (VIII) is severed as a treatment for intractable tinnitus, no assurance exists that the tinnitus will be eliminated. As a matter of fact, it may become more pronounced. In a similar vein, biofeedback can be instrumental in reducing stress, but it does not serve as a guarantee that all patients will react the same or receive the same benefit. For example, most biofeedback practitioners treating tinnitus will make some determination of its effectiveness after a given number of treatments. Failing to evidence improvement, the patient is referred to some other professional discipline, such as psychotherapy, for clinical management.

PITFALL

The use of biofeedback is not without some risks. Two potentially dangerous problems may arise from the use of biofeedback. A person with hypertension (high blood pressure) who is on medication to control it may reduce his blood pressure through biofeedback training to a point that is potentially dangerous. Unless a patient's blood pressure remains above a certain value, his or her medication can produce a toxic reaction. In addition, diabetic patients on prescribed medication may have some adverse reaction in the process of biofeedback.

In a recent study, Katajima and his associates (1998) reported on 55 tinnitus patients, 32 men and 23 women, who participated in biofeedback training. The training was administered to those who did not benefit from such conventional treatment as masker devices and various medications. The patient is told that the introduction of biofeedback training is not to immediately reduce the subjective loudness, but rather to improve one's ability to cope with the annoyance generated by the tinnitus and to improve the quality of life. The *Vernon Five Level Grading Scale* was administered to each subject. This scale consists of three tinnitus assessment areas to which the subject responded. They were (1) tinnitus loudness, (2) tinnitus annoyance, and (3) tinnitus interference with life activities. This is a 5-point scale, where *1* represents minimal difficulty and *5* indicates pronounced difficulty. All patients were given the Manifest Anxiety Scale (MAS), SDS (Self-rating Depression Scale), and CMI (Cornell Medical Index) tests to determine psychological state. Electromyographic levels were recorded before and after the daily practice schedule. Improvement was related to the amount of decrease in microvolts. The data showed, for example, that when the decrease in microvolts was less than 0.6 μV, biofeedback was considered to be effective. Relative to tinnitus loudness, biofeedback was effective in 42% of the subjects. Tinnitus annoyance was reduced in 80% of the patients, and tinnitus interference reduction was 44%. When the microvolt decrease was greater than 0.6 μV, 37% had a change in loudness judgment, 59% were less annoyed by the tinnitus, and 44% thought that tinnitus interference was less. Of interest was the fact that none of the psychological test results showed any significant effect from biofeedback training. Although not statistically analyzed, we stated that the kind and type of hearing disorder, when present, had negative influence on the effectiveness of biofeedback training. We did stress that patients having a negative attitude toward biofeedback were not good candidates for this type of training.

Biofeedback training reduces muscle tension, thus encouraging relaxation, which has a positive effect on one's perception of subjective tinnitus and an increased ability to cope more effectively. The question arises, therefore, whether chemical muscle relaxants would have the same effect. We know of no study that supports or contests this view. Such an investigation may be worth the time and effort.

Masker Therapy

The awareness of the masking of tinnitus through the application of external sounds is not recent or new. It is reasonably certain that Hippocrates, in 400 B.C., was referring to tinnitus when he was reported to have said, "Why is it that the buzzing in the ear ceases if one makes a sound?" In 1883, V. Urbantschitsch (Feldmann, 1995) used tuning forks to assess the frequency of tinnitus and determine their masking properties. Many historical references to masking exist, but it was not until the rudimentary experimentation by a physician named Spaulding (1903) that the investigation of the masking principle was organized. He used a piano keyboard in an attempt to match the perceived pitch of the tinnitus. When the piano note matched the pitch of the tinnitus, the same note would then be produced on a wind instrument. The intensity of the note would be sustained and increased until the offending tinnitus was masked. He was among the first to report the phenomenon of residual inhibition. He observed that some patients would experience complete relief from tinnitus after the external sound was removed. No mention was made of how long the periods of residual inhibition would last.

Jones and Knudsen (1928) described two procedures for treating the patient with tinnitus. The first was to present a sound to the ear similar to the tinnitus with sufficient intensity to mask it. As did Spaulding, they reported the presence of residual inhibition that lasted for short periods. The second procedure was to design a sound-producing system that could be placed on the nightstand for those patients with tinnitus who experience difficulty sleeping.

In 1979 Feldmann (1987) in Germany investigated the effects of certain sounds on the perception of tinnitus. He found that some sounds were more effective than others in producing the masking affect. He, too, observed the presence of residual inhibition. The reader should be aware that no one-to-one correspondence exists between the understanding of conventional masking as reported by Wegel and Lane (1924) and that observed when attempting to mask tinnitus with some external, acoustically complex sound or with simple pure tones.

Despite these early observations about the positive effects of masking, it was not until the work of Vernon (1977) that a much more formalized approach to tinnitus masking was formulated.

In 1976 a formal masker-use program was developed and introduced at the Oregon Health Sciences University by Dr. Jack Vernon, who served as director of the Oregon Hearing Research Laboratory. It was during his tenure that a wearable masker device was developed and used to treat the patient with tinnitus. Since that early and auspicious beginning, the use of wearable masker devices has served as one of the more popular and successful methods of providing relief from troublesome tinnitus. The rationale for the use of masker devices is that it is psychologically easier to deal with an external acoustic event than it is to deal with an acoustic-like sensation generated somewhere in the head. Furthermore, if residual inhibition occurs, the probability of successful use of masker devices is enhanced.

The masker concept is used by three approaches. In the first instance is the use of a *simple masker device*. The device generates a white noise and the patient has control over the intensity level of the noise. The output of the noise signal can be frequency shaped so that a certain frequency range can be enhanced or suppressed depending on the needs of the patient relative to achieving a masking affect. Frequency emphasis (shaping) can be done at the manufacturing site or by the practitioner by adjusting one or more potentiometers. In the second instance a *combination device* is used. This device has a hearing aid circuit and a noise-producing circuit. The rationale for a combination device is based on an abundance of clinical data (Vernon & Meikle, in press), which show that most patients who have tinnitus have hearing loss as well. This is not to imply that all persons who have hearing loss are logical hearing aid candidates, but many are. When hearing is reduced to the point where amplification is indicated, the clinician tries to resolve each of the issues by providing amplification to improve sound and speech awareness and a controlled masker sound to manage tinnitus.

Both the masker and hearing aid circuits are contained in the same housing, making it a rather simple task for the patient or clinician to adjust the level of the hearing aid and to obtain an acceptable level of masker noise. The two circuits of

the combination device are available in a behind-the-ear and an in-the-ear hearing aid configuration. Starkey Laboratory and General Hearing Instruments are the major manufacturers of tinnitus devices.

The third of these approaches is the use of *hearing aids only*. Discretion must be exercised in the selection of hearing aids as the chosen method for tinnitus patient management. In many cases in which the patient needs hearing aids to improve speech reception and recognition, the hearing aids provide sufficient masking of the tinnitus to dictate against the use of a combination device. That is, as long as the patient is using the hearing aids, tinnitus is controlled to the point where coping skills are enhanced. However, the probability that measurable residual inhibition, lasting more than a few seconds, will occur when the hearing aids are removed is very low. Our clinical experience suggests that most patients using hearing aids only to mask tinnitus do not report any extended residual inhibition after a period of use. We have noticed as well that in those cases where minimum masking level is low, individuals with hearing impairment who use amplification are usually successful in achieving masking. In some instances individuals may wear the hearing aids at night. For them, the amplification of soft environmental sounds is sufficient to maintain a masking effect.

The Tinnitus Evaluation for Determining Masker Use

No absolute method of tinnitus evaluation serves as an infallible predictor of success with masker devices. However, a number of clinical procedures relate directly to the selection, fitting, and evaluation of masker devices. Three individual procedures are normally used as follows:

- Determining the perceived pitch of the tinnitus
- Determining the subjective loudness of the tinnitus
- Assessing the amount of acoustic energy needed to achieve masking of the offending tinnitus

The means of measuring these values was covered earlier in this chapter, in the section "Assessment and Evaluation of Tinnitus."

After obtaining reliable measures of pitch and loudness, the clinician will choose a stimulus most likely to mask the patent's tinnitus. The more closely the masker sound is to the actual pitch of the tinnitus, the more effective is masker use. That is, if the pitch match is measured at 4000 Hz, a narrow band of noise, perhaps 2000 to 6000 Hz, can be more effective than a broader band of noise. Obviously, the more narrow the noise band, the less is the interference with the reception and discrimination of speech. Conversely, if a narrow band of noise, perhaps 200 to 2000 Hz, is used to mask a tinnitus pitch of 4000 Hz, it will not be as effective. One must add that these observations are not always manifest clinically. We have seen some patients with high-frequency tonal tinnitus who preferred a low-pass, narrow band of noise as the masking stimulus. No diagnostic predictor of what a given patient will determine to be the most effective masking stimulus exists. Although a pure tone signal may have been used in the tinnitus matching procedure, such a sound is rarely used for masking. A pure tone could become equally as disturbing as the ongoing tinnitus itself.

Johnson and colleagues (1989) first reported the results of a study in which the effectiveness of various instruments were used in the treatment of tinnitus. Again, Johnson (1998) reported the clinical results of 370 patients with tinnitus seen for treatment at the Oregon Hearing Research Laboratory. Of this population, hearing aids only were recommend for 51 subjects, tinnitus maskers were recommended for 65, and a total of 228 subjects received recommendations for a tinnitus instrument, an instrument that has both a hearing aid and a masker circuit in the same case, each with its own volume control. The recommendation to evaluate both a hearing aid and a tinnitus masker was made for 18 patients. Eight subjects were recommended to try both a tinnitus instrument and a tinnitus masker. After a trial period, a total of 133 subjects (36%) decided not to purchase the recommended device. Of the remaining number, the rate of success with the tinnitus masker was 35%. For the tinnitus instrument, the results were more gratifying in that the success rate improved to 71%.

Johnson reported that the superior success rate with the tinnitus instrument may be for the following reasons: (1) The patient has both tinnitus and a hearing loss and the tinnitus instrument is more effective in treating each of the conditions. (2) If the patient's tinnitus can be effectively masked by amplification only, but he or she has difficulty sleeping because of the tinnitus, the masker portion of the device can be used during the night. (3) For those patients who find amplification to be only partially effective as a masking source, then the masker portion of the device may be useful. He reports, further, that about 50% of those who use hearing aids are provided relief through the use of amplification only. This particular study would suggest that those patients with hearing impairment and tinnitus should be fitted with tinnitus instruments. Because this instrument has two separate volume controls, the patient can decide when and where to use the masker portion of the instrument.

Even though the results of this study failed to reach one's level of expectation with respect to the value of various tinnitus instruments, it is apparent that a rather sizable population of patients with tinnitus do benefit from their use.

In another study Von Wedel (1998) reported on 792 tinnitus patients. The study reported the results of tinnitus therapy using tinnitus maskers and hearing aids from May 1987 to April 1993. The study evaluated the effectiveness of tinnitus maskers and hearing aids in providing some relief for severe disabling chronic tinnitus. Three areas were investigated in this study: First was the masking effect during use, second was residual inhibition after the use of the device, and third was subjective scaling of the therapeutic efficiency. All subjects determined the frequency, duration, and time of use, regardless of the instrument being evaluated. When comparing hearing aids with masker devices, 62.7% of the subjects reported some partial masking produced by the hearing aids on the basis of the amplification of environmental sounds. For the same or similar environmental sounds the tinnitus masker was effective for only 18.5% of the participants. For 76.9% of those using a tinnitus masker device, complete masking was achieved. For the hearing-aid-only population, only 17% experienced complete masking of the tinnitus.

After an experimental trial period of at least 4 to 6 weeks, 18.7% purchased a hearing aid and about 6% purchased a masker device. After 1 year, the authors reported that the 7.4% return rate for hearing aids had increased to 19% for the masker devices. After 2 years, the return rate for masker devices was 24.7% and for hearing aids was reported to be 9.6%. However, regarding the incidence of complete or partial residual inhibition, the results were somewhat more encouraging. That is, 94.7% of those using hearing aids reported complete or partial residual inhibition, which lasted less than 30 seconds. For a very small segment of this population, 0.3%, residual inhibition lasted about 1 minute. The incidence of residual inhibition less than 30 seconds for the tinnitus masker group was 71.3%. However, 15.7% of the tinnitus masker group reported residual inhibition of more than 60 seconds. Thirteen percent had residual effects lasting 2 to 3 hours. It is obvious that the masker device is more effective in producing complete residual inhibition.

There are, then, differences of opinion regarding the clinical usefulness of maskers and hearing aids in the treatment of the tinnitus. Certainly, the studies reviewed all produced very dissimilar results. It is nonetheless evident that a number of patients with tinnitus benefit from the use of one or the other. One does not know all the causes for acceptance or rejection of masker devices or hearing aids in the treatment of tinnitus. A number of factors may be completely unrelated to the clinical usefulness of various instruments. Success may depend on the skill of the clinician in the evaluation and selection process. The ability of the clinician to effectively manage a patient can be, and often is, a major factor in acceptance or rejection. Oftentimes, patients are skeptical of the reported benefits of any clinical procedure. Patients need to know the limitations and advantages of masker devices. They need to know that such devices are not a cure-all and that success may be only partial. Yet even partial success may be of great importance to some and provide marked relief from tinnitus. Each patient must be given enough time to appraise the value of the device. We have seen a number of patients over the years whose first response to a masker device or tinnitus instrument was a negative one. Some patients, early on, viewed the masker sound equally as noxious as their tinnitus. After a period of use and counseling, many accepted the device as beneficial in providing sufficient relief so that coping with tinnitus was a much easier task.

The clinician should not ignore the contribution of masking devices in the treatment of tinnitus. No one therapeutic philosophy or process is sufficiently compelling to use it above all others. Because one is not certain of the cause of tinnitus regarding site of lesion or the various behaviors and attitudes manifested by those so afflicted, one should maintain an open mind relative to that which can and cannot be beneficial in ameliorating the negative emotional and behavioral effects of subjective tinnitus.

Habituation Therapy (Tinnitus Retraining Therapy)

Individuals can habituate to a number of external and internal stimuli. For example, one is not aware constantly of the ticking of a grandfather clock. Nor is one aware of the refrigerator motor, which periodically comes on to maintain a constant temperature. This ability to habituate to a stimulus is predicated on clinical observations that as long as the stimulus, or acoustic event, is not threatening or demanding of attention, it can be habituated to. For sounds requiring some sort of mental awareness or assessment, for whatever reason, habituation is very difficult, if not impossible.

Disabling, chronic tinnitus is one of those acoustic-like sensations to which the person has not habituated. This inability to habituate is because the patient cannot determine what is generating the tinnitus and therefore must attend to it. If the attention given to it creates uncertainty, fear, or promotes negative behaviors, then psychological and emotional problems may manifest themselves. If these things happen, the patient may have a great deal of difficulty dealing with the behaviors arising from the tinnitus. When tinnitus creates these problems, most persons will seek some sort of therapeutic intervention.

Tinnitus retraining therapy (TRT) is one of several approaches used in the treatment process. The goal of this approach is to make tinnitus a nonissue in one's life. TRT is not a method of "coping" or adjusting to life with tinnitus, but rather it is a means through which one does not need to cope. The basic assumption underlying the TRT process is that if one habituates to a given signal, it becomes a part of the subconscious mind and does not become part of conscious perception. When TRT is successful, tinnitus is no longer consciously perceived by the patient. Because one has habituated to its presence, coping strategies are unnecessary.

In the late 1980s Dr. Pawel Jastreboff at the University of Maryland/Baltimore School of Medicine developed a model of tinnitus on the basis of the knowledge that persons can habituate to external or internal stimuli. He referred to this as a *neurophysiological model of tinnitus*. It has been eloquently described by him and various colleagues in a number of meaningful articles (Jastreboff, 1990; Jastreboff et al, 1987, 1988, 1992, 1994, 1995b; Jastreboff & Hazel 1993; Jastreboff & Sasaki 1994).

The Jastreboff model is shown in Figure 23–1. First, there is the locus of tinnitus (*source*). Many practitioners think that the initial neurogenerating site for tinnitus lies within the cochlea. Wherever the neural generating site may be, an acoustic-like sensation is produced. If the generated sound is

considered to be nonthreatening or of little consequence to degrading the quality of life, subcortical activity (*detection*) of the brain "shunts" or prevents the sound from getting to the conscious awareness level. However, should the sound be deemed as having threatening consequences, subcortical activities are bypassed and attention is given to the tinnitus in some part of the cortex of the brain (*perception and evaluation*). For example, if the patient thinks that the presence of tinnitus portends progressive hearing loss, dire illness, tumor, or loss of one's sanity, tinnitus will not be habituated to.

If the perception and evaluation of tinnitus suggest debilitating results, the limbic system (*emotional associations*) becomes involved and strong, negative emotional behaviors are generated. These emotional responses create what David Burns (1980) defined as *cognitive distortions*. Unless one interrupts these negative behaviors through some positive and sustained therapy and counseling interaction, they will continue to dominate much of the patient's waking moments and interfere greatly with the quality of life. Not only do these emotional associations dictate behavior, they may give rise to reactions of the autonomic nervous system (*annoyance*) that mediate certain systemic functions. Jastreboff reasoned that a type of "vicious circle" is created, wherein the inability to rationally resolve why tinnitus is present leads to a sustained, negative reaction. That is, (1) the tinnitus has not been habituated to, (2) emotional associations that lead to negative behaviors, and (3) these behaviors generate annoyance and the cycle is repeated.

The Jastreboff model offers a cogent, scientifically and neurophysiologically based explanation of the processes involved in one's perception and reaction to tinnitus. Although the model is of value in understanding what is happening, an obvious need to use the model in developing a therapeutic approach contributes to the habituation process. The TRT method is based on the model and provides a therapeutic approach that has been instrumental in assisting the patient with tinnitus in achieving an enhanced quality of life.

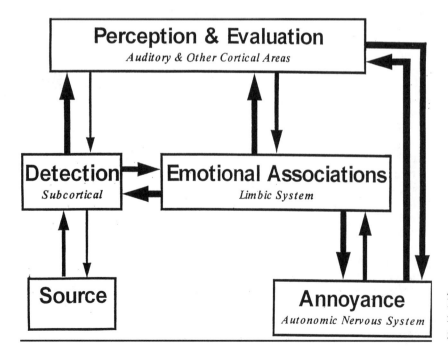

Figure 23–1 The Jastreboff neurophysiological model of tinnitus generation and self-perpetuation.

In developing the model, several well-established psycho-acoustic principles were invoked. From a neurophysiological point of reference, the brain interprets all sensory inputs (signals) in terms of contrast rather than absolute measures of magnitude. Early on, it was realized that for most patients with tinnitus, the contrast in the subjective loudness level of the tinnitus, compared with the level of the environmental background, was considerable. Because it is a less difficult task to perceive a dominant signal (tinnitus) in a milieu of environmental sounds, the ability of the brain to attend to it is a relatively easy task. Therefore, in the treatment process, a noise-generating device is used to artificially create a background of noise that is equal in loudness to the ongoing tinnitus. The rationale is that if the contrast between the tinnitus and the environmental background is reduced, the process of habituation is accelerated.

This concept of contrast reduction is shown in Figure 23–2. Note that the environmental background is shown at the bottom of the graph. The heavy dark line indicates the tinnitus level. It is evident that the perceived loudness of the tinnitus is greater than the environmental background. The intensity of noise produced by the noise generators is set at a point where the patient perceives it as being equally as loud as the tinnitus. This is referred to as the *mixing point*. Obviously, if the level of the noise generators were set to a level that masked the tinnitus, habituation would not take place. One cannot habituate to something that is not perceived.

From a treatment point of view, the patient is instructed to set the output level of the noise generators to achieve this mixing point. It is recommended that the devices be used for a minimum of 8 hours a day. Ideally, the noise generators should be worn during most waking hours to achieve maximum advantage in the shortest period of time. The output level of the devices is set each morning and is not changed during the day, regardless of changes in the subjective loudness of the tinnitus. Although the time to achieve maximum benefit may vary from patient to patient, 18 to 24 months is normal. This does not mean that one must wait this period of time before some change is noticed. We have seen patients who achieved subjective benefit only after a few weeks of noise generator use. For these patients, even though the tinnitus was still consciously perceived, their negative emotional responses were altered. A case in point is that of a 34-year-old woman who was in considerable emotional distress when first seen at our center. During the initial interview, she was in constant tears and was convinced she would be faced with this "terrible burden" all her life. After entering the TRT program, she was able to control her frequent emotional outbursts, even though the subjective loudness of tinnitus had not been altered appreciably.

Dr. Steve Nagler (personal correspondence, 1997), director of the Southeastern Center for Tinnitus and Hyperacusis, Atlanta, Georgia, states: "In TRT, the intimate bond between the limbic system and the tinnitus signal is cleaved by removing importance from the signal using a process called 'directive counseling.'" In essence, the use of *directive counseling* is an integral part of retraining therapy, and its importance to therapeutic success cannot be overstated. The value of directive counseling is that of having the patient participate in an extended discussion during which the meaning of tinnitus is explained through the use of illustrative materials. Such material may include pictorial representations of specific anatomical and physiological functions and the role each plays in the generation of tinnitus. The intent of these extended discussions is to "demystify" tinnitus. One wants to take the mystery and uncertainty out of tinnitus and present the information in such a manner that the patients' concerns about unfounded negative effects are reduced or eliminated.

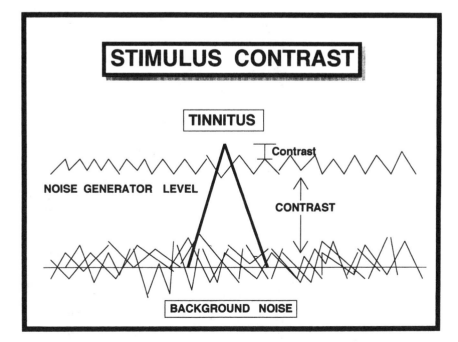

Figure 23–2 Tinnitus is easy to detect not because it is objectively loud but because it is louder than any background noise. The noise generator reduces the contrast between tinnitus and other sounds reaching the ear, making tinnitus harder to detect.

PITFALL

The TRT approach is much more than fitting noise generators to the ears and then forgetting the patient. If this is the attitude of some, both the clinician and the patient will be disappointed with the results. A difference exists between an intellectual acceptance of the principles underlying TRT and the emotional and behavioral changes that must come about to achieve success. Just because a rational approach to the treatment of tinnitus is presented, no automatic assurance is present that the patient will be able to embrace the therapeutic concepts and immediately change the ways in which they react to tinnitus. The therapy must account for the individual's mental and emotional strength. A positive need for an effective and ongoing counseling strategy exists.

Directive counseling is as much an art as it is a science. Effective patient management requires that both the patient and the clinician participate in the counseling effort. In that each participates, each benefits from the experience. The patient is benefited because he or she gains a greater understanding of the disorder and, therefore, deals with emotional responses to it in a more objective and intelligent manner. The clinician benefits because he or she learns more about human behavior and experiences a sense of accomplishment from making a positive contribution to the patient's well-being.

Seldom is a single session effective in altering the patient's perception of the negative aspects of tinnitus. To have the patient accept that tinnitus can be managed effectively and that habituation can and does occur may require directive counseling sessions over a period of 18 to 24 months. Each counseling session serves to reinforce positive attitudes that habituation can and does occur for those reasons discussed. Furthermore, counseling serves to guard against the patient giving up prematurely by concluding that TRT is ineffective.

One may set goals in the management of the directive counseling program. Without question, the more important ones are the following:

1. To have the patient gain a thorough understanding of the principles underlying the development and administration of TRT. His or her understanding should be based on rational and defensible data that can be presented objectively and be easily assimilated by the patient.

2. To have the patient diligently carry out all instructions relating to the use of the noise-generating devices.

3. To have the patient avoid silence. The reason for avoiding silence is rather straightforward. If the patient is in a quiet environment, the contrast between that environment and the ongoing tinnitus is at its maximum. The patient can use several means of avoiding silence. The patient can have a radio playing at an acceptable background level or keep a fan going. The sounds produced assist in reducing the contrast between the tinnitus and the environment and contribute to the rate with which habituation will occur.

4. To have the patient behave in such a manner that attention is not drawn constantly to the tinnitus. Whatever means the patient can devise to engage in activities that are pleasant and serve as positive means of distraction are most important in contributing to the success of TRT. The reason for this is rather apparent. If the patient is always, or frequently, assessing the present state of tinnitus, habituation is virtually impossible.

Each patient presents as a unique functioning individual who deals with adversity in a number of ways. Counseling strategies may differ, depending on the mental and emotional states of the patient. For example, patients who are obsessed with their tinnitus and its assumed negative effects may be more resistant to therapy than others. Such patients may require more frequent counseling sessions early on in the training program. Other patients may have difficulty accepting any therapeutic approach because they have developed a mind-set that has created suspicion and uncertainty. For these patients, more time may be required to establish a working rapport.

Whatever the personality type of the patient, the underlying philosophy of TRT must be emphasized. Until the patient embraces the inherent value of this approach, the more the emphasis is placed on the counseling process. The combined results of sound therapy and directive counseling are to have the patient habituate to the tinnitus and to the emotional responses generated by it. Usually we find positive changes in behavior first, even though the tinnitus has not been habituated to.

The authors do not claim that TRT works for everyone because certainly it does not. When one looks at the results presented by Jastreboff, 80% of those patients seen at the University of Maryland/Baltimore benefit from the program. Benefit is measured in the following way: Patients complete the same questionnaire before and after therapy. The answers for each are analyzed to determine the degree of success. For a given patient's treatment to be defined as successful, he or she must report a 30% decrease in the level of annoyance and a 20% decrease in the amount of time the patient is aware of his or her tinnitus. In addition, a percentage increase in the ability to perform tasks that could not be performed before tinnitus therapy must occur.

OTHER THERAPEUTIC APPROACHES

Space does not permit a lengthy description of other alternative forms of treatment. This all too brief overview of other treatment modalities is not to indict them or to relegate them to some substandard status as a form of therapeutic intervention. A decision had to be made regarding what treatment strategies would be explained in more detail and what strategies would be given less emphasis. We apologize to those readers who believe that too little emphasis was given to a specific form of treatment.

Among the therapies that have been used over the years, the use of *direct electrical stimulation* has received considerable attention. Electrical stimulation may be effective for some patients, but not others. The cause and magnitude of the hearing impairment may be related to the success of stimulation.

Staller (1998) reported that severity and type of tinnitus can be related to successful treatment, whereas in other reports neither of these factors appear to be related to successful treatment. In general, treatment was deemed successful if some reduction occurred in the subjective loudness of the tinnitus. Finally, some patients who received a cochlear implant experienced significant reduction in tinnitus loudness. Unfortunately, others noticed tinnitus onset after the cochlear implant.

Whatever mechanisms respond to an electrical stimulus, the positive result for some has been a most welcome change. We recommend articles by Ito and Sakakihara (1998) and Staller (1998) be reviewed to gain a greater appreciation of the benefits and limitations of electrical stimulation. Staller (1998) reviews some of the past and more current applications of electrical stimulation, its clinical usefulness, and subsequent effects on subjective tinnitus. Ito and Sakakihara (1998) discuss the effects of cochlear implant suppression on the subjective loudness of tinnitus.

Microvascular decompression surgery has been used for the treatment of tinnitus. The principle underlying this approach is based on the observation that blood vessel compression on the fifth cranial nerve can and does produce pain. One may hypothesize that blood vessel compression of the eighth nerve may produce tinnitus. The forces causing this compression are probably related to a sagging of the brain as a result of the aging process and arteriosclerosis, causing an elongation of the arteries. It is these two forces that generate vascular compression tinnitus. Microvascular decompression of the eighth nerve tends to ameliorate the effects of the two forces described here. However, many practitioners dispute the usefulness of this procedure for tinnitus relief, whereas some neurosurgeons do not believe that the potential benefit justifies the risk (Jastreboff, personal communication, 1998).

Dental problems are the cause of a specific type of tinnitus. Most reports suggest that jaw joint problems are primarily responsible. *Temporal mandibular joint (TMJ)* disorders can generate pain, discomfort, and tinnitus. It has been suggested that Pinto's ligament (Morgan, 1998), also referred to as the discomalleolar ligament or the anterior malleolar ligament, serves as the physical connection between the TMJ and the ear. Although the role played by Pinto's ligament has not been confirmed, ample evidence exists that treating TMJ problems can reduce the subjective loudness of tinnitus caused by dental disorder.

Holistic and homeopathic approaches have been used in treating a number of disorders, including tinnitus (Nagler, personal communication, 1998). However, significant differences exist between the two. Basically, holistic management of the patient assumes that an organism is much more than the sum of its parts. Any treatment plan, therefore, must demand that the individual be studied as a whole person. Rather than just assessing the effect of a specific medication or device acting on a specific disorder, the thoughts, actions, and behaviors of the patient must be taken into account.

The holistic approach certainly embraces the use of some form of counseling to assist the patient in understanding how thought processes could perpetuate or intensify the problem. For some, the dichotomy of oriental and occidental medicine or treatment strategy lies in the observation that holistic approaches are more akin to the oriental management of human disorders.

The principles underlying homeopathic approaches are entirely different than holistic principles. Perhaps, more simplistic than necessary, homeopathy is based on the canon, or law, of similia. That is, likes are cured by likes. In essence, substances that may cause certain symptomatic behaviors in normal healthy persons may be effective with persons having some particular disorder if given in small or highly diluted quantities. A significant body of information, based on scientific scrutiny, is lacking that a homeopathic approach is effective in the treatment of tinnitus (Nagler, 1997). The authors hasten to point out that anecdotal reports may suggest the benefit of this therapeutic method but are aware of only one very limited double-blind study to confirm benefits derived by the patient with tinnitus. This is despite the fact that the very nature of homeopathy lends itself easily to double-blind studies (Nagler, 1997). That single study (Simpson et al, 1995) contained internally contradictory results.

Other alternative treatments include *vitamin therapy, dietary controls, acupuncture, acupressure, chiropractic manipulation*, and a host of other interventions designed to treat the patient with tinnitus. As with many other treatment modalities for a host of common ills, the placebo effect is always possible. It cannot be underestimated as an effective ingredient in the treatment process. Human dynamics are such that one does not always know or understand those factors contributing to successful therapy. Patients who respond positively to a specific therapy may do so because they like and respond well to the therapist, feel some reduction of stress by virtue of having taken steps to do something about the problem, or receive empathetic support from friends and family.

HYPERACUSIS

It would be academically shallow to discuss tinnitus without some mention of hyperacusis. Although tinnitus and hyperacusis may be entirely separate neurophysiololgical entities, the mutual incidence of each is relatively high. That is, many persons experiencing tinnitus also complain of hyperacusis. Although many patients reporting hyperacusis have hearing loss, normal-hearing persons have hyperacusis in its moderate-to-severe form.

Hyperacusis is defined as a disproportionate growth in the subjective loudness of sounds. Vernon (1998) defines hyperacusis as "a collapse of loudness tolerance so that almost all sounds produce loudness discomfort, even though the actual sound intensity is well below that judged to be uncomfortable by others" (p. 223). Whatever the appropriate definition may be, those who have it cannot adjust to normal acoustic environments because of loudness discomfort. In the extreme, some patients isolate themselves in a sound-attenuated environment and fear to venture from that "safe place" for fear of encountering sounds that may produce severe discomfort or pain. As unusual as this behavior may appear, in the experience of the authors and from perusal of Internet discussion groups, it would seem to occur with a great deal of frequency.

A clinical entity referred to as "*phonophobia*," or the fear of sounds, also exists. Individuals so afflicted are fearful of being exposed to sounds that have caused pain or discomfort. As a result, they avoid many social contacts and experiences because of this fear. For example, patients fearing some unexpected encounter with offending sounds will wear earplugs or some other type of noise defender 24 hours a day. We have had more than one patient sitting in our clinic's quiet waiting room while wearing the same type of earmuffs the ground crews at airports use. Even the slightest change in their acoustic world may trigger an unpleasant and immediate reaction.

For some, hyperacusis may be much more debilitating than relentless, subjective tinnitus. The American Tinnitus Association conducted a survey of 112 persons having both tinnitus and hyperacusis. Of this number, 53% said that their hyperacusis was more debilitating than the tinnitus. Twenty-five percent of this population stated that each problem was equally disturbing. Of the remainder, 16% reported their tinnitus to be the most debilitating and 6% of the respondents were uncertain.

Many patients having hyperacusis reported some TMJ problem. In the same report by the American Tinnitus Association of the population of 112 persons, 65 indicated some TMJ symptom expressed in the following way: (1) 58% reported jaw problems; (2) 43% indicated jaw pain; (3) malocclusion or bite problems in 51%; (4) bruxism, or grinding of the teeth, in 52%; and (5) a clicking sensation in the jaw joint in 5%. Fullness in the ear was reported in 83% of the 112 persons reporting hyperacusis. Not unlike tinnitus, the neural mechanisms responsible for the onset and perpetuation of hyperacusis are not known. This phenomenon, too, awaits discovery and resolution.

The treatment of hyperacusis may take many forms. No common consensus exists among practitioners as to an infallible therapeutic approach. However, most agree that patients should not isolate themselves from normal environmental sounds. To do so invites disaster relative to increasing one's loudness tolerance. On the other hand, the patient should not have frequent exposure to loud sounds that induce discomfort and pain. The essence of therapy, therefore, is to devise a clinical scheme, whereby the patient understands the intent of the therapy and makes a sustained effort to carry out the established protocols.

The treatment of hyperacusis may vary from one clinician to another. The sought-after clinical goal is that of having the patient tolerate acoustic environments that, before the therapeutic process, could not be tolerated. This is not to suggest that one is attempting to have patients accept environments that would be uncomfortable to the normal-hearing person with normal sound tolerances. The intent is to have the patient gradually tolerate greater sound levels so that *normal* sound environments will not be uncomfortable.

Hyperacusis management relies on one of two approaches: ear protection and desensitization. Because hyperacusis is an abnormal sensitivity to day-to-day sounds, the most obvious management technique would be to reduce the perceived level of those sounds. The patient would protect his ears from whatever sounds he finds intolerable, be it traffic, office equipment, or conversation.

Hearing protection might solve the patient's immediate difficulty. However, it will only exacerbate the underlying problem. By continually keeping his ears protected from day-to-day sounds, the patient is creating an artificial hearing loss. The pathological neurological activity that causes the abnormal increase in hearing sensitivity will compensate for the artificial loss by further enhancing the internal gain of the auditory system. The result will be like that of a patient addicted to sleeping pills. The dose must be continually increased. Similarly, as the subcortical brain continues to enhance the internal sensitivity of the hearing system, ever greater and greater hearing protection is required. In the end the patient will constantly require hearing protection, even when in quiet, and will not be able to tolerate any activity outside a very quiet home.

We are not opposed to the use of ear defenders. Rather, we suggest they be used only when necessary. If the patient knows that an uncomfortable noise level is to be encountered or if unexpectedly an uncomfortable noise is experienced, ear defender use is justified. Micro-Tech has developed a hyperacusis instrument that is, in effect, a reverse hearing aid. Technically, it features an extreme compression ratio and a low compression kneepoint. The shell design uses a very tight fit and a soft earcanal, ensuring that the only sound entering the earcanal comes through the circuit. If the volume control is turned half on, a 2000 Hz, 50 dB SPL tone will receive just enough amplification to compensate for insertion loss. With the same volume control setting, a 70 dB SPL, 2000 Hz tone would be attenuated to only 62 dB SPL in the earcanal. A 90 dB input would have an output of only 70 dB SPL. The device is considered experimental. Nonetheless, it is available to any hearing aid dispenser or dispensing audiologist.

The advantage of such an instrument is tremendous. A hyperacusic patient might well be able to function normally in normal employment and social situations. The potential disadvantage of this approach is the same as that of using any other hearing protection. It could interfere with or prevent application of any retraining therapy that would produce a long-term result. Then again, the patient and clinician might be able to work together to very gradually increase the sound levels, thereby achieving auditory retraining.

CONCLUSIONS

The authors have described tinnitus and some of the clinical modalities that have been used in its treatment. It must be stated again that the cause of this disorder and its cure continue to escape discovery. A common consensus exists that the locus of tinnitus—the neural generating site(s)—lies somewhere within the auditory system of man. Continued investigation will ultimately result in the uncovering of the mysteries surrounding this problem.

In the interim, an urgent need to work with tinnitus patients and to assist them in dealing more effectively with the negative consequences that often arise still exists. Should one choose to work with these patients, a good deal more is involved than just an interest in the phenomenon of tinnitus itself. Some dedication to understanding the many issues surrounding the problem must be present. In the authors' view, one must maintain an open mind and resist the temptation to conclude that this or that clinical approach is the absolute answer. One must understand the rationale underlying any therapeutic approach and assess its relative importance for that individual patient. The administering of therapy is an undertaking that implies that both the clinician and patient are intimately involved in the process and that both benefit from it. The clinician benefits because of the professional satisfaction received and an advance in one's knowledge on the basis of that experience. The patient benefits because his or her quality of life has been altered for the better.

If the question is: Should audiologists become involved in the treatment process? the answer clearly is yes. For the audiologist, any malfunction of the human auditory system should be of concern. The audiologist is trained to understand and work with disorders affecting the auditory system. Tinnitus is a disorder of that system that affects millions of persons. The challenges and clinical frustrations are there to be dealt with. It is, however, these challenges and clinical frustrations that make the task a most rewarding one.

Appendix A
Tinnitus Severity Scale

Patient Name: _____   Date: _____

Please circle the answer that best describes your condition.

1. I am aware of my tinnitus:
   4—Always
   3—Usually
   2—Occasionally
   1—Never

2. I believe my tinnitus interferes with my hearing:
   4—Always
   3—Often
   2—Occasionally
   1—Never

3. As a result of my tinnitus, I am:
   4—Always irritable
   3—Often irritable
   2—Occasionally irritable
   1—Seldom/never irritable

4. When I have to take medication (sleeping pills and/or tranquilizers) because of my tinnitus, I am:
   4—Always upset
   3—Often upset
   2—Occasionally upset
   1—Never upset

5. My tinnitus has affected my nerves as follows:
   4—I've become an extremely nervous person.
   3—I've always been a nervous person, and the tinnitus is making me more nervous.
   2—I've never considered myself a nervous person, but my tinnitus sometimes makes me nervous.
   1—My tinnitus has no effect on my nerves.

6. My hearing loss interferes with my ability to communicate with others to the following degree:
   4—Always
   3—Often
   2—Occasionally
   1—Never

7. In my relationships with others, my tinnitus has:
   4—Made me change most of them
   3—Made me change many of them
   2—Made me change a few of them
   1—Had no effect on them

8. I am bothered by my tinnitus:
   4—Extremely
   3—Very much
   2—Slightly
   1—Not at all

9. I am worried about my ability to function:
   4—If my tinnitus stays the same.
   3—If my tinnitus becomes worse.
   2—If my tinnitus stays the same, I am not worried about my ability to function.
   1—I am not worried about my ability to function regardless of any change in my tinnitus.

10. Because of my tinnitus, my sleep is affected as follows:
    4—It takes me more than 1 hour to fall asleep, and I awaken during the night and can't get back to sleep quickly.
    3—It takes me more than 1 hour to fall asleep.
    2—I awaken in the middle of the night and can't get back to sleep quickly.
    1—I have no trouble sleeping.

11. My ability to concentrate is affected by my tinnitus:
    4—Always
    3—Usually
    2—Occasionally
    1—Never

12. Because of my hearing loss, my participation in group activities is affected as follows:
    4—Avoid
    3—Often avoid
    2—Occasionally avoid
    1—Never avoid

13. Regardless of how loud my tinnitus is, I am annoyed by it as follows:
    4—Always
    3—Often
    2—Only annoyed when it is loud
    1—Not annoyed

14. As a result of my tinnitus, I feel depressed:
    4—Always
    3—Usually
    2—Occasionally
    1—My tinnitus does not affect my moods.

15. Because of my tinnitus, my participation in outside activities is as follows:
    4—No longer participate
    3—Usually avoid them
    2—Occasionally avoid them
    1—Never avoid them

Appendix B
Tinnitus Handicap Inventory

Patient Name: _____ Date: _____

Instructions: The purpose of this scale is to identify difficulties that you may be experiencing because of your tinnitus. Please answer Yes, No, or Sometimes to each question. Please do not skip any questions.

1F.	Because of your tinnitus, is it difficult for you to concentrate?	YES	SOMETIMES	NO
2F.	Does the loudness of your tinnitus make it difficult for you to hear people?	YES	SOMETIMES	NO
3E.	Does your tinnitus make you angry?	YES	SOMETIMES	NO
4F.	Does your tinnitus make you feel confused?	YES	SOMETIMES	NO
5C.	Because of your tinnitus, do you feel desperate?	YES	SOMETIMES	NO
6E.	Do you complain a great deal about your tinnitus?	YES	SOMETIMES	NO
7F.	Because of your tinnitus, do you have trouble falling to sleep at night?	YES	SOMETIMES	NO
8C.	Do you feel as though you cannot escape your tinnitus?	YES	SOMETIMES	NO
9F.	Does your tinnitus interfere with your ability to enjoy social activities (such as going out to dinner, to the movies)?	YES	SOMETIMES	NO
10E.	Because of your tinnitus, do you feel frustrated?	YES	SOMETIMES	NO
11C.	Because of your tinnitus, do you feel that you have a terrible disease?	YES	SOMETIMES	NO
12F.	Does your tinnitus make it difficult for you to enjoy life?	YES	SOMETIMES	NO
13F.	Does your tinnitus interfere with your job or household responsibilities?	YES	SOMETIMES	NO
14E.	Because of your tinnitus, do you find that you are often irritable?	YES	SOMETIMES	NO
15F.	Because of your tinnitus, is it difficult for you to read?	YES	SOMETIMES	NO
16E.	Does your tinnitus make you upset?	YES	SOMETIMES	NO
17E.	Do you feel that your tinnitus problem has placed stress on your relationships with members of your family and friends?	YES	SOMETIMES	NO
18F.	Do you find it difficult to focus your attention away from your tinnitus and on other things?	YES	SOMETIMES	NO
19C.	Do you feel that you have no control over your tinnitus?	YES	SOMETIMES	NO
20F.	Because of your tinnitus, do you often feel tired?	YES	SOMETIMES	NO
21E.	Because of your tinnitus, do you feel depressed?	YES	SOMETIMES	NO
22E.	Does your tinnitus make you feel anxious?	YES	SOMETIMES	NO
23C.	Do you feel that you can no longer cope with your tinnitus?	YES	SOMETIMES	NO
24F.	Does your tinnitus get worse when you are under stress?	YES	SOMETIMES	NO
25E.	Does your tinnitus made you feel insecure?	YES	SOMETIMES	NO

From Newman et al (1996).

REFERENCES

BRUMMETT, R. E. (1995). A mechanism for tinnitus. In: J. Vernon, & A. Moller (Eds.), *Mechanisms of tinnitus* (pp. 7–10). Boston: Allyn & Bacon.

BRUMMETT, R. E. (1998). Are there any safe and effective treatments available to treat my tinnitus? In: J. Vernon (Ed.), *Tinnitus: Treatment and relief* (pp. 34–42). Boston: Allyn & Bacon.

BRUMMETT, R. E., JOHNSON, R., & SCHLEUNING, A. (1993). Alprazolam (Xanax) for tinnitus relief [Abstract 398]. *Association for Research in Otolaryngology, 2–6,134.*

BURNS, D. (1980). *Feeling good: The new mood therapy.* New York: Avon Books.

DOBIE, R., & SULLIVAN, M. (1998). Antidepressant drugs and tinnitus. In: J. Vernon (Ed.), *Tinnitus: Treatment and relief.* Boston: Allyn & Bacon.

FELDMANN, H. (1987). Masking of tinnitus. In: H. Feldmann (Ed.), *Proceedings of the III International Tinnitus Seminar,* Karlsrkuhe: Harsch Verlag.

FELDMANN, H. (1995). Mechanisms of tinnitus. In: J. Vernon, & A. Moller (Eds.), *Mechanisms of tinnitus* (pp. 43–51). Boston: Allyn & Bacon.

FISHER, E., PARIK, A., HARCOURT, J., & WRIGHT, A. (1994). The burden of screening for acoustic neuroma: Asymmetric otological symptoms in the ENT clinic. *Clinics in Otolaryngology, 19;19–21.*

GERKIN, G. M. (1995). Central auditory mechanisms and the generation of tinnitus. In: G. Reich, & J. Vernon (Eds.), *Proceedings of the Fifth International Tinnitus Seminar* (pp. 410–417). Portland, OR: American Tinnitus Association.

GROSSAN, M. (1989). The biofeedback program. In: R. Sandlin (Ed.), *The understanding and treatment of tinnitus.* Portland, OR: American Tinnitus Association.

GUTH, P. S. (1998). Drugs treatments for tinnitus at Tulane University School of Medicine. In: J. Vernon (Ed.), *Tinnitus: Treatment and relief* (pp. 55–59). Boston: Allyn & Bacon.

HALLAM, R. (1989). *Living with tinnitus.* Wellingborough, Northamptonshire, England: Thorsons Publishing Group.

HAWKINS, D. B. (1987). Description and validation of an LDL procedure designed to select SSPL 90. *Ear and Hearing, 8;162–169.*

HELLER, M. F., & BERGMAN, M. (1953). Tinnitus in normally hearing persons. *Annals of Otolaryngology, 62;73–83.*

HINDMARCH, I., BEAUMONT, G., BRANDON S., & LEONARD, B.E. (Eds.) (1990). *Benzodiazapines: Current concepts.* New York: John Wiley & Sons.

ITO, J., & SAKAKIHARA, J. (1998). Suppression of tinnitus by cochlear implant. In: J. Vernon (Ed.), *Tinnitus: Treatment and relief* (pp. 91–98). Boston: Allyn & Bacon.

JAKES, S., HALLAM, R., CHAMBERS, C., & HINCHCLIFFE, R. (1985). A factor analytical study of tinnitus complaint behavior. *Audiology, 24;195–206.*

JAKES, S., HALLAM, R., & HINCHCLIFF, C. (1988). A factor analytical study of tinnitus complaint behavior. *Audiology, 24;195–200.*

JASTREBOFF, P. (1990). Phantom auditory perception (tinnitus): Mechanisms of generation and perception. *Neurological Research, 8;221–254.*

JASTREBOFF, P. (1995a). Processing of the tinnitus signal within the brain. In: G. Reich, & J. Vernon (Eds.), *Proceedings of the Fifth International Tinnitus Seminar* (pp. 58–67). Portland, OR: American Tinnitus Association.

JASTREBOFF, P. (1995b). Tinnitus as a phantom perception: Theories and clinical implications. In: J. Vernon, & A. Moller (Eds.), *Mechanisms of tinnitus* (pp. 73–93). Boston: Allyn & Bacon.

JASTREBOFF, P., BRENNAN, J., COLEMAN, J., & SASAKI, C. (1988). Phantom auditory sensation in rats: An animal model for tinnitus. *Behavioral Neuroscience, 102;811–822.*

JASTREBOFF, P., BRENNAN, F., & SASAKI, C. (1987). Behavioral and electrophysiological animal model of tinnitus. In: H. Feldmann (Ed.), *Proceedings of the III International Tinnitus Seminar.* Karlsrkuhe: Harsch Verlag.

JASTREBOFF, P., BRENNAN, F., & SASAKI, C. (1989). Behavioral and electrophysiological animal model of tinnitus. In: H. Feldman (Ed.), *Proceedings of the IV Annual International Tinnitus Seminar* (pp. 45–49). Munster: Karlsruhe Karsch Verlag.

JASTREBOFF, P., & HAZEL, J. (1993). A neurophysiological approach to tinnitus: Clinical implications. *British Journal of Audiology, 27;7–17.*

JASTREBOFF, P., HAZELL, J., & GRAHAM, R. L. (1994). Neurophysiological model of tinnitus: Dependence of the minimal masking level on treatment outcome. *Hearing Research, 80;216–232.*

JASTREBOFF, P., IKNER, C., & HASSEN, A. (1992). An approach to the objective evaluation of tinnitus in humans. In: J. Aran, & R. Dauman (Eds.), *Proceedings of the Fourth International Tinnitus Seminar, Bordeaux, 1991.* Amsterdam: Kugler Publications.

JASTREBOFF, P., & SASAKI, C. (1994). An animal model of tinnitus: A decade of development. *American Journal of Otology, 15;19–27.*

JOHNSON, R. (1998). The masking of tinnitus. In: J. Vernon (Ed.), *Tinnitus: Treatment and relief* (pp. 164–174). Boston: Allyn & Bacon.

JOHNSON, R., BRUMMETT, R., & SCHLEUNING, A. (1993). Use of alprozalam for relief of tinnitus. *Archives of Otolaryngology–Head and Neck Surgery, 842–845.*

JOHNSON, R., GREIST, S., PRESS, L., STORTER, K., & LENTZ, B. (1989). A tinnitus masking program: Efficacy and safety. *Hearing Journal, 42(11);18–25.*

JONES, I., & KNUDSEN, V. (1928). Certain aspects of tinnitus, particularly treatment. *Laryngoscope, 38;597–611.*

KATAJIMA, K., YAMANA, T., UCHIDA, K., & KITAHARA, M. (1998). Biofeedback training for tinnitus control. In: J. Vernon (Ed.), *Tinnitus: Treatment and relief* (pp. 131–139). Boston: Allyn & Bacon.

LEVY, R., & ARTS, H. (1996). Predicting neuroradiologic outcome in patients referred for audiovestibular dysfunction. *American Journal of Neuroradiology, 17(9);1717–1724.*

LOOKWOOD, A., SALVI, R., COAD, M., TOWSLEY, M., WACK, D., & MURPHY, B. (1998). The functional neuroanatomy of tinnitus. *Neurology, 50;114–120.*

MEIKLE, M., JOHNSON, R., GRIEST, S., PRESS, L., & CHARNELL, M. (1995). Oregon Tinnitus Data Archive 95-01. *http://www.ohus.edu/ohrc-otda/*.

MELZACK, R. (1992). Phantom limbs. *Scientific American, 266*;120–126.

MORGAN, D. (1998). Tinnitus and the jaw joint (TMJ). In: J. Vernon (Ed.), *Tinnitus: Treatment and relief* (pp. 197–200). Boston: Allyn & Bacon.

NAGLER, S. (1997). Tinnitus and homeopathy—My view. *Tinnitus Today, 22*(3);10,11.

NEWMAN, C., JACOBSON, G., & SPITZER, J. (1996). Development of the tinnitus handicap inventory. *Archives of Otolaryngology–Head and Neck Surgery, 122*(2);143–148.

SCHULTZ, G., & MELZACK, R. (1991). The Charles Bonnet syndrome: Phantom visual images. *Perceptions, 20*;809–825.

SIMPSON, J., ATKIN, M., DONALDSON, I., & DAVIES, W. (1995). A double-blind trial of a homoeopathic remedy for tinnitus. In: G. Reich, & J. Vernon (Eds.), *Proceedings of the Fifth International Tinnitus Seminar* (pp. 92–97). Portland, OR: American Tinnitus Association.

SPAULDING, A. (1903). Tinnitus, with a plea for its more accurate musical notation. *Annals of Otology, 32*;263–272.

STALLER, S. (1998). Suppression of tinnitus with electrical stimulation. In: J. Vernon (Ed.), *Tinnitus: Treatment and relief* (pp. 77–90). Boston: Allyn & Bacon.

STYPULKOWSKI, P. (1989). Mechanisms of salicylate ototoxicity. *Journal of Hearing Research, 46*;113–145.

SWEETOW, R. (1989). Adjunctive approaches to tinnitus patient management. *Hearing Journal, 42*(11);38–43.

TYLER, R., & STOUFER, J. (1989). A review of tinnitus loudness. *Journal of Hearing, 42*(11);52–57.

VALENTE, M., PETEREIN, J., GOEBEL, J., & NEELY, J. (1995). Four cases of acoustic neuroma with normal hearing. *Journal of the American Academy of Audiology, 6*(3);203–210.

VERNON, J. (1975). Tinnitus. *Hearing Aid Journal, 13*(11):82–83.

VERNON, J. (1977). Attempts to relieve tinnitus. *Journal of the American Academy of Audiology, 2*;124–131.

VERNON, J. (ED.). (1998). *Tinnitus: Treatment and relief.* Boston: Allyn & Bacon.

VON WEDEL, S. (1998). Tinnitus masking with tinnitus maskers and hearing aids: A longitudinal study of efficacy from 1987 to 1993. In: J. Vernon (Ed.), *Tinnitus: Treatment and relief.* (pp. 187–192). Boston: Allyn & Bacon.

WALGER, M., VON WEDEL, H., CALERO, L., & HOENEN, S. (1995a). Effectiveness of low-power-laser and ginkgo therapy in patients with chronic tinnitus. In: G. Reich, & J. Vernon (Eds.), *Proceedings of the Fifth International Tinnitus Seminar* (pp. 96–98). Portland, OR: American Tinnitus Association.

WALGER, M. H., VON WEDEL, H., HOENEN, S., & CALERO, L. (1995b). Transmission of low-power-laser to the human cochlea. In G. Reich, & J. Vernon (Eds.), *Proceedings of the Fifth International Tinnitus Seminar* (pp. 99–100). Portland, OR: American Tinnitus Association.

WAYNER, D. (1998) Cognitive therapy and tinnitus: An intensive Weekend Workshop. In: J. Vernon (Ed.), *Tinnitus: Treatment and relief* (pp. 116–130). Boston: Allyn & Bacon.

WEGEL, R., & LANE, C. (1924). The auditory masking of one pure tone by another and its probable relation to the dynamics of the ear. *Physiology Review, 23*;266–285.

WITT, U., & FELIX, C. (1989). Selektive photo-biochemotherapie in der kombination laser und ginkgo-pflanzenextrakt nach der methode Witt. Neue altenativre moglichkeit bei innenohrsstorungen. *Informationsmaterial der Firma Felas Lasers GmbH*, Steinredder 1; 2409 Scharbeutz I, Germany.

PREFERRED PRACTICE GUIDELINES

Professionals Who Perform the Procedure(s)

▼ Clinical audiologists. For tinnitus retraining therapy, clinical audiologists who have been properly trained in the neurophysiological model of tinnitus developed by Dr. Pawel Jastreboff and in the therapy Dr. Jastreboff has developed from that model.

Expected Outcomes

▼ The patient will experience a significant decrease in the awareness of tinnitus.

▼ The patient will experience a significant decrease in the perceived interference in the quality of life caused by tinnitus.

▼ The patient will experience a significant decrease in the interference in daily activities from tinnitus.

▼ The patient will experience a significant decrease in the negative emotional distress caused by tinnitus.

▼ No instrument fitting shall put the patient at risk for hearing threshold shift.

▼ All instrument fittings shall be comfortable.

▼ The patient shall understand the rationale and protocol for his or her particular therapy.

Clinical Indications

▼ Therapy shall be initiated for patients who express significant handicap or emotional distress because of tinnitus.

Clinical Processes

▼ Patient interviews to determine the extent of handicap and/or emotional distress caused by tinnitus.

▼ In-depth audiological evaluation.

▼ When appropriate, medical referral.

▼ Measurements of the frequency and intensity of tinnitus.

▼ Measurement of loudness discomfort levels.

▼ Review of available tinnitus therapies with the patient.

▼ When appropriate, referral for medical, psychological or psychiatric evaluation, biofeedback, or other useful therapies.

▼ If masking is to be used, selection and setting of the masker frequency response and maximum output.

▼ If tinnitus retraining therapy is to be used, proper classification of the patient according to the protocols developed by Dr. Jastreboff.

▼ If tinnitus retraining therapy is to be used, directive counseling of the patient according to the protocols developed by Dr. Jastreboff. The directive counseling is to include frequent contact during the first 3 months of therapy.

▼ If tinnitus retraining therapy is to be used, selection of the proper protocol, based on appropriate classification, and training of the patient in that protocol.

▼ All therapies shall be performed only by properly trained and qualified persons.

Documentation

▼ All contact with the patient, whether in person or by telephone, fax, or E-mail, shall be fully documented.

▼ All instrument sales and fittings shall contain all documentation required by state and federal law.

Chapter 24

Future Trends in Amplification

H. Christopher Schweitzer

Outline

As the calendar moves rapidly toward a new millennium, much has been made of the triumph of twentieth-century technology and the wonders that must surely follow in the twenty-first century. The legendary baseball player and notorious word scrambler Yogi Berra once declared, "Making predictions is hard, especially when it's about the future!" Recognizing the obvious risks of recording predictions in print, this chapter will nevertheless propose some forecasts for amplification developments into the future. A fundamental assumption throughout this chapter will be the inevitable continued digitization of the hearing aid industry. It is my opinion that what began in the 1980s as laboratory experiments with power-hungry digital hearing aid prototypes followed by the introduction of small, computationally intensive completely-in-the-canal (CIC) digital hearing aids in the late 1990s will proceed long into the future. Yogi Berra notwithstanding, digital hearing aids will dominate the industry of the future for both technical and clinical reasons, some of which will be elaborated on later in the chapter.

THE SHRINKING TRANSISTOR

Amplification is fundamentally about power and power management. Acoustic and electrical power, adjusted and manipulated in wearable commercial devices, provide personal communication power for millions of hearing aid users.

Slightly more than 50 years ago three young scientists at Bell Laboratories were engaged in experiments that would dramatically transform power management in electronics, communications, and, unquestionably, hearing aids. The Nobel Prize in physics was awarded in 1956 to John Bardeen, Walter Brattain, and William Shockley for their invention of the transistor. Having poked two electrodes into a thin sliver of germanium, they observed a marvelous gain in power of almost 100 times over the input voltage from this curious "semiconductor," as it would be called. The course of hearing aid development would subsequently follow the continued refinement of the transistor, and virtually every segment of society would likewise feel the impact to a profound degree. It was clearly as profound a transformational event as the invention of the telephone by the man to whose memory their laboratory was named. Notably, one of the first commercial applications of the new transistor was an implementation to reduce the size of hearing aids in 1952 (Lybarger, personal communication, 1998; Preves, personal communication, 1998). By 1954, hearing aids had been almost entirely converted to transistorized designs for their amplification requirements.

The pace of the continued development of transistorized circuits has not slowed in the past 50 years but rather has grown exponentially. Although the focus of attention in recent decades has been on computers and microchips, sometimes lost to public awareness is that those elements are comprised of transistors . . . lots of them. The semiconductor industry is engaged in a furious race to embed continuously denser populations of transistors into microprocessors, and projections for the future are quite astounding. Computer chip maker Intel, in a cooperative developmental effort with Motorola, Advanced Micro Devices (AMD), and the U.S. Department of Energy, expects to be able to build processors with *1 billion transistors* by the end of the first decade of the 2000s (Goodwin, 1997). Such a chip is expected to operate at a clock speed of 10 gigahertz (compared with the fastest Pentium processors of today running at speeds approaching 400 megahertz). Perhaps even more astonishing, the new billion-transistor chip is also expected to deliver *100,000 million* instructions per second (MIPS)! This is an extraordinary projection, and one that has profound spillover ramifications for hearing aid systems whose use and value will increasingly

Audiology: Treatment. Edited by Valente, Hosford-Dunn, and Roeser. Thieme Medical Publishers, Inc., New York © 2000

depend on their ability to accomplish rapid computations without perceived delays. Conversely, the possibilities for the future of "computational management of hearing problems" is inexorably linked to such benchmarks as MIPS. Generally, developments in the huge global microprocessor industry invariably have a "trickle-down" effect on the pace of digital hearing aid hardware development.

The conversion of hearing aid processing to digital signal processing (DSP) is fairly well advanced, even exceeding earlier projections (Schweitzer, 1997a). Little reason exists to expect a backlash return to analog or digitally controlled analog (DCA) systems in the future. The present generation of DSP hearing aids, as of this writing, are considered genuinely advanced technologies and deliver tens to somewhere more than 100 MIPS. Progressively smaller and more computationally powerful chips, along with associated reductions of power requirements, point toward a steady progression of the number of possible MIPS in hearing aid–size packages. This argues that the next important advances in amplification for the hearing-impaired will be driven by the clinical elegance of the software. That is, the value of future systems will be in their ability to intelligently exploit this increasingly rapid computational stream, as expressed in MIPS. To extract meaningful listening patterns out of the flurry of sounds that often simultaneously arrive at the input to the hearing enhancement system requires fast

and elegant computation. This, of course, alludes to the "Holy Grail" of hearing aid design—the disambiguation of meaningful signal targets from noisy "jammers"—a process greatly confounded because listeners routinely vary their decision of what is a noise and what is signal (Schweitzer, 1997b), as illustrated in Figure 24–1.

Of course, increases in the number of transistors within a given area could only have been enabled by technologies that reduced transistor size while increasing their performance. As a general rule, such developments follow the well-known "Moore's law," named for the cofounder and chairman emeritus of Intel Corporation, Gordon Moore. Moore's law says that the number of transistors that can be drawn on a fixed circuit space doubles every 18 months. To illustrate the remarkable progress associated with such an exponential shrinkage, consider Figure 24–2, which uses various Intel chips as benchmarks, then projects forward into the future on the basis of projections by the above-mentioned consortium.

To accomplish such continued progress in microprocessors, physical constraints in transistor circuit lines, or electron channels, are targeted for massive research and development efforts. Reduction from the current 0.35 μm width of Pentinum processor features toward an incredible 0.10 μm width to produce the 1 billion transistor chips suggested previously are projected by 2007 (Goodwin, 1997). The 0.01 μm size represents a benchmark known as the "point one" barrier

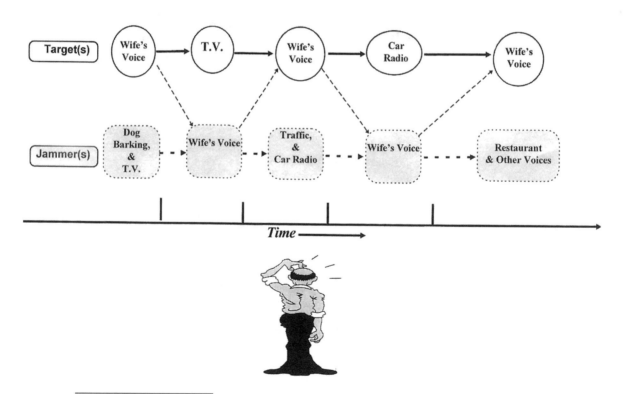

Figure 24–1 Example of the time-varying nature of an individual's determination of a particular sound as either a "signal" or a "noise." The same acoustic signature may at various times be a desired "target" sound or an undesired "jammer," depending on moment-to-moment decisions. (From *Seminars in Hearing*, Thieme, New York.)

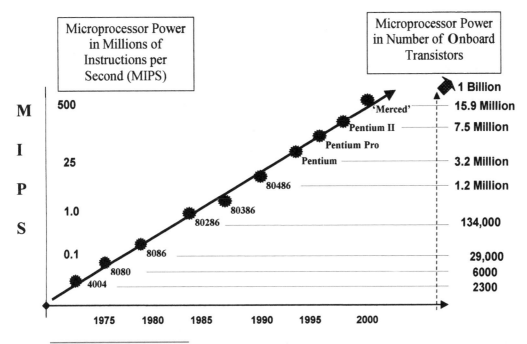

Figure 24–2   Illustration of the dramatic increases in microprocessors over less than 25 years.

and will be discussed further. Joint research by industry and the U.S. Department of Energy laboratories to develop an extreme ultra violet (EUV) advanced lithographic technique is expected to enable such an accomplishment in silicon wiring. Meanwhile, National Semiconductor Corporation was expecting in 1998 to reach 0.25 μm silicon features (Takahashi, 1997). This would enable 20 million transistors on a single chip, almost three times more than on an Intel Pentium II processor.

To illustrate how a pattern of progress in the larger semiconductor industry has a shaping influence on the much smaller hearing aid industry, consider some observations recently made by Gerald Popelka (1998). Dr. Popelka was involved in digital hearing aid research since the early 1980s as part of the development team at the Central Institute for the Deaf (CID) in St. Louis. Relying on his experience with technology advances from the CID work from 1981 to 1998, he tracked the progression of computerized hardware for use in hearing aids. He then extended forward another 17 years to the year 2015 and made some enticing predictions regarding further developments that will serve to augment further hearing aid progress.

Popelka proposed two ways to follow the development trend in hearing aid circuitry. In the first, he allowed power consumption and chip size to progressively decrease but kept the number of transistors constant. This would obviously be advantageous for consumers by extending battery life but would constrain computational power. On the basis of a 1-volt power supply, his development trend looked like the following:

	1981	1998	2015
Power consumption	2.0 mW	0.33 mW	0.03 mW
Processor chip size	50 mm²	1.5 mm²	0.015 mm²
Transistors	50 k	50 k	50 k
Speed	5 MIPS	5 MIPS	5 MIPS

Alternately, Popelka proposed that if designers chose to trade off power consumption for processing speed by maintaining the 2.0 mW power consumption with a 1-volt supply, he projected the following scenario:

	1981	1998	2015
Transistors	50 k	1.8 M	180 M
Speed	5 MIPS	30 MIPS	300 MIPS

In this second scenario, in which the numbers of calculations are vastly increased, the potential for truly exciting hearing aid applications emerges. With such prospects for hardware improvements, it remains a question of how cleverly software engineers can address the challenges of auditory impairment (Westerman & Sandlin, 1997).

FUNDAMENTAL CHANGES IN COMPUTING

The previous comments have all assumed the expanded dependency of hearing aid devices on microprocessors, which are, of course, miniature computers. In fact, it may be too early to demonstrate unambiguous clinical user benefits from such a conversion (to digital hearing aids). But an undeniable assumption is that development trends will continue to "digitize" the hearing aid industry (Kruger & Kruger, 1994; Schweitzer, 1997a; Westerman & Sandlin, 1997) because of both technical advantages and clinical flexibility. Moreover, existing advantages in digital circuit stability, noise floor superiority, and the prospect of greatly reduced feedback problems will join with fundamental production cost reductions to expand DSP chip construction for hearing aids. Last, expected declines in DSP chip power consumption will likely secure the eventual surpassing of any remaining advantages for analog designs.

Clearly, it is a reasonable expectation to foresee the continued shrinkage of the ubiquitous transistor, and likewise the microprocessors that are assembled from them. But what are the physical limits? The trajectory of component size reduction moves conceptually toward the quantum level, meaning chips approaching the size of atoms. That is the estimate of experts in the area of lithography, the process of etching the microscopic circuit lines on microchips (Davidson, 1997). As the manufacturing processes move forward from optical lithography to x-ray and the EUV method mentioned previously, the dimensions begin to approach the weird world of quantum physics. At such tiny sizes the movement of electrons becomes more difficult to predict and becomes controlled by principles of probability rather than the neat exactitudes of Newtonian physics. Furthermore, the basis of present computing is switching by use of tiny gates whose positions determine a "1" state or a "0" state. At dimensions less than 0.1 μm (known to the researchers as the "point one" limit) electrons could not be controlled by such gates—they would simply jump in an indeterminate manner or leak through the wired passages (Kaku, 1997). The "point one" limit also reflects the fact that as the number of transistors per area increases, as Moore's Law predicts, the dissipation of heat becomes increasingly problematic.

BEYOND SILICON

Because hearing aids are now so highly dependent on developments in the computer industry, it is worth additional discussion of advances there. Progress in so-called quantum computing raises the possibility that all current extensions of Moore's law could be vastly exceeded by significant exponents because the fundamental rules would have to change. Work at Hewlett-Packard's Quantum Structures Research Initiative, for example, suggests quantum computers would be stunningly faster than anything possible with transistor-based technology. One type of quantum computer might store information in hydrogen atoms. Hydrogen atoms have only a single electron. By firing microlasers at the hydrogen atom the electron could be switched back and forth between a high and low orbit, as in Figure 24–3. Such shifts in fundamental operations would greatly enhance the use of binary code now used in DSP. Progress in this area is advancing at an extremely rapid pace. It is important to recognize that just a few years ago mainstream physicists considered devices now in production virtually impossible.

Another variation of a quantum transistor involves vibrating quantum dots to selected resonances that correspond to bit codes of "1s" and "0s" with the prospect for many (perhaps a million) circuits operating simultaneously under the control of a single oscillating atom. Research at Texas Instruments implies such quantum transistor array concepts are crystallizing toward real implementations.

Other scientists at the frontiers of progress have suggested that the real future of computation might involve advances that surpass current binary computing and its dependency on silicon. Benyus (1997) writes extensively about numerous

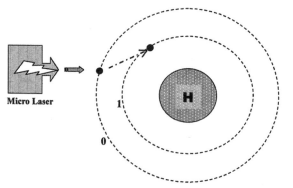

Hydrogen atom with a single electron and two possible orbits that could constitute a pair of binary states

Figure 24–3 Conceptual model of a "quantum computer," which uses a microlaser to force the single electron of a hydrogen atom to move between an outer and inner orbit, thus creating a binary state device.

biological computing approaches that are under investigation. Many such approaches accelerate computation dramatically past present binary silicon-based operations. Similarly, Kaku (1997) predicts the complete demise of silicon in the early twenty-first century. Kaku, a theoretical physicist who codiscovered String Theory, elaborates on the vast increases in computational power that could be derived from work with DNA-based computing. DNA molecules are considered ideal for molecular computing. They constitute only 0.3% of the volume of the nucleus of the cell, but pack more than 100 trillion times the information stored in present-day, high-power computers. Even the fastest silicon-chip computers calculate sequentially, that is, one number at a time, and they generate a nontrivial by-product, heat. DNA computers run much slower but can simultaneously process billions of numbers, and, of course, are much more energy efficient. This is possible because, unlike binary encoding, which uses only two symbols, "0" and "1", the DNA code consists of four symbols representing the four nucleic acids. (The reader may recall that a 3.6 billion string of the letters representing those chemicals is needed to spell out the code for a human being.) An ounce of DNA would reportedly be enough to construct a computer 100,000 times faster than the fastest supercomputer yet assembled.

Therefore, the development of DNA computing and other techniques that exploit molecular biological processes (hence using structures designed around carbon, rather than silicon) hold the promise of vast increases in parallel computing that would not require the traditional controls required in present computers. Processes under investigation at dozens of research centers on biologically based computing methods would potentially have the additional advantages of structural evolution. That is, unlike silicon-based hardware, the basic physical elements of organic computers could be expected to change with learning and thereby yield ever-increasing efficiencies and value. Such prospects certainly suggest profound advantages in the quest for ways to intelligently manage the delivery of spoken language for auditory purposes.

Another example of alternatives to silicon in nanotechnology with long-range relevance to hearing aid amplification is work at IBM's Zurich research laboratory with C60 molecules—carbon atoms shaped like geodesic soccer balls. Experiments have yielded fivefold increases in voltage applied by simply compressing these so-called buckyballs by 0.1 millionth of a millimeter. Strings of buckyballs (named for Buckminster Fuller, the inventor of the geodesic dome structure) could become the component basis for nanocomputers according to the Nobel Prize–winning discoverers of buckyballs.

Nanotechnologies are likely to influence hearing aids of the future in other ways as well. It may be expected that micromachined transducers can be used to construct both arrays of microphones and receivers to the advantage of hearing-impaired listeners. Microphone arrays are already understood to yield advantages in selecting a target out of a surround of undesirable acoustic competition (Kates & Weiss, 1996; Liu et al, 1997; Schweitzer & Krishnan, 1996). Figure 24–4 shows one interesting implementation of microphone array products development by Starkey Laboratories. The fig-

ure certainly suggests "future" in the look, but the device is a robust example of a highly directional system that can couple to existing hearing aids by means of modulating a magnetic field. Nanotechnologies might be used to shrink such arrays to much more desirable sizes. One might imagine considerably smaller microphones fastened into the folds of the external ear and equipped with tiny remote transmitters relayed to hearing aid processing units and receivers located further into the earcanals. Progress in nanotechnologies, including transducers, amplifiers, and radio technologies, suggests such a scenario is not unattainable (Bush-Vishniac, 1998; Rogers & Kaplan, 1998). A great deal of developmental work is directed toward integrating electronics entirely with transducer/sensors. Bush-Vishniac (1998) gives several reasons why the pace of progress in electromechanical devices is "escalating dramatically," as she put it. These include nearly instantaneous exchanges of information, shorter design times, the rise of small and mid-size niche companies, and the potential for major financial rewards in the worldwide market for extremely miniaturized devices.

Finally, work in "optical computing" should be mentioned, partly because it returns the reader to Bell Labs, where in 1990 a prototype optical computer was demonstrated. That work, which has been pursued in many other research centers, would yield devices operating with laser light crisscrossing within an optical cube. Light paths can cross and superimpose without interference, similar to the way multiple sounds can coexist by the principle of superposition. Hence, increases in computational speed, reductions in heat, and the elimination of present constraints for separate wire routes all propose great advantage for optical computers.

Of course, it is a long way from the advanced basic research laboratory to implementation in a hearing aid product. But the significance to the reader is that developments in the support industries of electronics and biomedical engineering create a wave of progress that lifts the rather small hearing aid industry, sometimes much faster than linear expectations.

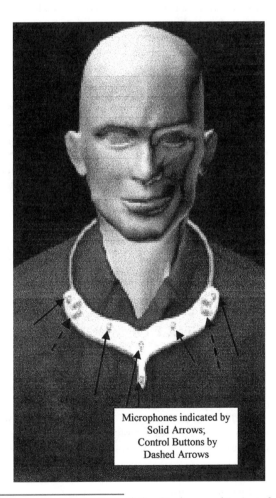

Figure 24–4 illustration caption:

Microphones indicated by Solid Arrows; Control Buttons by Dashed Arrows

Figure 24–4 Illustration of the Starkey multimicrophone array as worn around the neck. The soft, flexible material houses microphones arrayed in a manner that produces a strong directionality and associated spatial enhancement. Controls for the devices can also be seen. The signal is sent magnetically to hearing aids of any size and received by a telecoil.

TAPPING INTO RESEARCH IN THE BASIC SCIENCES

Returning to the opening lines of this chapter about the difficulty of future predictions, it is worth recalling how the course of technical progress is often decidedly nonlinear. Some breakthroughs emerge rapidly and smoothly accelerate. Others stumble and crawl far longer than first expectations, but then jump forward in a quantum leap. Dr. Lynn Huerta (1998) of the National Institute on Deafness and Other Communication Disorders drew attention in her discussion of "future developments in amplification" to the difficulties of making breakthrough predictions in bioengineering. She referred to bold published "expert estimates" of the amount of time needed to develop certain heart assist technologies promising it was only an 18-month challenge. It subsequently took some of the best biomedical researchers and clinicians 30 years to achieve those same technical objectives. Huerta also drew attention to some recent preliminary findings from basic research that could conceivably deliver dramatic, long-term yields in future generation hearing aid systems by scientists supported by the National Institutes of Health. Some of the work relates to biologically inspired computational approaches. A few examples that illustrate how basic science can translate into applied research include the following:

- The development of intelligent systems on the basis of biological models that can selectively amplify sounds in the presence of intense competing sounds. Specifically, a research group headed by Dr. Albert Feng at the Beckman Institute in Champaign-Urbana, Illinois, is using a model based on physiological studies in the auditory brain stem of the frog to develop a unique approach to addressing the problem of detecting signals in difficult and noisy situations.

- Development of a directionally sensitive microphone based on the structure and function of a parasitic fly ear. In this fly, the ears are so close together that interaural time and intensity differences are minute, yet these flies can localize sounds quite well. This group, headed by Drs. Ron Hoy and Ronald Miles at Cornell University in Ithaca, New York, and at the State University of New York, Binghamton, New York, is capitalizing on this unique structure to build a biologically based microphone specifically for use in hearing aids. The design promises to improve on existing directional microphones.

- Using animal preparations with hearing loss to develop signal processing algorithms that result in "normal" central auditory nervous system function. For example, a group at Johns Hopkins University in Baltimore, Maryland, headed by Dr. Murray Sachs, is specifically interested in using an animal model to develop signal processing algorithms to compensate for an induced hearing loss as measured at the level of the auditory nerve.

Efforts such as those just described in concert with the many other ongoing and new research programs give hope that better understanding of the function of normal and pathological auditory systems will lead to better strategies for providing appropriately designed signal-processing strategies. The route to genuine advances in hearing aid technologies has always benefited from the broad collateral developments in the basic sciences. That tendency is expected to continue in the future even as audiopathic science continues to mature and make its own bold steps into the new millennium.

PLATFORM DECISIONS

The first true digital hearing aids, both laboratory prototypes and commercial releases, were notably quite large because of the need to use commercially available DSP chips. Such body aid devices manufactured by Nicolet and Rion could not enjoy market success for that very reason. In the absence of small, "off-the-shelf," general-purpose DSP chips that could work at the low voltages (1.3 V) of hearing aids, designers of initial market releases of DSP small, head-worn hearing aids were generally forced to develop their own application-specific custom chips. In addition, they essentially had to choose between design architectures that used what could be described as either hardwired or softwired technologies for

their systems. Hardwired systems make use of proprietary processing algorithms in a fundamentally fixed processing architecture but allow adjustments of programmable parameters during the fitting. Such approaches characterize approaches used by Oticon, Siemens, and Widex in their products. Genuinely new processing strategies for such designs require a new integrated circuit (IC) and electronic module. Hardwired designs have an advantage, however, of small size and low current consumption, certainly nontrivial virtues for hearing aids.

Softwired DSP systems, in contrast (of which none are presently available but are expected soon from ReSound and Danavox from their AudioLogic development project), have the notable advantage of being able to readily implement new sound processing algorithms without requiring new IC development. However, this approach generally has the challenge of larger circuitry size and less economical current drain requirements. (See postscript.)

Some manufacturers have elected to build combination designs that include elements of both hardwired and softwire approaches (Philips, for example). The clinical and user advantages of greater processing flexibility in softwired DSP will arguably compel increasing resources to be directed toward improvements in the size and power constraints of these more open platform designs. Furthermore, major DSP chip manufacturers such as Texas Instruments, LSI, and Motorola may well make available in the future "off-the-shelf" DSP IC chips with the low power and small size requirements for hearing aid applications. Such a development would undoubtedly have a significant impact on the extent of DSP penetration into the hearing aid market as smaller companies, that are otherwise shut out for development cost reasons, could then feature digital products. Hence, the future may include a greater emphasis on open platforms, although controversy over the exact meaning of "open" will likely persist (Nielsen, 1997). Extensive introduction of such systems would both enable and simultaneously require clinicians to make fundamental signal processing design decisions that have previously been left to manufacturers.

CONVERGENCE OF MULTIPURPOSE COMMUNICATION DEVICES

It is almost inevitable that everything that exploits microprocessors will get smaller and more powerful in the future. Similarly, the use of microprocessors in more devices and new applications is fully expected. The uncertainly lies in the form and interaction of everyday devices as the continued shrinking of products like telephones and personal computers converge into single "fusion packages" (Pelton, 1998; Wilpon, 1998; Zimmerman, 1996). As Figure 24–5 suggests, the familiar wristwatch could evolve into a multipurpose control center that theoretically could operate wireless telephones, Web-linked communications, audiopathic augmentation (i.e., hearing aids), and language translation devices (Flanagan, 1998; Sagisaka, 1998), all housed in the same device that resembles a traditional hearing aid. Progress in wireless technologies (Stutzman &

TELECOMMUNICATION DEVICES

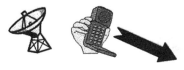

May Converge with

To Create New MULTI-PURPOSE *"FUSION" DEVICES*

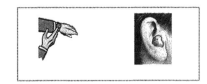

e.g., **Wristwatch controlled, Web-linked, head-worn, Speaker-Smart, Language Translation/Telephone/Hearing Aid/Radio/Computer Combination Devices**

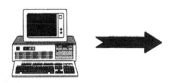

Microcomputers

+

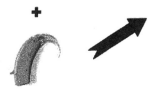

**Augmentative Devices
(i.e. HEARING AIDS)**

Figure 24–5   As technical advances enable more computation in smaller packages, a convergence of various personal communication devices may result in new "fusion" products that look strikingly like hearing aids. When needed, they could, in fact, be hearing aids but also serve as telephones, voice mail links, language translators, and more. Control for such devices could be accomplished by wristwatch systems.

Dietrich, 1998) will continue to make an impact on and reshape interpersonal life as communication tools become ever more pervasive.

Such a convergence of personal communication hardware may seem to be a peculiar blending of medical devices (hearing aids) with general purpose consumer products. From the standpoint of the consumer, hearing aids have always been communication devices, government labeling and regulation notwithstanding. It could be argued that hearing aids are essentially nothing more than short-range telecommunication devices with customized sound shaping. Once appropriate audiological diagnostics are accomplished, the fitting process could be conceptualized as an audio engineering (or engin-*ear*-ing task) that could conceivably be increasingly driven by the consumer (Schweitzer & Monroe, 1998).

Zimmerman (1996) has described the development of personal area network (PANs) technology that uses the body's electromagnetic field as a "wet wire" for interdevice communications. The body's natural salinity makes it an excellent conductor of electrical current. PAN technology uses this conductivity to create an external electric field that routes nanoamp and picoamp currents through the body to carry data. Zimmerman specifically mentions that head-mounted

PAN devices could include hearing aids. A unit no larger than a credit card might be kept in the pocket or worn as a wristwatch to communicate either to another device or to remote sensors. The applications under study at IBM Research Laboratories include the transfer of personal financial or medical data exchanges through simple handshake connections. Piezoelectric shoe inserts could be used to generate the small amount of power required for such systems. Certainly, obstacles related to data transmission rates may preclude a direct transfer of PAN technology, as presently conceived, to computationally sophisticated hearing aids. But it may be shortsighted to assume no other enabling breakthroughs can follow. A scan of the July 1998 special technology awards issue of *Discover* indicates that many impressive advances in computer hardware and electronics that could easily have an impact on future hearing aid fusion devices are discovered or developed almost monthly. Included were a tiny 35 mm fractal antenna, a microscopic electromechanical vibrating strip resonator (which may enable dramatic reductions in the size of wireless telephones), a method of using copper instead of aluminum in the microscopic wires of transistors, and a nonvolatile field effect transistor. The latter was discovered after the accidental overheating of an experimental capacitor, nicely illustrating how some developmental jumps are the result of serendipity, rather than intention. Clearly then, it is almost as dangerous to wager *against* the development of something as for it. Stephen Pinker (1997) makes this quite evident by including the following quotes in his discussion of the potential of artificial intelligence:

> "Heavier than air flying machines are impossible." (Lord Kelvin)

> "Man will never reach the moon, regardless of all future scientific advances." (Lee Deforest, inventor of the vacuum tube)

> "It is impossible to transmit the voice over wires, and were it possible to do so, it would be of no practical benefit." (1865 editorial in the *Boston Post*)

Of course, many other classic examples of blundered predictions for the future have been made, including the president of the American Medical Association discrediting the possibility of x-rays. Sometimes experts err on the conservative side; a 1949 issue of *Popular Mechanics* included the bold promise that "computers of the future will weigh no more than 1.5 tons." All this should suggest to the reader that trying to forecast what form future hearing aids will take might actually frame the wrong question. It is quite possible that traditional hearing aid forms may become the preferred package designs for a cluster of other products that are not intended for the hearing impaired. Indeed, the *Discover* magazine technology awards issue of 5 years ago (1993) featured a Bell Laboratories wireless phone of the future. It was entirely embodied in a case that to educated eyes looked exactly like a behind-the-ear hearing aid.

SIGNAL PROCESSING SOFTWARE

A persistent question, legitimately raised as hearing aid hardware has become increasingly complex and technically advanced, is whether such developments translate to genuine clinical benefit (Byrne, 1996). The answer, of course, is closely coupled to the software that is implemented in the computerized systems. DSP for hearing aids is fundamentally about software code that can manipulate the stream of acoustic events that arrive at the input of a system to the perceived benefit of the user. Will elegantly designed software solve the multiple and individually unique audiological problems identified by Moore (1996, 1998) that extend beyond simple threshold corrections? Will problems of impaired temporal processing and frequency selectivity be addressed adequately on an individualized basis in the hearing aids of the future?

Although theoretically those perceptual aberrations, and many others as described by Moore, should all be within the reach of well-designed software, as of yet little evidence has been produced. Clearly, parallel developments in diagnostics and fitting procedures must proceed to solidify the expected benefits from elegantly designed processing software algorithms. Westerman and Sandlin (1997), in their own attempt to forecast the future, indicated that "it is unlikely, if not impossible, that digital technology will restore an impaired auditory system to normal" (p. 59). But, as they also suggest, the potential for intelligent hearing systems is primarily a function of the cleverness of the software engineers. Needless to say, the continued input of auditory scientists and clinical researchers will be required to guide the software engineers.

Examples of the elegance and power of DSP approaches that computationally improve noisy signals are given in Figures 24–6 and 24–7 from work by Hermansen et al (1994). In this case a spectral sharpening strategy was implemented called PARTRAN, for parametric transformation. The algorithm was developed to address hearing problems presenting with threshold loss, widened critical bands, and loudness disturbances. As clearly seen in the figures, a decided speech signal sharpening and noise reduction is possible with this digital treatment. However, as with any laboratory development, its application in future wearable systems remains to be seen. On the other hand, as previously discussed in this chapter, the continued reduction of microprocessor size and power requirements, accompanied by simultaneous increasing increases in computational power, make it risky to rule out any development scenario.

Another interesting software design for severe hearing impairment is a frequency compression approach developed by RION engineers (Sakamoto et al, 1997). Figures 24–8 and 24–9 illustrate the application as applied to speech signals

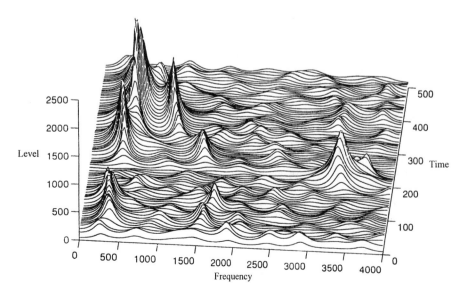

Figure 24–6 Three-dimensional representation of a single Danish word in a noisy condition before the digital PARTRAN treatment by Hermansen et al (1994). (Reproduced with permission from *Trends in Amplification* [1997], Woodland Publications, Inc., New York.)

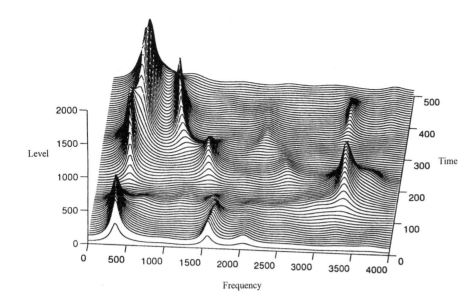

Figure 24–7 Same word as in Figure 24–5 after application of the PARTRAN algorithm showing impressive signal enhancement over the noise. (From Schweitzer [1997a], with permission.)

FREQUENCY COMPRESSION PROCESSING

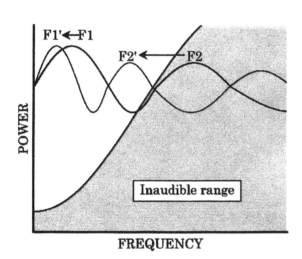

Figure 24–8 Frequency compression algorithm used in a digital hearing aid produced by RION in their HD-11 product. Formant 1 and 2 are shifted differentially as needed audiologically in this device, which allows users independent control over the amount of pitch shift for voiced and unvoiced speech sounds. (From Sakamoto et al [1997], with permission.)

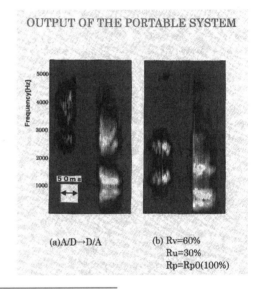

Figure 24–9 Spectrographic illustration of the downward shifting of the unvoiced consonant portion of the Japanese word /Sita/ spoken by a male talker. The compression of the high frequencies can be seen as greater than for the lower frequencies, showing a unique implementation of a digital processing algorithm for the auditorily impaired. (From Sakamoto et al [1997], with permission.)

that may contain energy too high in frequency for the listener. The real-time digital hearing aid system in which they have implemented the frequency compression algorithm shifts relevant content downward into the audible range. Their approach seems to have significantly different properties than previous attempts at "frequency transposition" by use of an analysis-synthesis technique known as PARCOR. The RION method uses a voice-generation model of speech to decide whether sounds are voiced or unvoiced to determine a sound discrimination coefficient. The algorithm simultaneously extracts the frequency envelope to analyze the pitch. Formants and fundamental frequency are treated separately as the PARCOR analysis-synthesis applies pitch-dependent compression. The compression for unvoiced sounds can be set separately from voiced sounds, and the commercial product allows the user to choose the amount of compression. This rather specialized digital hearing aid product is intended, of course, for listeners with rather severe hearing loss. Nevertheless, it is indicative of the kind of products that can be expected to increase in number in the future by implementing specialized DSP software solutions.

Another area of software development that could yield high dividends if successfully applied to hearing aid products is in the area of automatic speech recognition (ASR). Enormous resources are being applied to ASR for a multitude of commercial purposes from security, to automatic dictation, language translation, speech to text conversions, and computer interface control. *Business Week* (Gross et al, 1998) featured ASR as "the next big computer revolution." The pace of progress has been steady despite the rather daunting challenge of modeling enough of the human speech recognition process, a process long recognized as elusive and layered with redundancies, to succeed in diverse acoustic conditions.

Training software to handle the huge interspeaker and intraspeaker variations that accompany the rapidly changing and noise-degraded string of acoustic events requires tremendous computational power and elegantly designed software. But if a consumer could enter a command to the hearing aid system to sample a particular voice, like that of a teacher or lecturer, for some period of time, conceivably other inputs would be treated as rejectable noise for the duration of the command, providing decided situational benefit. One could imagine that the user's own voice could be simultaneously installed as a "passable" acoustic signature, so as not to disrupt one-on-one conversations in noisy environments. Perhaps, adjustable amounts of specific talker voice emphasis could be implemented, allowing the consumer to optimize the acoustic tunneling effect.

As suggested earlier, the use of such powerful and versatile tools in small, personal communication devices is likely to have appeal to many people without hearing loss or traditional needs for amplification. This fact alone could accelerate the pace of developmental efforts.

ANOTHER CONVERGENCE—CLINICIANS JOIN WITH CONSUMERS, PERCEPTION WITH PREDICTION

Through the second half of the twentieth century, hearing aid fittings have generally proceeded from the assumption that hearing aids are medical devices, and therefore a medical model of diagnosis-leads-to-prescription serves consumers well. But the insufficiencies of peripheral auditory maps to represent the complexities of personal preferences and the cognitive-linguistic variables that affect hearing aid use are well known. Prescription to the point of gross amplification design is certainly useful as a first step. But consumers have expressed a strong desire to directly participate in the processing and parameter adjustment (Schweitzer & Gerhardt, 1996), and a trend toward integrating subjective preferences into fittings is likely to emerge and augment the perceived improvements in future hearing aid technologies.

Evidence for such a trend comes from work in Germany. Geers et al (1997) have developed a systematic and compre-

hensive fitting approach proceeding from the assertion that audiological testing provides insufficient data for present and future hearing aid technologies. Their interactive method uses a touch screen to move from an interview component for identifying specific needs and preferences to a prescriptive component based within a NOAH module. Late in the procedure it introduces an interactive fine-tuning stage. The psychoacoustic model of the Geers systems makes use of fuzzy logic operations. Input values for the fuzzy logic optimization include the following:

- Signal parameters of natural acoustic samples
- Signal parameters as processed by the hearing system
- Audiological data of the hearing-impaired listener
- Psychoacoustic ratings of normal-hearing listeners for the acoustic samples
- Psychoacoustic ratings of the hearing-impaired listeners

The resulting output of the system yields a "HearNet" profile that includes dimensions such as speech intelligibility, comfort, distortion, tone quality, loudness, and noise acceptability. The output also generates the programmable hearing aid configurations. An example of a HearNet profile is given in Figure 24–10.

Haubold and Geers (1993) and Haubold (1996) and his colleagues in Germany have shown data of their total system approach, which they have dubbed A-Life 9000. Their findings support the supposition that significant improvements in perceived naturalness of sound and overall satisfaction can be achieved with their method of interactively involving the patient into the hearing aid design and customized fitting. Further developments that reduce the uncertainties of aligning the expanded digital signal processing possibilities with consumer desires will require an increased measure of trust in patient perceptions and new technical tools for that purpose (Schweitzer et al, 1999; Schweitzer and Haubold, 1999).

GREATER USE OF BINAURAL AND ACOUSTIC CUES IN DIAGNOSTICS AND REHABILITATION

A final area that deserves speculative mention for future forecasting is the extension of binaural testing and binaural hearing systems. Clinical audiology, of course, has been organized around the medical approach of dissection, which separates the two ears. Moreover, hearing aids have obviously been uncorrelated products, unable to communicate with one another in any kind of centralized processing system. But the auditory system is fundamentally about correlating the inputs of the two ears for purposes of localization and targeting desired signals from competing jammers (Bodden, 1997; Gilkey & Anderson, 1996; Yost & Dye, 1997). The advance of digital instrumentation has enabled a number of approaches toward virtual audiometric procedures that proceed from a binaural view of clinical audition (Besing & Koehnke, 1995; Koehnke & Besing, 1997; Nilsson et al, 1998; Vermiglio et al, 1998). Furthermore, hearing aid systems that use binaural

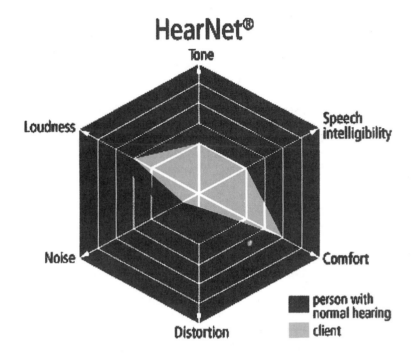

Figure 24–10   Output of the HearNet profile developed for Geers et al (1997) in Germany. As described in the text, the interactive A-Life 9000 system applies fuzzy logic to psychoacoustic ratings, lifestyle interviews, and other data to help patients interactively fine-tune their optimal hearing aid configuration.

cues to provide spatially selective advantages have been developed in the laboratory to the point of wearable prototypes (Liu et al, 1997; Schweitzer, 1997b). Such a system has already been implemented in a commercially available cochlear implant product (Margo et al, 1997). It is difficult to imagine that greater use of binaural clinical assessment tools and hearing systems will not follow the dual curves of reductions in digital processing chip size and increases in computational ability described earlier in this chapter.

The use of binaural processing approaches and the exploitation of acoustic cues derived from the pinna are both well established in the high-fidelity audio industry. Indeed, Hartmann (1998), in his discussion of head-related transfer functions (HRTFs), vital cues for robust directional audio, suggested lightly that in the future individuals may have their HRTFs measured in the process of purchasing virtual audio products. It seems inevitable that such fundamental aspects of human audition as phase and magnitude details, both interaural and intra-aural, will be put to greater advantage in clinical audiology, as well. If genuine benefits can be demonstrated in their application in advanced digital hearing aids, it is entirely conceivable that HRTFs and binaural interactions might be commonly obtained in the dispensing offices of the future. The Starkey Labs and House Ear Institute digital hearing aid development project seems to shows deliberate progress in that direction (Soli et al, 1996; Van Tassel, 1998).

CHALLENGES TO DISTRIBUTION

Distribution is one of the potential areas that technical progress could easily make an impact on, particularly with the total digitization of electronic systems and the interconnective web of the information age. It will become increasingly plausible, if not inevitable, that consumers will have the ability to download software for their hearing aid devices directly through their home computers by means of the World Wide Web. This could have a dramatic effect on audiological practice and the shape of professional hearing aid management.

It is well understood that the present aging population is increasingly computer literate and expectations for personalized value from information technologies can only expand. Already Philips has made some initial efforts to enable consumers to receive downloadable changes to their hearing aid systems (Staab et al, 1997), and it is difficult to imagine why further efforts would not be made as enabling hardware and software progress through broadband cable connections. It is certainly conceivable that government regulatory activities may intervene to shape the course of such developments. But if economic benefit is perceived with minimal consumer risk, a major reshaping of hearing aid distribution could be one of the net results of technology's inevitable advance. New entrants into the hearing aid industry, without a vested dispenser market to offend and/or lose, could proceed to approach distribution entirely on the basis of consumer-direct, Web-based marketing and product delivery. As of this writing many dozens of consumer-oriented Web pages are already on the Internet, many proposing direct purchase with a checkable FDA waiver form to decline the suggested medical examination. The Internet twist on "mail-order" hearing aids could have far more profound consequences than previous manifestations. Continued revisions in attitude toward hearing aids as communication devices rather than primarily medical devices as discussed earlier, could also influence the vector of change.

Claims by professionals of proprietary rights to hearing aid distribution may have little clout to deter such developments if major reductions in cost and efficiency should emerge as a consequence of new developments in product design and distribution alternatives. Hence, another scenario, beside a Web-based system of hearing aid software delivery, is one in which low-cost, digital hearing aids are available in retail department stores, pharmacies, and so forth with self-fitting technologies. Such a system could allow consumers to make interactive adjustments while listening to virtual representations of particular settings and sounds. The settings could be quickly loaded into small, user-attractive devices, with universal fit cases, or with adjustable-size components that in the process of automated coupling to the ear, may make measures of HRTFs and run a series of sound-processing optimization schemes.

Battery technologies could simultaneously advance in such a way that a sealed-in, advanced rechargeable, or even throw-away battery design, could be built into new low-cost products. In the case of a throw-away design, after 6 months or so the unit could be exchanged for a new one and the software simply transferred or updated, again at the same, nonaudiological, location. A blended scenario might have the purchase take place at such a discounted nonmedical facility, with all the software downloads proceeding at home after the consumer has returned.

Presumably pressure for such changes in distribution might be intercepted by vigilant professional organizations that manage to channel some control over fitting, adjustment, or validation through the audiological community. However distasteful some of these visions may seem to audiologists, it would seem dangerous to assume that technical progress in all other areas of hearing aid design and fitting systems will not also contain the seeds for significant changes in distribution as well. The role of hearing professionals may be substantially reshaped by the steady advance of technology.

CONCLUSIONS

In this chapter an attempt has been made to look forward into the future of amplification. Clearly, it has been suggested that the future will be a digital one. Although work to enable digital hardware to meet the requirements of hearing aid consumers is in progress, much is yet to be done toward the vast range of possibilities in signal processing software. It is expected that many specific applications will not wait long before introduction, followed by modification and advancement to the next generation. Changes in distribution and the fundamental assumptions about hearing aids as exclusively medical devices may also result from the advance of communication tools and information technologies.

Hearing aids are presently, and will continue to be, communication devices. As such, perhaps it is important to recall that ultimately, as expressed by Fujisaki (1998), communication is about linking one mind's thoughts into another person's mind. Although the form and processing capabilities of hearing aid hardware and software will continue to advance, accomplishing more and more in less and less space, the ultimate value for the future will be in the efficiency that the thoughts of one mind are relayed to another. If that fundamental goal is not achieved for individuals with impaired hearing, the great technical advances of the future will amount to little consequence.

POSTSCRIPT

As the calendar turns on the Millennium, Kurzweil (1999) makes the case that the pace of change is accelerating even more dramatically than suggested in this chapter. In fact, Kurzweil, inventor of reading machines, music synthesizers, and speech recognizers, even includes a future scenario with hearing aid chips ubiquitously implanted for use on a "demand basis." In the 15 months since this chapter was written, many comments are already obsolete as the pace of advances quickens. Notably, the Danavox and ReSound DSP chip developed by AudioLogic is indeed available in small size hearing aids. Furthermore, it is of such high fidelity quality that Web-based music companies in need of low-power, high-peformance audio amplifiers have incorporated the core in portable (MP3) players. That's quite an industrial reversal—that hearing aid amplifiers are now recruited into high fidelity applications. Yogi Berra certainly had it right. (Kurzweil, R. [1999]. *The age of spiritual machines*. New York: Viking Penguin.)

REFERENCES

BENYUS, J. (1997). How will we store what we learn? In: *Biomimicry: Innovations inspired by nature* (pp. 185–247). New York: William Morrow Co.

BESING, J., & KOEHNKE, J. (1995). A test of virtual auditory localization. *Ear and Hearing, 16*;220–229.

BODDEN, M. (1997). Binaural hearing and hearing impairment: Relations, problems, and proposals for solutions. *Seminars in Hearing, (18)*4;375–391.

BUSH-VISHNIAC, I. (1998). Trends in electromechanical transduction. *Physics Today, 51*(7);28–34.

BYRNE, D. (1996). Hearing aid selection for the 1990s: Where to? Key issues in hearing aid selection and evaluation. *Journal of the American Academy of Audiology, 7*(6);377–395.

DAVIDSON, K. (1997). Chip snip. *San Francisco Examiner*, Nov. 3.

FLANAGAN, J. (1998). *Junctures in speech communication*. Invited paper at the meeting of Acoustical Society of America, Seattle.

FUJISAKI, H. (1998). *Communications between minds: The ultimate goal of speech communication and the target of research for the next half-century.* Invited paper at the meeting of the Acoustical Society of America, Seattle.

GEERS, W., HAUBOLD, J., & SCHMALFUß, G. (1997). *Psychoacoustic based hearing aid fitting with complex acoustic signals.* Poster presentation at the second NIH/VA Hearing Aid Research and Development Conference, Bethesda, MD.

GILKEY, R., & ANDERSON, T. (Eds.). (1996). *Binaural and spatial hearing.* Hillsdale, NJ: Erlbaum.

GOODWIN, I. (1997). Intel, Motorola and Advanced Micro Devices enlist 3 DOE labs to develop new computer chip. *Physics Today, Oct. 85*, 86.

GROSS, N., JUDGE, P., PORT, O., & WILDSTROM, S. (1998). Speech technology is the next big thing in computing. *Business Week*, Special Report, Feb. 23.

HARTMANN, W. (1998). Head-related transfer functions. *Echoes, 8*(2);1–8.

HAUBOLD, J. (1996). A-life® 9000-individual optimization of hearing systems taking into account the acoustic environment. Hörbericht, GEERS Hörakustik Pub. 60/96:1–6.

HAUBOLD, J., & GEERS, W. (1993). *A-life—A modern hearing aid fitting procedure based on natural acoustic patterns* (pp. 497–504). Kolding, Denmark: Fifteenth Danavox-Symposium, Scanticon.

HERMANSEN, K., RUBAK, P., HARTMANN, U., & FINK, F. (1994). *Spectral sharpening of speech signals using the PARTRAN TOOL.* Paper presented at the Nordic Signal Processing Symposium, Alesund, Norway.

HUERTA, L. (1998). *Hearing aids, current status and future needs.* Panel presentation at the meeting of the American Academy of Audiology, Los Angeles.

KAKU, M. (1997). *Visions: How science will revolutionize the 21st century.* New York: Doubleday.

KATES, J., & WEISS, M. (1996). A comparison of hearing aid array-processing techniques. *Journal of the Acoustical Society of America, 99*;3138–3148.

KOEHNKE, J., & BESING, J. (1997). Clinical application of 3-D auditory tests. *Seminars in Hearing, 18*(4);345–355.

KRUGER, B., & KRUGER, F. (1994). Future trends in hearing aid fitting strategies: With a view towards 2002. In: M. Valente (Ed.), *Strategies for selecting and verifying hearing aid fittings* (pp. 300–342). New York: Thieme Medical Publishers, Inc.

LIU, C., FENG, A., WHEELER, B., O'BRIEN, W., BILGER, R., & LANSING, C. (1997). *A binaurally-based auditory processor effectively extracts speech in the presence of multiple competing sounds.* Poster presentation at the second NIH/VA Hearing Aid Research and Development Conference, Bethesda, MD.

MARGO, V., SCHWEITZER, C., & FEINMAN, G. (1997). Comparison of Spectra 22 performance in noise with and without an additional noise reduction preprocessor. *Seminars in Hearing, 18*(4);405–415.

MOORE, B. (1996). Perceptual consequences of cochlear hearing loss and their implications for the design of hearing aids. *Ear and Hearing, 17*;133–161.

MOORE, B. (1998). *Psychoacoustics of cochlear hearing impairment and the design of hearing aids.* Invited paper at the meeting of the Acoustical Society of America, Seattle.

NIELSEN, H. (1997). Defining "open platform" DSP. *Hearing Review, 5*(1);27

NILSSON, M., VERMIGLIO, A., & SOLI, S. (1998). *A comparison of signal detection, speech understanding, and sound localization performance.* Poster presentation at the meeting of the American Academy of Audiology meeting, Los Angeles.

PELTON, J. (1998). Telecommunications for the 21st century. *Scientific American, 278*(4);80–85.

PINKER, S. (1997). *How the mind works.* New York: Norton.

POPELKA, G. (1998). *Hearing aids, current status and future needs.* Panel presentation at the American Academy of Audiology meeting, Los Angeles.

ROGERS, A., & KAPLAN, D. (1998). Get ready for nanotechnology. *Newsweek, Special Issue*, The Power of Invention, February, 52,53

SAGISAKA, Y. (1998). *Recent advances in speech recognition for spontaneous speech translation.* Invited paper at the meeting of Acoustical Society of America, Seattle.

SAKAMOTO, S., GOTO, K., TATENO, M., & KAGA, K. (1997). *Development of a digital hearing aid with frequency compression processing based on the PARCOR analysis-syntheses technique.* Poster presentation at the second NIH/VA Hearing Aid Research and Development Conference, Bethesda, MD.

SCHWEITZER, C. (1997a). Development of digital hearing aids. *Trends in Amplification, 2*(2);41–77.

SCHWEITZER, C. (1997b). Application of binaural models to evaluate beamforming in digital hearing aids. *Seminars in Hearing, 18*(4);393–404.

SCHWEITZER, C., & GERHARDT, C. (1996). *Structured clinical "fine-tuning" strategy for binaural fitting of a Full Dynamic Range Compression, 3-channel programmable hearing aid.* Poster presentation at the meeting of the American Academy of Audiology meeting, Salt Lake City.

SCHWEITZER, C., & HAUBOLD, J. (1999). *Optimizing hearing aid fittings via an interactive model.* Instructional course presented at American Academy of Audiology convention, Miami Beach.

SCHWEITZER, C., & KRISHNAN, G. (1996). Application of beamforming to digital hearing aids. *Current Opinions in Head and Neck Surgery–Otolaryngology, 4*(5);335–339.

SCHWEITZER, C., & MONROE, T. (1998). *Self-adjusted determinations of loudness targets for speech.* Poster presentation at the meeting of the American Academy of Audiology meeting, Los Angeles.

SCHWEITZER, C., MORTZ, M., & VAUGHN, N. (1999). Perhaps not by prescription, but by perception. *Hearing Review, 3* (Suppl. on High Performance Hearing Solutions);58–62.

SOLI, S., GAO, S., & NILSSON, M. (1996). *An algorithm for enhancement of binaural hearing with hearing aids.* Paper presented at the meeting of Acoustical Society of America, Honolulu.

STAAB, W., EDMONDS, J., & GARCIA, H. (1997). Remote teleprogramming (RTP): Future directions in patient management. *Hearing Review*, (High Perform Hear Solutions, Vol. 2, Suppl.); pp. 50–52.

STUTZMAN, W., & DIETRICH, C. (1998). Moving beyond wireless voice systems. *Scientific American, 278*(4);92,93.

TAKAHASHI, D. (1997). PC-on-a-chip technology almost reality. *Wall Street Journal*, Nov. 23.

VAN TASSEL, D. (1998). New DSP instrument designed to maximize binaural benefits. *Hearing Journal, 51*(4);40–49.

VERMIGLIO, A., NILSSON, M., SOLI, S., & FREED, D. (1998). *Development of a virtual test of sound localization: The Source*

Azimuth Identification in Noise Test (SAINT). Poster presentation at the meeting of the American Academy of Audiology meeting, Los Angeles.

WESTERMAN, S., & SANDLIN, R. (1997). Digital signal processing: benefits and expectations. *Hearing Review* (High Perform Hear Solutions, Vol. 2, Suppl.);pp. 56–59.

WILPON, J. (1998). *Twenty-first century user interfaces within the telecommunications industry: Speech processing is the key.* Invited paper at the meeting of the Acoustical Society of America, Seattle.

YOST, W., & DYE, R. (1997). Fundamentals of directional hearing. *Seminars in Hearing, 18*(4);321–344.

ZIMMERMAN, T. (1996). Personal area networks: Near field intra-body communications. *MIT Media Lab Reports, 35*(3,4).

Chapter 25

Future Directions in Hearing Aid Selection and Evaluation

Dennis Byrne and Harvey Dillon

Outline

Several book chapters deal with future directions in amplification or some other aspect of audiology. What purpose is served by this type of writing? Is it just an indulgent exercise in crystal ball gazing or an opportunity to enthuse about the wonders of new technology? Enjoyable though such activities may be, taking a critical look at what lies ahead may also serve a practical purpose; if current trends are not heading in the right directions, we can start doing things to change them. The future depends on what is happening now, just as the current state of the art depends on what has been done in the past. By considering where current trends are leading, we can identify potential problems and important needs that are not receiving adequate attention. In other words, the practical value of considering the future is to help mold it to be what we want. This chapter is written from the practical orientation of repeatedly asking Where do we want to go? and comparing the answers with where current developments seem to be leading. We take it to mean that new technological developments should bring enormous benefits, but for their potential to be realized these developments need to be accompanied by appropriate research and clinical practices.

Almost 20 years ago, Byrne (1979) proposed a four-stage model of the hearing aid selection and evaluation process. This general model will provide a framework for organizing this chapter. The first stage of the process is "prescription," that is, deciding what amplification characteristics are required for the client. The second stage is "matching," which is finding the combinations of hearing aids, settings, and attachments that are expected to provide the prescribed amplification. This is followed by "verification" to check that the desired amplification has been achieved in the individual ear. Finally, the "evaluation" stage determines how effectively the aids are in alleviating the patient's hearing problems. This consists of outcomes measurements that may lead to, among other things, "fine-tuning" the hearing aid fittings if the outcomes are less successful than expected. Each of these stages will be considered with regard to the development and status of ideas and practices, current trends, issues, and future needs.

PRESCRIBING AMPLIFICATION— WHERE TO?

Development of Prescriptive Ideas

The development of hearing aid fitting procedures has been discussed by Sammeth and Levitt (adults) and Lewis (children) in Chapters 5 and 4, respectively, in this volume and in other publications (e.g., Byrne, 1983; Skinner, 1988; Studebaker, 1980). Here, it is worth reviewing some major trends to indicate how certain concepts may be relevant to future procedures.

Probably, the first concept of selective fitting was audiogram mirroring, that is, providing gain to equal the hearing loss at each frequency. It was soon found that the prescribed gain was more than was generally acceptable and the procedure was modified to provide gain equal to hearing threshold level (HTL) minus a constant (Knudsen & Jones, 1935). Thus mirroring was confined to shaping the frequency response curve to be the mirror image of the HTL curve. However, extreme high-frequency emphasis, even for the steepest of audiograms, was shown to be undesirable by the "Harvard" studies (Davis et al, 1947), and this has been confirmed by later research such as Skinner (1980) and Byrne (1986b). Although mirroring as such is no longer advocated, certain

Audiology: Treatment. Edited by Valente, Hosford-Dunn, and Roeser. Thieme Medical Publishers, Inc., New York © 2000

aspects of it occur in current procedures. The POGO II procedure (Schwartz et al, 1988), when applied to HTLs exceeding 60 dB, is a form of mirroring in that the formula could be expressed as gain = HTL − a constant, which is 30 dB (1/2 × 60 dB) at 1000, 2000, and 4000 Hz, 35 dB (1/2 × 60 dB + 5 dB) at 500 Hz, and 40 dB (1/2 × 60 dB + 10 dB) at 250 Hz. Formulas for fitting nonlinear hearing aids with low compression thresholds (<50 dB) may well include mirroring because this appears to be an appropriate theoretical approach for prescribing gain for low-level inputs. This is explicit in the "FIG6" procedure of Killion (1994); the prescribed gain, at each frequency, equals HTL minus 20 dB.

Prescriptive procedures based on the "half-gain" principle or on bisecting the dynamic range of hearing are of similar age to mirroring. Lybarger (1978) cites a 1930s' bisection procedure, and he attempted to patent the "half-gain rule" (Lybarger, 1944). This was stated in several slightly different forms such as gain equals half of HTL at all frequencies or gain equals half of HTL at 1000 Hz and higher frequencies but is somewhat less at the lower frequencies. When the half-gain rule is applied at any two frequencies, the frequency response slope between those frequencies will equal half of the audiogram slope between those frequencies. Thus a half-gain rule applied to various frequencies becomes a "half-slope" rule for prescribing frequency response. The half-gain rule and the half-slope rule, or some variation of it, have been the basis of many prescriptive formulas.

Watson and Knudsen (1942) proposed a procedure in which frequency response was prescribed to mirror the most comfortable listening level (MCL) curve, rather than the threshold curve. This general idea, with various modifications, has had several successors including the procedures of Shapiro (1976), Skinner et al (1982), and Cox (1983, 1988). The theory behind MCL and half-gain procedures is the same, namely both aim to amplify speech to the preferred listening level (PLL). Watson and Knudsen criticized an older procedure as trying to fit the frequency response curve, rather than the amplified signal, into the dynamic range of hearing. To do otherwise requires consideration of the input to the hearing aid, typically the long-term average speech spectrum (LTASS). Most recent procedures, whether of MCL or HTL type, either include adjustments for the LTASS or do something similar by providing, for a given HTL or MCL, less gain at the low frequencies where speech is more intense (Byrne et al, 1994) than at the mid and high frequencies. Although MCL-based procedures do not seem to be widely used for selecting linear amplification, the concept is an integral part of the several recent procedures that use loudness scaling for prescribing compression amplification. The curve of MCL across frequency will provide the basis for prescribing frequency response for an average level input.

In the 1950s and 1960s, little further development of prescriptive procedures occurred. From a current perspective, the most interesting new procedure may be that of Lybarger (1953), which used a half-gain rule for prescribing average gain but a quarter-slope rule for prescribing frequency response. The formula is similar to the later NAL-R procedure (Byrne & Dillon, 1986) and is the only other formula to use separate gain and slope rules.

A resurgence of interest in selective fitting occurred in the 1970s (Studebaker, 1980), continuing until the present. Several new prescriptive procedures were published (Berger et

al, 1978; Byrne & Tonisson, 1976; Shapiro, 1976), alongside a number of other articles on various aspects of aid fitting (Byrne, 1978, 1979; Byrne & Fifield, 1974; Gengel et al, 1971; Pascoe, 1975). Characteristics of the new procedures were that they included adjustments for the LTASS and that amplification was prescribed in terms of real-ear performance (Berger et al, 1978; Byrne & Tonisson, 1976). Further procedures followed, notably the CID (Skinner et al, 1982), the MSU (Cox, 1983, 1988), the POGO (McCandless & Lyregaard, 1983), the desired sensation level (DSL) (Seewald et al, 1985), and the NAL-R (Byrne & Dillon, 1986) procedures. Later, the POGO and NAL prescriptions were modified for severe hearing losses (Byrne et al, 1991; Schwartz et al, 1988). The modified POGO and NAL-R procedures are designated, respectively, POGO II and NAL-RP.

It can be seen from the preceding that many of the basic ideas of current prescriptive procedures had their origins in the 1930s and 1940s. Furthermore, the half-gain rule has now been validated by many studies as have other aspects of some procedures (reviews in Byrne, 1993; and Skinner, 1988).

Current Prescriptive Rationales
Prescribing Linear Amplification

Although linear prescriptive procedures do not provide a complete prescription for nonlinear amplification, their prescriptions should be appropriate for all types of aids for an average speech input level. Therefore, the well-established linear procedures provide a basis for comparison with current and future nonlinear procedures, and it is of interest to review certain features of the most widely used linear procedures that appear to be NAL-R, POGO II, and DSL. Although the three procedures are conceptualized and described in different ways, they are all of the same general type. They aim to amplify average conversational speech to a comfortable level, and to do this they provide a formula for prescribing gain from HTL at each frequency. Despite this commonality, the procedures result in substantially different prescriptions for some types of audiograms. The reason lies in the gain and slope rules embodied in the different formulas. These rules are summarized in Table 25–1.

A "whole" gain rule means that for every 1 dB increase in HTL, gain is increased by 1 dB; a "half-gain" rule means that for every 2 dB increase in HTL, gain is increased by 1 dB; a "two-thirds" gain rule means that every 3 dB increase in HTL is accompanied by a 2 dB increase in gain. Similarly, a "two-thirds" slope rule means that if the audiogram slope between two frequencies is increased by 3 dB, the frequency response slope is increased by 2 dB. As a note, it is a simplification to describe DSL as having a two-thirds gain rule because the rule for increasing gain as a function of HTL varies from 65% to 77% at different frequencies and becomes nonlinear at low HTLs. The gain and slope rules vary for the three procedures, and for NAL-RP and POGO II the rules change for severe hearing losses. The effects of using these three different rules may be summarized as follows.

For mild, flat hearing losses, all three procedures prescribe similar gain and frequency responses. For moderate, flat losses, all procedures prescribe a similar frequency response, but DSL prescribes more overall gain equivalent to using a higher

TABLE 25–1   Gain and slope rules used in NAL-RP, POGO II, and DSL (3.0) procedures

	Gain		Slope	
Procedure	<60–65dB	>60–65dB	<60–65 dB	>60–65 dB
NAL-RP	Half	Two-thirds	One-third	One-third or less
POGO II	Half	Whole	Half	Whole
DSL (3.0)	Two-thirds	Two-thirds	Two-thirds	Two-thirds

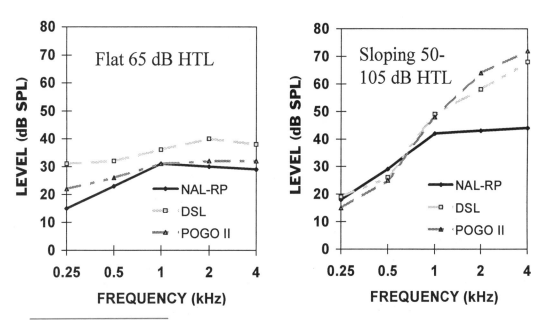

Figure 25–1   NAL-RP, DSL (3.0), and POGO II prescriptions for a flat hearing loss *(left panel)* and for a sloping high-frequency hearing loss *(right panel).*

volume control setting. For severe, flat losses, all procedures prescribe a similar frequency response, but DSL and POGO II prescribe more gain. For sloping, high-frequency audiograms, DSL and POGO II prescribe more high-frequency emphasis than does NAL-RP, especially so for severe, sloping losses. Some examples of the different prescriptions are shown in Figure 25–1.

Although NAL-RP, POGO II, and DSL are all well-established procedures, they yield very different prescriptions for some audiograms, notably for steeply sloping ones. How can such different procedures all provide acceptable hearing aid fittings? The answer is probably that, where the prescriptions differ substantially, the fittings actually differ less. For steep high-frequency losses, the gain provided at frequencies greater than 3000 Hz will be limited by what is obtainable, and this will usually be rather less than required for the NAL-RP prescription and far less than required to satisfy the DSL or POGO II prescriptions. Thus for this type of audiogram, the acceptability of POGO II and DSL prescriptions has never been tested. NAL research (Byrne, 1986a,b; Byrne & Cotton, 1988; Byrne et al, 1990a) has demonstrated that more high-frequency emphasis than that prescribed by the NAL-RP procedure is not desirable. This is consistent with other research, notably that of Skinner who concluded

that the difference in prescribed gain between 500 Hz and 2000 Hz should never exceed 35 dB (Skinner, 1980; 1988). The reason for making this point here is that future hearing aids may have less limitations than current hearing aids. It is therefore important to assess the validity of procedures even if some of the resulting prescriptions cannot be realized. Furthermore, our assessment of amplification requirements should guide the development of future hearing aids. In this context, how much high-frequency emphasis should hearing aids be designed to provide? The question, What is the best frequency response for a linear aid? is equivalent to What is the best frequency response *for an average input* for a nonlinear aid? A future need to agree on the answer to this question remains, given that current linear procedures provide varying answers.

Prescribing Nonlinear Amplification: Loudness Normalization

Over the past 10 years, various procedures have been proposed for prescribing nonlinear amplification. Several procedures have become well known and are described in Chapter 6 by Kuk. All these proposals are "armchair" procedures in that they are supported by logic rather than any significant body of research validating the procedure. The proposers of new procedures usually acknowledge the need for such validation (e.g., Cox, 1995).

Most new procedures are based on the idea of normalizing loudness, usually applied across the frequencies of speech and for overall level. One such procedure was the loudness growth in half-octave bands (LGOB) (Allen et al, 1990; Johnson et al, 1989; Pluvinage, 1989). More recent counterparts include FIG6 (Killion, 1994), IHAFF (Cox, 1995), DSL[i/o] (Cornelisse et al, 1995), RAB (Ricketts, 1996), and ScalAdapt (Kiessling et al, 1996). In introducing the IHAFF protocol, Mueller (1995) says that it is based on the "notion that when hearing aid processing is matched to the patient's loudness growth functions across frequencies, greatest user benefit will result" (p. 10). This procedure is implemented by measuring loudness growth functions at a minimum of two frequencies, whereas FIG6 and DSL[i/o] aim to normalize loudness using HTL-based prescriptive formulas.

Prescribing Nonlinear Amplification: Loudness Equalization and Other Rationales

Although DSL[i/o] has been presented as a loudness normalization procedure (Cornelisse et al, 1995), it is claimed that, by varying the formula, the procedure can also provide loudness equalization (Seewald et al, 1996). Certainly, the original DSL is based on an equalization rationale as are most of the recognized linear procedures. By this, we mean that all frequency bands of speech are amplified to be equally loud at a comfortable level or are amplified to MCL, which amounts to virtually the same thing (Byrne, 1986a).

A new NAL procedure, designated "NAL-NL1," has been designed for prescribing nonlinear amplification (Dillon et al, 1999). It is based on the concepts underpinning the three previous NAL procedures. The original (Byrne & Tonisson, 1976) and NAL-R (Byrne & Dillon, 1986) procedures aimed to equalize the loudness of all frequency bands of speech. It was reasoned that, for a comfortable listening level, equalization would maximize audibility over a wide frequency range. This, in turn, should maximize the capacity to understand speech, according to the articulation index (ANSI, 1969). However, it was found that although the NAL-R procedure (with extra gain for severe hearing losses) achieved its design of amplifying all frequency bands of speech to MCL (Byrne et al, 1990b), the prescribed frequency responses were not optimal for some severely hearing-impaired adults and children (Byrne et al, 1990a,c). When hearing loss was extreme at the high frequencies, it was preferable to make those frequencies less loud than the lower frequencies, which had better hearing. This principle was embodied in a new procedure, NAL-RP, in which the equalization rationale was modified so that relatively less audibility was provided at the high frequencies if the hearing loss was profound. The NAL-NL1 procedure is a further development of essentially the same ideas. It aims to maximize capacity to understand speech delivered at a soft, average, or loud level. The formula was derived from calculations combining a loudness model (Moore & Glasberg, 1999) with a modified form of the speech intelligibility index (SII), which is a new version of the articulation index. For

hearing losses that are not severe at any frequencies, NAL-NL1 approximates the loudness equalization rationale. When the hearing loss is severe at the high frequencies, those frequencies are amplified to be less loud than the other frequencies, which approximates the NAL-RP prescriptions for severe hearing losses. The theoretical justification for departing from loudness equalization, is increasing evidence for the need to allow for "hearing loss desensitization" (Ching et al, 1998; Hogan & Turner, 1998; Pavlovic, 1984; Pavlovic et al, 1987). Hearing loss desensitization will be discussed later in the context of audibility issues.

The fitting procedures recommended by manufacturers of advanced hearing aids exemplify a variety of concepts. Although the rationales may not always be explicit, it is clear that some imply neither normalization nor equalization. Thus a number of rationales for prescribing nonlinear amplification already exist. These need to be evaluated, as well as considering other possibilities for developing fitting rationales.

Prescribing Amplification for Multiple Memories

The rationale for using multiple memories, which exist in many programmable hearing aids, is that the optimal set of amplification characteristics may vary for different listening conditions or at different times in the same listening condition, depending on personal preferences. Research shows that a proportion of hearing aid users do have a use for multiple memories, depending partly on hearing loss characteristics and partly on the range of listening situations in which they need to use a hearing aid (Keidser, 1995; Kuk, 1992). If someone is a candidate for using multiple memories, the question arises of how to prescribe two or more sets of amplification characteristics.

To an extent, multiple memories and "adaptive" (compression) amplification are alternatives. For example, when a hearing aid wearer needs to communicate in traffic noise, it will probably be desirable to reduce the low-frequency amplification relative to that used in most other situations. This need could be met by providing a low-cut frequency response as an alternative memory or by using a bass increases at low levels (BILL)-type of compression system (i.e., one that provides more low-cut frequency response as input level increases). In theory, whenever the need for an amplification variation is related to a change in acoustic input (variations in overall level or spectra), it may be possible to meet that need by adaptive amplification. However, sometimes the need to vary amplification is related to changes in personal preferences rather than in acoustic input. For example, many situations exist where the predominant input would be speech. In some situations, such as talking with friends or at a meeting, the aid wearer may want to maximize speech intelligibility, whereas in other situations, such as in a public place surrounded by the conversation of strangers, intelligibility may be less important and a different type of amplification may be needed to provide the preferred sound quality. This is the type of need for which multiple memories are unique because only the person can decide what he or she wants to hear and what the importance of different sound qualities is at any particular time.

Considering the preceding points, it appears that multiple memories will continue to be useful for a proportion of hearing aid wearers. Therefore future needs in hearing aid prescription and evaluation include improving procedures for optimizing the use of multiple memories. It is possible to give some guidelines (Keidser et al, 1996), but our knowledge is far from complete with regard to who will benefit from having two or more memories and of how to decide what variations to provide. We need further research to more completely define the relationships between variations in acoustic conditions and the need to vary amplification. This will be relevant to the use of both multiple memories and adaptive hearing aids. We need further research to ascertain how people rate the various attributes of sound experience (e.g., speech intelligibility, tonal quality, listening comfort) and to determine how the relative importance of different attributes may vary among people and in different situations for the same person. Such research, of which there is very little, is relevant to a range of hearing aid evaluation issues, including the use of multiple memories.

Prescribing Maximum Output

Nearly all research on prescriptive fitting has focused on gain and frequency response, although some procedures include "armchair" formulas for prescribing maximum power output (MPO). Recent NAL publications describe a theoretically derived and experimentally validated procedure for prescribing MPO (Dillon & Storey, 1999; Storey et al, 1999). The procedure prescribes MPO from HTL measurements only.

CONTROVERSIAL POINT

Contrary to expectation, the NAL research indicated that the addition of loudness discomfort level (LDL) measurements did not significantly improve the prescription of MPO. In line with theoretical expectations, but contrary to a commonly expressed view, accuracy in MPO prescription is not very critical for mild hearing losses, but it becomes extremely important for severe losses.

So far, new developments in hearing aids have had only modest implications for MPO prescription. The use of low distortion-limiting systems may mean that MPO can be set slightly lower for some hearing aid wearers. However, for the more severe losses there remains the tricky problem of keeping MPO high enough to provide an adequate signal level but without permitting sounds to become uncomfortable. The use of low-level or medium-level input compression (discussed later) may reduce the importance of limiting. Indeed, it may prove most useful to treat the concept of MPO as part of a more general concept of maintaining listening comfort over a wide range of input levels. The future need may be to evaluate the effects of different combinations of compression types and to develop effective prescription methods.

Prescription and Validation Issues: Present and Future

Which Processing Strategies Work?

The first prescription issue that needs to be addressed is whether a particular type of amplification should *ever* be recommended. That is, does this type of amplification have advantages for *anybody*. Despite much research, our knowledge is still limited and the question has to be addressed again for each new type of processing that appears. Two problems lead to difficulties in obtaining conclusive answers to this question. The first is the choice of a suitable reference condition to compare the new processing with. It may be easy to demonstrate that the new processing is better than *something* else, but is that something the best alternative? For example, a well-fitted compression system may show a considerable advantage over a linear system with a flat frequency response, but the advantage may be less, or none at all, over a linear system with optimum frequency shaping. It needs to be shown that a new, usually more complex, processing system has advantages over the *best* alternative and that such advantages occur under realistic conditions of use. The second problem is the choice of adequate evaluation measures. The traditional speech recognition tests are rather insensitive for hearing aid evaluation purposes and may be incapable of demonstrating some of the advantages to be derived from new types of hearing aids. Evaluation measures will be discussed later. Here it may be noted that future progress will require improved evaluation measures even to answer the basic question of whether some particular types of processing have any advantages.

Who Can Benefit from a Particular Type, or Combination of Types, of Processing?

It may be that some types of processing can be beneficial for everybody. It is more likely, however, that any type of processing will have disadvantages, as well as possible advantages, even if the disadvantage is simply an extra cost for no benefit. Therefore, a prescription issue is how to choose the best type, or types, or processing for each individual. If multiple memories are used, the choice may be complicated because it may be desirable to use very different types of processing, rather than just variations of frequency response, in two or more memories. A future need is for more research comparing different types of processing with a view to determining how to choose the best type for particular hearing losses and needs.

What Should Be the Prescriptive Objectives?

A very basic question is What is the aim of providing one type of amplification rather than another? In what sense is a particular prescription "best"? In the past the usual answer has been to maximize speech intelligibility when the hearing aids are set for comfortable listening. That answer is a good start, but it is not adequate to cover all the desirable objectives of hearing aid prescription. If it were, the prescriptive problem would be simply to determine the optimum level and frequency response for speech intelligibility and use a high degree of slow-acting compression to keep all speech close to the optimum level. Although such a prescription has not been thoroughly tested, it is generally believed that an extremely narrow range of loudness variations would be unacceptable. The current loudness normalization procedures assume that a person with impaired hearing should experience the same range of loudness variations that a normally hearing person would in the same situation. Although we question that assumption, it does seem likely that a range of loudness variation is necessary for a natural auditory experience.

Speech intelligibility and loudness variations are not the only relevant prescriptive objectives. Other factors that are probably important include a natural experience of environmental sounds and music, the ability to detect and locate sounds, and natural feeling of spatial auditory perception. People with hearing loss experience difficulties localizing sounds (Noble et al, 1995), and the ways in which hearing aids are fitted can substantially affect sound localization (Byrne & Noble, 1998). The amplification required to optimize some objectives may differ from that required to optimize other objectives. For example, optimal speech intelligibility, especially under difficult conditions, will usually require more high-frequency emphasis than would be optimal for detecting and localizing sound. It is likely that the "best" amplification will be a compromise among optimizing various objectives that will assume varying degrees of importance for different people and at different times, depending on listening requirements and personal preferences. Killion (1982) argued that more consideration should be given to sound quality because hearing aids were providing most hearing aid users with good audibility and speech intelligibility. This is even more true today; the advantages of advanced hearing aids mostly relate to factors other than improved speech intelligibility. A major area of research need is to determine what prescriptive objectives are important and what compromises are likely to be preferred by individuals under particular circumstances.

Audibility and Speech Intelligibility

Although audibility has always been a central concept in prescribing amplification, its significance is still not properly appreciated. Audibility relates to all possible fitting objectives in that sounds that are inaudible cannot contribute to any aspect of auditory experience. The relationship of audibility to speech intelligibility is exemplified in the Articulation Index (AI), which is a method for estimating speech intelligibility from audibility (ANSI, 1969). The total audibility of speech is calculated by summing the audibility in each frequency band over the range from about 200 Hz to 6000 Hz. Audibility is maximal when the peak levels of the long-term average speech spectrum are 30 dB above HTL in each frequency band or are 30 dB above the level of any noise that exceeds HTL.

Over almost 50 years, attempts have been made to use the AI in either the development or evaluation of prescriptive procedures (e.g., Dugal et al, 1980; Fletcher, 1952; Humes, 1986; Rancovic, 1991). Some investigators have combined the AI with a loudness model to assess the effects on the AI of varying frequency response while loudness is held to a constant level (Leijon, 1989; Studebaker, 1992). The reason for

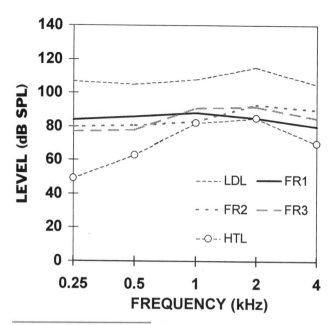

Figure 25–2   Example of peak levels of speech amplified by three frequency responses, with each adjusted to the preferred listening level.

maintaining a constant loudness is that a hearing aid wearer can be expected to adjust the hearing aid volume controls to provide the preferred loudness level, irrespective of what gain or frequency response has been prescribed. The general effect of varying frequency response is illustrated in Figure 25–2. The data are the peak levels of speech amplified with three frequency responses and with the overall gain adjusted to the preferred listening level for each frequency response.

Response 1 (FR1) provides more signal at the low frequencies at the expense of less signal at the high frequencies. Response 2 (FR2) provides the most high-frequency signal, but the least mid-frequency signal. Response 3 (FR3) provides the most mid-frequency signal but less low frequencies than response 1 and less high frequencies than response 2. The general point is that, for any given loudness level, increased audibility at some frequencies comes at the expense of less audibility at other frequencies. On the basis of the speech peak sensation levels (SLs) at each frequency, the AIs provided by each frequency response for speech at the preferred level could be calculated and would appear to provide a means of evaluating the relative effectiveness of different frequency responses. Unfortunately, such a simple method like a number of others (e.g., Mueller & Killion, 1990; Pavlovic, 1989) is not adequate. For sloping high-frequency hearing losses, the frequency response that gives the highest AI will have more high-frequency emphasis than the frequency response that provides the best speech intelligibility (Byrne, 1992). It is also necessary to account for "hearing loss desensitization" (HLD), which may be explained as follows. For severe hearing losses, the AI predicts better speech intelligibility than is achieved (Pavlovic et al, 1987). Furthermore, if the hearing loss is greatest at the high frequencies, a given SL at those frequencies will contribute less to intelligibility than the same amount of audibility at the lower frequencies (Pavlovic, 1984). An HLD adjustment has been used by Studebaker and Sherbecoe (1992). The importance for HLD, especially for determining the best amount of high-frequency emphasis, has been confirmed by Ching et al (1998) and Hogan and Turner (1998). These studies show that, when hearing loss is severe at the high frequencies, a given amount of audibility may contribute substantially less to speech intelligibility than might be supposed. The optimum amount of audibility may be considerably less than 30 dB SL and, in some instances, *any* audibility at the higher frequencies may be detrimental (Ching et al, 1998). The Ching et al data indicate that the HLD adjustment should be frequency-dependent and nonlinear. The latest AI procedure, now designated the SII (ANSI, Draft Standard, 1993), includes a speech level correction whereby the value of a particular amount of audibility is reduced for any frequency band where the level in that band is greater than the band level for speech with an overall level of 73 dB SPL. For speech that has been amplified to suit moderate and severe hearing losses, the speech level correction will have the same type of effect as an HLD adjustment. However, the standard speech level correction appears to be inadequate to account for HLD (Ching et al, 1998).

The general implications of HLD are that severe hearing losses and sloping high-frequency hearing losses require considerably less high-frequency emphasis than might seem logical or, indeed, is prescribed by some procedures, and that maximizing audibility, over a wide frequency range, is not always desirable. However, questions remain about the precise nature and size of HLD. For example, does the value of a given amount of audibility at one frequency depend only on the hearing level at that frequency or is it also influenced by the hearing at other frequencies, and to what extent does speech intelligibility depend on factors other than audibility? The significance of audibility for prescribing amplification is much less understood than is generally believed and is thus an important subject for future research.

Loudness Issues

No doubt exists that *some* aspects of loudness are vitally important for hearing aid prescription. Significant sounds need to be made audible but not uncomfortable. Loudness will be a major determinant of preferred gain levels. The relative loudness of different bands of speech will influence the total audibility of speech at the preferred overall loudness level. Loudness issues have assumed particular relevance because of the central role of loudness normalization in several recent prescriptive procedures. In procedures such as the Independent Hearing Aid Fitting Forum (IHAFF), normalization is advocated with respect to the overall loudness of sounds and the relative loudness of the various frequency bands of speech. Reasons exist why both these aspects of normalization are open to question (Byrne, 1996). Normalizing the relative loudness of speech bands is contrary to the rationale of most established linear procedures that are based on loudness equalization or something similar (e.g., NAL-R, DSL, CID). The evidence supporting those procedures argues against anything different, at least for an average input level. Indeed, normalizing loudness is not strictly

optimal for normally hearing people because in these listeners a degree of high-frequency emphasis improves the intelligibility of soft speech or speech in noise (Walker, 1996).

The logic of normalizing overall loudness is also debatable. Why should all people, including hearing aid wearers, experience sounds with precisely the same loudness? People normally experience a great range of sound levels and spectra, depending on voice levels, distance, and acoustic conditions. Provided that sounds are neither too soft to hear nor too loud to be comfortable, a wide range of loudness levels is acceptable. A good argument can be made for the desirability of experiencing a range of loudness levels (Killion, 1997), but there seems no reason why people in the same situation should experience exactly the same loudness sensations. Few audiologists would doubt the desirability of preventing sounds from becoming uncomfortable even though normally hearing people are sometimes subjected to uncomfortable levels. At the other end of the scale, why would a hearing aid wearer object if soft speech were a little louder? Furthermore, many people live and work in noisier environments than would have been common when our auditory systems were evolving. Hence no evolutionary argument exists that normal must be best.

Future research should focus on establishing what range of loudness levels hearing aid wearers prefer rather than assuming that the normal range is best. The preferred range may or may not turn out to be predictable from psychoacoustic measurements or other information such as the types of acoustic environments that the individual commonly encounters.

CONTROVERSIAL POINT

Despite the current popularity of normalizing loudness, it could prove that this concept has little or no relevance to prescribing amplification. This is an issue that only future research can resolve.

Are Laboratory Tests a Sufficient Basis for Prescription?

With current hearing aids, especially multiple memory types, it has become increasingly feasible to conduct field studies. That is, the patient can compare two or more amplification options over the range of situations normally experienced. This is fortunate because field trials may prove to be the only practical way of determining the optimal value for some parameters. Compression threshold (CT) seems to be in that category in that people do prefer different settings, and no obvious way of predicting needs from laboratory measurements exists (Dillon et al, 1998). It may be that some new parameters will need to be selected initially on a field trial basis but that, as knowledge accumulates, we shall eventually be able to develop prescriptive methods based on laboratory measures or other data available at the time of fitting. We predict that systematic field trials will play an increasing role in the fitting and "fine-tuning" of hearing aids.

Do People Need to Acclimatize to Hearing Aids?

Is a person's performance with a particular type of amplification likely to change after experience in using it? If so, how long does it take before performance and preferences stabilize? These questions are especially relevant to evaluation (discussed later), but they also have implications for prescription if the prescriptive method uses performance or preference data either in its derivation or clinical application. The issue has received considerable attention (Arlinger et al, 1996), but it is not possible to give a general answer about the importance of acclimatization. Undoubtedly, acclimatization can occur (Gatehouse, 1993), but the degree will depend on what type of amplification the person is getting used to. Experience with cochlear implants illustrates that it may take many months before it becomes clear how the implanted person can perform with the device (Tyler & Summerfield, 1996). Apparently, acclimatization may occur over several weeks even for a moderate change in frequency response (Gatehouse, 1993), although the bulk of research suggests that acclimatization effects are generally small (Turner et al, 1996). Some new types of processing (e.g., frequency transposition) will present a highly novel pattern of sound stimulation and consequently may, like cochlear implants, require a substantial period of acclimatization. For both research and clinical practice, any significant degree of acclimatization will incur problems that will need to be addressed and, with new developments in amplification, acclimatization may become an increasingly important issue.

With regard to prescription, one important question for future research is whether acclimatization has affected our assessment of amplification requirements. In particular, would people with severe hearing losses make more use of high-frequency information if they had been accustomed to hearing it better? Although it seems unlikely that acclimatization is a major factor, it is certainly possible that the optimal amount of high-frequency emphasis, as indicated by research, may be less than would have been found if the subjects had long-term experience with more high-frequency emphasis. This consideration may be especially applicable to children with severe hearing losses. At present, it seems safest to assume that the real-ear prescriptive requirements of children and adults do not differ. However, the issue remains to be resolved. Of course, the matching, verification, and evaluation processes are different for children because of their smaller ears and, sometimes, differences in the types of testing that can be managed (see Chapter 4 in this volume).

What Measurements Will Be Used in Future Prescriptions?

The measurements that will be needed for future prescriptions will depend on which fitting rationales prove to be valid and which measurements are effective for implementing those rationales.

Traditionally, the prescription of gain, frequency response, and MPO has been based on one or a combination of the measures, HTL, MCL, and LDL. The more popular gain and frequency response prescription procedures are based on HTL, although several MCL-based procedures have also been suggested. LDL has often been advocated as the main basis for

> **CONTROVERSIAL POINT**
>
> It seems unfortunate that the amplification requirements of children and adults are often considered completely separately. Some audiologists seem to forget that children are small adults. Research into amplification requirements, whether conducted with adults or children, should be considered to apply to both unless some good reason exists to suppose otherwise. Similarly, prescriptive procedures should apply to both groups unless future research demonstrates that they have different requirements.

prescribing MPO. The ULCL procedure of Cox (1983, 1988) may be considered a variation of an LDL or MCL procedure. MCL procedures do not seem to have ever become widely used, probably partly because HTL is an easier measurement and partly because MCL has never been shown to provide superior prescriptions. Indeed, it appears that inherently HTL and MCL are about equally predictive of amplification requirements (Byrne & Murray, 1985). More surprisingly, it has been shown recently (Storey et al, 1998) that HTL alone is virtually as good a predictor of MPO requirements as is the combination of HTL and LDL. This leads to the general point that although new, more difficult or more time-consuming measures may have good face validity, their use can only be justified if they can be shown to provide more effective prescriptions. We predict that HTL will continue to have a major role in new prescriptive procedures partly because audibility will always be a basic issue and partly because many other auditory abilities are at least somewhat predictable from HTL.

At present, it is common to advocate loudness scaling as the basis for prescribing compression amplification. This is exemplified in procedures such as LGOB (Allen et al, 1990), RELM (Humes et al, 1996), IHAFF (Cox, 1995), RAB (Ricketts, 1996), and ScalAdapt (Kiessling et al, 1996). The essence of such procedures is to construct a loudness growth curve at two or more frequencies by requiring the subject to indicate the sound levels that correspond to a series of loudness labels (typically five or more) ranging from "very soft" to" very loud" or "too loud." Despite the high level of interest in loudness scaling, there are three reasons to question whether it is likely to be widely adopted for clinical hearing aid fitting.

First, the use of loudness scaling would certainly complicate and extend the fitting process even though much effort has gone into devising relatively simple procedures (e.g., Cox et al, 1997). We wonder whether many audiologists will be willing to take the extra trouble considering the apparent reluctance to even do MCL measurements.

Second, loudness scaling results can be highly variable, depending on details of the measurement procedure, such as the range of presentation levels and labels used, whether the presentations are in an ascending or random order, or whether the testing is conducted through earphones or in the sound field. At best, a particular procedure may be reliable (Cox et al, 1997), but it cannot be assumed to give the same results as other, apparently equivalent, procedures. Thus any specific scaling procedure, rather than loudness scaling in general, would need to be demonstrated to be a valid predictor of amplification requirements.

Third, the most fundamental question is whether amplification requirements are closely related to loudness growth functions. The advocacy of loudness scaling is associated with promoting loudness normalization as the desirable prescriptive aim. If this aim is not accepted, no compelling argument exists for detailed measurements of loudness growth functions. There may be no point in using any loudness measurements or it may be sufficient to supplement HTL with just one or two loudness measurements such as ULCL. For the preceding reasons, it is doubtful whether the use of loudness scaling, for hearing aid prescription, will prove to be justified.

Future prescriptive procedures may make use of auditory tests other than those in current use. Speech recognition by listeners with impaired hearing cannot be fully explained by audibility, suggesting that other auditory abilities have a role (Ching et al, 1998). It is often suggested that frequency resolution should be related to speech recognition, but so far no strong correlation has been demonstrated after HTL is controlled for. Several studies (e.g., Byrne & Murray, 1985; Tyler et al, 1982) have shown high correlations between frequency resolution and HTL. Logically, frequency resolution may be a consideration for deciding how many bands should be used in a multiband hearing aid and in deciding what range each band should cover. Similarly, temporal resolution could be a consideration for choosing time constants and possibly compression ratios for compression systems. Although logical possibilities exist, no definite evidence is present that frequency or temporal resolution measures will prove useful for hearing aid prescription, much less any indication of precisely how they might be used.

It is also possible that more analytical types of speech recognition tests could find a role in future prescriptive procedures. Such tests could show how the perception of specific phonemes is influenced by variations in audibility in different frequency bands. Substantial research would be required to show whether this approach could lead to a practical prescriptive procedure and, if so, to develop such a procedure. Tests of sound localization can be useful in hearing aid prescription, especially in the choice of type of fitting (unilateral versus bilateral) and choice of earmold type (Byrne & Noble, 1998). Such measures could become a regular part of the prescription process.

So far, hearing aid prescription has made little use of any formal measures of listening environments, social needs, or personal preferences. We predict that some such measures may find increasing use in the future. To a degree, compression compensates for changes in listening environments in so far as these involve changing input levels to hearing aids. However, the desirable degree of compression could be influenced by how often very high or very low inputs are encountered. Communication needs could also be influential. For example, to what extent does the hearing aid wearer need to communicate when he or she is in a noisy environment? Furthermore, one person may give a high priority to maximizing understanding of speech relative to maximizing listening comfort; another person, or the same person at a different time, may give more priority to comfort. The "best" amplification for an individual, at any given time, may be a compromise in optimizing different auditory abilities, with priorities depending on individual needs and preferences.

The advent of multiple-memory hearing aids has drawn attention to the need to consider environments, needs, and preferences (Keidser et al, 1996). This experience may stimulate thinking about how such factors could be considered in other aspects of hearing aid prescription. Methods need to be developed for assessing these factors and for research into how they are related to amplification requirements. Some of the methods currently used for evaluation, such as the Abbreviated Profile of Hearing Aid Benefit (APHAB) (Cox & Alexander, 1995) and Client Oriented Scale of Improvement (COSI) (Dillon et al, 1997), may find application in the prescription process.

Prescription Requirements: Present and Future
Prescription Philosophy

Ideally, the first two stages of the hearing aid fitting process, prescription and matching, should be completely independent. That is, the amplification requirements of an individual should be determined without being constrained by what the currently available aids can do. The advantage of keeping the two processes distinct is that it is clear what compromises have had to be made. Such compromises may become unnecessary with further developments in hearing aids that may move closer to meeting requirements in an ideal way. Such developments will be discouraged if our knowledge of what is possible distorts our views of what is required. Sometimes prescriptive procedures are made more "practical" by adjusting them to match what is achievable, and sometimes such adjustments are erroneously assumed. For example, we note recent statements that, in modifying the NAL procedure to suit severe and profound losses, the high-frequency gain was *reduced to avoid acoustic feedback.* That would be totally opposed to our fitting philosophy; the NAL prescription is what it is because that is the requirement indicated by the research. If providing the appropriate amount of gain results in feedback, we must try to eliminate the feedback, not pretend that less gain is needed.

Any amplification characteristic that can be varied is potentially a prescription parameter. However, some parameter values (e.g., compression ratio [CR] of a compression limiting system) do not need to be varied for individuals because a parameter setting can be found that is suitable for everyone. Some other parameters may require only a limited degree of selection, perhaps switching a feature "on" for some people and "off" for the remainder. Only some parameters are individually prescribed in the sense that every significant variation among individuals requires a change in the prescription. Initial selection issues are to decide which parameters need to be prescribed and what is a suitable basis for prescribing each parameter.

Characteristics of Nonlinear Amplification

Virtually all modern hearing aids include some type or types of compression. These systems take many forms that may be classified according to whether the compression mostly affects low-level or high-level inputs, low-frequency or high-frequency sounds, and whether it is fast-acting or slow-acting

(Dillon, 1996). The simplest type of nonlinear amplification is compression limiting, which serves only to limit output but with much less distortion than does peak clipping. For some profound hearing losses, it may be desirable to avoid compression limiting to obtain the slightly higher output that is possible with peak clipping (Dawson et al, 1991). The prescription of limiting level (CT of a compression limiting system) is the same as prescribing MPO for a peak clipping aid. To provide effective limiting, CR must be high (>10:1) and attack time (Ta) must be fast (<5 ms); there is no reason why these parameters should be varied for individuals. Similarly, no apparent reason exists why release time (Tr) should be individually prescribed, although a good argument can be made for using a circuit that varies Tr according to the durational characteristics of the input (Killion, 1993).

For compression systems other than just limiting, CT and CR may become prescriptive parameters. Indeed, most of the rationales for using such systems require that one or both of those parameters be prescribed. Figures 25–3 and 25–4 show input/output (i/o) graphs for four compression systems designed on different rationales. However, an adequate picture of a compression system will require i/o graphs for several frequencies.

The left panel of Figure 25–3 shows *compression limiting (CL)*. As indicated earlier, the amplification is linear up to the limiting output level (~110 dB SPL), at which a very high degree of compression occurs. The right panel shows *wide dynamic range compression (WDRC)*. The rationale for this type of compression is to amplify a wide range of input sound levels to fall within the more limited dynamic range of a listener with a sensorineural hearing loss without requiring a range of input levels to map onto the same output level. CT corresponds to a low-input level (~40 dB SPL) and a moderate degree of compression (~2:1) is applied over the whole input range up to the limiting level (~110 dB SPL). The left panel of Figure 25–4 shows *low level compression (LLC)*. The CT, the first "kneepoint" of the function, also occurs at a low level (~40 dB SPL). Low and moderate inputs receive a moderate-to-high degree of compression (~3:1), but high input levels (i.e., those above the second kneepoint, ~80 dB SPL) are amplified linearly with relatively little, or even no, gain. This type of amplification is designed to normalize loudness. The right panel of Figure 25–4 shows what could be called *medium level compression (MLC)*, which differs from WDRC in that the CT is set at a higher level (>50 dB SPL). MLC may be considered appropriate if compression is viewed primarily for maximizing

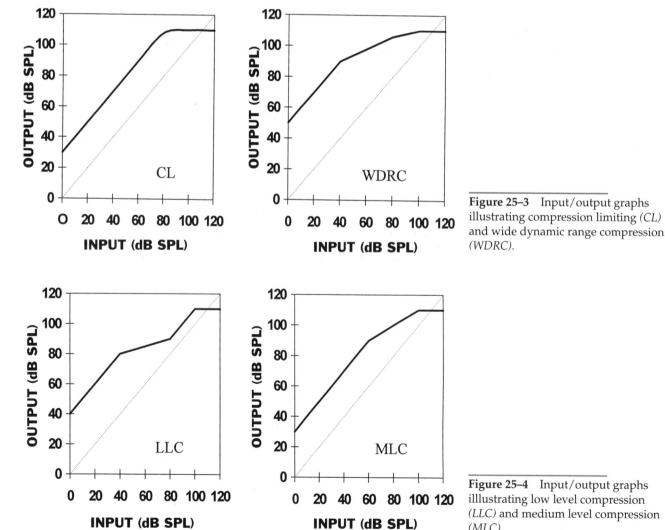

Figure 25–3 Input/output graphs illustrating compression limiting *(CL)* and wide dynamic range compression *(WDRC)*.

Figure 25–4 Input/output graphs illlustrating low level compression *(LLC)* and medium level compression *(MLC)*.

listening comfort rather than for normalizing loudness or making low-level sounds audible. (Restoring audibility for soft sounds is often a major part of the rationale of LLC or WDRC systems.) MLC is something between WDRC and CL. Although CL alone should prevent any sounds from exceeding LDL, most people have a range of somewhat lower levels that are higher than preferred. MLC can provide additional comfort by ensuring that nearly all sounds will remain close to, or less than, the preferred listening level rather than allowing a significant number of sounds to reach levels just below limiting. Although MLC has received little discussion, NAL research suggests that it may be preferred to WDRC by most hearing aid users, at least for single-channel hearing aids (Dillon et al, 1998).

Which Compression Characteristics Need to Be Prescribed?

The answer to which compression characteristics need to be prescribed depends on which type of compression system is favored, and therefore the long-term answer will depend on which types of compression are shown to be most effective. NAL research indicates that considerable variation exists in preferred CTs. Therefore, CT is a prescription parameter. Furthermore, the preferred CT is not predictable from HTL (Dillon et al, 1998). This is contrary to the loudness normalization rationale, which requires compression of all input levels that would result in audible sounds. Indeed, hearing aids designed to implement this rationale often have CT fixed at a low level. If a prescription is expressed in terms of the required gain for two or three input levels, the prescription can be met by various combinations of CT and CR. However, the amplification provided will vary in some respects for the different combinations that may, therefore, not be equally suitable. Thus CR as well as CT must be regarded as a prescription parameter.

The required compression characteristics and gain (for an average input level) may be frequency dependent. For example, a two-band system may require different CTs or CRs in each band. Indeed, some fitting rationales require different types of compression (e.g., WDRC in the low-frequency band combined with CL in the high-frequency band) in each band. Multiband systems often have adjustable crossover frequencies that then become another prescription parameter. Crossover frequencies are usually chosen according to the points of greatest change in the audiogram. For example, if the audiogram shows relatively good hearing up to 1000 Hz and significantly poorer hearing at 1500 Hz and higher frequencies, the crossover frequency for a two-band system would be placed around 1250 Hz.

Although comments have so far referred to fast-acting (syllabic) compression systems (Tr <100 ms), they are equally applicable to slow-acting compression systems (Tr >200 ms), either single or multiband. When applied to each channel of a multiband hearing aid, slow-acting compression reduces the range of long-term spectral shapes presented to the aid wearer, and reduces the range of overall levels. Automatic volume control (AVC) reduces the level differences between different talkers or the same talker speaking at one time in a loud voice and at another time in a soft voice. The use of AVC will reduce and possibly eliminate the need for syllabic compression (Stone et al, 1997). If syllabic compression is used

after AVC, the required amount of syllabic compression will be less because the long-term variations in input levels have already been reduced. The prescription of syllabic compression characteristics will, therefore, vary depending on whether it is used alone or after AVC.

Considering the preceding information, *how can we sum up the prescription needs for nonlinear amplification?* A comprehensive procedure, or set of procedures, for fitting nonlinear aids would include prescriptions for limiting level (MPO), gain, CT (and any higher kneepoint), and CR, and all are frequency dependent. It would also include a method for choosing the crossover frequencies for multiband systems. Rationales may be developed for prescribing some other parameters, such as attack or release times, but any comment on such possibilities would be highly speculative.

The required prescriptive parameters are illustrated in Figure 25–5, which is an example of a two-channel compression aid. The familiar parameter of MPO is represented by the limiting levels that could be different for each band. Multiband aids permit MPO to be prescribed on a frequency-by-frequency basis, which has been possible, but seldom implemented, with single-band circuits. The gain required for a typical input level is the same for a compression aid as for a linear aid because the compression is intended only as a means of dealing with higher than average or lower than average input levels. The difference between the gain for the two bands defines the frequency response for an average input.

The preceding example shows that a large part of the required prescription could be derived from an established linear procedure or by some equivalent method. However, it is still necessary to determine appropriate values for CT and CR, and it is not clear what the best bases for doing this are. Do these parameters need to be varied in numerous steps, or is it sufficient just to choose between two or three parameter settings? As suggested earlier, the basis for choosing CT could be the relative importance the aid wearer places on maximizing the audibility of soft sounds versus minimizing noise and minimizing the risk of acoustic feedback.

Loudness normalization procedures may provide a prescription for CR. However, the adequacy of such a prescription method depends on the validity of loudness normalization, which has been questioned (Byrne, 1996; Lunner et al, 1997). Therefore, a need exists for other methods for prescribing CR. One possibility could be based on determining the relative importance, for an individual, of maximizing listening comfort versus achieving the most natural sound quality. Consider the choice of CR for inputs that will be amplified to levels between the MCL level and the limiting level. A relatively high CR will maximize comfort by keeping more sounds close to the most comfortable level than would a lower CR. However, the dynamic range of sounds will be more restricted with the higher CR and that could result in a less natural sound quality. It seems likely that individuals will vary in the extent to which they value comfort versus quality, and if this can be assessed, it could provide a basis for prescribing CR.

In presenting this example, we are not advocating a new prescription procedure; rather, we are illustrating how one could be developed on principles that differ from those currently being propounded. The CT could be selected to be the best compromise between maximizing audibility and minimizing noise, whereas the CR could be the best compromise

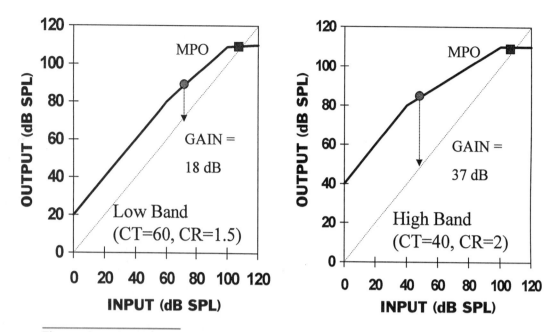

Figure 25–5 Prescription parameters for a two-band compression hearing aid. Frequency response is the difference between gain in the two bands for a given input leel. The crossover frequency could be, for example, 1250 Hz. The dotted line indicates "0" dB gain, and lines parallel to the dotted line indicate linear amplification.

for maximizing comfort while experiencing a good range of loudness variations.

The most obvious research need in hearing aid prescription is to develop and validate methods for prescribing CT and CR. It would also be desirable to examine the selection of crossover frequencies for multiband aids, although no obvious reason exists for questioning the current practice of choosing these to correspond to the points of greatest change in the audiogram. The prescription parameters discussed here may not be the ones that are familiar to audiologists who fit particular types of compression hearing aids. For some hearing aids and for some prescriptive formulas, the prescription takes the form of specifying gain and frequency response for two or more input levels. This is broadly equivalent to prescribing CT and CR together with gain for one input level. However, a prescription in the form of gain at two or three levels could be met with different combinations of CT and CR and these may not be equally suitable.

Signal Processing Aids

Some future aids, and to a limited extent some current aids, include types of signal processing other than compression. The most obvious examples are noise reduction, frequency transposition, and feedback cancellation. As a minimum, audiologists will need to decide whether to use a certain type of processing with a particular patient. For some types of processing this may be sufficient. For example, the operation of a particular noise-reduction scheme could depend entirely on physical characteristics of the environment (i.e., on the acoustic input). Other types of processing, such as frequency transposition, may require individual fitting in that the optimum processing parameter values may depend on the hearing loss. Thus the development of new types of processing will raise a series of fitting issues, the nature of which will

depend on how the processing works and on what advantages and disadvantages may occur.

Assistive Listening Devices

Many people use some form of assistive listening device, such as a TV aid or an FM aid (mainly in classrooms). Probably there are other people for whom assistive devices should be, but are not, considered. Research is needed on how to decide when an assistive device should be recommended and on how to choose an appropriate device or devices.

Prescription issues usually receive little consideration in relation to assistive devices. Stand-alone devices typically have few adjustment possibilities and no prescriptive fitting procedure. The fitting issue is partly avoided if the final stage of the amplification system is a personal hearing aid that has been individually fitted. Nonetheless, it is still necessary to check that the output of the aid is essentially the same (except with less noise) when operated with an assistive device as when on its own. For example, the frequency response of hearing aids in the telecoil mode is usually not the same as in the microphone mode (Upfold & Goodair, 1997). Such differences need to be recognized and, preferably, compensated for by adjustments to the assistive device.

Current Trends and Future Needs in Prescription
Development of Prescriptive Approaches and Fitting Confidence

As indicated earlier, several new prescriptive procedures are being suggested for fitting the new types of amplification that have recently become available. This section will examine these trends and address the questions of where hearing aid prescription seems to be going and where it should be going. However, before doing this, we offer a general reflection on how the state of the art develops with regard to hearing aid prescription. At certain times, audiologists fitting hearing aids have been confident about what they were doing, but at other times less so. The degree of confidence, at any given time, depends on two things. One is how many amplification options exist and hence the choices that need to be made; more choices leads to less confidence. The other factor is knowledge about how to use each fitting option; more knowledge means greater confidence. Over time, confidence tends to fluctuate because of a "seesawing" of the balance between the number of fitting options and knowledge of how to use them. In periods of rapid technological changes in hearing aids, the fitting options get ahead of the knowledge of how to use them. Any new hearing aid development tends to create uncertainty because it is seldom possible to be confident of how to use a new option until it has been available for clinical use and research. The danger is that in the rush to keep up with new technology, clinical fitting practices may become based simply on face validity or marketing hype, instead of having any solid scientific support.

The following sections examine three possible approaches for developing new fitting procedures for new types of hearing aids. One approach is to *develop a procedure around the capabilities of a particular device;* another is to *develop a procedure on the basis of a new rationale;* the third approach is to *extend or supplement an established rationale* to provide the basis for a new procedure. To varying extents, all three approaches are exemplified in current trends.

Device (Manufacturer)-specific Prescription Procedures

Most programmable and digital hearing aids are fitted with device-specific software. The software is used to calculate the required amplification and to program the aid to match the prescription. Inevitably, the particular way of programming the aid will be device-specific; that is, it will depend on the capabilities of the aid and how it can be achieved. However, two options for calculating the required amplification exist. Some fitting software includes one or more of the recognized generic prescription procedures, whereas other software provides a method devised by the manufacturer.

No intrinsic objection exists to the use of procedures developed by manufacturers. Such procedures could be based on research conducted by or for the manufacturer, possibly in collaboration with independent researchers. The procedures could be subjected to expert scrutiny through the normal publication and review processes, and they could be validated by independent research. Furthermore, procedures developed for particular devices could be used more generally.

However, both philosophical and scientific concerns are present, when procedures, whether developed by a manufacturer or anyone else, are not explicit and are not open to independent validation. The philosophical issue is that the audiologist who is responsible for fitting the patient is no longer deciding what amplification is best for that patient. Indeed, the audiologist may not know what amplification is being provided. It is therefore difficult to know whether the fitting formula is generally acceptable or whether it should be

varied for a particular individual. This type of concern has been expressed before in relation to the practice of selecting custom ITE aids by simply sending an audiogram to the manufacturer (Bratt & Sammeth, 1991). The scientific concern is that some manufacturers' fitting methods may not be very defensible or, at best, may be of unknown validity. Even when prescriptive methods are published, differences may exist between the method described and what is implemented in the manufacturer's software. Of course, the need for validation applies to *all* prescriptive procedures. The point being made here is that manufacturers' procedure may be less likely to be published and, if so, will not be accessible for validation studies.

The preceding comments should not be taken as being critical of manufacturers. Their fitting systems have been developed to meet a need, and the fitting of complex hearing aids is greatly facilitated by combining the software for prescribing amplification with that required to adjust the hearing aid. Nonetheless, this approach does have problems if the fitting system for a particular aid obliges the audiologist to use a particular prescription method. This is especially so if it is not clear how the method works or if it has not been validated.

Procedures Based on New Fitting Rationales

Most nonlinear fitting procedures that are not device-specific are based on the principle of normalizing loudness, applied across the frequencies of speech and for overall level (e.g., IHAFF, FIG6). Earlier, we have questioned this rationale, one reason being that it conflicts with the research evidence with respect to amplification requirements for an average input level. A possible disadvantage of any procedure based on a new rationale is that it may be unable make use of the knowledge gained from previous research. At present, the requirements for MPO, gain, and frequency response for an average-level input (65- to 70-dB SPL) are relatively well established. This knowledge is, in effect, disregarded when adopting a loudness normalization or any completely new rationale. This does not mean that such rationales cannot be validated, but the process must start from "scratch," rather than building on current knowledge. Having said this, it should be pointed out that no significant research has been done on amplification requirements for low-input or high-input levels. For these aspects of prescription, essentially choosing CTs and CRs, *all* procedures begin with untested assumptions.

Extending and/or Supplementing Current Prescriptive Rationales

The advantages of compression apply only to low-input levels (improved audibility) or high-input levels (improved comfort). For average-level inputs (65- to 70-dB SPL), compression and linear aids should provide the same amplification, and therefore it can be prescribed in the same manner. Thus a procedure such as NAL-R is appropriate for prescribing amplification for an average-input level for a compression hearing aid. The advantage of using such a procedure is that it has been thoroughly researched and it would take years of research to bring a new procedure to an equivalent state of validation. An average-level input, typically speech of 65- to 70-dB, is also the most common input level because it is the preferred listening level for communicating. Therefore, people try to arrange matters so that speech is received at around that level as much as possible (e.g., by moving closer to a talker or adjusting the volume of the TV). It is especially important to get the prescription correct for an average level because communicative functioning will depend heavily on listening to average level speech and less so on listening to soft or loud speech. As suggested by others (e.g., Kruger & Kruger, 1994), current fitting methods can provide a foundation that can be modified (extended) for fitting new types of hearing aids.

Valente et al (1997) have suggested the use of a modified NAL procedure as an interim measure, pending the development of validated prescriptive targets for nonlinear amplification. The NAL-R prescription is used for an average input and the gain prescriptions are increased or decreased for low and high inputs. The NAL-NL1 procedure does not actually use the NAL-RP prescriptions in its calculations, but it is based on the same rationale. Furthermore, in developing the new procedure, its prescriptions were compared with the NAL-RP prescriptions to ensure that reasonable agreement existed regarding the prescriptions for an average level and that the prescriptions for low and high levels were plausible in that they should show more and less gain, respectively. Some examples of these comparisons are illustrated in Figure 25–6, which shows NAL-NL1 prescriptions and NAL-RP prescriptions for a moderate flat hearing loss and a steeply sloping severe hearing loss.

The left panel of Figure 25–6 shows four prescriptive targets for a person with a sensorineural hearing loss and a flat 40 dB HTL audiogram. The targets are the insertion gain and frequency response prescribed by NAL-RP and the targets prescribed by NAL-NL1 for input levels of 50-, 70-, and 90-dB SPL. Predictably, the most gain is prescribed for the lowest (50 dB SPL) input level and the least gain is prescribed for the 90 dB SPL input level. The gain prescribed by NAL-NL1 for 70 dB SPL agrees reasonably with the NAL-RP prescription.

Indeed, NAL-RP could be expected to prescribe slightly more gain because the most typical input level would be 2- to 3-dB less than 70 dB SPL. The right panel of the figure shows the prescriptions for an audiogram having a constant, steep slope from 10 dB HTL at 250 Hz to 90 dB HTL at 4000 Hz. Again, most gain is prescribed by NAL-NL1 for the lowest input level and least for the highest input level. The NL 70 and NAL-RP prescriptions agree very closely except for a difference of 4 dB at 1000 Hz. For audiograms showing small losses at the low frequencies, no gain is needed for a high-input level and relatively little is needed for average-input or low-input levels to maximize the low-frequency contribution to speech intelligibility.

Although starting with an established procedure reduces the uncertainty in prescribing nonlinear amplification, procedures developed by that approach still need to be validated. The average input prescription is only as good as the linear procedure used to derive it, and room for debate about which procedure is most accurate still exists, especially about how much high-frequency emphasis should be provided for steeply sloping audiograms. For low (e.g., 50 dB SPL) and high levels (e.g., 80 dB SPL) more uncertainty exists because, although the prescriptions may be derived by extending established principles, the implementation of those principles may not be optimal. Furthermore, the rationale that is appropriate for an average input may not necessarily be best for lower or higher inputs. For example, NAL-NL1 uses the same rationale for prescribing for all input levels. That rationale, described earlier as a modified loudness equalization rationale, is implemented by calculating the gain and frequency response required to maximize the SII, modified to include a hearing loss desensitization factor, when speech inputs of all levels from 40- to 90-dB SPL are amplified to normal loudness. A rationale aiming to maximize speech intelligibility may not be applicable to high inputs for mild and moderate hearing losses because a range

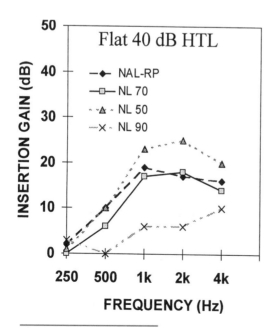
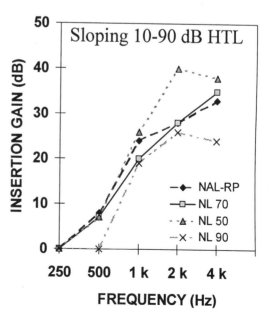

Figure 25–6 Examples of NAL-NL1 prescriptions, with NAL-RP prescription included for comparison.

of frequency-response characteristics should provide high intelligibility. Therefore, some additional basis may be required to decide which frequency response is best. One possibility suggested earlier could be to determine the best compromise between maximizing comfort and maximizing speech quality. Doubts were also outlined earlier about the appropriateness of normalizing overall loudness levels. These doubts are reinforced by the fact that amplifying an 80 dB input to normal loudness will often result in a *reduction* in SII compared with amplifying this input to a lower loudness level. These comments emphasize how little is known about amplification requirements for inputs substantially lower or higher than average. This is an additional reason for ensuring that the average level input prescription is soundly based on knowledge rather than supposition.

Validation of Prescriptive Rationales and Procedures

Any of the above approaches could lead to effective prescriptive procedures. The most important issue is that any procedure, regardless of how it is derived, must be validated by research. Such research needs to examine the validity of different prescriptive rationales, each of which could be used as the basis for a number of specific procedures. In addition, each procedure needs to be validated in its final form because, inevitably, sources of error will occur in the calculations, measurements, and assumptions needed to translate a rationale into a practical procedure. Procedures based on the same rationale can provide very different prescriptions for some patients because of differences in implementing the rationale. Furthermore, procedures having different rationales may, coincidentally, give similar prescriptions for some particular cases. A challenge for the future is to assess the validity of prescription concepts, such as normalizing loudness, independently of the validity of any particular procedure.

PEARL

Validation research tends to be difficult but is critical for progress in hearing aid prescription. It is relatively easy to dream up a plausible procedure but much more difficult, and personally threatening, to establish whether the procedure really works.

Future of Prescription

Recent increases in amplification options present new challenges for hearing aid prescription. Although numerous new prescriptive procedures are being proposed, relatively little research has been done on the basic issues relating to which rationales are best for fitting nonlinear amplification. Unfortunately, commercial success may sometimes be viewed as adequate validation which, in a sense, it may be from a manufacturer's point of view. However, that does not guarantee that audiologists are fulfilling their obligation to provide optimum amplification for each patient.

Although some dangers are present in current trends, we are optimistic that real progress will emerge through the combined

---

PITFALL

A danger exists that validation may be dismissed as too difficult, too expensive, or unnecessary. If this happens, audiologists may be forced to rely on plausible but unproven procedures or manufacturers' recommendations that may differ for every device, may have little research basis, or may use unspecified formulas.

---

efforts of research scientists, clinicians, and manufacturers. Among other things, such progress will require (a) more emphasis on validation research and correspondingly less readiness to accept plausible ideas as self-evidently correct, (b) recognition that *many* possible rationales and many ways of implementing each of them exist, (c) greater readiness to consider a wide range of possible prescription rationales, and (d) more research into the issues associated with all possible rationales.

MATCHING THE PRESCRIPTION

After amplification has been prescribed for an individual client, the next stage of the fitting process is to select hearing aids and combinations of settings and attachments that should provide the prescribed amplification. Although the principles of matching the prescription are the same for any type of hearing aid, the possibilities for accurate matching and the practicalities of achieving the best match are substantially different for programmable and digital aids than they have been for conventional aids. Matching procedures for current advanced hearing aids and future hearing aids will be discussed after briefly reviewing the matching procedures used with conventional aids.

Matching with Conventional Aids

Matching a prescription with a conventional hearing aid used to be relatively easy. As a first step, one would express the gain and MPO requirements in terms of 2-cc coupler measurements. One would then choose hearing aids that had the nonelectroacoustic features required for the subject (such as style, size, electrical input, telecoil), an appropriate average gain that allowed for an adequate reserve gain (~10- to 15-dB), a slope in the gain frequency response from 500 Hz to 2000 Hz that was approximately correct, and an MPO that approximately matched the target. Clinical judgment would be used to determine how large a vent should be included and whether an acoustic horn (for BTEs) should be ordered with the earmold. On the basis of either the measured coupler response or the measured real-ear response, the controls on the aid would be altered to arrive as close to the targets as possible. Because most hearing aids had three or less controls, adjustment of the aids was simple, and selection of the aids was not complicated by each hearing aid being able to be adjusted in a multitude of interacting ways.

Despite being simple, selecting hearing aids was not necessarily accurate. First, each aid was limited in flexibility. It is not possible to match gain simultaneously at a number of frequencies if only one tone control is adjusted. Even if hearing aids had two controls, such as a low-cut and a high-cut, neither of these was particularly useful if one wished to increase the gain at 4000 Hz, for example, or decrease the gain at 1000 Hz, for example, without appreciably affecting the gain at other frequencies. Even if aids were capable of matching a target exactly, no guarantee was present that the audiologist would choose these aids because the effects of vents and tubing (for BTEs) complicated the selection of hearing aids based on 2-cc coupler responses. These effects could be allowed for quantitatively, but the number of calculations needed was a disincentive, unless the audiologist had access to software that would perform these tasks. Matching for one required characteristic (e.g., adequate gain at high frequencies) often involved a compromise with some other desirable characteristics (e.g., freedom from occlusion, by using a large vent but without feedback occurring). Juggling in one's mind the quantitative information behind each of these things is very difficult, so a role for suitable software to assist in making the compromise has always been present. Software such as the Hearing Aid Selection Program (HASP) (Dillon et al, 1992) provides this assistance by performing the quantitative part of the process. Given that one particular fitting is unlikely to be best for all performance characteristics, some kind of weighting of the relative importance in achieving accuracy in matching each characteristic has to be done by the software, the audiologist, or both. The process is illustrated in Table 25–2, which shows the printout from the HASP hearing aid selection program.

The HASP program has been activated by entering the HTLs of the ear being fitted. The program then calculates the required gain and frequency response according to the NAL-RP formula and uses an additional formula to calculate the required MPO. Next, the program searches a database of information on the performance of various hearing aids, combined with the effects of different acoustic modifications, to identify the combinations that match the requirements most closely. Finally, the program ranks and lists the 15 to 20 combinations that provide the best matches. The ranking process considers several types of information and gives a different weight to each. The information in Table 25–2 shows

the ranking, from top to bottom, of various hearing aid/settings/acoustic modifications, selected from those available in the database. The audiologist, of course, may choose to weight them differently, and so choose an aid and settings that are not at the top of the list.

Several authors have advocated using acoustic information about the individual to make a more accurate estimate of the required coupler gain (Killion & Revitt, 1993; Mueller, 1989; Punch et al, 1990). Individual measurements of real-ear to coupler difference (RECD) and real-ear unaided response (REUR) do indeed allow the coupler gain needed to achieve an insertion gain target to be calculated with greater precision. Again, the extra complexity of the calculations needed makes it unlikely that this is done in practice, unless software is available to help. Examples include the DSL software and the NAL-NL1 nonlinear software. Alternately, some manufacturers of custom hearing aids allow the fitter to include information about RECD and REUR, and they make the appropriate corrections when aiming for a particular 2-cc target gain and SSPL.

Matching the nonlinear characteristics of a target (e.g., compression ratios and compression thresholds) was never an issue with conventional aids. First, having nonlinear targets is only a recent phenomenon. Second, conventional aids had few, if any, controls for adjusting nonlinear amplification parameters.

Matching with Programmable and Digital Aids

The advent of programmable and fully digital hearing aids is changing all that is involved in the matching process for several reasons. First, such hearing aids invariably have greater flexibility. Even if they use serial high-cut and low-cut filters, as with conventional hearing aids, they tend to include more filters per aid, and each filter tends to be more adjustable, in crossover frequency, slope, or both. Increasingly, hearing aids are using multiple parallel channels. Often this structure is justified by manufacturers on the basis that different compression characteristics can be selected within each band, although the evidence for or against this is scant indeed. The multichannel structure does, however, allow good flexibility of frequency-response adjustment, especially if it is combined

TABLE 25–2 To illustrate the matching process, this table shows some of the information provided by NAL's HASP for a sloping high-frequency audiogram

Aid Name	Tone	MPO Red. Steps	MPO Red. dB	Vent	Tube	Damper	Vdev	COF	F/B Margin
UNI UE-17	H	2	9	2mm	Libby4	None	–5	1.7	16
OTI 110-20	2	8		Occluded			–2	2.1	9
PHON 312-SC	00L	0	0	2mm			–2	2.0	8
PHON PSCC	8C	2	8	2mm	Libby4	680 N	–10	1.3	16

The program calculates the required gain, frequency response, and MPO, then, by searching a database, provides a list of the 20 most suitable aid options (only four shown here). The information, from *left to right,* is aid model; tone setting; MPO reduction (number of steps or dB below maximum); earmold vent; tubing (BTE only); damper (BTE only); volume deviation (amount by which volume control setting must be reduced or increased to provide prescribed average gain after allowing reserve gain of 15 dB for BTE or 10 dB for ITE); closeness of fit (rms deviation, across frequencies, between prescribed and obtained gain after equating average prescribed and obtained gains); feedback margin (extent to which gain could be increased before feedback is likely). The aids are listed in order of overall merit on the basis of a weighted average of the COF, Vdev, and F/B Mrgn figures.

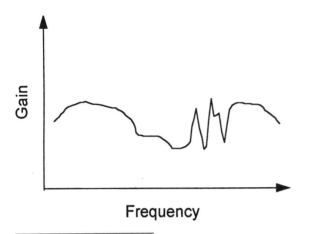

Figure 25–7 An example of the type of complex gain-frequency response shapes that can be obtained with IIR and FIR filters.

with traditional types of low-cut and high-cut filters or if four or more bands are present. With such structures, it becomes possible to alter the gain in a narrow frequency region without affecting the gain at all other frequencies.

Digital hearing aids have the potential to give a further leap in the accuracy and ease with which a target frequency response can be achieved. Digital filters can be made to have an arbitrary frequency-response shape, such as that shown in Figure 25–7, rather than a conventional low-pass, high-pass, or band-pass shape. Two basic classes of arbitrary shape digital filters exist. One is called a finite impulse response (FIR) filter and the other is called an infinite impulse response (IIR) filter. In the FIR filter the output is a weighted sum of the current input sample plus the previous n input samples, where n is referred to as the length of the filter or the number of taps in the filter. Filter lengths of 32 or 64 (they are usually powers of 2) are needed to make useful arbitrary response shape filters. In an IIR filter the output is the weighted sum of the current input, the past n input samples, and the past m output samples. IIR filters can achieve complex response shapes with far fewer taps (which equals n plus m). This means that they consume less power from the battery. They are, however, much harder to design and can accidentally become an oscillator if certain constraints are not observed. Such digital filters are likely to be used in the near future to accurately meet frequency-response targets, smooth out the peaks and troughs created by the transducers and the ear's acoustic properties, put notches in the gain frequency response and change the phase response to avoid feedback oscillations, and minimize the effects of background noise localized to particular frequency regions. Stay tuned, and learn the terminology now.

Programmable and digital hearing aids are also having a big effect on the ease with which nonlinear targets are being achieved. It is already common for multichannel hearing aids to have independent compressors in each channel. Each compressor can have its compression threshold adjusted, its compression ratio adjusted, or both. Each channel also has its gain for low-level stimuli and its saturation sound pressure level (SSPL) adjustable. For the most flexible hearing aids on the market, the accuracy with which nonlinear targets can

be achieved far surpasses our knowledge of what those targets should be, as outlined earlier.

The second impact of hearing aids being more flexible is that fewer hearing aids are required from any one manufacturer. This simplifies the selection task for the audiologist because it is much more likely that the audiologist will select the hearing aids most appropriate to the target the first time. Once it has been selected and the patient's details (at least the audiogram) entered into the fitting software, the hearing aid characteristics selected by the software are likely to result in a response close to the desired target. Of course, this assumes that the software also calculates the target. (Less desirably, the target can be directly entered by the audiologist.)

The increasingly sophisticated fitting software has made it more feasible to take into account an individual's RECD or REUR characteristics because it can do the necessary calculations once the data are entered. However, the increasingly flexible hearing aids have made it unnecessary to take these data into account. Whatever real-ear response is obtained on the first measurement, a more accurate match to a prescription is only minutes away if the hearing aid is adjusted by the audiologist or seconds away if it is adjusted automatically by the software. A few systems are already available that combine a hearing aid programmer with a real-ear gain analyzer. The ease and automation that these offer suggest that these will be the standard systems in the future, thus combining prescription, matching, and verification in one simple step.

VERIFYING HEARING AID FITTINGS

Verification means confirming that the prescribed hearing aid performance has been achieved in the ear being fitted. Verification is necessary because real-ear performance is not completely predictable from hearing aid measurements. The use of average correction figures (e.g., coupler response for flat insertion gain [CORFIG], or equivalently, REUR minus microphone location effects minus RECD) improves the likelihood that the matching procedure has been effective. However, a close match cannot be guaranteed because a proportion of individual ears will be substantially different from the average ear in terms of acoustic effects. Verification simply means that the prescription has been met. This is distinct from the further process of evaluation, which is concerned with determining how effective the fitting has been in meeting the client's needs.

Dating back at least to the 1940s (OSRD, 1946), it was realized that the performance of a hearing aid in an ear did not correspond precisely to the performance shown by measurements in a coupler. However, with rare minor exceptions, this fact was ignored in hearing aid selection methods developed before 1970. The situation began to change in the early 1970s with renewed interest in earmold venting and body baffle effects (Byrne, 1972; Erber, 1973). The development of the Knowles Electronics Mannikin for Acoustic Research (KEMAR) also raised awareness of real-ear factors even though a mannikin can simulate only average effects. Real-ear factors came to be considered in research (e.g., Pascoe, 1975) and, to a limited extent, in clinical procedures (Crouch & Pendry, 1975; Erber, 1973). The first hearing aid selection procedures to specifically include real-ear measurements (i.e., verification) were proposed by Byrne and Tonisson (1976) and Berger et al (1978). Both those procedures recommended prescription, followed by matching, followed by functional gain measurements to verify whether the prescribed real-ear performance had been obtained. This was followed by adjusting the fitting in those instances in which the measured performance was not an acceptable match to the prescription. Since the mid to late 1970s it has become the usual practice to recommend verification measures as part of the fitting process. Insertion gain measurements are the most common, but not the only, type of currently used verification measures.

Unresolved Issues in Verification
Insertion Gain versus Real-Ear Aided Response

Although this could equally have been called an unresolved issue in prescription or matching, it is not clear when one should attempt to prescribe, match, and verify a real-ear insertion response (REIR) and when one should prescribe, match, and verify a real ear aided response (REAR). The REIR indicates how much more sound is available at the earcanal in the aided condition than in the unaided condition, whereas the REAR indicates how much more sound is present at the eardrum than at some reference point in the sound field outside the head. Another way of looking at the difference is that REIR preserves the individual's REUR, whereas an REAR target does not. Assuming that the two approaches (REIR versus REAR) agree for a person with an average REUR, the differences will be greatest for those people who have REUR curves that are most different from average. These include infants, people with surgically altered earcanals, people with very short or long earcanals, and possibly people with extremely loose or tight eardrums. It seems that the preferred approach depends on which of these groups a particular patient belongs to. It is probably unreasonable to try and preserve the acoustic effects of something that has been caused by surgical intervention, so REAR is recommended for those groups. People with slightly aberrant REUR curves might be best served if their individual curves are preserved, particularly if they wear their hearing aids for part of the day only, so REIR is recommended for this group. Influencing this decision is the fact that for adults, REIR measurement is easier than REAR measurement because the probe tube does not need to be as close to the eardrum. Finally, for infants, measurement of REAR is easier because it is not a necessity to retain a probe tube within the unaided earcanal of a very mobile young person. Consequently, REAR is recommended for this group. For adults with average REUR curves, both procedures will produce the same result if done accurately, so REIR is recommended, again on the grounds of the measurements being easier. This last point, and choice of measurement type in general, is described in more detail in Dillon (in press). Modern selection procedures, such as DSL and NAL-NL1, allow the audiologist to specify either type of target. A practical problem is that few commecially available real-ear gain analyzers provide REAR targets or targets for nonlinear procedures. This situation is likely to change rapidly. Research is needed to resolve whether the recommendations given in this section are optimal, although it is not clear how the issue would be resolved, particularly in the case of the infants.

Real-Ear Gain Measurement with Complex Processing Schemes

Measurement of real-ear gain, using a probe microphone, has been the dominant method of verifying a prescription for most of the past decade. More recently, a few manufacturers of high-technology hearing aids have recommended that real-ear gain *not* be measured. Several possible reasons are behind this recommendation. The most likely is that the individual variations in achieving a desired target are much smaller than our current uncertainty about what those targets should be. In this circumstance there may seem to be little point in accurately adjusting a hearing aid to a target about which we are not confident.

CONTROVERSIAL POINT

We do not agree with the recommendation that real-ear gain not be measured for some advanced hearing aids. Our knowledge of nonlinear targets is rapidly improving, and a final verification measurement provides a check should any one of a large number of errors occur along the path from knowing the hearing loss through to the hearing aid being given particular settings.

A second reason for avoiding real-ear measurement is the hearing aid may react to the test signal in a different manner than it reacts to real speech. Some hearing aids, for instance, use the dynamics of the input signal to estimate whether an incoming signal is speech or noise and then alter their amplification characteristics accordingly. An unrealistic response to a standard test signal is only a temporary reason for not measuring real-ear performance. All that is necessary is that the test signal simulate whatever characteristic of the input signal that the aid responds to. Possibilities include pseudorandom noises with realistic crest factors, either with or without some form of amplitude modulation. Different test signals may well be needed for different processing strategies, and manufacturers should specify what characteristics are needed in a test signal such that realistic results will be obtained. In this age of real-time spectral analysis using fast Fourier transforms (FFT) and coherence measures between the output signal and the speech component of the input signal, real speech and real noise can be used if all else fails.

Self-Assessing, Self-Adjusting, and Self-Verifying Hearing Aids

Fitting hearing aids requires that hearing be assessed, targets calculated, the hearing aids be adjusted, the response verified, and the hearing aids be fine-tuned. In turn, this sequence of events requires that sounds be put into the earcanals and measured and that the patient's responses (detection of a signal, or loudness scaling) be communicated to the aid. Hearing aids and their associated fitting software can contain virtually all the instrumentation necessary to accomplish this. Already, pure tone generators have been built into digital hearing aids, so that the hearing aid generates the sound necessary to test the patient's threshold rather than an external audiometer and transducer. This approach has the advantage that the acoustic characteristics of the individual earcanal have partly been taken into account when threshold has been determined. Addition of another component to the hearing aids would complete the picture: a second microphone, monitoring the SPL generated by the hearing aids *within* the canal would allow threshold to be expressed as dB SPL in the canal and also allow the level of all amplified sounds to be expressed in the same units. Apart from assisting in the calculation of a more accurate target response, such a microphone could also be used to measure the real-ear aided gain of the hearing aids, could detect when the hearing aids have become faulty (Nowosielski et al, 1998), and may assist in detecting and removing feedback oscillations.

When coupled with suitable software, all that would be required of an audiologist is that the aid be physically fitted to the ear, with a suitable vent size included, and the responses of the subject (either detection of sounds if targets are based on thresholds or loudness ratings if based on individual loudness scales) be communicated to the fitting software. After this, the software could adjust the hearing aids, note the resulting response, and continue readjusting the hearing aids until the desired targets have been established.

Verifying Specific Signal Processing Strategies

As the number of signal processing strategies grows, so too will the variety of verification procedures needed. Most signal-processing strategies will need a specific verification method to show whether the strategy is working electronically as it should and, more importantly, whether it is working optimally, or at least sufficiently well, for that patient. Of course, if a strategy has no adjustable parameters (e.g., a directional microphone) and if using it carries no potential disadvantage, there would be no point in verifying whether it worked for an individual patient. It may be worth verifying electroacoustically that a directional microphone still has the degree of directionality expected from its specifications.

The following section provides information on the type of verification that might be appropriate to some new selection strategies.

Achievement of Fitting Rationale

Many of the new fitting procedures aim to normalize loudness at each frequency (e.g., FIG6, DSL[i/o], IHAFF). Although we do not agree that loudness normalization is an optimal strategy, if a hearing aid fitter considers it is worth achieving, then it is worth *verifying* that it is achieved. Verification could include loudness scaling with narrow band stimuli, although if this

was the method used to prescribe the hearing aid, such verification would really only ensure that a mistake had not happened during the prescription. Additional verification could include loudness scaling with broad-band stimuli (speech, noises, or combinations of these) or loudness balancing of two different narrow-band stimuli. It should not be assumed that the results of loudness balancing between stimuli would be predictable on the basis of loudness scaling of one stimulus at a time.

One new procedure (NAL-NL1) aims to maximize speech intelligibility. It would be totally impractical to verify this goal directly because that would involve measuring speech intelligibility with a number of alternative responses. A consequence of the new procedure, however, is that for a wide range of hearing losses loudness is made approximately constant across frequency for an input signal with spectral shape equal to the long-term average spectrum of speech. This consequence could at least be verified with suitably designed stimuli.

Reduction of Noise and Its Effects

With the advent of digital processing, several new methods of noise reduction are likely to emerge. Some of these may be directed toward reducing the effects of specific types of noise, such as low-frequency traffic rumble or steady machine noise. An obvious form of verification is to perform speech intelligibility or to obtain ratings of speech intelligibility in the presence of the target noise.

Feedback Reduction

Digital processing will certainly bring some new and effective methods for increasing gain before feedback oscillation occur. Verification of proper operation should be straightforward. The difference in achievable gain, with and without the reduction strategy operating, would indicate that it was working as intended. Verification of whether the particular strategy works well enough for that patient would merely consist of finding out how much more gain could be achieved for the patient (relative to the gain believed to be optimal) before feedback occurred. If an additional 10 dB of gain could be obtained without oscillation, the strategy would probably be appropriate. Of course, for nonlinear aids, gain decreases as input level increases, so gain would have to be measured at or below the compression threshold of the hearing aid.

Frequency Transposition

Frequency transposition is used to make high-frequency sounds audible, even though the patient may have no or poor hearing at those higher frequencies. An obvious form of verification would be to measure the aided thresholds at each input frequency. More detailed verification procedures would need to be matched to the prescription approach used to establish how the frequencies were transposed and how their levels were controlled. Verification of whether the patient could understand the transposed speech crosses the line into evaluation.

EVALUATING AND "FINE-TUNING" HEARING AID FITTINGS

The final stage of hearing aid fitting is evaluating its effectiveness in meeting the patient's needs. In what respects did the patient require help and how much help is he or she getting by using the hearing aid? What hearing difficulties remain and can they be alleviated by adjusting the hearing aid fitting or by other means? If the hearing aid is less effective than expected, this may prompt the audiologist to make some hearing aid adjustments, often referred to as "fine-tuning." This term is also used to cover adjustments made during the matching or verification stages to achieve a better match to the prescription. Evaluation has much broader purposes than simply identifying the need for fine-tuning. The audiologist needs to know how much a particular patient has been helped and which specific measures have been effective. This type of information, collected over a number of patients, may help the audiologist to decide what types of hearing aid fittings are likely to be effective for future patients and which problems are likely to be helped by specific measures (e.g., using open earmolds or providing multiple memories). Aside from this clinical "research," audiologists, along with all types of health professionals, are being called on increasingly to justify their management of individual patients and practices generally. At a broader level, managers of programs are being required to demonstrate successful outcomes to justify continued support.

Some form of evaluation has probably been practiced from the time the first hearing aids were fitted. This may be no more than asking the patient "How do your hearing aids sound?" either immediately after fitting or at a later follow-up. Indeed, the main form of evaluation used so far has probably been an informal inquiry into the patient's experiences and satisfaction and problems with the hearing aids. Until recently, the traditional American "hearing aid evaluation" procedure was the only commonly used formal evaluation procedure, although it was not used as an outcome measure, but more as a substitute for prescription. Nonetheless, the types of speech recognition tests developed for "hearing aid evaluation" have often been used for evaluation in research and, less frequently, in clinical practice. Another approach to evaluation is the use of structured questionnaires to replace or supplement informal inquiry. Some such questionnaires date back to the 1960s or early 1970s (High et al, 1964; Noble & Atherley, 1970). Although these early questionnaires could be used to evaluate hearing aid fittings, that application was not emphasized until the recent development of several new questionnaires (discussed later), some designed specifically to evaluate hearing aid outcomes. A further approach is the use of "quality" or "intelligibility" judgments, usually implemented by paired comparisons of amplified speech. Examples were suggested in the 1960s, but it is only over the last 15 years that this approach has received much research attention and that clinical procedures have been suggested (Byrne & Cotton, 1988). At present, a high level of interest exists in using self-assessment questionnaires as outcome measures and, to

a lesser extent, in using judgment procedures for fine-tuning. The following sections will discuss likely future developments in these areas and other possible evaluation measures.

Newer Trends and Future Possibilities
Speech Recognition

The idea of using speech tests to evaluate hearing aid fittings has a very long history (Carhart, 1946). The problems are well known: to choose one of two amplification characteristics, one has to use a speech test with sufficient items to make the random test-retest differences smaller than the likely difference between the true scores associated with each amplification condition. This is a serious problem when only two amplification conditions are present, and makes the use of speech recognition testing, for the purposes of fine-tuning, totally impractical when there are more conditions. To minimize this problem, speech tests rich in high-frequency speech cues have been suggested (Dennison & Kelly, 1978). The idea of using tests with items chosen to depend on particular frequency regions may have application to multichannel hearing aids. Such tests may allow the adequacy of audibility within each frequency region to be determined. A judicious choice of test items (and the response foils in a closed-set task), grouped into subscales, may allow speech tests sensitive to low-frequency and mid-frequency amplification to also be developed. If necessary, low-pass, band-pass, or high-pass filtering of the stimuli could increase the association between particular subscales and particular frequency regions. No matter how close the association between subscales and frequency regions, the fundamental limits on reliability imposed by the number of test items, as described by the binomial distribution, cannot be escaped. It is never likely that enough clinical time will be available to use speech recognition tests to reliably choose between two or three amplification conditions.

Ratings and Quality Judgments; Ease of Listening (Reaction Time)

Absolute ratings of speech quality or intelligibility and paired comparison preference judgments of speech quality or intelligibility have often been used in research studies over the last 15 years but have not been used clinically except in very informal ways. (The ubiquitous question How does that sound? when a hearing aid is first turned on is an informal absolute rating of quality, for example.)

Hearing aids are increasingly using devices and algorithms aimed at reducing the effects of background noise. These include directional microphones, switchable dual-microphone directional microphones, low-frequency compression circuits, and multichannel aids where the gain in each channel depends on the estimated signal and noise levels within each channel. These devices thus affect speech intelligibility and sound quality in different ways, and at present no validated rules exist for saying which patient requires which processing scheme under which acoustic conditions. Whenever there are no reliable rules for prescription, an increased emphasis must be placed on empirical evaluation and fine tuning. We would therefore expect increased use of more formal clinical evaluations using paired comparison ratings of sound quality or speech intelligibility. Such comparisons will require appropriate stimuli (e.g., continuous discourse against a variety of background noises) and knowledge of which types of noises and signal to noise ratios are most useful for examining the advantages of different processing schemes in the hearing clinic. Research aimed at acquiring this knowledge is urgently required, and such research will provide a start on forming prescriptive rules that may eventually make the subjective evaluations unnecessary.

Field Trials, Multimemory Aids, and Data Logging

Like speech testing, sound quality rating and paired comparison preference judgments become time consuming if many alternative conditions are to be compared. Clinical time costs money, so an alternative to gather such paired comparison data is to have the patient make the comparisons after leaving the hearing clinic. This is possible with multimemory hearing aids. Instead of providing just two or three programs, with the intent that these be the final programs used by the patient, hearing aids could have a greater number of programs, and the patient could find out, by trial and error, which programs work best in which circumstances. After a suitable listening period (such as two weeks), the most useful programs could be retained and the least useful programs replaced by other possibilities. Patients could report their preferences through a diary, or an electronic data logger within the hearing aids could indicate to the clinician how much time each program had been used for. Reprogramming of the aids could be done in a very short time and would not even require a visit to the clinic. Technically, the reprogramming could be done over the phone, although connecting the hearing aids to the phone by means of a suitable coupling device would be too confusing a task for a small proportion of patients. For these patients, an extended field trial evaluation period may not be feasible in any event.

Apart from minimizing clinical time, extended field trials have an important advantage: they evaluate different amplification characteristics in totally realistic conditions. Generally, it is possible to design a laboratory evaluation to either maximize or minimize the advantages of a processing scheme. For example, a directional microphone can be shown to be very effective when speech comes from in front of the person and noise comes from behind in nonreverberant conditions. It can be shown to have no advantage when speech and noise come from similar directions or when the reverberant intensity far exceeds the direct intensity of the speech. Under such conditions, the directional microphone may be worse than an omnidirectional microphone if it causes an unduly large low-frequency cut. Having the patients make their choices in their own environments takes away the uncertainty about whether simulations in the clinic are realistic.

Self-Assessment and Its Relation to Signal Processing

Self-assessment scales for measuring the benefit arising from hearing aids usually have subscales associated with particular acoustic conditions. For example, the Abbreviated Profile of Hearing Aid Benefit (APHAB; Cox & Alexander, 1995) has subscales called "Ease of Communication," "Background Noise," "Reverberation," and "Aversiveness of Sounds." Similarly, the Shortened Hearing Aid Performance Inventory for the Elderly

(SHAPIE; Dillon, 1994) has subscales called "Noise," "Reduced Cues," and "Miscellaneous." If scores for these subscales really reflect how much the hearing aids reduce disability in different environments and if signal processing schemes really do help differentially in different environments, there is great potential to use such self-assessment tools to improve hearing aid fittings. First, self-assessment tools that measure unaided disability in different environments (e.g., the unaided APHAB score) could be used to identify the need for different processing schemes. Second, self-assessment tools that measure reduction in disability could be used to see which of several processing schemes best reduced disability in the target situations. Whether the answers obtained from this process were more or less reliable than simply asking the patient which processing scheme was preferred in the situation is a matter for experimental investigation. So far, the only subscale that is clearly related to amplification characteristics is the "Aversiveness" subscale of APHAB, where a poor score is a clear indicator that SSPL is too high, and/or a more gradual form of compression is required for medium to high-level input sounds.

On a related topic, investigation is needed into whether hearing aid use, satisfaction, disability reduction, or handicap reduction is the most important measure against which the success of a signal processing scheme should be assessed. Suppose that a patient was given four different amplification schemes over successive weeks. The patient used scheme A for more hours per week than the others because it sounded pleasant and not fatiguing. Scheme B, however, resulted in the greatest disability reduction in that it made speech most intelligible, although it gave the speech a sound quality that the subject disliked. Scheme C best enabled the person to resume activities that he had previously ceased because of his hearing loss. Perhaps scheme C made low-level sounds more audible and it made bird-watching and hunting possible. Overall the patient expressed greatest satisfaction with scheme D because although it was not the best for any of the preceding attributes, it was reasonably good for all the atributes. Which scheme should we fit to such a person? An easy answer is four-program hearing aids. Another easy answer is hearing aids that adapt to each acoustic situation to the degree possible. However, such adaption may be limited because the hearing aid cannot know when intelligibility is a priority and when quality is a priority. Suppose, however, that no such adaptive hearing aids are available and that no single hearing aid has all four processing schemes (a very realistic assumption). This question illustrates a fundamental problem with our knowledge of self-assessment: We do not know what is the most important thing to measure. Measures of all four quantities (use, satisfaction, disability reduction, and handicap reduction) are available and often used, but we do not know which one is the most important to maximize, and we do not know how often maximizing one of these will conflict with maximizing the others. These are important areas for research.

Evaluating Spatial Hearing

Spatial aspects of hearing, unaided and aided, deserve and will probably receive more attention than they have in the past (Byrne & Noble, 1998). Improved localization of sound has long been regarded as an important advantage of bilateral fitting and such an advantage may also occur for completely-in-the-canal aids (Kochkin, 1996; Mueller & Ebinger, 1997). Improved aided localization has been demonstrated for fittings using certain types of ear molds rather than other types (Byrne et al, 1996, 1998; Noble et al, 1998). Hearing aids designed to improve binaural hearing are beginning to appear on the market. This increased attention to improving spatial hearing creates a need for evaluation to determine whether such improvement has actually occurred and what benefits it confers on the aid user.

One form of evaluation could be localization testing with an array of loudspeakers and suitable signal generating and switching equipment. Although such testing has not yet found a place in clinical practice, it would be feasible and useful (Byrne & Noble, 1998). Another possible measure would be self-assessment questionnaires containing questions about sound localization, externalization of sounds, and the general perception of correct spatial orientation. Where localization questions have been included in questionnaires, they have been found to correlate highly with overall disability as assessed by the remainder of the questionnaire (Noble & Atherly, 1970). Some indication also exists that disturbed localization is associated with adverse mental health effects (Eriksson-Mangold & Carlson, 1991). Speech recognition in noise tests, with the speech and noise from separate, possibly multiple, sources, may also give information on spatial hearing, although this may be difficult to assess separately from head shadow effects. Overall, we predict that spatial aspects of hearing will receive more attention in both the prescription and evaluation stages of the hearing aid fitting process.

Compatibility of Hearing Aids with Digital Telephones or other Electronic Devices

Increasingly, modern life involves the frequent use of electronic devices. Because some such devices have the potential to cause interference to hearing aids, audiologists will

need to consider whether the hearing aids they prescribe are compatible with the other electronic devices that the hearing aid wearer wishes to use or will come into close contact with. Indeed, the audiologist should be considering how other devices can be used, alone or in conjunction with hearing aids, to optimize the communicative efficiency of the patient.

At present, the one significant example of incompatibility is between hearing aids and digital mobile telephones. Very few hearing aids can be used with a digital mobile phone because, when the phone and hearing aid are brought close together, electromagnetic interference in the form of a moderate to loud "buzz" occurs (LeStrange et al, 1995). Certain measures, such as various types of shielding (LeStrange et al, 1995) and new microphones, can make hearing aids less susceptible (more immune) to electromagnetic interference and, consequently, more and more hearing aids will become usable with digital mobile phones. However, it is likely to be a long time, and perhaps will never happen, before all types of hearing aids can be used with all types of phones. The audiologist will therefore need to consider the immunity question in the hearing aid selection and evaluation process.

Phones of the future will be much more than phones. Increasingly, they will provide a range of communication facilities, with links to computers and fax machines. Furthermore, the mobile phone is just one example of an electronic device that will need to be used with hearing aids or will have potential to interfere with hearing aid use. We predict that in the near future the audiologist will need to be well informed about how to use hearing aids with, or near, a range of other devices and how to avoid interference problems.

CONCLUSIONS

In this chapter we have examined future directions in hearing aid prescription and evaluation by asking Where *should* we be going? and Are we heading in the right directions? Although the future is not entirely predictable or controllable, it will largely depend on what we decide to do now. At present, many current directions are very promising and exciting, others seem likely to be unproductive, and still other directions seem desirable but are largely neglected. We hope that some of the thoughts expressed in this chapter may suggest improved ways to shape the future. More generally, this amounts to saying that hearing aid prescription and evaluation, like any other field of scientific study, should be continually undergoing review and modification.

The time ahead is especially challenging because hearing aid technology is developing rapidly. This offers the audiologist a host of new amplification options but, unfortunately, knowledge of how to best use these options is limited. The challenge is to ensure that we do the research necessary to evaluate each option thoroughly to determine the benefits it provides to hearing aid wearers. The danger is that such research will be dismissed as too hard or too slow and that hearing aid fitting will become a pseudoscience mainly on the basis of marketing hype rather than experimental evidence.

Future research may focus on determining what the benefits of hearing aid fitting are and how each benefit can be achieved. Benefit must defined broadly to mean anything that makes a person with impaired hearing consider that it is better to wear hearing aids than not to or that one hearing aid is better than another. Traditionally, benefit has been defined narrowly, typically as meaning little other than improving hearing for speech. However, for most hearing aid users, the main exceptions being those with severe hearing losses, hearing aids provide good speech intelligibility in quiet and somewhat noisy conditions. For such hearing aid wearers, considerations of comfort, sound quality, or detection and localization of environmental sounds may become more important than minor differences in speech intelligibility. Although speech recognition will remain of paramount importance, many other aspects of auditory experience will require research to get a proper appreciation of hearing aid benefits and to provide a set of objectives for designing and fitting future hearing aids. In the speech recognition area the major challenges are to improve speech recognition in noise and to determine and to meet the requirements of people with severe hearing losses.

The future of hearing aid fitting and evaluation is challenging. It is up to us to decide what we want it to be and to make it happen.

REFERENCES

ALLEN, J.B., HALL, J.L., & PENG, P.S. (1990). Loudness growth in 1/2 octave bands (LGOB): A procedure for assessment of loudness. *Journal of the Acoustical Society of America, 88*;745–753.

AMERICAN NATIONAL STANDARDS INSTITUTE. (1969). *American national standards methods for the calculation of the Articulation Index* (ANSI S3.5-1969). New York: ANSI.

AMERICAN NATIONAL STANDARDS INSTITUTE. (1993). *American national standard methods for the calculation of the Speech Intelligibility Index* (ANSI S3.5-199x, Draft V3.1). New York: ANSI.

ARLINGER, S., GATEHOUSE, S., BENTLER, R.A., BYRNE, D., COX, R.M., DIRKS, D.D., HUMES, L., NEUMAN, A., PONTON, C., ROBINSON, K., SILMAN, S., SUMMERFIELD, A.Q., TURNER, C.W., TYLER, R.S., & WILLOT, J.F. (1996). Report of the Eriksholm workshop on auditory deprivation and acclimatization. *Ear and Hearing, 17*;87S–98S.

BERGER, K.W., HAGBERG, E.N., & RANE, R.L. (1978). *Prescription of hearing aids: Rationale, procedures, and results.* Kent, Ohio: Herald.

BRATT, G.W., & SAMMETH, C.A. (1991). Clinical implications of prescriptive formulas for hearing aid selection. In: G.A. Studebaker, F.H. Bess, & L.B. Beck (Eds.), *The Vanderbilt hearing-aid report II* (pp. 23–33). Parkton: York Press.

BYRNE, D. (1972). Some implications of body baffle for hearing aid selection. *British Journal of Audiology, 6*;86–91.

BYRNE, D. (1978). Selection of hearing aids for severely deaf children. *British Journal of Audiology, 12*;9–22.

BYRNE, D. (1979). Selective amplification: Some psychoacoustic considerations. In: F.H. Bess, B.A. Freeman, & J.S. Sinclair (Eds.), *Amplification in education* (pp. 260–285). Washington, DC: AG Bell.

BYRNE, D. (1983). Theoretical prescriptive approaches to selecting the gain and frequency response of a hearing aid. *Monographs in Contemporary Audiology, 4*(1);1–40.

BYRNE, D. (1986a). Effects of bandwidth and stimulus type on most comfortable loudness levels of hearing-impaired listeners. *Journal of the Acoustical Society of America, 80*; 484–493.

BYRNE, D. (1986b). Effects of frequency response characteristics on speech discrimination and perceived intelligibility and pleasantness of speech for hearing-impaired listeners *Journal of the Acoustical Society of America, 80*;494–504.

BYRNE, D. (1992). Key issues in hearing aid selection and evaluation. *Journal of the American Academy of Audiology, 3*;67–80.

BYRNE, D. (1993). Implications of National Acoustic Laboratories' (NAL) research for hearing aid gain and frequency response selection strategies. In: G.A. Studebaker, & I. Hochberg (Eds.), *Acoustical factors affecting hearing aid performance* (pp. 119–131). Boston: Allyn & Bacon.

BYRNE, D. (1996). Hearing aid selection for the 1990s: Where to? *Journal of the American Academy of Audiology, 7*;377–395.

BYRNE, D., & COTTON, S. (1988). Evaluation of the National Acoustic Laboratories' new hearing aid selection procedure. *Journal of Speech and Hearing Research, 31*;178–186.

BYRNE, D., & DILLON, H. (1986) The National Acoustic Laboratories' (NAL) new procedure for selecting the gain and frequency response of a hearing aid. *Ear and Hearing, 7*;257–265.

BYRNE, D., DILLON, H., TRAN, K., ARLINGER, S., WILBRAHAM, K., COX, R., HAGERMAN, B., HETU, R., KEI, J., LUI, C., KIESSLING, J., KOTBY, M.N., NASSER, N.H.A., ERIC LEPAGE KHOLY, W.A.H., NAKANISHI, Y., OYER, H., POWELL, R., STEPHENS, D., MEREDITH, R., SIRIMANNA, T., TAVARTKILADZE, G., FROLENKOV, G.I., WESTERMAN, S., & LUDVIDSEN, C. (1994). An international comparison of long-term average speech spectra. *Journal of the Acoustical Society of America, 96*;2108–2120.

BYRNE, D., & FIFIELD, D. (1974). Evaluation of hearing aid fittings for infants. *British Journal of Audiology, 8*;47–54.

BYRNE, D.J., & MURRAY, N. (1985). Relationships of HTLs, MCLs, LDLs and psychoacoustic tuning curves to optimal frequency response characteristics of hearing aids. *Australian Journal of Audiology, 7*;7–16.

BYRNE, D., & NOBLE, W. (1998). Optimizing sound localization with hearing aids. *Trends in Amplification, 3*(2);49–73.

BYRNE, D., NOBLE, W., & GLAUERDT, B. (1996). Effects of earmold type on ability to locate sounds when wearing hearing aids. *Ear and Hearing, 17*;218–228.

BYRNE, D., PARKINSON, A., & NEWALL, P. (1990a). Hearing aid gain and frequency response requirements of the severely/profoundly hearing-impaired. *Ear and Hearing, 11*;40–49.

BYRNE, D., PARKINSON, A., & NEWALL, P. (1990b). Comparisons of NAL and MCL based hearing aid frequency response prescriptions for severely/profoundly hearing-impaired clients. *Australian Journal of Audiology, 12*;1–9.

BYRNE, D., PARKINSON, A., & NEWALL, P. (1990c). Amplification for the severely hearing-impaired—Young and old. In: J.H. Jensen (Ed.), *Presbyacusis and other age related aspects* (pp. 455–464). Copenhagen: Stougaard Jensen.

BYRNE, D., PARKINSON, A., & NEWALL, P. (1991). Modified hearing aid selection procedures for severe/profound hearing losses. In: G. Studebaker, F. Bess, & L. Beck (Eds.), *The Vanderbilt hearing aid report II* (pp. 295–300). Maryland: York Press.

BYRNE, D., SINCLAIR, S., & NOBLE, W. (1998). Open ear mold fittings for improving aided auditory localization for sensorineural hearing losses with good high frequency hearing. *Ear and Hearing, 19;*62–71.

BYRNE, D., & TONISSON, W. (1976). Selecting the gain of hearing aids for persons with sensorineural hearing losses. *Scandinavian Audiology, 5;*51–59.

CARHART, R. (1946). Selection of hearing aids. *Archives of Otolaryngology, 44;*1–18.

CHING, T., DILLON, H., & BYRNE, D. (1998). Speech recognition of hearing impaired listeners. *Journal of the Acoustical Society of America, 103;*1128–1140.

CORNELISSE, L., SEEWALD, R.C., & JAMIESON, D.G. (1995). The input/output formula: A theoretical approach to the fitting of personal amplification. *Journal of the Acoustical Society of America, 97;*1854–1864.

COX, R. (1988). The MSU hearing instrument prescription procedure. *Hearing Instruments, 39*(1);6–10.

COX, R.M. (1983). Using ULCL measures to find frequency/gain and SSPL90. *Hearing Instruments, 34*(7);17–21, 39.

COX, R.M. (1995). Using loudness data for hearing aid selection: The IHAFF approach. *Hearing Journal, 48*(2);10–44.

COX, R.M., & ALEXANDER, G.C. (1995). The abbreviated profile of hearing aid benefit (APHAB). *Ear and Hearing, 16;*176–186.

COX, R.M., ALEXANDER, G.C., TAYLOR, I.M., & GRAY, G.A. (1997). The contour test of loudness perception. *Ear and Hearing, 18;*388–400.

CROUCH, J.D., & PENDRY, B.L. (1975). Otometry in clinical hearing aid dispensing. *Hearing Aid Journal, 28*(11);12, 42–48; 28(12)18,31–33.

DAVIS, H., STEVENS, S.S., & NICHOLS, R.H. (1947) *Hearing aids; An experimental study of design objectives.* Cambridge, MA: Harvard University Press.

DAWSON, P., DILLON, H., & BATTAGLIA, J. (1991). Output compression limiting for severe-profoundly deaf. *Australian Journal of Audiology, 13;*1–12.

DENNISON, L.B., & KELLY, B.R. (1978). High frequency consonant word discrimination lists in hearing aid evaluation. *Journal of the American Audiological Society, 4;*91–97.

DILLON, H. (1994). Shortened hearing aid performance inventory for the elderly (SHAPIE): A statistical approach. *Australian Journal of Audiology, 16;*37–48.

DILLON, H. (1996). Compression? Yes, but for low or high frequencies, for low or high intensities, and for what response times? *Ear and Hearing, 17;*287–307.

DILLON H. (In press). *Hearing aids.*

DILLON, H., BYRNE, D., & BATTAGLIA, J. (1992). Hearing instrument selection: By dispenser or computer. *Hearing Instruments, 43*(8);18–21.

DILLON, H. (1999). NAL-NLI: A new procedure for fitting nonlinear hearing aids. *Hearing Journal, 52*(4);10–16.

DILLON, H., JAMES, A., & GINIS, J. (1997). Client oriented scale of improvement (COSI) and its relationship to several other measures of benefit and satisfaction provided by hearing aids. *Journal of the American Academy of Audiology, 8;*27–43.

DILLON, H., & STOREY, L. (1998). National Acoustic Laboratories procedure for selecting the saturated sound pressure level of hearing aids: Theoretical prediction. *Ear and Hearing, 19;*255–266.

DILLON, H., STOREY, L., GRANT, F., PHILLIPS, A., SKELT, L., MAVRIAS, G., WOYTOWYCH, W., & WALSH, M. (1998). Preferred compression threshold with 2:1 wide dynamic range compression in everyday environments. *Australian Journal of Audiology, 20;*33–44.

DUGAL, R.L., BRAIDA, L.D., & DURLACH, N.I. (1980). Implications of previous research for the selection of frequency-gain characteristics. In: G.A. Studebaker & I. Hochberg (Eds.), *Acoustical factors affecting hearing aid performance* (pp. 119–131). Baltimore: University Park Press.

ERBER, N.P. (1973). Body-baffle and real-ear effects in the selection of hearing aids for deaf children. *Journal of Speech and Hearing Disorders, 38;*224–231.

ERIKSSON-MANGOLD, M., & CARLSON, S.G. (1991). Psychological and somatic distress in relation to perceived hearing disability, hearing handicap, and hearing measurements. *Journal of Psychosomatic Research, 35;*729–740.

FLETCHER, H. (1952). The perception of speech sounds by deafened persons. *Journal of the Acoustical Society of America, 24;*490–497.

GATEHOUSE, S. (1993). Role of perceptual acclimatization in the selection of frequency responses for hearing aids. *Journal of the American Academy of Audiology, 4;*296–306.

GENGEL, R.W., PASCOE, D., & SHORE, I. (1971). A frequency-response procedure for evaluating and selecting hearing aids for severely hearing-impaired children. *Journal of Speech and Hearing Disorders, 36;*341–353.

HIGH, W., FAIRBANKS, G., & GLORIG, A. (1964). Scale for self-assessment of hearing handicap (forms A and B). *Journal of Speech and Hearing Disorders, 29;*215–230.

HOGAN, C.A., TURNER, C.W. (1998). High frequency audibility: Benefits for hearing-impaired listeners. *Journal of the Acoustical Society of America, 104;*432–441.

HUMES, L. (1986). An evaluation of several rationales for selecting hearing aid gain. *Journal of Speech and Hearing Disorders, 51;*272–281.

HUMES, L.E., PAVLOVIC, C., BRAY, V., & BARR, M. (1996). Real-ear measurement of hearing threshold and loudness. *Trends in Amplification, 1;*121–135.

JOHNSON, J.S., PLUVINAGE, V, & BENSON, D. (1989). Digitally programmable full dynamic range compression technology. *Hearing Instruments, 40*(10);26–30.

KEIDSER, G. (1995). The relationship between various amplification schemes, listening conditions and hearing impairment. *Ear and Hearing, 16;*575–586.

KEIDSER, G., DILLON, H., & BYRNE, D. (1996). Guidelines for fitting multiple-memory hearing aids. *Journal of the American Academy of Audiology, 7;*406–418.

KIESSLING, J., SCHUBERT, M., & ARCHUT, A. (1996). Adaptive fitting of hearing instruments by category loudness scaling (ScalAdapt). *Scandinavian Audiology, 25;*153–160.

KILLION, M. (1982). Transducers, earmolds and sound quality considerations. In: G.A. Studebaker, & F. Bess (Eds.), *The Vanderbilt hearing aid report* (pp. 104–111). Upper Darby: Monographs in Contemporary Audiology.

KILLION, M. (1993). The K-Amp hearing aid: An attempt to present high fidelity for persons with impaired hearing. *American Journal of Audiology 2*;52–74.

KILLION, M. (1994). Fig6.WQ1: Loudness-based fitting formulae. *Handout at Jackson Hole Rendezvous*, Jackson, WY.

KILLION, M.C. (1997). A critique of four popular statements about compression. *Hearing Review, 4*(2);36,38.

KILLION, M.C., & REVITT, L. (1993). CORFIG and GIFROC: Real ear to coupler and back. In: G.A. Studebaker & I. Hochberg (Eds.), *Acoustical factors affecting hearing aid performance* (pp. 65–85). Boston: Allyn & Bacon.

KNUDSEN, V.O., & JONES, I.H. (1935). Artificial aids to hearing. *Laryngoscope, 45*;48–69.

KOCHKIN, S. (1996). Customer satisfaction and subjective benefit with high performance hearing aids. *Hearing Review, 3*(12); 16–26.

KRUGER, B., & KRUGER, F.M. (1994). Future trends in hearing aid fitting strategies: With a view towards 2020. In: M. Valente (Ed.), *Strategies for selecting and verifying hearing aid fittings* (pp. 300–342). New York: Thieme Medical Publishers.

KUK, F. (1992). Evaluation of the efficacy of a multimemory hearing aid. *Journal of the American Academy of Audiology, 3*;338–348.

LEIJON, A. (1989). *Optimization of hearing aid gain and frequency response for cochlear rearing losses.* Technical Report No. 189, School of Electrical and Computer Engineering. Gothenburg: Chalmers University of Technology.

LESTRANGE, R.L.J., BURWOOD, E., BYRNE, D., JOYNER, K.H., WOOD, M., & SYMONS, G.L. (1995). *Interference to hearing aids by the digital mobile telephone system, global system for mobile communications (GSM),* NAL Report No. 131. Sydney: Australian Hearing Services.

LUNNER, T., HELLGREN, J., ARLINGER, S., & ELBERLING, C. (1997). A digital filterbank hearing aid: Three processing algorithms—user preference and performance. *Ear and Hearing, 18*;373–387.

LYBARGER, S.F. (1944). *U.S. Patent Application* SN 543.278.

LYBARGER, S.F. (1953). *Basic manual for fitting radioear hearing aids.* Pittsburgh: Radioear Corp.

LYBARGER, S.F. (1978). Selective amplification—A review and evaluation. *Journal of the American Audiological Society, 3;* 258–266.

McCANDLESS, G.A., & LYREGAARD, P.E. (1983). Prescription of gain/output (POGO) for hearing aids. *Hearing Instruments, 34*(1);16–17,19–21.

MOORE, B.C.J, & GLASBERG, B.R. (1997). A model of loudness perception applied to cochlear hearing loss. *Auditory Neuroscience, 3*;289–311.

MUELLER, H.G. (1989). Individualizing the ordering of custom hearing instruments. *Hearing Instruments, 40*(2);18–22.

MUELLER, H.G. (1995). Editor's introduction. In: R.M. Cox, Using loudness data for hearing aid selection: The IHAFF approach. *Hearing Journal, 48*(2);10–44.

MUELLER, H.G., & EBINGER, K.A. (1997). Verification of the performance of CIC hearing aids. In: M. Chasin (Ed.), *CIC handbook* (pp. 101–126). San Diego: Singular.

MUELLER, H.G., & KILLION, M.C. (1990). An easy method for calculating the Articulation Index. *Hearing Journal 43*(9);14–17.

NOBLE, W., & ATHERLEY, G. (1970). The hearing measurement scale: A questionnaire assessment of auditory disability. *Journal of Audiological Research, 10*;229–250.

NOBLE, W., BYRNE, D., & TER-HORST, K. (1997). Auditory localization, detection of spatial separateness, and speech hearing in noise by hearing impaired listeners. *Journal of the Acoustical Society of America, 102*;2343–2352.

NOBLE, W., SINCLAIR, S., & BYRNE, D. (1998). Improvement in aided sound localization with open earmolds: Observations in people with high frequency hearing loss. *Journal of the American Academy of Audiology, 9*;25–34.

NOBLE, W., TER-HORST, K., & BYRNE, D. (1995). Disabilities and handicaps associated with impaired auditory localization. *Journal of the American Academy of Audiology, 6*;129–140.

NOWOSIELSKI, J., REDHEAD, T.J., & CASEY, N.J. (1998). A new direction in hearing aids—Self fitting and self controlled hearing aids. *13th National Conference of the Audiological Society of Australia,* May 1998, Sydney.

OSRD. (1946). *Hearing and hearing aids.* Harvard University Office of Scientific Research and Development. Report No. 4666. Cambridge, MA: Harvard University.

PASCOE, D.P. (1975). Frequency responses of hearing aids and their effects on speech perception of hearing-impaired subjects. *Annals of Otology, Rhinology, and Laryngology, 84* (Suppl. 23);1–40.

PAVLOVIC, C.V. (1984). Use of the Articulation Index for assessing residual auditory function in listeners with sensorineural hearing impairment. *Journal of the Acoustical Society of America, 75*;1253–1258.

PAVLOVIC, C.V. (1989). Speech spectrum considerations and speech intelligibility predictions in hearing aid evaluations. *Journal of Speech and Hearing Disorders, 54*;3–8.

PAVLOVIC, C.V., STUDEBAKER, G.A., & SHERBECOE, R.L. (1987). An articulation index based procedure for predicting the speech recognition performance of hearing-impaired individuals. *Journal of the Acoustical Society of America, 80*;50–57.

PLUVINAGE, V. (1989). Clinical measurement of loudness growth. *Hearing Instruments, 39*(3);28–32.

PUNCH, J., CHI, C., & PATTERSON, J. (1990). A recommended protocol for prescriptive use of target gain rules. *Hearing Instruments, 41*(4);12–19.

RANKOVIC, C.M. (1991). An application of the articulation index to hearing aid fitting. *Journal of Speech and Hearing Research, 34*;391–402.

RICKETTS, T.A. (1996). Fitting hearing aids to individual loudness perception measures. *Ear and Hearing, 17*;124–132.

SCHWARTZ, D., LYREGAARD, P.E., & LUNDH, P. (1988). Hearing aid selection for severe/profound hearing losses. *Hearing Journal, 41*(2);13–17.

SEEWALD, R.C., ROSS, M., & SPIRO, M.K. (1985). Selecting amplification characteristics for young hearing-impaired children. *Ear and Hearing, 6*;48–53.

SEEWALD, R.C., CORNELISSE, L.E., RAMJI, K.V., SINCLAIR, S.T., MOODIE, K.S., & JAMIESON, D.G. (1996). *DSL v4.0 for windows manual.* London, Ontario: University of Western Ontario.

SHAPIRO, I. (1976). Hearing aid fitting by prescription. *Audiology, 15*;163–173.

SKINNER, M.W. (1980). Speech intelligibility in noise induced hearing loss: Effects of high-frequency compensation. *Journal of the Acoustical Society of America, 67*;306–317.

SKINNER, M.W. (1988). *Hearing aid evaluation.* Englewood Cliffs, NJ: Prentice Hall.

SKINNER, M.W., PASCOE, D.P., MILLER, J.D., & POPELKA, G.R. (1982). Measurements to determine the optimal placement of speech energy within the listener's auditory area: A basis for selecting amplification characteristics. In: G.A. Studebaker, & F. Bess (Eds.), *The Vanderbilt hearing aid report* (pp. 161–169). Upper Darby: Monographs in Contemporary Audiology.

STONE, M.A., MOORE, B.C.J, WOJTCZAK, M., & GUDGIN, E. (1997). Effects of fast-acting high-frequency compression on the intelligibility of speech in steady and fluctuating background sounds. *British Journal of Audiology, 31;* 257–273.

STOREY, L., DILLON, H., YEEND, I., & WIGNEY, D. (1998). The National Acoustic Laboratories procedure for selecting the saturation sound pressure Level of hearing aids: Experimental validation. *Ear and Hearing, 19;*267–279.

STUDEBAKER, G.A. (1980). Fifty years of hearing aid research: An evaluation of progress. *Ear and Hearing, 1;*57–62.

STUDEBAKER, G.A. (1992). The effect of equating loudness on audibility-based hearing aid selection procedures. *Journal of the American Academy of Audiology, 3;*113–118.

STUDEBAKER, G.A., & SHERBECOE, R.L. (1992). LASR3 (SSB): A model for the prediction of average speech recognition performance of normal hearing and hearing-impaired persons. *Laboratory Report 92-02 Hearing Sciences Laboratory.* Memphis, TN; Memphis State University.

TURNER, C.W., HUMES, L.E., BENTLER, R.A., & COX, R.M. (1996). A review of past research on changes in hearing aid benefit over time. *Ear and Hearing, 17;*14S–28S.

TYLER, R.S., & SUMMERFIELD, A.Q. (1996). Cochlear implantation: Relationships with research on auditory deprivation and acclimatization. *Ear and Hearing, 17;* 38S-50S.

TYLER, R.S., SUMMERFIELD, Q., WOOD, E.J., & FERNANDES, M.A. (1982). Psychoacoustic and phonetic temporal processing in normal and hearing-impaired listeners. *Journal of the Acoustical Society of America, 72;*740–752.

UPFOLD, L., & GOODAIR, G. (1997). Noise and distance: A comparison of aided performance using microphone and telecoil inputs. *Australian Journal of Audiology, 19;*35–41.

VALENTE, M., POTTS, L.G., & VALENTE, M. (1997) Signal testing approaches. In: H. Tobin (Ed.), *Practical hearing aid selection and fitting* (pp. 75–93). Washington, DC: Department of Veterans Affairs, Rehabilitation Research and Development Service.

WALKER, G. (1996). The preferred speech spectrum of people with normal hearing and its relevance to hearing aid fitting. *Australian Journal of Audiology, 19;*1–8.

WATSON, N.A., & KNUDSEN, V.O. (1942). Selective amplification in hearing aids. *Journal of the Acoustical Society of America, 11;*406–419.

Chapter 26

Regeneration of the Auditory Pathway

Brenda M. Ryals

Outline

Ten years ago the discovery that birds could replace sensory hair cells in the inner ear was both exciting and puzzling. After nearly 50 years of studies of the inner ear in mammals, no evidence had been found that would lead anyone to suspect that the inner ear of any warm-blooded vertebrates might be able to regenerate or restore damaged or lost sensory hair cells. If no previous evidence was found in mammals, did it mean that we just had not looked hard enough? Or did it mean that birds were somehow special, perhaps retaining a capacity lost in higher order vertebrates? It was quickly determined that birds are unique in their ability to spontaneously regenerate or restore lost or damaged sensory cells within the auditory portion of the inner ear. Experiments similar to those performed in birds were performed in small mammals (e.g., rat, guinea pig), and no evidence of spontaneous regeneration or restoration of auditory hair cells was found. This *does not mean*, however, that no hope exists for the restoration of the sensory cells of the inner ear in mammals and humans. *It does mean*, though, that some factor or combination of factors will have to be provided to either stimulate a dormant capacity for self-repair or stimulate

mechanisms similar to those in birds to act in the mammalian inner ear.

The discovery of hair cell regeneration in birds has led to an entirely new field of investigation in hearing and deafness. Auditory scientists in laboratories around the world are actively involved in studying ways in which we may one day be able to restore lost or damaged sensory cells of the inner ear in mammals, including humans. New discoveries in molecular genetics, cell cycle, cell signaling, and cell-cell interactions are happening every day. The goal of this chapter is to provide *an overview of our current* understanding of the mechanisms underlying postmitotic hair cell regeneration, the behavioral consequences of hair cell regeneration, and to describe the potential impact of this research on prevention and/or treatment of hearing loss. To do this, it is first necessary to understand the normal developmental sequence of hair cell generation and differentiation within the cochlea. Thus the first section of this chapter will briefly review what we know about normal cell cycle division and differentiation.

Hair cell regeneration, to a large extent, is a recapitulation of these normal processes. The primary difference is that we are still unclear about what the "trigger" is that stimulates the cycle to begin again after maturity. We do know that, so far, hair cell regeneration only occurs after hair cell loss. Thus the second portion of this chapter will deal with our current understanding of the potential "triggers" for regeneration of hair cells and their reinnervation in the inner ear. Finally, the last section of the chapter will deal with the behavioral consequences of hair cell regeneration and future directions for research. Does hair cell regeneration "cure" deafness? What is the potential for triggering hair cell regeneration in humans? How might hair cell regeneration and cochlear implants work together? Providing an overview of current information in a field of research that is advancing so rapidly is a risky business. One always worries that some new advance will occur before publication of the textbook. Therefore, the intention of this chapter is to provide the clinician with a good background for interpretation of the exciting scientific and clinical advances to come.

THE CELL CYCLE

This section is not a summary of the embryogenesis of the inner ear. Excellent summaries of the development of the inner ear can be found in Rubel (1978), Romand (1983), and Pujol et

Audiology: Treatment. Edited by Valente, Hosford-Dunn, and Roeser. Thieme Medical Publishers, Inc., New York © 2000

al (1991). Instead, I will provide a brief overview of the factors known to occur in the generation and differentiation of hair cells within the inner ear. For those interested in a more in-depth discussion, the following references should prove informative: Lewis (1991), Corwin et al (1993), Rivolta (1997).

Hair cells are formed within the vestibular and cochlear portions of the inner ear from ectodermal cells in the otic placode. These cells undergo division (mitosis) and differentiation (full morphological development into a recognizable hair cell with stereocilia) early in development and do not continue to divide after they are fully formed (Ruben & Sidman, 1967). In other words, they are postmitotically quiet. The cell cycle that produced these fully differentiated cells is an ordered set of events, culminating in cell growth and division into two daughter cells. Because hair cell regeneration essentially repeats this early process, it is important to understand the fundamental cycles the cell goes through to form a new cell (daughter cell—these new cells are called daughter cells because they are the progeny of the first cell and they retain the ability to continue to divide if stimulated appropriately). Figure 26-1 is a diagram of the cell cycle. Each phase in the cycle represents a point at which the cell may remain until stimulated to enter the next stage. Fully developed hair cells have reached the point at which division has ceased to occur—they have "finished" the cycle. Cells may remain in G0 or G1 (G stands for "gap" in the cell cycle; G0 indicates no gap—the cell is quiet; G1 is the first gap, or the stage in which the cell is no longer quiet but is just starting to prepare to divide) until a "trigger" occurs that prompts them to enter the S stage. The S stage stands for "synthesis" and is the point at which DNA replication occurs (this is the phase in which the chromosomes split apart). Most cells that are stimulated to enter the S stage are said to then be "committed" to proceed to gap 2 (G2) and M (mitosis). G2 is the gap or pause

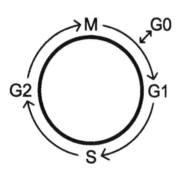

Figure 26–1   The cell cycle is an orderly set of events that culminates in cell division into two daughter cells. *G* stands for "gap" in the cell cycle. The stages of the cell cycle pictured here are G0-G1-S-G2-M. When cells are quiet, not getting ready to divide or grow, they are said to be in "G0" phase. The next gap in time, G1, represents the time when the cell is just beginning to get ready to divide. This stage is followed by the synthesis stage (*S*), when the DNA replicates within the nucleus of the cell. After DNA replication, another gap, G2, represents the period just before the cell finally divides into two separate cells. The *M* stage stands for "mitosis" and occurs when the nuclear chromosomes separate and two new cells are formed. Mitosis is the creation of two new cells with identical DNA from a single cell.

between synthesis and the onset of actual cell division (M). The time it takes to reach mitosis can vary, depending on the signals and the cell type. During mitosis the nuclear chromosomes separate and the cell divides to form two new cells.

How cell division is controlled is a very complex issue. For a more complete analysis of the features critical to cell cycle regulation, the reader is advised to refer to the December 1996 issue of *Science* (pp. 1643–1672) and the "Biology Project" at www.biology.arizona.edu. The following terms describe some of the features that are important in regulating the cell cycle:

PEARL

Regulation of the cell cycle has been a critical area of cancer research. Cancer is a disease in which regulation of the cell cycle goes wrong and normal cell growth and behavior are lost. Researchers involved in hair cell regeneration are learning a lot from cancer researchers about what postmitotic triggers might be and what "inhibiting" factors or genes are necessary to stop cell growth and division.

Cdk (cyclin-dependent kinase, adds phosphate to proteins): These are major control switches for the cell cycle. They can cause the cell to move from G1 to S or G2 to M.

MPF (maturation promoting factor): These include the Cdk and other proteins that trigger progression through the cell cycle.

Growth Factors: A multitude of growth factors have been found to promote cell division and growth. Among the growth factors likely important to hair cell regeneration are epithelial growth factors, nerve growth factors, and fibroblast growth factors.

p53: This is a protein that functions to inhibit or block the cell cycle if the DNA is damaged. If the damage is severe enough, this protein can cause cell death.

- *p53* levels increase in damaged cells, allowing time to repair DNA by blocking the cell cycle.
- *p53* mutation is the most frequent mutation, leading to tumor formation or uninhibited cell division.

p27: This is a protein that binds to CdK and blocks the cell from entry into S phase. Deficiencies in p27 may relate to increased cell division.

Ruben and Sidman (1967) investigated the cellular kinetics necessary for hair cell division and growth in normal mouse ears. Their findings demonstrated that the pattern of cell division and maturation is similar to that found in the neural tube. That is, when a cell enters S phase, its nucleus drops to the basement (i.e., basal) membrane; the nucleus then moves toward the lumen (i.e., lumenal) or "top" of the epithelium where mitosis occurs. Figure 26–2 illustrates this progression of the cell cycle as it occurs in the inner ear.

Once the cell has divided, other factors are critical for its appropriate differentiation or morphological maturity. Retinoic acid (RA) is one such factor. RA has been shown to influence hair cell proliferation and particularly maturation

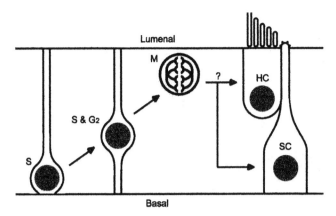

Figure 26–2 Diagram depicting the movement of a cell in the inner ear during early embryonic development. First the cell is stimulated to enter the cell cycle; when it reaches synthesis, S phase, the nucleus of the cell moves down toward the basilar membrane. As the cell progresses through the next stages (*S* and *G2*), the nucleus moves up; when it reaches the top of the sensory epithelium (lumen), the chromosomes separate (*M*, mitosis) and two new cells are formed (a hair cell [*HC*] and a support cell [*SC*]).

in mammals (Kelley et al, 1993; Lefebvre et al, 1993). When RA was added to cultures of mammalian inner ears that had damaged or missing hair cells, new hair cells appeared to replace those that were gone. After in-depth investigation, it appears that RA is most critical for cells that might need a trigger to fully differentiate rather than divide. In other words RA is crucial to the cells final "commitment" to be a "hair cell."

Genetic factors are certainly critical to the appropriate development and maturation of the inner ear hair cells (Steel et al, 1997). New advances in genetic research have shown that some of the unconventional (nonmusclelike) myosin genes (myosin VIIA, VI, and MYO15) are important for the appropriate formation of hair cell stereocilia bundles. The most common clinical manifestation of mutations on these genes is seen in patients with Usher's syndrome.

Finally, the interactions between hair cell final maturation (differentiation) and neural synapse formation is crucial. In many epithelia, including the inner ear, hair cells differentiate as innervation develops. For example, *inner* hair cells differentiate and are innervated before differentiation and innervation of *outer* hair cells. Many investigators have interpreted this evidence as indicating that full differentiation of hair cells depends on synapse formation or innervation (for review see Corwin & Warchol, 1991; Rubel, 1978). Other investigators have disputed this interpretation. Hair cells develop in the absence of innervation during regeneration from denervated lateral line organs, and mammalian hair cells differentiate in the absence of innervation in organ culture. An experiment by Corwin and Cotanche (1989) showed that otocysts denervated several days before hair cell formation, then transplanted to a membrane with no neural elements, developed normal patterns of hair cell stereocilia. Their interpretation was that hair cells can develop in the absence of innervation.

Questions still remain regarding the interactions between hair cells and innervation. Bohne and Harding (1992)

reported that nerve fibers continue to grow and appear to "seek" hair cell attachments in chinchilla inner ears with severe hair cell loss after noise exposure. Researchers using tissue culture techniques have shown that although hair cell formation can occur without innervation, formation and differentiation of hair cell patterns is much better in the presence of spiral ganglion cells. These issues are especially important to postmitotic hair cell regeneration. Can we stimulate hair cells to regenerate in the absence of auditory nerve fibers? This will almost certainly be the case in many congenitally deaf individuals. How many neurons, if any, are necessary? If hair cells can regenerate in the absence of local auditory neurons, will distant neurons "seek" them out? Will reinnervation occur after hair cell regeneration? How much "reinnervation" is necessary for functional recovery? These questions have been the focus of several studies on hair cell regeneration in birds. Some answers are found in the next two sections.

HAIR CELL REGENERATION—BIRDS

The Avian Basilar Papilla and the Mammalian Cochlea: Similarities and Differences

Figure 26-3 is a schematic representation of the auditory sensory epithelium (basilar papilla) in birds and mammals (organ of Corti).

Although the overall appearance of the avian basilar papilla is quite different from the mammalian organ of Corti, many similarities exist. These include the presence of tectorial membrane, two types of hair cells with stereocilia bundles, gradient of basilar membrane width from base to apex, and differential innervation patterns on the two hair cell types. The primary difference in the two auditory end organs is that the basilar papilla contains a continuous sheet of hair cells across its width from neural (tall hair cells) to abneural (short hair cells) edge, whereas the organ of Corti supports one distinct row of hair cells on the neural edge (inner hair cells) separated by the tunnel of Corti from three distinct rows of hair cells (outer hair cells) on the abneural edge. The supporting cells in the bird's cochlea are located in the same place as the supporting cells in the mammalian cochlea (i.e., just beneath the hair cells with their apical tops adjacent to the hair cell's apical tops). But the bird's supporting cells are not nearly so well differentiated as mammal's supporting cells. Several types of supporting cells are found in the mammalian cochlea (Deiters' cells, Claudius' cells, and inner phalangeal cells). Each of these supporting cells has a specific shape and position, but the supporting cells in the bird's cochlea are all similar in shape, and as far as we can tell, they are all capable of becoming hair cells under the right conditions.

Postmitotic Hair Cell Precursors—Cell Division

The first evidence that hair cells might be replacing themselves in the bird inner ear came unexpectedly from studies examining hair cell damage and loss after noise or drugs (Cotanche, 1987; Cruz et al, 1987). The primary purpose of both of these studies was to describe the aspects of hair cell damage and loss in birds after overstimulation with noise or drug toxicity. To the investigators' surprise, they both

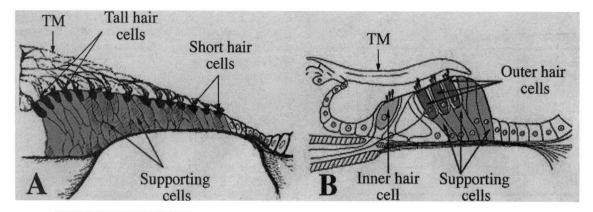

Figure 26–3 **(A)** Schematic representation of the sensory epithelium, or basilar papilla, in birds. Tectorial membrane *(TM)* is located above the hair cells. Tall hair cells are located on the neural or modiolar side of the epithelium and receive primarily afferent innervation from the auditory nerve (similar to inner hair cells in mammals **[B]**). Short hair cells are located on the abneural or non-modiolar side of the epithelium and receive primarily efferent innervation (similar to outer hair cells in mammals **[B]**). **(B)** Schematic representation of the sensory epithelium or organ of Corti in mammals. Tectorial membrane *(TM)* is located above the hair cells. Two types of hair cells, tectorial membrane and supporting cells, are found in the sensory epithelium of both birds and mammals.

noticed evidence of the recovery of either hair cell number (Cruz et al, 1987) or stereocilia bundles (Cotanche, 1987). This suggested that avian hair cells were capable of recovery from severe damage, but did not indicate whether this recovery was the result of the re-emergence of "lost or damaged" hair cells (hair cells that might have appeared to be gone, but in fact just could not be recognized as hair cells); through the addition of new cells replacing old ones;

> ### PITFALL
>
> **A lot of questions remain to be answered, but the prevailing dogma of no postmitotic addition of hair cells leads most to believe that the recovery of cell number or stereocilia is due to some recovery process not related to postmitotic activity.** *Researchers must be ever vigilant to confront current dogma whenever possible rather than allow the prevailing knowledge to limit their experimental choices.*

through new growth of stereocilia on old cells; or through some process of "conversion" of cells that previously were present but were not differentiated as hair cells. Fortunately, experiments could be performed to test for such cell division and differentiation in the inner ear. Two experiments were conducted simultaneously in two separate laboratories to determine whether this recovery was the result of replacement of lost hair cells through the addition of "new" hair cells (Corwin & Cotanche, 1988; Ryals & Rubel, 1988). Investigators injected a radioactive marker of thymidine (one of the four major nucleosides in DNA) to determine whether cells in the sensory epithelium had re-entered the cell cycle and divided to produce new hair cells after acoustic overstimulation and hair cell loss. When the

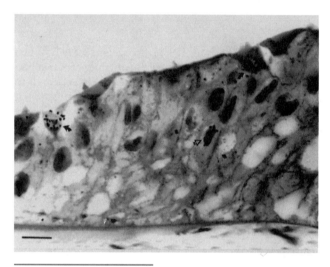

Figure 26–4 Photomicrograph of hair cells located with the damaged area of the basilar papilla after sound damage. Small black "dots" are seen over the nuclei of hair cells *(closed arrows)* and support cells *(open arrow)*. These "dots" are the radiographically labeled thymidine in the nuclear DNA, which divided to form these regenerated hair cells.

cochlear tissues were developed for autoradiography (a technique to view radioactively labeled cell nuclei indicating cell division/DNA synthesis), clearly labeled support cell and hair cell nuclei were found in the region of previous hair cell loss in the cochlea. No cells were labeled outside the region of cell damage or in control birds not exposed to acoustic overstimulation. These results strongly supported the idea that recovery of stereocilia bundles and hair cell number was a result of renewed postmitotic cell division in the damaged cochlea. Figure 26–4 is a photomicrograph showing hair cells and support cells with labeled nuclei in the basilar papilla of an adult quail.

These results indicated that hair cell regeneration is induced in a population of cells that are normally not dividing; acoustic trauma and subsequently hair cell loss stimulated these normally quiescent cells to re-enter the cell cycle. These studies, done in young chicks and adult quail, were repeated in senescent quail and the results showed that hair cell regeneration could be stimulated throughout life (Ryals & Westbrook, 1990). Further studies with ototoxic drugs to destroy hair cells showed evidence of cell division and postmitotic hair cell production as the mechanism for hair cell replacement (Lippe et al, 1991). The next question to be answered was Where do these new hair cells come from? Which cells are stimulated to re-enter the cell cycle to divide and become new hair cells?

The most likely candidate cell for new production of hair cells in the postembryonic inner ear are support cells that reside in the sensory epithelium near the hair cells themselves. Several studies have now shown that in normal avian vestibular end organs and in damaged auditory end organs, support cells divide and their descendants differentiate into new support cells and new hair cells (for review see Stone et al, 1998). Figure 26-5 is a cartoon adapted from Stone and Rubel (1996) depicting the cellular events that occur during hair cell regeneration after ototoxicity.

Hair cells die, are extruded from the sensory epithelium (this occurs after noise or ototoxicity), and undergo degeneration and death within the basilar papilla. In the region of hair cell loss all support cells expand their apical surfaces and some enter the cell cycle. The nuclei of dividing support cells migrate away from the basement membrane and undergo mitosis at the luminal surface (see similar cellular kinetics in Fig. 26–2 during embryogenisis). Postmitotic cells then differentiate into either other support cells or into hair cells. Some evidence exists (Stone & Cotanche, 1994) showing that cell division and differentiation may be either symmetrical (one support cell divides to form either two hair cells or two support cells) or asymmetrical (one support cell divides to form one support cell and one hair cell).

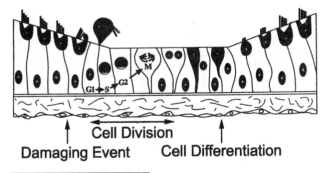

Figure 26–5 Cellular events during hair cell regeneration in the chick cochlea. After a damaging event (ototoxicity or noise), hair cells die and are extruded from the sensory epithelium. In the region of hair cell loss some support cells are stimulated to enter the cell cycle (G1-S-G2-M). The nuclei of dividing support cells migrate away from the basilar membrane and undergo mitosis at the lumenal surface (M). These new cells then differentiate into hair cells and are called regenerated hair cells. (Adapted from Stone and Rubel [1996], with permission.)

It may be that not all support cells are capable of serving as hair cell progenitors. All support cells in the chick basilar papilla seem to have the ability to re-enter the cell cycle (Bhave et al, 1995), but not all actually progress to S phase after hair cell loss (Robertson et al, 1996). This may mean that there are two or more classes of support cells; one that has reached final differentiation and cannot divide and one that can be stimulated to undergo mitosis. So far researchers have not been able to show that different classes of avian support cells are present. Certainly morphologically different support cells are present in the mammalian cochlea, and future studies of support cell classes in birds may prove instructive for the future stimulation of hair cell regeneration in mammals.

On the other hand, it could be that only one single class of support cells is present within the basilar papilla, but that an intrinsic signal restricts the proportion of cells that progress to mitosis after damage. One suspects that such an inhibitory signal could be necessary to retain the appropriate number and precise geometric organization of structures within the sensory epithelium. Proteins such as p53 and p27 (see preceding) have been shown to act in inhibiting cell cycle progression in other systems.

Postmitotic Hair Cell Precursors—Cell Conversion

Recent studies suggest there may be a subset of support cells in nonmammalian species that have the ability to directly differentiate into hair cells without undergoing cell division (for review see Stone et al, 1998). Figure 26-6 shows representative photomicrographs of regenerated hair cells labeled for postmitotic cell division and hair cells without labels that were formed by means of direct differentiation from support cell to hair cell. This direct differentiation from support cell to hair cell has been variously termed "direct transdifferentiation," "cell conversion," and "nonmitotic hair cell regeneration." The first evidence for nonmitotic hair cell regeneration was seen in amphibian lateral line organs (Balak et al, 1990) and later confirmed in bullfrog sacculus (Baird et al, 1996; Steyger et al, 1997) and chick basilar papilla (Adler & Raphael, 1996; Adler et al, 1997). Evidence for nonmitotic hair cell regeneration has primarily depended on transmission electron microscope (TEM) and light microscope analysis of intracellular properties showing morphological features of both hair cells and support cells without evidence of cell division (no evidence of DNA synthesis). Other studies have prevented cell division by injecting DNA synthesis blockers after hair cell loss and continued to find morphological evidence of new hair cell formation. *Thus two mechanisms seem responsible for the hair cell replacement* after trauma (or the ongoing hair cell proliferation in the nonmammalian vestibular system): *stimulation of support cell division and stimulation of support cell direct transdifferentiation.*

Potential Mechanisms for Triggering Postmitotic Hair Cell Regeneration and/or Conversion

The cellular events that stimulate hair cells to divide and form new hair cells are only just beginning to be understood. We

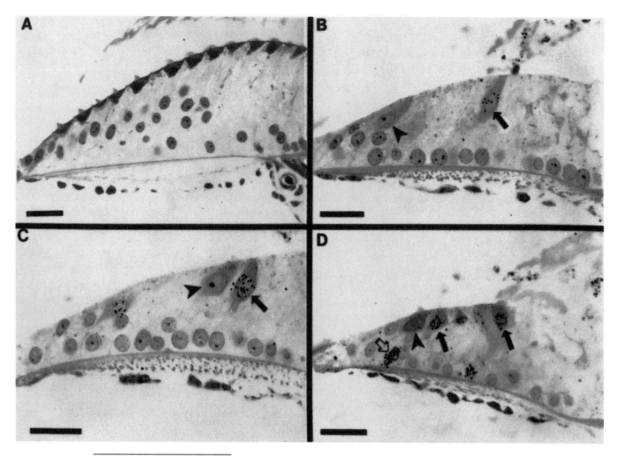

Figure 26–6   **(A)** Photomicrograph of section through normal chick cochlea. **(B)** Section through a chick cohclea 5 days after gentamicin injection. Two regenerating hair cells are seen, one labeled for postmititic division *(long arrow)* and one unlabeled *(arrowhead)*. **(C)** Section through a chick cochlea 5 days after gentamicin injection. As in **(B),** two characteristic regenerating hair cells are seen, one labeled *(long arrow)* and one unlabeled *(arrowhead)*. **(D)** Section through a chick cochlea 12 days after gentamicin injection. Two supporting cells are labeled *(open arrow)*. Three cells are present with the characteristic morphology of regenerating hair cells; two labeled *(long arrows)* and one unlabeled *(arrowhead)*. (Adapted from Robertson et al [1996], with permission.)

know that hair cell regeneration coincides in time and location with hair cell loss after trauma (drug, noise, laser induced). We also know that in the vestibular epithelium in birds, hair cell regeneration coincides with naturally occurring cell death and loss. This correspondence in space and time with cell death has led some investigators to postulate that there is something either about the death of an adjacent hair cell or the loss of contact with an adjacent hair cell that may be a triggering factor. Breaking the intercellular contacts between the damaged hair cells and the surrounding support cells could provide a mechanism for signaling a type of wound healing process similar to that which occurs after a cut in the skin. Cell-to-cell contacts can normally act to inhibit cell division. Changes in these contacts, by cutting the skin or extruding a hair cell, can release this mitotic inhibition and trigger cell division and replacement (Corwin & Warchol, 1991; Stone et al, 1998). Interestingly, when hair cells are lost in the mammalian organ of Corti, evidence has shown that a scar is formed by the subsequent contact of support cell to support cell. In other words, in the organ of Corti

disruption of cell-to-cell contacts does not trigger support cell division and hair cell formation (Roberson & Rubel, 1994; Sobkowicz et al, 1992). Investigations into the differences in the molecular cascade of events after hair cell–support cell contact disruption are needed to help researchers understand why birds respond with regeneration and mammals with scar formation.

Although the hypothesis that cell-to-cell contact signaling plays a role in triggering hair cell regeneration is reasonable, it seems likely that the signaling for repair and regeneration is complex and involves more than one signaling pathway. Studies of molecular events in the inner ear after trauma are difficult in the living animal. Thus in vitro models (that is, maintenance of the auditory sensory epithelium in a culture dish) have been developed to directly study the molecules that influence support cell mitosis in the inner ear. These studies have been instructive, revealing that diffusible molecules are probably intimately involved in triggering hair cell regeneration (Tsue et al, 1994; Warchol & Corwin, 1996). These diffusible factors (that is, factors or molecules that are scattered throughout the fluids in the inner ear) include specific proteins, growth factors, leukocytic cells, cell adhesion molecules, and gene influences on protein and protein receptors.

The case of direct, nonmitotic cell differentiation to form a new hair cell presents a somewhat different situation. Generally, differentiated cells, like support cells, retain their phenotype throughout life. However, direct, nonmitotic cell differentiation has been reported in other systems and the inner ear. Regulatory factors that trigger direct cell differentiation are not completely understood but seem to be similar to factors that can stimulate mitotic cell differentiation. For example, reports have shown that laminin and fibroblast growth factor can induce retinal pigment cells to nonmitotically differentiate to neuronal cells (Park & Hollenberg, 1991; Reh et al, 1987).

Researchers are far from understanding the complex cascade of events that drive a support cell to re-enter the cell cycle, divide and form a new hair cell, or directly convert to a new hair cell. It seems likely that multiple cellular events are required, including transcriptional activity in the case of mitosis, and a variety of cytoplasmic changes. Increased research using advanced molecular biological techniques will help to identify the additional molecules involved in hair cell regeneration. For more in-depth reviews on the issues involved in triggering hair cell regeneration, the reader may wish to refer to Oesterle and Rubel (1996), Corwin and Oberholtzer (1997), Cotanche (1997), Feghali et al (1998), and Stone et al (1998).

HAIR CELL REGENERATION—MAMMALS

As stated previously, examination of the organ of Corti in mammals after hair cell loss confirmed the earlier observation of no hair cell regeneration (Roberson & Rubel, 1994; Sobkowicz et al, 1992). The situation in the mammalian vestibular system has not been so clear. In 1993 two studies reported hair cell replacement in the vestibular sensory epithelium of mature mammals (Forge et al, 1993; Warchol et al, 1993). Forge and colleagues (1993) used scanning electron microscopy to analyze the utricle in guinea pigs several weeks after aminoglycoside-induced hair cell loss. They found evidence of immature-appearing stereociliary bundles and an increase in the number of bundles. Complementary studies by Warchol et al (1993) used in vitro techniques and DNA synthesis markers to reveal evidence of cell proliferation. They found a small number of labeled cells within the sensory epithelium both in human-cultured and guinea pig–cultured utricles. The presence of such cells in the sensory epithelium was taken as one indication of regenerated hair cells. However, before we can say, *unequivocally*, that new hair cells have been regenerated within the mammalian sensory epithelium, better markers specific to hair cells are needed. Although cell proliferation after damage in the mammalian utricle seems sure, we remain unclear as to whether this proliferation leads to true hair cell regeneration.

Because evidence exists for cell proliferation after damage in the mammalian vestibular system, many investigators

---

CONTROVERSIAL POINT

These labeled cells (Warchol et al, 1993) were located in the sensory epithelium and had morphological characteristics of immature hair cells (nucleus located toward the lumenal surface and immature stereocilia). There were, however, very few labeled cells. Other investigators have questioned whether this small number of labeled immature hair cells could account for the larger number of immature stereocilia bundles seen in vivo (Rubel et al, 1995). Subsequent studies have shown that direct nonmitotic differentiation of support cells may be a primary factor in increased hair cell number after ototoxic hair cell loss in mammalian vestibular epithelia (Li & Forge, 1997; Lopez et al, 1997).

have taken this system as a model for learning more about how we might stimulate cell proliferation and regeneration in the auditory system. Studies using in vitro (culture dish) techniques have shown that the addition of transforming growth factor and epidermal growth factor supplemented with insulin can increase cell division in support cells in the mature mammalian vestibular sensory epithelium. Other growth factors that show promise are fibroblast growth factor and insulin growth factor. Members of the transforming growth factor-beta family of growth factors, specifically TGF1, 2, 3, and 5, have been shown to be important for inhibiting sensory cell proliferation. Future studies are likely to focus on the role of these factors in stimulating differentiation and pattern formation and inhibiting mitosis.

PITFALL

Growth factors are mitogens. That is, they act to induce cell division. Studies using the introduction of specific growth factors into the mammalian inner ear, in vivo, have shown that although they can cause vestibular hair cell proliferation, they also stimulate proliferation of extrasensory cells (Kunz & Oesterle, 1998). Thus future efforts at stimulating hair cell regeneration in mammals cannot depend on signals for cell proliferation alone. Other signaling molecules involved in the inhibition of proliferation and/or differentiation and pattern formation must be present.

Investigators working in vitro have attempted to stimulate regeneration of mammalian auditory hair cells. An early report by Lefebvre et al (1993) indicated that RA might stimulate regeneration of auditory hair cells in neonatal rat cochlea maintained in culture. However, later investigations did not support a role for RA alone for the induction of auditory hair cell regeneration (Chardin & Romand, 1995). To date, cell proliferation has not been observed in normal or damaged organ of Corti from postnatal mammals. Some evidence of microvillar tufts resembling immature stereociliary bundles has been seen in young rats after drug-induced damage (Lenoir & Vago, 1997; Romand et al, 1996), suggesting that cells in the organ of Corti may attempt regeneration but fail to complete differentiation and eventually die. Further studies will undoubtedly focus on the origin of these cells in the organ of Corti and on why they fail to fully differentiate, as well as the cascade of molecular events necessary to stimulate regeneration and differentiation.

The Role of Genetic Research in Hair Cell Regeneration

New techniques for altering gene expression in the mammalian inner ear are beginning to give us a better understanding of the regulation of mitotic activity and hair cell generation in the inner ear. The most impressive advances in this area have come from investigations using either mutant mouse strains or mice in which a particular gene has been removed or "knocked out." Using the mutant "shaker" mouse strain, investigators have been able to determine a role for the myosin gene in hair cell and stereocilia development and maturation (Steele et al, 1997). Using mice with absent receptors for fibroblast growth factor-3 (FGF3-knock out), researchers have found that auditory and vestibular hair cells continue to be produced, suggesting that this receptor is not necessary for hair cell production and differentiation (Mansour, 1994; Ornitz et al, 1996).

Another technique that is likely to become quite useful in future attempts at stimulating hair cell regeneration in mammals is gene transfection. Successful gene transfer in the inner ear has been accomplished with adenovirus vectors into postmitotic cochlear hair cells (Dazert et al, 1997; Raphael et al, 1996; Weiss et al, 1997). This technique, developed by scientists interested in the potential for gene therapy, involves inserting a particular gene or gene product that encodes a relevant protein into the organ of interest. This gene is transported by the virus (the virus is simply the host and does not cause "sickness") to the cells of interest. Gene transfer has been successfully accomplished and shown to protect auditory hair cells in vitro and spiral ganglion cells in vivo from ototoxic injury (Ernfors et al, 1996; Low et al, 1996). Further studies using these techniques will doubtless have a role in the eventual stimulation of hair cell regeneration in the mammalian cochlea.

NEURAL CONSEQUENCES OF HAIR CELL REGENERATION

During hair cell embryogenesis, neural synapse formation occurs at almost the same time as final hair cell differentiation. Many investigators, as previously mentioned, have implied an either trophic (guiding) or tropic (maintaining) relationship between hair cells and auditory neurons. What happens then when hair cells are lost and then replaced in the mature inner ear?

All the work in auditory hair cell regeneration and reinnervation has been done in birds. Therefore, it is important to first define the normal neural innervation pattern for tall and short hair cells (see Fig. 26-3) within the avian basilar papilla. In general, tall hair cells receive primarily afferent innervation (similar to inner hair cells in mammals), and short hair cells receive primarily efferent innervation (similar to outer hair cells in mammals). Because both tall and short hair cells have been shown to have the capacity for regeneration, reinnervation necessarily involves both cell types.

The first study of the effects of hair cell regeneration on neural innervation analyzed changes in the number of afferent ganglion cell bodies (Ryals et al, 1989). This study found that the number of ganglion cells decreased after hair cell regeneration by as much as 27% even though the hair cell number had returned to within 96% of normal. This finding led investigators to wonder whether the number of synapses beneath the hair cells might also be changing after regeneration. Using longitudinal TEM analysis of tall and short hair cells after cochlear damage and hair cell regeneration, early studies attempted to determine innervation patterns on the newly repopulated sensory epithelium. A review of some of these studies may be found in Ryals and Dooling (1996).

Immediately after acoustic trauma, hair cells are extruded from the sensory epithelium; often neural terminals remain attached to the hair cells as they leave the epithelium, leaving the remaining dendrite behind. From 0 to 3 days after acoustic trauma, neural fibers can be seen throughout the epithelium. However, no synaptic contacts are seen on what appear to be "embryonic" or regenerated hair cells. By 4 days after acoustic trauma, hair cells could be observed with synaptic contacts. Other investigators (Duckert & Rubel, 1990) have observed nerve fibers in close association with presumptive hair cell precursors as early as 1 day after aminoglycoside administration. After 7 days of drug therapy, they report afferent nerve terminals in contact with both unerupted and erupted sensory cells.

Ryals and Westbrook (1994) obtained autoradiographic confirmation of both afferent and efferent neural synapse formation on both tall and short hair cells within 10 days of acoustic trauma. Regenerated tall and short hair cells identified by autoradiography ([³H]thymidine) were analyzed for their neural contacts with TEM. Seven autoradiographically labeled hair cells in semithin sections were positively identified in immediately adjacent thin serial sections. Labeled hair cells were morphologically similar to adjacent cells with no label and generally appeared to receive similar innervation (Fig. 26–7).

Regenerated short hair cells showed large chalice-shaped, efferent terminals; intermediate hair cells received both afferent and efferent innervation, and tall hair cells were contacted by two to three afferent terminals with synaptic specializations. These results provide conclusive evidence of both efferent and afferent synaptic contacts on newly regenerated hair cells of all types within 10 days of acoustic trauma.

In a separate experiment (Ryals et al, 1991a), TEM sections taken in a plane parallel to the basilar membrane were analyzed in both normal papillae and papillae exposed to acoustic trauma. Sixty-eight short hair cells and 107 tall hair cells were examined from two mature quail. Serial thin sections were taken over an area approximately 50% of length from the basal tip of the basilar papilla. Tall hair cells had an average of 1.86 (±1.07) afferent terminals and 0.27 (±0.52) efferent terminals, whereas short hair cells had an average of 0.21 (±0.44) afferents terminals and 1.13 (±0.83) efferent

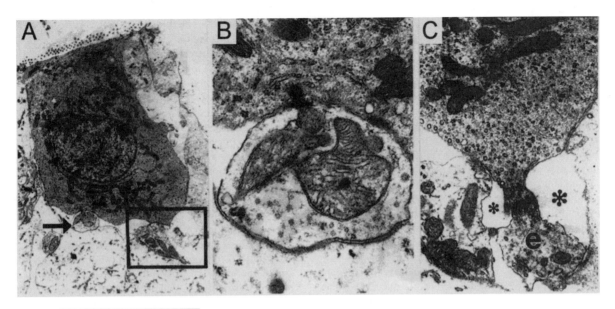

Figure 26–7 **(A)** TEM photomicrograph of positively identified ([³H]thymidine label) regenerated tall hair cell. Both afferent *(arrow)* and efferent *(outlined area)* terminals can be identified, ×4000. **(B)** Higher magnification of afferent terminal area indicated by arrow in **(A)**. Synaptic specializations and mitochondria are contained within the terminal cytoplasm, ×31,000. **(C)** High magnification of the next serial section outlined in **(A)**. Efferent *(e)* neural elements are surrounded by extracellular spaces (*), ×156,000.

terminals. Comparisons with studies in other avian species are difficult because the innervation patterns of hair cells are graded from basal to distal tip and from neural to abneural edge. In general, however, these findings in normal quail compare rather well with those in normal chicken and starling.

The basilar papillae from quail allowed to survive 12 to 20 weeks after acoustic trauma (1500 Hz pure tone at 115 dB SPL for 12 hours) were analyzed in the same manner just mentioned and compared with normal controls. Thirty-six tall hair cells and 56 short hair cells were examined in two animals. The number of afferent terminals on both short and tall hair cells was significantly reduced 12 to 20 weeks after acoustic trauma ($t = 3.345$, $P < .001$ for tall hair cells and $t = 2.458$, $P < .01$ for short hair cells). The distribution of afferent endings on tall hair cells also changed. In the control quail, more than 70% of the tall hair cells had one or two afferent endings, whereas in the noise-exposed quail only about 50% had one to two endings. The number and distribution of efferent terminals did not change significantly for either cell type.

In summary, these results show that newly regenerated hair cells receive both afferent and efferent innervation within 10 days of acoustic trauma. However, 3 to 5 months later, the distribution of afferent terminals has changed, and their number is significantly reduced. Because all hair cells appear mature 3 to 5 months after trauma, and because no autoradiographic confirmation of regenerated hair cells was attempted, it remains unclear whether this redistribution and reduction of afferent terminals occurred solely on regenerated hair cells.

The results of synaptic changes along with ganglion cell number decreases suggest that degeneration and reduction in afferent terminals and cell bodies occur after newly regenerated hair cells have formed mature-appearing synaptic efferent and afferent specializations. The process for maintaining innervation to the regenerated hair cells and to cells surviving acoustic trauma remains to be explained. At least three possibilities present themselves. One possibility is that the neural fiber and cell body degeneration occurs at the level of the regenerated hair cell. It may be that the terminals seen 10 days after acoustic trauma on regenerated hair cells begin to die over the next several days. This degeneration could occur if the hair cell was incapable of maintaining the neural synaptic specialization and/or if neurotrophic factors necessary for maintenance were insufficient over time. A corresponding situation has been reported during normal embryogenesis in chicks. Many more afferent synaptic endings are initially formed on new hair cells than ultimately survive. Similarly, Duckert and Rubel (1993) report that short hair cells regenerated in the basal tip of the papilla after ototoxicity initially show many more afferent synaptic contacts than survive over the subsequent 15 weeks. Our results coincide with this pattern of initial afferent synapse formation followed by later degeneration. This terminal degeneration becomes obvious at the cell body level by 3 to 6 months after trauma.

A second is that the neural degeneration occurs in terminals and cell bodies that were damaged by the acoustic trauma. If this were the case, it would seem that this degeneration should occur fairly rapidly. Changes in neural terminals, at the TEM level, earlier than 3 months after trauma have not been performed to date.

Finally, it may be that neural terminals not traumatized by acoustic overstimulation, but that lose their hair cell targets through hair cell extrusion, degenerate over time. It is possible that some hair cells are lost by an extrusion process that has little to do with direct acoustic overstimulation. In this case, neural terminals on these cells may not be overstimulated but would lose their hair cell contacts. Loss of hair cell contact may put these terminals at risk for degeneration and death. In any of these cases the presence of new, innervated hair cells does not seem sufficient to prevent neural terminal degeneration or to maintain the normal compliment of ganglion cell bodies within the auditory nerve over time.

More recent studies have used immunocytochemical staining techniques to analyze changes in innervation patterns throughout the basilar papilla. These studies can give a more generalized view because, unlike TEM studies, they are not limited to a small number of hair cells within a specific area of the basilar papilla. Their findings have generally corroborated the previous results showing innervation of both tall and short hair cells throughout the basilar papilla after hair cell regeneration (Ofsie & Cotanche, 1996; Ofsie et al, 1997). Studies with specific attention to efferent innervation have shown that the presence of efferent terminals does not seem to be necessary for regeneration and maturation of hair cells (Wang & Raphael, 1996) and that neural terminal damage and reinnervation is different as a function of type of injury (i.e., ototoxicity versus acoustic trauma) (Hennig & Cotanche, 1998). In general, it appears that the temporal course of functional recovery of hearing can be predicted on the basis of the temporal course of reinnervation.

BEHAVIORAL CONSEQUENCES OF HAIR CELL REGENERATION

The avian inner ear provides a useful model for the study of hair cell regeneration and recovery in the vertebrate ear, but the ultimate value of this regenerative capacity depends on whether it results in functional recovery of auditory and vocal behavior. In response to either acoustic trauma or insult from ototoxic drugs, both young and adult birds show a temporary period of hair cell loss and regeneration, usually culminating in considerable anatomical, physiological, and behavioral recovery within several weeks (see previous review references and Dooling et al, 1997; Ryals & Dooling, 1996; Ryals et al, 1991b). Behavioral recovery, as typically defined, only refers to a return of absolute auditory sensitivity to near pretrauma levels. Much less is known about the recovery of more complex auditory behavior and the effect of hearing loss and recovery on the production or recognition of learned vocalizations (Dooling et al, 1997; Manabe et al, 1998). Although evolutionarily distant from humans, birds provide the only animal model for restoring hearing by renewed sensory cell input and for examining the effect of such recovery on learned vocalizations. The question is whether a "new" auditory periphery results in sufficient functional recovery that a bird can again perceive, learn, and produce complex acoustic communication signals.

The following discussion is a summary of experiments (Dooling et al, 1997) designed to test whether a bird can discriminate among, and reliably classify, complex vocal signals after hair cell loss and regeneration. Furthermore, this summary will review findings from studies designed to also determine whether precision in vocal production is permanently affected by such temporary hearing loss.

Budgerigars (domesticated parakeets), learn new vocalizations throughout life, especially in response to changes in

their social milieu. Furthermore, these birds experience hair cell loss and threshold shift after administration of the ototoxic drug kanamycin. Experiments have shown that this threshold shift is followed, within several days or weeks, by hair cell regeneration and a gradual recovery to within 20 dB of normal auditory sensitivity (Dooling et al, 1997; Hashino et al, 1992). By 6 days of kanamycin injection virtually all the hair cells are missing in the basal 40% of the papilla. Hair cells begin to be replaced (regeneration) in the basal 40% during the following 6 days, whereas hair cell damage (swelling, stereocilia abnormalities) begins to be seen in the distal half of the papilla. Hair cell number is almost normal within 4 weeks of kanamycin cessation, and by 12 weeks hair cell number is within normal limits (±1 SD) (see Fig. 26–8).

Abnormalities similar to those reported in chicken hair cell stereocilia after ototoxic drug administration (Duckert & Rubel, 1993) remain in the basal portion of the papilla, even after 7 months. That is, even though hair cell number returns, stereocilia orientation and polarization patterns are abnormal in many of the new hair cells. The question then arises: How is hearing changed when hair cell number is renewed?

Pure Tone Absolute and Relative Threshold Changes

In the first experiment, budgerigars were trained by operant conditioning with food reward to detect and discriminate pure tones that varied in frequency and intensity (see Fig. 26–9).

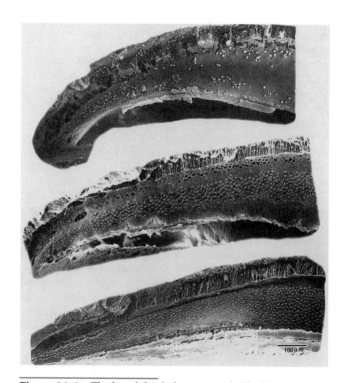

Figure 26–8   The basal (high-frequency) half of the inner ear of budgerigars killed after 8 days of injection with kanamycin (0 day survival), 14 days survival, and 28 days survival. Almost complete loss of hair cells is seen after 8 days of kanamycin injections; recovery is well under way by 14 days, and hair cell number is back to normal by 28 days after injections. (From Dooling et al [1997], with permission.)

Absolute Threshold Task

1. Operant conditioning and the method of constant stimuli

2. Peck observation key to present sound

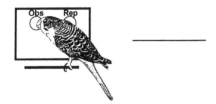

_____

3. Peck report key if sound is detected

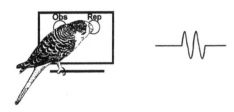

4. Bird tested at a single frequency each day in two 100-trial sessions with 30% of trials as sham trials

Discrimination Task

1. Operant conditioning and the method of constant stimuli with repeating background (1/500ms)

2. Peck observation key to present sound

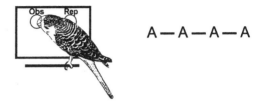

A — A — A — A

3. Peck report key if sound is detected

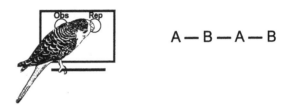

A — B — A — B

4. Bird tested in two 100-trial daily sessions
   This procedure is used for:
   a. frequency difference limens
   b. intensity difference limens
   c. discrimination among bird calls

Figure 26–9 Cartoons depicting the training of birds for behavioral testing of absolute and relative thresholds.

All birds showed absolute and differential thresholds that were within normal limits for this species. For testing absolute thresholds, the birds were trained to detect 300 ms pure tone pulses presented at the rate of 2/s. In difference threshold tests using the method of constant stimuli, birds were required to discriminate a change (in frequency or intensity) against a repeating background of tone pulses. Peak sound pressure levels for frequency, intensity, and call discrimination tests were set to a sensation level of 60 dB. Birds were then injected with the ototoxic drug kanamycin (200 mg/kg/day) for 8 to 10 days followed by a resumption of psychophysical testing at approximately biweekly intervals for the next 23 weeks. After kanamycin treatment, birds were tested on absolute thresholds at 1000 and 2860 Hz so that intensity and frequency difference limens could also be measured in these birds concurrently. Another set of birds was tested for absolute thresholds at octave intervals from 500 to 8000 Hz.

As expected, after extensive hair cell loss, absolute thresholds at all frequencies were elevated immediately after treatment with kanamycin but gradually recovered to within about 15- and 25-dB of preinjection thresholds at 1000 and 2860 Hz, respectively, by 8 weeks. Figure 26–10 shows absolute thresholds for 2860 Hz in one bird before, during, and after kanamycin injections. These findings are in general

agreement with previous reports of threshold recovery after ototoxicity (Hashino et al, 1992; Marean et al, 1995; Niemiec et al, 1994). Despite elevated absolute thresholds, difference thresholds for intensity and frequency were within normal limits at 1000 Hz and only moderately elevated at 2860 Hz 4 weeks after the cessation of injections.

Changes in Complex Sound Discrimination

Three of the above-mentioned birds were also tested on a pairwise discrimination task to discriminate among five natural, species-typical, contact calls and their synthetic analogs. In this test each call in the set served as both a background and a target a total of 10 times resulting in an "n" of twenty tests on each stimulus pair. Discrimination was essentially 100% _between_ contact call types, but performance varied considerably when birds were required to discriminate _within_ call types (i.e., discriminate a natural call from its synthetic analog or vice versa).

The relatively easy discriminations between contact calls from different birds (e.g., two natural calls of Fig. 26–11) were unaffected 4 weeks after kanamycin treatment. In contrast, the more difficult discriminations between a natural call and its synthetic analog (e.g., natural versus synthetic calls of Fig. 26–11A) were significantly impaired for several months

Effect of Kanamycin on Absolute Threshold

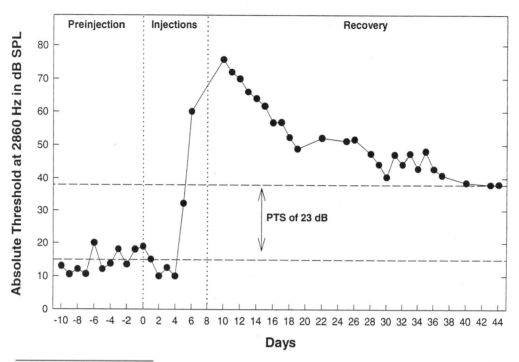

Figure 26–10 Absolute behavioral thresholds for one budgerigar before (preinjection) during, and after injection of 200 mg/kg kanamycin. Threshold elevation began on the sixth day of injections, reached its greatest elevation about 2 days after the last injection, and returned to within 23 dB of preinjection levels 6 weeks after injections.

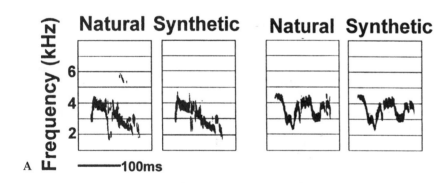

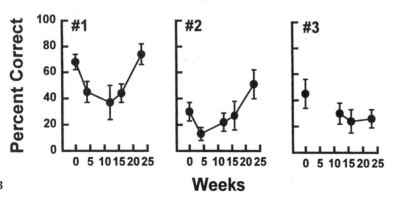

Figure 26–11 **(A)** Sonograms of natural contact calls recorded from two different birds and their synthetic analogs. **(B)** The percent correct for each of three budgerigars discriminating among the five natural contact calls and their synthetic analogs before treatment with kanamycin and at various times during recovery. The discrimination performance of two birds eventually returned to preinjection levels or better, whereas one bird was still significantly impaired even after 23 weeks of recovery. (From Dooling et al [1997], with permission.)

after treatment but improved to preinjection performance levels for two of the three birds (i.e., No. 1 and No. 2) only at 23 weeks of recovery (Fig. 26–11B).

The ability to discriminate among different complex vocalizations is not the same as the ability to recognize previously familiar vocalizations. This difference could be seen as analogous to the difference between closed-set and open-set recognition in speech discrimination testing. To test whether previously familiar sounds were recognized after hair cell loss and regeneration, birds were trained on a second task involving the classification of two different contact call types. In this task birds were trained on a go/no-go task to peck one LED (observation key) to hear one of two contact calls from an overhead loudspeaker. If the "Go" call was presented, the bird was required to peck a second LED (report key) within 2 seconds to obtain food. If the "No-go" call was presented, the bird was required to withhold responding on the report key for 2 seconds to avoid punishment, which consisted of extinguishing the chamber lights for 10 seconds and delaying the initiation of the next trial. Call recognition returned to a better than 75% correct level by approximately 1 month after kanamycin injections.

Taken together, these results indicate that hearing sensitivity and resolution returns to normal or nearly normal levels over time after hair cell loss and regeneration. Threshold sensitivity for pure tones returns more quickly than the ability to discriminate or recognize complex vocalizations.

Changes in Vocalization Patterns

The loss of hearing in humans can have a profound effect on the quality of speech and the quality of acoustic communication. To examine the effect of hair cell loss and regeneration on vocal production, three male budgerigars were trained by operant conditioning to produce different contact calls to two different LEDs. If the bird's call matched a spectral template stored in the computer, the bird was rewarded with food. A summary of the specific experimental details can be found in Dooling et al (1997).

Once the bird was responding reliably, a call was reinforced only when the call was sufficiently different (using the similarity index) from the previous call the bird produced. In this way the bird learned to produce at least two different contact calls to obtain food. These calls were stored as the template-to-be-matched in subsequent experiments with kanamycin.

Figure 26–12 shows template matching performance for the two call types before, during, and after an 8-day course of kanamycin in three different birds (Romeo, Miki, and Bert). Vocal behavior is impaired during kanamycin injections but recovers to previous performance levels within 10 to 15 days after kanamycin injections. The bird's ability to produce a vocal match to a stored contact call has recovered to preinjection levels of precision long before auditory recovery reaches asymptote at about 8 weeks.

These studies were the first to address recovery of the discrimination and perception of vocalizations after hair cell damage and regeneration and the first to track concomitant changes in the precision of vocal production. Both hearing and vocal production are severely affected when many hair

---

PEARL

These early studies in birds suggest that hair cell regeneration in humans will result in the return of both auditory sensitivity and speech discrimination for those who have heard before. Speech production should remain or return to normal performance levels. Further research will be needed to predict what the degree of hearing and speech performance may be for those patients with congenital or prelingual deafness.

---

cells are damaged or lost, but both behaviors return to normal or near normal over time.

Absolute thresholds and frequency and intensity difference limens recover considerably by 4 to 8 weeks. Discrimination and classification tests with vocal signals reveal instances of severe, prolonged perceptual deficits even with a full complement of new hair cells. These deficits also recover over time and with repeated testing and they can be at least partially offset by raising stimulus level. We conclude that, with sufficient time and training, the mature avian auditory system can accommodate input from a newly regenerated periphery sufficiently to allow for recognition of previously familiar vocalizations and the learning of new complex acoustic classifications.

Interestingly, although the precision of vocal production is initially affected by hearing loss from hair cell damage, this precision recovers long before the papilla is repopulated with new, functional hair cells. This suggests that, even in the absence of absolutely perfect auditory feedback, budgerigars, like humans, can also rely on long-term memory combined perhaps with feedback from other sensory systems to guide vocal production. Because both young and adult budgerigars deafened by cochlear removal show permanent changes in vocal output, the questions now should focus on how long the sensorimotor interfaces can do without appropriate sensory feedback before functional recovery in vocal production is no longer possible. The answer to this question, even in a bird, should have immediate relevance for treatment of hearing loss in humans and the timing of auditory prosthetic devices such as cochlear implants.

WHERE DO WE GO FROM HERE?

Basic Science

We are far from understanding the complex cascade of events that drives a support cell to re-enter the cell cycle, divide, and form a new hair cell or directly convert to a new hair cell. It seems likely that multiple cellular events are required, including transcriptional activity, in the case of mitosis, and a variety of cytoplasmic changes. Scientists will need to use new techniques in molecular genetics, cell signaling, and mechanisms of cell death to address the many complex issues involved. At this point, the most critical question remains open: Can auditory hair cell regeneration be stimulated in mammals/humans? Genetic and molecular factors critical to

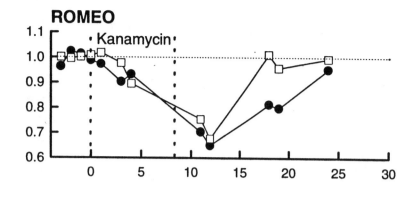

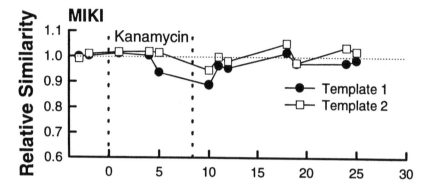

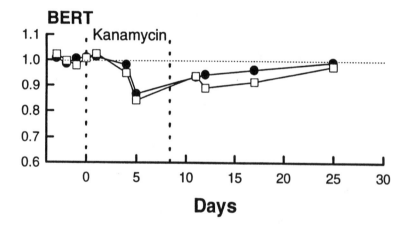

Figure 26–12   Relative similarity of contact calls produced by two birds to their respective templates before, during, and after injections with the ototoxic drug kanamycin. Kanamycin causes a decrease in the precision of vocal production in both birds, but this precision recovers within 5 to 15 days after the cessation of injections and well before the return of auditory function. (From Dooling et al [1997], with permission.)

answering this question include (1) the role of growth factors as potential triggers for cells that might be induced to re-enter the cell cycle, (2) the role of leukocysts in stimulating scar formation or wound healing mechanisms, (3) the role of cell adhesion molecules in influencing cell patterning, (4) gene influences on protein and protein receptors (such as p53 and p27) necessary for cell cycle stimulation and inhibition, and (5) intracellular signaling mechanisms involving various protein and protein kinases.

Finally, scientists will need to address questions of neural involvement and central auditory plasticity after hair cell regeneration. If hair cells can be regenerated in humans, what is the impact of the underlying cause? Are particular structures within the cochlea necessary for regeneration? How many hair cells need to be regenerated to restore function? How many neurons need to contact new hair cells to restore sensitivity and discrimination? What is the influence of onset

or duration of hearing loss to regeneration potential and hearing restoration?

Clinicians

Audiologists are faced with questions just as challenging as those faced by basic scientists. What is the best treatment strategy for our patients with sensorineural hearing loss? Just 10 years ago clinicians advising patients with sensorineural hearing loss had very few options. Because no medical treatment was available for sensorineural hearing loss, the option was clear; if the degree of hearing loss is sufficient, a hearing aid can be of benefit. The advent of cochlear implants changed the therapeutic world for those advising patients with severe-to-profound sensorineural hearing loss. "Tomorrow" the advent of hair cell regeneration may change that world further. For today stimulation of new hair cell growth in the human impaired ear remains elusive. Because we do not know the impact of either duration or onset of hearing loss on the potential for hair cell regeneration, it is important to advise patients to use current technology wisely. The goal we all hope to achieve is the best possible hearing today, while leaving the possibility open to new technologies for even better hearing tomorrow.

CONCLUSIONS

It is a tremendous leap from understanding hair cell regeneration and hearing recovery in birds to restoring hearing in patients with sensorineural hearing loss. However, our increased understanding of the underlying cellular, genetic, and molecular mechanisms of avian hair cell regeneration has put us on the road toward achieving a goal that just a decade ago was deemed impossible. The intention of this chapter was to provide the clinician with a good background for interpretation of the exciting scientific and clinical advances to come. Although the road ahead will be complex, the rewards are sure to be great. Current knowledge is burgeoning; future advances in knowledge are sure to come and with them the potential solution to the social isolation of lost communication.

REFERENCES

ADLER, H.J., KAMEDA, M., & RAPHAEL, Y. (1997). Further evidence for supporting cell conversion in the damaged avian basilar papilla. *International Journal of Developmental Neuroscience, 15;*375–385.

ADLER, H.J., & RAPHAEL, Y. (1996). New hair cells arise from supporting cell conversion in acoustically damaged chick inner ear. *Neuroscience Letters, 205;*17–20.

BAIRD, R.A., TEYGER, P.S., & SCHUFF, N.R. (1996). Mitotic and non-mitotic hair cell regeneration in the bullfrog vestibular otolith organs. *Annals of the New York Academy of Science, 781;*59–70.

BALAK, K.J., CORWIN, J.T., & JONES, J.E. (1990). Regenerated hair cells can originate from supporting cell progeny: Evidence from phototoxicity and laser ablation experiments in the lateral line system. *Journal of Neuroscience, 10;*2502–2512.

BHAVE, S.A., STONE, J.S., RUBEL, E.W., & COLTRERA, M.D. (1995). Cell cycle progression in gentamicin-damaged avian cochleas. *Journal of Neuroscience, 15;*4618-4628.

BOHNE, B.A., & HARDING, G.W. (1992). Neural regeneration in the noise-damaged chinchilla cochlea. *Laryngoscope, 102*(6); 693–703.

CHARDIN, S., & ROMAND, S. (1995). Regeneration and mammalian auditory hair cells [letter; comment]. *Science, 267* (5198);707–711.

CORWIN, J.T., & COTANCHE, D.A. (1988). Regeneration of sensory hair cells after acoustic trauma. *Science, 240;*1772–1774.

CORWIN, J.T., & COTANCHE, D.A. (1989). The development of location-specific hair cell stereocilia in denervated embryonic ears. *Journal of Comprehensive Neurology, 288;*529–537.

CORWIN, J.T., & OBERHOLTZER, J.C. (1997). Fish n' chicks: Model recipes for hair cell regeneration? *Neuron, 19*(5);951–954.

CORWIN, J.T., & WARCHOL, M.E. (1991). Auditory hair cells: Structure, function, development and regeneration. *Annual Review of Neuroscience, 14;*301–333.

CORWIN, J.T., WARCHOL, M.E., & KELLEY, M.W. (1993). Hair cell development. *Current Opinions in Neurobiology, 3*(1);32-37.

COTANCHE, D.A. (1987). Regeneration of hair sterociliary bundles in the chick cochlea following severe acoustic trauma. *Hearing Research, 30*(2–3);181–195.

COTANCHE, D.A. (1997). Hair cell regeneration in the avian cochlea. *Annals of Otology, Rhinology and Laryngology Supplement, 168;*9–15.

CRUZ, R.M., LAMBERT, P.R., & RUBEL, E.W. (1987). Light microscopic evidence of hair cell regeneration after gentamicin toxicity in chick cochlea. *Archives of Otolaryngology—Head and Neck Surgery, 113*(10);1058–1062.

DAZERT, S., BATTAGLIA, A., & RYAN, A.F. (1997). Transfection of neonatal rat cochlear cells in vitro with an adenovirus vector. *International Journal of Developmental Neuroscience, 15*(4–5);577–583.

DOOLING, R.J., RYALS, B.M., & MANABE, K. (1997). Recovery of hearing and vocal behavior after hair cell regeneration. *Proceedings of the National Academy of Science, 94;*14206–14210.

DUCKERT, L.G., & RUBEL, E.W. (1990). Ultrastructural observations on regenerating hair cells in the chick basilar papilla. *Hearing Research, 48*(1–2);161–182.

DUCKERT, L.G, & RUBEL, E.W. (1993). Morphological correlates of functional recovery in the chicken inner ear after gentamycin treatment. *Journal of Comprehensive Neurology, 331* (1);75–96.

ERNFORS, P., DUAN, M.L, ELSHAMY, W.M., & CANLON, B. (1996). Protection of auditory neurons from aminoglycoside toxicity by neurotrophin-3. *National Medicine, 2*(4);463–467.

FEGHALI, J.G., LEFEBVRE, P.P., STAEKER, H., KOPKE, R., FRENZ, D.A., MALGRANGE, B., LIU ,W., MOONEN, G., RUBEN, R.J., & VAN DE WATER, T.R. (1998). Mammalian auditory hair cell regeneration/repair and protection: A review and future directions. *Ear Nose and Throat Journal, 77*(4);276,280,282–285.

FORGE, A., LI, L., CORWIN, F.T., & NEVILL, G. (1993). Ultrastructural evidence for hair cell regeneration in the mammalian inner ear [see comments]. *Science, 259;*1616–1619.

HASHINO, E., TANAKA, Y., SALVI, R.J., & SOKABE, M. (1992). Hair cell regeneration in the adult budgerigar after kanamycin ototoxicity. *Hearing Research, 59;*46–58.

HENNIG, A.K., & COTANCHE, D.A. (1998). Regeneration of cochlear efferent nerve terminals after gentamycin damage. *Journal of Neuroscience, 18*(9);3282–3296.

KELLEY, M.W., XU, X.M., WAGNER, M.A., WARCHOL, M.E., & CORWIN, J.T. (1993). The developing organ of Corti contains retinoic acid and forms supernumerary hair cells in response to exogenous retinoic acid in culture. *Development, 119*(4);1041–1053.

KUNZ, A.L., & OESTERLE, E.C. (1998). Transforming growth factor alpha with insulin induces proliferation in rat utricular extrasensory epithelia. *Otolaryngology—Head and Neck Surgery, 118*(6);816–824.

LEFEBVRE, P.P., MALGRANGE, B., STAECKER, H., MOONEN, G., & VAN DE WATER, T.R. *(1993).* Retinoic acid stimulates regeneration of mammalian auditory hair cells. *Science, 260;*692–695.

LENOIR, M., & VAGO, P. (1997). Does the organ of Corti attempt to differentiate new hair cells after antibiotic intoxication in rat pups? *International Journal of Developmental Neuro-science, 15*(4–5);487–495.

Lewis J. (1991). Rules for the production of sensory cells. *Ciba Foundation Symposium, 160;*25–39.

Li, L., & Forge, A. (1997). Morphological evidence for supporting cell to hair cell conversion in the mammalian utricular macula. *International Journal of Developmental Neuroscience, 15*(4–5);433–446.

Lippe, W.R., Westbrook, E.W., & Ryals, B.M. (1991). Hair cell regeneration in the chicken cochlea following aminoglycoside toxicity. *Hearing Research, 56;*203–210.

Lopez, I., Honrubia, V., Lee, S.C., Schoeman, G., & Beykirch, K. (1997). Quantification of the process of hair cell loss and recovery in the chinchilla crista ampullaris after gentamicin treatment. *International Journal of Developmental Neuroscience, 15*(4-5);447–461.

Low, W., Dazert, S., Baird, A., Ryan, A.F. (1996). Basic fibroblast growth factor (FGF-2) protects rat cochlear hair cells in organotypical culture from aminoglycoside injury. *Journal of Cellular Physiology, 167*(3);443–450.

Manabe, K., Sadr, E.I., & Dooling, R.J. (1998). Control of vocal intensity in budgerigars *(Melopsittacus undulatus):* Differential reinforcement of vocal intensity and the Lombard effect. *Journal of the Acoustical Society of America, 103*(2);1190–1198.

Mansour, S.L. (1994). Targeted disruption of int-2 (fgf-3) causes developmental defects in the tail and inner ear. *Molecular Reproduction Development, 39*(1);62-67; discussion 67–68.

Marean, G.C., Cunningham, D., Burt, J.M., Beecher, M.D., & Rubel, E.W. (1995). Regenerated hair cells in the European starling: Are they more resistant to kanamycin ototoxicity than original hair cells? *Hearing Research, 82*(2);267–276.

Niemiec, A.J., Raphael, Y., & Moody, D.B. (1994). Return of auditory function following structural regeneration after acoustic trauma: Behavioral measures from quail. *Hearing Research, 75*(1–2);209–224.

Oesterle, E.C., & Rubel, E.W. (1996). Hair cell generation in vestibular sensory receptor epithelia. *Annals of the New York Academy of Science, 781;*34-46.

Ofsie, M.S., & Cotanche, D.A. (1996). Distribution of nerve fibers in the basilar papilla of normal and sound-damaged chick cochlea. *Journal of Comparative Neurology, 1;*370(3);281–294.

Ofsie, M.S., Hennig, A.K., Messana, E.P., & Cotanche, D.A. (1997). Sound damage and gentamicin treatment produce different patterns of damage to the efferent innervation of the chick cochlea. *Hearing Research, 112*(1–2);207–223.

Ornitz, D.M., Xu, J., Colvin, J.S., McEwen, D.G., MacArthur, C.A., Coulier, F., Gao, G., & Goldfarb, M. (1996). Receptor specificity of the fibroblast growth factor family. *Journal of Biological Chemistry, 271*(25);15292–15297.

Park, C.M., & Hollenberg, M.J. (1991). Induction of retinal regeneration in vivo by growth factors. *Developmental Biology, 148;*322–333.

Pujol, R., Lavigne-Rebillard, M., & Uziel, A. (1991). Development of the human cochlea. *Acta Otolaryngolegen Supplement (Stockholm), 482;*7–12.

Raphael, Y., Frisancho, J.C., & Roessler, B.J. (1996). Adenoviral-mediated gene transfer into guinea pig cochlear in vivo. *Neuroscience Letters, 207*(2);137–141.

Reh, T.A., Nagy, T., & Gretton, H. (1987). Retinal pigmented epithelial cells induced to transdifferentiate to neurons by laminin. *Nature, 330;*68–71.

Rivolta, M.N. (1997). Transcription factors in the ear: Molecular switches for development and differentiation. *Audiological Neurootology, 2;*36–49.

Robertson, D.W., Kreig, C.S., & Rubel, E.W. (1996). Light microscopic evidence that direct transdifferentiation gives rise to new hair cells in regenerating avian auditory epithelium. *Auditory Neuroscience, 2;*195–205.

Roberson, D.W., & Rubel, E.W. (1994). Cell division in the gerbil cochlea after acoustic trauma. *American Journal of Otology, 15*(1);28–34.

Romand, R. (1983). *Development of auditory and vestibular systems.* New York: Academic Press.

Romand, R., Chardin, S., & Le Calvez, S. (1996). The spontaneous appearance of hair cell-like cells in the mammalian cochlea following aminoglycoside ototoxicity. *Neuroreport, 8*(1);133–137.

Rubel, E.W. (1978). Ontogeny of structure and function in the vertebrate auditory system. In: M. Jacobson (Ed.), *Handbook of sensory physiology. IX: Development of sensory systems* (pp. 135–237). New York: Springer-Verlag.

Rubel, E.W., Dew, L.A., & Roberson, D.W. (1995). Mammalian vestibular hair cell regeneration. *Science, 267*(5198);701–707.

Ruben, R.J., & Sidman, R.L. (1967). Serial section radiography of the inner ear. Histological technique. *Archives of Otolaryngology, 86*(1);32–37.

Ryals, B.M., & Dooling, R.J. (1996). Changes in innervation and auditory sensitivity following acoustic trauma and hair cell regeneration in birds. In: R.J. Salvi, D. Henderson, F. Fiorino, & V. Colletti (Eds.), *Auditory plasticity and regeneration* (pp. 84–100). New York: Thieme Medical Publishers.

Ryals, B.M., & Rubel, E.W. (1988). Hair cell regeneration after acoustic trauma in adult Coturnix quail. *Science, 240;*1774–1776.

Ryals, B.M., Ten Eyck, B., & Westbrook, E.W. (1989). Continued ganglion cell loss after hair cell regeneration. *Hearing Research, 43;*81–90.

Ryals, B.M., & Westbrook, E.W. (1990). Hair cell regeneration in senescent quail. *Hearing Research, 50;*87–96.

Ryals, B.M., Westbrook, E.W. (1994). TEM analysis of neural terminals on autoradiographically identified regenerated hair cells. *Hearing Research, 72;*81–88.

Ryals, B.M., Westbrook, E.W., Spencer, R.F. (1991a). Hair cell re-innervation after acoustic trauma in Coturnix quail [abstract]. *Association for Research in Otology, 14;*338.

Ryals, B.M., Westbrook, E.W., Stoots, S., & Spencer, R.F. (1991b). Changes in the acoustic nerve after hair cell regeneration. *Experiments in Neurology, 115;*18–22.

Sobkowicz, H.M., August, B.K., & Slapnick, S.M. (1992). Epithelial repair following mechanical injury of the developing organ of Corti in culture: An electron microscopic and autoradiographic study. *Experiments in Neurology, 115*(1);44–49.

Steel, K.P., Mburu, P., Gibson, F., Walsh, J., Varela, A., Brown, K., Self, T., Mahony, M., Fleming, J., Pearce, A., Harvey, D., Cable, J., & Brown, S.D. (1997). Unraveling the genetics of deafness. *Annals of Otology, Rhinology, and Laryngology Supplement, 168;*59–62.

Steyger, P.S., Burton, M., Hawkins, J.R., Schuff, N.R., & Baird RA. (1997). Calbindin and parvalbumin are early markers of non-mitotically regenerating hair cells in the bullfrog vestibular otolith organs. *International Journal of Developmental Neuroscience, 15;*417–432.

STONE, J.S., & COTANCHE, D.A. (1994). Identification of the timing of S phase and the patterns of cell proliferation during hair cell regeneration in the chick cochlea. *Journal of Comprehensive Neurology, 341;*50–67.

STONE, J.S., OESTERLE, E.C., & RUBEL, E.W. (1998). Recent insights into regeneration of auditory and vestibular hair cells. *Current Opinion Neurology* 11;17–24.

STONE J.S., & RUBEL EW. (1996). Stimulating hair cell regeneration: On a wing and a prayer. *Nature Medicine, 2*(10); 1136–1139.

TSUE, T.T., OESTERLE, E.C., & RUBEL, E.W. (1994). Diffusible factors regulate hair cell regeneration the avian inner ear. *Proceedings of the National Academy of Science USA, 91;* 1584–1588.

WANG, Y., & RAPHAEL, Y. (1996). Re-innervation patterns of chick auditory sensory epithelium after acoustic overstimulation. *Hearing Research, 97*(1–2);11–18.

WARCHOL, M.E., & CORWIN, J.T. (1996). Regenerative proliferation in organ cultures of the avian cochlea: Identification of the initial progenitors and determination of the latency of the proliferative response. *Journal of Neuroscience, 16;*5466–5477.

WARCHOL, M.E., LAMBERT, P.R., GOLDSTEIN, B.J., FORGE, A., & CORWIN, J.T. (1993). Regenerative proliferation in inner ear sensory epithelia from adult guinea pigs and humans. *Science, 259;*1619–1622.

WEISS, M.A., FRISANCHO, J.C., ROESSLER, B.J., & RAPHAEL, Y. (1997). Viral-mediated gene transfer in the cochlea. *International Journal of Developmental Neuroscience, 15*(4–5);577–583.

INDEX